ADVANCES IN OPHTHALMOLOGY

Edited by **Shimon Rumelt**

Advances in Ophthalmology
Edited by Shimon Rumelt

Published by InTech
Janeza Trdine 9, 51000 Rijeka, Croatia

Publishing Process Manager Martina Durovic

Technical Editor Teodora Smiljanic

Cover Designer InTech Design Team

Additional hard copies can be obtained from orders@intechopen.com

Advances in Ophthalmology, Edited by Shimon Rumelt
p. cm.
ISBN 978-953-51-0248-9

For EU product safety concerns:
IN TECH d.o.o., Prolaz Marije Krucifikse Kozulić 3, 51000 Rijeka, Croatia,
info@intechopen.com or visit our website at intechopen.com.

Meet the editor

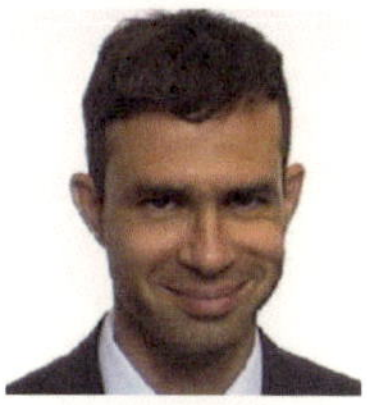

Dr Rumelt received his medical degree and diploma in ophthalmology from Tel Aviv University, Israel. He completed his ophthalmology residency program at Western Galilee - Nahariya Medical Center in Nahariya, Israel, and then an oculoplastics fellowship at Massachusetts Eye and Ear Infirmary, Boston, MA, and vitreoretinal fellowship at Boston University. He earned his Master's degree in Public Administration (Health Systems) from Clark University, Worcester, MA. Dr Rumelt is a senior ophthalmologist at the Western Galilee - Nahariya Medical Center and is engaged in various fields in ophthalmology. He is involved with clinical activities, surgery, research, teaching medical students, residents, and fellows.

Contents

Preface

This book covers selected topics in ophthalmology, providing a glimpse into the advancements in different aspects of the field. It is not aimed to cover the whole field of ophthalmology, and hopefully, more topics will be covered in future books. The book is intended for the general ophthalmologists, sub-specialists, researchers, residents, and fellows. It covers both basic and clinical concepts of ophthalmology. Each author incorporated his/her own perspectives on each topic adding his/her won theories, future trends, and research. Therefore, the book should enable researchers and clinicians to adopt new ideas for further basic research and clinical practice.

This book, arranged in a systematic approach, discusses first the general aspects of ophthalmology (surgery), and then disorders affecting different structures of the eye from the cornea and ocular surface backwards to the retina and the structures surrounding the globe. It is a product of a balance between the expedited publishing process and encompassing broad aspects of the field.

This book is a result of multi-national ophthalmologists from around the globe, with a common desire to take care of patients. Some of the authors have been involved for many years within this field, some are just at their beginning. Some authors are researches, others are clinicians. Some are world leaders, others will be. I hope that our readers will be as much a wide variety as our authors are.

The book is accessible online to allow free access to as many readers as possible, and is also available on print for those who do not have online access, or are interested in having their own hard copy. This will definitely contribute to the worldwide distribution of the knowledge on ophthalmology between researchers and clinicians.

I would like to acknowledge each and every one of the contributors for their excellent work on each chapter. Each one of them devoted time and effort to write a chapter, contributing to the success of this book and the advancement of ophthalmology. I would thank Ms. Martina Durovic and Mr. Jan Hyrat, the book Publishing Process Managers for their expert assistance in all the issues concerning this book, to Ms. Ana Nikolic, the Head of Editorial Consultants for her useful assistance, and for all for choosing me to be the editor of the book. My gratitude to the technical editors for arranging the book in a uniform format and for the publisher InTech, for undertaking this mission. Lastly, thanks to my family, teachers, and students from whom I studied throughout the years.

I hope that this book will be part of a series of books in all the sub-specialties of ophthalmology, and that it will be an example for global collaboration, not only between physicians, but also between everyone for the betterment of the humankind. I wish you, the reader, an enjoyable journey throughout ophthalmology and I hope that you will find the book interesting.

Shimon Rumelt, MD, MPA
Department of Ophthalmology,
Western Galilee – Nahariya Medical Center,
Nahariya,
Israel

Part 1

Basic Concepts in Ophthalmology

1

Lasers in Ophthalmology

Magdalena Zdybel, Barbara Pilawa and Anna Krzeszewska-Zaręba
Medical University of Silesia in Katowice
Poland

1. Introduction

Lasers emit electromagnetic waves of characteristic properties and energies (Gilmour, 2002; Krzeszewska & Zdybel, 2010; Podbielska et al., 2004; Sieroń et al., 1994; Ziętek, 2009). These specific features are used in the modern ophthalmology (Dick et al., 2010; Evans & Abrahamse, 2009; Gilmour, 2002; Schmidt-Erfurth, 2010; Seitz & Langenbucher, 2000; Soong & Malta, 2009). In this work we described theoretic problems of lasers as the quantum systems, the propagation of laser radiation, the lasers parameters and ranges of them. The historical data about laser apparatus and their applications are cited. The biophysical effects caused by laser radiation in biological structures during therapy are mentioned.

The applications of lasers in ophthalmology are widely taking to account. We described widely the two laser applications in ophthalmology which are connected with paramagnetic species and singlet oxygen. We chose these subjects, because of our experimental experience in spectroscopic studies of paramagnetic centers (Beberok et al., 2010; Buszman et al., 2003, 2005a, 2005b, 2006; Chodurek et al., 2003; Domagała et al., 2008; Latocha et al., 2004, 2005, 2006; Matuszczyk et al., 2004; Najder-Kozdrowska et al., 2009, 2010; Pilawa et al., 2002, 2003a, 2003b, 2005a, 2008c; Zdybel et al., 2009, 2010) and singlet oxygen O_2 with zero spin (Bartłomiejczyk et al., 2008; Latocha et al., 2008; Pilawa et al., 2005b, 2006, 2008a, 2008b). In this work the view of the information in scientific papers is done.

2. Lasers as the quantum systems – Basic theory

2.1 Energy levels

The quantum theory describes the energy levels of atoms and molecules (Glinkowski & Pokora, 1993; Sieroń et al., 1994; Ziętek, 2009). Electrons may move only between these levels, and these transitions are accompanied by emission or absorption of energy by the optical system. The emitted or the absorbed energies reveal the values related to the distances between the energy levels. The system will not absorb the energy, when the energy is lower or higher than the value of the energetic band between the levels. Energy levels of the optical active medium play an important role in laser irradiation. The energy levels of the materials used in laser construction determine the energy necessary to their excitation and the energy of emitted electromagnetic waves is dependent on these levels. The energy (E) of the electromagnetic waves produced by lasers is presented according to the formulas (Bartosz, 2006; Hatfield, 1976; Hewitt, 2001; Jaroszyk, 2008; Ziętek, 2009):

$$E = h\nu \quad (1)$$

$$E = hc/\lambda \quad (2)$$

where h is the Planck constant (h = 6,626 x 10^{-34} Js), c is the speed of the waves (c = 299 792 458 m/s), v is the frequency of electromagnetic waves in Hertz, λ is the wavelength in meters. The frequency and wavelength determine the color of laser radiation.

The emitted energy is fitted to the biological structures treated by the individual lasers, so the reason of the majority of lasers used in ophthalmology is understandable. Summing up, the lasers produce electromagnetic waves with the given energy correspond to the energy levels of their optical systems, and it interact on the specific tissues or cells.

2.2 Optical pumping

Condition of absolute emission of radiation by laser is the previous excitation of its active optical system e.g. molecules formed in this system (Glinkowski & Pokora, 1993; Sieroń et al., 1994; Ziętek, 2009). This excitation is called the optical pumping. Excitation of molecules in laser may be done by electromagnetic waves emitted by lamps, by heating or by energy of electrical field (Podbielska et al., 2004; Sieroń et al., 1994).

2.3 Inversion of electron location on the energy levels

As the result of the optical pumping of the quantum molecular system, higher amount of electrons are located on the levels of the higher energy than those of the lower energy (Glinkowski & Pokora, 1993; Podbielska et al., 2004; Sieroń et al., 1994; Ziętek, 2009). The continuous propagation of energy to the system of electrons in molecules causes that the electrons upon absorption of this energy moves to the higher energy levels. Afterwards they return to the lower energy states via relaxation processes. The time of electron-lattice relaxation processes depends on the molecular structure of the optical system in lasers. Electron-lattice relaxation is the transition of the electrons from the excited energy levels to the ground energy levels via magnetic interactions with diamagnetic lattice molecules (Stankowski & Hilczer, 2005; Wertz & Bolton, 1986). The long time of interactions of electrons with the lattice causes the mentioned above inversion. The pumped electrons stay on the higher energetic level and the former irradiation of the molecular system in laser do not pump electrons to the higher levels, because of their absence in the lower energy levels (Ziętek, 2009). The inversion of electrons location on levels is useful to the former effective stimulation emission of radiation in laser apparatus (Glinkowski & Pokora, 1993).

2.4 Stimulated emission of radiation

The name of the **LASER** apparatus comes from the roles of its work as the "**L**ight **A**mplification of **S**timulated **E**mission of **R**adiation" (Maiman, 1960). Two types of emission of electromagnetic waves, the spontaneous and stimulated emissions, are known (Bartosz, 2006; Hatfield, 1976; Hewitt, 2001; Jaroszyk, 2008; Krzeszewska & Zdybel, 2010; Morrish, 1970; Sieroń et al., 1994). Spontaneous emission is the ordinary effect of energy loosening by the excited electrons at the non defined moment. Spontaneous emission is the result of the principle that the optimal state of the system is the state with the lowest energy (Glinkowski & Pokora, 1993; Jóźwiak & Bartosz, 2008; Sieroń et al., 1994; Ziętek, 2009). The stimulated emission is the most important effect to produce laser irradiation. The scheme of stimulated emission of radiation is shown in Figure 1, which was prepared according to the definition of this effect presented in (Sieroń et al., 1994). The stimulated emission of radiation is the controlled effect of energy loosening by the electrons. Before the proper effect of stimulated emission the electron is excited, for example by pumped photons, to the higher energy level. After this the stimulated photon is emitted to the system and at this moment two photons of the same energy are emitted. The energy of the individual emitted photon is equal to the difference between energy of the excited and ground state energy levels. The amplification of the energy of radiation is the effect of emission of these two photons after absorption of one exciting photon by electron. The radiation comes from stimulated emission consist of photons of the same energy so of the same frequency. It means that laser produce monochromatic electromagnetic waves. Monochromatic electromagnetic waves are the same frequency waves (Ziętek, 2009).

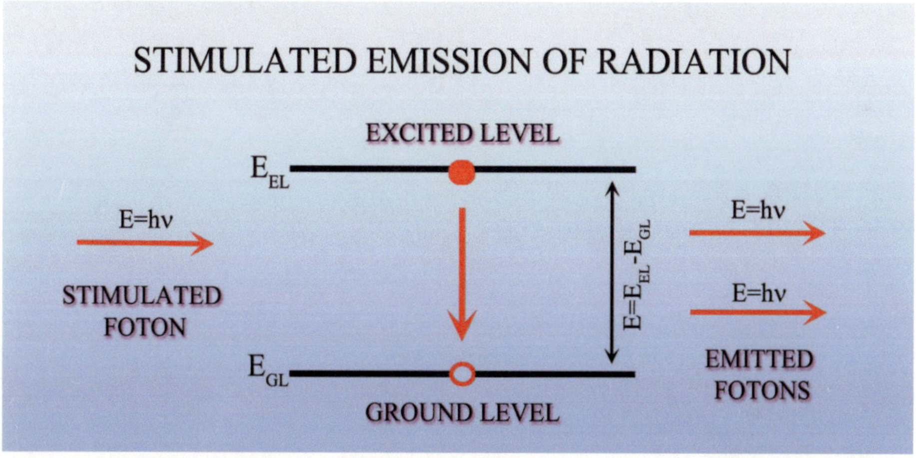

Fig. 1. The scheme of the stimulated emission of radiation prepared according to its definition in (Sieroń et al., 1994).

The exemplary way of the electrons between the three energy levels during laser action is described in work of Sieroń et al. (Sieroń et al., 1994). The main energy levels of electrons are the ground, non-stabile excited, and the quasi-stabile levels, respectively. Electrons are pumped by photons to the non-stabile level with the highest energy in this quantum system. Energy of the pumped photons is equal difference between energy of the non-stabile level and the ground level. Afterwards the electrons without radiation come to the quasi-stabile energy level located lower than the non-stabile level. During the optical pumping there is an increase in number of electrons on quasi-stabile level. At the moment dependent on the type of laser the effect of inversion of distribution of electrons in the energy levels occurs. The higher number of electrons stays on the quasi-stabile level than on the ground level with the lowest energy. The pumping is stopped then and the stimulating photons are sent to the electrons system. At the same time, at the moment of interactions of electrons with stimulated photons the stimulated emission appears. All the electrons located on the quasi-stabile energy level come to the ground energy level. The photons connected with the transition and the stimulated photons are irradiated. The emitted electromagnetic waves have properties of laser radiation, which are described in the next part of this chapter.

3. The properties of laser radiation

Laser radiation as electromagnetic waves differs from the light emitted by the ordinary lamp (Hewitt, 2001). The white light emitted from bulb is superposition of electromagnetic waves with frequencies and wavelengths corresponding to the background colors: red, orange, yellow, green, blue, and violet. The frequencies of the waves increase in the previously given order, and the wavelengths decreases in this manner. The summing of these electromagnetic waves of different colors gives the effect of white light. The component waves in the white light are not coherent. Coherent waves are the waves with the same phase shift (Ziętek, 2009). The component electromagnetic waves in the beam of white light are shown in Figure 2a constructed according to (Hewitt, 2001).

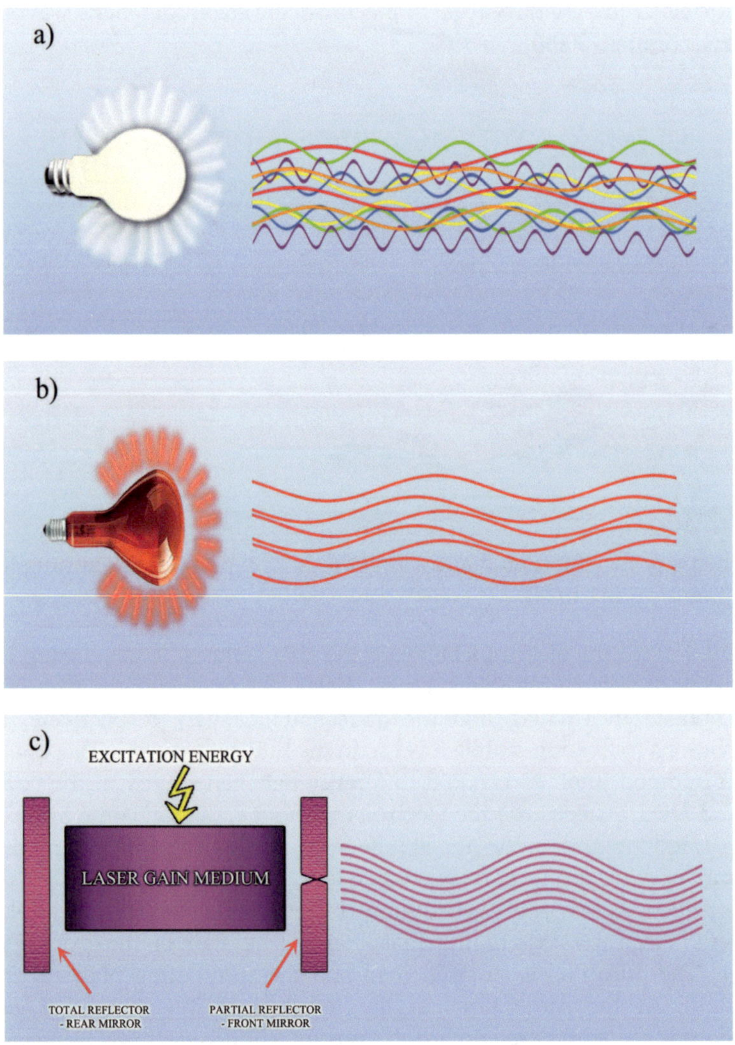

Fig. 2. The electromagnetic waves emitted by: the ordinary lamp produced the white light (a), the source of the monochromatic light (b), and laser (c). The scheme is prepared according to (Hewitt, 2001).

The monochromatic light from the lamp consists of electromagnetic waves of the same frequencies and the same wavelengths (Hewitt, 2001). The waves are not coherent. The electromagnetic waves in the beam of monochromatic light reveal different phases. The monochromatic and incoherent waves are presented in Figure 2b, which was prepared according to (Hewitt, 2001). The fine examples of monochromatic light are the red waves emitted by SOLLUX lamp (Hewitt, 2001).

Lasers produce monochromatic electromagnetic waves (Glinkowski & Pokora, 1993; Hewitt, 2001; Sieroń et al., 1994; Ziętek, 2009). The properties of laser radiation distinguish it from the ordinary white or monochromatic light (Figure 2c) (Hewitt, 2001). The laser waves are monochromatic and coherent. Contrary to white light, laser radiation is monochromatic and in the same phase.

Laser radiation differs from electromagnetic waves sending by the therapeutic BIOPTRON lamps (Straburzyńska-Lupa & Straburzyński, 2004). The BIOPTRON lamp produces electromagnetic waves of the same frequency, but they are incoherent (Figure 3) (Straburzyńska-Lupa & Straburzyński, 2004). The maxima and minima of energy appear on the area of the tissue exposed to coherent laser irradiation. The homogeneous distribution of energy on irradiated area is characteristic for BIOPTRON light.

Fig. 3. The electromagnetic waves emitted by BIOPTRON lamps. Prepared according to (Straburzyńska-Lupa & Straburzyński, 2004).

Laser electromagnetic waves in the environment propagate as perpendicular electric and magnetic fields (Hewitt, 2001). The ranges of wavelength of electromagnetic waves emitted by lasers are showed on figure 4. The values of the wavelengths are cited from (Gilmour, 2002; Ziętek, 2009). The biophysical and biological effects on tissues depend on the energy and the wavelengths of electromagnetic waves (Gilmour, 2002; Jaroszyk, 2008).

There are three basic effects of lasers on biological tissues: photochemical (photoablation and photoradiation), thermal (photocoagulation and photovaporation), and ionizing (photodisruption) (L'Esperance, 1983; Podbielska et al., 2004). The photochemical effects are the result of absorption of energy of laser radiation by molecules in tissues without their destruction. During photoablation the absorption of laser energy causes the increase of temperature of the tissues. Practically the photoablation is caused by the short laser pulses of high energy. Photoradiation is the effect which appears after the transition of the excited by laser molecules in tissues to the ground or the lower energy levels with accompanied radiation of electromagnetic waves. These electromagnetic waves may be responsible for biostimulation effects and tissue temperature rise. Thermal effects interact mainly by the increase of temperature of the tissues after laser irradiation. Photocoagulation causes the increase of temperature in tissues up to 80-90°C via absorption of the laser energy.

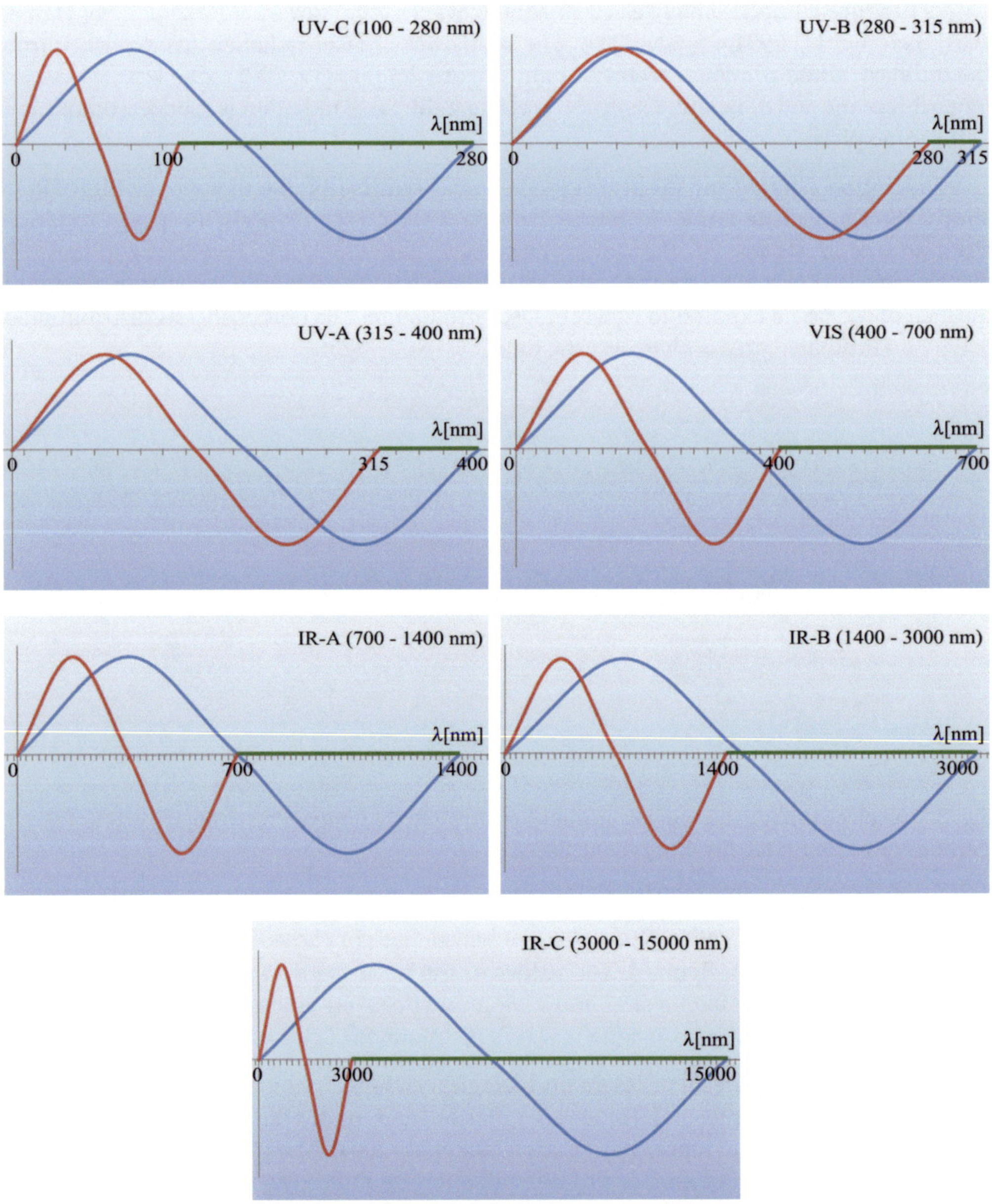

Fig. 4. The ranges of length of electromagnetic waves emitted by lasers. The values of the wavelengths (λ) are cited from (Gilmour, 2002; Ziętek, 2009).

The photocoagulation closes blood and lymphatic vessels, and causes of the necrosis of tissues. Photocoagulation denatures proteins and inactivates enzymes. The laser irradiation of high energy which causes the increase of temperature of the tissues up to 100-300°C is called as the photovaporation. The using of lasers with the high energy of pulse lead to photodisruption effects via ionization in tissues. The ionization is accompanied by the formation of shock waves. The photodisruption effects play an important role in the microsurgery of the front part of the eye.

UV-C and UV-B waves cause increase of pigmentation, burns and photokeratitis (Ziętek, 2009). UV-A waves cause burns, photosensitizing reactions, intensification of dark pigment production, and cataract (Ziętek, 2009). The visible light may destruct retina, lead to burn, and photosensitizing reaction. IR-A and IR-B waves may be responsible for burns and the others thermal destruction of epithelium and cataract. IR-B and IR-C waves may destruct cornea (Ziętek, 2009).

4. History of lasers application in ophthalmology

The history of lasers is connected with the basic theory of quantum radiation presented by Albert Einstein in 1916 (Wróblewski, 2006). This theory defines and characterizes spontaneous and stimulated emission of radiation by atoms. The method of optical pumping of atoms was discovered by Alfred Kastler and Jean Brossel in 1949 (Wróblewski, 2006) and in 1966 Kastler received the Nobel Prize. The inversion of electron localization on energy levels and the effect of stimulated emission of radiation were practically discovered by Edward Purcell and Robert Pound in 1950 (Wróblewski, 2006). In 1960 Theodore Harold Maiman constructed the ruby laser ($Al_2O_3:Cr^{3+}$) emitting light of 694 nm, which is still used in ophthalmology (Seitz & Langenbucher, 2000; Wróblewski, 2006; Ziętek, 2009). In Poland the first ruby laser was constructed by Zbigniew Puziewicz group from Military University of Technology in 1963 (Podbielska et al., 2004). The following types of lasers: helium-neon (He-Ne) (1150 nm), semiconducting, carbon dioxide (CO_2) (10600 nm), argon (476.5 nm, 488.0 nm, 514.5 nm), hydrogen (H_2) (102.5-123.9 nm), excimer (172 nm), and gallium nitride (GaN) (365 nm), were built in 1961, 1962, 1963, 1964, 1970, 1974, 1991, respectively (Ziętek, 2009). The krypton (647.1 nm, 568.2 nm, 530.8 nm) and neodymium: yttrium-aluminum-garnet (Nd:YAG) (1064 nm) lasers were introduced to clinical applications in 1972 and 1980, respectively (L'Esperance, 1983).

The ruby (694 nm) laser is used in the therapy of the following ocular structural defects: retinal tears, peripheral pigmentary degeneration and lattice degeneration of the retina (L'Esperance, 1983). Argon laser is used in the structural defects of the retina and choroid (L'Esperance, 1983). Krypton (647.1 nm) laser is mainly used in outer retinal structural diseases (L'Esperance, 1983). Krypton red laser photocoagulation is exemplary performed in retinal hemorrhagic diseases, retinal edematous diseases, pigment epithelial abnormalities (L'Esperance, 1983). Carbon dioxide laser is applied in operations with the high blood loss (L'Esperance, 1983).

In 1940 light was used in ophthalmology to coagulation of the retina by Gerd Meyer-Schwickerath (Seitz & Langenbucher, 2000). In Poland the first ruby (694 nm) laser coagulator to ophthalmology was constructed in 1965 (Podbielska et al., 2004). In 1961 Campbell applied confocal laser system to retinal coagulation. In 1971 argon laser was by the first used in eye surgery (Seitz & Langenbucher, 2000). In 1977 Nd:YAG (1064 nm) laser was used to microexplosion by Franz Fankhauser and Daniele Aron-Rosa. The history of lasers in ophthalmology is broadly described in the paper of Berthold Seitz (Seitz & Langenbucher, 2000).

5. Types of lasers using in ophthalmology

The group of lasers used in ophthalmology produces coherent electromagnetic radiation of different wavelengths (Dick et al., 2010; Evans & Abrahamse, 2009; Gilmour, 2002; Schmidt-Erfurth, 2010; Seitz & Langenbucher, 2000; Sieroń et al., 1994; Soong & Malta, 2009). Optical systems of ophthalmologic lasers are: CO_2, excimer, argon, tunable dye, Nd:YAG (Gilmour, 2002). Optical systems of excimer lasers contain molecules of dimmers of noble gases as argon fluoride (ArF), krypton fluoride (KrF) and xenon fluoride (XeF) (Ziętek, 2009).

The therapeutic effects as photocoagulation, photoablation, ablation via plasma, interact on eye structures. Photocoagulation is performed by the following lasers: blue-green (488-514 nm) and green (514 nm), argon, krypton red (647 nm), diode infrared (810 nm), Nd:YAG infrared (1064 nm) (Gilmour, 2002). Photoablation is carried on by lasers: excimer ultraviolet (193 nm), holmium: yttrium-aluminum-garnet (Ho:YAG) infrared (2060 nm), erbium: yttrium-aluminum-garnet (Er:YAG) infrared (2940 nm), and CO_2 infrared (10,600 nm). Ablation by plasma is done by pulsed infrared neodymium: yttrium lithium fluoride Nd:YLF (1053 nm) laser (Gilmour, 2002).

6. Parameters of lasers radiation using in ophthalmology

The power of laser is the energy emitted by laser during one second (L'Esperance, 1983; Sieroń et al., 1994). The lasers of low (4-5 mW), medium (6-500 mW), and high (above 500 mW) powers are used in medicine (Sieroń et al., 1994). The examples of lasers of low, medium and high powers are ruby, Nd:YAG, semiconducting (Podbielska et al., 2004; Ziętek, 2009). The lasers of low powers are called the soft lasers, and lasers which emit electromagnetic wave of high power are called hard lasers. The classification of lasers correspond to their irradiated power are shown in Figure 5 (Glinkowski & Pokora, 1993; Sieroń et al., 1994).

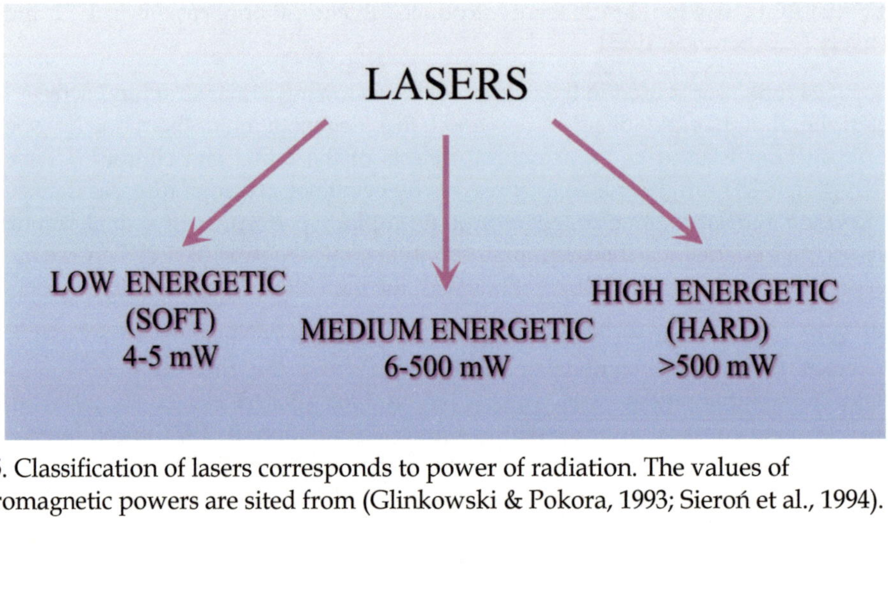

Fig. 5. Classification of lasers corresponds to power of radiation. The values of electromagnetic powers are sited from (Glinkowski & Pokora, 1993; Sieroń et al., 1994).

The biophysical effects in biological systems under laser irradiation are described by Sieroń et al. (Podbielska et al., 2004; Sieroń et al., 1994). Photochemical, thermal and acoustic effects appear during laser radiation propagation in biological samples. Photochemical reactions mainly exist in melanin biopolymers, enzymes, photosensitizers, and hemoglobin, which strongly absorb its energy. Thermal effects take place not only in the irradiated units, but they are also observed in the neighboring structures, because of thermal conductivity of the tissues. The lasers of the highest power cause heating, strong electric field, microplasma formation, increase of pressure, and as the result acoustic effects appear in the tissues.

The soft lasers with the low energy emitted to tissues during one second are used to biostimulation effects (Podbielska et al., 2004; Sieroń et al., 1994). The soft ruby lasers with low energy may be used to biostimulation (Podbielska et al., 2004). The light initiates and increases biochemical reactions. Lasers of medium power are applied in photodynamic therapy. Hard lasers are used to destruction of tissues mainly via thermal effects (Sieroń et al., 1994). Non-thermal effect of photo-destruction occurs in the irradiated structures, when the laser of high power interacts with biological system during the very short time (Podbielska et al., 2004; Sieroń et al., 1994). Free radicals may be produced by lasers of the three mentioned above ranges of power.

The power dose, time, methods, and pulse frequency should be taken to account during planning the laser therapy (Podbielska et al., 2004; Sieroń et al., 1994; Ziętek, 2009). The power, density of power, and density of energy should be correlated to the application of laser. Density of laser power I [W/m^2] is the power related to one square meter of the irradiated area. Density of laser energy H [J/m^2] is the power related to one square meter of the irradiated area (Podbielska et al., 2004; Sieroń et al., 1994; Ziętek, 2009).

7. Application of lasers in ophthalmology

The large amount of laser applications in ophthalmology is known. In that kind of medicine the excimer, argon, krypton, Er:YAG, Nd:YAG and semiconductor lasers are usually used (Dick et al., 2010; Evans & Abrahamse, 2009; Gilmour, 2002; Schmidt-Erfurth, 2010; Seitz & Langenbucher, 2000; Soong & Malta, 2009). The use of lasers in ophthalmology comes down to coagulate, cut and leads to photoablation. Laser radiation can reach the eyeball and focus on the retina and other locations within the eye without surgical intervention. The most common disease which are treated with laser light are glaucoma, cataract, retinal detachment, diabetic retinopathy (Fankhauser & Kwasniewska, 2003; Gilmour, 2002).

Glaucoma is an eye disease in which the optic nerve suffers damage (Chung & Guan, 2006; Eckert, 2010; Herdener & Pache, 2007; Hoffmann & Schulze, 2009; Juzych et al., 2004; Kanamori et al., 2006; Keicher & Stoffelns, 2010; Ngoi et al., 2005; Preußner et al., 2010; Schlote et al., 2008; Wilmsmeyer et al., 2006). It causes permanently decay of vision and if it is untreated it progresses to complete blindness. Glaucoma is often associated with increased pressure of the eye fluid (Gilmour, 2002). The cases in which there is constantly raise of intraocular pressure without any associated optic nerve damage are called ocular hypertension. In that case there is no glaucoma damage. The cases in which there is normal or low ocular pressure with typical for glaucoma visual field are called normal or low tension glaucoma. However, raised intraocular pressure is still the most significant risk factor for glaucoma progression. The permanent damage of the optic nerve and blindness are the effects of untreated glaucoma (Chung & Guan, 2006; Eckert, 2010; Herdener & Pache,

2007; Hoffmann & Schulze, 2009). There are two main categories of glaucoma - open or closed angle. First of them progresses much slower than the other and in this case patient can have any notice of vision lose. In the closed angle glaucoma, the symptoms of disease can appear rapidly (Chung & Guan, 2006). Gradual loss of vision occurs with open angle and chronic angle-closure glaucoma and with acute angle-closure glaucoma. That is why that kind of disorder it is recognized when the disease is quite advanced. In glaucoma once lost visual field cannot be recovered. There is about two percent chance of glaucoma progression in people with a family history of this eye disease. Both laser surgeries and conventional surgeries are performed to treat glaucoma. Selective laser trabeculoplasty (SLT) is one of the newest, efficient methods for the treatment of open angle glaucoma, pseudoexfoliative glaucoma and pigmentary glaucoma. In that kind of treatment Q switch Nd:YAG laser with a wavelength of 532 nm is usually used (Eckert, 2010; Gilmour, 2002). This laser affects on the cells of the trabecular meshwork but it does not cause any destruction or coagulation. The second method of laser treatment in glaucoma is argon laser trabeculoplasty (ALT). That method is focused on drainage correction of fluid from the eye. As a result the intraocular pressure is lower (Wilmsmeyer et al., 2006). In open angle glaucoma the drainage site of the eye does not function normally. In that disorder the iris is encircled by the trabecular meshwork of an eye. The increase of pressure is the result of difficult in drainage. In ALT therapy an argon laser beam is directed at the trabecular meshwork. As the effect the trabecular meshwork drain fluid more effectively (Eckert, 2010; Wilmsmeyer et al., 2006). Nd:YAG and argon lasers are used in iridotomy (L'Esperance, 1983). Argon lasers may be used in iridoplasty (L'Esperance, 1983).

Laser therapy is used in cataract too (Baratz et al., 2001; Çinal et al., 2007; Gilbert, 2011; Hille et al., 2001; Kanellopoulos & Group, 2001; Mahdavi, 2011; Shammas & Shammas, 2007; Verge´s & Llevat, 2003). The cataract is a disease that develops in the crystalline lens of an eye. It can block the passage of light and causes problems from slight to complete opacity. In age-related cataract the power of the lens may be increased, causing near-sightedness called myopia. The opacification of the lens may also reduce the perception of blue colors. Cataract typically progresses slowly and causes vision loss (Gilmour, 2002). That kind of disease potentially induces blinding if it is untreated. Cataract usually affects both eyes, but in most cases one eye is affected earlier than the other. A senile cataract which occurs in the elderly is characterized by an initial opacity and subsequent edema of the lens. One of the most popular cataract treatments nowadays is laser surgery, which uses light to dissolving cataract. The most popular method of cataract surgery is phacoemulsification. In that kind of treatment nucleus is cracking or chopping into smaller pieces. This fragmentation makes emulsification easier. Emulsification of the lens using the Er:YAG laser is very effective for performing small incision cataract surgery in eyes with soft and medium nuclei. The small ablation zones which are created during treatment can help prevent damage to surrounding ocular structures. The Er:YAG technique causes low ablation energy and does not result in thermal injury (Duran & Zato, 2001). Another method involves the removal of almost the entire natural lens while the elastic lens capsule is left intact to allow implantation of an intraocular lens. It is called conventional extracapsular cataract extraction (ECCE). That kind of treatment may be indicated for patients with very hard cataracts or other situations in which phacoemulsification is problematic. Increasingly to remove the pupillary membranes developed after ECCE is used Nd:YAG laser (Kozobolis et al., 1997). Intracapsular cataract extraction (ICCE) is rarely performed kind of cataract surgery, because of high rate of complications. It involves the removal of the lens and the surrounding lens capsule in one piece. After lens removal, an artificial plastic lens - implant is placed (Gilbert, 2011; Kanellopoulos & Group, 2001).

Lasers are also used in medical operations in the field of refractive eye surgery (Gilmour, 2002; Glinkowski & Pokora, 1993; Kim et al., 2011). The main aim of that kind of treatment is to achieve the correct relationship between the length of the eyeball and the power of its optical centers. This is possible by modifying the other shell knobs and intraocular tissues. Refractive surgery can eliminate the necessary of use the contact lenses or glass (Krzeszewska & Zdybel, 2010).

At the beginning of the development of refractive eye surgery procedures used CO_2 lasers (Glinkowski & Pokora, 1993; Kim et al., 2011). However, because of emerging adverse effects they were abandoned. Currently pulsed excimer laser emitting a beam with a wavelength of 193 nm is used during surgeries. The pulses from the beam which is transmitted last from 10 ns to 20 ns. This laser radiation penetrates the cornea to a depth of 1 µm leading to photoablation of the tissue (Krzeszewska & Zdybel, 2010). This is the most common refractive method nowadays. Excimer laser ablation is done under a partial-thickness lamellar corneal flap. While refractive surgery is becoming more affordable and safe, it may not be recommended for everybody. Patients that have medical conditions such as glaucoma, diabetes uncontrolled cardiovascular disease, autoimmune disease, pregnant women or people with certain eye disease are not good candidates for refractive surgery (Kim et al., 2011). Although the risk of complications is decreasing compared to the early days of refractive surgery, there is still a small chance for serious problems. It may appear vision problems such as double-vision, ghosting, halos, starbursts and dry-eye syndrome. Refractive surgery is used in myopia, hyperopia and astigmatism treatment (Gilmour, 2002; Seitz & Langenbucher, 2000).

Myopia is an eyes disease with a refractive defect (Gilmour, 2002). In that kind of disorder while accommodation relaxes, the collimated light produces image focus in front of retina. In other words it is a condition of the eye where the light that comes in does not directly focus on the retina. Because of that the image that one sees is out of focus when looking at a distant object but comes into focus when looking at a close object (Seitz & Langenbucher, 2000).

Hyperopia is a vision defect caused by an imperfection of an eye causing difficulty focusing on near objects and in extreme cases causing a sufferer to be unable to focus on objects at any distance. In that kind of disease power of the cornea and lens is insufficient and the image appears blurred (Gilmour, 2002).

Astigmatism is the visual defect, which is the result of an inability of the cornea to properly focus an image onto the retina. As the effect the image is blurred (Seitz & Langenbucher, 2000).

Laser subephithelial keratomileusis (LASEK) and laser in-situ keratomileusis (LASIK) processes are very common in laser surgery (Gilbert, 2011; Hille et al., 2001; Kanellopoulos & Group, 2001; Verge´s & Llevat, 2003). In LASEK which is the laser epithelial keratomileusis, the cornea's surface layer is treated with alcohol and peeled back to reshape the layer underneath. LASIK prevents most problems of postoperative pain, slow rehabilitation and corneal haze (Kanellopoulos & Group, 2001; Shammas & Shammas, 2007).

Lasers are also very useful tools in the management of malignant and benign intraocular lesions, nowadays. One of the most popular methods for small melanomas treatment is transpupillary thermotherepy (TTT) using 810 nm infrared laser. That kind of treatment can be used in medium and large melanomas as combination therapy with other treatment modalities (Gilmour, 2002).

The important application of lasers in the modern ophthalmology is their use in photodynamic therapy (PDT) (Podbielska et al., 2004). Photodynamic therapy was recently used to treat wet age-related macular degeneration (AMD). That kind of therapy was used for monitory of cases in AMD (Gilmour, 2002; Nakata et al., 2011). Now PDT is used in polypoidal choroidal vasculopathy (Akaza et al., 2007; Nakata et al., 2011; Podbielska et al., 2004). In PDT lasers with the medium range of electromagnetic radiation power are used (Podbielska et al., 2004). The molecules of photosensitizers and their excitation by laser play the most important role in this method. Laser radiation of the proper energy excites the photosensitizer molecules, which come to the next excited energy level, and after it comes to the lower energy level via sending the energy to the eye structures. The scheme of the processes in photodynamic therapy is presented in Figure 6. This scheme was prepared according to the work (Podbielska et al., 2004).

These optical processes form reactive free radicals and oxygen molecules O_2 in the singlet state in eye (Fig. 6) (Podbielska et al., 2004). Free radicals and oxygen molecules damage the pathologically changed structures in eye. Free radicals are the paramagnetic molecules containing unpaired electrons and the short lifetime characterize them, because of free radicals interactions with both dia- and paramagnetic molecules in tissues. Mainly the reactive oxygen species are formed upon laser irradiation during photodynamic therapy, especially hydroxyl radicals (OH) and superoxide radical anion ($O_2^{\cdot-}$) (Podbielska et al., 2004). Single oxygen molecules are diamagnetic, but this oxygen form is higher reactive than paramagnetic oxygen molecules in the ground state, because of the most molecules in the environment are diamagnetic, so the reactions between the similar units go easier (Bartosz, 2006; Podbielska et al., 2004).

Free radicals and singlet oxygen in the physiology are not expected, but their formation in the pathological state of organism during photodynamic therapy is the most important effect (Bartosz, 2006; Jóźwiak & Bartosz, 2008; Podbielska et al., 2004). Free radicals and singlet oxygen damage the pathologically changed tissue. The condition of laser irradiation should be fitted to the conditions of the highest formation of free radicals and singlet oxygen.

Free radicals (S = 1/2) may be directly detected by electron paramagnetic resonance (EPR) spectroscopy (Eaton et al., 1998; Jóźwiak & Bartosz, 2008; Kęcki, 1999; Kirmse & Stach, 1994; Morrish, 1970; Stankowski & Hilczer, 2005; Symons, 1987; Wertz & Bolton, 1986). Electron paramagnetic resonance effect is characteristic for unpaired electrons located in magnetic field of magnetic induction B (Stankowski & Hilczer, 2005; Symons, 1987; Wertz & Bolton, 1986). The electromagnet and the cavity of EPR spectrometer is presented in Figure 7. The Zeeman splitting of energy levels occurs in magnetic field. The spin magnetic moments orientations - parallel and anti-parallel to magnetic field are responsible for Zeeman Effect. Zeeman Effect is the effect of splitting of energy levels of unpaired electrons in the magnetic field as the result of parallel or non parallel electron magnetic moments orientations in this field (Stankowski & Hilczer, 2005; Wertz & Bolton, 1986). The quantization of magnetic moments of unpaired electrons with spin S in magnetic field results from the 2S + 1 (S, S-1, ..., -S) possible values of magnetic spin quantum number M_S. Energy of these states is given by the following formula (Stankowski & Hilczer, 2005; Wertz & Bolton, 1986):

$$E(M_S) = g\,\mu_B\,B\,M_S \tag{3}$$

where: E – energy, M_S – magnetic spin number, g – spectroscopic factor, μ_B – Bohr magneton, B – induction of magnetic field.

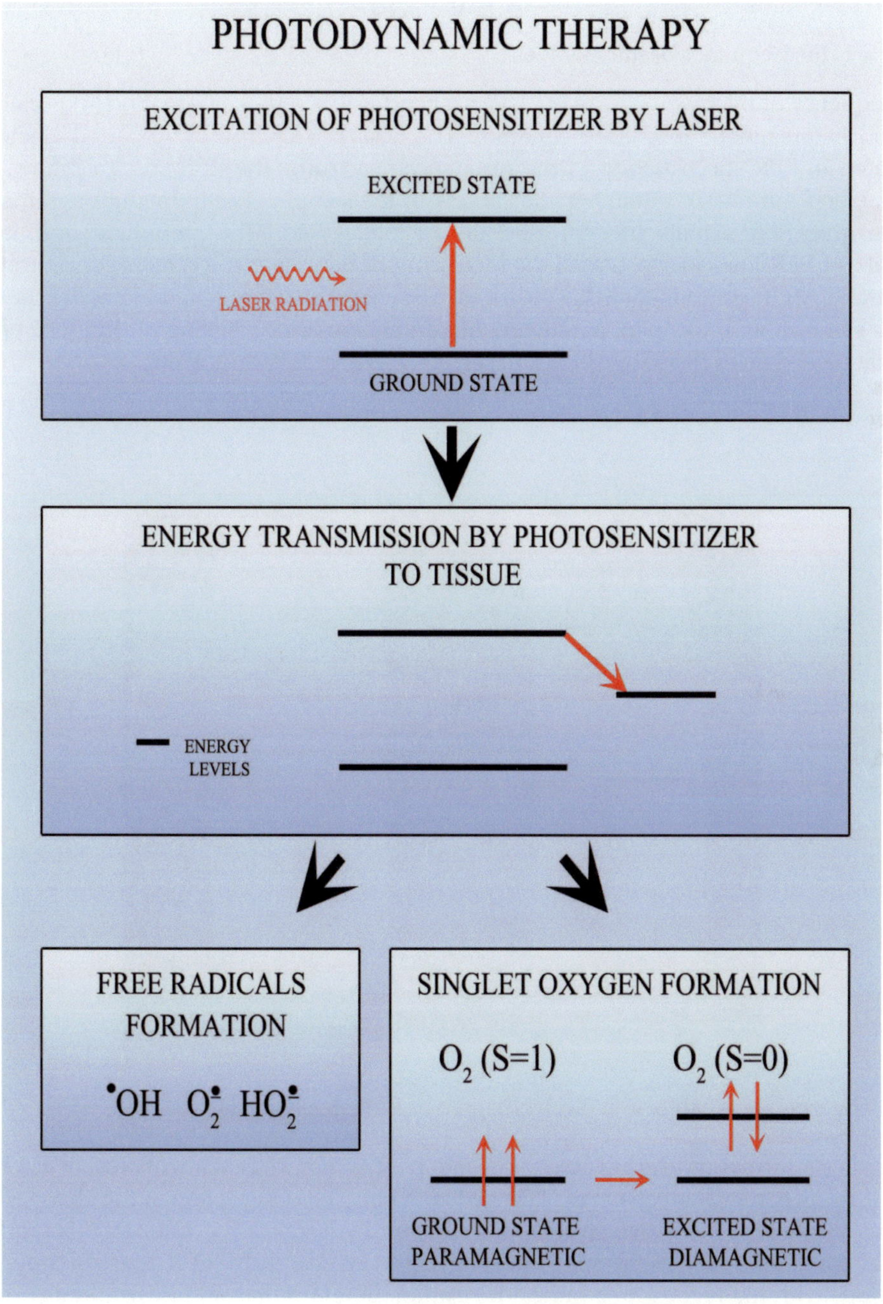

Fig. 6. Photodynamic therapy processes. Prepared according to (Podbielska et al., 2004).

Unpaired electrons are excited to the higher energy levels in magnetic field by microwaves (Stankowski & Hilczer, 2005; Symons, 1987; Wertz & Bolton, 1986). The energy of microwaves (hv) must be fitted to the distances between energy levels (ΔE) of unpaired electrons (Stankowski & Hilczer, 2005; Wertz & Bolton, 1986):

$$hv = \Delta E = g\ \mu_B\ B \quad (4)$$

where v is the frequency of microwaves.

The frequency of microwave from the basic X-band is 9.3 GHz. The equation (4) is called the electron paramagnetic resonance equation. The absorbed energy by unpaired electrons is presented in EPR spectroscopy as the resonance spectrum. The EPR spectra inform about the type and number of paramagnetic centers in the sample. The individual paramagnetic centers give EPR signals in characteristic magnetic field. The amplitude and integral intensity of EPR lines increase with the increasing of paramagnetic centers concentration in the sample. Multi-component EPR spectra as the superposition of several lines are measured for the samples with complex paramagnetic centers system consisting of different types of paramagnetic species (Stankowski & Hilczer, 2005; Wertz & Bolton, 1986).

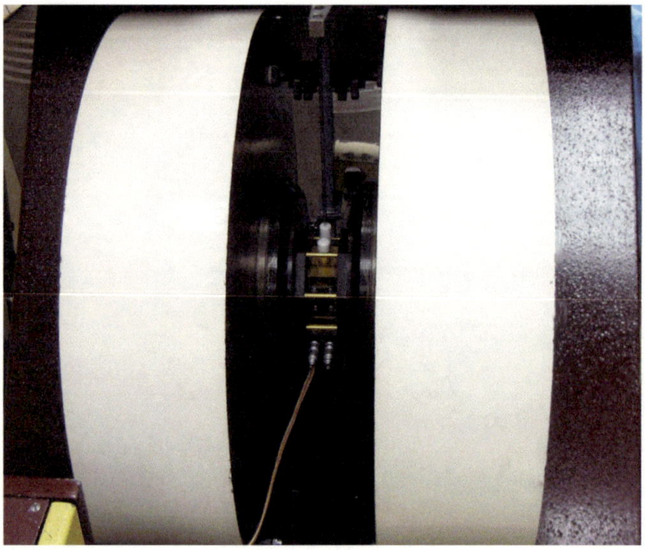

Fig. 7. The resonance cavity and electromagnet of EPR spectrometer.

Free radicals formation during laser irradiation of tumor cells with photosensitizers was studied by us earlier (Latocha et al., 2004, 2005, 2006). The observation of the changes of the amount of free radicals in eye structures irradiated by lasers is proposed in this work. The optimal conditions of PDT in ophthalmology may be search by EPR spectroscopy as the conditions with the highest free radical formation. Similar application was discussed by us for PDT of different tumor cells (Latocha et al., 2004, 2005, 2006).

The optimal conditions of photodynamic therapy are also accompanied by the highest formation of singlet oxygen. Singled oxygen as the diamagnetic molecule may be measured by EPR spectroscopy only by the use of oximetric probes. Oximetric probe is the paramagnetic sample which EPR spectrum strongly changes under changes of the concentration of singlet oxygen in its environment. Our previous results indicates that coal multi-ring aromatic samples may be used as the oximetric probes (Bartłomiejczyk et al., 2008; Latocha et al., 2008; Pilawa et al., 2005b, 2006, 2008a, 2008b). The coal oximetric probes were synthesized by Helena Wachowska group from Institute of Chemistry of Adam Mickiewicz University in Poznań (Poland). Scheme of the idea of application of EPR method and coal oximetric probe is shown in Figure 8. Coal paramagnetic probe contains chemical structures with unpaired electrons with the high probability of interactions with oxygen molecule O_2. Before laser irradiation paramagnetic molecules in the ground triplet state with spin of 1 mainly exist in the environment of the oximetric probe. Paramagnetic oxygen quenches EPR lines of coal probe. After laser irradiation the amount of paramagnetic oxygen molecules decreases, so the amplitudes of the EPR lines of coal probe increase. Under laser irradiation the paramagnetic oxygen molecules become diamagnetic, so the increase of the EPR line of coal probe is proportional to the singlet oxygen formation (Bartłomiejczyk et al., 2008; Latocha et al., 2008; Pilawa et al., 2005b, 2006, 2008a, 2008b). Such methods may be proposed in ophthalmology.

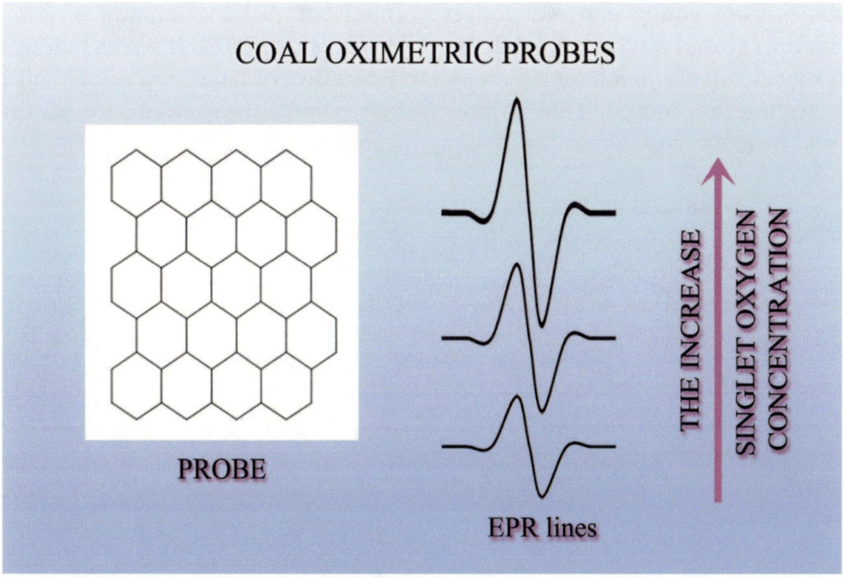

Fig. 8. Potential coal oximetric probe and the changes of its EPR line with increasing of singlet oxygen concentration in the environment.

Lasers in ophthalmology is used to the damage the eye structures via conducting of the energy from melanin biopolymer to them (Gilmour, 2002). Mainly eumelanins with the chemical structure presented in Figure 9 exist in eye (Bilińska et al., 2002; Pasenkiewicz-Gierula, 1990; Sarna, 1981; Zdybel, 2008).

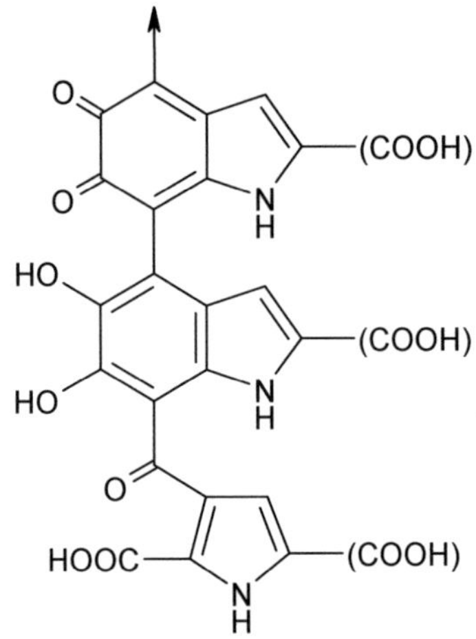

Fig. 9. The chemical structure of eumelanin polymer (Wakamatsu & Ito, 2002).

Melanins are the paramagnetic polymers with o-semiquinone free radicals with spin of 1/2 and biradicals with spin of 1 incorporated in their structure (Kozdrowska, 2006; Najder-Kozdrowska et al., 2009, 2010; Pilawa et al., 2004; Sarna, 1981; Zdybel, 2008). o-Semiquinone free radicals structure is presented in Figure 10 (Kozdrowska, 2006; Pasenkiewicz-Gierula, 1990; Sarna, 1981). Our earlier EPR studies of human retinal pigment epithelium melanosomes from young and old donors pointed out that the amount of free radicals depend on the age and method of irradiation (Bilińska et al., 2002). It seems that free radical reactions in melanin of eye influences on therapeutic effect of laser irradiation. This problem is the interesting proposition of the future electron paramagnetic resonance studies of free radicals and melanin biopolymer and laser application in ophthalmology.

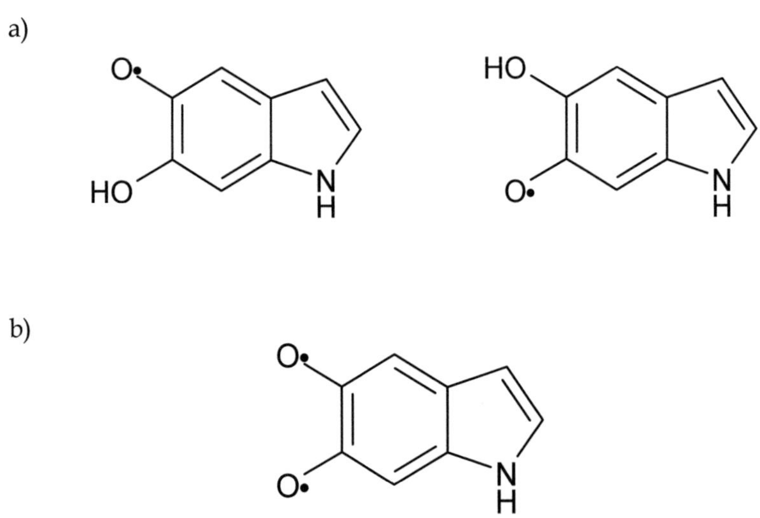

Fig. 10. o-Semiquinone free radicals (a) (Pasenkiewicz-Gierula, 1990; Sarna, 1981) and biradicals (b) (Kozdrowska, 2006) existing in melanin.

The second types of paramagnetic centers - biradicals in melanin were discovered in the last years (Kozdrowska, 2006; Najder-Kozdrowska et al., 2009, 2010; Pilawa et al., 2004; Zdybel, 2008). It is possible that biradicals of melanin could play the role in interactions of laser radiation with eye structures.

The free radicals and biradicals may be differentiated and detected by electron paramagnetic resonance spectroscopy (Kozdrowska, 2006; Najder-Kozdrowska et al., 2009, 2010; Pilawa et al., 2004; Zdybel, 2008). Integral intensities of EPR lines of free radicals and biradicals change differently with the increasing of the measuring temperature (Fig. 11) (Hatfield, 1976). Such dependences were obtained for melanin paramagnetic centers differ in spins (S: 1/2 and 1) (Hatfield, 1976; Kozdrowska, 2006; Najder-Kozdrowska et al., 2009, 2010; Pilawa et al., 2004; Zdybel, 2008).

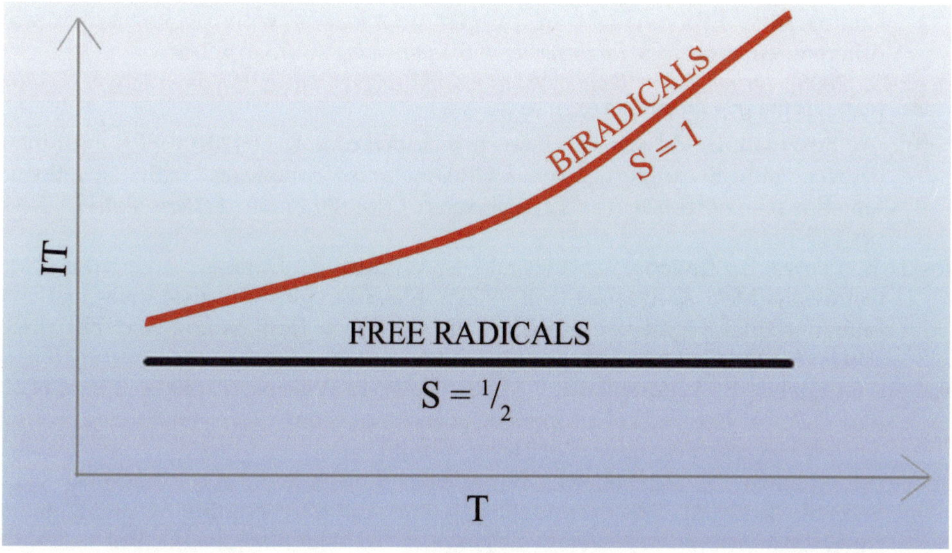

Fig. 11. Changes of integral intensity of EPR lines of free radicals (S = 1/2) and biradicals (S = 1) with the measuring temperature according to functions in (Hatfield, 1976).

The following theoretical functions for free radicals and biradicals in melanin were used (Hatfield, 1976; Kozdrowska, 2006; Zdybel, 2008):

$$IT = C \quad \text{for } S = ½ \tag{5}$$

$$IT = D/(3 + \exp(J/kT)) \quad \text{for } S = 1 \tag{6}$$

where: I - integral intensity of EPR lines, T - temperature, S - spin, k - Boltzmann constant, C, D, J - coefficients in the equations.

The electron paramagnetic resonance spectroscopy could be very useful in modern ophthalmology. EPR is the physical method of examination of paramagnetic species which does not damage the sample. The conditions of the laser therapy may be spectroscopically found and the reactions in the eye structures may be tested.

8. Acknowledgements

The EPR studies of paramagnetic centers in Department of Biophysics in 2011 are financially supported by Medical University of Silesia in Katowice, Poland; grant number KNW-1-086/P/1/0.

9. References

Akaza, E.; Yuzawa, M.; Matsumoto, Y.; Kashiwakura, S.; Fujita, K. & Mori R. (2007). Role of photodynamic therapy in polypoidal choroidal vasculopathy. *Japanese Journal of Ophthalmology*, Vol. 51, pp. 270-277

Baratz, K.H.; Cook, B.E. & Hodge D.O. (2001). Probability of Nd:YAG laser capsulotomy after cataract surgery in Olmsted County, Minnesota. *American Journal of Ophthalmology*. Vol.131, No.2, pp. 161-166, ISSN 0002-9394

Bartłomiejczyk, S.; Pilawa, B.; Krzesińska, M.; Pusz, S.; Zachariasz, J. & Wałach, W. (2008). Comparative EPR analysis of oxygen interactions with plants carbonized at different temperatures. *Engineering of Biomaterials*, Vol.73, pp. 1-3

Bartosz G. (2006). *Druga twarz tlenu. Wolne rodniki w przyrodzie*, Wydawnictwo Naukowe PWN, ISBN 978-83-01-13847-9, Warszawa

Beberok, A.; Buszman, E.; Zdybel, M.; Pilawa, B. & Wrześniok, D. (2010). EPR examination of free radical properties of DOPA-melanin complexes with ciprofloxacin, lomefloxacin, norfloxacin and sparfloxacin. *Chemical Physics Letters*, Vol.497, No.1-3, pp. 115-122

Bilińska, B.; Pilawa, B.; Zawada, Z.; Wylęgała, E.; Wilczok, T.; Dontsov, A.E.; Sakina, M.A.; Ostrovsky, M.A. & Ilyasova, V.B. (2002). Electron spin resonance investigations of human retinal pigment epithelium melanosomes from young and old donors. *Spectrochimica Acta A*,Vol.58, pp. 2257-2264

Buszman, E.; Pilawa, B.; Witoszyńska, T.; Latocha, M. & Wilczok, T. (2003). Effect of Zn^{2+} and Cu^{2+} on free radical properties of melanin from *Cladosporium cladosporioides*. *Applied Magnetic Resonance*, Vol.24, pp. 401-407

Buszman, E.; Pilawa, B.; Zdybel, M.; Wilczyński, S.; Gondzik, A.; Witoszyńska, T. & Wilczok, T. (2006). EPR examination of Zn^{2+} and Cu^{2+} binding by pigmented soil fungi *Cladosporium cladosporioides*. *Science of The Total Environment*, Vol.363, No.1-3, pp. 195-205

Buszman, E.; Pilawa, B.; Zdybel, M.; Wrześniok, D.; Grzegorczyk, A. & Wilczok, T. (2005a). EPR examination of Zn^{2+} and Cu^{2+} effect on free radicals in DOPA-melanin-netilmicin complexes. *Chemical Physics Letters*, Vol.403, No.1-3, pp. 22-28

Buszman, E.; Pilawa, B.; Zdybel, M.; Wrześniok, D.; Grzegorczyk, A. & Wilczok, T. (2005b). Paramagnetic center in DOPA-melanin-dihydrostreptomycin complexes. *Acta Physica Polonica A*, Vol.108, No.2, pp. 353-356

Chodurek, E.; Pilawa, B.; Dzierżęga-Lęcznar, A.; Kurkiewicz, S.; Świątkowska, L. & Wilczok, T. (2003). Effect of Cu^{2+} and Zn^{2+} ions on DOPA-melanin structure as analyzed by pyrolysis-gas chromatography-mass spectrometry and EPR spectroscopy. *Journal of Analytical and Applied Pyrolysis*, Vol.70, No.1, pp. 43-54

Chung, R.S.H. & Guan, A.E.K. (2006). Unusual visual disturbance following laser peripheral iridotomy for intermittent angle closure glaucoma. *Graefe's Archive for Clinical and Experimental Ophthalmology*, Vol.244, (October 2005), pp. 532–533

Çinal, A.; Demirok, A.; Yasar, T.; Yazicioglu, A.; Yener, H.I. & Kilic, A. (2007). Nd:YAG laser posterior capsulotomy after pediatric and adult cataract surgery. *Annals of Ophthalmology*, Vol.39, No.4, pp. 321-326, ISSN 1558-9951

Dick, H.B.; Elling, M. & Willert, A. (2010). Femtosecond laser in ophthalmology - A short overview of current Applications. *Medical Laser Application*, Vol.25, pp. 258–261

Domagała, W.; Pilawa, B. & Lapkowski, M. (2008). Quantitative in-situ EPR spectroelectrochemical stuidies of doping processes in poly(3,4-alkylenedioxythiophene)s: Part 1: PEDOT. *Electrochimica Acta*, Vol.53, No.13, pp. 4580-4590

Durán, S. & Zato, M. (2001). Erbium:YAG laser emulsification of the cataractous lens. *Journal of Cataract & Refractive Surgery*, Vol.27, pp. 1025-1032

Eaton, G.R.; Eaton, S.S. & Salikhov, K.M. (1998). *Foundations of modern EPR*, World Scientific, Singapore, New Jersey, London, Hong Kong

Eckert, S. (2010). Lasertrabekuloplastik in der Glaukomtherapie. *Der Ophthalmologe*, Vol.107, (December 2009), pp. 5–7

Evans, D.H. & Abrahamse, H. (2009). A review of laboratory-based methods to investigate second messengers in low-level laser therapy (LLLT). *Medical Laser Application*, Vol.24, pp. 201–215

Fankhauser, F. & Kwasniewska, S. (2003). *Lasers in Ophthalmology - Basic, Diagnostic and Surgical Aspects: A Review*, Kugler Publications, ISBN 90-6299-189-0, The Hague, The Netherlands

Gilbert, W.R. (2011). Advances in cataract surgery: A review for the non-ophthalmic physician. *Northeast Florida Medicine*, Vol.62, No.2, pp. 15-19

Gilmour, M.A. (2002). Lasers in ophthalmology. *The Veterinary Clinics Small Animal Practice*, Vol.32, pp. 649–672

Glinkowski, W. & Pokora, L. (1993). *Lasery w terapii*, Laser Instruments - Centrum Techniki Laserowej, Warszawa

Hatfield, W.E. (1976). Properties of magnetically condensed compounds, In: *Theory and applications of molecular paramagnetism*, Boudreaux E.A., pp. 357-369, John Wiley & Sons, New York, London, Sydney

Herdener, S. & Pache, M. (2007). Minimal-invasive Glaukomchirurgie: Excimer-Laser-Trabekulotomie. *Der Ophthalmologe*, Vol.104, (August 2007), pp. 730–732

Hewitt, P.G. (2001). *Fizyka wokół nas*, Wydawnictwo Naukowe PWN, ISBN 978-83-01-14718-1, Warszawa

Hille, K.; Hans, J.; Manderscheid, T.; Spang, S. & Ruprecht, K.W. (2001). Laser-flare bei kombinierter Katarakt- und Glaukomichirurgie. *Der Ophthalmologe*, Vol.98, pp. 47–53

Hoffmann, E.M. & Schulze, A. (2009). Glaukomdiagnostik mittels Scanning-Laser-Polarimetrie. *Der Ophthalmologe*, Vol.106, (August 2009), pp. 696–701

Jaroszyk, F. (2008). *Biofizyka*, PZWL, ISBN 978-83-20-03676-3, Warszawa

Jóźwiak, Z. & Bartosz, G. (2008). *Biofizyka. Wybrane zagadnienia wraz z ćwiczeniami.* Wydawnictwo Naukowe PWN, ISBN 978-83-01-14461-6, Warszawa

Juzych, M.S.; Chopra, V.; Banitt, M.R.; Hughes, B.A.; Kim, C.; Goulas, M.T. & Shin, D.H. (2004). Comparison of long-term outcomes of selective laser trabeculoplasty versus argon laser trabeculoplasty in Open-Angle Glaucoma. *American Academy of Ophthalmology*, Vol.111, No.10, (October 2004), pp. 1853-1859, ISSN 0161-6420

Kanamori, A.; Nagai-Kusuhara, A.; Escaño, M.F.T.; Maeda, H.; Nakamura, M. & Negi, A. (2006). Comparison of confocal scanning laser ophthalmoscopy, scanning laser polarimetry and optical coherence tomography to discriminate ocular hypertension and glaucoma at an early stage. *Graefe's Archive for Clinical and Experimental Ophthalmology*, Vol.244, (July 2005), pp. 58–68

Kanellopoulos, A.J. & Group, P.I. (2001). Laser cataract surgery. A prospective clinical evaluation of 1000 consecutive laser cataract procedures using the dodick photolysis Nd:YAG system. *Ophthalmology*, Vol.108, (April 2001), pp. 649-655, ISSN 0161-6420

Kęcki, Z. (1999). *Podstawy spektroskopii molekularnej*, Państwowe Wydawnictwo Naukowe, Warszawa

Keicher, A.S. & Stoffelns, B.M. (2010). Argon laser suture lysis following glaucoma filtering surgery - A short introduction to the procedure. *Medical Laser Application*, Vol.25, pp. 209-213

Kim, P.; Sutton, G.L. & Rootman D.S. (2011). Applications of the femtosecond laser in corneal refractive burgery. *Current Opinion in Ophthalmology*, Vol.22, pp. 238-244

Kirmse, R. & Stach, J. (1994). *Spektroskopia EPR. Zastosowania w chemii.* Uniwersytet Jagielloński, Kraków

Kozdrowska, L. (2006). *Właściwości centrów paramagnetycznych kompleksów DOPA-melaniny z kanamycyną i jonami miedzi(II)*, Rozprawa doktorska. Uniwersytet Zielonogórski, Zielona Góra

Kozobolis, V.P.; Pallikaris, I.G.; Tsambarlakis, I.G. & Vlachonikolis, I.G. (1997). Nd:YAG laser removal of pupillary membranes developed after ECCE with PC-IOL implantation. *Acta Ophthalmologica Scandinavica*, Vol.75, No.6, pp. 711-715

Krzeszewska, A. & Zdybel, M. (2010). Lasers and their application in medicine and pharmacy. *Scientific Review in Pharmacy*, Vol.6, pp. 24-31

Latocha, M.; Pilawa, B., Zdybel, M. & Wilczok, T. (2005). Effect of laser radiation on free radicals in human cancer G361 cells. *Acta Physica Polonica A*, Vol.108, No.2, pp. 409-412

Latocha, M.; Pilawa, B.; Kuśmierz, D.; Zielińska, A. & Nawrocka, D. (2006). Changes in free radicals system of *Imr-90* and *C-32* cells during photodynamic therapy. *Polish Journal of Environmental Studies*, Vol.15, No.4A, pp. 154-156

Latocha, M.; Pilawa, B.; Pietrzak, R.; Nowicki, P. & Wachowska, H. (2008). Conditions of photodynamic therapy of tumor cells examined by carbonized coal and EPR spectroscopy. *Engineering of Biomaterials*, Vol.73, pp. 4-6

Latocha, M.; Pilawa, E.; Chodurek, E.; Buszman, E. & Wilczok, T. (2004). Paramagnetic center in tumor cells. *Applied Magnetic Resonance*, Vol.26, pp. 339-344

L'Esperance, F.A. (1983). *Ophthalmic lasers. Photocoagulation, photoradiation, and surgery*, The C. V. Mosby Company, ISBN 0-8016-2823-7, St. Louis, Toronto, London

Mahdavi, S. (2011). Laser cataract surgery: the next new thing in ophthalmology. *Cataract & Refractive Surgery Today*, Vol.12, (March 2011), pp. 83-87

Maiman, T. (1960). Stimulated optical radiation in ruby. *Nature*, Vol.187, pp. 493-494

Matuszczyk, M.; Buszman, E.; Pilawa, B.; Witoszyńska, T. & Wilczok, T. (2004). Cd^{2+} effect on free radicals in *Cladosporium cladosporioides*-melanin tested by EPR spectroscopy. *Chemical Physics Letters*, Vol.394, No.4-6, pp. 366-371

Morrish, A.H. (1970). *Fizyczne podstawy magnetyzmu*, Państwowe Wydawnictwo Naukowe, Warszawa

Najder-Kozdrowska, L.; Pilawa, B.; Buszman, E.; Więckowski, A.B.; Świątkowska, L.; Wrześniok, D. & Wojtowicz, W. (2010). Triplet states in DOPA-melanin and in its complexes with kanamycin and copper Cu(II) ions. *Acta Physica Polonica A*, Vol.118, No.4, pp. 613-618

Najder-Kozdrowska, L.; Pilawa, B.; Więckowski, A.B.; Buszman, E. & Wrześniok, D. (2009). Influence of copper(II) ions on radicals in DOPA-melanin. *Applied Magnetic Resonance*, Vol.36, No.1, pp. 81-88

Nakata, I.; Yamashiro, K.; Yamada, R.; Gotoh, N.; Nakanishi, H,; Hayashi, H.; Tsujikawa, A.; Otani, A.; Ooto, S.; Tamura, H.; Saito, M.; Saito, K.; Iida, T.; Oishi, A.; Kurimoto, Y.; Matsuda, F. & Yoshimura N. (2011). Genetic variants in pigment epithelium-derived factor influence response of polypoidal choroidal vasculopathy to photodynamic therapy. *American Academy of Ophthalmology,* Vol.118, No.7, pp. 1408-1415

Ngoi, B.K.A.; Hou, D.X.; Koh L.H.K. & Hoh, S.T. (2005). Femtosecond laser for glaucoma treatment: a study on ablation energy in pig iris. *Lasers in Medical Science,* Vol.19, (January 2005), pp. 218–222

Pasenkiewicz-Gierula M. (1990). *Badanie struktury i dynamiki paramagnetycznych układów molekularnych o spinie s = 1/2 metodą elektronowego rezonansu paramagnetycznego (ERP),* Rozprawa habilitacyjna. Uniwersytet Jagielloński, Kraków

Pilawa, B.; Bartłomiejczyk, S.; Krzesińska, M.; Pusz, S.; Zachariasz, J. & Wałach, W. (2008a). Influence of oxygen O_2 on microwave saturation of EPR lines of plants carbonized at 650^{0}C and potential application in medicine. *Engineering of Biomaterials,* Vol.73, pp. 7-9

Pilawa, B.; Buszman, E.; Gondzik, A.; Wilczyński, S.; Zdybel, M., Witoszyńska, T. & Wilczok, T. (2005a). Effect of pH on paramagnetic centers in *Cladosporium cladosporioides. Acta Physica Polonica A,* Vol.108, No.1, pp. 147-150

Pilawa, B.; Buszman, E.; Wrześniok, D.; Latocha, M. & Wilczok, T. (2002). Application of EPR spectroscopy to examination of gentamicin and kanamycin binding to DOPA-melanin. *Applied Magnetic Resonance,* Vol.23, pp. 181-192

Pilawa, B.; Chodurek, E. & Wilczok, T. (2003a). Types of paramagnetic centres in Cu^{2+} complexes with model neuromelanins. *Applied Magnetic Resonance,* Vol.24, pp. 417-422

Pilawa, B.; Latocha, M.; Buszman, E. & Wilczok, T. (2003b). Effect of oxygen on spin-spin and spin-lattice relaxation in DOPA-melanin. Complexes with chloroquine and metal ions. *Applied Magnetic Resonance,* Vol.25, pp. 105-111

Pilawa, B.; Latocha, M.; Kościelniak, M.; Pietrzak, R. & Wachowska, H. (2006). Oxygen effects in tumor cells during photodynamic therapy. *Polish Journal of Environmental Studies,* Vol.15, No.4A, pp. 160-162

Pilawa, B.; Latocha, M.; Krzyminiewski, R.; Kruczyński, Z.; Buszman, E. & Wilczok, T. (2004). Effect of temperature on melanin EPR spectra. *Physica Medica,* Vol.1, pp. 96-98

Pilawa, B.; Latocha, M.; Ramos, P; Kościelniak, M.; Pietrzak, R. & Wachowska, H. (2008b). New paramagnetic probes and singlet oxygen formation in cells. *Current Topics in Biophysics,* Vol.31, pp. 10-15

Pilawa, B.; Pietrzak, R.; Wachowska, H. & Babeł, K. (2005b). EPR studies of carbonized cellulose - oxygen interactions. *Acta Physica Polonica A,* Vol.108, No.2, pp. 151-154

Pilawa, B.; Zdybel, M.; Latocha, M.; Krzyminiewski, R. & Kruczyński, Z. (2008c). Analysis of lineshape of black *Drosophila melanogaster* EPR spectra. *Current Topics in Biophysics,* Vol.31, pp. 5-9

Podbielska, H.; Sieroń, A. & Stręk, W. (2004). *Diagnostyka i terapia fotodynamiczna,* Wydawnictwo Medyczne Urban & Partner, ISBN: 83-87944-79-3, Wrocław

Preußner, P.R.; Ngounou, F. & Kouogan, G. (2010). Controlled cyclophotocoagulation with the 940 nm laser for primary open angle glaucoma in African eyes. *Graefe's Archive for Clinical and Experimental Ophthalmology,* Vol.248, (May 2010), pp. 1473–1479

Sarna T. (1981). Badanie struktury i właściwości centrów aktywnych melanin. *Zagadnienia Biofizyki Współczesnej,* Vol.6, pp. 201-219

Schlote, T.; Grüb, M. & Kynigopoulos, M. (2008). Long-term results after transscleral diode laser cyclophotocoagulation in refractory posttraumatic glaucoma and glaucoma in aphakia. *Graefe's Archive for Clinical and Experimental Ophthalmology*, Vol.246, (October 2007), pp. 405–410

Schmidt-Erfurth, U. (2010). Current concepts in the management of diabetic macular edema. *Johns Hopkins Advanced Studies in Ophthalmology*, Vol.7, No.2, (December 2010), pp. 52-59

Seitz, B. & Langenbucher, A. (2000). Lasers in ophthalmology. *The Lancet Perspectives*, Vol.356, (December 2000), pp. S26-S28

Shammas, H.J. & Shammas, M.C. (2007). No-history method of intraocular lens power calculation for cataract surgery after myopic laser in situ keratomileusis. *Journal of Cataract & Refractive Surgery*, Vol.33, pp. 31–36

Sieroń, A.; Cieślar, G. & Adamek M. (1994). *Magnetoterapia i laseroterapia. Podstawy teoretyczne. Oddziaływania biologiczne. Zastosowania kliniczne*, Śląska Akademia Medyczna, Katowice

Soong, H.K. & Malta, J.B. (2009). Perspective femtosecond lasers in ophthalmology. *American Journal of Ophthalmology*, Vol.147, No.2, pp. 189-197

Stankowski, J. & Hilczer, W. (2005). *Wstęp do spektroskopii rezonansów magnetycznych*, Wydawnictwo Naukowe PWN, Warszawa

Straburzyńska-Lupa, A. & Straburzyński, G. (2004). *Fizjoterapia*, Wydawnictwo Lekarskie PZWL, ISBN 83-200-2904-X, Warszawa

Symons, M. (1987). *Spektroskopia EPR w chemii i biochemii*, Państwowe Wydawnictwo Naukowe, Warszawa

Verge´s, C. & Llevat, E. (2003). Laser cataract surgery: Technique and clinical results. *Journal of Cataract & Refractive Surgery*, Vol.29, pp. 1339–1345

Wakamatsu, K. & Ito, S. (2002). Advanced chemical methods in melanin determination. *Pigment Cell Research*, Vol.15, No.3, pp. 174-183

Wertz, J.E. & Bolton, J.R. (1986). *Electron Spin Resonance Theory and Practical Applications*, Springer Verlag, ISBN 0-412-01161-1, New York, London

Wilmsmeyer, S.; Philippin, H. & Funk, J. (2006). Excimer laser trabeculotomy: a new, minimally invasive procedure for patients with glaucoma. *Graefe's Archive for Clinical and Experimental Ophthalmology*, Vol.244, (October 2006), pp. 670–676

Wróblewski, A.K. (2007). *Historia fizyki*, Wydawnictwo Naukowe PWN, ISBN 83-01-14635-1, Warszawa

Zdybel, M. (2008). *Złożony układ centrów paramagnetycznych kompleksów DOPA-melaniny z netilmicyną, jonami cynku(II) i miedzi(II)*, Rozprawa doktorska. Śląski Uniwersytet Medyczny, Katowice

Zdybel, M.; Pilawa, B.; Buszman, E. & Witoszyńska, T. & Cieśla, H. (2010). EPR studies of *Cladosporium cladosporioides* mecelium with flucytosine. *Current Topics in Biophysics*, Vol.3, pp. 271-275

Zdybel, M.; Pilawa, B.; Buszman, E. & Wrześniok, D. (2009). Zastosowanie spektroskopii EPR do badania melanin oraz kompleksów melanin z jonami metali i substancjami leczniczymi. *Farmaceutyczny Przegląd Naukowy*, Vol.6, No.6, pp. 42-46

Ziętek, B. (2009). *Lasery*, Wydawnictwo Naukowe Uniwersytetu Mikołaja Kopernika, ISBN 978-83-231-2345-3, Toruń

2

Microsurgical Techniques in Ophthalmology – Current Procedures and Future Directions

Pradeep Prasad[1,2], Allen Hu[1,2],
Robert Beardsley[1,2] and Jean-Pierre Hubschman[1,2]
[1]*Retina Division, Jules Stein Eye Institute,*
[2]*Department of Ophthalmology,*
David Geffen School of Medicine at University of California, Los Angeles, California,
USA

1. Introduction

Given the small dimensions of the human eye, ocular surgery demands the ability to both visualize and precisely manipulate delicate tissue within a microscopic space. Microsurgical technological advancements have rapidly changed the way in which ophthalmic microsurgery is performed and have provided for greater surgical efficiency and improved functional outcomes.

A thorough understanding of normal ocular anatomy is critical to define pathologic anatomic conditions, to delineate surgical goals, and to develop and utilize surgical tools to optimize patient outcomes. The anatomy of the eye and orbit can be broadly categorized as extraocular structures (including the eyelids, lacrimal gland, canalicular system, conjunctiva, and extraocular muscles) and intraocular structures, located within the globe of the eye. Intraocular structures are further grouped based on their location in the anterior or posterior segments of the eye (figure 1). The anterior segment consists of (from anterior to posterior): the cornea, anterior chamber, iris, and crystalline lens. The crystalline lens is suspended in place by hundreds of zonular fibers, which extend from the ciliary body to a thin capsule surrounding the lens. Contraction of the ciliary body changes the tension of the zonular fibers on the lens, allowing the lens to change its shape and focusing power. The cornea and lens are of particular importance as a majority of ophthalmic surgical interventions are performed on these structures, such as corneal transplantation, refractive corneal surgery, and cataract extraction.

The posterior segment of the eye consists of the vitreous humor (a clear gelatinous substance composed primarily of water, type II collagen, and hyaluronic acid), the neurosensory retina, the retinal pigment epithelium (which promotes the function and viability of the neurosensory retina), and the choroid (a vascular layer interposed between the retinal pigment epithelium and the sclera). The neurosensory retina is a highly organized extension of the central nervous system composed of photoreceptors and multiple layers of interconnected neurons. These neurons ultimately synapse on ganglion cells, whose axons coalesce into the optic nerve. Posterior segment ophthalmic surgery generally involves removal of the vitreous humor to: 1) relieve traction of the vitreous on the retina, 2) remove visually-significant opacities within the vitreous, or 3) to gain access to the retina or sub-retinal space for further surgical manipulation.

The origins of ophthalmic surgery date back as far as the sixth century B.C. when ancient Indian surgeons used curved needle-like instruments to dislodge a cataract, a technique termed "couching". Further contributions by Greek, Middle Eastern and European physicians provided detailed functional knowledge of the eye and intraocular structures.

Development of the surgical microscope further revolutionized ophthalmic microsurgery. Although initially little more that a binocular telescope worn by the surgeon, the modern ophthalmic microscope provides a well-lit binocular stereoscopic view with a high-level optical clarity (figure 2). Foot pedal controls allow the surgeon to adjust magnification (approximately 10-30x), illumination intensity, x-y axis movement and level of focus. Furthermore, both contact and non-contact lens based systems are now employed to provide a wide-angle stereoscopic view of the posterior segment. Indeed, the ophthalmic microscope has enabled precise visualization of both anterior and posterior segment structures making modern ophthalmic microsurgery possible. Two such ophthalmic surgeries, cataract extraction and pars plana vitrectomy, are described below in detail.

1.1 Cataract extraction

1.1.1 Technique overview

Over two million cataract extractions are performed yearly in the United States making it the most common ophthalmic surgery, and among the most frequently performed surgeries in any field. A "cataract" refers to a focal or diffuse opacification of the crystalline lens, a structure that is normally optically clear and measures approximately 10mm wide and 6mm deep. Opacities within the lens limit the normal focusing ability of the lens resulting in blurred vision. Although cataract formation is most commonly an age-related process, cataracts may form at any age due to a number of different etiologies including medications, systemic metabolic disease, and ocular trauma. Although many methods have been developed to remove cataracts, the most common technique employed in modern ophthalmic microsurgery is "phacoemulsification".

Standard phacoemulsification for cataract extraction typically begins with the creation of a 2.2 to 3 mm tunnel or wound in the peripheral cornea to gain access to the anterior chamber. The anterior chamber is stabilized during intraocular manipulation with an ophthalmic viscoelastic device (a clear, removable, gel-like substance composed primarily of water and hyaluronic acid). A circular opening is then created in the anterior face of the lens capsule, termed a "continuous curvilinear capsulorrhexis". With the lens contents now accessible, the tip of a handpiece connected to a phacoemulsification machine is placed within the anterior chamber. This handpiece performs three functions: 1) administration of ultrasonic energy to fracture the lens material into small pieces; 2) aspiration to remove the small lens particles; 3) irrigation of a saline-like solution to maintain the volume of the anterior chamber (Figure 3).

Once the lens material is successfully removed, a clear artificial lens is typically placed within the intact capsule of the lens. Although early intraocular lenses were composed of rigid polymethylmethacrylate (PMMA) requiring enlargement of the corneal wound for intraocular placement, modern intraocular lenses are composed of silicone or acrylic, both of which are biologically inert and can be folded and placed into the eye through a small corneal incision.

2. Principles of phacoemulsification

The fluid dynamics of phacoemulsification require constant fluid irrigation into the anterior chamber to maintain normal depth while lens material is aspirated. Due to the small volume of the anterior chamber, fluid circulation during phacoemulsification is critical to ensure efficient removal of the cataract while preventing complications due to anterior chamber collapse. Indeed, if outflow, or aspiration through the handpiece is allowed to exceed inflow, or irrigation, even for a fraction of a second, anterior chamber instability may result in unintended damage to intraocular tissue.

The formula that governs fluid flow during phacoemulsification surgery is Poiseuille's law:

$$Q = \Delta P \pi r^4 / 8 \eta L,$$

where Q is flow rate, ΔP is the pressure gradient, r is the radius of instrument tip, η is fluid viscosity, and L is length of the tubing. Given that the viscosity of the fluid and length of the tube are constant, flow is essentially proportional to the change in pressure and radius of the tubing.

In the case of phacoemulsification surgery, ΔP is the pressure gradient between the infusion pressure and the vacuum driving aspiration. The source of fluid inflow is a bottle of balanced salt solution, the height of which can be adjusted relative to the patient's eye to control infusion pressure. Fluid outflow is dependent on the vacuum level generated by the machine. The surgeon can control both the infusion pressure and vacuum or aspiration.

3. Phacoemulsificaiton instruments

The primary tool of phacoemulsification is the handpiece (figure 4). The tip of this tool delivers ultrasonic energy to break up the lens, aspirate fluid and lens material, and provide inflow of fluid to the anterior chamber. The handpiece is connected to a machine that regulates the aspiration pressure, the infusion pressure, and the intensity of the ultrasonic energy delivered by the handpiece. The design of the handpiece tip varies with respect to the angle and size of the lumen. Steeper tip bevels (less angled) provide better cutting ability into dense lens nuclear material whereas flatter tip bevels provide a larger surface area for improved aspiration of large lens fragments.

Modern phacoemulsification machines also employ foot pedal controls with at least three positions that allow the surgeon to control the fluidics of phacoemulsification. The first position typically provides irrigation only, which cools the handpiece and keeps the anterior chamber formed. The second position, in addition to irrigating, engages the aspiration mode at a constant or variable rate, depending on the settings selected by the surgeon. In the third position, ultrasound energy is delivered in addition to irrigation and aspiration. Many other microsurgical instruments are also utilized in conjunction with the phacoemulsification probe to facilitate manipulation of the lens material and to improve the efficiency of cataract extraction.

Ultrasonic power for phacoemulsification is generated by applying a time-varying electric field across a piezoelectric crystal in the phacoemulsification handpiece. The oscillating crystal deforms in response to the electric field, resulting in the conversion of electrical to mechanical energy. Oscillation of the tip occurs at a preset frequency that varies from 27 kHz to 60 kHz. The amplitude of the movement, or stroke length, ranges from 50 μm to 100 μm and is modulated when the phacoemulsification power is changed. As the tip retracts, a vacuum is created resulting in the formation of "cavitation bubbles". When the bubbles implode, they release heat and shock waves that fracture the lens material. Phacoemulsification power can also be modulated by varying the duty cycle; the period of time when the phacoemulsification power is being delivered. Varying the duty cycle allows for efficient administration of phacoemulsification energy to promote fracturing of lens material while minimizing excess heat and energy that may damage the cornea or other intraocular structures.

4. Phacoemulsification systems

While there are a variety of phacoemulsification machine manufacturers and configurations, they all generate the required vacuum and aspiration based on one of two pump types: Venturi and peristaltic.

A peristaltic system (figure 5) utilizes a series of rollers to displace fluid, producing flow in a compressible tube that is wound tightly around a rotating wheel. As the wheel turns, a segment of fluid trapped between two rollers is moved, resulting in more fluid being drawn into the tubing. Therefore, the flow rate is directly proportional to the speed of the rotary mechanism. Significant vacuum is generated only when the tip is occluded. The surgeon sets a desired flow rate and vacuum limit. The flow rate determines how rapidly the vacuum builds up when the handpiece tip is occluded and flow is restricted.

The Venturi pump (figure 6) utilizes the Venturi effect to create vacuum. The Venturi effect refers to the creation of vacuum secondary to the flow of a fluid (typically nitrogen or air in a phacoemulsification machine) over an opening. Thus, a Venturi pump allows a given vacuum level to be generated immediately, without occlusion of the phacoemulsification tip as is required in the peristaltic system. As such, flow cannot be directly modulated and is dependent on the vacuum level generated. The Venturi system provides the surgeon with near instantaneous vacuum levels and potentially higher flow rates.

5. Femtosecond laser technology and the future of phacoemulsification

In the near future, a new application of an existing technology may alter the way in which cataract surgery is performed. The femtosecond laser is a device that emits coherent optical pulses with a wavelength of 800nm and duration on the order of 10^{-15} seconds. It has been used extensively in ophthalmology due to its ability to alter delicate tissue in a precise and predictable way. In addition to its precision, the femtosecond laser can cut tissue with practically no heat development. Clinical trials utilizing the femtosecond laser to perform the incisional steps of cataract surgery, including cornea wound creation, capsulorrhexis creation, and disassembly of the lens are currently ongoing. Future applications of this laser may allow many steps of phacoemulsification to be automated, thus minimizing risk and error while increasing surgical efficiency.

5.1 Vitreoretinal surgery

5.1.1 Basic techniques

Vitreoretinal surgery, in its modern form, is a minimally invasive technique similar to laparoscopic surgery whereby small entry ports or trocars are placed on the surface of the eye to gain surgical access to intraocular structures. A variety of instruments including surgical manipulators, illuminating probes, laser probes, and infusing and aspirating devices can be placed through the trocars for a variety of surgical procedures. The trocars are placed at a safe anatomic entry point, the pars plana, located within a narrow band around the eye 3 to 4 mm posterior to the corneoscleral junction. This space lies just posterior to the highly vascularized ciliary body but anterior to the retina. Placing trocars too far anteriorly or posteriorly can lead to significant complications and surgical failure.

The vitreous body, a clear gelatinous structure located between the crystalline lens and the retina, occupies approximately 80% of the volume of the human eye. It is mainly composed of water (99%), collagen fibrils (type II collagen), and hyaluronic acid. The vitreous gel is integral in the pathogenesis of many posterior segment diseases. For example, in diabetic retinopathy, bleeding into the vitreous cavity can severely reduce visual acuity since dense hemorrhages can become loculated within the vitreous body. In some instances where the hemorrhage does not dissipate on its own, vitrectomy is necessary to remove the vitreous and blood. The vitreous body is adherent to a number of structures in the posterior segment including tight adhesions over the optic disc, the macula, retinal blood vessels and the ora serrata (a band which straddles the anterior retina and the pars plana where the vitreous and retina are anatomically fused and cannot be surgically separated). Thus, vitreous removal must be performed in a precise and controlled fashion to minimize excessive traction of the retina, which may result in complications such as retinal tears and detachment. Although the vitreous plays an important role in ocular development *in utero,* removal of the vitreous in the adult eye has no deleterious effects on the health of the retina. Once vitrectomy is performed, the vitreous cavity is typically replaced by the surgeon with balanced salt solution, which is eventually replaced by the eye with aqueous humor. Therefore, the vitreous body does not reform once it is removed.

5.2 Principles of vitreoretinal surgery

Surgery within the posterior segment of the eye is bound by the same principles as anterior segment surgery: the volume of the eye must be maintained as material is removed. Adding complexity to vitreoretinal surgery is the difficulty in visualization of the posterior segment during intraocular surgical maneuvers. External illumination is generally inadequate to visualize the retina and, despite advances in modern lens systems, the surgeon's view of the retinal periphery can be limited while operating near the posterior pole.

The first pars plana vitrectomy was performed by Robert Machemer in 1970 using a 17-gauge (1.42 mm diameter) one-port system that combined an infusion cannula and vitreous cutter in one handpiece. Since that time, numerous innovations have improved the efficiency and outcomes of this procedure and led to the development of the modern 3-port 20-gauge pars plana vitrectomy. In this procedure, three 20-gauge sclerotomies are created within the pars plana. One sclerotomy is used to anchor a cannula that infuses balanced salt solution into the posterior cavity while the vitrectomy is performed, thus maintaining intraocular pressure. The remaining ports are used for the vitrectomy probe and a light probe to remove the vitreous and illuminate intraocular structures respectively. Following removal of the vitreous, the sclerotomy can be used to introduce other instruments such as intraocular forceps and laser probes to further manipulate and treat the retina (figure 7).

Visualization during pars plana vitrectomy is performed using the operating microscope in conjunction with a contact lens (which can be held by the assistant or sewn onto the eye at the corneoscleral junction) or a non-contact lens viewing system. Direct contact visualization systems allow for greater field of view and enhanced three-dimensional perception. Non-contact lens viewing systems are easier to use and do not require an assistant or additional surgical maneuvers to anchor the lens to the ocular surface, but sacrifice some field of view and three-dimensional perception.

5.3 Vitrectomy instruments

The basic tools of pars plana vitrectomy are a vitreous cutter, illuminating device, laser probe, various tissue manipulators such as micro-forceps for delicate intraocular work, and an infusion cannula to maintain intraocular pressure. The workhorse of pars plana vitrectomy is the vitreous cutter, whose basic function is to remove the vitreous in a controlled fashion. Because the vitreous is a semi-solid structure with adhesions to the retina, simple aspiration of the vitreous results in excess traction on the retina. To minimize such traction, the vitrectomy probe is designed with both an aspiration port and a cutting mechanism to aspirate a small volume of vitreous into the handpiece and to cut and remove it. High cut speeds allow for incremental removal of small amounts of vitreous while minimizing tractional forces of the vitreous on the retina. Lower cut speeds result in removal of larger volumes of vitreous, thereby increasing the rate at which vitreous is removed. Most modern high-speed (600-5000 cuts per minute) vitrectomy probes are pneumatically driven with a side-cutting guillotine port near the tip of the instrument (figure 8).

Most vitrectomy machines are equipped with a built-in light source employing either yellow or white light from a halogen or metal-halide light source. The light probe, a fiberoptic cable encased in a plastic handpiece, is connected to the light source and can function as a separate instrument or, in some cases, can be combined with the infusion cannula to simultaneously illuminate and irrigate the posterior segment. A recent innovation has been the introduction of a xenon light source, which can provide bright illumination through a narrow probe. This has facilitated the performance of smaller gauge surgery and eliminated light wavelengths under 400 nm that can be phototoxic to the retina.

Many surgical instruments have been developed to facilitate surgical procedures on the macula. The macula is located at the center of the posterior pole of the retina and has the highest concentration of photoreceptors. It is responsible for fine central visual acuity needed for such tasks as reading, driving and other activities of daily living. Pars plana vitrectomy may be required to treat a variety of macular diseases including epiretinal membranes, macular holes, vitreo-macular traction, and hemorrhagic age-related macular degeneration. Instruments used to manipulate and treat the macula include a variety of micro-forceps (e.g. end-grasping and pick forceps), scissors, needles and cannulas.

The intraocular laser probe allows for minimally invasive and precise ablation of retinal tissues and is used in a wide variety of surgical procedures. Similar to the light probe, the "endolaser" probe is also a fiber-optic cable encased in a plastic handpiece. The intensity of the laser ablation is controlled by the surgeon by modulating the power and duration of the laser as well as by altering the distance of the probe tip to the retina. Intraocular laser is typically employed for two key purposes: 1) to treat retinal tears by creating a fibrous scar between the retina and the underlying choroid thus preventing fluid in the eye from collecting underneath the retina; and 2) to ablate non-perfused or ischemic retinal tissue (as in diabetic retinopathy and other occlusive retinal vascular diseases) to decrease the pathologic production of growth factors that result in retinal neovascularization, intraocular hemorrhage and retinal edema.

5.4 Vitrectomy systems

Vitrectomy machines, similar to phacoemulsification machines, are complex devices that drive the vitreous probe cutter, provide irrigation at an adjustable level to control intraocular pressure, aspirate and remove intraocular material, and provide a light source for intraocular illumination. Many of these functions are controlled via foot pedal by the surgeon, similar to the previously-described phacoemulsification machine.

Two major types of systems are used to drive the vitrectomy probe cutter: electric guillotine and pneumatic guillotine. The electric guillotine employs an electric drive motor with a sinusoidal transmission, translating the rotary motion of an electric motor shaft to the linear guillotine motion of the cutter tip. The profile of motion of the guillotine remains constant as the cut rate is altered. That is to say, the duty cycle, or ratio of time the cutter port is open or closed, remains constant regardless of the cut rate.

The second type of handpiece, which is pneumatically driven, uses pulses of air or gas to close the cutter tip. The pneumatically-driven guillotine is attached to a diaphragm. When a pulse of air is delivered, the diaphragm and guillotine extend, closing the cutter tip and completing a cut. The guillotine then retracts to its original position either through a spring mechanism or through a "dual drive" system where an additional pulse of air pushes the guillotine back, thus opening the cutter tip. In the spring mechanism, as the cut rate is increased, the duration of open time per cut decreases, while the closed time remains constant (decreasing the duty-cycle). The "dual drive" system allows for improved duty cycle compared with the spring mechanism, but the duty cycle still decreases at high cut rates.

6. Current directions

Recent advances in vitreous surgery have resulted in the development of smaller instruments: the 23- and 25-gauge transconjunctival suture-less vitrectomy systems (figure 9). A standard 20-gauge (0.9 mm diameter) vitrectomy requires removal of the conjunctiva and sutures to close the sclerotomies used to access the posterior segment. 23-gauge (0.6 mm diameter) and 25-gauge (0.5 mm diameter) entry wounds, when constructed properly, are small enough to self-seal and thus can be placed through the conjunctiva and sclera without the need for closing sutures. To allow for easy entry and exit of surgical instruments during vitrectomy and to align the entry holes in the conjunctiva and sclera, a 23- or 25-gauge trocar is placed at the site of the desired sclerotomy. The trocar consists of two components: a polyimide cannula and a polymer hub. The polyimide cannula maintains the transconjunctival and transcleral tunnel through which surgical instruments are passed. The polyimide cannula material provides both strength and flexibility, allowing the cannula wall to be thin while avoiding collapse or buckling. The polymer hub is the part of the trocar visible on the surface of the eye and prevents the trocar from sliding into the vitreous cavity. The hub has a central hole that is continuous with the cannula, allowing for instruments to be inserted into the vitreous cavity.

Many surgeons believe the potential advantages of smaller gauge, suture-less techniques include shortened operative time and faster patient recovery. However, the reduction in port diameter results in reduced flow rates compared with 20-gauge cutters, and therefore, smaller-gauge surgery may require more time to remove the same amount of vitreous or may be inadequate to remove dense or highly organized vitreous. Other concerns with suture-less techniques include the increased risk of post-operative hypotony and infection if the sclerotomies are not constructed properly.

7. The future of ophthalmic surgery – Robot-assisted microsurgery?

With recent innovations in engineering and the demands for increasingly precise and efficient ophthalmic microsurgery, the next major advancement in ophthalmic surgery may be the integration of mechanization and robotics into ophthalmic microsurgical techniques. The potential benefits of robotic surgery in ocular surgery include increased precision, reduction of human error, task automation and the capacity for remote surgery.

Guerrouad and Vidal described one of the first ocular robotic systems in 1989. Named the "Stereotaxical Microtelemanipulator" (SMOS), it provided relatively good range of motion for basic surgical tasks but the technology was too premature at that time to raise tangible interest for further development. In the 1990s, Steve Charles and researchers at Northwestern University demonstrated the use of robotic platforms for ophthalmic surgery with precise position measurement and fine incremental motion but these prototypes were limited by the complexity of its software control and the need for increased robotic responsiveness to human controls.

Presently, the Food and Drug Administration has approved the *da Vinci* Surgical System (Intuitive Surgical, Sunnyvale, CA), which has become the most commonly employed robotic platform in human surgery (figure 10). Although it has been used in the fields of general surgery, urology, gynecology and cardiac surgery, its use in ophthalmic surgery is in its early phases. Preliminary studies have demonstrated good robot arm responsiveness to human controls for external and intraocular surgical tasks. However, the remote center of motion (pivot point) and limited range of motion of the robot arm make intraocular manoeuvrability difficult with excessive distortion of the globe of the eye. Furthermore, while the visualization system of the *da Vinci* system is adequate for extraocular and some anterior segment surgical procedures, posterior segment surgery is hampered by a limited field of view. Finally, the surgical instruments of the *da Vinci* instruments are not well-suited to ophthalmic microsurgery due to their bulkiness. Recent studies have better defined the range of motion required for robot-assisted ophthalmic surgery and further refinements to the robot surgery platform are underway to make this technology a tangible option in the near future.

Ocular robotic surgery poses a myriad of unique challenges and the application of this technology will undoubtedly require many stages of evolution. Further work will be required to continue to integrate traditional surgical techniques with new devices to bring the advantages of robotics to the field of ophthalmology.

8. Conclusion

Ophthalmic microsurgery has rapidly evolved in recent history as advances in medical device technology have led to the development of numerous minimally invasive procedures for the treatment of ocular diseases. The multi-disciplinary integration of technology and knowledge from the fields of biomaterials, optics, lasers, ultrasonics and pneumatics have helped to refine the surgical tools available to ophthalmic surgeons, increasing their efficiency and surgical outcomes. As life expectancy and the prevalence of various systemic diseases continue to rise, so too will the burden of ocular disease. Further advances to better address these demands will undoubtedly lead to novel surgical techniques and devices, expanding the role of ophthalmic surgery to undiscovered heights.

9. References

American Academy of Ophthalmology. Basic and Clinical Science Course: Lens and Cataract. Basic Principles of Ophthalmic Surgery. San Francisco: American Academy of Ophthalmology, 2006.

American Academy of Ophthalmology. Basic and Clinical Science Course: Retina and Vitreous. San Francisco: American Academy of Ophthalmology, 2006.

American Academy of Ophthalmology. Basic and Clinical Science Course: Fundamentals and Principles of Ophthalmology. San Francisco: American Academy of Ophthalmology, 2006.

Apple, DJ. Sims, J. Harold Ridley and the Invention of the Intraocular Lens. Survey of Ophthalmology 1996 Feb; 40(4): 279-292.

Beebe DC . The lens. In PL Kaufman, A Alm, eds., Adler's Physiology of the Eye, 10th ed., pp. 117–158. St. Louis: Mosby, 2003.

Bourla, D. H., J. P. Hubschman, et al. (2008). Feasibility study of intraocular robotic surgery with the da Vinci surgical system. Retina 28(1): 154-8.

Charles S, Das H, Ohm T, et al. Dexterity-enhanced telerobotic microsurgery. Proc IEEE Int Conf Adv Robot 1997;July:5–10

Charles S. Debating the pros and cons of 23-g vs 25-g vitrectomy: the pros of 25-g vitrectomy. Retina Physician 2006; 3: 24–25.

Devgan, U. Phaco Fundamentals for the Beginning Phaco Surgeon. Bausch and Lomb Ophthalmology World Report Series, 2009: 1-54.

Georgescu, D., A. F. Kuo, et al. (2008). A fluidics comparison of Alcon Infiniti, Bausch & Lomb Stellaris, and Advanced Medical Optics Signature phacoemulsification machines. Am J Ophthalmol 145(6): 1014-1017.

Guerrouad, A. and D. Jolly (1989). Automatic analysis of weariness during a micromanipulation task by SMOS. IEEE Conference Proceeding 3: 906-907

Guerrouad, A. and P. Vidal (1989). SMOS: stereotaxical microtelemanipulator for ocular surgery. IEEE Conference Proceeding 3 879-880.

Guerrouad, A. and P. Vidal (1991). Advantage of computer aided teleoperation (CAT) in microsurgery. IEEE Conference Proceeding 1: 910- 914.

Hubschman, J. P., J. L. Bourges, et al. The Microhand': a new concept of micro-forceps for ocular robotic surgery. Eye 2010 Feb; (24(2): 364-367

Hubschman, J. P., J. L. Bourges, et al. Effect of Cutting Phases on Flow Rate in 20-, 23-, and 25-Gauge Vitreous Cutters. Retina 2009: Oct; 29(9): 1289-93.

Jensen, P. S., K. W. Grace, et al. (1997). Toward robot-assisted vascular microsurgery in the retina. Graefes Arch Clin Exp Ophthalmol 235(11): 696-701.

Machemer R, Parel JM, Norton EW. Vitrectomy: a pars plana approach: technical improvements and further results. Trans Am Acad Ophthalmol Otolaryngol 1972; 76: 462–466.

Nagy Z, Takacs A, Filkorn T, Sarayba M. Initial clinical evaluation of an intraocular femtosecond laser in cataract surgery. J Refract Surg 2009 Dec;25(12):1053-60.

O'Malley C, Heintz Sr RM. Vitrectomy with an alternative instrument system. Ann Ophthalmol 1975; 7: 585–588: 91–94.

Siebel, Barry. Phacodynamics: Mastering the Tools and Techniques of Phacoemulsification Surgery. New Jersey: Slack Incorporated, 2005.

Son, J., J. L. Bourges, et al. Quantification of intraocular surgery motions with an electromagnetic tracking system. Stud Health Technol Inform 2009; 142: 337-9.

Tsirbas, A., C. Mango, et al. Robotic ocular surgery. Br J Ophthalmol 2007; 91(1): 18-21.

Williams, GA. 25-, 23-, or 20-gauge instrumentation for vitreous surgery? Eye 2008; 22: 1263–1266.

Zabriskie, Norman. The Operating Microscope and Surgical Loupes. American Academy of Ophthalmology. Basic and Clinical Science Course: Basic Principles of Ophthalmic Surgery. Basic Principles of Ophthalmic Surgery. San Francisco: American Academy of Ophthalmology, 2006.

3

Transient Receptor Potential (TRP) Channels in the Eye

Zan Pan[1], José E. Capó-Aponte[2,3] and Peter S. Reinach[3]
[1]*Margaret Dyson Vision Institute, Weill Cornell Medical College, New York, NY,*
[2]*Visual Sciences Branch, U.S. Army Aeromedical Research Laboratory, Fort Rucker, AL,*
[3]*Department of Biological Science, State University of New York, College of Optometry, New York, NY, USA*

1. Introduction

The first member of transient receptor potential (TRP) channel superfamily was discovered in photoreceptors of *Drosophila* over 30 years ago.[1] Since then this protein superfamily has been extensively characterized based on exponential increases in the number of publications related to TRP channels. With 28 TRP homologous genes identified in mammals, TRP channels have been detected in both neural and non-neural tissues.

In humans, 27 different TRP genes are classified into two groups and six different subfamilies based on their amino acid homology and phenotypes associated with mutant genes. The genes of TRP channel in Group 1 and Group 2 are only distantly related. The Group 1 of TRP genes are comprised of TRPC (canonical), TRPM (melastatin), TRPV (vanilloid) channel subfamilies, with TRPA (ankyrin) being more recently assigned to this group.[2] Such categorization is based on their resemblance to the amino acid sequence of the *Drosophila* TRP channel. The nomenclature of TRP channel genes in Group 2 is based on the human phenotypes generated by the mutation of the founding genes of each subfamily, including polycystic kinase disease (PKD) and mucolipidosis type IV (MCOLN, mucolipin). Their encoded proteins have also been referred to as TRPP (polycystin) and TRPML (mucolipin), respectively (Figure 1).

The TRP superfamily is evolutionally conserved from nematodes to mammals.[3] The common features of TRP channels are six putative transmembrane spanning domains and a cation-permeable pore formed by a short hydrophobic region between transmembrane domains 5 and 6. They are configured as homo- or hetero-tetramers to form non-selective cation channels (Figure 2). Their permeability ratios to Ca^{2+}/Na^{+} vary significantly among individual members. TRPV5 and TRPV6 channels exhibit a Ca^{2+}/Na^{+} permeability ratio of greater than 100, indicating high Ca^{2+} selectivity.[4] In contrast, TRPM4 and TRPM5 channels are impermeable to Ca^{2+} but are selective for monovalent cations (Na^{+}, K^{+}).[5, 6] Such intra-family variability is unique to the TRP channel superfamily whereas most other ion channel families have little difference in ionic permeability within a family.[7]

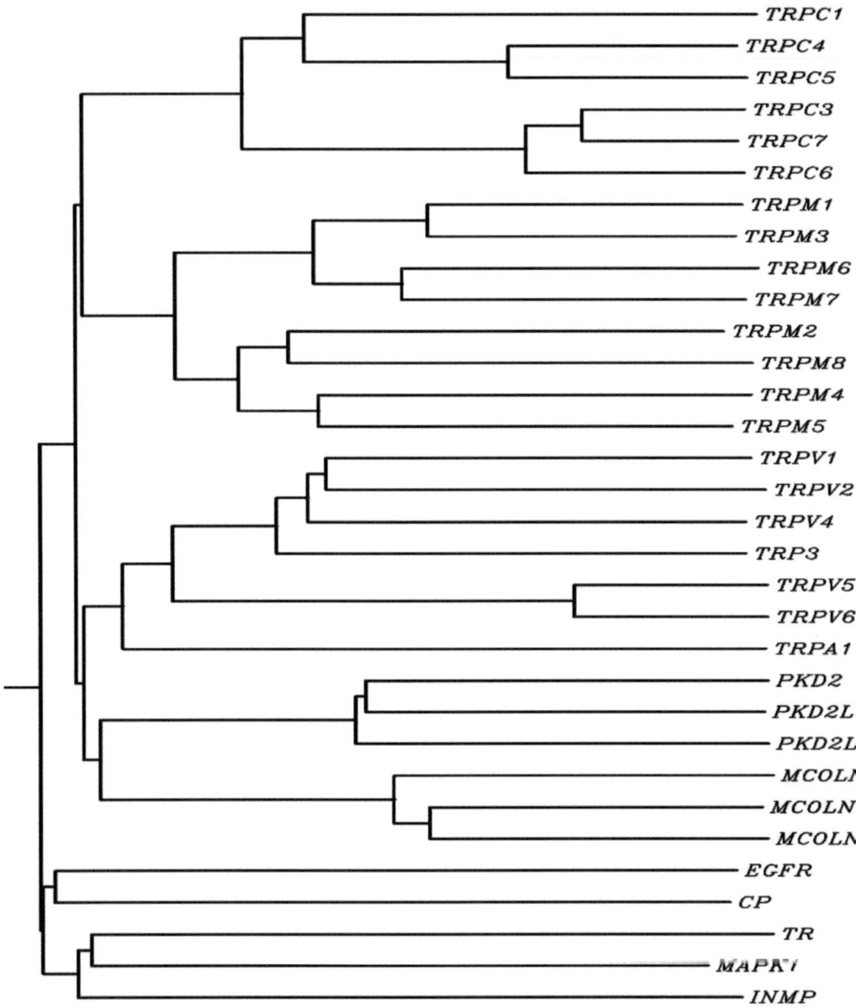

Fig. 1. Human TRP channel superfamily dendrogram. Random proteins bound to the plasma membrane (i.e., EGF receptor, EGFR), endoplasmic reticulum (i.e., calreticulin precursor, CP), mitochondria (thioredoxin reductase, TR), cytosolic protein (i.e., mitogen-activated protein kinase 1, MAPK1) and nuclear membrane (i.e., inner nuclear membrane protein, INMP) are shown to illustrate that PKD and MCOLN are evolutionarily related to TRP channels or are the results of convergent evolution. The dendrogram shows that PKD and MCOLN belong to the TRP channel superfamily, since random genes extend from branches distinct from the TRP channel superfamily.[8]

TRP channel subfamilies in Group 1 share substantial sequence homology in the transmembrane domain 6. What divides each subfamily is differences in their intracellular domains. TRPC, TRPV and TRPA channels contain ankyrin repeats near the intracellular N-terminal domain, whereas the TRPC and TRPM channels subfamilies possess proline-rich 'TRP domain' in the region of the C-terminal near the putative transmembrane segment. TRPM6 and TRPM7 channels have a protein kinase domain in the C-terminal.

The TRPC subfamily consists of seven genes (TRPC1–7) in mammals, but TRPC2 channel is a pseudogene in humans. TRPC channels are widely expressed in multiple systems. TRPC4, TRPC5, TRPC6 and TRPC7 channels are identified in the various ocular tissues of mammals.[9-12] The TRPM channel subfamily comprises eight genes (TRPM 1–8), of which three encode channel-like proteins and five non-channel proteins. TRPM1 channels are expressed in retinas and TRPM8 channels in corneas.[13, 14] The TRPV channels subfamily contains six members (TRPV1–6). TRPV1, TRPV2, TRPV3 and TRPV4 channels are expressed in the cornea whereas TRPV1, TRPV2, TRPV5 and TRPV6 channels are expressed in the retina.[15-20] The TRPA channel subfamily has only one member, TRPA1.

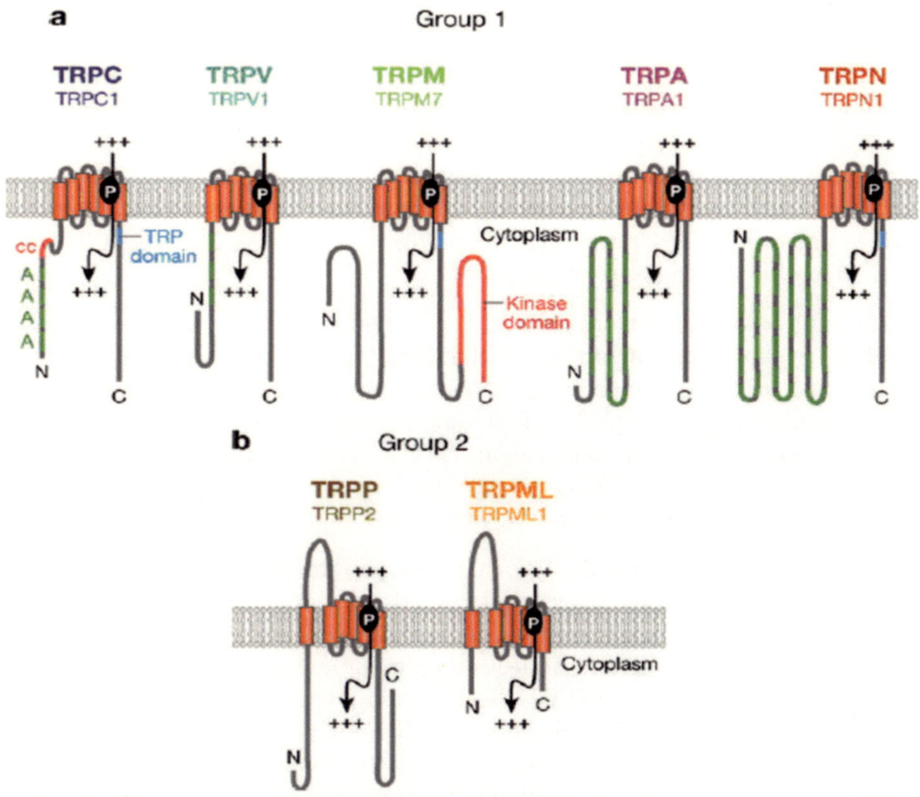

Fig. 2. Domain structure of the TRP channel superfamily. There are five TRP channel subfamilies in Group 1 (TRPN, no mechanoreceptor potential C channels are expressed in mammals) (a) and two TRP channel subfamilies in Group 2 (b). All subfamilies contain a six-transmembrane domain unit with a cation-permeable pore between domains 5 and 6. Four of such units are assembled as a homo- or hetero-tetramer to form a TRP channel. Domain indications: ankyrin repeats (A), coiled-coil domain (cc), protein kinase domain (TRPM6 and TRPM7 channels only), cation-permeable pore (P), transmembrane (TM) domain, cation-permeable (+++), TRP channels domain (TRPC and TRPM channels only), large extracellular loop between transmembrane domains 1 and 2 (TRPP and TRPML channels only). Adapted with permission from Venkatachalam and Montell.[21]

TRPP and TRPML channel subfamilies belong to Group 2. They contain limited sequence homology to TRP channels in Group 1, although such resemblance to classical TRP channels is still larger than those of random genes (e.g., EGFR, INMP) (Figure 1). TRPP channel proteins share 25 percent amino acid sequence homology to TRPC3 and TRPC6 channels over a region including transmembrane domains 4 and 5 and the hydrophobic pore loop between domains 5 and 6. TRPML channel proteins consist of three small proteins compared with other TRP channel proteins. Homology of their amino acid sequence with TRPC channels proteins is restricted to the region spanning transmembrane domains 4 to 6 (amino acids 331 to 521). TRP channels in Group 2 have a unique large extracellular loop between their first and second transmembrane domains. They are named as TRP channels based on the six transmembrane domains that they contain and function as cation-permeable channels.

The activation mechanisms of TRP channels are unique in that there are a diverse host of stimuli that can activate TRP channels and exhibit sharp differences in stimulatory modes even within each TRP channel subfamily. TRP channels were initially recognized as sensory mechanisms to a variety of stimuli, ranging from light, temperature, osmotic pressure, smell, taste, mechanical stress and acidity. There is also increasing awareness of their roles in mediating wound healing, inflammation, apoptosis and excretion. These channels are sensitive to intracellular and extracellular messengers, as well as declines in the calcium content of intracellular calcium stores (ICS).

Their activation following conformation changes modulates Ca^{2+}/Na^{+} cell permeability ratios, which is dependent on TRP channel subunit composition. Transient increases in intracellular calcium concentration trigger intracellular activation of mediators including: 1) phospholipase C (PLC) by coupled GTP-binding protein, leading to stimulation of store-operated Ca^{2+} channels; 2) transactivation of EGF tyrosine receptors through MMP-mediated HB-EGF shedding.[4, 10, 16] The physiological significance of TRP channel expression is indicated by the finding that TRP channel mutations are linked to human diseases.[22]

There is compelling evidence that the TRP channel superfamily plays a critical role in ocular homeostasis and pathogenesis. Functional importances of TRP isotypes expressed in different ocular tissues are multi-faceted. Their activation is essential for retaining corneal deturgescence and clarity, mediating aqueous humor outflow through trabecular meshwork and ciliary body as well as inducing light sensation in retina. Mutation of TRP channels is associated with ocular pathological phenotypes either due to loss of its homeostatic role or over-activation of its function. The realization of the importance of TRP channel has prompted much research effort to investigate novel strategies for regulating TRP channels function in a number of ocular diseases.

2. Roles of TRP channels in corneal sensation and wound healing

Continuous renewal of corneal epithelial layer is essential to maintain corneal transparency. The intact epithelium not only offers a smooth and clear optical surface, but also provides corneal barrier function. This property protects the underlying stroma from swelling and pathogenic invasion. Should such protection become compromised by ocular surface diseases, outcomes can range from mild symptoms, such as irritation, photophobia, to severe consequences including corneal opacity, ulceration and even perforation. TRP channel functions have been indicated to associate with maintaining corneal sensation and integrity. Corneas express ample collection of TRP channel isotypes in various mammalians. There are TRPC1, TRPC3, TRPC4, TRPC6 and TRPC7 as well as TRPV1–4 channels in the corneal epithelium, TRPV1-4 in the corneal endothelium, TRPV1, TRPA1, and TRPM8 in the corneal nerves.[10, 15-17, 23, 24, 25-27] These channels are involved in corneal regenerative, protective and sensory mechanisms.

TRPC4 channels protein is localized in plasma membranes of cultured human corneal epithelial cells (HCEC) and mediate epidermal growth factor (EGF)-promoted epithelial proliferation. They are activated by EGF-induced depletion of ICS content in the endoplasmic reticulum. This depletion occurs as a consequence of stimulation of PLC activity which results in increases in inositol 1,4,5-trisphosphate (IP3) formation. This response leads to declines in ICS content and activation of TRPC4 store operated channel (SOC) function. Its activation induces intracellular Ca^{2+} influx leading to stimulation of downstream signalling cascades. They include the mitogen activated protein kinase (MAPK) cascade composed of ERK, JNK and p38 casettes as well as protein kinase A (PKA), protein kinase C (PKC), JAK/STAT and PI3-K/AKT/GSK-3. All of their activations contribute to the control of increases in cell survival and proliferation elicited by EGF. The importance of TRPC4 channels activation to mediate EGF-induced mitogenic responses is indicated by the finding that knockdown of its gene expression in HCEC eliminated the mitogenic response to EGF.[10]

TRPV1 channel expression was first identified on the ophthalmic branch of the trigeminal nerve. More recently, the functional expression of this channel was also identified in the corneal epithelial and endothelial layers. A hallmark of its activity is that the vanilloid compounds (such as capsaicin isolated from hot chilli pepper), hyperosmolarity, acidity (pH below 6) and high temperatures (above 43°C) stimulate TRPV1 channels. In the mouse corneal epithelium, severe chemical injury to corneal epithelium induces TRPV1 channel activation leading to dysregulated inflammation, scarring and loss of corneal transparency. On the other hand, its activation stimulates in HCEC proliferation and migration through EGF receptor (EGFR) transactivation.[28] The involvement of TRPV1 channel activation in inducing these diverse responses is indicated by the finding that in homozygous TRPV1 knockout mice the wound healing response to an alkali burn does not result in losses of corneal transparency. Similarly, TRPV1 channel activation in some types of dry eye disease resulting from exposure to hyperosmolar tears may account for chronic inflammation since TRPV1 channels activation caused by exposure to a hyperosmolar challenge induced large increases in a host of proinflammatory cytokines (e.g., IL-6, IL-8, TNFα and IL-1β) and chemoattractants (e.g., MCP-1) in HCEC. On the other hand, pre-exposure to a selective TRPV1 channel antagonist obviated all of these responses, suggesting that TRPV1 channels are potential drug target for the treatment of dry eye syndrome because suppression of its activation may reduce ocular surface inflammation.[16, 23]

In contrast with TRPV1, its cohort, TRPV4 channel reacts to a different spectrum of stresses. Unlike TRPV1, which is thought to only be activated by a hyperosmolar stress, TRPV4 channels may instead be an osmosensor for a hypoosmolar challenge.[17] Such a stress is encountered by the cornea during exposure to fresh water (e.g., swimming, bathing, use of some eye drops). This hypotonic exposure results initially in corneal epithelial swelling due to obligatory water influx in order to reach equilibration between the cell interior and surface tears. However, excessive swelling can lead to cell lysis. To counter the initial swelling, corneal epithelial cells mediate regulatory volume decrease (RVD) behavior by stimulating volume-sensitive potassium and chloride channels as well as potassium-chloride co-transporter (KCC) activity to restore isotonic cell volume through osmotically coupled net fluid efflux.

TRPV1–4 channel isoforms also serve as thermosensors over defined temperature ranges in the corneal epithelium. In addition, TRPV3 channel activation, either by temperatures above 33°C or by its selective agonist, carvacrol, not only contributes to thermosensation, but also accelerates epithelial wound recovery by enhancing cell survival, proliferation and migration.[15, 29] TRPV1–3 and TRPC4 channels are also expressed in corneal endothelial cells.[9, 30] TRPV1–3 channels are sensitive to temperatures from 25 to 40°C, similar to their epithelial counterparts.

TRP channels play an important role in mediating corneal sensations. The cornea has the highest sensory nerve density of any tissue in the body. The corneal sensory nerves originate from the ophthalmic branch of the trigeminal ganglion and are responsible for eliciting nociception to thermal, chemical and mechanical stimuli.[31] TRPV1 channels colocalize with substance P (SP) and calcitonin-gene-related peptide (CGRP) in the ophthalmic branch of the trigeminal nerve indicating their role in eliciting nociceptive perception. This realization makes TRPV1 channel tenable as a potential drug target for treating neurotrophic keratopathy.[31, 32] Additionally, the TRPM8 channel contributes to corneal cold sensation and basal tear secretion required to maintain corneal surface hydration.[14, 33]

Taken together, these studies on the corneal epithelial, endothelial cells and corneal nerves indicate that functional expression of TRP channels are essential for maintaining corneal transparency and eliciting adaptive responses to stresses. This indicates the importance of further studies on TRP channel regulation since such insight may lead to novel strategies for treating corneal diseases and better management of ocular surface inflammatory pain.

3. Roles of TRP channels in glaucoma

Some members of the TRPC and TRPV channel subfamilies are expressed in trabecular meshwork, ciliary muscle and retinal ganglion cells.[34, 35] Their roles have been associated with regulating intraocular pressure through modulation of aqueous humor flows and ganglion cell survival. The trabecular meshwork contains contractile elements whose tension modulation changes fluid drainage rate from the anterior chamber into the Canal of Schlemm. The contractile state of trabecular meshwork is governed by tension imparted from the ciliary muscle and possibly trabecular meshwork itself.[35, 36] The trabecular meshwork and the ciliary muscle act as functional antagonists. Such opposition is evident since ciliary muscle contraction leads to relaxation of the trabecular meshwork with subsequent increases in fluid outflow whereas trabecular meshwork contraction has the opposite effect.[35] Malfunction of trabecular meshwork and ciliary muscle contractility often leads to ocular hypertension and glaucoma.[37] Their contractile states are modulated by changes in intracellular Ca^{2+} concentration and Ca^{2+} channel activity. Specifically, increases in cytoplasmic Ca^{2+} resulting from the stimulation of TRP channels enhance contractility. Other types of Ca^{2+} channels that regulate intracellular Ca^{2+}concentration include L-type voltage-gated Ca^{2+} channels, receptor operated Ca^{2+} channels and store-operated calcium entry (SOCE) pathways. In bovine trabecular meshwork cells, TRPC1 and TRPC4 channels are implicated in the formation of heteromeric SOCE channels which contribute to rises in cytoplasmic Ca^{2+} store and therefore trabecular meshwork contractility during exposure to bradykinin or endothelin-1.[4]

Similarly TRPC1, TRPC3, TRPC4 and TRPC6 channels are also present in ciliary muscle cells. The ciliary muscle is densely innervated by parasympathetic nerves that stimulate muscle contraction through acetylcholine-mediated muscarinic receptor stimulation on neighboring muscle cells. Such activation leads to a surge in intracellular Ca^{2+} concentration resulting in membrane voltage depolarization via receptor-operated non-selective cation channels. TRPC1, TRPC3, TRPC4 and TRPV6 channels are considered as potential candidates for such channels as they are co-localized with muscarinic receptor type 3 in ciliary muscle fibres.[38, 39]

Modulation of TRPC channel activity in turn alters aqueous humor outflow and therefore intraocular pressure through changes in trabecular meshwork contractility. The dual localization of TRPC channels on ciliary muscles and trabecular meshwork cells suggests that strategies targeted towards their selective modulation may prove to be advantageous in providing better control of intraocular pressure in patients with ocular hypertension or glaucoma. Such an outcome is possible once there is definitive identification of the TRP channels subtypes on each of these tissues. At this point, it may be possible to maximize fluid outflow rates by selectively decreasing trabecular meshwork resistance through a decrease in its contractile state. Accordingly, additional studies are needed to map the TRP channels subtypes and characterize their mechanisms of regulation in the ciliary muscle and trabecular meshwork.

Chronic intraocular hypertension is a risk factor which in some cases can induce glaucoma due to damage to retinal ganglion cells. Such damage can result from either increased hydrostatic pressure, declines in retrograde neutrophin flow, ischemic or oxidative stress. Irreversible loss of retinal ganglion cells leads to gradual and often insidious vision impairment and possible blindness. Elevated intraocular pressures can activate TRP channels in retinal ganglion cells. TRP channel sensitivity to hydrostatic pressure has been described in the bladder, lungs and skin.[40-42] Sappington et al. showed *in vitro* that exposure of retinal ganglion cells to elevated hydrostatic pressure induced transient rises of intracellular Ca^{2+} accumulation due to TRPV1 channel activation. This effect promoted apoptosis of retinal ganglion cells whereas suppression of TRPV1 channel activation protected retinal ganglion cells from pressure-induced death.[34] Recently, similar stresses were identified to stimulate TRPV4 channel and induce apoptosis in retinal ganglion cells.[43] The increased levels of cytoplasmic Ca^{2+} are the underlying mechanism leading to retinal ganglion cells apoptosis.[44] Ca^{2+}-dependent calcineurin and calpain are a phosphatase and a protease, respectively, that trigger apoptosis signalling. Both of them induce cytochrome c release from mitochondria and trigger pro-apoptotic signalling. In contrast, the TRPV1 channel in the retinal microglia appears to have a retinoprotective effect. Retina microglia cells are essential to neuronal homeostasis and provide innate immunity for retina to defend against pathogenic infiltration. Exposure of microglia to chronic stress is associated with various neurodegenerative diseases, including retinal dystrophies. TRPV1 channel activation in the cultured retinal microglia cells by hydrostatic pressure induces increases in IL-6 and TNF-α release through transient rises in intracellular Ca^{2+} levels. Rises in IL-6 suppress pro-apoptotic signalling pathways and cell death.[45] Therefore, provided strategies can be devised to selectively induce increases in microglial TRPV1 channels expression, TRPV1 channels may be a potential drug target in managing pressure-induced retinal ganglion cell loss in glaucoma.

4. Possible roles of TRP channels in cataract development

Maintenance of intracellular Ca^{2+} levels is imperative to crystalline lens clarity.[46] Lenses with cortical cataracts have intracellular Ca^{2+} levels that are above those in the physiological range.[47] Accordingly, a better understanding of the mechanisms mediating control of lens intracellular Ca^{2+} levels is pertinent for identifying economical and novel drug strategies to preserve lens transparency or slow cataract progression.

As previously described, store-operated calcium entry (SOCE) channels are composed of TRP subunits and are heterogeneously expressed in the lens epithelial cells. Epithelial cells in the lens equatorial region have higher SOCE expression than that in the central anterior region. This difference is attributable to the fact that the size of the intracellular calcium storage is larger in the equatorial than the central anterior epithelial cells.[48] The higher intracellular Ca^{2+} load in the equatorial epithelium is required for its more rapid proliferative rate than other parts of the lens epithelium. However, the equatorial epithelium is more susceptible to damage that can induce cortical cataracts since the development of such cataracts is associated with Ca^{2+} overload in the lens epithelial cells. The identity of the TRP channels isoforms constituting SOCE channels is elusive since drugs that modulate SOCE channels activity have poor selectivity for each of the different TRP subunits in the TRPV and TRPC channel subfamilies. For example, the inhibitory effects of lanthanum are used as a criterion to distinguish between SOCE and TRPC channel involvement in the development of cataract. At lower concentrations (i.e., in the nanomolar range), lanthanum inhibits SOCE channels, whereas at higher concentrations it blocks TRPC-containing channels.[49, 50] However, this approach is problematic because a cut-off between lanthanum concentration ranges having the inhibitory effect on either SOCE or TRPC channel is poorly defined. Another complication is that, in the micromolar range, Ca^{2+} influx is potentiated through TRPC4- and TRPC5-containing pathways. Nevertheless, the current understanding is that SOCE channels are the major pathway for Ca^{2+} influx in the lens. Better insight into the specific involvement of TRP channels dysfunction in cataractogenesis will be clarified once either more selective Ca^{2+} channel modulators become available or genetic approaches are employed to selectively modulate levels of TRP channel isoform expression.

5. Roles of TRP channels in retinopathy

TRP channels are abundantly expressed in the entire retinal layer including the retinal pigment epithelium (RPE), photoreceptors, retinal ganglion cells, Müller cells, and microglia. Initially, TRP channel-mediated phototransduction was identified in *Drosophila* and 13 of the known 28 homologues of the mutant insect channels were next identified in the mammalian retina.[51] For example, the TRPC channels in mammals are most closely related to the *Drosophila* TRP channels. The difference is that in mammals the six TRPC subfamily genes (i.e., trpc 1, 3–7) encode seven proteins (TRPC1–7 channels), since TRPC2 is a pseudogene.

In *Drosophila* retinal photoreceptors, TRPC channels lead to photoexcitation. Light absorption converts rhodopsin to active metarhodopsin, which activates PLC. PLC hydrolyzes phosphatidylinositol 4,5-bisphosphate (PIP_2) to IP_3 and diacylglycerol (DAG). DAG can be degraded to release polyunsaturated fatty acids and protons. TRPC channel activation occurs as a consequence of phosphoinositide depletion and acidification resulting from PLC-induced PIP_2 hydrolysis and proton release associated with IP_3 formation.[34] TRPC channel activation by phosphoinositide metabolites suggests that these channels are part of the light-sensing mechanism for *Drosophila,* but their role in humans is still unclear.

TRP channel dysfunction has been implicated in mammalian retinopathy. Mutation of TRPM1 channels in ON bipolar cells has been linked to autosomal-recessive congenital stationary night blindness (CSNB), a heterogeneous group of retinal disorders characterized by non-progressive impaired night vision and variable decreased visual acuity.[52] On the other hand, Wang et al. reported that TRPC6 channel activation has a neuroprotective effect on retinal ischemia-reperfusion (IR) injury in the rat.[53] Following IR, the expression of TRPC6 channels decreases in retinal ganglion cells. Activation of TRPC6 channels before IR reduces retinal ganglion cell losses whereas suppression of TRPC6 channels has an opposite effect. Such protection by TRPC6 channels of retinal ganglion cells is dependent on brain-derived neurotrophic factor (BDNF) signalling.

The RPE layer has essential roles in sustaining normal retinal function. It regulates the hydration and ionic composition of the subretinal space, as well as rod outer segment function. RPE also secretes cytokines that are essential for retinal health. TRPV5 and TRPV6 expressions were identified *in vitro* in the human RPE, implicating that these two most calcium-selective channels of the TRP channel superfamily contribute to the regulation of the subretinal space calcium composition accompanying light/dark transitions.[19] TRPV2 channels were shown in another study to control RPE release of vascular endothelial growth factor (VEGF). Insulin-like growth factor-1 (IGF-1) is a TRPV2 channel activator that selectively induces the intracellular Ca^{2+} transients required for inducing VEGF release. Control of this response is needed to reduce retinal neovascularization, since wet age-related macular degeneration (AMD) is decreased or stabilized by treatment with anti-VEGF antibodies. These results suggest that reducing TRPV2 channels activity may provide another option for managing wet AMD.[54]

6. Summary

TRP channels are involved in ocular sensory and cellular functions. In mammals, TRP channel subunit proteins are encoded by 27 genes and are classified into two groups and six different subfamilies, based on differences in amino acid sequence homology. Group 1 and Group 2 of TRP channels are only remotely related, but share similar cation channel-forming structures of six transmembrane domains. Their cation selectivity and activation mechanisms are very diverse and depend on individual TRP channel. TRP channel activation induces a host of responses to variations in ambient temperature, pressure, osmolarity and pH. In addition, their activation by injury induces inflammation, neovascularization, pain and cell death, as well as wound healing. There is emerging interest in characterizing their roles in inducing ocular surface disease, glaucoma, cataracts and retinopathy. Such efforts could lead to the identification of novel drug targets for improving management of many ocular diseases.

7. References

[1] Minke B. Drosophila mutant with a transducer defect. *Biophys Struct Mech* 1977;3:59-64.

[2] Clapham DE. TRP channels as cellular sensors. *Nature* 2003;426:517-524.

[3] Harteneck C, Plant TD, Schultz G. From worm to man: three subfamilies of TRP channels. *Trends Neurosci* 2000;23:159-166.

[4] Montell C. The TRP superfamily of cation channels. *Sci STKE* 2005;2005:re3.

[5] Launay P, Fleig A, Perraud AL, Scharenberg AM, Penner R, Kinet JP. TRPM4 is a Ca2+-activated nonselective cation channel mediating cell membrane depolarization. *Cell* 2002;109:397-407.

[6] Hofmann T, Chubanov V, Gudermann T, Montell C. TRPM5 is a voltage-modulated and Ca(2+)-activated monovalent selective cation channel. *Curr Biol* 2003;13:1153-1158.

[7] Voets T, Janssens A, Droogmans G, Nilius B. Outer pore architecture of a Ca2+-selective TRP channel. *J Biol Chem* 2004;279:15223-15230.

[8] Pan Z, Yang H, Reinach PS. Transient receptor potential (TRP) gene superfamily encoding cation channels. *Hum Genomics* 2011;5:108-116.

[9] Xie Q, Zhang Y, Cai Sun X, Zhai C, Bonanno JA. Expression and functional evaluation of transient receptor potential channel 4 in bovine corneal endothelial cells. *Exp Eye Res* 2005;81:5-14.

[10] Yang H, Mergler S, Sun X, et al. TRPC4 knockdown suppresses epidermal growth factor-induced store-operated channel activation and growth in human corneal epithelial cells. *J Biol Chem* 2005;280:32230-32237.

[11] Warren EJ, Allen CN, Brown RL, Robinson DW. The light-activated signaling pathway in SCN-projecting rat retinal ganglion cells. *Eur J Neurosci* 2006;23:2477-2487.

[12] Da Silva N, Herron CE, Stevens K, Jollimore CA, Barnes S, Kelly ME. Metabotropic receptor-activated calcium increases and store-operated calcium influx in mouse Muller cells. *Invest Ophthalmol Vis Sci* 2008;49:3065-3073.

[13] Oancea E, Vriens J, Brauchi S, Jun J, Splawski I, Clapham DE. TRPM1 forms ion channels associated with melanin content in melanocytes. *Sci Signal* 2009;2:ra21.

[14] Madrid R, Donovan-Rodriguez T, Meseguer V, Acosta MC, Belmonte C, Viana F. Contribution of TRPM8 channels to cold transduction in primary sensory neurons and peripheral nerve terminals. *J Neurosci* 2006;26:12512-12525.

[15] Mergler S, Garreis F, Sahlmuller M, Reinach PS, Paulsen F, Pleyer U. Thermosensitive transient receptor potential channels (thermo-TRPs) in human corneal epithelial cells. *J Cellular Physiol (in press)* 2010.

[16] Pan Z, Wang Z, Yang H, Zhang F, Reinach PS. TRPV1 Activation is Required for Hypertonicity Stimulated Inflammatory Cytokine Release in Human Corneal Epithelial Cells. *Invest Ophthalmol Vis Sci (in press)* 2010.

[17] Pan Z, Yang H, Mergler S, et al. Dependence of regulatory volume decrease on transient receptor potential vanilloid 4 (TRPV4) expression in human corneal epithelial cells. *Cell Calcium* 2008;44:374-385.

[18] Sappington RM, Calkins DJ. Contribution of TRPV1 to microglia-derived IL-6 and NFkappaB translocation with elevated hydrostatic pressure. *Invest Ophthalmol Vis Sci* 2008;49:3004-3017.

[19] Kennedy BG, Torabi AJ, Kurzawa R, Echtenkamp SF, Mangini NJ. Expression of transient receptor potential vanilloid channels TRPV5 and TRPV6 in retinal pigment epithelium. *Mol Vis* 2010;16:665-675.

[20] Leonelli M, Martins DO, Kihara AH, Britto LR. Ontogenetic expression of the vanilloid receptors TRPV1 and TRPV2 in the rat retina. *Int J Dev Neurosci* 2009;27:709-718.
[21] Venkatachalam K, Montell C. TRP channels. *Annu Rev Biochem* 2007;76:387-417.
[22] Nilius B, Voets T, Peters J. TRP channels in disease. *Sci STKE* 2005;2005:re8.
[23] Zhang F, Yang H, Wang Z, et al. Transient receptor potential vanilloid 1 activation induces inflammatory cytokine release in corneal epithelium through MAPK signaling. *J Cell Physiol* 2007;213:730-739.
[24] Yang H, Sun X, Wang Z, et al. EGF stimulates growth by enhancing capacitative calcium entry in corneal epithelial cells. *J Membr Biol* 2003;194:47-58.
[25] Yamamoto Y, Hatakeyama T, Taniguchi K. Immunohistochemical colocalization of TREK-1, TREK-2 and TRAAK with TRP channels in the trigeminal ganglion cells. *Neurosci Lett* 2009;454:129-133.
[26] Salas MM, Hargreaves KM, Akopian AN. TRPA1-mediated responses in trigeminal sensory neurons: interaction between TRPA1 and TRPV1. *Eur J Neurosci* 2009;29:1568-1578.
[27] Bang S, Kim KY, Yoo S, Kim YG, Hwang SW. Transient receptor potential A1 mediates acetaldehyde-evoked pain sensation. *Eur J Neurosci* 2007;26:2516-2523.
[28] Yang H, Wang Z, Capo-Aponte JE, Zhang F, Pan Z, Reinach PS. Epidermal growth factor receptor transactivation by the cannabinoid receptor (CB1) and transient receptor potential vanilloid 1 (TRPV1) induces differential responses in corneal epithelial cells. *Exp Eye Res* 2010;91:462-471.
[29] Yamada T, Ueda T, Ugawa S, et al. Functional expression of transient receptor potential vanilloid 3 (TRPV3) in corneal epithelial cells: involvement in thermosensation and wound healing. *Exp Eye Res* 2010;90:121-129.
[30] Mergler S, Valtink M, Coulson-Thomas VJ, et al. TRPV channels mediate temperature-sensing in human corneal endothelial cells. *Exp Eye Res* 2010;90:758-770.
[31] Murata Y, Masuko S. Peripheral and central distribution of TRPV1, substance P and CGRP of rat corneal neurons. *Brain Res* 2006;1085:87-94.
[32] Okada Y, Reinach PS, Kitano A, Shirai K, Kao WW, Saika S. Neurotrophic keratopathy; its pathophysiology and treatment. *Histol Histopathol* 2010;25:771-780.
[33] Parra A, Madrid R, Echevarria D, et al. Ocular surface wetness is regulated by TRPM8-dependent cold thermoreceptors of the cornea. *Nat Med* 2010;16:1396-1399.
[34] Sappington RM, Sidorova T, Long DJ, Calkins DJ. TRPV1: contribution to retinal ganglion cell apoptosis and increased intracellular Ca2+ with exposure to hydrostatic pressure. *Invest Ophthalmol Vis Sci* 2009;50:717-728.
[35] Wiederholt M, Thieme H, Stumpff F. The regulation of trabecular meshwork and ciliary muscle contractility. *Prog Retin Eye Res* 2000;19:271-295.
[36] Wiederholt M. Direct involvement of trabecular meshwork in the regulation of aqueous humor outflow. *Curr Opin Ophthalmol* 1998;9:46-49.
[37] Weinreb RN, Khaw PT. Primary open-angle glaucoma. *Lancet* 2004;363:1711-1720.
[38] Salmon MD, Ahluwalia J. Discrimination between receptor- and store-operated Ca(2+) influx in human neutrophils. *Cell Immunol* 2010;265:1-5.
[39] Sugawara R, Takai Y, Miyazu M, Ohinata H, Yoshida A, Takai A. Agonist and antagonist sensitivity of non-selective cation channel currents evoked by muscarinic receptor stimulation in bovine ciliary muscle cells. *Auton Autacoid Pharmacol* 2006;26:285-292.

[40] Goto M, Ikeyama K, Tsutsumi M, Denda S, Denda M. Calcium ion propagation in cultured keratinocytes and other cells in skin in response to hydraulic pressure stimulation. *J Cell Physiol* 2010;224:229-233.

[41] Yin J, Kuebler WM. Mechanotransduction by TRP channels: general concepts and specific role in the vasculature. *Cell Biochem Biophys* 2010;56:1-18.

[42] Birder LA. TRPs in bladder diseases. *Biochim Biophys Acta* 2007;1772:879-884.

[43] Ryskamp DA, Witkovsky P, Barabas P, et al. The polymodal ion channel transient receptor potential vanilloid 4 modulates calcium flux, spiking rate, and apoptosis of mouse retinal ganglion cells. *J Neurosci* 2011;31:7089-7101.

[44] Qu J, Wang D, Grosskreutz CL. Mechanisms of retinal ganglion cell injury and defense in glaucoma. *Exp Eye Res* 2010;91:48-53.

[45] Sappington RM, Chan M, Calkins DJ. Interleukin-6 protects retinal ganglion cells from pressure-induced death. *Invest Ophthalmol Vis Sci* 2006;47:2932-2942.

[46] Duncan G, Williamsa MR, Riacha RA. Calcium, cell signalling and cataract. *Progress in Retinal and Eye Research* 1994;13:623-652.

[47] Duncan G, Bushell AR. Ion analyses of human cataractous lenses. *Exp Eye Res* 1975;20:223-230.

[48] Rhodes JD, Russell SL, Illingworth CD, Duncan G, Wormstone IM. Regional differences in store-operated Ca2+ entry in the epithelium of the intact human lens. *Invest Ophthalmol Vis Sci* 2009;50:4330-4336.

[49] Gwack Y, Srikanth S, Feske S, et al. Biochemical and functional characterization of Orai proteins. *J Biol Chem* 2007;282:16232-16243.

[50] Nilius B, Owsianik G, Voets T, Peters JA. Transient receptor potential cation channels in disease. *Physiol Rev* 2007;87:165-217.

[51] Gudermann T, Mederos y Schnitzler M. Phototransduction: keep an eye out for acid-labile TRPs. *Curr Biol* 2010;20:R149-152.

[52] van Genderen MM, Bijveld MM, Claassen YB, et al. Mutations in TRPM1 are a common cause of complete congenital stationary night blindness. *Am J Hum Genet* 2009;85:730-736.

[53] Wang X, Teng L, Li A, Ge J, Laties AM, Zhang X. TRPC6 channel protects retinal ganglion cells in a rat model of retinal ischemia/reperfusion-induced cell death. *Invest Ophthalmol Vis Sci* 2010;51:5751-5758.

[54] Cordeiro S, Seyler S, Stindl J, Milenkovic VM, Strauss O. Heat-Sensitive Trpv Channels Regulate Vegf-a Secretion in Retinal Pigment Epithelial Cells. *Invest Ophthalmol Vis Sci* 2010;51:6001-6008.

Part 2

Cornea and Ocular Surface

4

Recent Advances in Mucosal Immunology and Ocular Surface Diseases

De-Quan Li[1,*], Zuguo Liu[2], Zhijie Li[1,3], Zhichong Wang[4] and Hong Qi[5]
[1]*Ocular Surface Center, Cullen Eye Institute, Department of Ophthalmology, Baylor College of Medicine, Houston, TX,*
[2]*Xiamen Eye Institute, Xiamen University, Xiamen,*
[3]*Key Laboratory for Regenerative Medicine of Ministry of Education and Department of Ophthalmology, Jinan University, Guangzhou,*
[4]*State Key Laboratory of Ophthalmology, Zhongshan Ophthalmic Center, Sun Yat-sen University, Guangzhou,*
[5]*Department of Ophthalmology, Peking University Third Hospital, Beijing,*
[1]*USA*
[2,3,4,5]*China*

1. Introduction

The mucosa, a mucus-secreting membrane, is linings of surface and cavities that are exposed to the external environment and internal organs. The mucosal immune system has a unique anatomy and physiology, which provides protection to an organism's various mucous membranes from invasion by potentially pathogenic microbes. It provides three main functions: protecting the mucus membrane against infection, preventing the uptake of antigens, microorganisms, and other foreign materials, and moderating the organism's immune response to that material. The mucosal epithelium forms the initial interface between the environment and host, and functions not only as a barrier but also as a sensor providing bidirectional communication with other resident mucosal lymphoid cells with the capacity to respond to pathogenic microbes and other injurious agents.

It has become increasingly clear that epithelial cells play important roles not only in host defense and inflammation, but also in regulation of immune responses. The mammalian immune system is comprised of two branches, the innate immune system and the adaptive immune system, that work in tandem to provide resistance to infection. The innate immune cells, represented primarily by monocytes, macrophages, dendritic cells and granulocytes, are the first line of host defense and are responsible for immediate recognition and control of microbial invasion. In contrast, the adaptive immune system, represented by B and T lymphocytes, has a delayed response, which is characterized by clonal expansion of cells that bind to a highly specific antigen and have immunological memory [1]. Substantial new evidence now indicates that epithelial cells are central participants, as initiators, mediators and regulators, in the innate and adaptive immune responses, as well as in the transition from innate immunity to adaptive immunity.

---

* Corresponding Author

This new concept has been recently generated from studies mainly in skin and airway epithelial cells. In addition to its function as a physical barrier, human skin has been shown to be an important immune organ displaying various defense mechanisms, which can be divided into three major functional compartments: natural epithelial defense, innate immunity and antigen-elicited adaptive immunity [2-4]. Airway epithelial cells have been recognized to be at the interface of innate and adaptive immunity [5-7]. Airway epithelial cells produce antimicrobial host defense molecules and proinflammatory cytokines and chemokines in response to microbial pathogens. Recruitment of immune cells, including dendritic cells, T cells and B cells into the proximity of epithelium results in the enhancement of adaptive immunity through interactions with epithelial cells. Epithelial cells are also responsible for mucus production in both protective immune responses and allergic airway inflammatory diseases. The crucial roles of epithelial cells in the innate and adaptive immune responses for host defense have also been recognized in other epithelia, including gastrointestinal mucosa [8-10] and ocular surface [11-13]. This chapter is focused on recent advances of this new concept that mucosal epithelium plays a central role in initiating and regulating innate and adaptive immune responses in ocular inflammatory diseases, based on literature review and our new findings. These novel breakthroughs in mucosal immunology would facilitate new therapeutic strategies for treating ocular inflammatory diseases.

2. Toll-like receptors and ocular mucosal innate immunity

The innate immune response relies on evolutionarily ancient germline-encoded receptors, the pattern recognition receptors (PRRs) [14], which recognize highly conserved microbial structures (Table 1). PRRs recognize microbial components, known as pathogen-associated molecular patterns. A breakthrough in the understanding of the ability of innate immune system to rapidly recognize pathogens occurred with the discovery of the Toll-like receptors (TLRs), which is the most important family among the PRRs. At least 10 human TLRs have been identified to date. Each TLR has unique ligand specificity. In general, TLRs 1, 2, 4, 5 and 6 present on the cell plasma membrane and respond to a variety of components of bacteria and fungi (Table 1); and TLRs 3, 7, 8 and 9 mainly present on endosomal membranes inside cells and recognize viral nucleic acids [12]. Among 4 types of transmembrane proteins structurally, TLRs are single-pass type I transmembrane proteins with leucine rich repeats in the extracellular domain for ligand recognition, and a Toll/IL-1 receptor (TIR) domain in the cytoplasmic portion for intracellular signaling [12, 15-17]. TLRs are expressed on immune cells that are most likely to first encounter microbes, such as neutrophils, monocytes, macrophages, and dendritic cells [15]. Ligand recognition by TLRs facilitates the dimerisation of TLRs that triggers the activation of signaling pathways, which originates from the cytoplasmic TIR domain, and culminates in the activation of the nuclear transcription factor NF-κB (nuclear factor kappa-light-chain-enhancer of activated B cells), which leads to the expression of pro-inflammatory molecules, such as TNF-α, IL-1β, IL-6 [16, 18-20]. In addition to innate immune cells, an array of TLRs is expressed by epithelial cells at interfaces between host and environment including that of the skin [2, 21], respiratory tract [5, 6], gastrointestinal tract [9], and ocular surface [12, 13]. Strategic expression of TLRs at such host/environment interfaces appears to play an important role in the first line of defense against microbial invasion at these sites.

TLR	Microbial components	Ligands used for study
TLR1/TLR2	Triacylated lipopeptide (LP)	Pam3CSK4 (1-100 μg/ml)
TLR2*	Bacterial lipoprotein	
	Peptidoglycan	peptidoglycan-BS (1-50 μg/ml)
	lipoteichoic acid	LTA-SA (0.1-10 μg/ml)
	Zymosan (fungi)	Zymosan (1-100 μg/ml)
TLR3	Double stranded RNA (viruses dsRNA)	Poly I:C (5-50 μg/ml)
TLR4	LPS (Gram negative bacteria)	LPS (1-50 μg/ml)
	Bacterial HSP60	
	Respiratory syncytial virus coat protein	
TLR5	Flagellin (flagellated bacteria)	Flagellin-ST (1-25 μg/ml)
TLR6/TLR2	Diacylated lipopeptides	FSL-1 (0.1-10 μg/ml)
TLR7	Imidazoquinolone antiviral drug	Imiquimod (R837, 1-50 μg/ml)
TLR8	Single stranded RNA (viruses ssRNA)	ssRNA40 (0.1-10 μg/ml)
	Imidazoquinolone antiviral drug	
TLR9	Unmethylated CpG motifs of bacterial DNA	C-CpG-ODN (1-50 μg/ml)
TLR10	Unknown	

* TLR2 forms heterodimers with TLR1 and TLR6: TLR1 associates with TLR2 to recognize tri-acyl lipopeptides; TLR6/TLR2 heterodimer recognizes diacyl lipopeptides.

Table 1. Human Toll-like receptors (TLRs) and their microbial ligands

Ocular mucosal epithelial cells have been identified to express an array of functional TLRs [12, 13]. The production of pro-inflammatory cytokines, chemokines and antimicrobial peptides is stimulated via TLR2 by corneal epithelial cells exposed to yeast zymosan [22] and peptidoglycan of Staphylococcus aureus [23]. This pathway may have a role in the pathogenesis of Gram positive bacterial keratitis. Signaling through TLR9 appears important in P. aeruginosa keratitis, and silencing TLR9 signaling reduces inflammation, but likely contributes to decreased bacterial killing in the cornea [24]. Stimulation of TLR3 can induce the expression of proinflammatory cytokines, chemokines and antiviral genes that help to defend the cornea against viral infection [25, 26]. However, the distinctive role of ligand-stimulated TLR signaling in epithelium on regulation of innate and adaptive immunity remains to be elucidated.

3. Ocular epithelial cytokine TSLP links innate and adaptive immunity via Th2 inflammatory responses

Compelling evidence has been recently provided that thymic stromal lymphopoietin (TSLP) represents a key initiator of allergic inflammation at the interface of epithelial and dendritic cells, and TSLP may have a determinant role in the initiation and maintenance of the allergic immune response in atopic dermatitis and asthma [27-31]. Skin-derived TSLP was found to trigger progression from epidermal-barrier defects to asthma, the atopic march, in mice [31, 32].

TSLP is a 140-amino acid IL-7-like 4-helix bundle cytokine that was first isolated from a murine thymic stromal cell line and shown to support B-cell development in the absence of IL-7 [33]. Mouse and human TSLP share a poor homology of 43% amino acid identity. The human TSLP gene is localized in chromosome 5q22, not far from the gene cluster encoding for all the Th2 cytokines, IL-4, IL-5 and IL-13 [34]. The TSLP receptor (TSLPR) complex consists of a TSLP binding chain and the IL-7 receptor α chain (IL-7Rα). Like TSLP, human and mouse TSLPR share approximately 40% amino acid identity. By interacting with the heterodimeric receptor TSLPR/IL-7Rα, TSLP appears to initiate phosphorylation of signal transducer and activator of transcription (STAT) 3 and STAT-5 [27, 35].

It was demonstrated that epithelial cell-derived TSLP could strongly activate human myeloid dendritic cells to mature dendritic cells that produce OX40 ligand (OX40L) in the absence of IL-12 to induce an inflammatory Th2 response characterized by high level of pro-inflammatory cytokine TNF-α with low level of anti-inflammatory cytokine IL-10, distinct from the regulatory Th2 responses characterized by low TNF-α and high IL-10 production [27, 28]. This suggests that TSLP represents a key initiator of allergic inflammation at the interface of epithelial cells and dendritic cells. TSLP was also demonstrated to direct the innate phase of allergic immune responses through activating mast cells. Therefore, TSLP and OX40L may represent important targets for intervention in the initiation of allergic inflammatory responses.

Epithelial cells appear to be the major potential producer of TSLP in both mice and humans, although fibroblasts, smooth muscle cells, and mast cells all have the potential to produce TSLP [35, 36]. The expression of TSLP by epithelial cells has been recently shown to be stimulated by microbial ligands, inflammatory and Th2 cytokines [37-39]. Using ocular mucosal epithelium as a model, Li and associates [40] have evaluated the expression and production of TSLP by primary human corneal epithelial cells in response to 11 extracted or synthetic microbial components that are ligands of TLRs 1-9 (Table 1). As shown in Figure 1A, TSLP expression and production were found to be largely induced by the ligands to TLRs 3, 5 and 6, which were polyinosinic-polycytidylic acid (polyI:C), flagellin and FSL-1, respectively, representing viral dsRNA and the bacterial components flagellin and lipopeptides. PolyI:C and flagellin, the major TSLP inducers, stimulated TSLP production to 67- and 19-fold, respectively. The TSLP mRNA reached the peak levels rapidly in 4 hours in response to these ligands. The specificity of this response was confirmed when respective antibody against TLR3 or TLR5 significantly blocked TSLP expression induced by polyI:C and flagellin, respectively. The pattern of TLR-dependant TSLP induction indicates that human corneal epithelial cells are able to rapidly initiate an innate immune response to virus or bacteria through TLR-mediated pathways. TSLP was also moderately induced by pro-inflammatory cytokines at both mRNA and protein levels. TNF-α or IL-1β induced a concentration dependent increase in the TSLP mRNA and protein, but their stimulatory effects were much weaker than that of polyI:C and flagellin, which stimulated TSLP protein production over 15- and 4-fold higher, respectively, than TNF-α. These data suggest that TSLP induction is mainly through a TLR-dependant innate immune response to microbes in human ocular epithelium.

IL-4 and IL-13, the major cytokines secreted by Th2 cells, not only moderately induced TSLP mRNA and protein, but also strongly synergized with microbial ligands, such as polyI:C, or pro-inflammatory cytokine TNF-α to promote TSLP expression and production (Figure 1B). This synergized induction of TSLP was further confirmed in an ex vivo experiment model using fresh human corneal epithelial tissues (Figure 1C). These findings demonstrate that adaptive immunity-derived Th2 cytokines are capable of amplifying the TSLP expression and production by the corneal epithelium, which in turn has the capability of priming Th2 cell differentiation through dendritic cell activation [27, 28]. These findings suggest that blocking TSLP could be a novel strategy for treatment of allergic diseases or other TSLP-driven conditions.

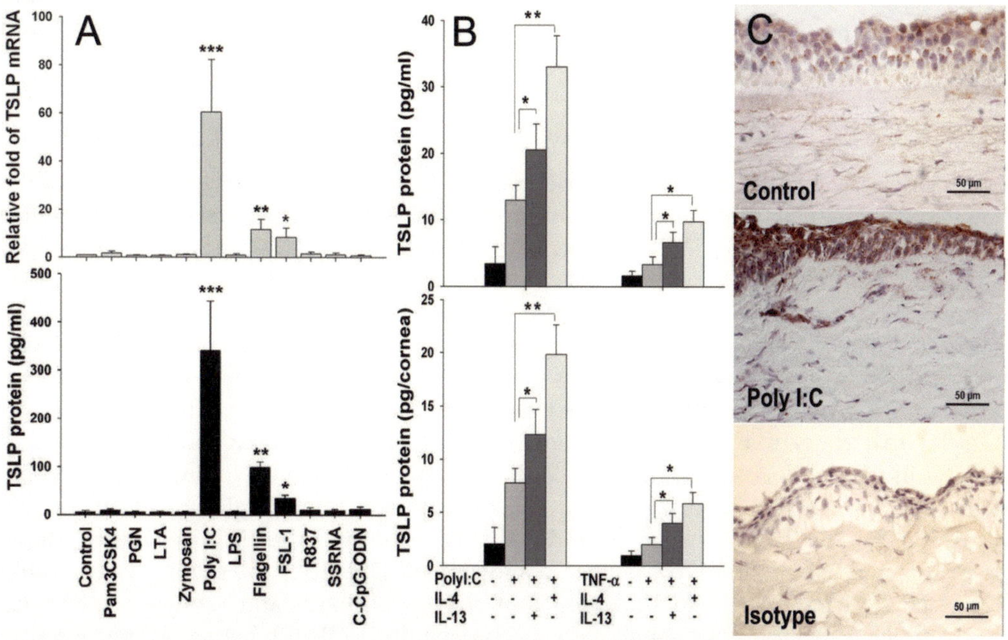

Fig. 1. TLR-mediated induction of TSLP by microbial ligands, TNF-α and Th2 cytokines. **A.** TSLP induction in HCECs. The confluent primary HCECs were incubated with 50µg/ml polyI:C or 10µg/ml of Pam3CSK4, peptidoglycan (PGN), LTA, Zymosan, LPS, flagellin, FSL-1, R837, single stranded RNA (ssRNA40) or C-CpG-ODN for 4 hours for TSLP mRNA expression by RT-qPCR, or for 48 hours for TSLP protein in the culture supernatants by ELISA; **B.** TSLP induction in an ex vivo model of human corneal tissues. A fresh corneoscleral tissue was cut into 4 equal size pieces. Each quarter of corneal tissue was placed into a well of 8-chamber slides in 150 µl of serum-free SHEM medium without or with polyI:C (50 µg/ml) or TNF-α (20 ng/ml) in the presence of IL-4 or IL-13 (100 ng/ml) for 24 hours. The culture supernatants were used for TSLP ELISA. Results shown are mean ± SD of 3 independent experiments. * $p < 0.05$; ** $p < 0.01$; *** $P < 0.001$. **C.** The corneal tissues were prepared for cryosections for TSLP immunohistochemical staining with isotype IgG as negative control.

Although the recognition of different ligands by specific TLRs leads to activation of an intracellular signaling cascade in a myeloid differentiation primary response gene 88 (MyD88)-dependent or independent fashion, all TLRs share NF-κB signal transduction pathways for activation of the transcription factors [20]. TNF-α is also well known to promote activation of the NF-κB signaling pathway [41]. TSLP induction has been observed through NF-κB activation in airway epithelial cells [30] and synovial fibroblasts [42]. As evaluated by Western blot analysis and immunofluorescent staining, NF-κB was found to be dramatically activated in corneal epithelial cells exposed to polyI:C, flagellin or TNF-α for 4 hours. This activation was evidenced by nuclear translocation of p65 protein, one of the two proteins in NF-κB heterodimer. This p65 nuclear translocation and TSLP induction, stimulated by polyI:C, flagellin or TNF-α were markedly blocked by TLR3, TLR5 or TNF-α specific antibody, respectively, and also by quinazoline, a NF-κB activation inhibitor [40]. These findings confirm that TSLP is mainly induced by microbial components, proinflammatory cytokines and Th2 cytokines in human corneal epithelial cells via TLR and NF-κB signaling pathways, suggesting that epithelium-derived TSLP links the innate and adaptive immune responses,

4. TSLP/OX40L/OX40 signaling initiates Th2-dominant allergic conjunctivitis

Allergic diseases like seasonal allergy, asthma, atopic dermatitis, affect up to 20-30% of the population in industrialized countries, and up to 50% of these individuals reporting ocular allergic manifestations [43-45]. The incidence of allergies has increased steadily over the past 30 years. Th2-dominant hypersensitivity is a major contributor to allergic inflammatory diseases, but the underlining mechanism for initiation of this adaptive immune disorder by mucosal epithelia remains a relative mystery. The molecular triggers for Th2 allergic inflammation were not clear until studies identified a novel epithelium-derived pro-allergic cytokine TSLP, which activates myeloid dendritic cells (DCs) to produce OX40 ligand (OX40L) that triggers a Th2 inflammatory response. TSLP has been identified as a key initiator in the development of human allergic disease [31, 46, 47], including asthma, atopic dermatitis and allergic conjunctivitis, a triad of common atopic IgE-dependent allergic diseases [48]. The direct link between TSLP expression and the pathogenesis of atopic dermatitis and asthma in vivo has been demonstrated [29]. TSLP was found to be highly expressed by keratinocytes in skin lesions of atopic dermatitis and was associated with dendritic cell activation in situ [49]. Evidence associating TSLP with human asthma has also been reported [29, 32]. Patients suffering from one member of the triad often show symptoms of one or both of the other members, suggesting a common genetic or initiating element in these diseases [31].

Using a well characterized murine model of experimental allergic conjunctivitis (EAC) induced by short ragweed (SRW) pollen [50, 51], Li and colleagues observed that the repeated topical challenges with ragweed pollen allergen generated typical signs of allergic conjunctivitis in the pollen-sensitized BALB/c mice, which developed lid edema, conjunctival redness, chemosis, and tearing, as well as frequent scratching of the eye lids [52]. They found that TSLP mRNA expression was significantly upregulated in the corneal and conjunctival epithelia from mice sensitized and challenged with pollen when compared with phosphate buffered saline (PBS) alone and untreated normal controls. Immunohistochemical staining confirmed an increase in TSLP production in the eyes challenged with SRW pollen. As shown in Figure 2A, the corneal and conjunctival epithelia in EAC BALB/c mice displayed much stronger TSLP staining throughout the entire epithelium, especially the superficial epithelial layers of the conjunctiva, than the PBS-treated control. These data indicate the stimulated TSLP mRNA expression and protein production by ocular surface epithelia in the SRW-induced EAC murine model.

The accumulation of CD11c positive ($CD11c^+$) dendritic cells on the ocular surface was detected in this EAC model by reverse transcription and quantitative real-time polymerase

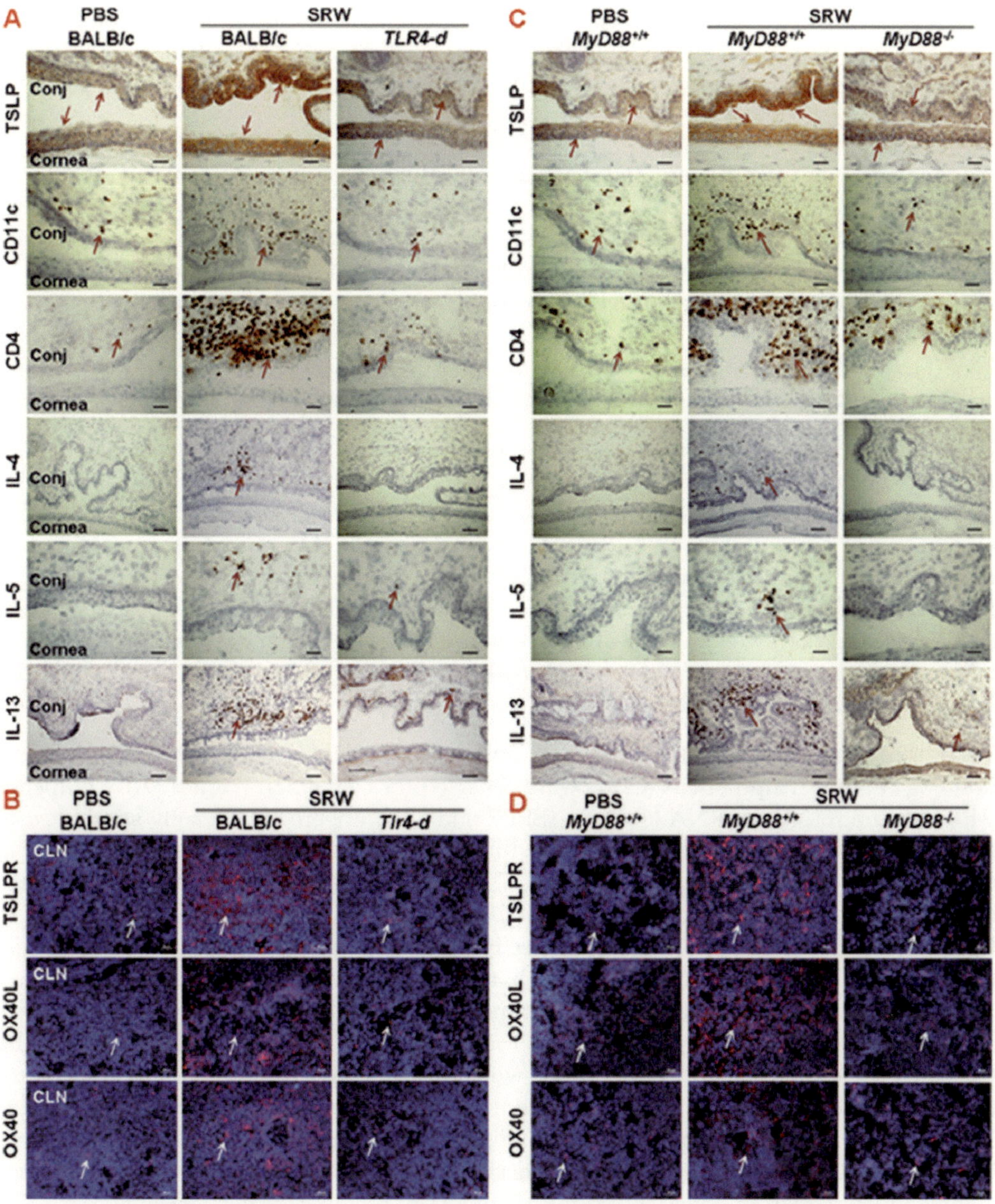

Fig. 2. The stimulated production of TSLP signaling proteins and Th2-dominant inflammation in SRW-induced EAC model requires TLR4 and MyD88. **Top panel**: The representative images showing immunohistochemical staining of epithelial TSLP, markers for dendritic (CD11c) and T cells (CD4), and Th2 cytokines (IL-4, IL-5 and IL-13) on cornea and conjunctiva (Conj) of wild type and *Tlr4* deficient BALB/c mice challenged by SRW pollen, with PBS-treated mice as controls (**A**), and of C57BL/6 based wild type *MyD88*$^{+/+}$ and knockout *MyD88*$^{-/-}$ mice challenged by SRW pollen, with PBS-treated mice as controls (**C**). **Bottom panel**: The representative images showing immunofluorescent staining of TSLP activated signals, TSLPR, OX40L and OX40 on cervical lymph nodes (CLN) of wild type and

Tlr4 deficient BALB/c mice challenged by SRW pollen with PBS-treated mice as controls (**B**), and of C57BL/6 based wild type *MyD88*$^{+/+}$ and knockout *MyD88*$^{-/-}$ mice challenged by SRW pollen, with PBS-treated mice as controls (**D**). Bar: 20μm; Arrows: red or red brown positive staining signals.

chain reaction (RT-qPCR) and immunostaining. The increased mRNA levels of CD11c, TSLPR and OX40L were observed in ocular surface, especially in conjunctival tissues, where their transcripts increased to 4-10 fold, respectively ($P< 0.05$ or <0.01), from SRW pollen-challenged mice, compared with PBS controls. The large amount of CD11c$^+$ dendritic cells was accumulated in the ocular surface of the pollen challenged eyes, primarily in the stroma subjacent to the conjunctival epithelia, in EAC mice, but not in the control mice treated with PBS (Figure 2A). These results suggest that ocular surface was infiltrated with TSLP activated dendritic cells that express TSLPR and produce OX40L in the EAC mice.

Th2-dominant inflammatory response was clearly observed on ocular surface in the mice challenged by pollen. The infiltration of T lymphocytes was evidenced by the increased CD4 mRNA expression and a markedly increased number of CD4 immunopositive (CD4$^+$) cells in the ocular surface, especially in the conjunctiva, of EAC mice (Figure 2A), when compared with PBS control mice. These CD4$^+$ T cells appear to be Th2 lineage because the transcripts of three key Th2 cytokines, IL-4, IL-5 and IL-13, were all found to be expressed at significantly higher levels in corneal and conjunctival tissues from the EAC mice than the PBS controls. Immunostaining data confirmed that the IL-4, IL-5 and IL-13-producing Th2 cells were largely infiltrated in conjunctival stroma (Figure 2A).

To confirm the TSLP signaling in SRW pollen-induced EAC mice, the ocular surface draining cervical lymph nodes (CLN) were collected for evaluation (Figure 3A). Compared with PBS controls, the mRNA levels of TSLPR and OX40L were significantly stimulated to 7.5 and 4.1 fold respectively (both $P<0.01$) while CD11c expression only slightly increased in CLN from EAC mice, indicating CD11c$^+$ DCs were markedly activated by ocular surface epithelia-derived TSLP. The mRNA levels of OX40 (3.4 fold, $P<0.05$) and Th2 cytokines, IL-4, IL-5 and IL-13 (13.2, 12.8 and 5.5 fold, respectively, all $P<0.01$), significantly increased while CD4 expression was not changed in the CLN from EAC mice, indicating naive CD4$^+$ T cells were largely differentiated to Th2 cells that might be primed by OX40L produced by TSLP activated dendritic cells [28]. The increased TSLPR$^+$, OX40L$^+$ and OX40$^+$ cells in the draining CLN of the pollen challenged EAC mice were further confirmed by immunofluorescent staining that showed dramatically increased immunoreactivity of these 3 signaling proteins at cell membrane and cytoplasm in CLN (Figure 2B). All these results demonstrate that TSLP/OX40L/OX40 signaling plays a critical role in the development of Th2-dominant allergic inflammation in pollen induced EAC model in BALB/c mice, suggesting that TSLP signaling molecules could be novel therapeutic targets to treat allergic inflammatory disease.

5. Cutting edge breakthrough: Short ragweed pollen triggers ocular allergic inflammation through TLR4-dependent innate immune response

Although there have been numerous studies on the development of allergen-induced inflammation, the mechanisms leading to resolution of allergic inflammation remain poorly understood. This represents an important knowledge gap and potential challenge because failure to resolve allergen driven inflammation potentially leads to recurrent or chronic allergic diseases. Pollen, a ubiquitous allergen, affects a large population of allergic patients. Pollen is the trigger of seasonal rhinitis, conjunctivitis and asthma, as well as an exacerbating factor of atopic dermatitis. However, the underlying molecular mechanism by which pollen induces Th2-dominant allergic inflammation via epithelial innate immunity pathways is largely unknown. Substantial evidence now indicates that epithelial cells are central participants in innate and adaptive immune responses [4, 5, 7]. Based on the observation that we and other groups have made [40, 53, 54] that TSLP is mainly induced via TLR mediated innate response in epithelia exposed to microbial products, we hypothesized that pollen, such as Ambrosia artemisiifolia short ragweed (SRW), the most widespread plant in North America, may serve as a functional TLR4 agonist that induces production of a proallergic cytokine TSLP via innate immune response to trigger Th2-dominant allergic inflammation. To uncover the novel phenomenon and molecular signaling pathways involved in pollen induced allergic inflammation, a comprehensive set of experiments has been conducted using a well-characterized murine model of allergic conjunctivitis induced by SRW pollen in BALB/c, TLR4 deficient and MyD88 knockout mice, as well as a murine topical ocular surface challenge model and a culture model of primary human corneal epithelial cells exposed to an aqueous extract of defatted SRW pollen.

TLR-mediated TSLP induction has been recognized [39, 53, 54]. We have demonstrated that TSLP was largely induced by specific TLR ligands in human corneal epithelial cells [40]. MyD88 is a universal adapter protein necessary for response to all TLRs except TLR3 [55, 56]. *Tlr4*-deficient (*Tlr4*-d, C.C3-Tlr4Lps-d/J) and MyD88 knockout (*MyD88*$^{-/-}$) mice have been used to identify TLR4 mediated signaling [57, 58]. To explore whether SRW pollen stimulates TSLP through TLR4-dependent innate response, we sensitized and topically challenged the wild-type BALB/c, *Tlr4*-d (Jackson Laboratory, Bar Harbor, ME) and *MyD88*$^{-/-}$ mice (gifts from Dr. Shizuo Akira, Research Institute for Microbial Disease, Osaka University, Japan) with SRW pollen.

Compared with wild-type BALB/c mice, the ocular allergic signs, stimulated TSLP/OX40L/OX40 signaling and Th2-dominant inflammatory response by ocular mucosa, especially conjunctival tissues, were dramatically reduced or eliminated in BALB/c based *Tlr4*-d mice. As shown in Figure 3A, the mRNA levels of TSLP, OX40L, OX40 and Th2 cytokines (IL-4, IL-5 and IL-13) were significantly stimulated in cornea, conjunctiva and draining CLN from wild-type BALB/c, but not in those from *Tlr4*-d mice. The immunostaining results confirmed that SRW pollen did not stimulate TSLP and its downstream molecules or a Th2 response in ocular mucosal tissues (Figure. 2A) and draining CLN (Figure. 2B) of *Tlr4*-d mice. These findings suggest that TLR4-dependent TSLP signaling was involved in the SRW pollen induced allergic inflammation.

The SRW topical challenges triggered the typical allergic signs and scratching behavior in wild type *MyD88*$^{+/+}$ mice, although less severe than BALB/c mice. The expression of TSLP and its signaling molecules, TSLPR, OX40L and OX40, as well as Th2 cytokines IL-4, IL-5 and IL-13 was significantly stimulated in the cornea, conjunctiva and CLN from SRW challenged wild type *MyD88*$^{+/+}$ mice at both mRNA (Figure. 3B) and protein levels (Figure 2C, 2D). Clinical allergic signs and stimulated production of TSLP signaling molecules (TSLPR, OX40L and OX40) and Th2 cytokines (IL-4, IL-5 and IL-13) were dramatically reduced or eliminated in SRW challenged *MyD88*$^{-/-}$ mice as evaluated by RT-qPCR (Figure

3B) and immunostaining (Figure 2C, 2D). These findings suggest that MyD88 pathway is involved in the TLR4-dependent TSLP signaling induced by SRW pollen.

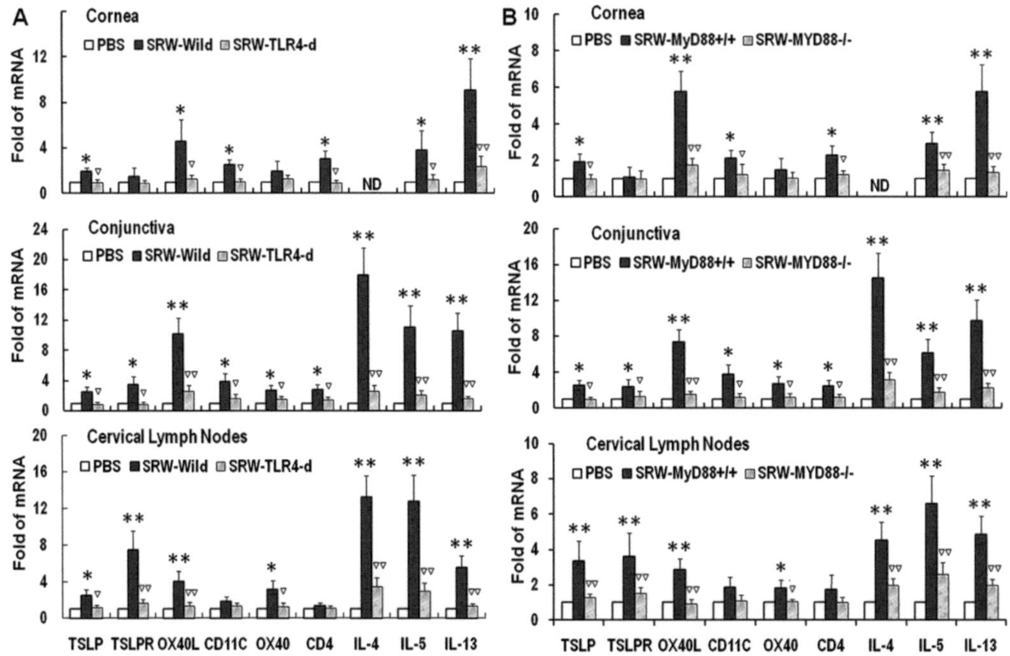

Fig. 3. The stimulated expression of TSLP signaling molecules and Th2 cytokines in SRW-induced EAC model requires TLR4 and MyD88. The mRNA expression of proallergic cytokine TSLP, its downstream signals in dendritic (TSLPR, OX40L, & CD11c) and T cells (OX40 & CD4), as well as Th2 cytokines (IL-4, IL-5 and IL-13) by corneal epithelium, conjunctiva and cervical lymph nodes in wild type and *Tlr4* deficient BALB/c mice sensitized and topically challenged by SRW with PBS-treated mice as controls (**A**), and in C57BL/6 based wild type $MyD88^{+/+}$ and knockout $MyD88^{-/-}$ mice, sensitized and topically challenged by SRW pollen, with PBS-treated mice as controls (**B**). The mRNA levels are presented as relative fold in EAC mice over the controls, which were evaluated by RT and real-time qPCR using TaqMan gene expression assay system with GAPDH as an internal control. Results shown are the Mean ± SD of four independent experiments. *$P<0.05$, **$P<0.01$; $n=4$, compared with PBS controls; ▽P<0.05, ▽▽P<0.01, n=4, compared with wild type mice.

To confirm that SRW pollen directly stimulates TSLP production by ocular mucosal epithelia through TLR4-dependent innate immunity pathway, we created a topical challenge murine model using an aqueous extract of defatted SRW pollen (SRWe) at 150μg/5μl/eye for 4-24 hours. TSLP mRNA was induced as early as 4 hours and reached peak levels at 8 hours, and TSLP protein levels increased in 24 hours in ocular epithelia exposed to SRWe. As shown in Figure 4 A & B, SRWe significantly stimulated TSLP mRNA by 2 fold in corneal and conjunctival epithelia (Both $P<0.05$), and its protein levels by 3.2 fold (from 150.2±37.6 pg/mg cellular protein to 480.00±89.6 pg/mg) in cornea epithelia and 2.2 fold (from 128.6±29.8 pg/mg to 281.6±19.3 pg/mg) in conjunctiva in BALB/c mice when compared with untreated or PBS-treated controls. The SRWe-stimulated TSLP were significantly decreased at both mRNA and protein levels by TLR4 blocker, a rat anti-mouse TLR4 antibody, but not by its isotype rat IgG2a.

The SRWe topical challenge did not increase TSLP mRNA (Figure 4C) and protein levels (Figure 4D) in corneal and conjunctival epithelia of *Tlr4-d* mice. Similarly, a TLR4 agonist lipopolysaccharides (LPS, 5μg/5μl/eye) stimulated TSLP production by corneal and conjunctival epithelia in BALB/c mice, but not in *Tlr4-d* mice. Furthermore, we applied this topical challenge model to MyD88 knockout mice and their wild type controls. SRWe

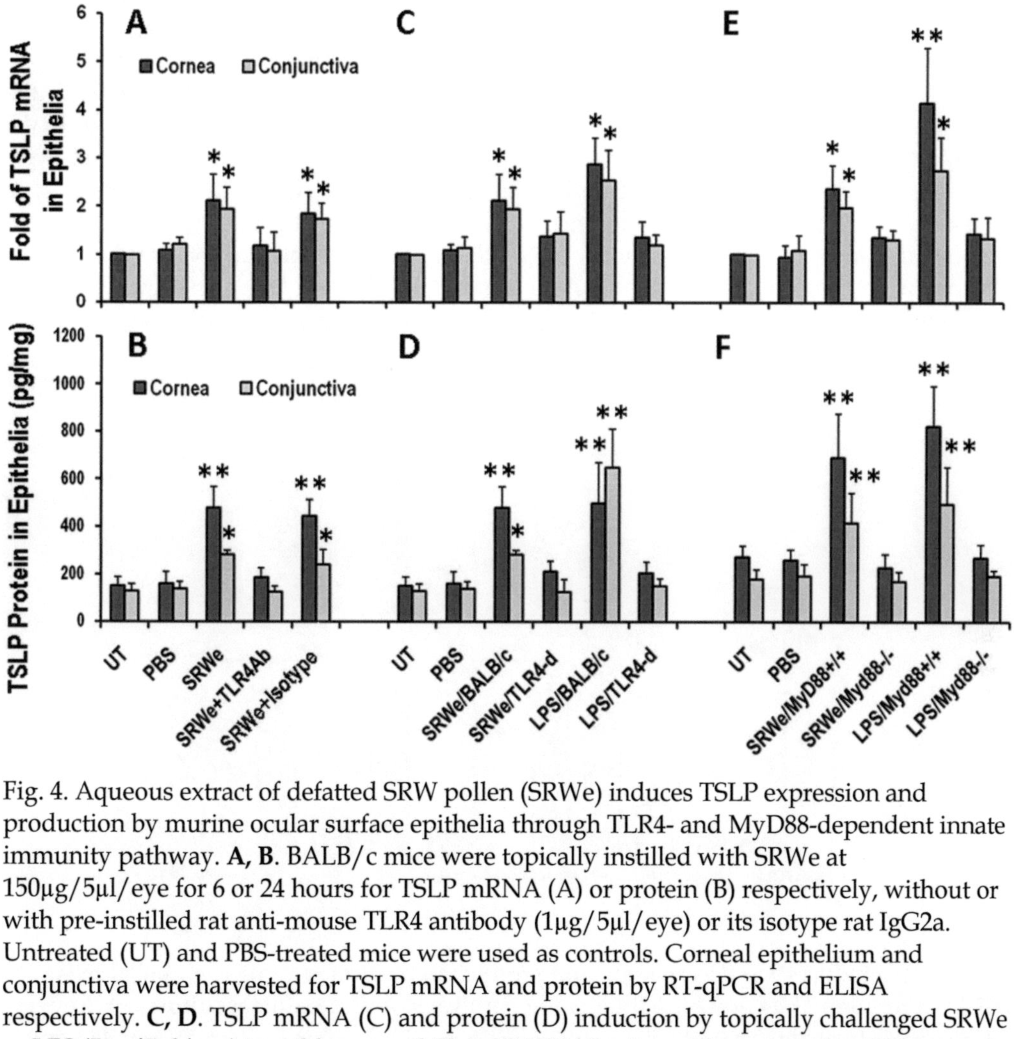

Fig. 4. Aqueous extract of defatted SRW pollen (SRWe) induces TSLP expression and production by murine ocular surface epithelia through TLR4- and MyD88-dependent innate immunity pathway. **A, B**. BALB/c mice were topically instilled with SRWe at 150μg/5μl/eye for 6 or 24 hours for TSLP mRNA (A) or protein (B) respectively, without or with pre-instilled rat anti-mouse TLR4 antibody (1μg/5μl/eye) or its isotype rat IgG2a. Untreated (UT) and PBS-treated mice were used as controls. Corneal epithelium and conjunctiva were harvested for TSLP mRNA and protein by RT-qPCR and ELISA respectively. **C, D**. TSLP mRNA (C) and protein (D) induction by topically challenged SRWe or LPS (5μg/5μl/eye) in wild type and *Tlr4-d* BALB/C mice, with untreated or PBS-treated mice as controls. **E, F.** TSLP mRNA (E) and protein (F) induction by topically challenged SRWe or LPS in wild type $MyD88^{+/+}$ and knockout $MyD88^{-/-}$ mice, with untreated or PBS-treated mice as controls. Results shown are the Mean ± SD of four independent experiments. *P<0.05, **P<0.01; n=4, compared with PBS controls.

promoted TSLP production by ocular epithelia at both mRNA (Figure 4E) and protein levels (Figure 4F) only in *MyD88*$^{+/+}$ mice, but not in *MyD88*$^{-/-}$ mice, a similar pattern to that observed following LPS topical challenge. Taken together, these data demonstrated that SRWe directly stimulates TSLP production by ocular mucosal epithelia via a TLR4-dependent innate pathway.

To explore whether this phenomenon occurs in humans, we investigated TSLP expression in human corneal epithelium. TSLP mRNA was upregulated at 4 hours and its protein was detected at 24 hours in human corneal epithelial cells (HCECs) exposed to SRWe, which is consistent with our previous report [40]. TSLP induction at mRNA (Figure 5A) and protein levels (Figure 5B) was concentration-dependently stimulated by SRWe in primary HCECs. TSLP protein was barely detectable (4.83±1.60 pg/ml) in the supernatant of normal HCEC cultures. SRWe at 10μg/ml increased the TSLP protein to 48.92±4.23 pg/ml (P<0.01), the levels comparable to that stimulated by 10ng/ml of TNF-α in HCECs [40]. The SRWe (10μg/ml)-stimulated TSLP mRNA was significantly blocked by pre-incubation of cells with 10μg/ml of neutralizing monoclonal antibody against human TLR4, but not by its isotype mouse IgG2a k (Figure 5C). Furthermore, SRWe stimulated TSLP expression was also significantly inhibited by quinazoline, a NF-κB Activation Inhibitor (Figure 5C). These findings were confirmed by detection of increased TSLP protein levels as shown in Figure 5D. These data demonstrate that SRW induces TSLP production in human corneal epithelial cells through TLR4 and NF-κB innate signaling pathways.

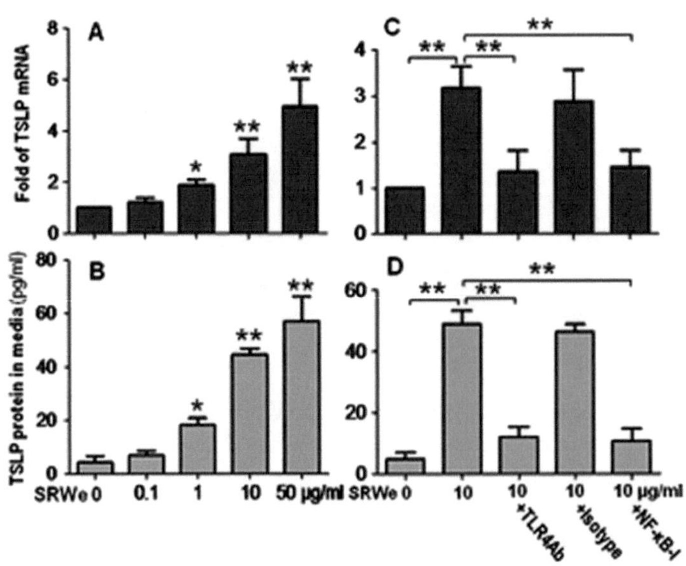

Fig. 5. SRWe induces TSLP expression and production by human corneal epithelial cells (HCECs) through TLR4 and NF-κB signaling pathways. **A, B.** Confluent cultures of primary HCECs were treated with 0.1 to 50 μg/ml of SRWe for 4 hours for TSLP mRNA or 48 hours for TSLP protein in the supernatants. **C, D.** HCECs were pre-incubated with mouse TLR4 antibody (10μg/ml), isotype mouse IgG2a k, or NF-κB activation inhibitor quinazoline (NFkB-I, 10μM) for 1 hour before adding 10μg/ml SRWe for 4 hours for TSLP mRNA or 48 hours for TSLP protein in the supernatants. Results shown are the Mean ± SD of four independent experiments. *P<0.05, **P<0.01; n=4.

Traditionally, TLRs recognize conserved microbial components as ligands or agonists. Recent studies have revealed that TLR4 recognizes a wider variety of ligands than previous thought. In addition to its first identified ligand, bacterial LPS, TLR4 was found to recognize certain viral proteins such as the F protein from respiratory syncytial virus and mouse mammary tumor virus. Not limited to pathogen-associated molecular patterns (PAMP), TLR4 responds to human endogenous structural proteins derived from tissue injury or during inflammation, the damage-associated molecular patterns (DAMP), such as type III repeat extra domain A of fibronectin, oligosaccharides of hyaluronic acid, human heat-shock protein Hsp60 and Hsp70 (see review [59]). A few reports have revealed the potential for protein extracts from plants and herbs to activate TLR4, such as taxol, an antitumor agent derived from the Yew plant [60], and aqueous extract of Rhodiola imbricata rhizome, a medicinal plant [61].

In conclusion, we have for the first time uncovered a novel phenomenon and a unknown mechanism that short ragweed pollen, serving as a functional TLR4 agonist, induces TSLP/OX40L/OX40 signaling to trigger Th2-dominant allergic inflammation via TLR4-dependent innate immunity pathways [62]. These novel findings shed light on the understanding of innate mucosal epithelial immunity involved in allergic inflammation, and may create new therapeutic targets to cure allergic disease.

6. Epithelium-derived interleukin 33 initiates allergic inflammation

The IL-1 receptor family has several members, including the classical IL-1 receptor (IL-1R) and the IL-18 receptor (IL-18R). In 1989, one member of the family, ST2, a protein encoded by IL-1 receptor-like 1 (IL-1RL1) gene, was identified as an orphan receptor [63]. Investigation into the function of ST2 revealed its participation in inflammatory processes, particularly regarding mast cells, type 2 $CD4^+$ T helper cells and the production of Th2-associated cytokines. In fact, ST2 was characterized as a specific cellular marker that differentiated Th2 from Th1 T cells. Clinical and experimental observations led to the association of ST2 with disease entities such as asthma, pulmonary fibrosis, rheumatoid arthritis, collagen vascular diseases and septic shock [64]. In 2005, the discovery of IL-33 as a ST2 ligand provided new insights into ST2 signaling [65]. By binding to ST2 receptor, IL-33 can activate Th2 cells and mast cells to secrete the proinflammatory and Th2 cytokines and chemokines that lead to severe pathological changes in mucosal organs [66].

IL-33 is produced mainly by epithelial and endothelial cells, fibroblast, and others [66-68]. IL-33 expression has been found to be up-regulated by stimulation with inflammatory cytokines, TNF-α and IL-1β [69]. However, the expression and regulation of IL-33 by mucosal surface epithelia has not been well elucidated. Using fresh donor corneal tissues and primary HCECs, we recently observed that IL-33 is mainly expressed by epithelium and largely induced by microbial products through TLR and NF-κB signaling pathways [70]. The findings suggest that the mucosal epithelial cell-derived cytokine IL-33 may play an important role in allergic inflammatory diseases through innate immune responses.

As shown in Figure 6A, IL-33 expression and production were largely induced by polyI:C, lipopolysaccharides (LPS), flagellin, FSL-1 and R837, the ligands for TLR3, -4, -5, -6 and -7, representing viral dsRNA and the bacterial components flagellin and lipopeptides, respectively. PolyI:C and flagellin were major IL-33 inducers, stimulating IL-33 production by 7- and 4-fold, respectively, with the peak mRNA levels at 8 hours by HCECs. The IL-33 induction by these 2 ligands was further confirmed using an ex vivo donor corneal tissue model (Figure 6B). The specificity of TLR-dependent response by HCECs was also confirmed when an antibody against TLR3 or TLR5 significantly inhibited IL-33 expression by polyI:C or flagellin respectively (Figure 6C). The pattern of TLR-dependent IL-33 induction indicates that HCECs are able to rapidly initiate an innate immune response to virus or bacteria, and play an important role in allergic inflammatory disease.

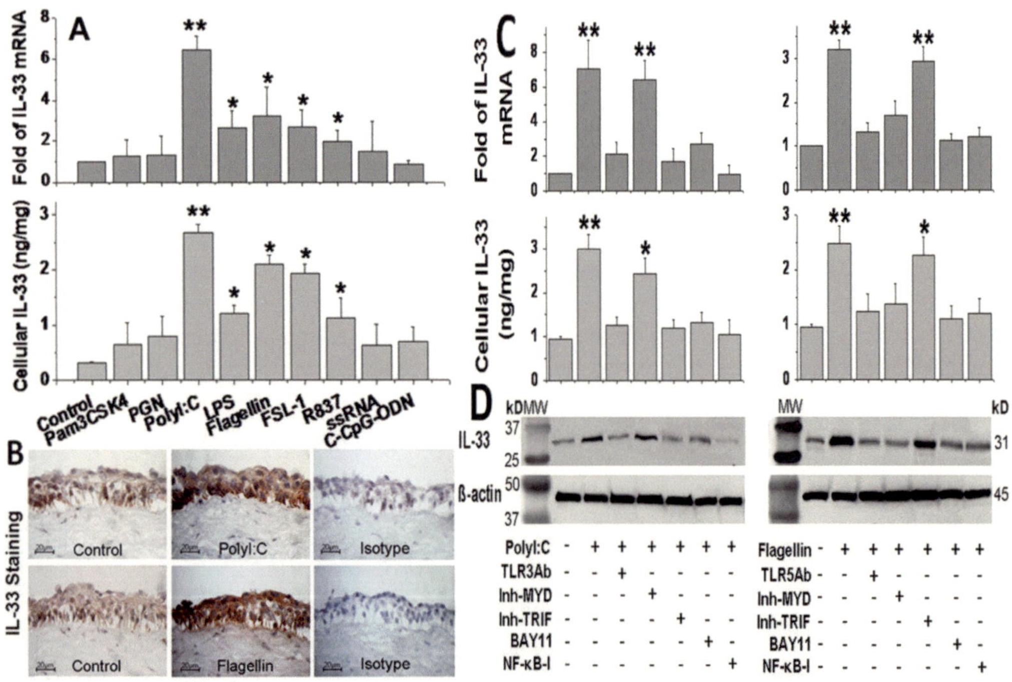

Fig. 6. TLR-dependent induction of IL-33 by microbial ligands in human corneal epithelium. **A.** IL-33 mRNA and protein levels induced by primary human corneal epithelial cells (HCECs) exposed to 50μg/ml polyI:C or 10μg/ml of Pam3CSK4, peptidoglycan (PGN), polyI:C, LPS, flagellin, FSL-1, R-837, ssRNA40 or C-CpG-ODN for 8 or 48 hours, evaluated by quantitative real-time PCR or ELISA, respectively. Results shown are the mean ± SD of four independent experiments. *P< 0.05; **P < 0.01. **B.** The immunohistochemical staining showing IL-33 induction in an ex vivo human corneal tissues by polyI:C (50μg/ml) or flagellin (10μg/ml) for 24 hours with isotype IgG as a negative control. **C.** TLR and NF-κB signaling pathways involved in IL-33 induction by polyI:C or flagellin in HCECs exposed to polyI:C (50μg/mL) or flagellin (10μg/mL) in the absence or presence of preincubated rabbit TLR3Ab (10μg/mL), TLR5Ab (10μg/mL), BAY11-7082 (10μM) or quinazoline (10μM) for 1 hour, and Pepinh-MYD (40μM) or Pepinh-TRIF (40μM) for 6 hours. The cultures treated by ligands for 8 hours for IL-33 mRNA, or for 48 hours for IL-33 protein by ELISA and by Western blot with β-actin as control (**D**). Results shown are the mean ± SD of four independent experiments. *P< 0.05; **P < 0.01.

IL-33 is an extracellular inflammatory cytokine while it also acts as a nuclear transcription factor [71]. It has been shown that IL-33 is mainly localized to the nucleus of endothelial cells and bound to chromatin. IL-33 mRNA is primarily translated and synthesized in vivo as a 30-kDa precursor, a pro-IL-33 protein. As a member of IL-1 super family and like IL-1 and

IL-18, pro-IL-33 protein sequence does not have a signal peptide that directs it for secretion via the ER–Golgi pathway [66, 72]. Like pro-IL-1β, human pro-IL-33 was reported to be cleaved by caspase-1 to generate active form, an 18-kDa fragment (mature IL-33), which is sufficient to activate signaling via the IL-33 receptor ST2. Recombinant mature IL-33 has been known to induce Th2-associated cytokines and inflammatory cytokines via its receptor, ST2 [72, 73]. However, processing of pro-IL-33 in vivo has not been clarified yet. It is not clear whether caspase-1 cleavage of pro-IL-33 occurs in vivo and whether, as for IL-1β, this cleavage is a prerequisite for IL-33 secretion and bioactivity.

Our data have showed that no significantly changes of IL-33 protein levels can be detected by ELISA in the culture supernatants, other than in cell lysate, of the HCECs. IL-33 protein levels significantly increased in the cell lysate, but not in the culture supernatants, of HCECs exposed to polyI:C or flagellin for 24-48 hours, when compared with the untreated control. However, the stimulated cellular IL-33 protein was released outside the cells into culture supernatant after co-incubation with ATP for additional 30 minutes, as evaluated by ELISA and Western blot analysis [70]. The finding supports a notion that caspase 1-dependant activation may involved in the release and secretion of IL-33 protein since ATP has been known to activate caspase-1 through triggering the P2X7 receptor [74]. Further studies are necessary to clarify the underlining mechanism.

As shown in Figure 6C evaluated by RT-qPCR and ELISA, as well as in Figure 6D by Western blotting, synthetic dsRNA polyI:C-induced IL-33 mRNA expression and protein production were markedly blocked by TLR3 antibody and TIR-domain-containing adaptor inducing interferon (TRIF) inhibitory peptide (Pepinh-TRIF), but not by TLR5 antibody or MyD88 inhibitory peptide (Pepinh-MYD), while extracted bacterial component flagellin-induced IL-33 production was dramatically suppressed by TLR5 antibody and Pepinh-MYD, but not by TLR3 antibody or Pepinh-TRIF, in corneal epithelial cells. The stimulated IL-33 induction by polyI:C or flagellin were also significantly blocked by IκB-α inhibitor BAY11-7082 or NF-κB activation inhibitor quinazoline. Further study has shown that NF-κB was dramatically activated with p65 protein nuclear translocation in corneal epithelial cells exposed to polyI:C or flagellin for 4 hours, as evaluated by Western blot analysis and immunofluorescent staining. BAY 11 selectively inhibits the phosphorylation and degradation of IκB-α, blocked the nuclear translocation of NF-κB p65 protein. NF-κB activation inhibitor quinazoline also blocked the p65 nuclear translocation. These findings demonstrate a novel phenomenon that a newly defined pro-allergic cytokine IL-33 is largely induced by microbial components through TLR and NF-κB signaling pathways in human corneal epithelium. This suggests that human ocular mucosal epithelium plays an important role in initiating Th2-dominant allergic inflammation via innate immune responses.

In a clinical study, we have tested conjunctival impression cytology specimens obtained from 8 patients with active atopic conjunctivitis and 8 normal subjects by RT-qPCR (Figure 7). The mRNA levels of TSLP, TSLPR, OX40L, OX40, IL-33 and ST2 were found to be significantly elevated in the atopic group compared with the normal control subjects, suggesting a potential role of TSLP/TSLPR/OX40L/OX40 and IL-33/ST2 signaling pathways in allergic conjunctivitis (Figure 7A). In SRW pollen induced EAC mice, the transcripts and proteins of IL-33, ST2, and IL-1 receptor accessory protein (IL1RAP) were also found to be significantly increased in the corneal epithelium, conjunctiva and CLN, as evaluated by RT-qPCR (Figure 7B) and immunostaining (Figure 7C). IL-33, ST2 and TLRs could become novel biomarkers and molecular targets for the intervention to treat allergic inflammatory diseases.

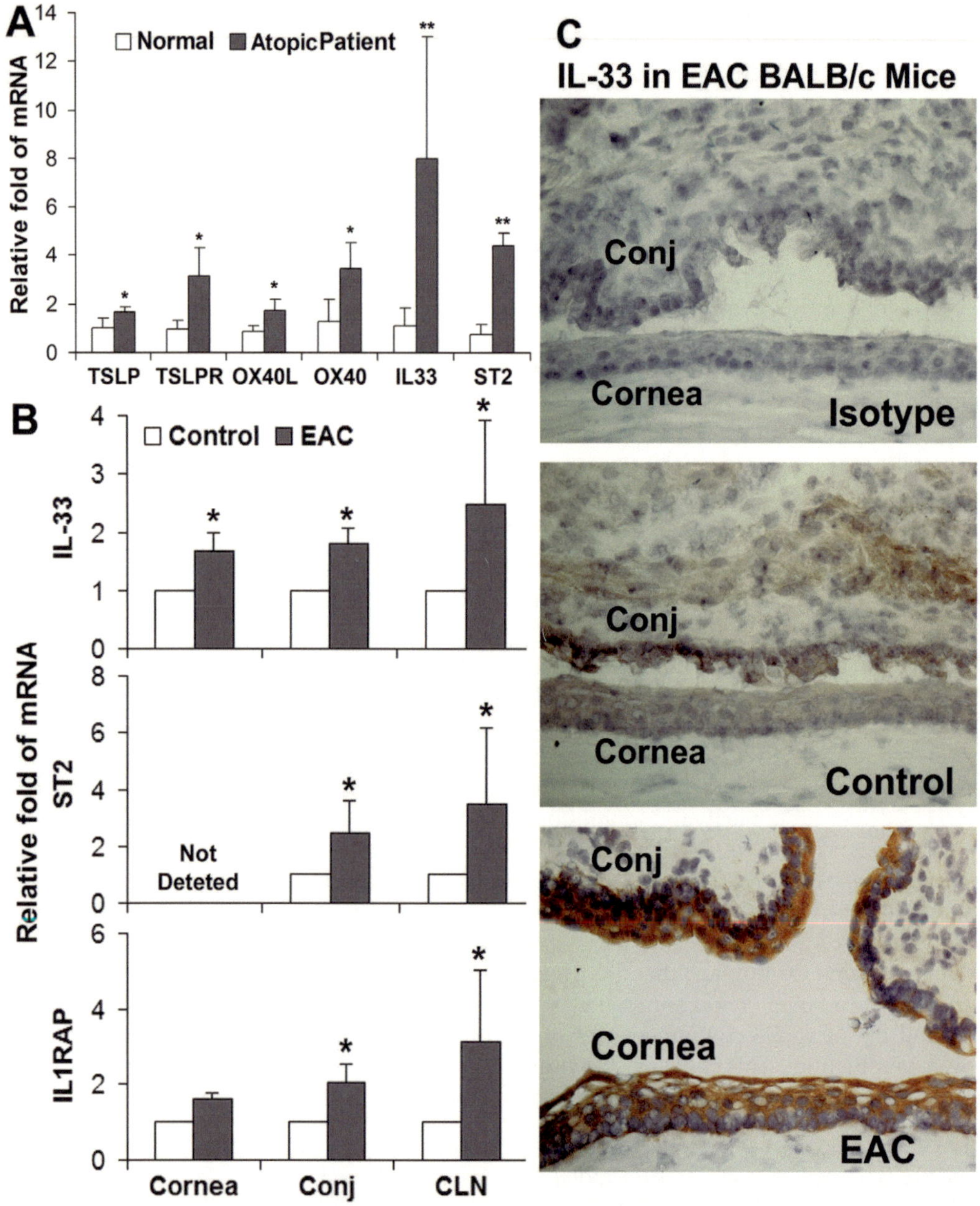

Fig. 7. The role of IL-33 in allergic disease. **A.** Elevated mRNA levels of TSLP and IL-33 signaling molecules in conjunctiva of atopic patients compared with normal subjects by RT-qPCR. * $P<0.05$, ** $P<0.01$, n=8. **B.** The mRNA levels of IL-33, ST2 and IL1RAP in corneal epithelium (Cornea), conjunctiva (Conj) and cervical lymph nodes (CLN) of in BALB/c mice with PBS-treated mice as controls. * $P<0.05$, n=3. **C.** Immunostaining images showing the stimulated IL-33 in ocular surface of EAC BALB/c mice with untreated mouse control and isotype IgG negative control.

7. Th17 pathway links innate and adaptive immunity

Th17 has been recently identified as a new T helper cell subset. $CD4^+$ T helper (Th) cells now include three different types based on their cytokine signatures: interferon-γ (IFN-γ)-secreting Th1, IL-4, -5, and -13-secreting Th2 [75], and IL-17-producing Th17 cells [76]. Th17 cells have been recognized to be key effector T cells in a variety of human inflammatory and autoimmune diseases as well as experimental animal models [77, 78]. The IL-17 family includes 6 members (IL17A-F). IL-17A (also known as IL-17) and IL-17F are the founding members of the IL-17 cytokine family. The genes encoding IL-17A and IL-17F are localized in the same chromosomal region in mice and in humans. But IL-17F has significantly weaker biological activity than IL-17A [79, 80]. IL-17E, also known as IL-25, is produced by Th2 cells and mast cells. In contrast, IL-17B, IL-17C and IL-17D have not been well investigated [81, 82]. The receptor for IL-17A (IL-17R or IL-17RA) is a single-pass transmembrane protein of approximately 130 kDa. Four additional receptors (IL-17RB-RE) have been identified, but are not well characterized. IL-17RC was recently identified to be a receptor for IL-17F [83]. It has been reported that Th17 cells also produce IL-22 [84, 85] and CC-chemokine attractant ligand 20 (CCL20) [86] in mice and humans. Therefore, distinct from Th1 and Th2 cells, Th17 cells produce a unique and expanding array of pro-inflammatory cytokines.

Compelling evidence has demonstrated that the differentiation of Th17 cells from naïve $CD4^+$ T cells is initiated by cytokines IL-6 or TGF-β, and expanded by cytokines IL-23, IL-1β and IL-21. IL-6 or TGF-β was proposed as a major initiator necessary for Th17 differentiation [87-89]. IL-23 was the first cytokine shown to selectively regulate IL-17 expression [90, 91], but it might not be required for the initial differentiation of Th17 cells in vivo [92]. Recently, IL-1β was found to promote Th17 cell development and proliferation in the presence of TGF-β and IL-6 [88]. IL-21, produced by activated T cells and natural killer (NK) cells [93], may be required for full commitment of Th17 cells [94, 95]. Hence IL-23, IL-1β and IL-21 may possibly maintain and expand the differentiated Th17 cells in the presence of IL-6 and TGF-β [88]. Furthermore, STAT3 has been found to mediate the initiation of Th17 cell differentiation by these inducing cytokines [87]. Activation of STAT3 induces the expression of retinoic-acid-receptor-related orphan receptor-α (RORα) and RORγt [96], two transcription factors that promote the Th17-cell-associated gene-expression program, leading to the production of IL-17, IL-17F, IL-22 and CCL20.

Using peripheral $CD4^+$ T cell isolated from mouse spleen and cervical lymph nodes, our team evaluated the differential effects of these inducing cytokines in promoting Th17 differentiation [97]. The results showed that IL-6 and TGF-β1, only minimally induced IL-17 production at both mRNA and protein levels. In the presence of IL-6 and TGF-β1, IL-23 was the strongest stimulator of the Th17 signature cytokines IL-17A and IL-17F, IL-22, and chemokine CCL20, as well as STAT3 among the 3 expanding cytokines IL-23, IL-1β and IL-21. In the 4 cytokine system, IL-1β stimulated much higher levels of IL-17 family cytokines, 1.5-2 fold greater than IL-21 in the presence of TGF-β1, IL-6 and IL-23. These findings suggest that TGF-β1 and IL-6 initiate low level differentiation of Th17 cells; and their maintenance and development need other expanding factors, among which IL-23 plays a potent role and IL-1β amplifies this expansion further in Th17 differentiation [97].

A variety of mucosal epithelia have been found to produce Th17 inducing cytokines, including TGF-β1, IL-6, IL-23, and IL-1β [98, 99]. IL-1β is a well recognized proinflammatory cytokine produced by mucosal epithelia in response to stress, infection or wounding. In an attempt to mimic known stressors of the ocular surface, we measured production of Th17 inducing cytokines in cultured HCECs in response to hyperosmotic stress, microbial components and inflammatory cytokines.

The ocular surface epithelium is subjected to hyperosmotic stress in dry eye conditions. Exposure of human epithelial cells to hyperosmotic stress has been noted to activate mitogen-activated protein kinase pathways and stimulate production of pro-inflammatory cytokines, such as IL-1β, TNF-α, and IL-8 [100]. We have also observed that TGF-β1, IL-6 and IL-23 were highly induced in the corneal epithelium in response to hyperosmotic stress.

We evaluated the expression and production of Th17-inducing cytokines by HCECs in response to 9 extracted or synthetic microbial components that are ligands of TLRs 1-9, respectively. TGF-β1, IL-6, IL-23, and IL-1β expression and production were found to be largely induced by polyI: C, flagellin, and R837, the respective ligands for TLRs3, 5 and 7, representing viral or bacterial infections. Among these TLR agonists, polyI:C was the strongest stimulator of Th17 inducing cytokines by HCECs.

Hyperosmotic stress and microbial components also promoted production of pro-inflammatory cytokines including TNF-α, which plays an important role in ocular surface disease [100, 101]. Consequently, TNF-α stimulus was found to markedly induce TGF-β1, IL-6, IL-23, and IL-1β.

Based on our findings that among TLR ligands, polyI:C is the potent stimulator of Th17 inducing cytokines, and that TNF-α is a representative pro-inflammatory factor, we evaluated the Th17 inducing capacity of conditioned media (CM) of HCECs treated with polyI:C and TNF-α [97]. It has been observed that Th17 cell differentiation was significantly stimulated in $CD4^+$ T cells exposed to the 50% conditioned media of HCECs challenged by polyI:C (CM-polyI:C) or TNF-α (CM-TNF-α) when compared with media from untreated cultures.

As shown in Figure 8A-E, the mRNA levels of IL-17A, IL-17F, IL-22, CCL-20 and STAT3 were significantly higher in $CD4^+$ T cells treated with CM-polyI:C or CM-TNF-α for 4 days compared with the control medium or conditioned media of HCEC culture without any stressors (CM-Control, all $P<0.05$, n=3). IL-17 protein levels in the supernatants of $CD4^+$ T cells exposed to CM-polyI:C or CM-TNF-α for 4 days (Figure 8F) were also significantly higher than the media (both $P<0.01$, n=3) and CM ($P<0.05$, n=3) controls. Furthermore, the number of IL-17-producing cells differentiated from $CD4^+$ T cells, determined by ELISPOT bioassay (Figure 8G, 8H), displayed the same pattern to the induction of IL-17 mRNA and protein. The numbers of IL-17-producing cells were stimulated by CM-polyI:C or CM-TNF-α, to the levels similar to that seen in the 3-cytokine system (TGF-β1+IL-6+IL-23), suggesting that cytokines in the conditioned media of HCECs exposed to polyI:C or TNF-α were capable to promote Th17 cell expansion to levels induced by IL-6+TGF-β1+IL-23. It suggests that the Th17 cells can be indeed promoted by factors produced by corneal epithelium in response to a variety of inflammatory stimuli [97].

8. Th17-mediated inflammation in dry eye

Dry eye is the second most common problem of patients seeking eye care, and is characterized by eye irritation symptoms and blurred vision. The prevalence of dry eye

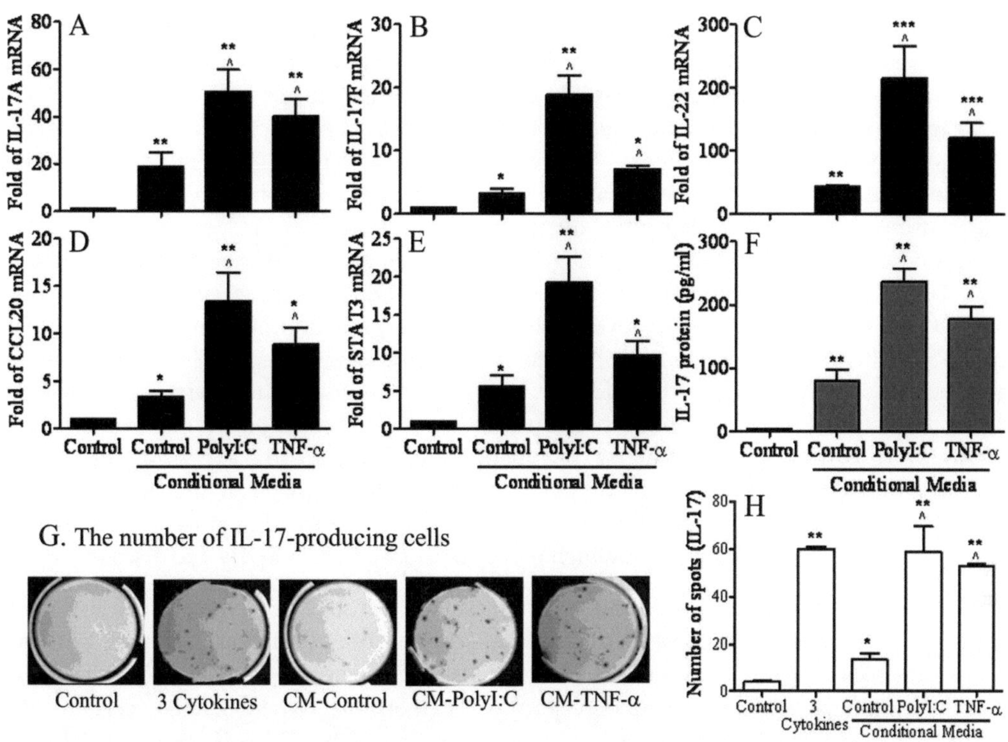

Fig. 8. Induction of Th17 differentiation of murine CD4+ T cells cultured in RPMI media containing 50% conditioned media (CM) of HCECs. **A-E.** Real-time PCR data showing the relative fold of mRNA of Th17 associated cytokines (IL-17A, IL-17F, IL-22, CCL-20) and regulator STAT3 in CD4+ T cells incubated for 4 days with 50% of conditioned media of HCECs irritated by polyI:C (CM-PolyI:C) or TNF-α (CM-TNF-α) for 48 hrs. **F.** Luminex immunobead assay showing IL-17 concentration in the supernatant of CD4+ T cells receiving the same treatment for 4 days. **G & H.** ELISPOT bioassay showing the spots/$3x10^5$ cells/well, representing the numbers of IL-17-producing T cells, in CD4+ T cells treated with CM-PolyI:C, CM-TNF-α, or 3 cytokines (TGF-β1+IL-6+IL-23) for 7 days. Results shown are mean ± SD of 3-5 independent experiments. *, $P < 0.05$; **, $P < 0.01$; ***, $P < 0.001$ each treated groups vs. media control. ^, $P < 0.05$; ^^, $P < 0.01$; ^^^, $P < 0.001$ CM-PolyI:C or CM-TNF-α groups vs. CM-control group.

increases with age, 6% at the age of 40, and 15-25% in the population over the age of 65. Among dry eye patients, 11% have been estimated to have the systemic autoimmune condition Sjögren's syndrome, a severe and potentially blinding condition. Dry eye is a potent stimulus of both innate and adaptive immune systems. At the nexus of the dry eye inflammatory/immune response is the dynamic interplay between the ocular surface epithelia and bone marrow derived immune cells. On the one hand, the ocular surface epithelial cells play a key initiating role in this inflammatory reaction, while on the other hand they are targets of cytokines that are produced by activated T cells that are recruited to the ocular surface in response to dry eye.

Dry eye has been demonstrated to cause inflammation of the ocular surface, evidenced by increased levels of inflammatory cytokines (IL-1, IL-6, and TNF-α) in the tear fluid, corneal and conjunctival epithelium, and an increased infiltration of dendritic cells and T lymphocytes in the conjunctiva [102-105]. Recently, increased levels of IL-17, IL-23 and IL-6 were found in saliva and salivary glands biopsies obtained from patients with the severe autoimmune dry eye condition, Sjögren's syndrome [106]. The increased matrix metalloproteinase (MMP) 9 and disrupted barrier function were observed in human [107] and murine dry eye [108]. Recently, our group has found increased expression of Th17 associated cytokines and IL-17-producing cells in human and experimental murine dry eye [108, 109]. Increased expression of Th17 cytokine IL-17A was observed in corneal and conjunctival epithelia of the dry eye mice. Since IL-17A is produced by T cells, not by epithelial cells, the Th17 reaction of the ocular surface is likely due to $CD4^+$ T cells, which have previously been found to infiltrate ocular surface tissues following experimental desiccating stress [110, 111]. Antibody neutralization of IL-17 ameliorated experimental dry eye-induced corneal epithelial barrier dysfunction and decreased the expression of MMP-3 and -9 [108]. These findings provide clear evidence that changes in the ocular surface environment, such as Th17-inducing cytokines, following desiccating stress are capable of inducing Th17 differentiation [112], which plays an important role in dry eye disease.

Th17 differentiation was also found to be mediated through a dendritic cell-mediated pathway. DCs have an important function in Th17 cell differentiation. They are antigen-presenting cells specialized to activate $CD4^+$ T cells and through their interaction with $CD4^+$ T cells to initiate primary immune responses. Furthermore, when primed, certain DCs express a high-level of Th17 inducing cytokines, including IL-6, TGF-β, IL-23 and IL-1 [113].

We found that efficient differentiation of $CD4^+$ T cells to IL-17 producers required the combination of ocular surface epithelium from dry eye mice and dendritic cells. $CD4^+$ T cells that were co-cultured with ocular epithelial explants from desiccating stress-induced dry eye mice and dendritic cells were found to express increased mRNA levels of Th17 cytokines (IL-17A, IL-17F, IL-22) and chemokine (C-C motif) ligand 20 (CCL20) (Figure 9A), as well as to produce and release IL-17A (Figure 9B & 9D), but not Th1 cytokine IFN-γ (Figure 9C). Exposure of dendritic cells to conditioned media from ocular surface explants of dry eye mice did not sufficiently activate these cells to promote T cell differentiation. The possible explanations for these findings include the need for direct contact between these cells, more efficient activation of cytokines such as TGF-β1 produced by the ocular surface epithelial cells or insufficient concentrations of Th17 inducing factors in the explants conditioned media.

The transcription factor RORγt was identified as a candidate master regulator that drives Th17 cell lineage differentiation [96]. Expression of RORγt is induced by TGF-β or IL-6, and overexpression of γt was found to promote Th17-cell differentiation when both Th1- and Th2-cell differentiations were blocked. In a model of experimental autoimmune encephalomyelitis, mice with RORγt-deficient T cells were found to have attenuated autoimmune disease and lacked tissue-infiltrating Th17 cells [96]. We found robust up-regulation (up to 100 fold) of the level of Th17 cell transcription factor-RORγt in T cells co-cultured with desiccated ocular surface tissues and dendritic cells (Figure 9E). This provides further evidence of the potent Th17 prone environment induced by desiccation.

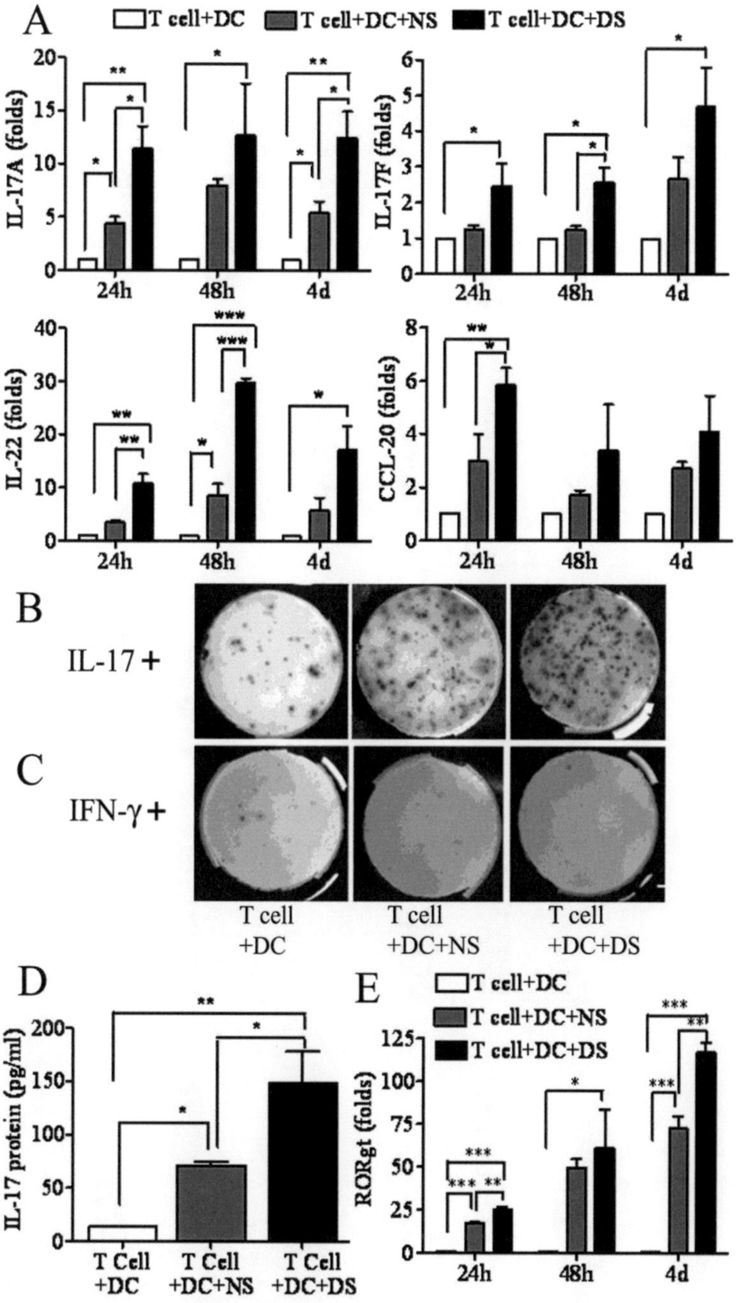

Fig. 9. Th17 differentiation of CD4+ T cells induced by the co-culture with dendritic cells (DCs) in the presence of cornea and conjunctival tissues of C57BL/6 mice subjected to desiccating stress. A. Real-time PCR data showing the relative mRNA expression (*x*-fold) of Th17 cytokines (IL-17A, IL-17F, IL-22, CCL-20) in CD4+ T cells ($3x10^5$ cells/ well) co-cultured for 1, 2, 4 days with DCs (T cell+DC), or with DCs and cornea and conjunctival explants from non-stressed control mice (T cell+DC+NS) or from mice desiccating stressed for 10-day (T

cell+DC+DS), (n=4). B & C. ELISPOT bioassay showing the numbers of IL-17 or IFN-γ-producing cells in these 3 groups. D. IL-17 concentration in the supernatant of CD4+ T cells co-cultured with DCs for 4 days in absence or presence of corneal and conjunctival explants from non-stressed and 10 day desiccating stressed mice. E. Real-time PCR showing the relative mRNA expression of RORγt in CD4+ T cells co-cultured for 1, 2, 4 days in 3 conditions. Data are presented as mean ± SD of 3 or 4 independent experiments. *P<0.05, **P<0.01, ***P<0.001.

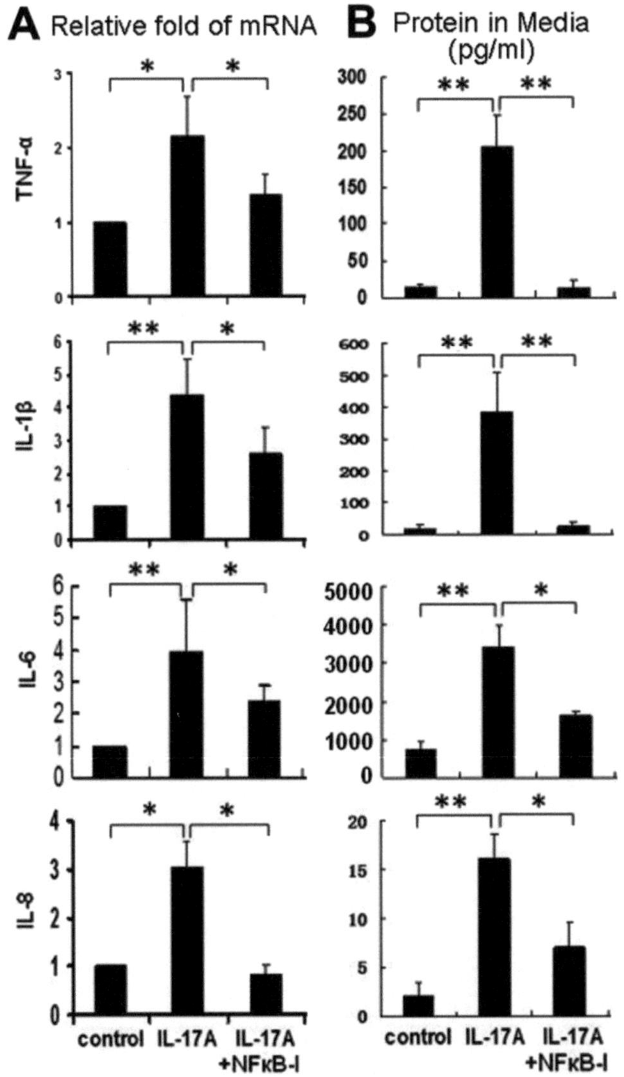

Fig. 10. The inflammatory effects of IL-17 on HCECs. Primary HCECs (5×10^5 cells/well) were treated with recombinant human IL-17A at 10 ng/ml for 4-48 hours with or without NF-κB activation inhibitor quinazoline (NFκB-I, 5μM). The pro-inflammatory cytokines (TNF-α, IL-1β and IL-6) and chemokine IL-8 were measured by RT-qPCR for mRNA (**A**) and by ELISA or Luminex immunobead assays in culture supernatants (**B**). Results shown are mean ± SD of 4 independent experiments. * $P < 0.05$, ** $P < 0.01$.

IL-17 producing T cells are distinct from Th1 cells. Analysis of the expression of transcription factors showed clearly that IL-17-producing T cells expressed neither GATA-3 nor T-bet and its target Hlx, which were typically expressed by IFN-γ-producing Th1 cells [88]. In the T cells co-cultured with desiccated ocular surface tissues and dendritic cells, we observed the lower expression of Th1 associated factors (IL-2, T-bet) and Th2 associated factors (IL-4, IL-13, GATA-3). There was no change in production of IFN-γ and IL-12 transcripts as well as in the number of IFN-γ-producing $CD4^{+}T$ cells in this co-culture system. Taken together, these findings indicate that desiccating stress may selectively promote the Th17 pathway, a finding that is consistent with the increased level of IL-17 in dry eye disease [108].

IL-17 initiates pro-inflammatory effects by binding to the IL-17 receptor (IL-17R), which is expressed by a variety of cell types including epithelial, endothelial, and fibroblastic stromal cells [81, 114]. As shown in Figure 10, recombinant human IL-17A (10 ng/ml) significantly increased mRNA levels (2-4 fold) of proinflammatory cytokines (TNF-α, IL-1β and IL-6) and chemokine IL-8 expressed by HCECs. These stimulatory responses to IL-17A were confirmed by 4-7 fold increases at protein levels. The stimulated production of these inflammatory cytokines and chemokine was significantly suppressed at both mRNA (all $P<0.05$, n=4) and protein levels ($P<0.05$ or 0.01) by NF-κB activation inhibitor quinazoline [115], indicating NF-κB pathway is involved in the inflammatory effect of IL-17 on mucosal epithelium.

These findings demonstrate that desiccating stress stimulates the expression and production of Th17 inducing cytokines by corneal and conjunctival epithelia, and that desiccation creates an environment promoting Th17 differentiation through a dendritic cell-mediated pathway. We hypothesize that Th17 inducing cytokines produced by the ocular epithelium may participate in Th17 differentiation in three ways: (1) activation of immature dendritic cells on the ocular surface; (2) direct transfer to the lymph node in lymphatic liquid; or (3) direct promotion of differentiated Th17 cells that infiltrate the ocular surface.

9. Conclusion

This chapter focused on recent breakthroughs in ocular mucosal immunology, including the discoveries of TLR signaling in innate immunity, novel epithelium-derived pro-allergic cytokines TSLP and IL-33, and a new Th17 cell population in adaptive immunity. One of important breakthroughs is a discovery of a novel mechanism by which short ragweed pollen, serving as a functional TLR4 agonist, induces TSLP/OX40L/OX40 signaling to trigger Th2-dominant allergic inflammation via TLR4-dependent innate immunity pathways. All these advances provide compelling evidence that mucosal epithelium actively participate, as initiators, mediators and regulators, in innate and adaptive immune responses for host defense, in addition to physical barrier function. These novel signaling molecules may be critical for allergic, inflammatory and autoimmune diseases on mucosal ocular surface, and may become potential molecular targets for new therapies to treat these ocular diseases.

10. Abbreviations used in this chapter

CLN: cervical lymph nodes; **DAMP**: damage-associated molecular patterns; **DC**: dendritic cell; **dsRNA**: double stranded RNA; **EAC**: experimental allergic conjunctivitis; **HCECs**:

human corneal epithelial cells; **IL**: interleukin; **MyD88**: myeloid differentiation primary response gene 88; *MyD88$^{-/-}$*: *MyD88* knockout mice; **LPS**: lipopolysaccharide; **NF-κB**: nuclear factor kappa B; **PBS**: phosphate buffered saline; **PGN**: peptidoglycan; **PAMP**: pathogen-associated molecular patterns; **PCR**: polymerase chain reaction; **polyI:C**: polyinosinic-polycytidylic acid; **PRR**: pattern recognition receptor; **R837**: imiquimod; **RT-qPCR**: reverse transcription and quantitative real-time PCR; ROR: retinoic-acid-receptor-related orphan receptor; **SRW**: short ragweed; **SRWe**: aqueous extract of defatted short ragweed pollen; **ssRNA**: single stranded RNA; **TGF-β**: transforming growth factor; **Th1**: T helper cell type 1; **Th17**: T helper cell producing IL-17 family; **Th2**: T helper cell type 2; **TLR**: Toll-like receptor; *Tlr4-d*: *Tlr4* gene deficient; **TRIF**: TIR-domain-containing adaptor inducing interferon; **TSLP**: thymic stromal lymphopoietin; **TSLPR**: TSLP receptor.

11. References

[1] Hoebe K, Janssen E, Beutler B. The interface between innate and adaptive immunity. *Nat Immunol.* 2004;5:971-974.
[2] Meyer T, Stockfleth E, Christophers E. Immune response profiles in human skin. *Br J Dermatol.* 2007;157 Suppl 2:1-7.
[3] Buchau AS, Gallo RL. Innate immunity and antimicrobial defense systems in psoriasis. *Clin Dermatol.* 2007;25:616-624.
[4] Wollenberg A, Klein E. Current aspects of innate and adaptive immunity in atopic dermatitis. *Clin Rev Allergy Immunol.* 2007;33:35-44.
[5] Kato A, Schleimer RP. Beyond inflammation: airway epithelial cells are at the interface of innate and adaptive immunity. *Curr Opin Immunol.* 2007;19:711-720.
[6] Mayer AK, Dalpke AH. Regulation of local immunity by airway epithelial cells. *Arch Immunol Ther Exp (Warsz).* 2007;55:353-362.
[7] Schleimer RP, Kato A, Kern R, Kuperman D, Avila PC. Epithelium: at the interface of innate and adaptive immune responses. *J Allergy Clin Immunol.* 2007;120:1279-1284.
[8] Muller CA, Autenrieth IB, Peschel A. Innate defenses of the intestinal epithelial barrier. *Cell Mol Life Sci.* 2005;62:1297-1307.
[9] Ishihara S, Rumi MA, Ortega-Cava CF, Kazumori H, Kadowaki Y, Ishimura N, Kinoshita Y. Therapeutic targeting of toll-like receptors in gastrointestinal inflammation. *Curr Pharm Des.* 2006;12:4215-4228.
[10] Sharma R, Young C, Neu J. Molecular modulation of intestinal epithelial barrier: contribution of microbiota. *J Biomed Biotechnol.* 2010;2010:305879.
[11] Hazlett LD. Role of innate and adaptive immunity in the pathogenesis of keratitis. *Ocul Immunol Inflamm.* 2005;13:133-138.
[12] Kumar A, Yu FS. Toll-like receptors and corneal innate immunity. *Curr Mol Med.* 2006;6:327-337.
[13] Chang JH, McCluskey PJ, Wakefield D. Toll-like receptors in ocular immunity and the immunopathogenesis of inflammatory eye disease. *Br J Ophthalmol.* 2006;90:103-108.
[14] Akira S, Uematsu S, Takeuchi O. Pathogen recognition and innate immunity. *Cell.* 2006;124:783-801.
[15] Takeda K, Kaisho T, Akira S. Toll-like receptors. *Annu Rev Immunol.* 2003;21:335-376.
[16] Trinchieri G, Sher A. Cooperation of Toll-like receptor signals in innate immune defence. *Nat Rev Immunol.* 2007;7:179-190.
[17] Gay NJ, Gangloff M. Structure and function of Toll receptors and their ligands. *Annu Rev Biochem.* 2007;76:141-165.

[18] Vercammen E, Staal J, Beyaert R. Sensing of viral infection and activation of innate immunity by toll-like receptor 3. *Clin Microbiol Rev.* 2008;21:13-25.
[19] Liu J, Buckley JM, Redmond HP, Wang JH. ST2 negatively regulates TLR2 signaling, but is not required for bacterial lipoprotein-induced tolerance. *J Immunol.* 2010;184:5802-5808.
[20] Kawai T, Akira S. Signaling to NF-kappaB by Toll-like receptors. *Trends Mol Med.* 2007;13:460-469.
[21] Miller LS, Modlin RL. Toll-like receptors in the skin. *Semin Immunopathol.* 2007;29:15-26.
[22] Li DQ, Zhou N, Zhang L, Ma P, Pflugfelder SC. Suppressive effects of azithromycin on zymosan-induced production of proinflammatory mediators by human corneal epithelial cells. *Invest Ophthalmol Vis Sci.* 2010;51:5623-5629.
[23] Kumar A, Zhang J, Yu FS. Innate immune response of corneal epithelial cells to Staphylococcus aureus infection: role of peptidoglycan in stimulating proinflammatory cytokine secretion. *Invest Ophthalmol Vis Sci.* 2004;45:3513-3522.
[24] Huang X, Barrett RP, McClellan SA, Hazlett LD. Silencing Toll-like receptor-9 in Pseudomonas aeruginosa keratitis. *Invest Ophthalmol Vis Sci.* 2005;46:4209-4216.
[25] Kumar A, Zhang J, Yu FS. Toll-like receptor 3 agonist poly(I:C)-induced antiviral response in human corneal epithelial cells. *Immunology.* 2006;117:11-21.
[26] Ueta M, Hamuro J, Kiyono H, Kinoshita S. Triggering of TLR3 by polyI:C in human corneal epithelial cells to induce inflammatory cytokines. *Biochem Biophys Res Commun.* 2005;331:285-294.
[27] Liu YJ. Thymic stromal lymphopoietin and OX40 ligand pathway in the initiation of dendritic cell-mediated allergic inflammation. *J Allergy Clin Immunol.* 2007;120:238-244.
[28] Liu YJ, Soumelis V, Watanabe N, Ito T, Wang YH, Malefyt RW, Omori M, Zhou B, Ziegler SF. TSLP: an epithelial cell cytokine that regulates T cell differentiation by conditioning dendritic cell maturation. *Annu Rev Immunol.* 2007;25:193-219.
[29] Holgate ST. The epithelium takes centre stage in asthma and atopic dermatitis. *Trends Immunol.* 2007;28:248-251.
[30] Lee HC, Ziegler SF. Inducible expression of the proallergic cytokine thymic stromal lymphopoietin in airway epithelial cells is controlled by NFkappaB. *Proc Natl Acad Sci USA.* 2007;104:914-919.
[31] Demehri S, Morimoto M, Holtzman MJ, Kopan R. Skin-derived TSLP triggers progression from epidermal-barrier defects to asthma. *PLoS Biol.* 2009;7:e1000067.
[32] Zhang Z, Hener P, Frossard N, Kato S, Metzger D, Li M, Chambon P. Thymic stromal lymphopoietin overproduced by keratinocytes in mouse skin aggravates experimental asthma. *Proc Natl Acad Sci U S A.* 2009;106:1536-1541.
[33] Sims JE, Williams DE, Morrissey PJ, Garka K, Foxworthe D, Price V, Friend SL, Farr A, Bedell MA, Jenkins NA, Copeland NG, Grabstein K, Paxton RJ. Molecular cloning and biological characterization of a novel murine lymphoid growth factor. *J Exp Med.* 2000;192:671-680.
[34] Quentmeier H, Drexler HG, Fleckenstein D, Zaborski M, Armstrong A, Sims JE, Lyman SD. Cloning of human thymic stromal lymphopoietin (TSLP) and signaling mechanisms leading to proliferation. *Leukemia.* 2001;15:1286-1292.
[35] Reche PA, Soumelis V, Gorman DM, Clifford T, Liu M, Travis M, Zurawski SM, Johnston J, Liu YJ, Spits H, de Waal MR, Kastelein RA, Bazan JF. Human thymic stromal lymphopoietin preferentially stimulates myeloid cells. *J Immunol.* 2001;167:336-343.

[36] Soumelis V, Reche PA, Kanzler H, Yuan W, Edward G, Homey B, Gilliet M, Ho S, Antonenko S, Lauerma A, Smith K, Gorman D, Zurawski S, Abrams J, Menon S, McClanahan T, de Waal-Malefyt RR, Bazan F, Kastelein RA, Liu YJ. Human epithelial cells trigger dendritic cell mediated allergic inflammation by producing TSLP. *Nat Immunol.* 2002;3:673-680.
[37] Allakhverdi Z, Comeau MR, Jessup HK, Yoon BR, Brewer A, Chartier S, Paquette N, Ziegler SF, Sarfati M, Delespesse G. Thymic stromal lymphopoietin is released by human epithelial cells in response to microbes, trauma, or inflammation and potently activates mast cells. *J Exp Med.* 2007;204:253-258.
[38] Bogiatzi SI, Fernandez I, Bichet JC, Marloie-Provost MA, Volpe E, Sastre X, Soumelis V. Cutting Edge: Proinflammatory and Th2 cytokines synergize to induce thymic stromal lymphopoietin production by human skin keratinocytes. *J Immunol.* 2007;178:3373-3377.
[39] Kato A, Favoreto S Jr, Avila PC, Schleimer RP. TLR3- and Th2 cytokine-dependent production of thymic stromal lymphopoietin in human airway epithelial cells. *J Immunol.* 2007;179:1080-1087.
[40] Ma P, Bian F, Wang Z, Zheng X, Chotikavanich S, Pflugfelder SC, Li DQ. Human corneal epithelium-derived thymic stromal lymphopoietin links the innate and adaptive immune responses via TLRs and Th2 cytokines. *Invest Ophthalmol Vis Sci.* 2009;50:2702-2709.
[41] Mohan RR, Mohan RR, Kim WJ, Wilson SE. Modulation of TNF-alpha-induced apoptosis in corneal fibroblasts by transcription factor NF-kappaB. *Invest Ophthalmol Vis Sci.* 2000;41:1327-1336.
[42] Ozawa T, Koyama K, Ando T, Ohnuma Y, Hatsushika K, Ohba T, Sugiyama H, Hamada Y, Ogawa H, Okumura K, Nakao A. Thymic stromal lymphopoietin secretion of synovial fibroblasts is positively and negatively regulated by Toll-like receptors/nuclear factor-kappaB pathway and interferon-gamma/dexamethasone. *Mod Rheumatol.* 2007;17:459-463.
[43] Stern ME, Siemasko KF, Niederkorn JY. The Th1/Th2 paradigm in ocular allergy. *Curr Opin Allergy Clin Immunol.* 2005;5:446-450.
[44] Niederkorn JY. Immune regulatory mechanisms in allergic conjunctivitis: insights from mouse models. *Curr Opin Allergy Clin Immunol.* 2008;8:472-476.
[45] Buc M, Dzurilla M, Vrlik M, Bucova M. Immunopathogenesis of bronchial asthma. *Arch Immunol Ther Exp (Warsz).* 2009;57:331-344.
[46] Ying S, O'Connor B, Ratoff J, Meng Q, Fang C, Cousins D, Zhang G, Gu S, Gao Z, Shamji B, Edwards MJ, Lee TH, Corrigan CJ. Expression and cellular provenance of thymic stromal lymphopoietin and chemokines in patients with severe asthma and chronic obstructive pulmonary disease. *J Immunol.* 2008;181:2790-2798.
[47] Matsuda A, Ebihara N, Yokoi N, Kawasaki S, Tanioka H, Inatomi T, de Waal MR, Hamuro J, Kinoshita S, Murakami A. Functional role of thymic stromal lymphopoietin in chronic allergic keratoconjunctivitis. *Invest Ophthalmol Vis Sci.* 2010;51:151-155.
[48] Kay AB. Allergy and allergic diseases. First of two parts. *N Engl J Med.* 2001;344:30-37.
[49] Komine M. Analysis of the mechanism for the development of allergic skin inflammation and the application for its treatment:keratinocytes in atopic dermatitis - their pathogenic involvement. *J Pharmacol Sci.* 2009;110:260-264.
[50] Magone MT, Chan CC, Rizzo LV, Kozhich AT, Whitcup SM. A novel murine model of allergic conjunctivitis. *Clin Immunol Immunopathol.* 1998;87:75-84.

[51] Stern ME, Siemasko K, Gao J, Duong A, Beauregard C, Calder V, Niederkorn JY. Role of interferon-gamma in a mouse model of allergic conjunctivitis. *Invest Ophthalmol Vis Sci.* 2005;46:3239-3246.

[52] Zheng X, Ma P, de Paiva CS, Cunningham MA, Hwang CS, Pflugfelder SC, Li DQ. TSLP and downstream molecules in experimental mouse allergic conjunctivitis. *Invest Ophthalmol Vis Sci.* 2010;51:3076-3082.

[53] Le TA, Takai T, Vu AT, Kinoshita H, Chen X, Ikeda S, Ogawa H, Okumura K. Flagellin Induces the Expression of Thymic Stromal Lymphopoietin in Human Keratinocytes via Toll-Like Receptor 5. *Int Arch Allergy Immunol.* 2010;155:31-37.

[54] Kinoshita H, Takai T, Le TA, Kamijo S, Wang XL, Ushio H, Hara M, Kawasaki J, Vu AT, Ogawa T, Gunawan H, Ikeda S, Okumura K, Ogawa H. Cytokine milieu modulates release of thymic stromal lymphopoietin from human keratinocytes stimulated with double-stranded RNA. *J Allergy Clin Immunol.* 2009;123:179-186.

[55] Johnson AC, Heinzel FP, Diaconu E, Sun Y, Hise AG, Golenbock D, Lass JH, Pearlman E. Activation of toll-like receptor (TLR)2, TLR4, and TLR9 in the mammalian cornea induces MyD88-dependent corneal inflammation. *Invest Ophthalmol Vis Sci.* 2005;46:589-595.

[56] Piggott DA, Eisenbarth SC, Xu L, Constant SL, Huleatt JW, Herrick CA, Bottomly K. MyD88-dependent induction of allergic Th2 responses to intranasal antigen. *J Clin Invest.* 2005;115:459-467.

[57] Akira S, Hoshino K, Kaisho T. The role of Toll-like receptors and MyD88 in innate immune responses. *J Endotoxin Res.* 2000;6:383-387.

[58] Tsuji RF, Hoshino K, Noro Y, Tsuji NM, Kurokawa T, Masuda T, Akira S, Nowak B. Suppression of allergic reaction by lambda-carrageenan: toll-like receptor 4/MyD88-dependent and -independent modulation of immunity. *Clin Exp Allergy.* 2003;33:249-258.

[59] Fasciano S, Li L. Intervention of Toll-like receptor-mediated human innate immunity and inflammation by synthetic compounds and naturally occurring products. *Curr Med Chem.* 2006;13:1389-1395.

[60] Kawasaki K, Akashi S, Shimazu R, Yoshida T, Miyake K, Nishijima M. Mouse toll-like receptor 4.MD-2 complex mediates lipopolysaccharide-mimetic signal transduction by Taxol. *J Biol Chem.* 2000;275:2251-2254.

[61] Mishra KP, Ganju L, Chanda S, Karan D, Sawhney RC. Aqueous extract of Rhodiola imbricata rhizome stimulates Toll-like receptor 4, granzyme-B and Th1 cytokines in vitro. *Immunobiology.* 2009;214:27-31.

[62] Li D-Q, Zhang L, Pflugfelder SC, de Paiva CS, Zhang X, Zhao G, Zheng X, Su Z, Qu Y. Short ragweed pollen triggers allergic inflammation via TLR4-dependent TSLP/OX40L/OX40 signaling pathways. J Allergy Clin. Immunol. 2011;128: 1318-1325.e2

[63] Tominaga S. A putative protein of a growth specific cDNA from BALB/c-3T3 cells is highly similar to the extracellular portion of mouse interleukin 1 receptor. *FEBS Lett.* 1989;258:301-304.

[64] Kakkar R, Lee RT. The IL-33/ST2 pathway: therapeutic target and novel biomarker. *Nat Rev Drug Discov.* 2008;7:827-840.

[65] Eiwegger T, Akdis CA. IL-33 links tissue cells, dendritic cells and Th2 cell development in a mouse model of asthma. *Eur J Immunol.* 2011;41:1535-1538.

[66] Schmitz J, Owyang A, Oldham E, Song Y, Murphy E, McClanahan TK, Zurawski G, Moshrefi M, Qin J, Li X, Gorman DM, Bazan JF, Kastelein RA. IL-33, an interleukin-

1-like cytokine that signals via the IL-1 receptor-related protein ST2 and induces T helper type 2-associated cytokines. *Immunity.* 2005;23:479-490.
[67] Moussion C, Ortega N, Girard JP. The IL-1-like cytokine IL-33 is constitutively expressed in the nucleus of endothelial cells and epithelial cells in vivo: a novel 'alarmin'? *PLoS One.* 2008;3:e3331.
[68] Smith DE. IL-33: a tissue derived cytokine pathway involved in allergic inflammation and asthma. *Clin Exp Allergy.* 2009.
[69] Allam JP, Bieber T, Novak N. Dendritic cells as potential targets for mucosal immunotherapy. *Curr Opin Allergy Clin Immunol.* 2009;9:554-557.
[70] Zhang L, Lu R, Zhao G, Pflugfelder SC, Li DQ. TLR-mediated induction of pro-allergic cytokine IL-33 in ocular mucosal epithelium. *Int J Biochem Cell Biol.* 2011;43:1383-1391.
[71] Haraldsen G, Balogh J, Pollheimer J, Sponheim J, Kuchler AM. Interleukin-33 - cytokine of dual function or novel alarmin? *Trends Immunol.* 2009;30:227-233.
[72] Hayakawa M, Hayakawa H, Matsuyama Y, Tamemoto H, Okazaki H, Tominaga S. Mature interleukin-33 is produced by calpain-mediated cleavage in vivo. *Biochem Biophys Res Commun.* 2009;387:218-222.
[73] Talabot-Ayer D, Lamacchia C, Gabay C, Palmer G. Interleukin-33 is biologically active independently of caspase-1 cleavage. *J Biol Chem.* 2009;284:19420-19426.
[74] Krishnan J, Selvarajoo K, Tsuchiya M, Lee G, Choi S. Toll-like receptor signal transduction. *Exp Mol Med.* 2007;39:421-438.
[75] Mosmann TR, Coffman RL. TH1 and TH2 cells: different patterns of lymphokine secretion lead to different functional properties. *Annu Rev Immunol.* 1989;7:145-173.
[76] Dong C. Diversification of T-helper-cell lineages: finding the family root of IL-17-producing cells. *Nat Rev Immunol.* 2006;6:329-333.
[77] Komiyama Y, Nakae S, Matsuki T, Nambu A, Ishigame H, Kakuta S, Sudo K, Iwakura Y. IL-17 plays an important role in the development of experimental autoimmune encephalomyelitis. *J Immunol.* 2006;177:566-573.
[78] Hwang SY, Kim HY. Expression of IL-17 homologs and their receptors in the synovial cells of rheumatoid arthritis patients. *Mol Cells.* 2005;19:180-184.
[79] Chang SH, Dong C. A novel heterodimeric cytokine consisting of IL-17 and IL-17F regulates inflammatory responses. *Cell Res.* 2007;17:435-440.
[80] Williams IR. CCR6 and CCL20: partners in intestinal immunity and lymphorganogenesis. *Ann N Y Acad Sci.* 2006;1072:52-61.
[81] Moseley TA, Haudenschild DR, Rose L, Reddi AH. Interleukin-17 family and IL-17 receptors. *Cytokine Growth Factor Rev.* 2003;14:155-174.
[82] Gaffen SL, Kramer JM, Yu JJ, Shen F. The IL-17 cytokine family. *Vitam Horm.* 2006;74:255-282.
[83] Kuestner RE, Taft DW, Haran A, Brandt CS, Brender T, Lum K, Harder B, Okada S, Ostrander CD, Kreindler JL, Aujla SJ, Reardon B, Moore M, Shea P, Schreckhise R, Bukowski TR, Presnell S, Guerra-Lewis P, Parrish-Novak J, Ellsworth JL, Jaspers S, Lewis KE, Appleby M, Kolls JK, Rixon M, West JW, Gao Z, Levin SD. Identification of the IL-17 receptor related molecule IL-17RC as the receptor for IL-17F. *J Immunol.* 2007;179:5462-5473.
[84] Liang SC, Tan XY, Luxenberg DP, Karim R, Dunussi-Joannopoulos K, Collins M, Fouser LA. Interleukin (IL)-22 and IL-17 are coexpressed by Th17 cells and cooperatively enhance expression of antimicrobial peptides. *J Exp Med.* 2006;203:2271-2279.

[85] Zheng Y, Danilenko DM, Valdez P, Kasman I, Eastham-Anderson J, Wu J, Ouyang W. Interleukin-22, a T(H)17 cytokine, mediates IL-23-induced dermal inflammation and acanthosis. *Nature.* 2007;445:648-651.

[86] Hirota K, Yoshitomi H, Hashimoto M, Maeda S, Teradaira S, Sugimoto N, Yamaguchi T, Nomura T, Ito H, Nakamura T, Sakaguchi N, Sakaguchi S. Preferential recruitment of CCR6-expressing Th17 cells to inflamed joints via CCL20 in rheumatoid arthritis and its animal model. *J Exp Med.* 2007;204:2803-2812.

[87] Yang XO, Panopoulos AD, Nurieva R, Chang SH, Wang D, Watowich SS, Dong C. STAT3 regulates cytokine-mediated generation of inflammatory helper T cells. *J Biol Chem.* 2007;282:9358-9363.

[88] Veldhoen M, Hocking RJ, Atkins CJ, Locksley RM, Stockinger B. TGFbeta in the context of an inflammatory cytokine milieu supports de novo differentiation of IL-17-producing T cells. *Immunity.* 2006;24:179-189.

[89] Mangan PR, Harrington LE, O'Quinn DB, Helms WS, Bullard DC, Elson CO, Hatton RD, Wahl SM, Schoeb TR, Weaver CT. Transforming growth factor-beta induces development of the T(H)17 lineage. *Nature.* 2006;441:231-234.

[90] Murphy CA, Langrish CL, Chen Y, Blumenschein W, McClanahan T, Kastelein RA, Sedgwick JD, Cua DJ. Divergent pro- and antiinflammatory roles for IL-23 and IL-12 in joint autoimmune inflammation. *J Exp Med.* 2003;198:1951-1957.

[91] Zhou L, Ivanov II, Spolski R, Min R, Shenderov K, Egawa T, Levy DE, Leonard WJ, Littman DR. IL-6 programs T(H)-17 cell differentiation by promoting sequential engagement of the IL-21 and IL-23 pathways. *Nat Immunol.* 2007;8:967-974.

[92] Langrish CL, Chen Y, Blumenschein WM, Mattson J, Basham B, Sedgwick JD, McClanahan T, Kastelein RA, Cua DJ. IL-23 drives a pathogenic T cell population that induces autoimmune inflammation. *J Exp Med.* 2005;201:233-240.

[93] Leonard WJ, Spolski R. Interleukin-21: a modulator of lymphoid proliferation, apoptosis and differentiation. *Nat Rev Immunol.* 2005;5:688-698.

[94] Korn T, Bettelli E, Gao W, Awasthi A, Jager A, Strom TB, Oukka M, Kuchroo VK. IL-21 initiates an alternative pathway to induce proinflammatory T(H)17 cells. *Nature.* 2007;448:484-487.

[95] Nurieva R, Yang XO, Martinez G, Zhang Y, Panopoulos AD, Ma L, Schluns K, Tian Q, Watowich SS, Jetten AM, Dong C. Essential autocrine regulation by IL-21 in the generation of inflammatory T cells. *Nature.* 2007;448:480-483.

[96] Ivanov II, McKenzie BS, Zhou L, Tadokoro CE, Lepelley A, Lafaille JJ, Cua DJ, Littman DR. The orphan nuclear receptor RORgammat directs the differentiation program of proinflammatory IL-17+ T helper cells. *Cell.* 2006;126:1121-1133.

[97] Zheng X, Bian F, Ma P, de Paiva CS, Stern M, Pflugfelder SC, Li DQ. Induction of Th17 differentiation by corneal epithelial-derived cytokines. *J Cell Physiol.* 2010;222:95-102.

[98] Aujla SJ, Dubin PJ, Kolls JK. Th17 cells and mucosal host defense. *Semin Immunol.* 2007;19:377-382.

[99] Holtta V, Klemetti P, Sipponen T, Westerholm-Ormio M, Kociubinski G, Salo H, Rasanen L, Kolho KL, Farkkila M, Savilahti E, Vaarala O. IL-23/IL-17 immunity as a hallmark of Crohn's disease. *Inflamm Bowel Dis.* 2008;14:1175-1184.

[100] Li D-Q, Luo L, Chen Z, Kim HS, Song XJ, Pflugfelder SC. JNK and ERK MAP kinases mediate induction of IL-1beta, TNF-alpha and IL-8 following hyperosmolar stress in human limbal epithelial cells. *Exp Eye Res.* 2006;82:588-596.

[101] Barton K, Monroy DC, Nava A, Pflugfelder SC. Inflammatory cytokines in the tears of patients with ocular rosacea. *Ophthalmology.* 1997;104:1868-1874.

[102] Corrales RM, Villarreal A, Farley W, Stern ME, Li DQ, Pflugfelder SC. Strain-related cytokine profiles on the murine ocular surface in response to desiccating stress. *Cornea.* 2007;26:579-584.

[103] Turner K, Pflugfelder SC, Ji Z, Feuer WJ, Stern M, Reis BL. Interleukin-6 levels in the conjunctival epithelium of patients with dry eye disease treated with cyclosporine ophthalmic emulsion. *Cornea.* 2000;19:492-496.

[104] Solomon A, Dursun D, Liu Z, Xie Y, Macri A, Pflugfelder SC. Pro- and anti-inflammatory forms of interleukin-1 in the tear fluid and conjunctiva of patients with dry-eye disease. *Invest Ophthalmol Vis Sci.* 2001;42:2283-2292.

[105] Pflugfelder SC, de Paiva CS, Li DQ, Stern ME. Epithelial-immune cell interaction in dry eye. *Cornea.* 2008;27 Suppl 1:S9-11.

[106] Nguyen CQ, Hu MH, Li Y, Stewart C, Peck AB. Salivary gland tissue expression of interleukin-23 and interleukin-17 in Sjogren's syndrome: findings in humans and mice. *Arthritis Rheum.* 2008;58:734-743.

[107] Chotikavanich S, de Paiva CS, Li DQ, Chen JJ, Bian F, Farley WJ, Pflugfelder SC. Production and Activity of Matrix Metalloproteinase-9 on the Ocular Surface Increase in Dysfunctional Tear Syndrome. *Invest Ophthalmol Vis Sci.* 2009; 50:3203-3209.

[108] de Paiva CS, Chotikavanich S, Pangelinan SB, Pitcher JD, III, Fang B, Zheng X, Ma P, Farley WJ, Siemasko KF, Niederkorn JY, Stern ME, Li DQ, Pflugfelder SC. IL-17 disrupts corneal barrier following desiccating stress. *Mucosal Immunol.* 2009;2:243-253.

[109] Chauhan SK, El AJ, Ecoiffier T, Goyal S, Zhang Q, Saban DR, Dana R. Autoimmunity in dry eye is due to resistance of Th17 to Treg suppression. *J Immunol.* 2009;182:1247-1252.

[110] de Paiva CS, Villarreal AL, Corrales RM, Rahman HT, Chang VY, Farley WJ, Stern ME, Niederkorn JY, Li DQ, Pflugfelder SC. Dry eye-induced conjunctival epithelial squamous metaplasia is modulated by interferon-gamma. *Invest Ophthalmol Vis Sci.* 2007;48:2553-2560.

[111] Stern ME, Siemasko KF, Gao J, Calonge M, Niederkorn JY, Pflugfelder SC. Evaluation of ocular surface inflammation in the presence of dry eye and allergic conjunctival disease. *Ocul Surf.* 2005;3:S161-S164.

[112] Zheng X, de Paiva CS, Li DQ, Farley WJ, Pflugfelder SC. Desiccating stress promotion of Th17 differentiation by ocular surface tissues through a dendritic cell-mediated pathway. *Invest Ophthalmol Vis Sci.* 2010;51:3083-3091.

[113] Shainheit MG, Smith PM, Bazzone LE, Wang AC, Rutitzky LI, Stadecker MJ. Dendritic cell IL-23 and IL-1 production in response to schistosome eggs induces Th17 cells in a mouse strain prone to severe immunopathology. *J Immunol.* 2008;181:8559-8567.

[114] Molesworth-Kenyon SJ, Yin R, Oakes JE, Lausch RN. IL-17 receptor signaling influences virus-induced corneal inflammation. *J Leukoc Biol.* 2008;83:401-408.

[115] Bian F, Qi H, Ma P, Zhang L, Yoon KC, Pflugfelder SC, Li DQ. An immunoprotective privilege of corneal epithelial stem cells against Th17 inflammatory stress by producing glial cell-derived neurotrophic factor. *Stem Cells.* 2010;28:2172-2181.

5

Trafficking of Immune Cells in the Cornea and Ocular Surface

Yureeda Qazi,
Aslihan Turhan and Pedram Hamrah
Cornea Service, Massachusetts Eye and Ear Infirmary,
Department of Ophthalmology, Harvard Medical School
USA

1. Introduction

The role of immuno-inflammatory responses in the cornea and ocular surface has continuously been evolving over the past decades and has been becoming the center stage for therapeutic approaches for many diseases. In fact, the relevance of inflammation as a significant component in the pathophysiology of most acute and chronic forms of corneal and ocular surface diseases (e.g., microbial keratitis, allergy, and dry eye syndrome) has become evident. Both local and systemic immunomodulation with anti-inflammatory agents have been used successfully in improving these conditions or bringing these conditions under control. Thus, understanding the cellular and molecular mechanisms by which the ocular surface participates in immuno-inflammatory disorders is crucial for a more rational clinical approach to treating these diseases.

There are several unique anatomical and physiological features of the cornea and ocular surface as compared to other tissues in the body, which translate into specific mechanisms by which they are involved in both inciting and expressing immunity, as well as preventing unnecessary inflammation. There are a very large number of immune and inflammatory disorders that involve the cornea and ocular surface. Control of leukocyte entry and migration within the cornea and ocular surface is thus vital to regulate protective and pathological responses. While local control of pathogens is dependent on the ability of immune cells to access and operate within these sites, too much inflammation can be deleterious and lead to loss of vision. In this chapter, the current knowledge on the coordinated migratory events that regulate leukocyte trafficking in the cornea and ocular surface are discussed. The aim is to first provide an overview of the contribution of resident bone marrow (BM)-derived cells of the cornea and ocular surface. Second, the role of infiltrating leucocytes in some of the innate defense mechanisms will be discussed. Third, we will provide a summary of the mechanisms that dictate immune cell trafficking to the cornea and ocular surface in response to inflammation. Finally, we will discuss trafficking mechanisms of antigen presenting cells from the cornea and ocular surface to draining lymph nodes where the immune responses are initiated.

2. Role of leukocytes in disease

2.1 Overview of resident leukocytes

The cornea and ocular surface have constant and direct contact with the external world. This necessitates a powerful and intrinsic immune surveillance system involved in their natural defense. Resident ocular tissue elements together with circulating bone marrow-derived cells are important components of this system, delicately balancing defense and tolerance under steady sate conditions. The ocular surface consists of three distinct anatomical regions: the cornea, limbus, and the conjunctiva. These regions function both in concert and independently against microbial, immunogenic and traumatic insults.

Antigen presenting cells (APCs) and in particular dendritic cells (DCs) orchestrate the immune response through their capacity to capture, process and subsequently present antigens. APCs serve as the principal immune sentinels to the foreign world. They can be divided into 'professional' and 'nonprofessional' types. While the latter are found among nonlymphoid tissues (e.g., vascular endothelial or some tissue epithelial cells), professional APC are BM-derived, and form an integral part of the immune system. Professional APCs include DCs (including epithelial Langerhans cells; LCs), macrophages, and B cells, although DCs are the most potent APCs. Expression of major histocompatibility class II (MHC-II) antigens on DCs, whose primary function is to distinguish between self and non-self, plays an integral role in antigen recognition and presentation. DCs have a dual function as key regulators of T cell immunity and tolerance induction to both self and foreign antigens. Precursor and progenitor DCs constitutively repopulate normal tissues from the bloodstream, and are recruited in elevated numbers to sites of inflammation. A second type of DC precursors is constituted by peripheral blood monocytes that are recruited during an inflammation.

DCs originate from bone marrow hematopoietic stem cells. (Traver et al., 2000; Wu et al., 2001) DC progenitors are not restricted to the BM and can be found in multiple locations. These progenitors can differentiate into DC upon challenge in peripheral tissues. Fully differentiated DC are found in healthy tissues as immunologically immature cells, being able to sample foreign antigens, but not able activate T cells. Although rare in numbers in the circulation, one fully mature DC is capable to interact with ten thousand T cells per day.(O'Keeffe et al., 2003) DC consist of several distinct populations that can be differentiated by surface and intracellular phenotypic markers, immunological function, and anatomic location. Irrespective of their phenotype and immunological role, DC exert their activity in the eye remote from their place of origin, where they utilize their advanced migratory skills for navigation. Currently, factors leading to the development from precursor DC to differentiated mature DC are still largely unknown. It has been shown that depending on the environmental cues, different forms of DC may be generated.(Naik et al., 2006) Further, while in lymphoid as well as in some non-lymphoid organs,(Kabashima et al., 2005; Merad et al., 2002) DC have been shown to proliferate locally, it is yet unclear whether resident corneal DC have the same proliferative potential, or are alternatively replenished through circulating DC. The diverse functions of DC in immune regulation depend on the diversity of DC subsets and lineages and on the functional plasticity of DCs at their immature stage.

Over the last several decades, the search for corneal APC, largely reliant on their presumed and universal MHC-II expression, had led to the dogma that APC are essentially absent in the central corneal. This absence of corneal APC was assumed to be a critical component of corneal immune privilege. However, this paradigm has now shifted with the demonstration of a diverse population of resident APC over the last years.(Hamrah et al., 2003a; Hamrah et al., 2003b, c) Dendritic cells, the sentinels of the immune system, were recently discovered to reside not only in the peripheral cornea, but also in the centreal cornea (**Fig 1**).(Hamrah et al., 2003c; Hamrah et al., 2002b; Liu et al., 2002) While a large number of DC are MHC class II+ in the periphery, a large population of MHC class II-*negative* immature/precursor DC are present both in the central epithelium and stroma.(Hamrah et al., 2003c; Hamrah et al., 2002b) Immature DC do neither express major histocompatibility complex (MHC)-II nor costimulatory molecules unless they are incited by cytokines. Thus, in contrast to other organs, where terminally differentiated populations of resident DC and/or macrophages outnumber colonizing precursors, large numbers of DCs within the cornea remain in an undifferentiated state.

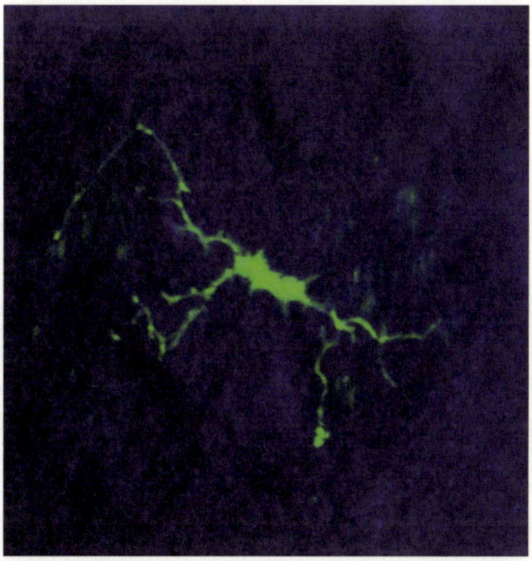

Fig. 1. Dendritic Cell in central corneal epithelium in CD11c-Yellow fluorescent protein (YFP) transgenic mouse

The constitutive presence of these DCs in the cornea focuses now attention on the cornea as a participant in immune and inflammatory responses, rather than the cornea being essentially a collagenous tissue that simply responds to the activity of infiltrating cells. Other immune cells that populate the cornea and ocular surface are T cells, B cells, macrophages, plasma cells, and neutrophils (PMN). Further, macrophages and neutrophils together with natural killer (NK) cells, initially constitute the primary innate immune response, while DCs, T cells and B cells largely play a role in the secondary, adaptive response.(Janeway C, 2004) While the primary innate immune response is non-specific, rapid, and lacks memory, the secondary adaptive immune response is slower, but highly specific. Further, T and B cell responses maintain immunological memory, such that any following encounters with the same antigen will lead to rapid and robust immune responses.

2.2 Microbial keratitis

2.2.1 Herpes simplex virus type-1 (HSV-1)

HSV-1, is a member of the α-herpesviridae family of double-stranded DNA (dsDNA) viruses.(Shukla & Spear, 2001) HSV-1 infections are prevalent both in the developed and developing countries with a higher and earlier onset of seroconversion in population groups of lower socioeconomic status.(Whitley & Roizman, 2001) 60% to 90% of the global adult population is infected with this pathogen, with a remarkably high prevalence of approximately 90% in the United States.(Carr et al., 2001; Whitley & Roizman, 2001) The two main forms of ocular HSV-1 infections are epithelial keratitis, and immune stromal keratitis.(Thomas, J. & Rouse, 1997) In the West, HSV-1 is also the leading cause of blindness secondary to recurrent infection, corneal stromal inflammation (herpes stromal keratitis; HSK), stromal thinning, neovascularisation and scarring.(Dana, M. R. et al., 2000)

The ocular surface, through several means, is able retard host invasion by external pathogens. The tear film which forms the outermost layer of the ocular surface presents the first barrier to viral invasion.(Farris, 1998) Some of the anti-viral factors in the tear film include, but are not limited to, tear film proteins such as lysozyme, immunoglobulin A (IgA), lactate dehydrogenase (LDH), complement proteins, amylase, peroxidase, as well as interferons alpha (IFNα) and beta (IFNβ). (Babu et al., 1995; Chatterjee et al., 1984; Chen et al., 1994) Since herpes viruses rely on replication and dissemination in metabolically active cells (Schang et al., 1998; Schang et al., 2000), the terminally differentiated outer layers of the corneal epithelium act as both a physical and metabolic barrier against viral entry. In the event of a breach in the integrity of the corneal epithelium, the virion attaches to epithelial cells via interaction of its surface glycoproteins with cognate receptors, (Campadelli-Fiume et al., 2007; Shukla et al., 1999; Spear, 2004) leading to either attachment, surfing and fusion of the virion envelope to the host cell plasma membrane, or, via endocytosis of the nucleocapsid into the host cell cytoplasm. Having intercepted the barriers to entry, HSV-1 inhibits its host's programmed cell death, assembles its immune-defying, host-crippling machinery to invade, replicate and infect the cornea, nerves and eventually the trigeminal ganglion where the virus maintains lifelong latency, leading to recurrent infections and potentially irreversible damage to the corneal tissue.(Akhtar & Shukla, 2009; Whitley & Roizman, 2001) Transmission may occur through cell lysis and shedding of viral progeny or cell-to-cell spread of the virion. Once the host corneal epithelial layers are penetrated, HSV replicates in the corneal epithelial cells. Following host infection, the outcome of viral latency or resolution has been shown to be dependent on the initial viral load.(Kintner & Brandt, 1995).

Cytokines are low molecular weight proteins produced by various resident corneal cells such as epithelial cells, stromal cells, and APCs.(Torres & Kijlstra, 2001) They are responsible for recruiting inflammatory and immune cells via cell-to-cell signalling through autocrine, paracrine and endocrine pathways, thus promoting tissue damage.(Balkwill & Burke, 1989) As the disease course changes, expression profiles of cytokines follow suit. During the early phase of HSK, the cornea expresses interleukin (IL)-1α, interferon (IFN)-γ and IL-2, whereas IL-4 is expressed later, indicating that the Th1 T cell response is required for induction of HSK. (Babu et al., 1995; Niemialtowski & Rouse, 1992b) (Heiligenhaus et al., 1999) While IL-2 may be responsible for incurring destructive effects on the stroma, IL-2 knockout mice are more prone to severe HSV infection, which is ameliorated by providing recombinant IL-2 treatment, hence indicating that the Th1 T cell response not only plays a role in tissue destruction, but also plays a protective role against HSV-1 invasion.(Ghiasi et al., 1999) Paradoxically, IFN-γ has also been implicated in the clearance of virus from the cells thus reducing latency, (Bouley et al., 1995; Smith et al., 1994) (Hendricks et al., 1991) yet driving immunopathogenesis as exemplified by the reduction in HSK severity following neutralisation of IFN-γ titres beforehand. (Hendricks et al., 1992b; Niemialtowski & Rouse, 1992a, b) Among the array of cytokines produced, IL-1 is particularly pertinent to corneal melting by induction of LC migration into the cornea thereby priming the tissue for further destruction. In order to combat the effects of IL-1, human corneal epithelium and stroma constitutively express interleukin-1 receptor antagonist (IL-1 RA), which helps maintain corneal immune privilege.(Dana, M. R. et al., 1998; Kennedy et al., 1995) Finally, while proinflammatory cytokines contribute to the augmentation of the immune response, vascular endothelial growth factor (VEGF) secreted by polymorphonuclear (PMN) cells, and local epithelial cells, contributes to corneal neovascularization in HSK.(Lee, S. et al., 2002; Zheng, M. et al., 2001)

Chemokines are specific, small cytokines of 8-10 kDa and can be classified according to their structure and function. Structurally, they fall into four families, the two most important of which are the CXC (alpha) and CC (beta) families. The CC and CXC chemokines are named based on intervening residues between their amino (N)-terminal cysteine amino acids. Hence, the CC family of chemokines have two adjacent cysteine amino acids near the N-terminus without an intervening residue. However, in the CXC family of chemokines, these N-terminal cysteine residues are separated by an amino acid "X", thus their "CXC" salutation. Chemokine receptors (CCR) CCR1, CCR2, CCR5, CXC chemokine receptor (CXCR) CXCR2 and their ligands (CCL/CXCL) have a well-defined role in HSV. Viral replication leads to expression of chemokines such as macrophage inflammatory protein (MIP)-1α/CCL3, KC/CXCL1, MIP-1β/CCL4, MIP-2/CXCL2, monocyte chemotactic protein (MCP)-1/CCL2 and lymphotactin/XCL1. (Thomas, J. et al., 1998) (Wolpe et al., 1989) Of these, MIP-1 α /CCL3 plays the most pivotal role in causing stromal inflammation, possibly by recruiting neutrophils and T cells as seen in experimental studies on murine corneas.(Tumpey et al., 1998; Wolpe et al., 1988) Furthermore, CXCR3 and its ligands, namely, monokine induced by gamma interferon (MIG)/CXCL9, interferon gamma-induced protein 10 (IP-10)/CXCL10 and interferon-inducible T-cell alpha chemoattractant (I-TAC)/ CXCL11 may also contribute to the development of a protective, anti-viral immune response seen in the cornea following HSV-1 infection. (Carr et al., 2008; Wuest & Carr, 2008) These chemokines may form potential targets for therapy in HSK.

It is well established that primary infection with HSV-1 incites both a localized innate immune response, and systemic immunity through the adaptive arm of the immune cascade. The localized innate immune response involves PMNs, natural killer (NK) cells, and macrophages, with the adaptive immune response involving DCs and T cells.(Brandt & Salkowski, 1992; Ghiasi et al., 2000; Hendricks & Tumpey, 1990; Meyers-Elliott & Chitjian, 1981; Niemialtowski & Rouse, 1992a; Pepose, 1991; Tullo et al., 1983; Tumpey et al., 1996) Clinically, the collection of these cells is seen as infiltrates in the corneal stroma. Within 48 hours following infection, PMN cells, which constitute the first line of defense, are recruited to the cornea by means of the limbus vasculature, following a multi-step adhesion cascade, including selectins, integrins, and chemokines.(Thomas, J. et al., 1997) A cytokine and chemokine response by recruited PMN cells, including tumor necrosis factor (TNF-α),(Daheshia et al., 1998) then quickly translates into recruitment of other cells to the site of infection. Additionally, toll-like receptors (TLRs) expressed on the corneal epithelium and stroma, recognise pathogens and their activation leads to generation of both an innate and acquired adaptive immune responses. Of particular note are TLRs 3, 4, 7, and 9 which mediate an anti-viral response to corneal epithelial infection with HSV-1 (Redfern & McDermott) Binding of the pathogen to TLRs causes release of cytokines and chemokines which provide alert signals to draw in inflammatory cells such as neutrophils and lymphocytes. TLR activation also induces resident corneal APCs to express MHC-II and costimulatory molecules thus engaging the acquired immune response.(Hamrah & Dana, 2007) The anti-viral immune response of TLR7 has been successfully tested in clinical trials treating HSV following the success of Imiquimod, an FDA-approved TLR7 agonist used in the treatment of infection with the human papilloma virus (HPV).(Miller, R. L. et al., 2008) Despite encouraging results of TLR agonist therapy for HSV, one must exercise caution in their use since excessive TLR stimulation can lead to an unfavourably strong immune response with much damage to bystander cells and tissues of the eye.

Langerhans cells have been found in abundance near the limbus and are recruited to the site of inflammation within a few days in the wake of HSV-1 infection.(Streilein et al., 1979) (Asbell & Kamenar, 1987; Hendricks et al., 1992a) There they process the viral antigens for presentation to naïve T-helper (Th0) cells in draining lymph nodes. These Th0 cells mature into Th1 or Th2 cells depending upon the type of cytokines, prostaglandins and costimulatory molecules released by LCs and cells of the innate immune system.(Torres & Kijlstra, 2001) The extent of stromal damage in HSK is affected by the density of LCs in the cornea.(Asbell & Kamenar, 1987; Hendricks et al., 1992a; Jager et al., 1991; Jager et al., 1992; Miller, J. K. et al., 1993) Virally-induced migration or maturation of LCs in the cornea precedes the development of HSK. Induction of LC migration into the central cornea before HSV-1 infection results in an accelerated and enhanced delayed type hypersensitivity (DTH) response to HSV-1 antigens, and an increased severity of HSK. On the contrary, depletion of DCs reduces the incidence and severity of HSK, suggesting a role for DCs in the induction of a T cell response. These findings have led to the conclusion that HSV-1 infection results in *de novo* migration of LCs from the limbus, which in turn might play a role in the immunopathology of HSK through presentation of antigens to T cells in the infected cornea. Thus, patients that have a higher density of corneal LCs are likely to get more severe forms of HSK, which highlights the role of LCs as a potential therapeutic target in HSK.

HSK has been studied extensively using mouse models of disease and $CD4^+$ T helper 1 (Th1) cells have been purported to be key mediators in the immunopathogenesis of corneal HSV-1 infection. (Hendricks, 1997; Streilein et al., 1997) In mice depleted of CD4+ cells, HSK development and progression was prevented or retarded, whereas depletion of CD8+ cells either made no difference or made the severity of HSK worse. (Newell et al., 1989a; Newell et al., 1989b) Corticosteroids, which are commonly prescribed in addition to antiviral therapy in HSK, work partially via inhibition of CD4+ T-cell response and are thus effective in controlling inflammatory damage to the eye. Among other local tissue factors, the kind of T-helper response generated is orchestrated by a fine balance between cytokines IL-12 and IFN-α, and IL-4 and IL-10, which mature Th0 cells into Th1 or Th2 respectively. (Torres &

Kijlstra, 2001) The predominant expression of cytokines IL-2 and IFN- α in HSK further corroborates the role of CD4+ Th1 immune response in HSK pathogenesis.(Hendricks et al., 1992b; Niemialtowski & Rouse, 1992b) The role of Th2 cells in HSK is far more controversial and inconclusive. While some groups state that Th2 cells have negligible involvement in HSK, (Niemialtowski & Rouse, 1992a, b) others either ascribe Th2 cells as inducers of HSK, (Foster et al., 1993; Jayaraman et al., 1993) or ascribe their role to convalescent phase of HSK.(Jayaraman et al., 1993) There is however one caveat; the kind of response generated is also driven by the strain of HSV-1. Corneal infections with the reticuloendotheliosis (RE) strain of HSV-1 are predominantly CD4+ driven, whereas the relatively less neuroinvasive (KOS) strain recruits and activates CD8+ T cells. (Hendricks & Tumpey, 1990; Newell et al., 1989a; Russell et al., 1984) T cell mediated delayed type hypersensitivity eventually is critical for the elimination of the virus. After this point circulating memory T and B lymphocytes continuously scan the cornea.

The suggested T-cell mediated immune response in HSK, is supported by the fact that specific HSV epitopes have been shown to mount an immune response by generation of autoreactive T cells. (Zhao et al., 1998) Murine studies of chronic HSK further demonstrated that despite clinical signs of active disease and lesions, 10-15 days post viral inoculation, viral antigens and messenger RNA (mRNA) were undetectable in the corneas of these mice.(Babu et al., 1996) Furthermore, Avery and colleagues performed elegant experiments, demonstrating that transfer of autoreactive $CD4^+$ T cells to into athymic mice infected with HSV-1, results in the development of HSK.(Avery et al., 1995) However, there is ongoing debate regarding the source of antigenic response elicited in HSK. Verjans et al. have shown that T cells harvested and cultured from HSK donor corneas failed to show reactivity against human corneal antigens.(Verjans et al., 2000) Moreover, human studies to date have been inconclusive and it has been hypothesised that a variable clinical spectrum of disease in patients with recurrent HSK may either be due to a heterogeneous immune response to the HSV epitopes, or, to heterogeneity in the expression of corneal autoantigens in the host.(Ellison et al., 2003)

Based on the ability of HSV-1 to circumvent the immune response and maintain latency, along with the complexity of immune players that orchestrate signalling cascades leading to a spectrum of disease seen clinically, it is challenging for clinicians to treat HSK effectively. Attempts towards immunomodulation of HSK have been made, ranging from induction of apoptosis in T cells by amniotic membrane transfer,(Bauer et al., 2009) to suppression of chemotaxis and activation of CD4+T cells by targeting chemokine receptors.(Komatsu et al., 2008; Lee, S. K. et al., 2008). However, with an evolving and deeper understanding of the molecular mediators of HSV-1 infection, new molecular targets may provide platforms for emerging therapies.

2.2.2 Pseudomonas keratitis

One of the most important organisms in the group of bacterial keratitides is the Gram-negative bacterium *Pseudomonas aeruginosa. P. aeruginosa* is an opportunistic pathogen, which like other microbes, requires a breach in the corneal surface for infection.(Hazlett et al., 1978) Such infections are typically seen in individuals who wear contact lenses for extended periods of time, and in nosocomial or tropical settings stemming from the ability of the bacterium to grow in any niche without much nutritional support.(Hazlett, 2004)

Pseudomonal keratitis is highly invasive and can lead to corneal perforation within 24-48 hours post-infection.(Jones, 1973) Pseudomonal infections of the cornea are marked by inflammation and necrosis; there is a suppurative stromal infiltrate, coagulative necrosis, epithelial edema, a mucopurulent exudate, and in some cases a paracentral corneal ring infiltrate that can be seen in addition to a hypopyon.(Hazlett, 2004) One of the main host factors that is the culprit for a stromal meltdown is the massive recruitment of neutrophils, which release lysosomal enzymes and oxidative compounds, digesting collagen of the stromal extracellular matrix. (Carubelli et al., 1990; Nicas & Iglewski, 1985; Trinkaus-Randall et al., 1991; Van Horn et al., 1978; Weiss, 1989) IL-6, one of the cytokines expressed within 24 hours of *P.aeruginosa* invasion, may be involved in recruitment of PMNs to the site of inflammation by upregulating the expression intercellular adhesion molecule-1 (ICAM-1), a key molecule involved in migration of neutrophils.(Cole et al., 1999; Youker et al., 1992) Integrin-mediated neutrophil migration is a critical phenomenon that occurs not only within the proteoglycan matrix, but also among stromal keratocytes which express adhesion molecules.(Burns et al., 2005)

The rapid spread of infection in the early stages of disease has been attributed in part to a delayed response from the responsible TLRs, TLR-2, -4 and -5, which are expressed at a later stage in the disease thus leading to a delay in activation of both the innate and adaptive arms of the immune response. (Jin et al.) Using a murine model of pseudomonal keratitis, Sun and colleagues demonstrated that *P.aeruginosa* activates expression of TLR-4/5 on resident corneal bone marrow-derived macrophages, inducing transcription of chemokines and cytokines such as KC/CXCL1, as well as IL-1α and IL-1β. Subsequent recruitment of neutrophils into the corneal stroma leads to destruction of *P.aeruginosa*. The produced IL-1 has a positive feedback effect by activating the IL-1 receptor in macrophages and other cells of the cornea, thus ensuring a sustained response against the bacteria.(Sun et al.) While a sustained immune response favours reducing bacterial load, it is also associated with bystander local tissue damage from dysregulation of cytokines and chemokines as seen by elevated expression of TNF- α , MIP-2/CXCL2, IL-1α but low levels of IL-10.(Zhou et al.) It is evident that the role of a prompt and efficient immune response is critical in curtailing the spread and severity of pseudomonal keratitis, and eventually in preventing loss of vision. However, the caveat to a robust immune response remains the collateral damage incurred to surrounding cells and tissues.

From a therapeutic standpoint, TLRs make interesting molecular targets. Particularly, TLR-9 is one of the first in its class to be expressed when the cornea is invaded by *P. aeruginosa*. Huang and colleagues used RNA interference (RNAi) to knockdown TLR-9 in mice which resulted in decreased corneal opacity, fewer corneal perforations, with decreases in PMNs, inductors of the Th1 pathway IFN-γ and IL-12, and mediators of chemotaxis IL-1 β and MIP-2/CXCL2, but higher bacterial titers than controls.(Huang et al., 2005) Further, when mice were either depleted of $CD4^+$ T cells or received IFN- γ neutralising antibodies prior to inoculation, they were spared corneal perforation and had a reduced DTH response, corroborating the role of a CD4+ T-cell mediated immunopathogenesis of this disease.(Kwon & Hazlett, 1997) Cytokines released by CD4+ T cell and LC result in infiltration of higher numbers of PMN, eventually leading to increased corneal.(Hazlett et al., 2001; Hazlett et al., 2002) While some propose that in order to minimise this collateral damage to ocular tissues, therapies should consider directing the immune response from

CD4+/Th1 mediated towards a Th2 pathway, (Kijlstra, 1994) others are of the opinion that it is the balance between pro-and anti-inflammatory mediators that is of greater significance in pseudomonal keratitis. (Hazlett, 2004) (O'Callaghan et al., 1996)

2.2.3 Fungal keratitis

Fungal keratitis is a vision-threatening infection and has seen a recent continual rise in incidence, with a spike during 2005-2006, following *Fusarium* contamination of a commercial contact lens solution. The three most common risk factors for fungal keratitis are contact lens use, trauma and penetrating keratoplasty. (Yildiz et al.) (Iyer et al., 2006) Filamentous fungi form the majority of causative organisms with *Fusarium* (41%), *Candida* (14%), *Aspergillus* (12%) and *Curvularia* (12%) being among the top contenders.(Iyer et al., 2006; Jurkunas et al., 2009) Fungal infections of the cornea, if not treated immediately and managed appropriately, can rapidly lead to corneal ulceration, perforation, corneal neovascularisation, loss of vision and possibly, loss of the eye. (Yuan & Wilhelmus, 2009) (Thomas, P. A. & Geraldine, 2007) It is thus imperative to understand the molecular underpinnings of fungal keratitis, especially the involvement of immune players, for a more thorough understanding towards devising novel and efficacious treatment modalities.

Contact lens wear can compromise the integrity of the corneal epithelium, making it susceptible to fungal invasion. It is known that contact lens wear can induce a subclinical host immune response with recruitment of LCs into the cornea. (Sankaridurg et al., 2000) TLRs on APCs, such as LCs or macrophages, recognize fungi, thereby activating the innate and adaptive immune response to clear the infection.(Barton & Medzhitov, 2003; Johnson et al., 2005) Hu et al. demonstrated the importance of macrophages through depletion of these cells, showing the contribution of macrophages in two different fungal infection models 5 and 7 days following infection. In this study development of more severe keratomycosis in mice depleted of macrophages points the contribution of macrophages in limiting fungal disease. (Hu et al., 2009) *In vitro* studies have shown that inactivated hyphae of *Fusarium solani* upregulate gene expression of TLRs-2, 3, 4 and 6, along with protein expression of TLRs 2 and 4 with resultant increases in cytokine expression of IL-6 and IL-8. The importance of TLR-4 in modulating the host defense mechanisms to fungi, especially *Fusarium* keratitis, has been demonstrated by several groups. In an experimental model of infectious keratitis, it was observed that resolution of *Fusarium* keratitis involved activation of both the innate immune response along with the adaptive arm through TLR-4.(Sun et al.) In another murine study, inoculation in knockout models of TLR-4, lead to impaired host anti-fungal defense mechanisms, decreased production of CXCL1 with subsequent decreased recruitment of neutrophils into the cornea, as well as uncontrolled fungal growth and eventually corneal perforation (Tarabishy et al., 2008) On the contrary, hydrocortisone treatment *in vitro* leads to a TLR-mediated increase in resistance to *Fusarium solani* with a concomitant increase in IL-6 expression by human corneal endothelial cells (HCEC).(Jin et al., 2007)

Similarly, in humans, fungal keratitis secondary to *Aspergillus* and *Candida* species also rely on human corneal TLRs 2 and 4 for hosting an immune response.(Mambula et al., 2002; Netea et al., 2002; Netea et al., 2003) TLRs 2 and 4 recognise fungal zymosan and mannan, leading to an expected increase in the production of IL-6 and IL-1β when challenged with *Aspergillus*, which is diminished by knocking down these innate receptors, confirming the putative role of TLRs 2 and 4 in Aspergillus keratitis.(Guo & Wu, 2009) In a recent study from the same group investigated the effect of targeting TLR2 by a small interfering RNA (siRNA) construct applied subconjunctively and topically to the cornea, showed that suppressing TLR2 expression in the cornea results in a decrease in neutrophil infiltration, allowing the cornea to preserve its morphological integrity. Suppressing TLR2 expression also caused a decrease in TNF-α, IL-1β, IL-6, IL-12, monocyte chemoattractant protein (MCP-1)/CCL2 and macrophage inflammatory protein (MIP-2)/CXCL2 expression. Immunomodulation by targeting TLR2 might be a treatment approach in fungal keratitis to avoid damage to the cornea by an immune response.(Guo et al.) *Aspergillus fumigatus* also induces IL-10 expression, and taken together, these cytokines attract and direct PMNs into the cornea, inciting innate immunity.(Redfern & McDermott) Thus, in addition to anti-fungal therapy, modulating fungus-specific TLR responses and controlling the host's immune response to the patient's advantage, is an exciting avenue to explore in the field of molecular anti-fungal therapy towards quicker resolution of infection with minimal residual damage.

2.2.4 *Acanthamoeba* keratitis

Acanthamoeba keratitis (AK) is a resilient, vision-threatening infection of the cornea. *Acanthamoeba* is an ubiquitous protozoa, which is exceptionally difficult to treat. Infection with *Acanthamoeba* either resolves spontaneously, or, as often seen, results in progressive infection and eventual corneal melting, suggesting a role of the immune system in its pathophysiology. Corneal transplantation is indicated in cases of severe infection, however, reinfection can commonly occur due to the presence of *Acanthamoeba* cysts within the host graft bed. Reinfection and recrudescence indicates the absence of memory against this parasite, and hence a poor activation of the adaptive arm of the immune response. *Acanthamoeba species* exist freely in the environment and on certain mucosal surfaces of healthy individuals.(Alizadeh et al. 1996; Niederkorn et al. 1999) Two of the most critical risk factors for AK include contact lens use and corneal trauma.(Niederkorn et al. 1999) Trophozoites attach to the surface of the contact lens which are then introduced to the ocular surface. Integrity of the host immune machinery predicts the severity of infection and incidence of disease as patients with AK have lower tear levels of IgA against *Acanthamoeba* antigens as compared to healthy controls, implicating the role of mucosa-mediated immunity in AK. (Alizadeh et al. 2001) The unique resilience of the double-layered cellulose wall of *Acanthamoeba* cysts, which are resistant to extreme temperatures, UV and gamma irradiation, underlies the challenges of treating AK. Systemic immunization to *Acanthamoeba* antigens does not confer immunity unlike mucosa-induced immunity.

Once the trophozoites invade the corneal epithelium through dislodgement of the epithelial cells caused by contact-lens induced microabrasions, there is a TLR-4-mediated immune response in corneal epithelial cells with release of cytokines IL-8 and TNF-α as shown in rats (Ren and Wu 2011). The innate immune response is activated with recruitment of neutrophils and macrophages. Macrophages are believed to be pivotal to the resolution of AK. They have a chemotactic response to the pathogen, and bear an inherent ability to kill the trophozoites *in vivo*. This phenomenon can be demonstrated by the depletion of macrophages in Clodronate treated animals which develop severe, chronic AK. (Stewart et al. 1992; van Klink et al. 1996) Although cysts are more difficult to eradicate, macrophages forming the first line of defence in AK may also attack *Acanthamoeba* cysts by direct phagocytosis as seen *in vitro* (Hurt et al. 2003). Like macrophages, neutrophils also form the first-line defence against both *Acanthamoeba* cysts and trophozoites, but demonstrate a more robust and efficient response. They are found in large numbers in corneas with AK, where they clear the protozoan using myeloperoxidase-dependent killing. Neutrophils are important both in the prevention and resolution of AK.(Hurt et al. 2003; Clarke et al. 2005).

The most convincing and potent response from the adaptive arm of the immune system is the secretion of IgA antibody. IgA antibody promotes neutrophil-mediated killing of trophozoites hence preventing adhesion of the trophozoites to the corneal epithelium. Furthermore, it shuts down the corneal melt-down plant of the trophozoites by inhibiting mannose-induced cytopathic protein 133 (MIP-133)-induced digestion of the corneal epithelium and stroma. The role of corticosteroids in the treatment of AK remains controversial. This issue arises from the contrary effects of dexamethasone on the eye; on the one hand they help in the resolution of AK-associated ocular inflammation, but on the other hand, they induce excystment of dormant cysts leading to recrudescence. Thus, targeting MIP-133 offers an attractive target in the therapy of AK. Earlier detection of disease by visualization of cysts in the cornea using *in vivo* confocal microscopy (IVCM) may offer an advantage in the management of AK.(Kumar et al. 2010) Through a more sensitive approach in the detection and consequent treatment of AK, the prognosis may be improved leading to fewer cases of corneal melting and associated complications.

2.3 Corneal transplantation

Corneal transplantation is the most common form of solid tissue transplantation with approximately 45,000 cases being performed annually in the United States alone.(CCTS, 1992; Niederkorn, 1999; Streilein, 1999) Unlike other solid tissue transplants, corneal allotransplants enjoy immune privilege, and neither require standard human leukocyte antigen (HLA) matching, nor permanent systemic immunosuppression. First time recipients of corneal allografts enjoy a 2-year graft survival rate of greater than 90% if the recipient corneal bed is avascular and free of inflammation.(Niederkorn, 1990) Corneal immune privilege is attributed to: (a) an avascular corneal bed which prevents recruitment of immune cells and leukocytes to the graft site, thus preventing recognition of non-self HLA antigens; (b) lack of lymphatic vessels, which eliminates transport and presentation of non-self HLA antigens and egress of APCs to T cells in draining lymph nodes, thus decreasing sensitisation (c) paucity of mature $MHC\text{-}II^+/HLA\text{-}DR^+$ resident corneal dendritic cells, including LC, thus decreasing direct presentation of unmatched HLA antigens to T cells; (d) constitutive expression of Fas ligand (CD95; FasL), which programs cell death of activated Fas^+ T cells; (e) local ocular production of immunomodulatory neuropeptides and factors in aqueous humour such as transforming growth factor beta (TGF)-β_2 and alpha-melanocyte stimulating hormone (α -MSH), which inhibits alloantigen-driven T cell activation and DTH.(Dana, M. R. et al., 2000; Dua & Azuara-Blanco, 1999; Griffith et al., 1995; Jager et al., 1995; Niederkorn, 1990; Niederkorn et al., 1989; Streilein, 1993, 1995; Stuart et al., 1997; Thiel et al., 2009)

Neovascularization of the corneal graft greatly increases the rate of rejection.(Alldredge & Krachmer, 1981; Maguire et al., 1994) As per guidelines of the Collaborative Corneal Transplantation Studies, the recipient cornea is considered "high-risk" if there is stromal vascularisation in two or more quadrants preoperatively.(1992) The other factors which lead to graft rejection include growth of lymphatic vessels into the cornea, thereby establishing drainage to the cervical lymph nodes;(Hamrah et al., 2002a) migration of LCs into the cornea; maturation of resident LCs and DCs of the cornea, which can then serve as APCs;(Dekaris et al., 1999; Hamrah & Dana, 2007; Hamrah et al., 2002b; Liu et al., 2002) increased expression of cytokines IL-1 and TNF- α , which lead to recruitment of neutrophils, suppression of anterior chamber-associated immune deviation (ACAID), maturation of corneal APCs, upregulation of vascular adhesion molecules, and recruitment of leukocytes.(Dana, M. R. & Streilein, 1996; Dana, R., 2007; Hamrah et al., 2007; Pepose et al., 1985; Streilein et al., 1996; Yamagami et al., 1999; Zhu, S. et al., 1999; Zhu, S. N. & Dana, 1999)

The process of corneal transplant rejection includes an induction phase, called the "afferent" arm, and an expression phase, called the "efferent" arm. In the afferent arm, the host becomes sensitized to the donor antigens by APCs (e.g., MHC class II-positive DC, LC, macrophages, etc.) that present antigens to T cells in draining lymph nodes. This sensitization process involves two different pathways. The *direct* pathway, which involves *donor* APCs that sensitize the host *directly* when T cells recognize the donor class II MHC, thus generating direct alloreactive T cells, and the *indirect* pathway, which involves *host* APCs that migrate to the graft, take up donor antigens, process it, migrate to draining lymph nodes, and then present their antigens to T cells. Host sensitization to donor antigens of corneal grafts occurs through both pathways of sensitization, especially in high-risk corneal grafting. Further, the critical role of draining cervical lymph nodes in the process of allosensitization has been clearly demonstrated by recent studies. Upon arrival in the lymph nodes, APCs upregulate surface expression of co-stimulatory molecules, secrete cytokines, leading to activation of T cells. The subsequent efferent phase is then responsible for the actual rejection of the graft. This phase consists of the proliferation of alloreactive T cells in lymphoid organs, migration of these cells to the cornea, and the development of "memory" that can assist the alloimmune response in case of repeated exposure to the same antigens. Both $CD8^+$ cytotoxic T lymphocyte (CTL) and $CD4^+$ T helper (Th) cells have been implicated in the rejection process. Th1 cells uniquely secrete IL-2, IFN-γ, and lymphotoxin, and have the purpose of eradicating offending pathogens by promoting inflammation. Th2 cells secrete IL-4 and IL-10, suppress Th1 cells, and promote B cell differentiation, leading to the production of antibodies. $CD4^+$ Th1 cells are the primary mediators of the efferent arm and act directly as effector cells and not as helper cells in corneal graft rejection. IL-2, secreted by these cells, stimulates the activation and proliferation of other T and B cells, whereas IFN-γ activates macrophages and induces expression of class II antigens in the donor tissue. The role of $CD8^+$ T cells in the rejection of allogeneic corneal grafts remains controversial. While $CD8^+$ T cells can contribute to graft rejection, corneal grafts can still be rejected in their absence, hence making $CD8^+$ T cells sufficient but not necessary for graft rejection.

A major factor directing the recruitment of T cells and other leukocytes into grafts are chemokines. Surgical trauma induces release of early cytokines such as TNF-α and IL-1 by corneal epithelial cells. These cytokines in turn stimulate the production of early neutrophil- and macrophage-attractant chemokines, including MIP-2/CXCL2, MCP-1/CCL2, regulated upon activation normal T-cell expressed and secreted protein (RANTES)/CCL5, MIP-1α/CCL3, MIP-1β/CCL4 and eotaxin/CCL11, especially after high-risk corneal transplantation.(Flynn et al., 2008; Yamagami et al., 2005; Yamagami et al., 2000; Yamagami et al., 1999) While early chemokines direct non-antigen-specific leukocytes to the graft, late chemokines as stated above produced by the graft and infiltrating leukocytes recruit alloantigen-primed T cells into the graft. In addition, recipients of high-risk transplants express very high levels of the IP-10/CXCL10 chemokine. Chemokines function together with other molecular mediators including integrins and adhesion molecules to direct the immune response toward the graft. Therapeutic endeavours seek to inhibit either or both arms of the immune response to prolong graft survival. Regulatory T cells ($Foxp3^{+}T_{regs}$) have been shown to promote graft survival by inhibiting alloimmunity in draining lymph nodes as opposed to altering to the effector arm of the immune response.(Chauhan et al., 2009; Cunnusamy et al.; Tang & Bluestone, 2008) Measures devised to enhance graft survival should essentially revolve around three main goals: (a) to prevent induction of alloimmune response, (b) to inhibit or deplete immune effector cells, and, (c) to induce tolerance to specific alloantigens.(Niederkorn, 2002)

2.4 Dry Eye Disease

Dry eye disease (DED) is one of the most common diagnoses made in ophthalmic practice. DED affects millions of people around the world. It is more prevalent in women than men and is of inflammatory etiology.(Calonge et al.; 2007b) In epidemiologic studies conducted by Schaumberg and colleagues, they found a prevalence of 5.7% in women aged 50 years or younger, and 9.8% in women aged 75 years or above.(Schaumberg et al., 2003) Patients usually present with ocular irritation and in severe cases, there may be accompanying ocular pain, punctate keratopathy and filamentary keratitis.(Pflugfelder, 1998) The definition of DED has been modified over the years to integrate evolving concepts of the involvement of tear film hyperosmolarity, inflammation of the ocular surface, and the effects of DED on vision. In 2007, the International Dry Eye Workshop (DEWS) defined DED as: "a multifactorial disease of the tears and ocular surface that results in symptoms of discomfort, visual disturbance, and tear film instability with potential damage to the ocular surface. It is accompanied by increased osmolarity of the tear film and inflammation of the ocular surface."(DEWS, 2007a)

Clinically, DED can be categorised into (a) aqueous deficient and, (b) evaporative dry eye. (Lemp, 1995) Aqueous deficient DED consists of disorders that affect the lacrimal functional unit (LFU). The term "lacrimal functional unit" was coined in 1998 by Stern and group, comprising the ocular surface, lacrimal glands, associated innervation, and neuroendocrine factors.(Stern et al., 1998; Stern et al., 2004) The clinical diagnosis of DED is made using a combination of examination techniques, including Schirmer's test, tear film osmolarity, and fluorescein tear break-up time (fTBUT). A reading of less than 15mm on the Schirmer's strip in conjunction with elevated tear film osmolarity (>315 mOsm) is indicative of decreased tear production, hence, suggestive of aqueous-deficient DED. When fTBUT is less than 10 seconds, there is increased suspicion of evaporative DED. Diseases that lead to aqueous deficient dry eye disease include Sjögren's syndrome and non-Sjögren's autoimmune conditions. Whereas, evaporative dry eye is due to diseases that affect the production, quality and distribution of the tear film lipid layer, namely, meibomian gland dysfunction (MGD) and chronic blepharitis.(Barabino & Dana, 2007; Calonge et al.) It has been demonstrated that regardless of the etiology of dry eye, inflammation of the ocular surface and homing of immune cells to the target tissue, are hallmarks of DED. These immuno-inflammatory processes are culprits of corneal and conjunctival damage leading to the presenting symptoms.(Barabino & Dana, 2007; Dana, M. R. & Hamrah, 2002)

Recent evidence suggests a role for chemokines in the pathogenesis of dry eye syndromes. Increased RNA levels of IL-8, which is chemotactic for neutrophils, are found in the conjunctival epithelium of Sjogren's syndrome patients compared to controls. Furthermore, increased levels of select chemokines in the lacrimal glands of nonobese diabetic (NOD) mice, an animal model of Sjogren's syndrome, have been detected. NOD mice are a murine model for type-1 insulin-dependent diabetes with an autoimmune component. They represent a murine model of Sjogren's syndrome based on the similar histopathological picture of sialoadenitis. These mice have lymphocytic infiltration of not just the pancreas but also the submandibular and lacrimal glands. Both RANTES/CCL5 and IP-10/CXCL10 gene transcripts are detected in lacrimal glands at 8 weeks of age increased markedly during the course of active disease, concomitant with induction of their receptors CCR1, CCR5 and CXCR3. The examination of lacrimal glands indicated that lymphocytes in the inflammatory infiltrates are responsible for the production of these chemokines. Moreover, anti-RANTES treatment significantly reduced inflammation in the lacrimal glands of these mice. Further, patients with DED have a significant increase in the number of ocular surface cells that express CCR5, the receptor for RANTES/CCL5 and MIP-1β/CCL4. These data suggest that a better understanding of the role of chemokines and chemokine receptors in DES could open new doors for development of molecular strategies for immune modulation in this common disorder.

Numerous studies have demonstrated the enhanced expression of pro-inflammatory cytokines (e.g., IL-1, IL-6, IL-8, TNF-α) mRNA and protein by the ocular surface epithelium or tear film. The increase of these proinflammatory cytokines can lead to epithelial cell proliferation, keratinization, and angiogenesis, and thereby could link ocular surface disease with a number of lid margin disorders, such as rosacea, characterized by inflammation. In addition, IL-1 may lead to upregulation of matrix proteases, including collagenases, and thereby exacerbate stromal pathology as well as alter the paracrine effect of other cytokines on resident DCs, macrophages, fibroblasts, and epithelial cells by altering the matrix milieu in which these cytokines bind their respective receptors. Corneal epithelial cells respond to stress signals by producing cytokine mediators of inflammation such as TNF- α , IL-1β, IL- 8 and MMPs.(Li et al., 2006; Luo et al., 2004) Subsequently, maturing resident and recruited DC carry antigen to the draining lymph nodes to present and activate T cells. T cell-mediated responses have recently been shown to play a center stage in DED. Th1 cells recognize antigenic peptides in association with MHC class II molecules on the surface of APC, and release pro-inflammatory cytokines that increase vascular permeability and recruit further inflammatory cells to the site of injury. Due to the nonspecific nature of cell recruitment employed by CD4+ Th1 cells, inflammation can be severe with damage to bystander tissue. More recently, Th 17 associated cytokines and IL 17 producing cells have been found in the ocular surface epithelium of dry eye patients and it has been hypothesized that epithelial cells subjected to desiccating conditions promote DC to secrete IL-6, IL-23 and TGF-β, which in turn induce Th17 cells.(Zheng, X. et al.)

3. Leukocyte trafficking

Trafficking signals finely control the movement of distinct subsets of immune cells into and out of specific tissues. Leukocyte extravasation from blood to tissue, including that of APC and T cells, usually occurs through a multistep process, involving adhesion molecules and chemokines. Because the accumulation of leukocytes in tissues contributes to a wide variety of diseases, these 'molecular codes' provide new targets for inhibiting tissue-specific inflammation. However, immune cell migration is also critically important for the delivery of protective immune responses to tissues. Therefore, the challenge lies in identifying trafficking molecules that will specifically inhibit key cell subsets that drive disease processes without affecting the migration of leukocytes required for protective immunity.

Adhesion molecules can be categorized according to their structure or function. Four major families are distinguished structurally: the selectins, the sialomucins, the integrins, and the Ig superfamily. Leukocyte tethering and rolling, mediated typically by three selectins, L-selectin, E-selectin and P-selectin, are the first steps in the process of leukocyte binding to vascular endothelium. Two selectins, P- and E-selectin, are expressed on activated endothelium, whereas L-selectin is found on leukocytes. L-selectin is involved in the homing of T cells to lymphoid tissues but is also expressed on other leukocytes, where it participates in inflammation. E-selectin is expressed on corneal vascular endothelium, whereas P-selectin is expressed on inflamed vascular endothelium and by certain leukocytes. P-selectin glycoprotein ligand-1 (PSGL-1) binds all three selectins and is expressed on peripheral blood DC.

In the cornea, studies in both human and animal models of disease have confirmed that cell adhesion molecules are closely associated with the development of herpetic keratitis, and corneal allograft rejection. P- and E-selectin have been shown to mediate neutrophil recruitment to the cornea in studies using P/E-selectin knockout mice. Integrins are found on most cell types. Two subfamilies are most important for leukocyte migration: the α4 (CD49) and the β2 (CD11/CD18) integrins. Four distinct members of β2 integrins exist, three of which are expressed by DC. Vascular endothelial ligands for these molecules are members of the immunoglobulin superfamily. Leukocyte arrest in venules requires *in situ* activation of at least one of the four main integrins: VLA-4 (binds to VCAM-1), α4β7 (binds to MadCAM-1), Mac-1(binds to ICAM-1) and LFA-1 (binds to ICAM-1 and 2). VCAM-1 has been shown to be present on monocytes and vascular endothelial cells during corneal inflammation. Arguably the most important ligand for β2 integrins is ICAM-1, which is expressed on many cell types and is strongly upregulated upon exposure to inflammatory cytokines in the cornea and on limbal endothelial cells, deletion of which has been shown to suppress corneal graft rejection.

Chemokine receptors regulate leukocyte retention within tissues. The migration of leukocytes to inflammatory sites depends on a cascade of discrete events mediated, in part, by chemokines and their receptors. Numerous chemokines have now been described during inflammation, including CCL3/MIP-1α, CCL4/MIP-1β, and CCL5/RANTES, ligands for CCR1 and CCR5; CCL2/MCP-1, a ligand for CCR2; CCL22/MDC and CCL17/TARC, ligands for CCR4; CCL20/MIP-3α, the ligand for CCR6; CXCL8/IL-8, a ligand for CXCR1 and CXCR2; CXCL1/KC, CXCL2/MIP-2, and CXCL5/ENA-78, ligands for CXCR2; CXCL9 /MIG, CXCL10/IP10 and CXCL11/ITAC, ligands for CXCR3. In addition, constitutively expression of CCLs 2-5,CXCL10, and CCL27/CTACK, a ligand for CCR10 have been described in the normal cornea. Which of these chemokines is relevant in recruitment, retention and egrees of corneal APC, is unclear. Little is known about the constitutive recruitment of DC and macrophage precursors into peripheral tissues in the absence of inflammation. APC function and migratory behavior are related to rapid and coordinated *switching* in chemokine receptor expression by these cells, allowing them to coordinate migratory routes and biological function. During inflammation, CCL2, CCL5, and CXCL8 are produced to attract immature DC that express CXCR4 and CCR4 respectively. In addition, these DC are ideally suited for recruitment to inflammatory sites by their expression of functional receptors for inflammation-induced chemokines, such as CCR1, CCR2, CCR3, CCR5 and CXCR1.

Inflammatory signals induce resident corneal DCs to undergo maturation. Upon maturation, DCs downregulate pattern recognition receptors necessary for surveillance of antigens and upregulate CCR7, a receptor important in the homing of DCs to the lymph nodes. Maturing CCR7+ DCs then enter CCL21-expressing lymphatic vessels and travel to the draining lymph nodes where CCR7 ligands, namely, CCL19/EBI1 ligand chemokine (ELC) and CCL21/secondary lymphoid tissue chemokine (SLC), are produced. In addition, after fluorescein isothiocyanate (FITC) painting (dendritic cell migration assay), CXCR4 inhibition has been shown to impair LC and dermal DC migration to draining LNs, indicating that both CCR7 and CXCR4 make independent contributions to the egress of DCs from resident tissue to the lymph nodes. DC migration into and along afferent lymphatics occurs through a series of steps, including (1) mobilization, (2) detachment, (3) interstitial migration, (4) entry into the afferent lymphatics, and (5) transit via lymph. Recent data have shown that lymphatic endothelial cells upregulate E-selectin, chemokines (CCL5, CCL20, and CXCL5), and adhesion molecules (ICAM-1 and VCAM-1) after cytokine stimulation *in vitro* or *in vivo*. Once in the draining lymph nodes, antigen-loaded mature DCs activate naive T cells, which then proliferate and enter the blood and migrate back to the site of inflammation. In the cornea, CCR5 and CX3CR1, but not CCR1 are partially involved in the recruitment of MHC-II$^+$ LCs. How the central immature LC or stromal APC populations are recruited is not known, although the recently demonstrated constitutive expression of CCR2 on stromal BM-derived cell subsets, implicates a role for this chemokine. Further, both vascular endothelial growth factor (VEGFR)-3 and CCR7 are partially implicated in the egress of stromal DCs. APC recruitment to the cornea is likely complex, highly regulated and dependent on recruitment signals that are either tissue-specific or inflammation-induced, or both.

4. Conclusion

The cornea and ocular surface are constantly exposed to environmental pollutants and irritants, microbes, and other potentially noxious agents. Since from an evolutionary standpoint the scope of the host defense mechanisms against these stimuli should be narrow, that is to say adequately effective to protect the eye against the potential harm from these agents and yet tempered enough not to lead to unwanted damage, the eye has developed many mechanisms to effect and regulate its response to environmental challenges. Identification of the critical pathways of cell migration to and from the cornea will provide new molecular targets for pharmacological intervention in inflammatory, infectious, alloimmune and autoimmune diseases and may lead to novel highly specific strategies for immunotherapy, through modulation of APC and T cell migration and function. Few effective anti-inflammatory drugs have emerged over the last decades in the ophthalmic field and an urgent need for new drugs exists, as many inflammatory diseases are inadequately responsive to current medications.

5. References

Akhtar, J. & Shukla, D. (2009). Viral entry mechanisms: cellular and viral mediators of herpes simplex virus entry. *FEBS J.* 276: 7228-7236.

Alizadeh, H., Niederkorn, J.Y., McCulley, J.P., in: Pepose, J.S., Holland, G.N., Wilhelmus, K.R. (Eds.), Ocular Infection and Immunity, Mosby, St. Louis, 1996, pp. 1062e1071.

Alizadeh H, Apte S, El-Agha MS, Li, L. Hurt, M. Howard, K. Cavanagh, H. D. McCulley, J. P. Niederkorn, J.Y. (2001) Tear IgA and serum IgG antibodies against Acanthamoeba in patients with Acanthamoeba keratitis. *Cornea.* 20:622-627.

Alldredge, O.C. & Krachmer, J.H. (1981). Clinical types of corneal transplant rejection. Their manifestations, frequency, preoperative correlates, and treatment. *Arch Ophthalmol.* 99: 599-604.

Asbell, P.A. & Kamenar, T. (1987). The response of Langerhans cells in the cornea to herpetic keratitis. *Curr Eye Res.* 6: 179-182.

Avery, A.C., Zhao, Z.S., Rodriguez, A., Bikoff, E.K., Soheilian, M., Foster, C.S., & Cantor, H. (1995). Resistance to herpes stromal keratitis conferred by an IgG2a-derived peptide. *Nature.* 376: 431-434.

Babu, J.S., Kanangat, S., & Rouse, B.T. (1995). T cell cytokine mRNA expression during the course of the immunopathologic ocular disease herpetic stromal keratitis. *J Immunol.* 154: 4822-4829.

Babu, J.S., Thomas, J., Kanangat, S., Morrison, L.A., Knipe, D.M., & Rouse, B.T. (1996). Viral replication is required for induction of ocular immunopathology by herpes simplex virus. *J Virol.* 70: 101-107.

Balkwill, F.R. & Burke, F. (1989). The cytokine network. *Immunol Today.* 10: 299-304.

Barabino, S. & Dana, M.R. (2007). Dry eye syndromes. *Chem Immunol Allergy.* 92: 176-184.

Barton, G.M. & Medzhitov, R. (2003). Toll-like receptor signaling pathways. *Science.* 300: 1524-1525.

Bauer, D., Wasmuth, S., Hennig, M., Baehler, H., Steuhl, K.P., & Heiligenhaus, A. (2009). Amniotic membrane transplantation induces apoptosis in T lymphocytes in murine corneas with experimental herpetic stromal keratitis. *Invest Ophthalmol Vis Sci.* 50: 3188-3198.

Bouley, D.M., Kanangat, S., Wire, W., & Rouse, B.T. (1995). Characterization of herpes simplex virus type-1 infection and herpetic stromal keratitis development in IFN-gamma knockout mice. *J Immunol.* 155: 3964-3971.

Brandt, C.R. & Salkowski, C.A. (1992). Activation of NK cells in mice following corneal infection with herpes simplex virus type-1. *Invest Ophthalmol Vis Sci.* 33: 113-120.

Burns, A.R., Li, Z., & Smith, C.W. (2005). Neutrophil migration in the wounded cornea: the role of the keratocyte. *Ocul Surf.* 3: S173-176.

Calonge, M., Enriquez-de-Salamanca, A., Diebold, Y., Gonzalez-Garcia, M.J., Reinoso, R., Herreras, J.M., & Corell, A. (2010). Dry eye disease as an inflammatory disorder. *Ocul Immunol Inflamm.* 18: 244-253.

Campadelli-Fiume, G., Amasio, M., Avitabile, E., Cerretani, A., Forghieri, C., Gianni, T., & Menotti, L. (2007). The multipartite system that mediates entry of herpes simplex virus into the cell. *Rev Med Virol.* 17: 313-326.

Carr, D.J., Harle, P., & Gebhardt, B.M. (2001). The immune response to ocular herpes simplex virus type 1 infection. *Exp Biol Med (Maywood).* 226: 353-366.

Carr, D.J., Wuest, T., & Ash, J. (2008). An increase in herpes simplex virus type 1 in the anterior segment of the eye is linked to a deficiency in NK cell infiltration in mice deficient in CXCR3. *J Interferon Cytokine Res.* 28: 245-251.

Carubelli, R., Nordquist, R.E., & Rowsey, J.J. (1990). Role of active oxygen species in corneal ulceration. Effect of hydrogen peroxide generated in situ. *Cornea.* 9: 161-169.

Chatterjee, S., Lakeman, A.D., Whitley, R.J., & Hunter, E. (1984). Effect of cloned human interferons on the replication of and cell fusion induced by herpes simplex virus. *Virus Res.* 1: 81-87.

Chauhan, S.K., Saban, D.R., Lee, H.K., & Dana, R. (2009). Levels of Foxp3 in regulatory T cells reflect their functional status in transplantation. *J Immunol.* 182: 148-153.

Chen, S.H., Oakes, J.E., & Lausch, R.N. (1994). Synergistic anti-herpes effect of TNF-alpha and IFN-gamma in human corneal epithelial cells compared with that in corneal fibroblasts. *Antiviral Res.* 25: 201-213.

Clarke DW, Alizadeh H, Niederkorn, J.Y. (2005). Failure of Acanthamoeba castellanii to produce intraocular infections. *Invest Ophthalmol Vis Sci.* 46:2472-2478.

Cole, N., Bao, S., Willcox, M., & Husband, A.J. (1999). Expression of interleukin-6 in the cornea in response to infection with different strains of Pseudomonas aeruginosa. *Infect Immun.* 67: 2497-2502.

Cunnusamy, K., Chen, P.W., & Niederkorn, J.Y. (2011). IL-17A-Dependent CD4+CD25+ Regulatory T Cells Promote Immune Privilege of Corneal Allografts. *J Immunol.* 186: 6737-6745.

Daheshia, M., Kanangat, S., & Rouse, B.T. (1998). Production of key molecules by ocular neutrophils early after herpetic infection of the cornea. *Exp Eye Res.* 67: 619-624.

Dana, M.R., Dai, R., Zhu, S., Yamada, J., & Streilein, J.W. (1998). Interleukin-1 receptor antagonist suppresses Langerhans cell activity and promotes ocular immune privilege. *Invest Ophthalmol Vis Sci.* 39: 70-77.

Dana, M.R. & Hamrah, P. (2002). Role of immunity and inflammation in corneal and ocular surface disease associated with dry eye. *Adv Exp Med Biol.* 506: 729-738.

Dana, M.R., Qian, Y., & Hamrah, P. (2000). Twenty-five-year panorama of corneal immunology: emerging concepts in the immunopathogenesis of microbial keratitis, peripheral ulcerative keratitis, and corneal transplant rejection. *Cornea.* 19: 625-643.

Dana, M.R. & Streilein, J.W. (1996). Loss and restoration of immune privilege in eyes with corneal neovascularization. *Invest Ophthalmol Vis Sci.* 37: 2485-2494.

Dana, R. (2007). Comparison of topical interleukin-1 vs tumor necrosis factor-alpha blockade with corticosteroid therapy on murine corneal inflammation, neovascularization, and transplant survival (an American Ophthalmological Society thesis). *Trans Am Ophthalmol Soc.* 105: 330-343.

Dekaris, I., Zhu, S.N., & Dana, M.R. (1999). TNF-alpha regulates corneal Langerhans cell migration. *J Immunol.* 162: 4235-4239.

Dua, H.S. & Azuara-Blanco, A. (1999). Corneal allograft rejection: risk factors, diagnosis, prevention, and treatment. *Indian J Ophthalmol.* 47: 3-9.

Ellison, A.R., Yang, L., Cevallos, A.V., & Margolis, T.P. (2003). Analysis of the herpes simplex virus type 1 UL6 gene in patients with stromal keratitis. *Virology.* 310: 24-28.

Farris, R. (1998). Abnormalities of the tears and treatment of dry eyes. in *The Cornea* (ed. HE Kauffman, B.B., MB McDonald), pp. p109-130. Butterworth-Heinemann, Boston.

Flynn, T.H., Mitchison, N.A., Ono, S.J., & Larkin, D.F. (2008). Aqueous humor alloreactive cell phenotypes, cytokines and chemokines in corneal allograft rejection. *Am J Transplant.* 8: 1537-1543.

Foster, C.S., Rodriguez Garcia, A., Pedroza-Seres, M., Berra, A., Heiligenhaus, A., Soukiasian, S., & Jayaraman, S. (1993). Murine herpes simplex virus keratitis is accentuated by CD4+, V beta 8.2+ Th2 T cells. *Trans Am Ophthalmol Soc.* 91: 325-348; discussion 349-350.

Ghiasi, H., Cai, S., Perng, G.C., Nesburn, A.B., & Wechsler, S.L. (2000). The role of natural killer cells in protection of mice against death and corneal scarring following ocular HSV-1 infection. *Antiviral Res.* 45: 33-45.

Ghiasi, H., Cai, S., Slanina, S.M., Perng, G.C., Nesburn, A.B., & Wechsler, S.L. (1999). The role of interleukin (IL)-2 and IL-4 in herpes simplex virus type 1 ocular replication and eye disease. *J Infect Dis.* 179: 1086-1093.

Griffith, T.S., Brunner, T., Fletcher, S.M., Green, D.R., & Ferguson, T.A. (1995). Fas ligand-induced apoptosis as a mechanism of immune privilege. *Science.* 270: 1189-1192.

Group, T.C.C.T.S.R. (1992). The collaborative corneal transplantation studies (CCTS). Effectiveness of histocompatibility matching in high-risk corneal transplantation. The Collaborative Corneal Transplantation Studies Research Group. *Arch Ophthalmol.* 110: 1392-1403.

Guo, H., Gao, J., & Wu, X. (2011). Toll-like receptor 2 siRNA suppresses corneal inflammation and attenuates Aspergillus fumigatus keratitis in rats. *Immunol Cell Biol.*

Guo, H. & Wu, X. (2009). Innate responses of corneal epithelial cells against Aspergillus fumigatus challenge. *FEMS Immunol Med Microbiol.* 56: 88-93.

Hamrah, P. & Dana, M.R. (2007). Corneal antigen-presenting cells. *Chem Immunol Allergy.* 92: 58-70.

Hamrah, P., Huq, S.O., Liu, Y., Zhang, Q., & Dana, M.R. (2003a). Corneal immunity is mediated by heterogeneous population of antigen-presenting cells. *J Leukoc Biol.* 74: 172-178.

Hamrah, P., Liu, Y., Zhang, Q., & Dana, M.R. (2003b). Alterations in corneal stromal dendritic cell phenotype and distribution in inflammation. *Arch Ophthalmol.* 121: 1132-1140.

Hamrah, P., Liu, Y., Zhang, Q., & Dana, M.R. (2003c). The corneal stroma is endowed with a significant number of resident dendritic cells. *Invest Ophthalmol Vis Sci.* 44: 581-589.

Hamrah, P., Yamagami, S., Liu, Y., Zhang, Q., Vora, S.S., Lu, B., Gerard, C.J., & Dana, M.R. (2007). Deletion of the chemokine receptor CCR1 prolongs corneal allograft survival. *Invest Ophthalmol Vis Sci.* 48: 1228-1236.

Hamrah, P., Zhang, Q., & Dana, M.R. (2002a). Expression of vascular endothelial growth factor receptor-3 (VEGFR-3) in the conjunctiva--a potential link between lymphangiogenesis and leukocyte trafficking on the ocular surface. *Adv Exp Med Biol.* 506: 851-860.

Hamrah, P., Zhang, Q., Liu, Y., & Dana, M.R. (2002b). Novel characterization of MHC class II-negative population of resident corneal Langerhans cell-type dendritic cells. *Invest Ophthalmol Vis Sci.* 43: 639-646.

Hazlett, L.D. (2004). Corneal response to Pseudomonas aeruginosa infection. *Prog Retin Eye Res.* 23: 1-30.

Hazlett, L.D., McClellan, S., Barrett, R., & Rudner, X. (2001). B7/CD28 costimulation is critical in susceptibility to Pseudomonas aeruginosa corneal infection: a comparative study using monoclonal antibody blockade and CD28-deficient mice. *J Immunol.* 166: 1292-1299.

Hazlett, L.D., McClellan, S.A., Rudner, X.L., & Barrett, R.P. (2002). The role of Langerhans cells in Pseudomonas aeruginosa infection. *Invest Ophthalmol Vis Sci.* 43: 189-197.

Hazlett, L.D., Rosen, D.D., & Berk, R.S. (1978). Age-related susceptibility to Pseudomonas aeruginosa ocular infections in mice. *Infect Immun.* 20: 25-29.

Heiligenhaus, A., Bauer, D., Zheng, M., Mrzyk, S., & Steuhl, K.P. (1999). CD4+ T-cell type 1 and type 2 cytokines in the HSV-1 infected cornea. *Graefes Arch Clin Exp Ophthalmol.* 237: 399-406.

Hendricks, R.L. (1997). An immunologist's view of herpes simplex keratitis: Thygeson Lecture 1996, presented at the Ocular Microbiology and Immunology Group meeting, October 26, 1996. *Cornea.* 16: 503-506.

Hendricks, R.L., Janowicz, M., & Tumpey, T.M. (1992a). Critical role of corneal Langerhans cells in the CD4- but not CD8-mediated immunopathology in herpes simplex virus-1-infected mouse corneas. *J Immunol.* 148: 2522-2529.

Hendricks, R.L. & Tumpey, T.M. (1990). Contribution of virus and immune factors to herpes simplex virus type I-induced corneal pathology. *Invest Ophthalmol Vis Sci.* 31: 1929-1939.

Hendricks, R.L., Tumpey, T.M., & Finnegan, A. (1992b). IFN-gamma and IL-2 are protective in the skin but pathologic in the corneas of HSV-1-infected mice. *J Immunol.* 149: 3023-3028.

Hendricks, R.L., Weber, P.C., Taylor, J.L., Koumbis, A., Tumpey, T.M., & Glorioso, J.C. (1991). Endogenously produced interferon alpha protects mice from herpes simplex virus type 1 corneal disease. *J Gen Virol.* 72 (Pt 7): 1601-1610.

Hu, J., Wang, Y., & Xie, L. (2009). Potential role of macrophages in experimental keratomycosis. *Invest Ophthalmol Vis Sci.* 50: 2087-2094.

Huang, X., Barrett, R.P., McClellan, S.A., & Hazlett, L.D. (2005). Silencing Toll-like receptor-9 in Pseudomonas aeruginosa keratitis. *Invest Ophthalmol Vis Sci.* 46: 4209-4216.

Hurt M, Proy V, Niederkorn JY, Alizadeh H. (2003) The interaction of Acanthamoeba castellanii cysts with macrophages and neutrophils. *J Parasitol.* 89:565-572.

Iyer, S.A., Tuli, S.S., & Wagoner, R.C. (2006). Fungal keratitis: emerging trends and treatment outcomes. *Eye Contact Lens.* 32: 267-271.

Jager, M.J., Atherton, S., Bradley, D., & Streilein, J.W. (1991). Herpetic stromal keratitis in mice: less reversibility in the presence of Langerhans cells in the central cornea. *Curr Eye Res.* 10 Suppl: 69-73.

Jager, M.J., Bradley, D., Atherton, S., & Streilein, J.W. (1992). Presence of Langerhans cells in the central cornea linked to the development of ocular herpes in mice. *Exp Eye Res.* 54: 835-841.

Jager, M.J., Bradley, D., & Streilein, J.W. (1995). Immunosuppressive properties of cultured human cornea and ciliary body in normal and pathological conditions. *Transpl Immunol.* 3: 135-142.

Janeway C, T.P., Walport M, Shlomchik M. (2004). *Immunobiology*. Garland Science.

Jayaraman, S., Heiligenhaus, A., Rodriguez, A., Soukiasian, S., Dorf, M.E., & Foster, C.S. (1993). Exacerbation of murine herpes simplex virus-mediated stromal keratitis by Th2 type T cells. *J Immunol.* 151: 5777-5789.

Jin, X., Lin, Z., & Xie, X. (2010). The delayed response of Toll-like receptors may relate to Pseudomonas aeruginosa keratitis exacerbating rapidly at the early stages of infection. *Eur J Clin Microbiol Infect Dis.* 29: 231-238.

Jin, X., Qin, Q., Tu, L., Zhou, X., Lin, Y., & Qu, J. (2007). Toll-like receptors (TLRs) expression and function in response to inactivate hyphae of Fusarium solani in immortalized human corneal epithelial cells. *Mol Vis.* 13: 1953-1961.

Johnson, A.C., Heinzel, F.P., Diaconu, E., Sun, Y., Hise, A.G., Golenbock, D., Lass, J.H., & Pearlman, E. (2005). Activation of toll-like receptor (TLR)2, TLR4, and TLR9 in the mammalian cornea induces MyD88-dependent corneal inflammation. *Invest Ophthalmol Vis Sci.* 46: 589-595.

Jones, D.B. (1973). Early diagnosis and therapy of bacterial corneal ulcers. *Int Ophthalmol Clin.* 13: 1-29.

Jurkunas, U., Behlau, I., & Colby, K. (2009). Fungal keratitis: changing pathogens and risk factors. *Cornea.* 28: 638-643.

Kabashima, K., Banks, T.A., Ansel, K.M., Lu, T.T., Ware, C.F., & Cyster, J.G. (2005). Intrinsic lymphotoxin-beta receptor requirement for homeostasis of lymphoid tissue dendritic cells. *Immunity.* 22: 439-450.

Kennedy, M.C., Rosenbaum, J.T., Brown, J., Planck, S.R., Huang, X., Armstrong, C.A., & Ansel, J.C. (1995). Novel production of interleukin-1 receptor antagonist peptides in normal human cornea. *J Clin Invest.* 95: 82-88.

Kijlstra, A. (1994). The role of cytokines in ocular inflammation. *Br J Ophthalmol.* 78: 885-886.

Kintner, R.L. & Brandt, C.R. (1995). The effect of viral inoculum level and host age on disease incidence, disease severity, and mortality in a murine model of ocular HSV-1 infection. *Curr Eye Res.* 14: 145-152.

Komatsu, K., Miyazaki, D., Morohoshi, K., Kuo, C.H., Kakimaru-Hasegawa, A., Komatsu, N., Namba, S., Haino, M., Matsushima, K., & Inoue, Y. (2008). Pathogenesis of herpetic stromal keratitis in CCR5- and/or CXCR3-deficient mice. *Curr Eye Res.* 33: 736-749.

Kumar RL, Cruzat A, Hamrah P. (2010). Current state of in vivo confocal microscopy in management of microbial keratitis. *Semin Ophthalmol.* 25:166-170.

Kwon, B. & Hazlett, L.D. (1997). Association of CD4+ T cell-dependent keratitis with genetic susceptibility to Pseudomonas aeruginosa ocular infection. *J Immunol.* 159: 6283-6290.

Lee, S., Zheng, M., Kim, B., & Rouse, B.T. (2002). Role of matrix metalloproteinase-9 in angiogenesis caused by ocular infection with herpes simplex virus. *J Clin Invest.* 110: 1105-1111.

Lee, S.K., Choi, B.K., Kang, W.J., Kim, Y.H., Park, H.Y., Kim, K.H., & Kwon, B.S. (2008). MCP-1 derived from stromal keratocyte induces corneal infiltration of CD4+ T cells in herpetic stromal keratitis. *Mol Cells.* 26: 67-73.

Lemp, M.A. (1995). Report of the National Eye Institute/Industry workshop on Clinical Trials in Dry Eyes. *CLAO J.* 21: 221-232.

Li, D.Q., Luo, L., Chen, Z., Kim, H.S., Song, X.J., & Pflugfelder, S.C. (2006). JNK and ERK MAP kinases mediate induction of IL-1beta, TNF-alpha and IL-8 following hyperosmolar stress in human limbal epithelial cells. *Exp Eye Res.* 82: 588-596.

Liu, Y., Hamrah, P., Zhang, Q., Taylor, A.W., & Dana, M.R. (2002). Draining lymph nodes of corneal transplant hosts exhibit evidence for donor major histocompatibility complex (MHC) class II-positive dendritic cells derived from MHC class II-negative grafts. *J Exp Med.* 195: 259-268.

Luo, L., Li, D.Q., Doshi, A., Farley, W., Corrales, R.M., & Pflugfelder, S.C. (2004). Experimental dry eye stimulates production of inflammatory cytokines and MMP-9 and activates MAPK signaling pathways on the ocular surface. *Invest Ophthalmol Vis Sci.* 45: 4293-4301.

Maguire, M.G., Stark, W.J., Gottsch, J.D., Stulting, R.D., Sugar, A., Fink, N.E., & Schwartz, A. (1994). Risk factors for corneal graft failure and rejection in the collaborative corneal transplantation studies. Collaborative Corneal Transplantation Studies Research Group. *Ophthalmology.* 101: 1536-1547.

Mambula, S.S., Sau, K., Henneke, P., Golenbock, D.T., & Levitz, S.M. (2002). Toll-like receptor (TLR) signaling in response to Aspergillus fumigatus. *J Biol Chem.* 277: 39320-39326.

Merad, M., Manz, M.G., Karsunky, H., Wagers, A., Peters, W., Charo, I., Weissman, I.L., Cyster, J.G., & Engleman, E.G. (2002). Langerhans cells renew in the skin throughout life under steady-state conditions. *Nat Immunol.* 3: 1135-1141.

Meyers-Elliott, R.H. & Chitjian, P.A. (1981). Immunopathogenesis of corneal inflammation in herpes simplex virus stromal keratitis: role of the polymorphonuclear leukocyte. *Invest Ophthalmol Vis Sci.* 20: 784-798.

Miller, J.K., Laycock, K.A., Nash, M.M., & Pepose, J.S. (1993). Corneal Langerhans cell dynamics after herpes simplex virus reactivation. *Invest Ophthalmol Vis Sci.* 34: 2282-2290.

Miller, R.L., Meng, T.C., & Tomai, M.A. (2008). The antiviral activity of Toll-like receptor 7 and 7/8 agonists. *Drug News Perspect.* 21: 69-87.

Naik, S.H., Metcalf, D., van Nieuwenhuijze, A., Wicks, I., Wu, L., O'Keeffe, M., & Shortman, K. (2006). Intrasplenic steady-state dendritic cell precursors that are distinct from monocytes. *Nat Immunol.* 7: 663-671.

Netea, M.G., Van Der Graaf, C.A., Vonk, A.G., Verschueren, I., Van Der Meer, J.W., & Kullberg, B.J. (2002). The role of toll-like receptor (TLR) 2 and TLR4 in the host defense against disseminated candidiasis. *J Infect Dis.* 185: 1483-1489.

Netea, M.G., Warris, A., Van der Meer, J.W., Fenton, M.J., Verver-Janssen, T.J., Jacobs, L.E., Andresen, T., Verweij, P.E., & Kullberg, B.J. (2003). Aspergillus fumigatus evades immune recognition during germination through loss of toll-like receptor-4-mediated signal transduction. *J Infect Dis.* 188: 320-326.

Newell, C.K., Martin, S., Sendele, D., Mercadal, C.M., & Rouse, B.T. (1989a). Herpes simplex virus-induced stromal keratitis: role of T-lymphocyte subsets in immunopathology. *J Virol.* 63: 769-775.

Newell, C.K., Sendele, D., & Rouse, B.T. (1989b). Effects of CD4+ and CD8+ T-lymphocyte depletion on the induction and expression of herpes simplex stromal keratitis. *Reg Immunol.* 2: 366-369.

Nicas, T.I. & Iglewski, B.H. (1985). The contribution of exoproducts to virulence of Pseudomonas aeruginosa. *Can J Microbiol.* 31: 387-392.

Niederkorn, J.Y. (1990). Immune privilege and immune regulation in the eye. *Adv Immunol.* 48: 191-226.

Niederkorn, J.Y. (1999). The immunology of corneal transplantation. *Dev Ophthalmol.* 30: 129-140.

Niederkorn JY, Alizadeh H, Leher H, McCulley JP. (1999) The pathogenesis of Acanthamoeba keratitis.*Microbes Infect.* 1:437-443.

Niederkorn, J.Y. (2002). Immunology and immunomodulation of corneal transplantation. *Int Rev Immunol.* 21: 173-196.

Niederkorn, J.Y., Peeler, J.S., Ross, J., & Callanan, D. (1989). The immunogenic privilege of corneal allografts. *Reg Immunol.* 2: 117-124.

Niemialtowski, M.G. & Rouse, B.T. (1992a). Phenotypic and functional studies on ocular T cells during herpetic infections of the eye. *J Immunol.* 148: 1864-1870.

Niemialtowski, M.G. & Rouse, B.T. (1992b). Predominance of Th1 cells in ocular tissues during herpetic stromal keratitis. *J Immunol.* 149: 3035-3039.

O'Callaghan, R.J., Engel, L.S., Hobden, J.A., Callegan, M.C., Green, L.C., & Hill, J.M. (1996). Pseudomonas keratitis. The role of an uncharacterized exoprotein, protease IV, in corneal virulence. *Invest Ophthalmol Vis Sci.* 37: 534-543.

O'Keeffe, M., Hochrein, H., Vremec, D., Scott, B., Hertzog, P., Tatarczuch, L., & Shortman, K. (2003). Dendritic cell precursor populations of mouse blood: identification of the murine homologues of human blood plasmacytoid pre-DC2 and CD11c+ DC1 precursors. *Blood.* 101: 1453-1459.

Pepose, J.S. (1991). Herpes simplex keratitis: role of viral infection versus immune response. *Surv Ophthalmol.* 35: 345-352.

Pepose, J.S., Gardner, K.M., Nestor, M.S., Foos, R.Y., & Pettit, T.H. (1985). Detection of HLA class I and II antigens in rejected human corneal allografts. *Ophthalmology.* 92: 1480-1484.

Pflugfelder, S.C. (1998). Advances in the diagnosis and management of keratoconjunctivitis sicca. *Curr Opin Ophthalmol.* 9: 50-53.

Redfern, R.L. & McDermott, A.M. (2010). Toll-like receptors in ocular surface disease. *Exp Eye Res.* 90: 679-687.

Russell, R.G., Nasisse, M.P., Larsen, H.S., & Rouse, B.T. (1984). Role of T-lymphocytes in the pathogenesis of herpetic stromal keratitis. *Invest Ophthalmol Vis Sci.* 25: 938-944.

Sankaridurg, P.R., Rao, G.N., Rao, H.N., Sweeney, D.F., & Holden, B.A. (2000). ATPase-positive dendritic cells in the limbal and corneal epithelium of guinea pigs after extended wear of hydrogel lenses. *Cornea.* 19: 374-377.

Schang, L.M., Phillips, J., & Schaffer, P.A. (1998). Requirement for cellular cyclin-dependent kinases in herpes simplex virus replication and transcription. *J Virol.* 72: 5626-5637.

Schang, L.M., Rosenberg, A., & Schaffer, P.A. (2000). Roscovitine, a specific inhibitor of cellular cyclin-dependent kinases, inhibits herpes simplex virus DNA synthesis in the presence of viral early proteins. *J Virol.* 74: 2107-2120.

Schaumberg, D.A., Sullivan, D.A., Buring, J.E., & Dana, M.R. (2003). Prevalence of dry eye syndrome among US women. *Am J Ophthalmol.* 136: 318-326.

Shukla, D., Liu, J., Blaiklock, P., Shworak, N.W., Bai, X., Esko, J.D., Cohen, G.H., Eisenberg, R.J., Rosenberg, R.D., & Spear, P.G. (1999). A novel role for 3-O-sulfated heparan sulfate in herpes simplex virus 1 entry. *Cell.* 99: 13-22.

Shukla, D. & Spear, P.G. (2001). Herpesviruses and heparan sulfate: an intimate relationship in aid of viral entry. *J Clin Invest.* 108: 503-510.

Smith, P.M., Wolcott, R.M., Chervenak, R., & Jennings, S.R. (1994). Control of acute cutaneous herpes simplex virus infection: T cell-mediated viral clearance is dependent upon interferon-gamma (IFN-gamma). *Virology.* 202: 76-88.

Spear, P.G. (2004). Herpes simplex virus: receptors and ligands for cell entry. *Cell Microbiol.* 6: 401-410.

Stern, M.E., Beuerman, R.W., Fox, R.I., Gao, J., Mircheff, A.K., & Pflugfelder, S.C. (1998). The pathology of dry eye: the interaction between the ocular surface and lacrimal glands. *Cornea.* 17: 584-589.

Stern, M.E., Gao, J., Siemasko, K.F., Beuerman, R.W., & Pflugfelder, S.C. (2004). The role of the lacrimal functional unit in the pathophysiology of dry eye. *Exp Eye Res.* 78: 409-416.

Stewart GL, Kim I, Shupe K, Alizadeh, H. Silvany, R. McCulley, J. P. Niederkorn, J. Y. (1992) Chemotactic response of macrophages to Acanthamoeba castellanii antigen and antibody-dependent macrophage-mediated killing of the parasite. *J Parasitol.* ;78:849-855.

Streilein, J.W. (1993). Tissue barriers, immunosuppressive microenvironments, and privileged sites: the eye's point of view. *Reg Immunol.* 5: 253-268.

Streilein, J.W. (1995). Immunological non-responsiveness and acquisition of tolerance in relation to immune privilege in the eye. *Eye (Lond).* 9 (Pt 2): 236-240.

Streilein, J.W. (1999). Immunobiology and immunopathology of corneal transplantation. *Chem Immunol.* 73: 186-206.

Streilein, J.W., Bradley, D., Sano, Y., & Sonoda, Y. (1996). Immunosuppressive properties of tissues obtained from eyes with experimentally manipulated corneas. *Invest Ophthalmol Vis Sci.* 37: 413-424.

Streilein, J.W., Dana, M.R., & Ksander, B.R. (1997). Immunity causing blindness: five different paths to herpes stromal keratitis. *Immunol Today.* 18: 443-449.

Streilein, J.W., Toews, G.B., & Bergstresser, P.R. (1979). Corneal allografts fail to express Ia antigens. *Nature.* 282: 326-327.

Stuart, P.M., Griffith, T.S., Usui, N., Pepose, J., Yu, X., & Ferguson, T.A. (1997). CD95 ligand (FasL)-induced apoptosis is necessary for corneal allograft survival. *J Clin Invest.* 99: 396-402.

Sun, Y., Chandra, J., Mukherjee, P., Szczotka-Flynn, L., Ghannoum, M.A., & Pearlman, E. (2010). A murine model of contact lens-associated fusarium keratitis. *Invest Ophthalmol Vis Sci.* 51: 1511-1516.

Sun, Y., Karmakar, M., Roy, S., Ramadan, R.T., Williams, S.R., Howell, S., Shive, C.L., Han, Y., Stopford, C.M., Rietsch, A., & Pearlman, E. TLR4 and TLR5 on corneal macrophages regulate Pseudomonas aeruginosa keratitis by signaling through MyD88-dependent and -independent pathways. *J Immunol.* 185: 4272-4283.

Tang, Q. & Bluestone, J.A. (2008). The Foxp3+ regulatory T cell: a jack of all trades, master of regulation. *Nat Immunol.* 9: 239-244.

Tarabishy, A.B., Aldabagh, B., Sun, Y., Imamura, Y., Mukherjee, P.K., Lass, J.H., Ghannoum, M.A., & Pearlman, E. (2008). MyD88 regulation of Fusarium keratitis is dependent on TLR4 and IL-1R1 but not TLR2. *J Immunol.* 181: 593-600.

Thiel, M.A., Kaufmann, C., Coster, D.J., & Williams, K.A. (2009). Antibody-based immunosuppressive agents for corneal transplantation. *Eye (Lond).* 23: 1962-1965.

Thomas, J., Gangappa, S., Kanangat, S., & Rouse, B.T. (1997). On the essential involvement of neutrophils in the immunopathologic disease: herpetic stromal keratitis. *J Immunol.* 158: 1383-1391.

Thomas, J., Kanangat, S., & Rouse, B.T. (1998). Herpes simplex virus replication-induced expression of chemokines and proinflammatory cytokines in the eye: implications in herpetic stromal keratitis. *J Interferon Cytokine Res.* 18: 681-690.

Thomas, J. & Rouse, B.T. (1997). Immunopathogenesis of herpetic ocular disease. *Immunol Res.* 16: 375-386.

Thomas, P.A. & Geraldine, P. (2007). Infectious keratitis. *Curr Opin Infect Dis.* 20: 129-141.

Torres, P.F. & Kijlstra, A. (2001). The role of cytokines in corneal immunopathology. *Ocul Immunol Inflamm.* 9: 9-24.

Traver, D., Akashi, K., Manz, M., Merad, M., Miyamoto, T., Engleman, E.G., & Weissman, I.L. (2000). Development of CD8alpha-positive dendritic cells from a common myeloid progenitor. *Science.* 290: 2152-2154.

Trinkaus-Randall, V., Leibowitz, H.M., Ryan, W.J., & Kupferman, A. (1991). Quantification of stromal destruction in the inflamed cornea. *Invest Ophthalmol Vis Sci.* 32: 603-609.

Tullo, A.B., Shimeld, C., Blyth, W.A., Hill, T.J., & Easty, D.L. (1983). Ocular infection with herpes simplex virus in nonimmune and immune mice. *Arch Ophthalmol.* 101: 961-964.

Tumpey, T.M., Chen, S.H., Oakes, J.E., & Lausch, R.N. (1996). Neutrophil-mediated suppression of virus replication after herpes simplex virus type 1 infection of the murine cornea. *J Virol.* 70: 898-904.

Tumpey, T.M., Cheng, H., Cook, D.N., Smithies, O., Oakes, J.E., & Lausch, R.N. (1998). Absence of macrophage inflammatory protein-1alpha prevents the development of blinding herpes stromal keratitis. *J Virol.* 72: 3705-3710.

Van Horn, D.L., Davis, S.D., Hyndiuk, R.A., & Alpren, T.V. (1978). Pathogenesis of experimental Pseudomonas keratitis in the guinea pig: bacteriologic, clinical, and microscopic observations. *Invest Ophthalmol Vis Sci.* 17: 1076-1086.

Van Klink F, Taylor WM, Alizadeh H, Jager MJ, van Rooijen N, Niederkorn JY. (1996) The role of macrophages in Acanthamoeba keratitis. *Invest Ophthalmol Vis Sci.* 37:1271-1281.

Verjans, G.M., Remeijer, L., Mooy, C.M., & Osterhaus, A.D. (2000). Herpes simplex virus-specific T cells infiltrate the cornea of patients with herpetic stromal keratitis: no evidence for autoreactive T cells. *Invest Ophthalmol Vis Sci.* 41: 2607-2612.

Weiss, S.J. (1989). Tissue destruction by neutrophils. *N Engl J Med.* 320: 365-376.

Whitley, R.J. & Roizman, B. (2001). Herpes simplex virus infections. *Lancet.* 357: 1513-1518.

Wolpe, S.D., Davatelis, G., Sherry, B., Beutler, B., Hesse, D.G., Nguyen, H.T., Moldawer, L.L., Nathan, C.F., Lowry, S.F., & Cerami, A. (1988). Macrophages secrete a novel heparin-binding protein with inflammatory and neutrophil chemokinetic properties. *J Exp Med.* 167: 570-581.

Wolpe, S.D., Sherry, B., Juers, D., Davatelis, G., Yurt, R.W., & Cerami, A. (1989). Identification and characterization of macrophage inflammatory protein 2. *Proc Natl Acad Sci U S A.* 86: 612-616.

WorkShop, I.D.E. (2007a). The definition and classification of dry eye disease: report of the Definition and Classification Subcommittee of the International Dry Eye WorkShop (2007). *Ocul Surf.* 5: 75-92.

WorkShop, I.D.E. (2007b). The epidemiology of dry eye disease: report of the Epidemiology Subcommittee of the International Dry Eye WorkShop (2007). *Ocul Surf.* 5: 93-107.

Wu, L., D'Amico, A., Hochrein, H., O'Keeffe, M., Shortman, K., & Lucas, K. (2001). Development of thymic and splenic dendritic cell populations from different hemopoietic precursors. *Blood.* 98: 3376-3382.

Wuest, T.R. & Carr, D.J. (2008). Dysregulation of CXCR3 signaling due to CXCL10 deficiency impairs the antiviral response to herpes simplex virus 1 infection. *J Immunol.* 181: 7985-7993.

Yamagami, S., Hamrah, P., Zhang, Q., Liu, Y., Huq, S., & Dana, M.R. (2005). Early ocular chemokine gene expression and leukocyte infiltration after high-risk corneal transplantation. *Mol Vis.* 11: 632-640.

Yamagami, S., Isobe, M., & Tsuru, T. (2000). Characterization of cytokine profiles in corneal allograft with anti-adhesion therapy. *Transplantation.* 69: 1655-1659.

Yamagami, S., Miyazaki, D., Ono, S.J., & Dana, M.R. (1999). Differential chemokine gene expression in corneal transplant rejection. *Invest Ophthalmol Vis Sci.* 40: 2892-2897.

Yildiz, E.H., Abdalla, Y.F., Elsahn, A.F., Rapuano, C.J., Hammersmith, K.M., Laibson, P.R., & Cohen, E.J. (2010). Update on fungal keratitis from 1999 to 2008. *Cornea.* 29: 1406-1411.

Youker, K., Smith, C.W., Anderson, D.C., Miller, D., Michael, L.H., Rossen, R.D., & Entman, M.L. (1992). Neutrophil adherence to isolated adult cardiac myocytes. Induction by cardiac lymph collected during ischemia and reperfusion. *J Clin Invest.* 89: 602-609.

Yuan, X. & Wilhelmus, K.R. (2009). Corneal neovascularization during experimental fungal keratitis. *Mol Vis.* 15: 1988-1996.

Zhao, Z.S., Granucci, F., Yeh, L., Schaffer, P.A., & Cantor, H. (1998). Molecular mimicry by herpes simplex virus-type 1: autoimmune disease after viral infection. *Science.* 279: 1344-1347.

Zheng, M., Deshpande, S., Lee, S., Ferrara, N., & Rouse, B.T. (2001). Contribution of vascular endothelial growth factor in the neovascularization process during the pathogenesis of herpetic stromal keratitis. *J Virol.* 75: 9828-9835.

Zheng, X., de Paiva, C.S., Li, D.Q., Farley, W.J., & Pflugfelder, S.C. Desiccating stress promotion of Th17 differentiation by ocular surface tissues through a dendritic cell-mediated pathway. *Invest Ophthalmol Vis Sci.* 51: 3083-3091.

Zhou, Z., Wu, M., Barrett, R.P., McClellan, S.A., Zhang, Y., & Hazlett, L.D. (2010). Role of the Fas pathway in Pseudomonas aeruginosa keratitis. *Invest Ophthalmol Vis Sci.* 51: 2537-2547.

Zhu, S., Dekaris, I., Duncker, G., & Dana, M.R. (1999). Early expression of proinflammatory cytokines interleukin-1 and tumor necrosis factor-alpha after corneal transplantation. *J Interferon Cytokine Res.* 19: 661-669.

Zhu, S.N. & Dana, M.R. (1999). Expression of cell adhesion molecules on limbal and neovascular endothelium in corneal inflammatory neovascularization. *Invest Ophthalmol Vis Sci.* 40: 1427-1434.

6

Keratoconus Layer by Layer – Pathology and Matrix Metalloproteinases

Dasha Nelidova and Trevor Sherwin
Department of Ophthalmology, Faculty of Medical and Health Sciences, University of Auckland, Auckland New Zealand

1. Introduction

Keratoconus is an ectatic disease in which the cornea develops a conical shape due to thinning of the collagenous corneal stroma. Characteristic morphological features seen on slit lamp examination are well described. This overview describes the recent advances in our understanding of keratoconic pathology, focussing particularly on the matrix metalloproteinase hypothesis of keratoconus disease progression.

2. The diversity and complexity of keratoconus

Keratoconus is a corneal ectatic disease where the cornea assumes a conical shape due to thinning of the corneal stroma, inducing irregular astigmatism and myopia and leading to marked impairment of vision[1]. Keratoconus typically starts at puberty and progresses until the third or fourth decade of life; alternatively it may commence later and arrest at any age. This disease is associated with several conditions, particularly those which encourage eye rubbing.

The mechanism of disease progression has long been the subject of intense research; however, research is complicated by the large degree of variation in clinical features between patients. *Forme fruste* or sub-clinical forms of the disease, likely contribute to the differences in reported incidence are estimated to occur between 50 and 230 per 100,000 of the general population[1]. There are also significant geographical variations. New Zealand, for example, has an unusually high prevalence of keratoconus. 50% of corneal transplants performed in New Zealand are due to this debilitating disease, compared with 30% in Australia[2] and 20% in the UK[3].

3. Clinical signs of keratoconus

The first adequate description of keratoconus, setting it aside from other ectatic conditions, was advanced by Nottingham in 1854 in his treatise 'Practical observations on conical cornea: and on the short sight, and other defects of vision connected with it'[4].

In 1943 Berliner[5] listed the seven distinct features of keratoconus as classified by Von der Heydt and Appelbaum:

1. Thinning of the cornea at the apex of the cone
2. Reflex from the endothelial cup
3. Striae
4. Irregular superficial opacities or scars
5. Ruptures in Descemet's membrane
6. Increased visibility of the nerve fibres and
7. Fleischer's ring.

These morphological features became incorporated by Duke-Elder[6] into the 1965 text 'System of Ophthalmology', which went on to describe keratoconus as a disease which can be recognised by:

1. A thinning of the cornea at the apex of the cone from one half to one fifth of its normal dimensions
2. An endothelial reflex in the central portion of the cornea at the peak of the cone
3. Vertical lines in the deeper layers of the stroma
4. An increased visibility of the nerve fibres which form a network of grey lines interspersed with small dots
5. Fleischer's ring, a line running round the base of the cone
6. Ruptures of Descemet's membrane of characteristic appearance
7. Ruptures in Bowman's membrane in advanced cases producing superficial linear scars.

Rabinowitz[1] lists the following clinical signs which may be present individually or in combination in moderate to advanced keratoconus:

'Stromal thinning (centrally or paracentrally, most commonly inferiorly or inferotemporally); conical protrusion; an iron line partially or completely surrounding the cone (Fleischer's ring); and fine vertical lines in the deep stroma and Descemet's membrane (Vogt's striae)... Other accompanying signs might include epithelial nebulae, anterior stromal scars, enlarged corneal nerves and increased intensity of the corneal endothelial reflex and subepithelial fibrillary lines.'

Since then advances in corneal topographical assessment have greatly aided the diagnosis of early disease. Prior to topography, forme fruste keratoconus was harder to recognise as patients do not necessarily have symptoms or observable clinical signs in these early stages.

4. Antero-posterior review of morphological changes in keratoconus

Pathological and histopathological abnormalities have been documented in every layer of the keratoconic cornea and this has previously been reviewed by our laboratory[7]. The following represents a layer by layer summary of keratoconic morphological variations reported.

4.1 Epithelium

Ex vivo histological analysis of keratoconic corneas has demonstrated significant thinning of the central epithelium[8]. Central epithelial thinning was significantly greater in those corneas which also had breaks in the Bowman's layer, however, the authors thought it likely that differences in the integrity of Bowman's layer could nevertheless be considered to be manifestations of the same disease process. Subsequent studies report thickened epithelia in keratoconus[9,10] or else no difference in epithelial thickness between keratoconus and normal controls[11].

In vivo confocal microscopy studies of the epithelium demonstrate morphological alterations in the area of the keratoconic corneal apex. Elongated superficial epithelial cells, arranged in a whorl-like fashion, can be observed. Near Bowman's membrane highly reflective changes and fold-like structures are visible[12]. These *in vivo* pathological features may well reflect the oedematous disruptions of basal epithelial integrity in keratoconus.

Apoptotic changes have also been detected in epithelia of keratoconic samples. TUNEL positive epithelial cells were confined to the superficial epithelium of normal corneas while extending further down in keratoconic corneas[9].This is supported by the work which reported that intense TUNEL labelling was present in the basal epithelia of fifteen out of sixteen keratoconic corneas examined[13].

The keratoconic basement membrane assumes an irregular appearance and breaks in places[14]. It also undergoes a change in composition[15,16] that cannot be explained by scarring alone. Laminin-1 and laminin-5 staining was shown to be irregular and thickened at defect sites, however monoclonal antibodies against the $\alpha 2$ and $\beta 2$ chains did not react[15]. Type IV collagen $\alpha 1$ and $\alpha 2$ reactivity was also only found in the defect regions of keratoconic or scarred corneas[15]. Immunostaining for type VII collagen was patchily localised to the basement membrane defects[15]. Integrin $\beta 4$ staining which was positive in the basement membrane and the lateral and apical cell membranes of the epithelial cells, was found to be discontinuous in keratoconic corneas[15]. It has been suggested that a process similar to wound healing might account for such differences in structure. Basement membrane alterations may affect critical interactions of the corneal epithelium with the underlying basement membrane, as well as cell-matrix interactions and matrix organization in the stroma[16].

4.2 Nerve fibres

Increased visibility of nerve fibres by slit lamp biomicroscopy has been demonstrated in keratoconus. Corneal nerves pass between the stroma and epithelium at sites of early degradative change[17]. Keratocytes wrap around the nerves as they pass through an otherwise acellular Bowman's layer[17]. Localised nerve thickenings develop in the epithelium and stress epithelial architecture[17].

4.3 Bowman's layer

Scanning electron microscopy has found defects and ruptures in Bowman's layer to varying degrees in all keratoconic corneas examined[18]. Discontinuities in Bowman's layer are sometimes accompanied by distortion of the stroma beneath the defect[15] or alternatively, direct contact between epithelial and stromal cells[19]. Rather than being seen throughout the affected cornea, such abnormalities of the extracellular matrix are usually confined to several loci, suggesting a localised focus of disease progression.

4.4 Stroma - Collagen lamellae and keratocytes

The thickness of collagen lamellae in keratoconus is unaltered, but the number of lamellae appears to be significantly reduced compared to normal tissue[20]. There is no difference in interfibrillar spacing between keratoconus and control corneas, conclusively demonstrating that stromal thinning in keratoconus is not due to closer packing of the fibrils in the stroma.

There is some evidence for a progressive loss of lamellae from the stroma, for example, a reduction in the volume of proteoglycan along the collagen fibrils has been found in keratoconus[21]. Low angle x-ray scattering has shown that the orientation of collagen fibrils within lamellae is also altered in the disease[22]. It is likely that these changes reflect the presence of a degradative process or alternatively, insufficient repair mechanisms. Biochemical analyses of stromal matrix components are inconclusive: Critchfield and co-workers[23] described decreased collagen and total protein levels in keratoconic tissue by western blotting. Radda et al.[24] found a 5% increase in type I collagen in keratoconus; while Zimmermann et al.[25] found no differences in collagen composition.

Keratoconus is also associated with changes in keratocyte morphology as well as loss of keratocyte density[11, 12]. Keratocytes may be lost though apoptosis[9,13], however, as apoptosis was not seen in all keratoconic samples analysed it was proposed that such cells might not be detected if at the time of analysis the tissue was in a period of keratoconic remission. An alternative explanation suggests that because keratoconus is diagnosed on the basis of clinical findings, there may be several diseases with differing pathophysiological mechanisms that produce the phenotypic change that is referred to as keratoconus.

Keratocyte density was lowest in the anterior-most part of the stroma[12]. Whilst there may be a significant decrease in the density of keratocytes in the stroma immediately underneath Bowmans' membrane, the remaining keratocytes are far from quiet. Such keratocytes and their pseudopodia are oriented apically towards the overlying epithelium and their activated state is reflected by the abundance of rough endoplasmic reticulum within the cells[26].

Studies of the peripheral keratoconic cornea also show discrete incursions of fine keratocytic processes into Bowman's membrane[10]. These processes were often observed in conjunction with posterior collapse of epithelial cells into the Bowman's layer[10].

4.5 Descemet's membrane

Ruptures and folds in Descemet's membrane are common in keratoconus[14]. The origin of these ruptures is unclear as several studies of extracellular matrix proteins have revealed no differences in the levels of collagens, laminin, entactin or perlecan between keratoconus and normal tissue[19,25]. The appearance of the defects in Descemet's membrane may well be associated with environmental factors such as eye rubbing and may lead to the development of hydrops[1].

4.6 Endothelium

The endothelium may be normal in keratoconus or may demonstrate intracellular dark structures, pleomorphisms or elongation of cells[1]. Scanning slit confocal microscopy and ultrasound biomicroscopy in living patients with keratoconus revealed central detachment of Descemet's membrane and endothelium from the posterior part of the stroma[27]. Ruptures in Descemet's membrane may directly lead to endothelial cell loss by triggering cell membrane perforation, loss of cell contents and edema[28]. Alternatively apoptosis may account for decreased endothelial cell density[13].

4.7 Evidence from recurrence of keratoconus

The recurrences of keratoconus in patients after penetrating keratoplasty[29] suggest either a recurrence of the host disease in the graft or else represent transmission of undiagnosed keratoconus from the donor cornea[30]. Histological examination of corneal buttons from patients undergoing repeated penetrating keratoplasty revealed structural changes compatible with a diagnosis of keratoconus in all the examined corneas[31]. Recurrence of keratoconus characteristics may be attributed to graft repopulation by the recipient cells, ageing of the grafted tissue, or both. However a recent study from our own laboratory failed to find evidence of recurrence of keratoconus in patients undergoing regraft surgery[32].

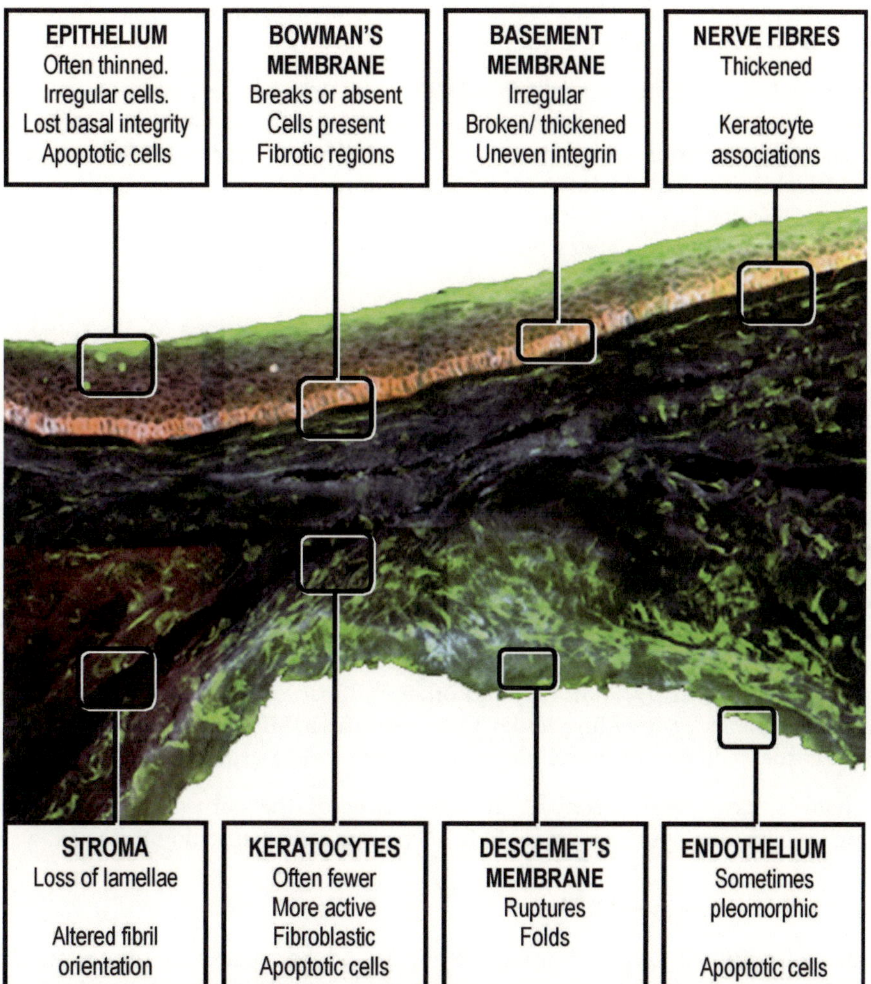

Fig. 1. A diverse range of morphological changes have been described in every layer of the keratoconic cornea. An antero-posterior section of a keratoconic cornea labelled with CellTracker green to highlight cellular morphology and integrin α3β1 labelling the basal epithelium in red helps to summarise characteristic histopathological abnormalities by corneal layer.
Figure reproduced by permission from Wiley-Blackwells[7]

5. Pathology to pathogenesis

The diversity of pathologies described for keratoconus are likely to represent temporal differences in the progression of the disease, positional differences relative to the apical centre of maximum damage and reflect a variety of pathophysiological diseases which make up the clinical pigeonhole of keratoconus.

Matrix metalloproteinases (MMPs) have long been suspected of mediating the pathological progression of keratoconus. The cornea is 70% collagen by weight and the reduced collagen content of the keratoconic cornea suggests a degraded extracellular matrix[23]. Extracellular matrix breakdown is, however, only a small component of the MMP repertoire of activity. Nevertheless, this function is essential for normal remodeling, leading to the constitutive expression of MMPs in healthy tissues.

Various models emphasise the role of MMPs in disease, for example, as mediators of connective tissue destruction in arthritis[33]. Consistent with such an involvement is the MMP hypothesis of keratoconus which proposes that MMPs are over-expressed in the disease while MMP inhibitors may be down-regulated, shifting the balance towards excessive tissue destruction. Over the last decade many studies have set out to measure the levels of MMPs and their inhibitors by a variety of techniques yet over-expression of MMPs or presence of active forms has not been found consistently[34].

It is important to consider that the relative balance between various MMPs could be more significant than absolute concentrations. This is relevant given that MMPs often undergo intermolecular interactions with each other to achieve activation from the latent form or to target MMP action to a particular site such as the cell surface. Paradoxically, tissue inhibitors of matrix metalloproteinases (TIMPs) can associate with pro form MMPs to trigger proteolytic activity[33]. Tissue degradation in thinning disorders, such as keratoconus, also involves the expression of inflammatory mediators, including proinflammatory cytokines and cell adhesion molecules[35], which modulate MMP activity and are themselves modulated by it.

The MMP family includes more than 25 members that make up five families based on their substrate preference: collagenases (MMP-1, MMP-8, and MMP-13), stromelysins (MMP-3, MMP-10), matrilysins (MMP-7, MMP-26), gelatinases (MMP-2, MMP-9), membrane type MMPs (MPP-14 to MMP-17, MMP-24) and others[36]. Most are synthesised by resident cells, some are brought in by invading leukocytes. Specific MMPs appear in specific locations within the cornea[36], likely due to cellular and soluble factors particular to the layer.

MMP changes have been described in every layer of the cornea in keratoconus. The following is a layer by layer summary of MMP changes reported within the last 15 years.

5.1 Tear film and increased MMP-9

Tear film composition reflects ocular surface events and tears may therefore be considered a vehicle for some of the pathogenic protagonists of keratoconus. Unfortunately, the cellular origin of any such molecules cannot be determined conclusively as both corneal and non-corneal secretions will be represented in the tear fluid.

In 2000 the presence of collagen degradation products was reported in the tears of patients with keratoconus[37]. The detected telopeptides were presumed to be of corneal origin but the authors conceded that serum and conjunctiva were also potential sources. The conjunctival epithelium is indeed altered in keratoconus. Elevation of lysosomal enzyme levels has been found in corneal and conjunctival epithelium[38] though such enzymes are mostly involved with lipid metabolism, rather than turnover of proteins or connective tissues. Lipids, however, are crucial to the integrity of the tear film and indeed, chronic ocular desiccation and aqueous tear deficiency can produce inferior corneal steepening and high astigmatism resembling keratoconus[39].

More recently, the levels of interleukin-6 (IL-6), tumour nectosis factor-α (TNF-α), and MMP-9 in the tear fluid of keratoconic patients were measured by enzyme linked immunoadsorbent assay and were found to be significantly higher than in normal subjects[40]. Increases in the levels of these molecules may be intermittent, but sufficient to provoke slowly progressive ectasia[40]. No significant differences in the concentrations of adhesion molecules inter cellular adhesion molecule-1 (ICAM-1) and vascular cell adhesion protein-1 (VCAM-1) were detected and other proteinases were not measured[40].

In most cases, keratoconus initially affects only one eye and later the ectasia may progress to include both eyes. Lema et al. followed up their initial work by measuring the concentrations of IL-6, TNF-α and MMP-9 in thirty patients with unilateral keratoconus - one eye diagnosed with keratoconus and the other eye having subclinical disease. IL-6 and TNF-α levels were found to be raised in both eyes in patients with asymmetric keratoconus, however, only TNF-α was significantly higher in the keratoconic eye, with respect to the subclinical one. Increased MMP-9 levels were found in keratoconic eyes only[35].

TNF-α has been shown to upregulate MMP-9 expression in human corneal epithelial cells[41] and such proinflammatory cytokines are present at the ocular surface even in the absence of inflammation[42]. Interestingly, increased concentrations of cytokines are found in tears from various ocular allergic disease states[43]. While atopy is associated with keratoconus[44], multivariate analysis has shown that the contribution to pathogenesis likely occurs from the eye rubbing encouraged by the itch of atopy rather than from chemical mediators associated with atopy itself[45].

The keratoconic ocular surface is characterised by a disorder of tear quality, decreased corneal sensitivity, conjunctival squamous metaplasia and higher fluorescein and rose bengal staining scores, all of which seem to relate to the extent of keratoconus progression[46]. In that respect the ocular surface is not unlike that of dry eye. It has been shown that inflammation plays an important role in both of these conditions and MMP-9 is found in the tears of both[40,47].

In fact MMP-9 accumulation has been demonstrated in several other disorders with an inflammatory basis, for example, in tears of patients with peripheral ulcerative keratitis, herpetic keratitis and Sjogren's syndrome[48].

Among the MMPs, MMP-9 is of central importance in cleaving epithelial basement membrane components and tight junction proteins that maintain corneal epithelial barrier function[47]. MMP-9 belongs to the gelatinase group of metalloproteinases that degrade denatured collagen; native collagens type IV, V, and VII; and elastin[47]. Expression of MMP-9 by ocular surface epithelia in normal healthy eyes is low. Indeed, MMP-9 knockout mice show significantly less alteration of epithelial barrier function in response to experimental desiccating stress than do wild-type mice, an effect abrogated by topical application of MMP-9 to the ocular surface[49].

5.2 Whole cornea studies and decreased TIMP-1

Studies have also assessed levels of various degradative enzymes in whole processed keratoconic corneas. This research was triggered by observations that cultured human dermal fibroblasts exposed to reactive oxygen species go on to upregulate MMP-1 and MMP-2 mRNA while downregulating TIMP-2 mRNA[50,51]. Thus oxidative stress was thought to be a contributing factor to the pathogenesis of keratoconus by promoting, amongst others, degradative activity.

Kenney et al. measured RNA levels by semi-quantitative reverse transcription-polymerase chain reaction (RT-PCR) and Southern blot. MMP-1, -2, -7, -9, -14, TIMP-2 and TIMP-3 mRNA levels did not differ between normal and keratoconic corneas[52]. There was, however, a 1.8 fold decrease in TIMP-1 mRNA and 2.8 fold decrease in TIMP-1 protein in keratoconus[52].

Decreased TIMP-1 may account for the high gelatinase activity and increased apoptosis of keratoconus. It has been proposed that TIMP-1 curtails the activity of MMP-2, the major protease of the corneal stroma. Unlike the constitutively expressed TIMP-2, TIMP-1 is an inducible inhibitor generally confined to the corneal epithelium[53]. Its synthesis seems to be upregulated in stromal cell cultures from scarred keratoconic corneas[53]. Apart from its anti-proteinase role TIMP-1 prevents TIMP-3 mediated stromal cell apoptosis[53]. Dysequilibrium in the TIMP-1/TIMP-3 system can thus, at least partially, account for the keratoconic condition.

It is likely that changes in MMP and TIMP systems are also present in several other eye diseases. For example, diabetic retinopathy corneas contain higher levels of MMP-3 and MMP-10 mRNA as measured by RT-PCR compared with keratoconic corneas[54]. This is thought to account for the various basement membrane and extracellular matrix alterations in the cornea of diabetic retinopathy.

5.3 Epithelium and increased MMP-1

Collier et al. performed peroxidase immunohistochemistry and determined that MMP-14 (MT1-MMP) was significantly elevated in the epithelium of keratoconic corneas compared to eye bank controls, while MMP-2 was not[55]. This was surprising given that MMP-14 was previously shown to activate latent MMP-2 as well as being able to degrade matrix molecules directly. MMP-14 forms a tri-molecular complex on the cell surface with MMP-2 and TIMP-2 in a complex sequence[55]. The timing of this interaction and concentrations of component molecules determine whether the MMP-14 active site is exposed and available for MMP-2 activation and matrix degradation[55].

It was also noted that the expression of MMP-14 in control corneas varied considerably from virtually none to pronounced levels, raising the possibility that the enzyme is expressed in response to any minor inflammatory or other pathological event.

Subsequent work failed to detect a significant difference in either MMP-2 or MMP-14 between keratoconic and normal epithelium[56], instead reporting higher levels of MMP-13 in the keratoconic epithelium compared to healthy specimens[56]. TNF-α and IL-1β increase corneal epithelial MMP-13 synthesis[57] while MMP-13 has been shown to activate MMP-9 *in vitro*[58]. The temporal and spatial correlation between MMP-13, MMP-9 and corneal re-epithelialisation suggests that MMP-13 plays a role in corneal reepithelialisation after injury[59]. MMP-13 activation seems to be much more prominent in bullous keratopathy than keratoconus[60].

Several studies report increased MMP-1 expression in keratoconus. The epithelia of healthy corneas and corneas with post LASIK keratectasia display nearly absent immunolabelling for MMP-1, whereas strong labelling occurs in the epithelium and stroma of keratoconic specimens[56,61,62]. MMP-1 is able to degrade many non-collagenous components of the extracellular matrix, including fibronectin, laminin, and basement membrane glycoproteins, but first and foremost, it cleaves native interstitial collagens types I and III[62].

MMP-1 can be effectively induced by the extracellular matrix metalloproteinase inducer (EMMPRIN), which is a member of the immunoglobulin superfamily of adhesion molecules[62]. In keratoconus, EMMPRIN expression was found in all layers of the cornea, especially in histopathologically altered areas, however, the distribution of MMP-1 did not totally overlap with histologically apparent corneal damage and EMMPRIN expression[62]. This may be because EMMPRIN upregulates other MMPs (MMP-2, MMP-3) in stromal fibroblasts. In areas of destruction EMMPRIN-inducible MMPs, other than MMP-1, may be participating in the local pathological process.

MMP-8 seems to be down-regulated in keratoconic epithelium compared to normal controls[56]. MMP-8 plays a paradoxical role in tissues, on the one hand being able to cleave collagens despite the presence of TIMPs and on the other controlling the inflammatory load in tissues by downregulating the polymorphonuclear (PMN) burden[63]. Unlike other MMPs epithelial MMP-8 is not upregulated by TNF-α and IL-1β[57]. Such MMPs may contribute to the pathogenesis of keratoconus by proteolytic modulation of proinflammatory cytokines or chemokines or the generation of apoptotic signals for inflammatory and corneal cells.

5.4 Stroma

Despite much research, contradictory reports preclude any conclusive statement on the contribution of specific MMPs to histopathological hallmarks found in the keratoconic corneal stroma.

In one study MMP-1, -2 and -13 immunolabelling was noted to be greater in keratoconic samples compared to normal controls while no difference in MMP-8 or MMP-14 immunolabelling was observed[56]. In another study, keratoconic immunolabelling for MMP-1, -2 and -3 resembled that of the normal cornea and post LASIK keratectasia[61] while peroxidase immunohistochemistry performed by Collier's group showed that MMP-14 was significantly elevated in the keratoconic stroma[55].

Stromal tissue layer supernatant showed no significant difference in MMP-2, MMP-9, pro MMP-13 and TIMP-1 concentrations between bullous keratopathy and keratoconus[60]. Keratocyte cultures from normal and keratoconic corneas also showed no significant changes in mRNA levels for MMP-1, -2, -3, TIMP-1, or TIMP-2[64]. Only TIMP-1 protein was decreased, prompting a three-fold increase in the MMP-2/TIMP-1 ratio in keratoconus[64].

Yet stromal cell cultures performed by Smith et al. found MMP-2 to be over-expressed in clear keratoconic and scarred keratoconic corneas[65]. The quantities of TIMP-1 and TIMP-2 in normal and clear keratoconic cultures were similar. Scarred keratoconic cultures over-expressed TIMP-1[65]. In these cultures the cells remained healthy and the extent of stress induced MMP-2 activation was low[65]. For this reason, in addition to inhibiting MMP activity, upregulated TIMP-1 production may be a feature of corneal scar tissue cells that are refractory to dying. Alternatively, TIMP-1 may prevent cell death that is conceivably initiated by upregulated TIMP-3 production and sequestration in the extracellular matrix[65].

5.5 Endothelium with Descemet's

There are only a few studies assessing MMP changes specific to Descemet's membrane and endothelium. The endothelial monolayer often gets damaged or lost as the result of tissue handling making studies technically difficult. It was noted that endothelial cells and Descemet's membrane were pathologically altered in keratoconus and EMMPRIN was expressed next to areas of histological damage without, however, any evidence of MMP-1 expression in the area[62]. Mackiewicz et al. did not detect a difference in MMP-1, -13 and -14 between keratoconus and healthy controls but did report more MMP-2 in the endothelium and Descemet's of keratoconus and less MMP-8 in the same layers compared to normal controls[56]. Endothelial tissue supernatant showed no significant difference in MMP-2, MMP-9, pro MMP-13 and TIMP-1 concentrations between bullous keratopathy and keratoconus[60].

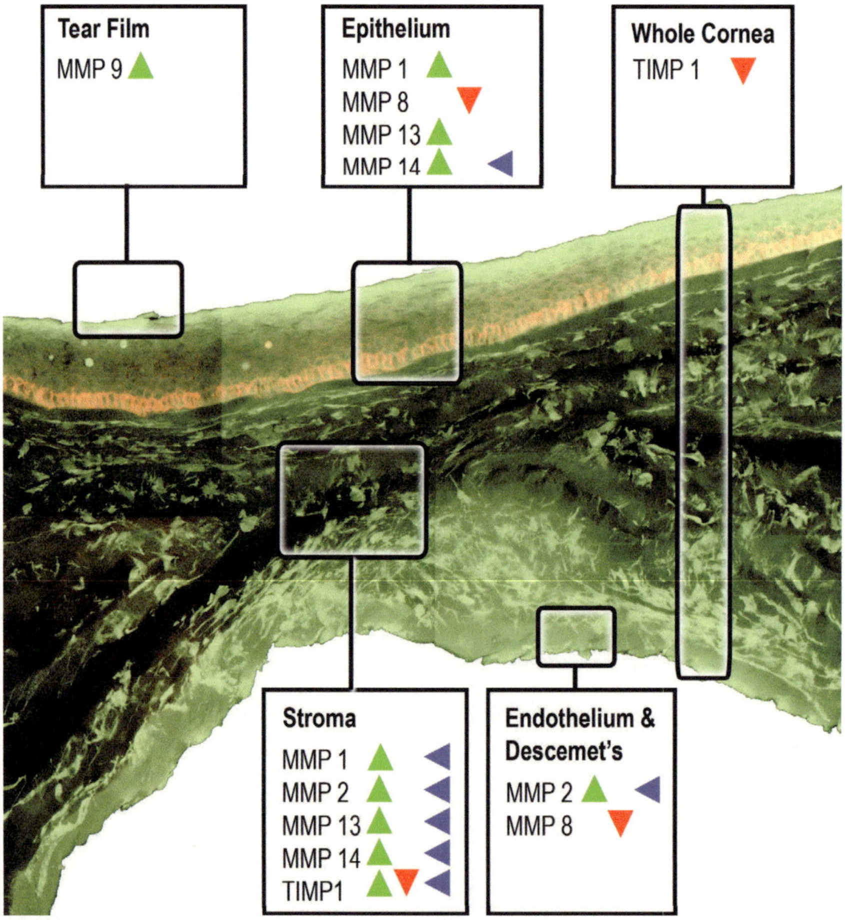

Fig. 2. Matrix metalloproteinase (MMP) and tissue inhibitor of matrix metalloproteinase (TIMP) changes have been described in every layer of the keratoconic cornea. Again, an antero-posterior section of a keratoconic cornea illustrated the MMP and TIMP molecules whose expression have been reported as altered in keratoconus. Green arrows represent increased expression, whilst red represents reported decreased expression and blue no change. It is evident in several cases that reported expression profiles are cotradictory.

6. Conclusion

MMPs are a group of proteolytic enzymes that are able to degrade the main components of the extracellular matrix and corneal membranes. Owing to these activities, MMPs are widely assumed to have a central role in the pathogenesis of keratoconus. However, studies have shown that MMPs can also handle substrates distinct from extracellular matrix proteins, influencing cell processes such as apoptosis. Proteolytic modulation of proinflammatory cytokines or chemokines or the generation of apoptotic signals for resident and inflammatory cells may prove to be as important in mediating keratoconus progression as purported extracellular matrix degradation.

The involvement of proteases in keratoconus has been the subject of much research; however, the exact nature of proteolytic phenomena that contribute to keratoconus progression remains unclear. Studies have described upregulation of MMP-1, MMP-2, MMP-9, MMP-13 and MMP-14 in keratoconus, yet this has not been seen consistently. Other authors report no change in MMP levels or else a downregulation of MMP-8 or TIMP-1. Increased activity of other proteinases such as cathepsins[66] likely contributes to the structural deterioration seen in keratoconus.

For MMP inhibition or TIMP upregulation to be considered a valid therapeutic target for amelioration of the disease process it is important to know exactly which MMPs are culpable. However, due to complex inter-molecular interactions between individual members of the MMP family, the ratios between various MMPs may turn out to be more significant to keratoconus pathogenesis than absolute concentrations of specific MMPs. The ability to measure multiple MMPs in a single corneal specimen is therefore necessary in order to understand the interplay of proteinases within the cornea. Tear fluid analysis affords the opportunity to investigate keratoconus protagonists in the earlier stages of the disease, a significant advantage over end-stage corneal tissue analysis. MMP changes are seen in many other corneal diseases, suggesting that MMP activation may be a nonspecific response to corneal insult. Indeed, the observed changes in inflammatory mediators or MMP levels within the cornea can in fact be epiphenomena of changes in corneal structure[35]. It is also possible that several diseases, with differing pathophysiology produce the phenotypic changes that are called keratoconus, accounting for the difference in proteinase profiles of examined keratoconic samples.

7. References

[1] Rabinowitz YS. Keratoconus. Surv Opthalmol. 1998; 42:297-319.
[2] Williams KA, Muehlberg SM, Lewis RF, Coster DJ. How succesful is corneal transplantation? A report from the Australian corneal graft register. Eye (Lond). 1995; 9:219-227.
[3] Vail A, Gore SM, Bradley BA, Easty DL, Rogers CA. Corneal transplantation in the United Kingdom and Northern Ireland. Brit J Ophthalmol. 1993; 77:650-6.
[4] Nottingham J. Practical observations on conical cornea: and on the short sight, and other defects of vision connected with it. 1854; London, John Churchill.
[5] Berliner ML. Biomicroscopy of the eye. 1943; New York, Paul B Hoeber Inc.
[6] Duke-Elder S. System of Ophthalmology. Vol VIII Diseases of the outer eye. 1965; London, Henry Kimpton.
[7] Sherwin T, Brookes NH. Morphological changes in keratoconus: pathology or pathogenesis. Clin Experiment Ophthalmol. 2004; 32(2):211-7.

[8] Scroggs MW, Proia AD. Histopathological variation in keratoconic corneas. Cornea. 1992; 11:553-559.
[9] Kim W-J, Rabinowitz YS, Meisler DM, Wilson SE. Keratocyte apoptosis associated with keratoconus. Exp Eye Res. 1999; 69:475-481.
[10] Sherwin T, Brookes NH, Loh I-P, Poole CA, Clover GM. Cellular incursion into Bowman's membrane in the peripheral cone of the keratoconic cornea. Exp Eye Res. 2002; 74:473-482.
[11] Erie JC, Patel SV, McLaren JW, Nau CB, Hodge DO, Bourne WM. Keratocyte density in keratoconus: A confocal microscopy study. Am J Ophth. 2002; 134:689-695.
[12] Somodi S, Hahnel C, Slowik C, Richter A, Weiss DG, Guthoff R. Confocal in vivo microscopy and confocal laser scanning fluorescence microscopy in keratoconus. Ger J Ophthalmol. 1997; 5:518-525.
[13] Kaldawy RM, Wagner J, Ching S, Seigel GM. Evidence of apoptotic cell death in keratoconus. Cornea. 2002; 21:206-209.
[14] Teng CC. Electron microscope study of the pathology of keratoconus: Part I. Am J Ophthalmol. 1963; 55:19-47.
[15] Tuori AJ, Virtanen I, Aine E, Kalluri R, Miner JH, Uusitalo HM. The immunohistochemical composition of corneal basement membrane in keratoconus. Curr Eye Res. 1997; 16:792-801.
[16] Cheng EL, Maruyama I, SundarRaj N, Sugar J, Feder RS, Yue BY. Expression of type XII collagen and hemidesmosome-associated proteins in keratoconus corneas. Curr Eye Res. 2001; 22:333-340.
[17] Brookes NH, Loh I-P, Clover GM, Poole CA, Sherwin T. Involvement of corneal nerves in the progression of keratoconus. Exp Eye Res. 2003; 77:515-524.
[18] Sawaguchi S, Fukuchi T, Abe H, Kaiya T, Sugar J, Yue, BT. Three dimensional scanning electron microscopic study of keratoconus corneas. Arch Ophthalmol. 1998; 116:62-68.
[19] Kenney MC, Nesburn AB, Burgeson RE, Butkowski RJ, Ljubimov AV. Abnormalities of the extracellular matrix in keratoconus corneas. Cornea. 1997; 16:345-51.
[20] Takahashi A, Nakayasu K, Okisaka S, Kanai A. Quantitative analysis of collagen fibres in keratoconus. Acta Soc Ophthalmol Jap. 1990; 90:1068-73.
[21] Fullwood NJ, Tuft SJ, Malik NS, Meek KM, Ridgway AEA, Harrison RJ. Synchrotron X-ray diffraction studies of keratoconus corneal stroma. Invest Ophthalmol Vis Sci. 1992; 33:1734-41.
[22] Daxer A, Fratzl P. Collagen fibril orientation in the human corneal stroma and its implication in keratoconus. Invest Ophthalmol Vis Sci. 1997; 38:1289-90.
[23] Critchfield JW, Calandra AJ, Nesburn AB, Kenney MCR. Keratoconus I. Biochemical Studies. Exp Eye Res. 1988; 46:953-64.
[24] Radda TM, Menzel EJ, Freyler H, Gnad HD. Collagen types in keratoconus. Graefes Arch Clin Exp Ophthalmol. 1982; 218:262-6.
[25] Zimmermann DR, Fischer RW, Winterhalter KH, Witmer R, Vaughan L. Comparative studies of collagens in normal and keratoconus corneas. Exp Eye Res. 1988; 46:431-42.
[26] Rock ME, Moore MN, Anderson JA, Binder PS. 3-D computer models of human keratocytes. CLAO J. 1995; 21:57-60.
[27] Wygledowska-Promienska D, Rokita-Wala I, Gierek-Ciaciura S, Piatek-Koronowska G. The alterations in corneal structure at III/IV stage of keratoconus by means of confocal microscopy and ultrasound biomicroscopy before penetrating keratoplasty. Klinika Oczna. 1999; 101:427-432.
[28] Jongebloed WL, Dijk F, Worst JG. Keratoconus morphology and cell dystrophy: a SEM study. Documenta Ophthalmologica. 1989; 72:403-409.

[29] Bechrakis N, Blom ML, Stark WJ, Green WR. Recurrent keratoconus. Cornea. 1994; 13:73-77.
[30] Krivoy D, McCormick S, Zaidman GW. Postkeratoplasty keratoconus in a nonkeratoconus patient. Am J Ophthalmol. 2001; 131:653-654.
[31] Bourges J-L, Salvoldelli M, Dighiero P, Assouline M, Pouliquen Y, BenEzra D, Renard G, Behar-Cohen F. A clinical and histologic follow up analysis of donor grafts. Ophthalmol. 2003; 110:1920-1925.
[32] Brookes NH, Niederer RL, Hickey DG, McGhee CNJ, Sherwin T. Recurrence of keratoconic pathology in penetrating keratoplasty buttons originally transplanted for keratoconus. Cornea. 2009; 28: 688-693.
[33] Brinckerhoff CE, Matrisian LM. Matrix metalloproteinases: a tail of a frog that became a prince. Nat Rev Mol Cell Biol. 2002; 3(3):207-14.
[34] Collier SA. Is the corneal degradation in keratoconus caused by matrix-metalloproteinases? Clin Experiment Ophthalmol. 2001; 29(6):340-4.
[35] Lema I, Sobrino T, Durán JA, Brea D, Díez-Feijoo E. Subclinical keratoconus and inflammatory molecules from tears. Br J Ophthalmol. 2009; 93(6):820-4.
[36] Fournié PR, Gordon GM, Dawson DG, Edelhauser HF, Fini ME. Correlations of long-term matrix metalloproteinase localization in human corneas after successful laser-assisted in situ keratomileusis with minor complications at the flap margin. Arch Ophthalmol. 2008; 126(2):162-70.
[37] Abalain JH, Dossou H, Colin J, Floch HH. Levels of collagen degradation products (telopeptides) in the tear film of patients with keratoconus. Cornea. 2000; 19:474–6.
[38] Fukuchi T, Yue BY, Sugar J, Lam S. Lysosomal enzyme activities in conjunctival tissues of patients with keratoconus. Arch Ophthalmol. 1994; 112(10):1368-74.
[39] De Paiva CS, Harris LD, Pflugfelder SC. Keratoconus-like topographic changes in keratoconjunctivitis sicca. Cornea. 2003; 22(1):22-4.
[40] Lema I, Durán JA. Inflammatory molecules in the tears of patients with keratoconus. Ophthalmology. 2005; 112(4):654-9.
[41] Li DQ, Lokeshwar BL, Solomon A, Monroy D, Ji Z, Pflugfelder SC. Regulation of MMP-9 production by human corneal epithelial cells. Exp Eye Res. 2001; 73:449–59.
[42] Sonoda S, Uchino E, Nakao K, Sakamoto T. Inflammatory cytokine of basal and reflex tears analysed by multicytokine assay. Br J Ophthalmol. 2006; 90(1):120-2.
[43] Cook EB. Tear cytokines in acute and chronic ocular allergic inflammation. Curr Opin Allergy Clin Immunol. 2004; 4(5):441-5.
[44] Jacq PL, Sale Y, Cochener B, Lozach P, Colin J. Keratoconus, changes in corneal topography and allergy. Study of 3 groups of patients. J Fr Ophtalmol. 1997; 20(2):97-102.
[45] Bawazeer AM, Hodge WG, Lorimer B. Atopy and keratoconus: a multivariate analysis. Br J Ophthalmol. 2000; 84(8):834-6.
[46] Dogru M, Karakaya H, Özçetin H, Ertürk H, Yücel A, Ozmen A, Baykara M, Tsubota K. Tear function and ocular surface changes in keratoconus. Ophthalmology. 2003; 110:1110–8.
[47] Chotikavanich S, de Paiva CS, Li de Q, Chen JJ, Bian F, Farley WJ, Pflugfelder SC. Production and activity of matrix metalloproteinase-9 on the ocular surface increase in dysfunctional tear syndrome. Invest Ophthalmol Vis Sci. 2009; 50(7):3203-9.
[48] Smith VA, Rishmawi H, Hussein H, Easty DL. Tear film MMP accumulation and corneal disease. Br J Ophthalmol 2001; 85:147–53.
[49] Pflugfelder SC, Farley W, Luo L, Chen LZ, de Paiva CS, Olmos LC, Li DQ, Fini ME. Matrix metalloproteinase-9 knockout confers resistance to corneal epithelial barrier disruption in experimental dry eye. Am J Pathol. 2005; 166(1):61-71.
[50] Brenneisen P, Briviba K, Wlaschek M, Wenk J, Scharffetter-Kochanek K. Hydrogen peroxide (H2O2) increases the steady-state mRNA levels of collagenase/MMP-1 in human dermal fibroblasts. Free Radic Biol Med. 1997; 22(3):515-24.

[51] Kawaguchi Y, Tanaka H, Okada T, Konishi H, Takahashi M, Ito M, Asai J. The effects of ultraviolet A and reactive oxygen species on the mRNA expression of 72-kDa type IV collagenase and its tissue inhibitor in cultured human dermal fibroblasts. Arch Dermatol Res. 1996; 288(1):39-44.
[52] Kenney MC, Chwa M, Atilano SR, Tran A, Carballo M, Saghizadeh M, Vasiliou V, Adachi W, Brown DJ. Increased levels of catalase and cathepsin V/L2 but decreased TIMP-1 in keratoconus corneas: evidence that oxidative stress plays a role in this disorder. Invest Ophthalmol Vis Sci. 2005; 46(3):823-32.
[53] Matthews FJ, Cook SD, Majid MA, Dick AD, Smith VA. Changes in the balance of the tissue inhibitor of matrix metalloproteinases (TIMPs)-1 and -3 may promote keratocyte apoptosis in keratoconus. Exp Eye Res. 2007 Jun; 84(6):1125-34.
[54] Saghizadeh M, Brown DJ, Castellon R, Chwa M, Huang GH, Ljubimova JY, Rosenberg S, Spirin KS, Stolitenko RB, Adachi W, Kinoshita S, Murphy G, Windsor LJ, Kenney MC, Ljubimov AV. Overexpression of matrix metalloproteinase-10 and matrix metalloproteinase-3 in human diabetic corneas: a possible mechanism of basement membrane and integrin alterations. Am J Pathol. 2001; 158(2):723-34.
[55] Collier SA, Madigan MC, Penfold PL. Expression of membrane-type 1 matrix metalloproteinase (MT1-MMP) and MMP-2 in normal and keratoconus corneas. Curr Eye Res. 2000; 21(2):662-8.
[56] Mackiewicz Z, Määttä M, Stenman M, Konttinen L, Tervo T, Konttinen YT. Collagenolytic proteinases in keratoconus. Cornea. 2006; 25(5):603-10.
[57] Li DQ, Shang TY, Kim HS, Solomon A, Lokeshwar BL, Pflugfelder SC. Regulated expression of collagenases MMP-1, -8, and -13 and stromelysins MMP-3, -10, and -11 by human corneal epithelial cells. Invest Ophthalmol Vis Sci. 2003; 44(7):2928-36.
[58] Knäuper V, Smith B, López-Otin C, Murphy G. Activation of progelatinase B (proMMP-9) by active collagenase-3 (MMP-13). Eur J Biochem. 1997; 248(2):369-73.
[59] Ye HQ, Maeda M, Yu FS, Azar DT. Differential expression of MT1-MMP (MMP-14) and collagenase III (MMP-13) genes in normal and wounded rat corneas. Invest Ophthalmol Vis Sci. 2000; 41(10):2894-9.
[60] Predović J, Balog T, Marotti T, Gabrić N, Bohac M, Romac I, Dekaris I. The expression of human corneal MMP-2, MMP-9, proMMP-13 and TIMP-1 in bullous keratopathy and keratoconus. Coll Antropol. 2008; 32 Suppl 2:15-9.
[61] Meghpara B, Nakamura H, Macsai M, Sugar J, Hidayat A, Yue BY, Edward DP. Keratectasia after laser in situ keratomileusis: a histopathologic and immunohistochemical study. Arch Ophthalmol. 2008; 126(12):1655-63.
[62] Seppälä HP, Määttä M, Rautia M, Mackiewicz Z, Tuisku I, Tervo T, Konttinen YT. EMMPRIN and MMP-1 in keratoconus. Cornea. 2006; 25(3):325-30.
[63] Owen CA, Hu Z, Lopez-Otin C, Shapiro SD. Membrane-bound matrix metalloproteinase-8 on activated polymorphonuclear cells is a potent, tissue inhibitor of metalloproteinase-resistant collagenase and serpinase. J Immunol. 2004; 172(12):7791-803.
[64] Kenney MC, Chwa M, Opbroek AJ, Brown DJ. Increased gelatinolytic activity in keratoconus keratocyte cultures. A correlation to an altered matrix metalloproteinase-2/tissue inhibitor of metalloproteinase ratio. Cornea. 1994; 13(2):114-24.
[65] Smith VA, Matthews FJ, Majid MA, Cook SD. Keratoconus: matrix metalloproteinase-2 activation and TIMP modulation. Biochim Biophys Acta. 2006; 1762(4):431-9.
[66] Zhou L, Sawaguchi S, Twining SS, Sugar J, Feder RS, Yue BY. Expression of degradative enzymes and protease inhibitors in corneas with keratoconus. Invest Ophthalmol Vis Sci. 1998; 39(7):1117-24.

7

Corneal Surgical Techniques

Miroslav Vukosavljević, Milorad Milivojević and Mirko Resan
Eye Clinic, Military Medical Academy, Belgrade, Serbia

1. Introduction

1.1 History of corneal refractive surgery

There is a long history of corneal refractive surgery. Leonardo Da Vinci in 1508 said the theory of refractive errors. The first systematic analysis of the nature and results of refractive errors came from Francis Cornelius Donders. His classic treatise, "On the anomalies of accommodation and refraction of the eye", outlined the fundamental principles of physiological optics. Ironically, in this treatise, Donders railed against surgical attempts to correct refractive errors by altering the corneal shape. In 1885 Hjalmar Schiotz performed corneal incision to correct astigmatism. Modern refractive surgery extended corneal reshaping to treat myopia and astigmatism. Throughout the 1930s and 1940s, Sato published several reports, describing his attempts to refine incisional refractive surgery with anterior and posterior corneal incisions. The Russian ophthalmologist, Fyodorov later developed a systematic process of anterior radial keratotomy and treated thousands of myopic patients with greater predictability. Lamellar surgery was first introduced by Jose Barraquer. He invented keratoplasty procedures that involved the transplantation of corneal tissue of a size different from the host size to alter the curvature of cornea. He also invented a series of lamellar procedures and developed a formula that represented the relationship between the added corneal thickness and the change in refractive power, later called Barraquer's law of thickness. The transition from incisional to ablative laser refractive surgery arose with the development of Excimer laser technology. Excimer lasers use argon fluoride gases to emit ultraviolet laser pulses. Taboda and Archibald reported the use of the Excimer laser to reshape the corneal epithelium in 1981. In 1983, Trokel and colleagues showed how the Excimer laser could be used to ablate bovine corneal stroma. In 1985, Seiler did the first Excimer laser treatment in a blind eye. He later did the first Excimer laser astigmatic keratotomy. In 1989, McDonald and colleagues did the first photorefractive keratectomy on a seeing eye with myopia. Jose Barraquer's pioneering work, including the use of lamellar procedures to subtract corneal stromal tissue and the development of the first microkerotomes, set the stage for laser in situ keratomileusis (LASIK) surgery. Ruiz and Rowsey modified Barraquer's technique to perform keratomileusis in situ with a geared automated microkeratome. In the early 1990s, Pallikaris and colleagues and Buratto and colleagues independently described a technique that combined two existing technologies: the microkeratome and the Excimer laser. Pallikaris coined the term LASIK for this new technique, which has become a widely used refractive technique worldwide (1).

1.2 Introduction

Astigmatism is a unique refractive error that causes reduced visual acuity and produces symptoms of glare, monocular diplopia, asthenopia, and distortion. The control and correction of astigmatism has been a topic of great interest to cataract, refractive and corneal surgeons.

Corneal refractive surgical techniques that can correct astigmatism are: incisional surgical techniques, such as arcuate keratotomy and limbal relaxing incisions; laser-assisted *in situ* keratomileusis (LASIK); and surface ablation techniques, such as photorefractive keratectomy (PRK), *trans*-epithelial PRK (tPRK), laser-assisted subepithelial keratomileusis (LASEK), epi-LASIK and Intralase.

Arcuate keratotomy is an incisional surgical technique in which arcuate incisions of approximately 95% depth are made in the corneal midperipheral 7,0 mm zone placed in the steep meridian(s). Arcuate keratotomy was used to correct naturally occuring astigmatism, but it is now used primarily to correct postkeratoplasty astigmatism. Limbal relaxing incisions are incisions set at approximately 600 μm depth, or 50 μm less than the thinnest pachymetry at the limbus, and placed just anterior to the limbus. Limbal relaxing incisions are used to manage astigmatism during or after phacoemulsification and intraocular lens (IOL) implantation (2).

LASIK is a lamellar laser refractive surgical technique in which the Excimer laser ablation is done under a partial-thickness lamellar corneal flap. The lamellar flap could be made with a microkeratome or with a femtosecond laser. The microkeratome uses an oscillating blade to cut the flap after immobilization of the cornea with a suction ring. Microkeratomes from several companies cut the lamellar flaps with either superior or nasal hinges, and can cut to depths of 100–200 μm. A femtosecond laser has been developed that can etch lamellar flaps within the cornea stroma at a desired corneal depth. The femtosecond laser provides more accuracy in flap thickness than previous methods; the microkeratome cuts can vary widely in depth. The ablation might either correct sphere and cylinder error, or is wavefront-guided. After the ablation has been completed, the stromal bed is irrigated and the corneal flap is repositioned (3).

Surface ablation is a generic term referring to the application of Excimer laser directly on the anterior stromal surface. The epithelium is removed in order for the Excimer laser to be applied to the stroma. There are several ways in which the epithelium can be separated from Bowmans layer. The epithelium can be fashioned as a flap and replaced (as in LASEK and epi-LASIK) or removed (as in PRK). Surface ablation techniques are continuously evolving in order to achieve better results with faster visual recovery and less pain (4).

LASIK and PRK are the most commonly used refractive surgical methods worldwide.

2. Laser in situ keratomileusis (LASIK)

Laser in situ keratomileusis (LASIK) is the most commonly used refractive surgical method worldwide. This method employs two technologies: Excimer laser and microkeratome. Excimer (acronym for excited dimer) laser is an ultraviolet gas laser (argon-fluoride, ArF) with wavelength of 193 nm, which achieves photoablative effect on tissue of corneal stroma.

First, microkeratome cuts through the cornea and make intrastromal flap on hinge. Flap has a diameter from 8 to 10 mm and its thickness can be 100-180 μm, but usually 100-130 μm (about 15-35% of total corneal thickness). Then the flap is lifted and the corneal stroma exposed to the Excimer laser, and stroma is remodeled according to the type of ametropia and its values. On the end of Excimer laser the flap is repositioned and for a short time have stable position without of need for sutures (5). Postoperative visual rehabilitation is rapid. Sixteen hours after LASIK the majority of patients are reaching 97% of the preoperative best corrected visual acuity (6).

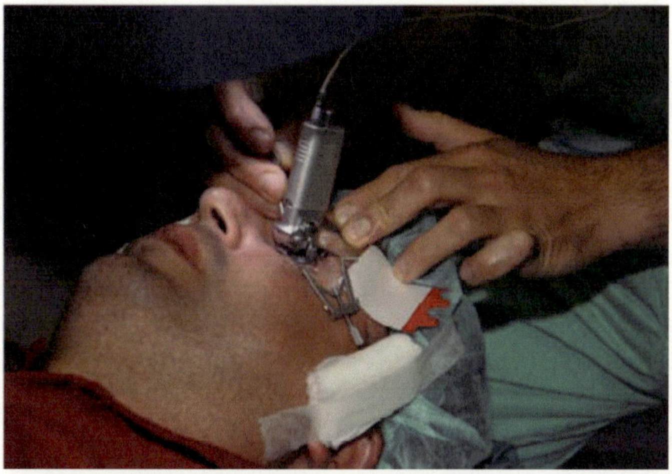

Fig. 1. Placing of suction ring and microkeratome on the eye (5).

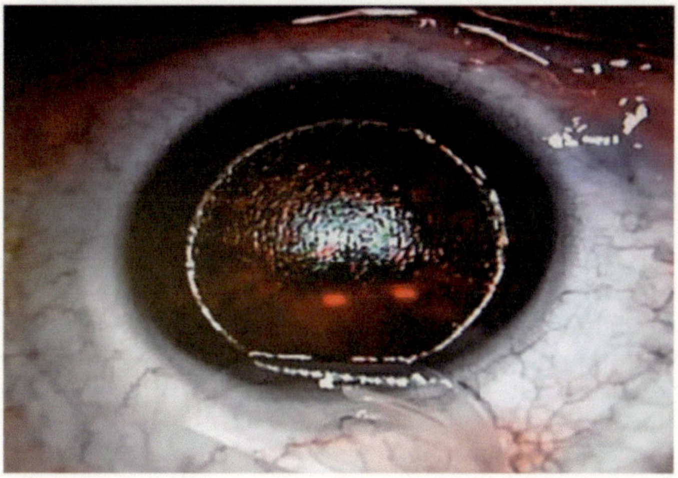

Fig. 2. Flap is created and corneal stroma prepared for Excimer laser ablation (5).

The American Academy of Ophthalmology (AAO) recommended the indications for LASIK: myopia up to - 10 Dsph, hyperopia up to + 4 Dsph, and astigmatism up to 4 Dcyl (7).

The contraindications for Excimer laser refractive surgery including LASIK and PRK are general and ophthalmic. General are: immunological diseases (autoimmune, collagen vascular, immune deficiency); pregnancy or breast feeding; the tendency to form keloids; diabetes; and systemic administration of isotretionin or amiodarone. Ophthalmic are: dry eye; neurotrophic keratitis; herpes zoster ophthalmicus / keratitis herpetica; glaucoma; ectatic corneal dystrophy (keratoconus, keratoglobus); highly irregular astigmatism; uveitis, diabetic retinopathy; progressive retinal disease and previously performed radial keratotomy (8).

The complications of LASIK include: intraoperative and postoperative complications. The intraoperative complications or flap related complications (9) are: wrong ablation, flap loss, buttonhole flap (hole in the flap), thin flap, brief flap, free cap (flap amputation), corneal bleeding, epithelial defects and corneal perforation (very rare). The postoperative complications (10) are: infections, dislocation of the flap, flap folding (striae), diffuse lamellar keratitis (sands of the Sahara), epithelial ingrowth, corneal ectasia, regression, intraflap fluid accumulation and paradoxical hypotony.

Each candidate for LASIK should be at least 21 years of age and must have a stable refractive error in the period of two years. Preoperative evaluation of each candidate includes: general and ophthalmic history; autorefractokeratometry; uncorrected visual acuity (UCVA) and best corrected visual acuity (BCVA); Schirmer test; review of the eye anterior segment on slit-lamp; applanation tonometry; review of the eye fundus in a wide pupil; imaging of corneal topography and aberrometry. The following formula to evaluate whether a candidate can safely perform LASIK is:

Central pachymetry – flap thickness - ablation depth = residual stromal thickness of the cornea

As a limit value for residual stromal thickness of the cornea (residual stromal bed) after cutting and effects of Excimer laser 300 μm are taken; as a critical value for steep corneal meridian (steep K) <39 or > 47 D are taken; as a limit value for elevation of the posterior corneal surface 50 μm are taken (5).

Numerous studies confirm the effectiveness of LASIK for the correction of astigmatism. Stojanovic and Nitter evaluated safety, efficacy, predictability, and stability in the treatment of myopic astigmatism with LASIK and PRK using the 200 Hz flying-spot technology of the Excimer laser. This retrospective study included 110 eyes treated with LASIK and 87 eyes treated with PRK that were available for evaluation at 6 and 12 months. The mean preoperative spherical equivalent (SE) was −5.35 diopters (D) ± 2.50 (SD) (range −1.13 to −11.88 D) in the LASIK eyes and −4.72 ± 2.82 D (range −1.00 to −15.50 D) in the PRK eyes. The treated astigmatism was 4.00 D in both groups. None of the eyes lost 2 or more lines of best spectacle-corrected visual acuity. Seventy-seven percent of the LASIK eyes and 78% of the PRK eyes achieved an uncorrected visual acuity of 20/20 or better; 98% in both groups achieved 20/40 or better. In conclusion, Excimer laser was safe, effective, and predictable and with LASIK and PRK the results are stable when treating low to moderate myopia and astigmatism up to 4.0 D (11). Ditzen et al evaluated safety, predictability, efficacy, and stability of LASIK for spherical hyperopia and hyperopia with astigmatism. This retrospective study analyzed the results of 23 eyes of 23 patients who had LASIK for spherical hyperopia (preoperative astigmatism $\leq$0.75 D) and 44 eyes of 44 patients who had LASIK for hyperopia with astigmatism. In group 1 (spherical hyperopia), mean preoperative spherical equivalent refraction was +4.88 ± 2.13 D (range +2.13 to +9.63 D); in group 2 (hyperopic astigmatism), +4.33 ± 2.15 D (range +0.50 to +9.50 D). One year after LASIK, mean spherical equivalent refraction was +0.30 ± 0.90 D (range -0.75 to +2.50 D) in group 1 and +0.29 ± 1.27 D (range -3.25 to +3.25 D) in group 2. In group 1, no eyes lost two or more lines, and one eye (6%) lost one line of best spectacle-corrected visual acuity at 1 year. In group 2, one eye (4%) lost one line and one eye (4%) lost more than two lines at 1 year. Uncorrected visual acuity of 20/40 or better was achieved in 83% (group 1) vs. 62% (group 2) at 1 year. In conclusion, LASIK seemed to be safe and effective for hyperopia and hyperopia with astigmatism for corrections up to +6.00 D (12). Albarran-Diego et al evaluated bitoric LASIK for the correction of mixed astigmatism. This prospective study included 28 eyes of 21 patients with mixed astigmatism who had bitoric LASIK. Six months after bitoric LASIK, the mean UCVA was 0.70 ± 0.23 (SD). The percentage of eyes with a UCVA of 20/40 or better was 78.6% and of 20/20, 21.4%. There was a statistically significant increase in the mean BCVA from 0.71 ± 0.19 before surgery to 0.83 ± 0.15 at 6 months. Three eyes (10.7%) lost 1 line of BCVA. The mean preoperative astigmatism of −4.04 ± 1.13 diopters (D) was reduced to −0.67 ± 0.79 D after surgery (13).

3. Photorefractive keratectomy (PRK)

Photorefractive keratectomy (PRK) is still a successful method in certain indications and now is used worldwide as PRK or as its modification - LASEK and EpiLASIK. All methods for its performance require use of Excimer laser (14).

PRK is superficial ablative method because the Excimer laser thinner and reshapes the anterior part of the corneal stroma just below Bowman's membrane. This provides greater residual stromal thickness, and thus strengthens the biomechanical strength of the cornea. But, ablation of front stroma, especially through a layer of Bowman's membrane, causing aggressive response in wound healing, which may result in frequent appearance of subepithelial clouding (haze) and scarring compared with LASIK. Recovery after PRK is slower and more painful compared with LASIK. One to four days after the intervention most of the patients have a transient low-intensity pain. Postoperative visual rehabilitation is a little longer and lasts several weeks (1,15).

Certain situations may favor PRK over LASIK in particular safety issues due to the absence of flap related complications in PRK. These situations include: predisposition for contact injury (e.g. those involved in martial arts or boxing); anterior basement membrane (BM) dystrophy; epithelial sloughing during LASIK in the fellow eye; thin corneas in which the residual stromal bed would be less than 250–300 mm; deep set eyes or a small palpebral aperture (poor exposure for the microkeratome); previous surgery involving the conjunctiva (e.g. glaucoma drainage bleb, scleral buckle); and moderate dry eye before surgery. In addition, flat (< 41 D) or steep corneas (> 48 D), with the risk of free, thin, incomplete or buttonholed flaps, may be better suited to PRK. It is desirable to avoid suction and iatrogenically raising the IOP during LASIK, as in patients with glaucoma or a risk of poor optic nerve perfusion, PRK procedure would be preferred (15).

In PRK the first step is corneal epithelium removing (mechanically with knife-hockey or rotating brush; or by chemical abrasion with 20% ethanol), then the corneal stroma is exposed to the effects of Excimer laser which thins and reshapes it according to the type of ametropia and its values and after that therapeutic soft contact lens is applied for 5 days.

The American Academy of Ophthalmology (AAO) recommended the next indications for PRK: myopia up to - 8 Dsph, hyperopia up to + 4 Dsph, and astigmatism up to 4 Dcyl (7). Large corrections (ablation depth greater than 100 μm) are considered for adjunctive 0,02% mitomycin C (MMC) because of the increased risk of postoperative haze and regression (16).

Complications of PRK include: subepithelial haze, corneal scarring, ectasia and regression.

Each candidate for PRK should be at least 21 years of age and must have a stable refractive error in the period of two years. Preoperative evaluation of each candidate includes: general and ophthalmic history; autorefractokeratometry; uncorrected visual acuity (UCVA) and best corrected visual acuity (BCVA) in each eye; Schirmer test; examination of the eye anterior segment on slit-lamp; applanation tonometry; examination of the eye fundus in a wide pupil; imaging of corneal topography and aberrometry. As a limit value for residual stromal thickness of the cornea (residual stromal bed) is 300 μm. The critical value for steep corneal meridian (steep K) is <39 or > 47 D and the limit value for elevation of the posterior corneal surface is 50 μm (5).

Numerous studies have investigated the effectiveness of PRK in the correction of astigmatism. Haw and Manche evaluated the safety and efficacy of PRK for the treatment of primary compound myopic astigmatism. Ninety three eyes from 56 patients with a mean spherical equivalent of −4.98 ± 1.80 diopters (range, −1.75 to −8.5) underwent photoastigmatic refractive keratectomy and were followed for 2 years. Fifty-six eyes (94.9%) had an uncorrected visual acuity of 20/40 or greater, whereas 34 eyes (57.6 %) demonstrated an uncorrected visual acuity of 20/20 or greater. One eye (1.7%) lost 2 or more lines of best spectacle-corrected visual acuity (17). Nagy et al evaluated the results of PRK using Gaussian flying spot technology in the treatment of hyperopia and hyperopic astigmatism. Two hundred eyes were evaluated with 12-month follow-up. Eyes were divided into four groups: group 1 (spherical hyperopia up to +3.50 D and astigmatism less than 1.00 D, n=62); group 2 (hyperopia up to +3.50 D and astigmatism of 1.00 D or more, n=44); group 3 (hyperopia greater than +3.50 D and astigmatism less than 1.00 D, n=56); and group 4 (hyperopia greater than +3.50 D and astigmatism of 1.00 D or more, n=38). In group 1, 82.2% (51/62 eyes) were within ±0.50 D of target refraction; 88.7% (55/62 eyes) had 20/20 or better uncorrected visual acuity; 1.6% (1/62 eye) lost two or more lines. In group 2, 68.1% (30/44 eyes) were within ±0.50 D; 77.2% (34/44 eyes) had 20/20 or better uncorrected visual acuity; 9.1% (4/44 eyes) lost two or more lines of spectacle-corrected visual acuity. In group 3, 76.8% (43/56 eyes) were within ±0.50 D; 78.6% (44/56 eyes) had 20/20 or better uncorrected visual acuity; 5.4% (3/56 eyes) lost two or more lines of spectacle-corrected visual acuity. In group 4, 42% (16/38 eyes) were within ±0.50 D; 60.5% (23/38 eyes) had 20/20 or better uncorrected visual acuity; 15.8% (6/38 eyes) lost two or more Snellen lines. In conclusion PRK was most safe and effective for low hyperopia (18).

4. Trans-epithelial photorefractive keratectomy (tPRK)

In this method, the Excimer laser is used to ablate the epithelium in addition to then ablating the underlying stroma. The cornea undergoes an epithelial ablation within a fixed diameter. The operating room lights are turned off as blue fluorescent light is emitted whereas epithelium is ablated. Once the blue fluorescence disappears, this indicates that the epithelium has been removed. Accuracy with this method is dependent upon regular epithelial thickness across the diameter treatment zone and also similar epithelial thicknesses between different eyes. This technique can produce variable results when laser surface enhancement is proposed after previous refractive surgery due to areas of epithelial hyperplasia causing variable epithelial thickness (15).

5. Laser-assisted subepithelial keratomileusis (LASEK)

LASEK is a surgical procedure that combines certain elements of both LASIK and PRK to improve the risk/benefit ratio. Diluted alcohol is used to loosen the epithelial adhesion to the corneal stroma. The loosened epithelium is moved aside from the treatment zone as a hinged sheet. Laser ablation of the subepithelial stroma is performed before the epithelial sheet is returned to its original position. The main rationale for combining elements of LASIK and PRK to LASEK is to avoid the flap-related LASIK complications and the slow visual recovery and haze risk of PRK. LASEK may avoid several of the inherent complications, including free caps, incomplete pass of the microkeratome, flap wrinkles, epithelial ingrowth, flap melt, interface debris, corneal ectasia, and diffuse lamellar keratitis, after LASIK and postoperative pain, subepithelial haze, and slow visual rehabilitation after PRK. Current ophthalmic literature does not provide the specific indications, visual outcomes, complications, and limitations of LASEK (19). Bilgihan et al. evaluated the efficacy, predictability, and safety of LASEK for treatment of high myopia with astigmatism. LASEK was performed in 61 eyes of 36 consecutive patients with myopic spherical equivalent refraction of -6.00 to -10.00 D using the Aesculap-Meditec MEL60 Excimer laser. Ninety-six percent of eyes achieved 20/40 or better uncorrected visual acuity (UCVA) at 1 month. At 12 months, 64% of eyes achieved 20/20 and 92% achieved 20/40 or better UCVA. Two eyes lost 2 lines of best spectacle-corrected visual acuity (BSCVA) at 6 or 12 months. Accuracy of correction was ±0.50 D from emmetropia in 82% of eyes, and ±1.00 D in 90% at 12 months (20). Taneri et al evaluated the visual outcomes and complications in low to moderate levels of myopia and astigmatism treated with LASEK. One hundred seventy-one eyes of 105 patients were studied. Preoperatively, the mean spherical equivalent was -2.99 diopters (D) ± 1.43 (SD) and the mean cylinder -0.78 ± 0.73 D. One week postoperatively, 96% of eyes had a UCVA of 20/40 or better but definitive visual recovery took more than 4 weeks in some eyes. Approximately 95% of eyes were within ±1.0 D of emmetropia after 4 to 52 weeks; the remaining 5% did not show major deviations. At 4 to 52 weeks, only 1 eye was overcorrected by more than 1.0 D of manifest refraction (21).

6. Epithelial laser in situ keratomileusis (Epi-LASIK)

Epi-LASIK has proved to be a suitable procedure, especially in patients with active lifestyles or occupations, eyes with thin corneas without ectatic disorders, and patients with moderate dry-eye syndrome. In epi-LASIK, an epithelial flap is created with the help of a special microkeratome. The epithelial flap is repositioned on the cornea after photoablation. It has been postulated that compared with conventional laser-assisted subepithelial keratectomy (LASEK), in which an epithelial flap is created after the epithelium is exposed to an alcohol solution, cell viability of the epithelial sheet is better in epi-LASIK surgery, in which mechanical separation is performed with a microkeratome. The quality of the epithelial separation is crucial for the success of the procedure because stromal lacerations or remaining islands of basal epithelial cells would reduce the optical quality of the cornea after photoablation (22).

Factor	PRK	LASEK	EPI-LASIK	LASIK
Range of correction	Low to moderately high			Low to moderately high
Postoperative pain	Mild to moderate 24–72 hours			Minimum 12 hours
Postoperative medications	1–3 months			1 week
Functional vision recovery	3 to 7 days			<24 hours
Refractive stability achieved	3 weeks to 3 months			1 week to 3 months
Specific complications	Haze formation, scarring	Haze formation, scarring	Haze formation, scarring, incomplete epithelial flap, stromal incursions	Free caps, incomplete pass of microkeratome, flap wrinkles, epithelial ingrowth, flap melt, interface debris, corneal ectasia, diffuse lamellar keratitis
Dry-eye sensitive	1 to 6 months			1 to 12 months
Thin corneas or wide pupils	Often not contraindicated			May be contraindicated depending on amount of intended correction
Special (relative) indications	Thin corneal pachymetry, wide scotopic pupil, LASIK complications in fellow eye, predisposition to trauma, keratoconus suspect (irregular astigmatism), glaucoma suspect, recurrent erosion syndrome, dry-eye syndrome, basement membrane disease			Concern about postoperative pain, requirement of rapid visual recovery
Special (relative) contraindications	Concern about postoperative pain, requirement of rapid visual recovery	Concern about postoperative pain, requirement of rapid visual recovery	Concern about postoperative pain, requirement of rapid visual recovery, glaucoma, scleral buckle, deep-set eyes, small palpebral fissure	Thin corneas, wide pupils, recurrent erosion syndrome, glaucoma, scleral buckle, deep-set eyes, small palpebral fissure

Fig. 3. Widely accepted relative differences between PRK, LASEK, epi-LASIK, and LASIK (23).

7. Femtosecond laser in laser in situ keratomileusis

In the early 1960s, Barraquer introduced the concept of lamellar refractive procedures. In the 1990s, Pallikaris et al. and Buratto et al. conceived of techniques combining lamellar procedures with Excimer laser ablation. These advances led to the development of modern laser in situ keratomileusis (LASIK) procedures. LASIK has several advantages over PRK when performed properly in appropriate eyes. These include faster visual recovery, less discomfort after surgery, and milder and more predictable wound healing with less risk for corneal stromal opacity (haze). Lamellar corneal flap formation is the critical step in successful LASIK surgery. Improper flap formation, including improper flap geometry, decentration, irregularity of the cut, and epithelial damage, can lead to myriad LASIK complications. Considerable progress has been made over the years in producing safer instruments for LASIK flap formation since the Automated Corneal Shaper was adapted to LASIK. Thus, more reliable and safer mechanical microkeratomes contributed to the explosive growth of refractive surgery over the past 15 years. Despite these advances, complications such as incomplete or partial flaps, free flaps, buttonholes, and small irregular flaps continue to plague refractive surgeons who perform LASIK with a microkeratome. There are also significant limitations to the eyes that can safely have lamellar flap formation performed with a mechanical microkeratome, including corneas that are too steep (likely to have buttonhole flaps), too flat (likely to have small diameter flaps), or relatively thin (more likely to have low residual stromal bed) (Fig. 4).

Decentered flaps
Irregular-shaped flaps
Incomplete flaps
Button-hole flaps
Flap laceration
Epithelial defects
Limited hinge location, 1 or 2 sites per head (nasal or superior)
Poor flap thickness predictability, SD of flap thickness ±20 to 40 μm
Wide range of flap thickness for a given attempted thickness (up to 200 μm range)
Achieved mean thickness less than the labeled head
Sensitive to preoperative corneal curvature: steeper corneas create thinner flaps
Sensitive to preoperative corneal thickness: thicker corneas create thicker flaps[20,21]
Menicus-shaped flaps: thinner centrally than peripherally
Highly variable hinge length
Flap thickness dependent on translation speed: faster translation creates thinner flaps
Blade quality affects results: second eye use of same blade associated with thinner flaps
Gap width of microkeratome head variable affecting flap thickness predictability
Anterior chamber perforation (older models)

Fig. 4. Corneal complications reported with conventional microkeratomes (24).

The femtosecond laser became available for LASIK flap formation approximately 10 years ago. Since the early femtosecond laser models were introduced, considerable progress has been made in improving flap geometry and limiting complications of LASIK performed with the laser. This has led to increasing popularity of LASIK performed with the femtosecond laser, to the point that different sources estimate that 30% to 50% of LASIK procedures in the United States in 2008 were performed using a femtosecond laser. Recently, new femtosecond laser models were introduced. These include the Femtec (20/10 Perfect Vision AG), the Femto LDV (Zeimer Group), the Visu-Max (Carl Zeiss Meditec) and commonly used IntraLase 60 kHz femtosecond laser (Abbott Medical Optics, Inc.). All 4 commercially available femtosecond laser systems use ultrashort pulses of laser and produce corneal tissue cutting using a photodisruption process. To create the lamellar flap, the IntraLase laser generates pulses of femtosecond laser at a near-infrared (1053 nm) wavelength and delivers closely spaced 3 mm spots, which are focused at variable depths to photodisrupt stromal tissue. When a high peak power is reached, hot plasma is generated, initiating a process of tissue ionization that is commonly called laser-induced optical breakdown. The hot plasma expands in shock waves and creates an intrastromal cavitation bubble composed primarily of water and carbon dioxide. Multiple cavitation bubbles coalesce, and an intrastromal cleavage plane is created. The laser delivers a series of pulses in a specified pattern to create the lamellar intrastromal cut and then extends the cleavage to the surface with a side cut to complete the flap (25). Stonecipher et al. reported the refractive results after LASIK for high myopia and cylinder at one center with one surgeon comparing two laser platforms. A total of 206 eyes of 121 patients were treated for -6.00 to -12.00 diopters (D) of spherical equivalent refractive error with up to 3.00 D of cylinder. All eyes underwent LASIK with the ALLEGRETTO WAVE 200-Hz (n=141) or 400-Hz (n=65) laser (Alcon Laboratories Inc). Corneal flaps were created with the IntraLase femtosecond laser (Abbott Medical Optics) at an intended thickness of 100 or 110 μm in all cases. At 3- and 6-month follow-up in the 200-Hz group, 77% (109/141) and 86% (121/141) of eyes, respectively, were within ±0.50 D of intended correction. In the 400-Hz group, 98.5% (64/65) and 100% (65/65) of eyes were within ±50 D of intended correction at 3 and 6 months postoperatively. At 3- and 6-month follow-up, 84% (119/141) and 77% (109/141) of eyes, respectively, in the 200-Hz group and 80% (52/65) and 92% (60/65) of eyes, respectively, in the 400-Hz group had 20/20 or better uncorrected distance visual acuity. At 6-month follow-up, refractive predictability and visual acuity were statistically superior in eyes in the 400-Hz group (chi square, P<.01). No eyes underwent retreatment as a secondary procedure during the time of analysis (26).

8. Refractive laser surgery in children

The use of Excimer laser vision correction in children is controversial because their eyes and refractive state continue to change. More studies on the growing eye and the effect of Excimer laser on the pediatric corneal endothelium are needed before the effect of refractive surgery in the pediatric age group can be fully understood (27).

Traditional methods of correcting and rehabilitating the refractive status of children with high myopia, myopic anisometropic amblyopia, hyperopia, hyperopic anisometropic amblyopia or significant astigmatism include glasses and contact lenses combined with some form of occlusion or optical penalization therapy. However, some children may not improve with these traditional forms of treatment because of aniseikonia, compliance issues, or both. This is especially true when children have concurrent medical diagnoses such as autism, cerebral palsy, developmental delay, Down syndrome, or other associated ocular disorders (eg, corneal, retinal, and optic nerve problems). So, in such children traditional optical refractive correction is often not successful (28, 29).

In the past ten years, refractive laser surgery techniques have been shown to be a good last-resort treatment in children who have failed with traditional treatment approaches. There are numerous reports of the successful performance of PRK, LASIK and LASEK in children when conventional therapy failed.

Autrata and Rehurek evaluated the visual and refractive results of multizonal PRK for high myopic anisometropia and contact-lens intolerance in children. Twenty-one patients aged 7 to 15 years with high myopic anisometropia had multizonal PRK in the more myopic eye and were retrospectively analyzed. The scanning-slit Nidek EC-5000 Excimer laser was used. The safety, efficacy, predictability, and stability of the procedure were evaluated. Long-term binocular vision outcome was analyzed. All patients completed a 4-year follow-up. The mean preoperative spherical equivalent (SE) refraction was - 8.93 diopters (D) ± 1.39 (SD) (range - 6.75 to - 11.75 D) and the mean postoperative SE was – 1.66 ± 0.68 D (range -

0.50 to - 2.75 D). The mean preoperative uncorrected visual acuity (UCVA) of 0.034 ± 0.016 increased to 0.35 ± 0.15 postoperatively. The mean preoperative best spectacle-corrected visual acuity (BSCVA) was 0.53 ± 0.19 and changed to 0.64 ± 0.16 postoperatively. No eye lost a line of BSCVA; 9 eyes gained 1 line, and 5 eyes gained 2 lines. No eye had + 3 haze. There were no significant complications. In conclusion, PRK was safe and effective in correcting high myopic anisometropia in children who were contact-lens intolerant (30).

Yin et al. assessed the efficacy of LASIK in facilitating amblyopia management of children from 6 to 14 years old, with high hyperopic and myopic anisometropia. Between 2000 and 2005, 42 children with high hyperopic anisometropic amblyopia and 32 children with high myopic anisometropic amblyopia underwent LASIK to reduce their anisometropia. LASIK was performed under topical or general anesthesia. Follow-up ranged from 6 months to 3 years, the averages of which were 17,45 months in the hyperopic group and 18,31 months in myopic group. Hyperopic anisometropia correction ranged from + 3.50 D to + 7.75 D, and the mean postoperative anisometropia was +0.56 ± 0.75 D at 3 years. Myopic anisometropia correction ranged from -15.75 to - 5.00 D and the mean postoperative anisometropia at 3 years was - 2.20 ± 1.05 D. The best-corrected visual acuity for distance and reading in the myopic group improved from 0.4 ± 0.25 and 0.58 ± 0.27, respectively, before surgery to 0.59 ± 0.28 and 0.96 ± 0.35, respectively, 3 years after surgery. In the hyperopic group, best-corrected visual acuity for distance and reading improved from 0.23 ± 0.21 and 0.34 ± 0.32, respectively, before surgery to 0.53 ± 0.31 and 0.80 ± 0.33, respectively, 3 years after surgery. Study shows that LASIK is an alternative method for correcting high hyperopic and myopic anisometropia. The proportion of patients who had stereopsis increased from 19.1% preoperatively to 46.7% postoperatively in the hyperopic group and from 19% to 89% in the myopic group. In conclusion, LASIK reduced high hyperopic and myopic anisometropia in children, thus facilitating amblyopia management and improving their visual acuity and stereopsis (31).

Astle et al. assessed the refractive, visual acuity, and binocular results of LASEK for anisomyopia, anisohyperopia, and anisoastigmatia in children with various levels of amblyopia secondary to the anisometropic causes. Retrospective review was of 53 children with anisometropia who had LASEK to correct the refractive difference between eyes. All LASEK procedures were performed using general anesthesia. Patients were divided into 3 groups according to their anisometropia as follows: myopic difference greater than 3.00 diopters (D), astigmatic difference greater than 1.50 D, and hyperopic difference greater than 3.50 D. The children were followed for at least 1 year. The mean age at treatment was 8.4 years (range 10 months to 16 years). The mean preoperative anisometropic difference was 6.98 D in the entire group, 9.48 D in the anisomyopic group, 3.13 D in the anisoastigmatic group, and 5.50 D in the anisohyperopic group. One year after LASEK, the mean anisometropic difference decreased to 1.81 D, 2.43 D, 0.74 D, and 2.33 D, respectively, and 54% of all eyes were within ± 1.00 D of the fellow eye, 68% were within ± 2.00 D, and 80% were within ± 3.00 D. Preoperative visual acuity and binocular vision could be measured in 33 children. Postoperatively, 63.6% of children had an improvement in best corrected visual acuity (BCVA) and the remainder had no noted change. No patient had a reduction in BCVA or a loss in fusional ability after LASEK. Of the 33 children, 39.4% had positive stereopsis preoperatively and 87.9% had positive stereopsis 1 year after LASEK. In conclusion, LASEK is an effective surgical alternative to improve visual acuity in anisometropic children unable to tolerate conventional methods of treatment or in whom these methods fail (32).

9. References

[1] Sakimoto T, Rosenblatt MI, Azar DT. Laser eye surgery for refractive errors. The Lancet 2006; 367 (9520): 1432-1447.

[2] American Academy of Ophthalmology. Incisional Corneal Surgery. In: American Academy of Ophthalmology. Refractive surgery, Section 13, 2010-2011. Singapore: American Academy of Ophthalmology; 2010. p. 67-71.

[3] American Academy of Ophthalmology. Photoablation. In: American Academy of Ophthalmology. Refractive surgery, Section 13, 2010-2011. Singapore: American Academy of Ophthalmology; 2010. p. 109-146.

[4] American Academy of Ophthalmology. Photoablation. In: American Academy of Ophthalmology. Refractive surgery, Section 13, 2010-2011. Singapore: American Academy of Ophthalmology; 2010. p. 92-109.

[5] Vukosavljević M, Milivojević M, Resan M, Cerović V. Laser in situ keratomyleusis (LASIK) for correction of myopia and hypermetropia – our one year experience Vojnosanitet Pregl 2009; 66 (12): 979–984.

[6] Giessler S, Duncker GIW. Short-term visual rehabilitation after LASIK. Graefes Arch Clin Exp Ophthalmol 2001; 239 (8): 603-608.

[7] American Academy of Ophthalmology. Patient Evaluation. In: American Academy of Ophthalmology. Refractive surgery, Section 13, 2010-2011. Singapore: American Academy of Ophthalmology; 2010. p. 41-58.

[8] Young JA, Kornmehl EW. Preoperative evaluation for refractive surgery. In: Yanoff M, Duker JS. Ophthalmology. St. Louis: Mosby; 2004. p. 133-136.

[9] Probst LE. Intraoperative complications. In: Probst LE. Lasik: a color atlas and surgical synopsis. Thorofare, NJ: Slack Incorporated; 2001. p. 211-232.

[10] Probst LE. Early and late postoperative complications. In: Probst LE. Lasik: a color atlas and surgical synopsis. Thorofare, NJ: Slack Incorporated; 2001. p. 257-297.

[11] Stojanovic A, Nitter TA. 200 Hz flying-spot technology of the LaserSight LSX excimer laser in the treatment of myopic astigmatism: six and 12 month outcomes of laser in situ keratomileusis and photorefractive keratectomy. *J Cataract Refract Surg* 2001; 27 (8): 1263- 1277.

[12] Ditzen K, Fiedler J, Pieger S. Laser in situ Keratomileusis for Hyperopia and Hyperopic Astigmatism Using the Meditec MEL 70 Spot Scanner. *J Refract Surg* 2002; 18: 430-434.

[13] Albarran-Diego C, Munoz G, Montes-Mico R, Alio JL. Bitoric laser in situ keratomileusis for astigmatism. *J Cataract Refract Surg* 2004; 30 (7): 1471-1478.

[14] Grabner G. Die entwicklung der refraktiven chirurgie. Spektrum Augenheilkd 2009; 23 (3): 187–192.

[15] Reynolds A, Moore JE, Naroo SA, Moore CBT, Shah S. Excimer laser surface ablation – a review. Clin Experiment Ophthalmol 2010; 38 (2): 168-182.

[16] Hashemi H, Taheri SM, Fotouhi A, Kheiltash A. Evaluation of the prophylactic use of mitomycin C to inhibit haze formation after photorefractive keratectomy in high myopia: a prospective clinical study. BMC Ophthalmol 2004; 4: 12.

[17] Haw WW, Manche EE. Photorefractive keratectomy for compound myopic astigmatism. *Am J Ophthalmol* 2000; 130 (1): 12-19.

[18] Nagy ZZ, Munkacsy G, Popper M. Photorefractive Keratectomy Using the Meditec MEL 70 G-scan Laser for Hyperopia and Hyperopic Astigmatism. J *Refract Surg* 2002; 18: 542-550.

[19] Taneri S, Zieske JD, Azar DT. Evolution, techniques, clinical outcomes and pathophysiology of LASEK : review of the literature. Surv Ophthalmol 2004; 49: 576–602.

[20] Bilgihan K, Hondur A, Hasanreisoglu B. Laser subepithelial keratomileusis for myopia of -6 to -10 diopters with astigmatism with the MEL60 laser. J Refract Surg 2004; 20: 121-126.

[21] Taneri S, Feit R, Azar DT. Safety, efficacy, and stability indices of LASEK correction in moderate myopia and astigmatism. J Cataract Refract Surg 2004; 30: 2130-2137.

[22] Herrmann WA, Hillenkamp J, Hufendiek K et al. Epilaser in situ keratomileusis: comparative evaluation of epithelial separation with 3 microkeratomes. J Cataract Refract Surg 2008; 34: 1761–1766.

[23] Taneri S, Weisberg M, Azar DT. Surface ablation techniques. J Cataract Refract Surg 2011; 37: 392–408.

[24] Binder PS. One thousand consecutive IntraLase laser in situ keratomileusis flaps. J Cataract Refract Surg 2006; 32: 962–969.

[25] Saloma MQ, Wilson SE. Femtosecond laser in laser in situ keratomileusis. J Cataract Refract Surg 2010; 36: 1024–1032.

[26] Stonecipher KG, Kezirian GM, Stonecipher M. LASIK for -6.00 to -12.00 D of myopia with up to 3.00 D of cylinder using the ALLEGRETTO WAVE: 3- and 6-month results with the 200- and 400-Hz platforms. J Refract Surg 2010; 26: 814-818.

[27] American Academy of Ophthalmology. Refractive Surgery in Ocular and Systemic Disease. In: American Academy of Ophthalmology. Refractive surgery, Section 13, 2010-2011. Singapore: American Academy of Ophthalmology; 2010. p. 203-222.

[28] Astle WF, Huang PT, Ereifej I, Paszuk A. Laser-assisted subepithelial keratectomy for bilateral hyperopia and hyperopic anisometropic amblyopia in children. J Cataract Refract Surg 2010; 36:260–267.

[29] Astle WF, Fawcett SL, Huang PT, Alewenah O, Ingram A. Long-term outcomes of photorefractive keratectomy and laser-assisted subepithelial keratectomy in children J Cataract Refract Surg 2008; 34: 411–416.

[30] Autrata R, Rehurek J. Clinical results of excimer laser photorefractive keratectomy for high myopic anisometropia in children: Four-year follow-up. J Cataract Refract Surg 2003; 29: 694–702.

[31] Yin ZQ, Wang H, Yu T, Ren Q, Chen Li. Facilitation of amblyopia management by laser in situ keratomileusis in high anisometropic hyperopic and myopic children. J AAPOS 2007; 11: 571–576.

[32] Astle WF, Rahmat J, Ingram AD, Huang PT. Laser-assisted subepithelial keratectomy for anisometropic amblyopia in children: Outcomes at 1 year. J Cataract Refract Surg 2007; 33: 2028–2034.

Part 3

Refraction and Refractive Correction

8

Incidence of Refractive Error and Amblyopia Among Young Adults – A Hospital Based Study

Ashok Kumar Narsani[1], Shafi Muhammad Jatoi[1], Mohan Perkash Maheshwari[2] and Khairuddin Shah[1]
[1]*Department of Ophthalmology, Liaquat University Eye Hospital, Hyderabad Sindh,*
[2]*Department of Pharmacology, Baqai Medical University, Karachi Sindh, Pakistan*

1. Introduction

Visual impairment remains a major public health problem world wide, with an estimated 161 million people with visual impairment, of whom 37 million are blind.[1] Uncorrected or inadequately corrected refractive errors have been shown to be a major cause of visual impairment in population-based studies[2-6]. While amblyopia is a significant cause of unilateral reduced visual acuity in a population aged 40 years and older.[7]

Genetic factors are thought to play a role in development of refractive errors. It has been established that myopia clusters within families, and familial high myopia (refraction of -6 diopter {D} or less) has been linked to long arm regions on chromosomes 7, 12 and 18[8,9]. Environmental risk factors have also been associated with refractive errors, myopia or hypermetropia. Education[10,11] and near-work[12] are both strongly associated with increasing severity of myopia.

In different parts of Asia such as in India, the Andhra Pradesh Eye Disease Study shows 15.2%[13] prevalence rate of myopia (spherical equivalent {SE} at least -1.0D). While study in a 15,068 Singapore military recruits aged 16 to 25 years, the prevalence rates of myopia (SE at least -0.5 D) were much higher with some racial variation, 82.2% in Chinese, 68.8% in Indians, and 65.0% in Malays[14]. Similar high rates of myopia (SE at least -0.25 D; 84%) were present in 16 to 18 years old Chinese children in Taiwan[15]. In Pakistan the prevalence rates of myopia, hypermetropia, astigmatism (with SE worse than –0.5 D, greater than +0.5D, and greater than 0.75D respectively) was 36.5%, 27.1%, and 37%, respectively in adults aged 30 years or more in the National Blindness and Visual Impairment Survey.[16]

In United states, the Baltimore eye survey[17] and Beaver Dam study[18] showed the prevalence rates of myopia (SE at least -0.5 D) were 28.1% in white adults aged 40 years or more and 26.2% in adults aged 43 to 84 years respectively.

Amblyopia is a frequent cause of unilateral or bilateral blindness. The prevalence of amblyopia ranges from 0.73% to 3.06%[7] in previous studies. However, the epidemiology of amblyopia among this region of Asia is not well described and may be different from other because of difference in distribution of refractive error or strabismus.

AIM: To assess the incidence of refractive error and associated amblyopia among young adult.

2. Methodology

2.1 Subjects

This six months study was conducted from June 2008 to November 2008 at tertiary referral center Liaquat University Eye Hospital, Hyderabad Sindh, Pakistan. Three thousand four hundred fifty two patients were included and examined in out patients department with age ranged from 20-40 years. The proportion of men and women was 1:0.54. Both rural and urban residents were evaluated. After taking written consent all subjects underwent a comprehensive ophthalmic examination, and a standardized form was used to extract the data, including the following variables: demographic information, best corrected visual acuity, types of refractive error including myopia, hypermetropia, astigmatism and amblyopia.

2.2 Methods

Monocular visual acuity was determined with current spectacle prescription if any. Pinhole acuity was assessed in eyes with presenting visual acuity <20/20. Non-cycloplegic auto-refraction followed by subjective refinements was performed in all subjects. The best corrected visual acuity was recorded. Refraction data was based on subjective refraction. Only the right phakic eye of each subject was considered for refractive error evaluation and amblyopia evaluated bilaterally.

Amblyopia was defined as best-corrected visual acuity of 20/40 or worse in the absence of any pathological cause. Hypermetropia was defined as a SE greater than +0.5 diopter sphere (DS)[17-21]. Emetropia was defined as a SE between -0.50 and +0.50 DS[20]. Myopia was defined as a SE worse than -0.50 DS[17--21] and a SE or worse than -5.00 DS[19] was classified as high myopia. Astigmatism correction was prescribed in minus cylinder format, and astigmatism was defined as cylindrical error worse than -0.50 diopter cylinder (DC) in any axis. The axis of any cylinder component was classified as with the rule (WTR) if the minus cylinder axis was within 15° of 180°, against the rule (ATR) for minus cylinder axis within 15° of 90°, or oblique (other than WTR or ATR)[22].

3. Results

Of the 3452 patients, 847 (24.54 %) patients had best corrected visual acuity 20/40 or better and remaining 2605 (75.46%) had less than 20/40 due to different anterior and posterior segment eye pathologies, or amblyopia.

Out of the 847 patients 525 (15.20 %) were phakic in right eye, and remaining 322 (9.32%) were pseudophakic. For refractive error the result was analyzed for only 15.20%

phakic ametropic patients. While for amblyopia all patients who met the criteria were evaluated.

There were 341 (64.95% of phakic ametropic patients) male and 184 (35.05%) were female. The age range from 20 to 40 years **(Table 1),** mean age being 26±3.9 years. The mean age of men and women was 28±3.9 and 24±6.3 years respectively (statistically significant at $P<0.001$). The mean refractive error was 0.75D.

Hypermetropia was found in 185 (35.24% of phakic ametropic) patients (Table 1). The mean age of hypermetropia was 26.31±4.51 years. Which was not significantly different from that of entire population ($P=0.5476$). There were 121 men (23.04% of total ametropic) and 64 women (12.19%). Man had significantly higher prevalence of hypermetropia than women ($P<0.001$).

Three hundred and fifteen (60% of phakic ametropic) patients had myopia (Table 1). The mean age of myopes was 23.69±3.98 years. Which was significantly lower than the entire population ($P<0.001$). There were 205 (39.05%) men and 110 (20.95%) women. The man had a significantly higher prevalence of myopia than did the women ($P<0.001$)

Twenty five (4.76%) patients of the study population were high myopes (Table 1). Among which 15 patients were males and 10 were females. The mean age among high myopes was 22. 50±3.25 years. Which was also significantly lower than the entire population ($P<0.0002$). However there was no significant different between the mean age of myopes and high myopes ($P=0.1632$).

Two hundred and fifteen (25.38 % of phakic ametropic) patients had astigmatism worse than -0.5 DC. The males were 134 (62.32%) of total astigmatic patients and remaining were females. The man had a significantly higher prevalence of astigmatism than women ($P<0.001$). One hundred and forty two (66.04%) patients had ATR astigmatism, 52 (24.18%) had WTR astigmatism and 21 (9.76%) had oblique astigmatism. The prevalence of against the rule astigmatism increased significantly with age ($P=0.007$).

The incidence of associated unilateral amblyopia was in 19 (3.62%) of phakic ametropic patients (Table 2). Ten (52.63%) patients were male and 09 (47.37%) were females. Amblyopia was not found to be significantly different by age ($p=0.1312$) group and gender ($p=0.1211$). Anisometropia was more common in amblyopic cases (41.75%) compared to the normal population (5.91%), and 69% of amblyopic eyes had visual acuity worse than 20/60. However, two amblyopic patients had strabismus in addition to anisometropia, but the prime reason of both conditions was anisometropia. While none of the case of bilateral amblyopia were seen in this study.

Age (yrs)	Hypermetropia		Myopia		High myopia		Total (%)
	M	F	M	F	M	F	
21-25	38	21	48	25	7	4	143 (27.23)
26-30	29	17	65	27	5	4	147 (28.00)
31-35	27	10	49	32	0	1	119 (22.68)
36-40	27	16	43	26	3	1	116 (22.09)
Total	121	64	205	110	15	10	525 (100)

Table 1. Age and type of refractive error

Age (yrs)	Frequency of amblyopia		Total (%)
	Male	Female	
21 -25	2	2	4 (21.04)
26 -30	3	2	5 (26.32)
31 -35	2	3	5 (26.32)
36 -40	3	2	5 (26.32)
Total	10	9	19 (100)

Table 2. Demography of amblyopia

4. Discussion

The incidence of hypermetropia in this study was 35.24% of total 525 phakic ametropic patients. In contrast to Andhra Paeye disease study (APEDS)[13], Barbados eye study[20], and several other studies[17,18] hypermetropia decrease with increasing age in our study

The incidence of myopia and high myopia in this study was 60% and 4.76% of the phakic ametropic patients and decreased with age. The Attebok et al[18], Wang et al[11], Katz et al[17] reported a significant trends of decreasing myopia with age. However the Chennai glaucoma study[3], Barbodos[20] study reported increase of myopia with age and also have an association of nuclear sclerosis with myopia. Saw[22], Guggenheim et al[23] and Dan et al[24] reported environmental influence such as near work, night lighting and ultraviolet exposure may be responsible for ageing of the crystalline lens and associated myopia. In contrast to population based studies from Australia[18], Singapore[19], and Indonesia[25], the incidence of myopia was more in males than females in our study.

The incidence of astigmatism in this study was 25.38% and increased significantly with age. The same has been reported from Chenni[3], Australia[18], Singapore[19], and Indonesia[25]. ATR astigmatism in this study was predominant that made the 66.04% of the total ametropic patients. In relation to the Chennai[3] study the incidence of ATR astigmatism significantly increased with age and WTR astigmatism decreased with age in our study. Gudmundsdottir et al[26], Pensyl et al[22] and Goss et al[28] reported same and the reason for this could be increased lid laxity with age causing flattening of vertical corneal meridian thereby decreasing WTR astigmatism and increased ATR astigmatism.

In this study the incidence, of associated amblyopia was 3.62% of phakic ametropic patients, which was less than Goel B.S[29] study in which amblyopia was reported 5.97%. One thing common in both were higher rate of amblyopia in ametropic then general population. In contrast to Karki JKD[30] study amblyopia was not found significantly different by age and gender in this study.

In conclusion, 15.20% of people had refractive error and 3.62% has the amblyopia. The prevalence of myopia was 60% and decreased with age. Hypermetropia was more common among men. The prevalence of astigmatism was 25.38%. It was interesting to note that against the rule astigmatism in contrast to other studies was observed more often (66.04%) in this study. Though the above study represent the regional population of limited age (20-40 years), but the differences in the pattern of refractive error in this study leads us to believe that genetic, racial, environmental and occupational influences may play an important role.

5. References

[1] Resnikoff S, Pascolini D, Etya'ale D, et al. Global data onvisual impairment in the year 2002. *Bull World Health Organ*.2004;82:844 -51.

[2] Munoz B, West SK, Rubin GS, Schein OD, Quigley HA, Bressler SB, Bandeen-Roche K. Causes of blindness and visual impairment in a population of older Americans. The Salisbury Eye Evaluation Study. *Arch Ophthalmol.* 2002;118:819–825.

[3] Foran S, Wang JJ, Mitchell P. Causes of incident visual impairment. *Arch Ophthalmol.* 2002;120:613–619.

[4] Weih LM, VanNewkirk MR, McCarty CA, Taylor HR. Age-specific causes of bilateral vision impairment. *Arch Ophthalmol.* 2000;118:264–269.

[5] VanNewkirk MR, Weih L, McCarty CA, Taylor HR. Cause-specific prevalence of bilateral visual impairment in Victoria, Australia. The Visual Impairment Project. *Ophthalmology.* 2001;108:960–967.

[6] Munoz B, West SK, Rodriguez J, Sanchez R, Broman AT, Snyder R, Klein R. Blindness, visual impairment and the problem of uncorrected refractive error in a Mexican-American population: Proyecto VER. *Invest Ophthalmol Vis Sci.* 2002;43:608–614.

[7] Brown SA, Weih LM, Fu CL, Dimitrov P, Taylor HR, McCarty CA. Prevalence of amblyopia and associated refractive errors in an adult population in Victoria, Australia. *Ophthalmic Epdimol* .2000;7:249-58.

[8] Naiglin L, Gazagne C, Dallongeville F, Thalamas C, Idder A, Rascol O, Malecaze F, Calvas P. A genome wide scanfor familial high myopia suggests a novel locus on chromosome7q36. *J Med Genet.* 2002;39:118–124.

[9] Young TL, Ronan SM, Drahozal LA, Wildenberg SC, Alvear AB, Oetting WS, Atwood LD, Wilkin DJ, King RA. Evidence that a locus for familial high myopia maps to chromosome 18p. *Am J Hum Genet.*1998;63:109–119.

[10] The Framingham Offspring Eye Study Group. Familial aggregation and prevalence of myopia in the Framingham Offspring Eye Study. *Arch Ophthalmol.* 1996;114:326–332.

[11] Wang Q, Klein BE, Klein R, Moss SE. Refractive status in the Beaver Dam Eye Study. *Invest Ophthalmol Vis Sci.* 1994;35:4344–4347.

[12] Midelfart A, Aamo B, Sjohaug KA, Dysthe BE. Myopia among medical students in Norway. *Acta Ophthalmol.* 1992;70:317-322.

[13] Dandona R, Dandona L, Naduvilath TJ, Srinivas M, McCarty CA, Rao GN. Refractive errors in an urban population in Southern India: the Andhra Pradesh Eye Disease Study. *Invest Ophthalmol Vis Sci.* 1999;40:2810–2818.

[14] Wu HM, Seet B, Yap EPH, Saw SM, Lim TH, Chia KS. Does education explain ethnic differences in myopia prevalence? A population-based study of young adult males in Singapore. *Optom Vis Sci.* 2001;78:234–239.

[15] Luke LK L, Yung-Feng S, Chong-Bin T, Chien-Jen C, Loung-An L, Port-Tying H, Ping-Kang H. Epidemiologic study of ocular refraction among schoolchildren in Taiwan in 1995. *Optom Vis Sci.* 1999;76:275–281.

[16] Jadoon MZ, Dineen B, Bourne RRA, Shah SP, Khan MA,. Johnson GJ, Gilbert CE, Khan MD. Refractive Errors in the Adult Pakistani Population: The National Blindness and Visual Impairment Survey. *Ophthalmic Epidemiol* 2008;15:183-190.

[17] Katz J, Tielsch JM, Sommer A. Prevalence and risk factors forrefractive error in an adult inner city population. *Invest Ophthalmol Vis Sci.* 1997;38:334–340.

[18] Attebo K, Ivers RQ, Mitchell P. Refractive errors in an older population: The Blue Mountains eye study. *Ophthalmology.* 1999;106:1066–1072.

[19] Wong TY, Foster PJ, Hee J, Pin Ng T, Tielsch JM, Chew SJ, Johnson GJ and Seah SKL. Prevalence and risk factors of refractive errors in adult Chinese in Singapore. *Invest Ophthalmol Vis Sci.* 2000;41:2486–2494.

[20] Wu SY, Nemesure B, Leske MC. Refractive errors in a black adult population: The Barbados Eye Study. *Invest Ophthalmol Vis Sci.* 1999;40:2179–2184.

[21] Gwiazda J, Scheiman M, Mohindra I, Held R. Astigmatism in children: changes in axis and amount from birth to six years. *Invest Ophthalmol Vis Sci.* 1984;25:88–92.

[22] Saw SM. A synopsis of the prevalence rates and enviromental risk factors for myopia. *Clin Exp Optom.* 2003;86:289-294.

[23] Guggenheim JA, Hill C, Yam TF. Myopia, genetics and ambient lighting at night in a UK sample. *Br J Ophthalmol.* 2003;87:580-582.

[24] Dong X, Dong, Ayala M, Lofgren S, Soderberg PG. Ultraviolet radiation induced catract: age and maximum acceptable dosage. *Invest Ophthalmol Vis Sci.* 2003;44:1150-1154.

[25] Saw SM, Gazzard G,Koh D, Farook M, Widjaja D, Lee J, Donald T. H. Tan DTH . Prevalence rates of refractive errors in Sumarta, Indonesia. *Invest Ophthalmol Vis Sci.* 2002;43:3174-3180.

[26] Gudmundsdottir E, Jonasson F, Jonsson V, Stefansson E, Sasaki H, Sasaki K. "With the rule" astigmatism is not the rule in the elderly. *Acta Ophthalmol.* 2000;78:642-646.

[27] Pensyl CD, Harrson RA, Simpson P, Waterbor JW. Distribution of astigmatism among sioux Indians in South Dakota. *J Am Optom Assoc.* 1997;68:425-431.

[28] Goss DA. Meridonial Analysis of with the rule astigmatism in Oklahoma *Indians. Optom Vis Sci.* 1989;66:281-287.

[29] Goel.B.S, Amblyopia: modern concept and management. In current topics in ophthalmology. I Gupta, A.K (ED), B.I Churchil Livingstone New Dehli, 1993, p 145.

[30] Karki KJD Prevalence of Amblyopia in ametropia in clinical set up. *Katmandu University Medical Journal.* 2006;4;470-73.

9

Myopia, Light and Circadian Rhythms

John R. Phillips, Simon Backhouse and Andrew V. Collins
Department of Optometry and Vision Science, The University of Auckland
New Zealand

1. Introduction

Myopia has been investigated scientifically for over a century but the search for an effective remedy has been manifestly unsuccessful. The prevalence of myopia in developed societies has now risen to about 30% in USA (Vitale, Sperduto et al. 2009) and up to 70% in some Asian centres (Lin, Shih et al. 2004). In addition to the socio-economic burden of providing optical corrections for myopia, common myopia limits career choice and increases the risk of glaucoma and cataract. High myopia also increases the risk of retinal detachment, chorio-retinal degeneration and subsequent visual impairment (Saw, Gazzard et al. 2005). Both genetic and environmental factors have been implicated in the aetiology of myopia. Children with myopic parents have a higher than normal risk of developing myopia (Mutti, Mitchell et al. 2002) and twin studies show a higher level of concordance of common myopia in monozygotic compared to dizygotic twins (Dirani, Chamberlain et al. 2006). However, the rapid rise in myopia prevalence over recent decades argues strongly that changing environmental factors also play an important role in the aetiology of myopia.

In the early 1900s Fuchs asserted '*The following means are advised to put a stop to the extension of myopia in schools. First, the excess of work which many scholars have at present to struggle with should be reduced'.... 'Instruction ought not to begin too early (if possible not before the completion of the sixth year) and more time should be allotted to bodily exercise, especially in the open air, than has hitherto been the case.*' (Duane 1919). Although the long-held view that myopia primarily results from too much near-work is now regarded as an over-simplification, several recent studies support Fuchs's idea that outdoor activity may have an important role in protecting against myopia.

There have been many attempts to inhibit the progression of myopia in children. More recently, these have included treatment with antimuscarinic agents such as atropine eye-drops (Chua, Balakrishnan et al. 2006) and optical devices including multifocal spectacle lenses (Gwiazda, Hyman et al. 2003), dual-focus contact lenses (Anstice and Phillips 2011) and orthokeratology (Kakita, Hiraoka et al. 2011). However, none of these approaches entirely arrests myopia progression in the long term and the vast majority of myopia is managed by optical correction alone. Although conventional optical corrections including refractive surgery restore acuity, they do not prevent the abnormal enlargement of the myopic eye, so children with myopia remain at increased risk of ocular disease later in life.

In this review we examine evidence from human and animal studies that one aspect of outdoor activity, namely exposure to natural light, may reduce the prevalence and progression of myopia. We focus on the timing of light exposure in relation to the circadian cycle and on the potential roles of dopamine and melatonin in control of ocular growth and refractive development.

2. Human myopia and light

2.1 Outdoor activity

Current epidemiological research, as quantified by validated surveys, supports the idea that time spent in outdoor activities has a beneficial effect in reducing myopia prevalence in children and young adults (Jones, Sinnott et al. 2007; Rose, Morgan et al. 2008a; Rose, Morgan et al. 2008b). Whether the effect derives predominantly from increased natural light exposure or increased activity (e.g. sport) or from greater viewing distances outdoors has yet to be ascertained. An association between greater physical activity and reduced myopia progression has been reported in university students (Jacobsen, Jensen et al. 2008) although this association may have been confounded by other factors in the outdoor environment where much of the activity took place. Other studies have found an association between increased outdoor hours and lower myopia even when time spent playing sport outdoors was excluded (Rose, Morgan et al. 2008a). Moreover, indoor sport appears to have no beneficial effect (Rose, Morgan et al. 2008a; Dirani, Tong et al. 2009) suggesting that physical activity alone cannot account for the effect of outdoor activity. Whether the increased viewing distance typically associated with being outdoors has a positive effect in reducing myopia is unknown. The idea that time spent outdoors may act beneficially by substituting for time spent in near and mid-working distance activities seems not to be the case (Rose, Morgan et al. 2008a). In relation to distance viewing outdoors, the accommodative demand for viewing beyond about 6 metres is minimal. Indoor environments, particularly in city apartments, inevitably restrict viewing distance and typically include low dioptric stimuli for accommodation over the peripheral visual field (Charman 2011). However, the most obvious difference between spending time outdoors and time indoors is in light exposure. The spectral composition of light outdoors includes large amounts of ultraviolet (UV) and infrared (IR) in addition to light in the visible spectrum. Indoors, the UV portion of the spectrum is largely absent and if incandescent lighting is used the composition of the light is often biased towards the red end of the spectrum. Light intensity indoors is rarely more than 800 lux, whereas outdoor light intensity is around 50,000 lux on a sunny, blue-sky day and is rarely less than 5,000 lux, even when overcast. The cumulative light exposure for one hour spent outdoors is thus very much greater than for one hour spent indoors (Backhouse, Ng et al. 2011). This increased light exposure during the day is generally believed to be the most likely basis for the beneficial effect of outdoor activity in reducing myopia prevalence (Rose, Morgan et al. 2008a).

2.2 Light at night

Between birth and 2 years of age, the normal eye grows very rapidly, with axial length increasing at a rate of about 2 mm/year before slowing to about 0.1 mm/year until the eye reaches adult size (Larsen 1971). It has been suggested that environmental influences acting in this early period of rapid eye growth may potentially affect refractive development later in life. Quinn et al. (Quinn, Shin et al. 1999) investigated the effects of light exposure early in life on refractive status later in childhood. Their study, which was based on a questionnaire completed by parents of children aged 2-16 years (median 8 years) on their child's night-time light-exposure, reported a strong, dose-dependent association between the prevalence of myopia at the time of the study and night-time lighting conditions experienced by the children before the age of 2 years. Remarkably, 55% of children who slept with the room lights on developed myopia whereas 34% of children who slept with night-lights, and 10% of children who slept in darkness, had developed myopia at the time of the study. On the statistical strength of their findings, the authors suggested that the absence of a daily period of darkness could be a precipitating factor in the later development of myopia. A similar study (Czepita, Goslawski et al. 2004) also reported increased prevalence of myopia in children who had experienced ambient light at night before the age of 2 years. However, several studies in different parts of the world, also based on parental questionnaires, have reported no difference in prevalence of myopia in children sleeping in darkness or with ambient light at night before the age of 2 years (USA (Gwiazda, Ong et al. 2000; Zadnik, Jones et al. 2000), Asia (Saw, Zhang et al. 2002), UK (Guggenheim, Hill et al. 2003)). Both studies from the USA found associations between the number of myopic parents in the family and nursery lighting experienced by the child before the age of 2 years, suggesting that the results obtained by Quinn et al. may have been confounded by the uncontrolled effect of parental myopia. However, exposure to light at night may also affect the refractive development of young adults. A study of law students (Loman, Quinn et al. 2002) reported an association between increased myopia progression during law school with less daily exposure to darkness (i.e. more artificial light at night).

2.3 Season of birth

Further evidence for the influence of light exposure early in life on later refractive error comes from studies on the effect of season of birth (and by implication perinatal photoperiod) on adult refractive status. In a study population of 276,911 adolescents born in Israel (Mandel, Grotto et al. 2008), moderate and severe myopia prevalence varied by birth month, with the summer months (June/July) being associated with a higher myopia prevalence than the winter months (December/January). Moreover, increasing photoperiod was associated with increasing myopia prevalence in a dose-dependent pattern. Mild myopia was not associated with either season of birth or photoperiod. Birth during the summer was also found to be significantly associated with high myopia in a UK study (McMahon, Zayats et al. 2009) but no association was found between postnatal photoperiod and prevalence of myopia in adulthood. Seasonal variations in photoperiod are particularly extreme above the Arctic Circle. However, in a study of Finnish military conscripts (Vannas, Ying et al. 2003) no associations between myopia prevalence and birth month, global irradiance at birth month or daily hours of darkness during the birth month were found, although there was a trend towards higher prevalence of myopia among conscripts living above the Arctic Circle.

The human data on light exposure and refractive development suggest that increased day-time outdoor light exposure is associated with reduced myopia prevalence whereas increased night-time exposure to artificial light may be associated with increased myopia development - a case of day-light good, night-light bad. The remainder of this review examines the underlying processes which could explain why perturbations in the daily light-dark cycle may affect eye growth and refractive development.

3. Light and animal models of myopia

Animal studies have shown that a diurnal light:dark photoperiod is required for the normal refractive development of the eye in chicks (Li, Troilo et al. 1995; Stone, Lin et al. 1995), tree shrews (Norton, Amedo et al. 2006) and Rhesus monkeys (Smith, Bradley et al. 2001). In normal chick eyes there is a diurnal growth rhythm in which greatest eye elongation occurs during the day with reduced growth rates at night (Weiss and Schaeffel 1993; Nickla, Wildsoet et al. 1998). The choroid also demonstrates a similar diurnal rhythm in which the choroid thins during the day and thickens at night (Papastergiou, Schmid et al. 1998). In eyes deprived of form vision in order to induce myopia, a phase shift occurs in the relationship between the axial length and choroidal rhythms such that peak axial growth occurs earlier than in normal eyes (Nickla, Wildsoet et al. 1998).

3.1 Effect of constant light

Rearing chicks under constant light with open eyes produces hyperopia, due to corneal flattening resulting in shallow anterior chambers (Li, Troilo et al. 1995; Stone, Lin et al. 1995). While the anterior chamber becomes shallower, the vitreous chamber lengthens, resulting in no net change in axial length at 2 weeks of age. Continued rearing of chicks in constant light beyond 2 weeks produces macrophthalmos (Oishi, Lauber et al. 1987). The final refractive state may be hyperopic despite the development of significantly deeper vitreous chambers (Li, Troilo et al. 1995). In form-deprived eyes, constant light also produces hyperopia despite overall longer axial lengths and enlarged vitreous chambers in both axial and equatorial directions; (Stone, Lin et al. 1995).

While rearing chicks under continuous light produces hyperopia, the effect is dependent on the level of ambient illumination. Thus, higher light intensities are correlated with higher degrees of hyperopia, lower corneal power and increased vitreous chamber depth. Cohen et al. (Cohen, Belkin et al. 2008) reported that chicks raised under continuous illumination at 10,000 lux for 90 days developed a hyperopic mean refraction of +11.97D, while those raised under 50 lux resulted in an emmetropic mean refraction of +0.63D. An illumination level of 500 lux also produced a relatively high hyperopic outcome of +7.90D. While vitreous chamber depth was positively correlated with light intensity, overall axial length did not vary significantly between groups due to the corneal flattening associated with increasing light intensity, resulting in an overall hyperopic refraction at the moderate and high illumination levels (Cohen, Belkin et al. 2008).

Monkeys raised under continuous light conditions (Smith, Bradley et al. 2001) do not exhibit the increase in ocular growth typically found in the chick. Rhesus monkeys raised under continuous light for 6 months developed hyperopic refractions similar in magnitude to animals raised under normal diurnal light cycles. However, the refractions were more variable in outcome, with some animals developing axial anisometropia and low myopia (Smith, Bradley et al. 2001). The authors cautioned that the animals may have been able to re-establish at least a partial diurnal cycle by shielding their eyes during sleep with their arms, although no significant difference in behaviour was observed (Smith, Bradley et al. 2001).

3.2 Effect of constant darkness

Rearing chicks in complete darkness also produces hyperopia irrespective of whether a diffusing goggle is worn (Gottlieb, Fugate-Wentzek et al. 1987). The degree of hyperopia produced is approximately double that of normal chicks by 42 days. In contrast, tree shrews placed in continuous darkness eventually exhibit a myopic shift in refraction (Norton, Amedo et al. 2006). Although the animals initially stabilise at a low degree of hyperopia following 16 days of normal visual experience after eye opening, a subsequent period of 10 days of continuous darkness results in vitreous elongation and a myopic refraction (Norton, Amedo et al. 2006). While both chicks and tree shrews exhibit ocular growth under constant darkness, the significant corneal flattening which produces hyperopia in chicks does not occur in the tree shrew. Conversely, raising rhesus monkeys in continuous darkness appears to interfere with the emmetropisation process such that they retain their relatively high hyperopic neonatal refractions (Guyton, Greene et al. 1989).

Gottlieb et al. (Gottlieb, Fugate-Wentzek et al. 1987) proposed that two mechanisms may combine under dark-rearing in chicks to produce the hyperopic outcome: a visual deprivation mechanism which triggers enlargement of the eye, as occurs in form-deprivation myopia, and a second photoperiod-related mechanism which results in corneal flattening.

A phase advance in the cycle of eye growth is found in chicks raised under constant darkness which is associated with an overall increase in axial growth and choroidal thinning (Nickla, Wildsoet et al. 2001). As the rhythms in choroidal thinning and axial growth persist under constant darkness, they must be circadian in origin, rather than simply diurnal in response to external light-dark cycles (Nickla, Wildsoet et al. 2001). Nickla (Nickla 2006) provides further evidence for the role of a phase shift in the temporal relationship between axial length and choroidal thickness cycles in the control of ocular growth in a study comparing recovery from form-deprivation, myopic defocus and hyperopic defocus in chicks. It appears that where the treatment requires a decrease in ocular growth (such as recovery from form-deprivation) the axial length and choroidal rhythms shift into phase. The mechanism by which such a phase shift might influence ocular growth is not certain, although it has been proposed that the variation in thickness of the choroid may regulate diffusion of a signal molecule from the retina to the sclera, or may act as a mechanical scaffolding against the influence of diurnal intra-ocular pressure changes on the sclera (Nickla 2006).

3.3 Diurnal modulation of illumination

In order to determine the minimum period of darkness within the diurnal light:dark cycle that is required for normal eye growth, Li et al. (Li, Howland et al. 2000) investigated the effect of various periods of darkness from zero (constant light) to a standard 12:12 h light:dark cycle in chicks. They found that at least 4 hours darkness per diurnal cycle produced a normal emmetropisation response in the chick (Li, Howland et al. 2000). Further investigations demonstrated that the 4 hours of darkness was most effective in blocking the effects of excess light exposure when presented in a single period at the same time of day, rather than at random times or as multiple periods totalling 4 hours (Li, Howland et al. 2000). Li et al. (Li, Howland et al. 2000) concluded that this period of darkness may be sufficient to entrain the intrinsic circadian clock of the avian retina (Morgan and Boelen 1996). The requirement for periods of darkness during a diurnal cycle in order to produce normal eye growth in chicks has a potential corollary in humans. As noted earlier, the use of night lights in children's bedrooms under the age of 2 years has been associated with the development of myopia in later life (Quinn, Shin et al. 1999).

Diurnal modulation of ambient illumination rather than the need for periods of total darkness may be the significant requirement for normal emmetropisation in chicks. Liu et al. (Liu, Pendrak et al. 2004) reared chicks under light:dark, light:dim and constant light cycles with the aim of investigating the effect of ambient lighting at night on emmetropisation. The irradiance of the light phase was 1500 μW/cm^2, while the dim phase varied between 0.01 and 500 μW/cm^2. The eyes of chicks raised under light:dark and light:dim cycles had comparable ocular refractions and dimensions. Conversely, rearing under constant light levels from 1 μW/cm^2 (~0.3 lux) to 1500 μW/cm^2 (~500 lux) produced the typical shallow anterior chamber and hyperopic shift in refraction as found previously in chicks. These results imply that the modulation of light levels during a diurnal cycle may be of more importance in the maintenance of the normal emmetropisation response than the absolute light (or dark) levels. Consequently, the use of light:dim diurnal cycles may be a more pertinent paradigm for study as it more closely approximates the typical urban environment with artificial lighting at night (Liu, Pendrak et al. 2004).

3.4 Amplitude modulation of illumination

Recent animal investigations support the fundamental hypothesis that light exposure is the mediator of the antimyopiagenic effect of outdoor activity (Rose, Morgan et al. 2008a). Experiments in chicks have shown that exposure to high ambient light levels, either artificial or natural, modifies the development of experimental myopia due to either visual form deprivation using translucent occluders, or induced defocus using spectacle lenses (Ashby, Ohlendorf et al. 2009; Ashby and Schaeffel 2010). While exposure to high illumination levels of 15,000 lux for 5 hours per day significantly reduced form-deprivation myopia by around 60%, in lens-induced myopia the rate of compensation for the induced defocus was modified, but not the final degree of refractive error produced (Ashby and Schaeffel 2010). The normal emmetropisation process in chicks can also be directly influenced by ambient light levels: raising animals under low light levels (50 lux) produced myopic refractive outcomes on average, while high light levels (10,000 lux) produced hyperopic refractive outcomes (Cohen, Belkin et al. 2011).

In form-deprivation experiments in chicks, exposure to high artificial light (15,000 lux) indoors or natural light (30,000 lux) outdoors for 15 minutes per day with occluders removed was sufficient to produce a statistically significant decrease in axial myopia beyond that produced by the removal of the occluders under normal laboratory light levels (500 lux) (Ashby, Ohlendorf et al. 2009). The antimyopiagenic effect of high illumination levels was also demonstrated under constant occluder wear conditions where a significant decrease in axial myopia development was also demonstrated in chicks raised under 15,000 lux for 6 hours per day when compared to animals raised under 50 or 500 lux (Ashby, Ohlendorf et al. 2009). As the antimyopiagenic effect occurred during continuous occluder wear the authors conclude that the effect cannot be due to a reduction in image blur resulting from pupil constriction as these animals did not receive clear form vision at any time in the occluded eye. It has been suggested that high ambient illumination levels may affect the diurnal variation in retinal dopamine, which is disrupted in form-deprivation in chicks (Weiss and Schaeffel 1993), with the proposal that the chick retina has a graded release of dopamine under high illumination levels which results in a retardation of myopia development (Ashby, Ohlendorf et al. 2009). The intra-vitreal administration of a dopamine antagonist (spiperone) blocked the protective effect of high illumination levels against form-deprivation myopia in chicks (Ashby and Schaeffel 2010) further supporting the hypothesis that this neurotransmitter is intrinsically involved in the control of the emmetropisation mechanism (Ashby and Schaeffel 2010; Mao, Liu et al. 2010; Nickla, Totonelly et al. 2010).

3.5 Chromaticity and refractive development

The contribution of the chromatic component of light to refractive development has been investigated in a number of animal models including chicks (Rucker and Wallman 2009), fish (Kroger and Wagner 1996) and guinea pigs (Long, Chen et al. 2009). Guinea pigs raised under long-wavelength light (peak at 760 nm) reportedly develop a significant degree of myopia, associated with a significant increase in vitreous chamber depth, over a period of 4 weeks when compared to animals raised under mixed-wavelength light (unfiltered halogen lamps) (Long, Chen et al. 2009). The myopiagenic effect of long-wavelength light was reversed by allowing the animals to recover under mixed-wavelength light conditions for two weeks, after which there was no significant difference in refraction (Long, Chen et al. 2009).

One possible explanation for the effect of wavelength on refractive outcome is based on the intrinsic chromatic aberration of the vertebrate eye (Mandelman and Sivak 1983) which could provide a sign-of-defocus signal for emmetropisation (Flitcroft 1990) as the long and short wavelength components would produce relative hyperopic and myopic defocus of the retinal image respectively. For example, in a comparison of the effects of raising guinea pigs under equiluminant short wavelength light (430 nm) or middle wavelength light (530 nm), Liu et al. (Liu, Qian et al. 2011) demonstrated that after 12 weeks the 530 nm group was less hyperopic due to faster vitreous elongation, while the 430 nm group was more hyperopic following slower vitreous elongation. The difference in refraction between the groups (4.50 D) exceeded the longitudinal chromatic aberration of the guinea pig eye (approximately 1.5 D) at the selected wavelengths, which was possibly due to additional accommodative effects produced by the monochromatic illumination (Seidemann and Schaeffel 2002), or by wavelength-dependent alteration of retinal or retinal pigment epithelium growth signals (Liu, Qian et al. 2011).

4. Light and circadian rhythms

The role of illumination level and the requirement for periodic light:dark cycles during normal refractive development points to a role for the intrinsic circadian clock and the associated dopamine-melatonin cycle in the control of eye growth (Cahill and Besharse 1995; Witkovsky 2004; Iuvone, Tosini et al. 2005). The presumed role of circadian rhythms, which persist in constant darkness independent of the diurnal light:dark cycle, is to regulate the timing of biological events so as to optimise the metabolic function and energy use of the organism (Roenneberg and Foster 1997; Levi and Schibler 2007).

4.1 The circadian pacemaker

Although the control of the circadian rhythm is a complex, multivariate process, it has been known for some time that light plays a pivotal role (Iuvone, Tosini et al. 2005). The underlying circadian rhythm is controlled by a circadian clock, through the expression of "clock genes" and their products, and entrainment cues known as zeitgebers ("time givers") which influence the timing of these rhythms (Roenneberg and Foster 1997; Iuvone, Tosini et al. 2005). The primary, central time keeping clock in the body is the suprachiasmatic nucleus (SCN) of the hypothalamus (Roenneberg and Foster 1997). The primary input to the SCN is from the retina via the retinohypothalamic tract (RHT) (Simonneaux and Ribelayga 2003), which makes light the primary zeitgeber for entrainment of the circadian rhythm (Roenneberg and Foster 1997). While input via the RHT is not necessary for the generation of a circadian rhythm (evidenced by the free running nature of the SCN rhythm), it is necessary for the entrainment of the circadian rhythm to the normal light:dark cycle (Inouye and Kawamura 1979).

4.2 The light entrainment pathway

The traditional view of the photosensitive retinal organisation is of a dual photoreceptor system comprising both rods and cones. However, circadian entrainment has been found to originate from a small subset of retinal ganglion cells, the intrinsically photosensitive retinal ganglion cells (ipRGCs) (Berson, Dunn et al. 2002; Hattar, Liao et al. 2002). The photopigment melanopsin, first described in melanophores on frog skin and subsequently found in the inner retina of a number of mammals including humans, provides the ipRGCs with this photosensitivity (Provencio, Rodriguez et al. 2000; Hattar, Liao et al. 2002). Melanopsin has an action spectrum that peaks around 480 nm (Berson, Dunn et al. 2002). However, studies in melanopsin-knockout mice showed that melanopsin is not essential for light entrainment of the circadian pacemaker, but improves the magnitude of the response (Ruby, Brennan et al. 2002). It transpires that the melanopsin-containing ipRGCs also receive input from the traditional rod and cone photoreceptors (Perez-Leon, Warren et al. 2006). There is a loss of photo-entrainment, but a persistence of pattern vision, in animals without functional ipRGCs providing definitive support for the role of the ipRGCs in the entrainment of the circadian system by light (Guler, Ecker et al. 2008). The entrainment of the circadian system in mammals is thus mediated by the ipRGCs as a balance between intrinsic photoreception enabled by melanopsin and input from the traditional retinal photoreceptors. In chicks melanopsin is found in both the retina and the pineal gland, indicating light can entrain the circadian pacemaker through both retinal (via ipRGCs) and direct pineal routes (Torii, Kojima et al. 2007; Neumann, Ziegler et al. 2008).

The SCN, working as a central master clock, controls the circadian timing of the organism through a multisynaptic pathway. The SCN projects to neurones in the paraventricular hypothalamic nucleus, which synapse preganglionic sympathetic neurons in the intermediolateral cell column, stimulating postganglionic sympathetic neurons in the superior cervical ganglion, before finally providing sympathetic input to the pineal gland (Larsen, Enquist et al. 1998). The main circadian mediator from the pineal gland is melatonin, a hormone first isolated from bovine pineal glands and named for its ability to lighten the melanocytes in frog skin (Lerner, Case et al. 1958). Melatonin acts through melatonin receptors in a diverse range of tissues, performing a variety of roles in circadian entrainment, endocrine functions, cardiovascular responses, the immune system, and ocular physiology (Alarma-Estrany and Pintor 2007).

4.3 Melatonin precursors

Melatonin (N-acetyl-5-methoxytryptamine) is a circadian hormone produced through a pathway involving four precursor intermediaries (Fig. 1.). All of the components necessary for the production of melatonin are active within the pineal gland, which is the main site of production (Axelrod 1974; Zawilska, Skene et al. 2009). The first step is the conversion of the dietary amino acid tryptophan to 5-hydroxytryptophan by the enzyme tryptophan hydroxylase (TPH); the second step involves the conversion of 5-hydroxytryptophan to serotonin via the enzyme aromatic L-amino acid decarboxylase (AADC); serotonin is converted in the third step to N-acetylserotonin by the enzyme arylalkylamine-N-acetyltransferase (AANAT); the final step is the O-methylation of N-acetylserotonin to melatonin by the enzyme hydroxyindole-O-methyltransferase (HIOMT). The rate limiting enzyme in the production of melatonin is widely thought to be AANAT, although recent work suggests that HIOMT may be the crucial limiting factor (Liu and Borjigin 2005). The precursor components of melatonin synthesis also show inherent circadian rhythms of production (Axelrod 1974). The retina is another significant producer of melatonin in some animals, providing the basis for a peripheral clock in addition to the central clock of the pineal gland (Iuvone, Tosini et al. 2005)

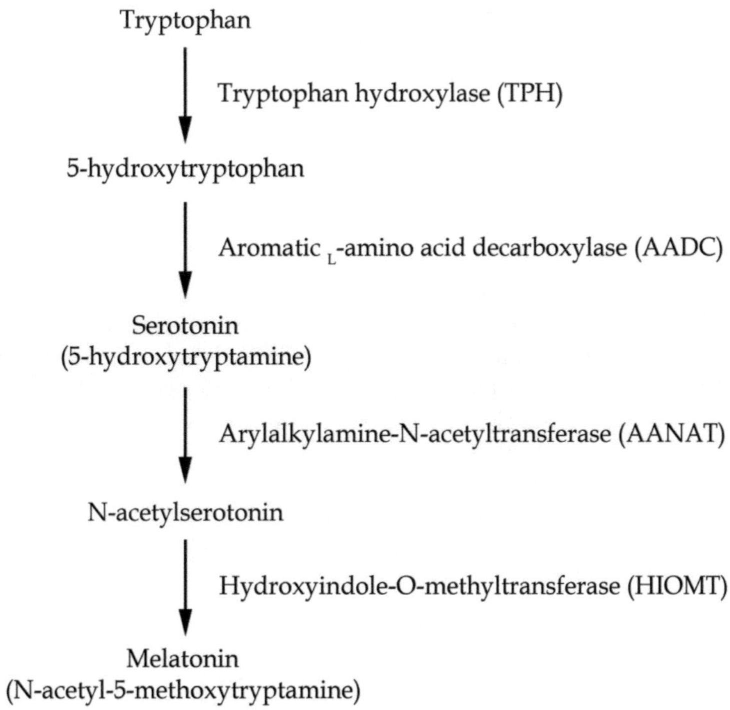

Fig. 1. Melatonin production pathway showing the precursor compounds and the enzymes involved.

4.4 Circadian melatonin rhythms

In the majority of species studied to date, whether they are diurnally or nocturnally active, there is a circadian secretion pattern of melatonin with high levels present at night and low levels during the day (Zawilska, Skene et al. 2009). The onset of darkness following a period of light leads to an increase in pineal AANAT and melatonin levels in phase with each other (Wilkinson, Arendt et al. 1977). However, there appears to be a refractory period for dark-induced melatonin rises such that darkness during periods when the organism is expecting it to be light does not induce the rise (Binkley, Macbride et al. 1975). Three distinct patterns of nocturnal melatonin production have been described in mammals: Type A is uncommon and represents a peak in melatonin late in the dark phase (e.g. Syrian hamster and house mouse); Type B is most common and shows peak melatonin expression occurring around midnight (e.g. rat, guinea pig, and human); and Type C which is also common and shows elevated melatonin levels for most of the dark phase (e.g. sheep and cat) (Zawilska, Skene et al. 2009). The human melatonin cycle, like that of animals (Tast, Love et al. 2001), can be entrained to variations in the light:dark cycle. When the light:dark cycle is phase-shifted by 12 hours, the human rhythm in melatonin secretion re-entrains to the new dark phase over a period of 5 to 7 days (Lynch, Jimerson et al. 1978).

4.5 Light and melatonin suppression

Darkness is required for the rise in melatonin, as animals kept in constant light show a reduction or complete loss of melatonin synthesis (Perlow, Reppert et al. 1980). However, the factor mediating the entrainment of the melatonin rhythm appears to be light exposure. Presentation of light during the dark phase, when melatonin levels are elevated, results in a rapid suppression of production and a reduction in serum melatonin concentration (e.g. (Illnerova, Backstrom et al. 1978; Rollag, O'Callaghan et al. 1978)). Human melatonin suppression by light is intensity dependant, with brighter light leading to greater levels of melatonin suppression (McIntyre, Norman et al. 1989; Zeitzer, Dijk et al. 2000). Suppression to near daytime levels (67% suppression) is achieved with 1000 lux (McIntyre, Norman et al. 1989), while a half maximal suppression response can be seen between approximately 50 and 130 lux (Zeitzer, Dijk et al. 2000). This light induced suppression also shows an inverse correlation with duration, such that longer durations of light require lower intensities of light to induce suppression (Aoki, Yamada et al. 1998). However, independent of light level there appears to be an asymptote for melatonin suppression after around 60 minutes of light exposure (Figueiro, Rea et al. 2006). Interestingly the melatonin suppression by light appears to be sensitised/desensitised by the amount of light received during the day prior, such that less light exposure (as experienced during winter months) results in much greater melatonin suppression for a given amount of light at night (Smith, Schoen et al. 2004; Higuchi, Motohashi et al. 2007).

The action spectrum for melatonin suppression shows peak effect between 446 and 477 nm (Brainard, Hanifin et al. 2001; Thapan, Arendt et al. 2001). The light response of the melanopsin containing ipRGCs mirrors that of the melatonin suppression action spectrum, indicating that these cells are the likely mediators of the response (Berson, Dunn et al. 2002). Circadian photo-entrainment also appears to be mediated by a peak action spectrum response from the same blue wavelength portion of the spectrum (Hattar, Lucas et al. 2003). These responses are also seen in humans, although a greater response is seen when polychromatic light is used instead of monochromatic light at peak melanopsin sensitivity, suggesting melanopsin may not be solely responsible and that rod and cone input also play a role (Revell and Skene 2007). Despite uncertainty as to the exact cellular input driving the circadian entrainment, it is clear that the blue end of the spectrum is important. Interestingly, exposure to the blue part of the spectrum also appears to suppress myopia development in guinea pigs (e.g. (Liu, Qian et al. 2011; Wang, Zhou et al. 2011)).

Wang et al. (Wang, Zhou et al. 2011) raised guinea pigs under blue light (480 nm), green light (530 nm) and broadband white light. After 10 days the levels of melatonin in the pineal glands were significantly lower in both the blue light and white light groups when compared to the green light group. This difference existed in both daytime (10 am) and night-time (10 pm) samples. The green-light group were also about 2 D more myopic, had greater axial lengths and greater vitreous depths than the other groups. Furthermore the green-light group exhibited reduced expression of retinal melanopsin mRNA and reduced levels of melanopsin protein. MT1 receptor mRNA expression was higher in both the retina and sclera of the green-light group. Overall this study demonstrated a clear link between wavelength of illumination, refractive error development and modulation of the melatonin pathway in guinea pigs.

4.6 Light as a zeitgeber

Light is the primary zeitgeber for the entrainment of the circadian system (Roenneberg and Foster 1997). Phase response curves have shown that the timing of light exposure is critical to circadian responses to light (Daan and Pittendrigh 1976). When light is presented at the beginning of the subjective night there is a phase delay of the subsequent activity-rest cycle, while light presented at the end of the subjective night leads to a phase advance. Presentation of light during the subjective day has little effect on the phase response curve, suggesting the twilight zones of dusk and dawn are the key times for entrainment (Roenneberg and Foster 1997). The phase shifting effect of light also affects the timing of the dim light melatonin onset (the increase in melatonin levels at night) (Lewy, Sack et al. 1985). Bright light in the evening delays dim light melatonin onset while bright light in the morning advances it. Bright light presented both in the morning and evening gives an intermediate response between delay and advance (Lewy, Sack et al. 1987). Exposure to bright light results in immediate melatonin suppression, but longer exposure of greater intensity is required to entrain the pacemaker (Hashimoto, Nakamura et al. 1996). However, dim light exposure at the appropriate time and for a long enough period has also been shown to entrain the circadian system (Zeitzer, Dijk et al. 2000). The importance of the timing of the signal for entrainment has a parallel in form-deprivation myopia wherein removal of the occluder for 40 minutes in the evening is more effective at reducing the induced myopia than if the occluder is removed in the morning (Ohngemach, Feldkaemper et al. 2001).

4.7 Photoperiodism and photoperiodic history

Photoperiodism, the adaptation of an organism's physiological functions to changes in season, is thought to be determined by both the absolute photoperiod length and by changes (either increasing or decreasing) in photoperiod length (Goldman 2001). Three main hypotheses to explain the influence of melatonin on this phenomenon exist: the duration, coincidence, and amplitude hypotheses.

The duration hypothesis proposes that the duration of night-time melatonin release is used as a signal encoding day length, with a shorter duration melatonin signal indicating long day/short night periods and vice versa (Simonneaux and Ribelayga 2003). In pinealectomised animals, short duration infusion of melatonin replicates a long day reproductive response while long duration infusion replicates a short day response (e.g.

(Bittman and Karsch 1984; Maywood, Buttery et al. 1990)). The coincidence hypothesis proposes that there is a coincidence between a sensitive period for signal detection and the presence of the melatonin signal. Infusion of melatonin at specific circadian time points in pinealectomised individuals suggests a critical period of sensitivity either at the onset of the dark phase (Gunduz and Stetson 2001), or at a specific time after the initial melatonin rise (Pitrosky, Kirsch et al. 1995). More recent work suggests that the coincidence timing effect of melatonin acts through clock gene expression oscillations (for review see (Hazlerigg and Wagner 2006)). While the amplitude hypothesis, which proposes that the peak amplitude of melatonin secretion is the signal for seasonal timing, is often discussed (e.g. (Simonneaux and Ribelayga 2003)), very little experimental data exists to back it up. Thus duration and timing of circadian signals may be more important than signal amplitude for circadian entrainment.

During periods of intermediate day-length between the winter and summer solstices a single day-length signal is insufficient to determine whether the days are becoming longer or shorter, so photoperiodic history, based upon the length of the preceding days, is used. The photoperiodic history appears to rely on the summation of recent photoperiod information over a number of days (Prendergast, Gorman et al. 2000), and the prenatal photoperiod actually appears to modify the postnatal day-length threshold which controls the maximal rate of development (Shaw and Goldman 1995). The ability of the perinatal photoperiodic history to influence future development rates may explain the observed season of birth effect in human refractive development (see Section 2.3).

5. Peripheral clocks

In addition to the master central circadian clock, peripheral systems and indeed individual cells also possess clocks (reviewed by (Balsalobre 2002)). Of these the retina, which also provides the main entrainment cue for the central clock, constitutes the most relevant peripheral clock for refractive development. The retina is a highly circadian tissue, showing rhythms in a variety of functions including visual sensitivity, the electroretinogram response, rod outer segment disc shedding, melanopsin mRNA expression, melatonin synthesis, and dopamine synthesis (for excellent reviews see (Iuvone, Tosini et al. 2005; Tosini, Pozdeyev et al. 2008)).

5.1 Retinal melatonin

Melatonin is synthesised in the retina in a circadian manner, independent of the SCN, in both non-mammalian (Cahill and Besharse 1992; Thomas, Tigges et al. 1993) and mammalian (Tosini and Menaker 1996) vertebrates. The retinal photoreceptors appear to be the source of this retinal melatonin production, with AANAT and HIOMT activity having been localised mainly to these cells, and only minimal activity in the inner nuclear layer and ganglion cells (Guerlotte, Greve et al. 1996; Coon, Del Olmo et al. 2002). Moreover, melatonin continues to be produced despite partial or complete destruction of the inner retina (Cahill and Besharse 1992; Thomas, Tigges et al. 1993). Human and primate retinas appear to be missing activity of the HIOMT enzyme, with expression of HIOMT mRNA in such small quantities that it contributes little to the production of melatonin (Bernard, Donohue et al. 1995; Coon, Del Olmo et al. 2002). However, labelling and activity of HIOMT in human photoreceptors has been demonstrated (Wiechmann and

Hollyfield 1987), although this has not been repeated by other groups. It has been postulated that N-acetylserotonin might take the place of a local melatonin signal in the retina of humans and primates (Iuvone, Tosini et al. 2005), or that the signal is provided by circulating melatonin levels (Osol and Schwartz 1984). Interestingly, human RPE and ciliary body also synthesise melatonin (Martin, Malina et al. 1992; Zmijewski, Sweatman et al. 2009).

5.2 Central and retinal dopamine rhythms

Dopamine is a neurotransmitter that has a multitude of roles, such as in learning and movement (Witkovsky 2004). Plasma dopamine levels in humans show a circadian rhythm in concentration that is phase-shifted relative to melatonin by approximately 180 degrees, peaking in the light phase and reaching lowest levels during the dark phase (Sowers and Vlachakis 1984). Primates (Perlow, Gordon et al. 1977), rats (Schade, Vick et al. 1995), and birds (Kang, Thayananuphat et al. 2007) also show these circadian rhythms in dopamine production; high in light, low in dark, and out of phase with melatonin. In pinealectomised rats the administration of melatonin suppresses dopamine expression in a dose-dependent manner (Khaldy, Leon et al. 2002).

Dopamine also has many roles in the retina, for example in light adaptation and cell death, as well as a potential role in ocular growth (Witkovsky 2004). As in the brain, retinal dopamine shows a diurnal rhythm with peak levels during the day and low levels during the night in non-human vertebrates (Nowak, Zurawska et al. 1989; Megaw, Boelen et al. 2006), and in human retinas (Di Paolo, Harnois et al. 1987). The diurnal variation in dopamine levels persists in constant darkness in mice, indicating that it has a circadian rhythm of release (Doyle, Grace et al. 2002), although others have found no circadian rhythm but a light activated fluctuation in retinal dopamine (Melamed, Frucht et al. 1984).

5.3 Light and dopamine

Dopamine is released from the perfused retina on exposing it to light (Kramer 1971), and light also stimulates retinal dopamine synthesis and turnover (Iuvone, Galli et al. 1978; Cohen, Hadjiconstantinou et al. 1983). Moreover, the light-activated rise in dopamine levels in the retina is much greater than the rise seen with the underlying circadian rhythm in constant darkness (Megaw, Boelen et al. 2006), and the metabolism of dopamine in the light is much greater than in the dark (Parkinson and Rando 1983; Megaw, Boelen et al. 2006). Furthermore, the intensity of light appears to be important for dopamine release and synthesis in the retina, with maximal stimulation and saturation of the response occurring between 32 to 80 lux in rats (Proll, Kamp et al. 1982; Brainard and Morgan 1987).

It transpires that change in light, in the form of flicker, is a more potent stimulus to dopamine release than constant light levels. This effect has been shown in several species, with increasing release rates seen with increasing stimulus presentation rates, and an increase in dopamine release above that seen with constant light alone (Kramer 1971; Weiler, Baldridge et al. 1997). Flickering light appears to increase dopamine release two to three times that of basal release levels. High frequency flicker at 6 Hz has also been shown to inhibit both form-deprivation myopia and lens-induced myopia in the chick (Schwahn and Schaeffel 1997). The degree of suppression is correlated with the length of the dark phase of the flicker duty cycle (Schwahn and Schaeffel 1997). This may be due to increased retinal dopamine levels as 2 hours of exposure to flickering light at 10 Hz was shown to restore the rate of dopamine synthesis under form-deprivation conditions in chicks, possibly due to increased transcription of the tyrosine hydroxylase gene in dopaminergic amacrine cells (Luft, Iuvone et al. 2004).

5.4 Dopamine and melatonin

When light is presented during the dark phase there is a rapid suppression of melatonin and an increase in dopamine to normal daytime levels (Adachi, Nogi et al. 1998). Interestingly, in knockout mice that do not produce melatonin there is a loss of the circadian dopamine rhythm when the animals are maintained in constant darkness, but the rhythm is restored on administering exogenous melatonin (Doyle, Grace et al. 2002). These results are intriguing as they show that in the absence of melatonin a normal dopamine rhythm can be maintained by light exposure in a rhythmic light:dark cycle, but that melatonin can, in the absence of a light driven zeitgeber, also influence dopamine rhythms. Indeed there is a complex interaction between melatonin and dopamine in the retina with mutual inhibitory effects between the two compounds. Intra-vitreal injection of dopamine into the eye at night suppresses melatonin while the injection of melatonin during the day suppresses dopamine (Adachi, Nogi et al. 1998). Melatonin leads to an increase in AANAT activity in the retina and a decrease in dopamine levels (Nowak, Zurawska et al. 1989; Nowak, Kazula et al. 1992), while dopamine inhibits retinal AANAT activity and melatonin release (Iuvone and Besharse 1986; Tosini and Dirden 2000).

As melatonin production has not been demonstrated in the human retina, endogenous melatonin released from the pineal gland potentially acts in the retina. Indeed high levels of melatonin are found in human retinas, and intraperitoneal injection of melatonin in mice leads to an increase in retinal melatonin levels (Osol and Schwartz 1984; Doyle, Grace et al. 2002). In chicks the pineal gland has been shown to have a significant influence over both expression of the dopamine D_2-receptor mRNA and dopamine release in the retina (Ohngemach, Feldkaemper et al. 2001). Dopamine has also been shown to increase the expression of melanopsin mRNA via a D_2-receptor pathway in ipRGCs (Sakamoto, Liu et al. 2005).

6. Dopamine, melatonin and refractive development

6.1 Dopamine

Retinal dopamine levels are reduced during the induction of form-deprivation myopia in the chick (Stone, Lin et al. 1989), rhesus monkey (Iuvone, Tigges et al. 1991) and guinea pig (Mao, Liu et al. 2010). In the chick, this reduction is due to a decreased rate of dopamine synthesis during the light phase of the diurnal light:dark cycle (Stone, Lin et al. 1989). The use of modified translucent occluders demonstrates that retinal dopamine levels inversely correlate with the degree of axial elongation (Stone, Pendrak et al. 2006). Retinal dopamine levels exhibit a bidirectional response to retinal blur in chicks, with lens-induced myopia decreasing and hyperopia increasing the levels respectively (Guo, Sivak et al. 1995) although this effect is not universally reported (Bartmann, Schaeffel et al. 1994). The increase in retinal dopamine associated with the slowing of axial growth in lens-induced hyperopia parallels recovery from form-deprivation myopia in the chick where a similar relationship between dopamine level and axial growth is reported (Pendrak, Nguyen et al. 1997).

The role of dopamine in the control of ocular growth is further supported by the demonstration that ocular administration of dopamine agonists can inhibit the axial growth and myopic refractions produced by form-deprivation in chicks (Rohrer, Spira et al. 1993; Nickla, Totonelly et al. 2010) and primates (Iuvone, Tigges et al. 1991). Also, extraocular administration of the dopamine precursor levodopa by intraperitoneal injection in guinea pigs raises retinal dopamine content and reduces the development of myopia during form-deprivation (Mao, Liu et al. 2010). The relationship between retinal dopamine pathways and lens-induced myopia is less certain. At dosages sufficient to suppress form-deprivation myopia in chicks, development of lens-induced myopia was not suppressed by intra-vitreal injections of 6-hydroxy dopamine, a drug which inhibits dopaminergic pathways (Schaeffel, Hagel et al. 1994). Conversely the non-specific dopaminergic agonist apomorphine has been shown to block negative lens-induced myopia in other chick studies (Schmid and Wildsoet 2004; Nickla, Totonelly et al. 2010).

Investigations using dopamine receptor subtype-specific agonists and antagonists have shown that the antimyopiagenic effect of dopamine is primarily mediated by D_2 receptors. For example, in form-deprivation in chicks, the protective effects of the non-specific dopaminergic agonist apomorphine were blocked by the D_2 specific antagonist spiperone, but not by the D_1 specific antagonist SCH-23390 (Rohrer, Spira et al. 1993).

In lens-induced myopia in chicks, both apomorphine (non-selective) and quinpirole (D_2 specific) agonists prevent the axial elongation and development of myopia associated with hyperopic defocus (Nickla, Totonelly et al. 2010). The effect is associated with an initial period of choroidal thickening, which is implicated in the inhibition of ocular growth either by the action of the choroid as a diffusion barrier to a growth signal or as an additional mechanical resistance to the effects of intraocular pressure (Nickla 2006). The D_2 antagonist spiperone is not as effective in abolishing the protective effect of periodic lens removal as has been previously found for the removal of form-depriving diffusers in chicks (McCarthy, Megaw et al. 2007). This may suggest a partial role for D_1 receptors in the control of ocular growth (Nickla, Totonelly et al. 2010).

6.2 Melatonin

While experimental evidence supports the role of retinal dopamine in the control of ocular growth and in the protective effect of light on myopia development, the role of melatonin, with which it is intrinsically linked in a counterphase cycle, is less certain (Cahill and Besharse 1995; Witkovsky 2004; Iuvone, Tosini et al. 2005).

Evidence for the role of an intrinsic melatonin rhythm in the control of eye growth is provided by Li and Howland (Li and Howland 2003) who demonstrated that the use of an opaque hood preventing light reaching the pineal gland for 12 hours per day is sufficient to significantly reduce the development of constant-light hyperopia in chicks. Covering one eye alone with an opaque occluder for 12 hours also partially prevented hyperopia development in the fellow eye under constant light conditions. The conclusion was that the eyes and pineal gland act as independent photoreceptors able to entrain the melatonin circadian rhythm which is protective against the effects of constant light on eye growth (Li and Howland 2003).

While diurnal retinal melatonin rhythms appear unaffected during form-deprivation (Hoffmann and Schaeffel 1996), the intra-vitreal injection of melatonin at relatively high doses (1000 μg) increases the level of form-deprivation myopia induced in the chick (Schaeffel, Bartmann et al. 1995; Hoffmann and Schaeffel 1996). Although retinal melatonin content was sampled twice a day (day and night) during monocular occlusion, and an expected diurnal variation in melatonin was found, no significant difference was found between the occluded and non-occluded eyes (Hoffmann and Schaeffel 1996). While the authors concluded that melatonin was not a significant component of the ocular growth control mechanism in form-deprivation in chicks a number of factors may have colluded to disguise the role of melatonin in form-deprivation myopia. These include the timing of the intra-vitreal injection of melatonin (between 2:00-3:00 pm) which may have occurred during a refractory period where the system was less sensitive, or that the duration (rather than the amplitude) of the nocturnal melatonin pulse may have been altered under form-deprivation conditions (see Section 4.7).

Rada and Wiechmann (Rada and Wiechmann 2006) demonstrated that the intraperitoneal injection of melatonin in chick at the beginning of each dark phase of the diurnal light cycle during a 5 day period of form-deprivation altered ocular growth patterns in both the form-deprived and control eyes. In form-deprived eyes, melatonin injection resulted in a significant reduction in anterior chamber depth, while vitreous chamber depth only exhibited a non-significant trend towards increased growth. The choroidal thickness was also significantly reduced in this group when compared to the sham-treatment group. The study also demonstrated the presence of melatonin receptors Mel(1A), Mel(1B) and Mel(1C) in the cornea, choroid, sclera, and retina of the chick. A diurnal rhythm in the expression of these receptors was identified where Mel(1C) expression was highest in the early morning around the onset of the light phase, while Mel(1A) and Mel(1B) expression was highest around the onset of the dark phase in the evenings. Rada and Wiechmann (Rada and Wiechmann 2006) concluded that the presence of melatonin receptors and diurnal rhythms of receptor expression, along with the effects of exogenous melatonin, suggests a significant role for melatonin in the control of ocular growth, and by extension, in the control of refractive development.

7. Conclusion

Recent human epidemiological studies propose that light exposure mediates the antimyopiagenic effect of outdoor activity. However, light may also have a causative role in myopia development when it is presented at an inappropriate time. Animal investigations demonstrate that light is a potent modulator of ocular growth and associated rhythms, including the interplay between dopamine and melatonin. One question is whether the effect of light on refractive development primarily acts through modification of circadian rhythms, or through some other intensity or wavelength dependent mechanism.

If the effect is circadian in origin, is there an optimal period for presenting light in order to control ocular growth and prevent myopia? Both constant light and constant dark disrupt ocular growth in animals and result in refractive error development. This can be ameliorated by either pharmacological interventions or controlled light exposure which re-establish more typical circadian rhythms. Light at night disrupts the normal circadian rhythm, rapidly decreasing melatonin and increasing dopamine, which potentially upsets the normal balance in ocular growth. As bright light presented in the middle of the day does not affect the timing of the circadian rhythm, presentation of a light signal during the twilight zones (dawn and dusk) is the most potent circadian zeitgeber. We hypothesise that the phase-advancing properties of morning light would be the most effective means of regulating the dopamine-melatonin circadian rhythm for the purposes of myopia control.

If the effect is not circadian in origin, then does the timing of the light signal matter or is it the nature of the stimulus (intensity and/or wavelength) that is important? Time spent outdoors leads to a significantly greater light dose than that received indoors, resulting in greater melatonin suppression and an increase in retinal dopamine. Additionally, the blue light spectral bias of outdoor light preferentially stimulates the melanopsin-containing ipRGCs, which would also lead to greater melatonin suppression. Both the intensity and wavelength of outdoor light favour increased retinal dopamine levels at the expense of melatonin. We hypothesise that it is this bias towards retinal dopamine production when outdoors that influences human refractive development, because increased dopamine has antimyopiagenic effects in animal experiments.

While the adage 'day-light good, night-light bad' in relation to refractive development is appealing, the true relationship between light and myopia is likely to be far more complex, with intricate interactions between the circadian cycle and the timing, intensity, and wavelength of the light exposure.

8. Acknowledgements

Simon Backhouse was supported by the New Zealand Association of Optometrists Education and Research Fund.

9. References

Adachi, A., T. Nogi, et al. (1998). "Phase-relationship and mutual effects between circadian rhythms of ocular melatonin and dopamine in the pigeon." *Brain Res* 792(2): 361-369.

Alarma-Estrany, P. and J. Pintor (2007). "Melatonin receptors in the eye: location, second messengers and role in ocular physiology." *Pharmacol Ther* 113(3): 507-522.

Anstice, N. S. and J. R. Phillips (2011). "Effect of dual-focus soft contact lens wear on axial myopia progression in children." *Ophthalmology* 118(6): 1152-1161.

Aoki, H., N. Yamada, et al. (1998). "Minimum light intensity required to suppress nocturnal melatonin concentration in human saliva." *Neurosci Lett* 252(2): 91-94.

Ashby, R., A. Ohlendorf, et al. (2009). "The effect of ambient illuminance on the development of deprivation myopia in chicks." *Invest Ophthalmol Vis Sci* 50(11): 5348-5354.

Ashby, R. S. and F. Schaeffel (2010). "The effect of bright light on lens compensation in chicks." *Invest Ophthalmol Vis Sci* 51(10): 5247-5253.

Axelrod, J. (1974). "The pineal gland: a neurochemical transducer." *Science* 184(144): 1341-1348.

Backhouse, S., H. Ng, et al. (2011). Light exposure patterns in children: a pilot study. Proceedings of the 13th International Myopia Conference, Tübingen, Germany, *Optom Vis Sci* 88(3): 395-403.

Balsalobre, A. (2002). "Clock genes in mammalian peripheral tissues." *Cell Tissue Res* 309(1): 193-199.

Bartmann, M., F. Schaeffel, et al. (1994). "Constant light affects retinal dopamine levels and blocks deprivation myopia but not lens-induced refractive errors in chickens." *Vis Neurosci* 11(2): 199-208.

Bernard, M., S. J. Donohue, et al. (1995). "Human hydroxyindole-O-methyltransferase in pineal gland, retina and Y79 retinoblastoma cells." *Brain Res* 696(1-2): 37-48.

Berson, D. M., F. A. Dunn, et al. (2002). "Phototransduction by retinal ganglion cells that set the circadian clock." *Science* 295(5557): 1070-1073.

Binkley, S., S. E. Macbride, et al. (1975). "Regulation of pineal rhythms in chickens: refractory period and nonvisual light perception." *Endocrinology* 96(4): 848-853.

Bittman, E. L. and F. J. Karsch (1984). "Nightly duration of pineal melatonin secretion determines the reproductive response to inhibitory day length in the ewe." *Biol Reprod* 30(3): 585-593.

Brainard, G. C., J. P. Hanifin, et al. (2001). "Action spectrum for melatonin regulation in humans: evidence for a novel circadian photoreceptor." *J Neurosci* 21(16): 6405-6412.

Brainard, G. C. and W. W. Morgan (1987). "Light-induced stimulation of retinal dopamine: a dose-response relationship." *Brain Res* 424(1): 199-203.

Cahill, G. M. and J. C. Besharse (1992). "Light-sensitive melatonin synthesis by Xenopus photoreceptors after destruction of the inner retina." *Vis Neurosci* 8(5): 487-490.

Cahill, G. M. and J. C. Besharse (1995). "Circadian rhythmicity in vertebrate retinas: Regulation by a photoreceptor oscillator." *Prog Retin Eye Res* 14(1): 267-291.

Charman, W. N. (2011). "Myopia, posture and the visual environment." *Ophthalmic Physiol Opt* 31(5):494-501

Chua, W. H., V. Balakrishnan, et al. (2006). "Atropine for the treatment of childhood myopia." *Ophthalmology* 113(12): 2285-2291.

Cohen, J., M. Hadjiconstantinou, et al. (1983). "Activation of dopamine-containing amacrine cells of retina: light-induced increase of acidic dopamine metabolites." *Brain Res* 260(1): 125-127.

Cohen, Y., M. Belkin, et al. (2008). "Light intensity modulates corneal power and refraction in the chick eye exposed to continuous light." *Vision Res* 48(21): 2329-2335.

Cohen, Y., M. Belkin, et al. (2011). "Dependency between light intensity and refractive development under light-dark cycles." *Exp Eye Res* 92(1):40-46.

Coon, S. L., E. Del Olmo, et al. (2002). "Melatonin synthesis enzymes in Macaca mulatta: focus on arylalkylamine N-acetyltransferase (EC 2.3.1.87)." *J Clin Endocrinol Metab* 87(10): 4699-4706.

Czepita, D., W. Goslawski, et al. (2004). "Role of light emitted by incandescent or fluorescent lamps in the development of myopia and astigmatism." *Med Sci Monit* 10(4): CR168-171.

Daan, S. and C. S. Pittendrigh (1976). "A Functional Analysis of Circadian Pacemakers in Nocturnal Rodents. II. The Variability of Phase Response Curves." *J Comp Physiol* 106(3): 253-266.

Di Paolo, T., C. Harnois, et al. (1987). "Assay of dopamine and its metabolites in human and rat retina." *Neurosci Lett* 74(2): 250-254.

Dirani, M., M. Chamberlain, et al. (2006). "Refractive errors in twin studies." *Twin Res Hum Genet* 9(4): 566-572.

Dirani, M., L. Tong, et al. (2009). "Outdoor activity and myopia in Singapore teenage children." *Br J Ophthalmol* 93(8): 997-1000.

Doyle, S. E., M. S. Grace, et al. (2002). "Circadian rhythms of dopamine in mouse retina: the role of melatonin." *Vis Neurosci* 19(5): 593-601.

Duane, A. (1919). *Fuch's Textbook of Ophthalmology*. Philadelphia, Lippincott.

Figueiro, M. G., M. S. Rea, et al. (2006). "Circadian effectiveness of two polychromatic lights in suppressing human nocturnal melatonin." *Neurosci Lett* 406(3): 293-297.

Flitcroft, D. I. (1990). "A neural and computational model for the chromatic control of accommodation." *Vis Neurosci* 5(6): 547-555.

Goldman, B. D. (2001). "Mammalian photoperiodic system: formal properties and neuroendocrine mechanisms of photoperiodic time measurement." *J Biol Rhythms* 16(4): 283-301.

Gottlieb, M. D., L. A. Fugate-Wentzek, et al. (1987). "Different visual deprivations produce different ametropias and different eye shapes." *Invest Ophthalmol Vis Sci* 28(8): 1225-1235.

Guerlotte, J., P. Greve, et al. (1996). "Hydroxyindole-O-methyltransferase in the chicken retina: immunocytochemical localization and daily rhythm of mRNA." *Eur J Neurosci* 8(4): 710-715.

Guggenheim, J. A., C. Hill, et al. (2003). "Myopia, genetics, and ambient lighting at night in a UK sample." *Br J Ophthalmol* 87(5): 580-582.

Guler, A. D., J. L. Ecker, et al. (2008). "Melanopsin cells are the principal conduits for rod-cone input to non-image-forming vision." *Nature* 453(7191): 102-105.

Gunduz, B. and M. H. Stetson (2001). "A test of the coincidence and duration models of melatonin action in Siberian hamsters: the effects of 1-hr melatonin infusions on testicular development in intact and pinealectomized prepubertal Phodopus sungorus." *J Pineal Res* 30(2): 97-107.

Guo, S. S., J. G. Sivak, et al. (1995). "Retinal dopamine and lens-induced refractive errors in chicks." *Curr Eye Res* 14(5): 385-389.

Guyton, D. L., P. R. Greene, et al. (1989). "Dark-rearing interference with emmetropization in the rhesus monkey." *Invest Ophthalmol Vis Sci* 30(4): 761-764.

Gwiazda, J., L. Hyman, et al. (2003). "A randomized clinical trial of progressive addition lenses versus single vision lenses on the progression of myopia in children." *Invest Ophthalmol Vis Sci* 44(4): 1492-1500.

Gwiazda, J., E. Ong, et al. (2000). "Myopia and ambient night-time lighting." *Nature* 404(6774): 144.

Hashimoto, S., K. Nakamura, et al. (1996). "Melatonin rhythm is not shifted by lights that suppress nocturnal melatonin in humans under entrainment." *Am J Physiol* 270(5 Pt 2): R1073-1077.

Hattar, S., H. W. Liao, et al. (2002). "Melanopsin-containing retinal ganglion cells: architecture, projections, and intrinsic photosensitivity." *Science* 295(5557): 1065-1070.

Hattar, S., R. J. Lucas, et al. (2003). "Melanopsin and rod-cone photoreceptive systems account for all major accessory visual functions in mice." *Nature* 424(6944): 76-81.

Hazlerigg, D. G. and G. C. Wagner (2006). "Seasonal photoperiodism in vertebrates: from coincidence to amplitude." *Trends Endocrinol Metab* 17(3): 83-91.

Higuchi, S., Y. Motohashi, et al. (2007). "Less exposure to daily ambient light in winter increases sensitivity of melatonin to light suppression." *Chronobiol Int* 24(1): 31-43.

Hoffmann, M. and F. Schaeffel (1996). "Melatonin and deprivation myopia in chickens." *Neurochem Int* 28(1): 95-107.

Illnerova, H., M. Backstrom, et al. (1978). "Melatonin in rat pineal gland and serum; rapid parallel decline after light exposure at night." *Neurosci Lett* 9(2-3): 189-193.

Inouye, S. T. and H. Kawamura (1979). "Persistence of circadian rhythmicity in a mammalian hypothalamic "island" containing the suprachiasmatic nucleus." *Proc Natl Acad Sci U S A* 76(11): 5962-5966.

Iuvone, P. M. and J. C. Besharse (1986). "Dopamine receptor-mediated inhibition of serotonin N-acetyltransferase activity in retina." *Brain Res* 369(1-2): 168-176.

Iuvone, P. M., C. L. Galli, et al. (1978). "Light stimulates tyrosine hydroxylase activity and dopamine synthesis in retinal amacrine neurons." *Science* 202(4370): 901-902.

Iuvone, P. M., M. Tigges, et al. (1991). "Effects of apomorphine, a dopamine receptor agonist, on ocular refraction and axial elongation in a primate model of myopia." *Invest Ophthalmol Vis Sci* 32(5): 1674-1677.

Iuvone, P. M., G. Tosini, et al. (2005). "Circadian clocks, clock networks, arylalkylamine N-acetyltransferase, and melatonin in the retina." *Prog Retin Eye Res* 24(4): 433-456.

Jacobsen, N., H. Jensen, et al. (2008). "Does the level of physical activity in university students influence development and progression of myopia? - A 2-year prospective cohort study." *Invest Ophthalmol Vis Sci* 49(4): 1322-1327.

Jones, L. A., L. T. Sinnott, et al. (2007). "Parental history of myopia, sports and outdoor activities, and future myopia." *Invest Ophthalmol Vis Sci* 48(8): 3524-3532.

Kakita, T., T. Hiraoka, et al. (2011). "Influence of overnight orthokeratology on axial elongation in childhood myopia." *Invest Ophthalmol Vis Sci* 52(5): 2170-2174.

Kang, S. W., A. Thayananuphat, et al. (2007). "Dopamine-melatonin neurons in the avian hypothalamus controlling seasonal reproduction." *Neuroscience* 150(1): 223-233.

Khaldy, H., J. Leon, et al. (2002). "Circadian rhythms of dopamine and dihydroxyphenyl acetic acid in the mouse striatum: effects of pinealectomy and of melatonin treatment." *Neuroendocrinology* 75(3): 201-208.

Kramer, S. G. (1971). "Dopamine: A retinal neurotransmitter. I. Retinal uptake, storage, and light-stimulated release of H3-dopamine in vivo." *Invest Ophthalmol* 10(6): 438-452.

Kroger, R. H. and H. J. Wagner (1996). "The eye of the blue acara (Aequidens pulcher, Cichlidae) grows to compensate for defocus due to chromatic aberration." *J Comp Physiol A* 179(6): 837-842.

Larsen, J. S. (1971). "The sagittal growth of the eye. IV. Ultrasonic measurement of the axial length of the eye from birth to puberty." *Acta Ophthalmol* 49(6): 873-886.

Larsen, P. J., L. W. Enquist, et al. (1998). "Characterization of the multisynaptic neuronal control of the rat pineal gland using viral transneuronal tracing." *Eur J Neurosci* 10(1): 128-145.

Lerner, A. B., J. D. Case, et al. (1958). "Isolation of Melatonin, the Pineal Gland Factor That Lightens Melanocytes." *J Am Chem Soc* 80(10): 2587-2587.

Levi, F. and U. Schibler (2007). "Circadian rhythms: mechanisms and therapeutic implications." *Annu Rev Pharmacol Toxicol* 47: 593-628.

Lewy, A. J., R. L. Sack, et al. (1987). "Antidepressant and circadian phase-shifting effects of light." *Science* 235(4786): 352-354.

Lewy, A. J., R. L. Sack, et al. (1985). "Immediate and delayed effects of bright light on human melatonin production: shifting "dawn" and "dusk" shifts the dim light melatonin onset (DLMO)." *Ann N Y Acad Sci* 453: 253-259.

Li, T. and H. C. Howland (2003). "The effects of constant and diurnal illumination of the pineal gland and the eyes on ocular growth in chicks." *Invest Ophthalmol Vis Sci* 44(8): 3692-3697.

Li, T., H. C. Howland, et al. (2000). "Diurnal illumination patterns affect the development of the chick eye." *Vision Res* 40(18): 2387-2393.

Li, T., D. Troilo, et al. (1995). "Constant light produces severe corneal flattening and hyperopia in chickens." *Vision Res* 35(9): 1203-1209.

Lin, L. L., Y. F. Shih, et al. (2004). "Prevalence of myopia in Taiwanese schoolchildren: 1983 to 2000." *Ann Acad Med Singapore* 33(1): 27-33.

Liu, J., K. Pendrak, et al. (2004). "Emmetropisation under continuous but non-constant light in chicks." *Exp Eye Res* 79(5): 719-728.

Liu, R., Y. F. Qian, et al. (2011). "Effects of different monochromatic lights on refractive development and eye growth in guinea pigs." *Exp Eye Res*. 92(6):447-453

Liu, T. and J. Borjigin (2005). "N-acetyltransferase is not the rate-limiting enzyme of melatonin synthesis at night." *J Pineal Res* 39(1): 91-96.

Loman, J., G. E. Quinn, et al. (2002). "Darkness and near work: myopia and its progression in third-year law students." *Ophthalmology* 109(5): 1032-1038.

Long, Q., D. Chen, et al. (2009). "Illumination with monochromatic long-wavelength light promotes myopic shift and ocular elongation in newborn pigmented guinea pigs." *Cutan Ocul Toxicol* 28(4): 176-180.

Luft, W. A., P. M. Iuvone, et al. (2004). "Spatial, temporal, and intensive determinants of dopamine release in the chick retina." *Vis Neurosci* 21(4): 627-635.

Lynch, H. J., D. C. Jimerson, et al. (1978). "Entrainment of rhythmic melatonin secretion in man to a 12-hour phase shift in the light/dark cycle." *Life Sci* 23(15): 1557-1563.

Mandel, Y., I. Grotto, et al. (2008). "Season of birth, natural light, and myopia." *Ophthalmology* 115(4): 686-692.

Mandelman, T. and J. G. Sivak (1983). "Longitudinal chromatic aberration of the vertebrate eye." *Vision Res* 23(12): 1555-1559.

Mao, J., S. Liu, et al. (2010). "Levodopa inhibits the development of form-deprivation myopia in guinea pigs." *Optom Vis Sci* 87(1): 53-60.

Martin, X. D., H. Z. Malina, et al. (1992). "The ciliary body - the third organ found to synthesize indoleamines in humans." *Eur J Ophthalmol* 2(2): 67-72.

Maywood, E. S., R. C. Buttery, et al. (1990). "Gonadal responses of the male Syrian hamster to programmed infusions of melatonin are sensitive to signal duration and frequency but not to signal phase nor to lesions of the suprachiasmatic nuclei." *Biol Reprod* 43(2): 174-182.

McCarthy, C. S., P. Megaw, et al. (2007). "Dopaminergic agents affect the ability of brief periods of normal vision to prevent form-deprivation myopia." *Exp Eye Res* 84(1): 100-107.

McIntyre, I. M., T. R. Norman, et al. (1989). "Human melatonin suppression by light is intensity dependent." *J Pineal Res* 6(2): 149-156.

McMahon, G., T. Zayats, et al. (2009). "Season of Birth, Daylight Hours at Birth, and High Myopia." *Ophthalmology*. 116(3):468-473

Megaw, P. L., M. G. Boelen, et al. (2006). "Diurnal patterns of dopamine release in chicken retina." *Neurochem Int* 48(1): 17-23.

Melamed, E., Y. Frucht, et al. (1984). "Dopamine turnover in rat retina: a 24-hour light-dependent rhythm." *Brain Res* 305(1): 148-151.

Morgan, I. G. and M. K. Boelen (1996). "A retinal dark-light switch: a review of the evidence." *Vis Neurosci* 13(3): 399-409.

Mutti, D. O., G. L. Mitchell, et al. (2002). "Parental myopia, near work, school achievement, and children's refractive error." *Invest Ophthalmol Vis Sci* 43(12): 3633-3640.

Neumann, T., C. Ziegler, et al. (2008). "Multielectrode array recordings reveal physiological diversity of intrinsically photosensitive retinal ganglion cells in the chick embryo." *Brain Res* 1207: 120-127.

Nickla, D. L. (2006). "The phase relationships between the diurnal rhythms in axial length and choroidal thickness and the association with ocular growth rate in chicks." *J Comp Physiol A Neuroethol Sens Neural Behav Physiol* 192(4): 399-407.

Nickla, D. L., K. Totonelly, et al. (2010). "Dopaminergic agonists that result in ocular growth inhibition also elicit transient increases in choroidal thickness in chicks." *Exp Eye Res* 91(5): 715-720.

Nickla, D. L., C. Wildsoet, et al. (1998). "Visual influences on diurnal rhythms in ocular length and choroidal thickness in chick eyes." *Exp Eye Res* 66(2): 163-181.

Nickla, D. L., C. F. Wildsoet, et al. (2001). "Endogenous rhythms in axial length and choroidal thickness in chicks: implications for ocular growth regulation." *Invest Ophthalmol Vis Sci* 42(3): 584-588.

Norton, T. T., A. O. Amedo, et al. (2006). "Darkness causes myopia in visually experienced tree shrews." *Invest Ophthalmol Vis Sci* 47(11): 4700-4707.

Nowak, J. Z., A. Kazula, et al. (1992). "Melatonin increases serotonin N-acetyltransferase activity and decreases dopamine synthesis in light-exposed chick retina: in vivo evidence supporting melatonin-dopamine interaction in retina." *J Neurochem* 59(4): 1499-1505.

Nowak, J. Z., E. Zurawska, et al. (1989). "Melatonin and its generating system in vertebrate retina: circadian rhythm, effect of environmental lighting and interaction with dopamine." *Neurochem Int* 14(4): 397-406.

Ohngemach, S., M. Feldkaemper, et al. (2001). "Pineal control of the dopamine D2-receptor gene and dopamine release in the retina of the chicken and their possible relation to growth rhythms of the eye." *J Pineal Res* 31(2): 145-154.

Oishi, T., J. K. Lauber, et al. (1987). "Experimental myopia and glaucoma in chicks." *Zoolog Sci* 4: 455-464.

Osol, G. and B. Schwartz (1984). "Melatonin in the human retina." *Exp Eye Res* 38(2): 213-215.

Papastergiou, G. I., G. F. Schmid, et al. (1998). "Ocular axial length and choroidal thickness in newly hatched chicks and one-year-old chickens fluctuate in a diurnal pattern that is influenced by visual experience and intraocular pressure changes." *Exp Eye Res* 66(2): 195-205.

Parkinson, D. and R. R. Rando (1983). "Effect of light on dopamine turnover and metabolism in rabbit retina." *Invest Ophthalmol Vis Sci* 24(3): 384-388.

Pendrak, K., T. Nguyen, et al. (1997). "Retinal dopamine in the recovery from experimental myopia." *Curr Eye Res* 16(2): 152-157.

Perez-Leon, J. A., E. J. Warren, et al. (2006). "Synaptic inputs to retinal ganglion cells that set the circadian clock." *Eur J Neurosci* 24(4): 1117-1123.

Perlow, M. J., E. K. Gordon, et al. (1977). "The circadian variation in dopamine metabolism in the subhuman primate." *J Neurochem* 28(6): 1381-1383.

Perlow, M. J., S. M. Reppert, et al. (1980). "Photic regulation of the melatonin rhythm: monkey and man are not the same." *Brain Res* 182(1): 211-216.

Pitrosky, B., R. Kirsch, et al. (1995). "The photoperiodic response in Syrian hamster depends upon a melatonin-driven circadian rhythm of sensitivity to melatonin." *J Neuroendocrinol* 7(11): 889-895.

Prendergast, B. J., M. R. Gorman, et al. (2000). "Establishment and persistence of photoperiodic memory in hamsters." *Proc Natl Acad Sci U S A* 97(10): 5586-5591.

Proll, M. A., C. W. Kamp, et al. (1982). "Use of liquid chromatography with electrochemistry to measure effects of varying intensities of white light on DOPA accumulation in rat retinas." *Life Sci* 30(1): 11-19.

Provencio, I., I. R. Rodriguez, et al. (2000). "A novel human opsin in the inner retina." *J Neurosci* 20(2): 600-605.

Quinn, G. E., C. H. Shin, et al. (1999). "Myopia and ambient lighting at night." *Nature* 399(6732): 113-114.

Rada, J. A. and A. F. Wiechmann (2006). "Melatonin receptors in chick ocular tissues: implications for a role of melatonin in ocular growth regulation." *Invest Ophthalmol Vis Sci* 47(1): 25-33.

Revell, V. L. and D. J. Skene (2007). "Light-induced melatonin suppression in humans with polychromatic and monochromatic light." *Chronobiol Int* 24(6): 1125-1137.

Roenneberg, T. and R. G. Foster (1997). "Twilight times: light and the circadian system." *Photochem Photobiol* 66(5): 549-561.

Rohrer, B., A. W. Spira, et al. (1993). "Apomorphine blocks form-deprivation myopia in chickens by a dopamine D2-receptor mechanism acting in retina or pigmented epithelium." *Vis Neurosci* 10(3): 447-453.

Rollag, M. D., P. L. O'Callaghan, et al. (1978). "Serum melatonin concentrations during different stages of the annual reproductive cycle in ewes." *Biol Reprod* 18(2): 279-285.

Rose, K. A., I. G. Morgan, et al. (2008a). "Outdoor activity reduces the prevalence of myopia in children." *Ophthalmology* 115(8): 1279-1285.

Rose, K. A., I. G. Morgan, et al. (2008b). "Myopia, lifestyle, and schooling in students of Chinese ethnicity in Singapore and Sydney." *Arch Ophthalmol* 126(4): 527-530.

Ruby, N. F., T. J. Brennan, et al. (2002). "Role of melanopsin in circadian responses to light." *Science* 298(5601): 2211-2213.

Rucker, F. J. and J. Wallman (2009). "Chick eyes compensate for chromatic simulations of hyperopic and myopic defocus: evidence that the eye uses longitudinal chromatic aberration to guide eye-growth." *Vision Res* 49(14): 1775-1783.

Sakamoto, K., C. Liu, et al. (2005). "Dopamine regulates melanopsin mRNA expression in intrinsically photosensitive retinal ganglion cells." *Eur J Neurosci* 22(12): 3129-3136.

Saw, S. M., G. Gazzard, et al. (2005). "Myopia and associated pathological complications." *Ophthalmic Physiol Opt* 25(5): 381-391.

Saw, S. M., M. Z. Zhang, et al. (2002). "Near-work activity, night-lights, and myopia in the Singapore-China study." *Arch Ophthalmol* 120(5): 620-627.

Schade, R., K. Vick, et al. (1995). "Circadian rhythms of dopamine and cholecystokinin in nucleus accumbens and striatum of rats - influence on dopaminergic stimulation." *Chronobiol Int* 12(2): 87-99.

Schaeffel, F., M. Bartmann, et al. (1995). "Studies on the role of the retinal dopamine/melatonin system in experimental refractive errors in chickens." *Vision Res* 35(9): 1247-1264.

Schaeffel, F., G. Hagel, et al. (1994). "6-Hydroxy dopamine does not affect lens-induced refractive errors but suppresses deprivation myopia." *Vision Res* 34(2): 143-149.

Schmid, K. L. and C. F. Wildsoet (2004). "Inhibitory effects of apomorphine and atropine and their combination on myopia in chicks." *Optom Vis Sci* 81(2): 137-147.

Schwahn, H. N. and F. Schaeffel (1997). "Flicker parameters are different for suppression of myopia and hyperopia." *Vision Res* 37(19): 2661-2673.

Seidemann, A. and F. Schaeffel (2002). "Effects of longitudinal chromatic aberration on accommodation and emmetropization." *Vision Res* 42(21): 2409-2417.

Shaw, D. and B. D. Goldman (1995). "Influence of prenatal and postnatal photoperiods on postnatal testis development in the Siberian hamster (Phodopus sungorus)." *Biol Reprod* 52(4): 833-838.

Simonneaux, V. and C. Ribelayga (2003). "Generation of the melatonin endocrine message in mammals: a review of the complex regulation of melatonin synthesis by norepinephrine, peptides, and other pineal transmitters." *Pharmacol Rev* 55(2): 325-395.

Smith, E. L., 3rd, D. V. Bradley, et al. (2001). "Continuous ambient lighting and eye growth in primates." *Invest Ophthalmol Vis Sci* 42(6): 1146-1152.

Smith, K. A., M. W. Schoen, et al. (2004). "Adaptation of human pineal melatonin suppression by recent photic history." *J Clin Endocrinol Metab* 89(7): 3610-3614.

Sowers, J. R. and N. Vlachakis (1984). "Circadian variation in plasma dopamine levels in man." *J Endocrinol Invest* 7(4): 341-345.

Stone, R. A., T. Lin, et al. (1995). "Photoperiod, early post-natal eye growth, and visual deprivation." *Vision Res* 35(9): 1195-1202.

Stone, R. A., T. Lin, et al. (1989). "Retinal dopamine and form-deprivation myopia." *Proc Natl Acad Sci U S A* 86(2): 704-706.

Stone, R. A., K. Pendrak, et al. (2006). "Local patterns of image degradation differentially affect refraction and eye shape in chick." *Curr Eye Res* 31(1): 91-105.

Tast, A., R. J. Love, et al. (2001). "The pattern of melatonin secretion is rhythmic in the domestic pig and responds rapidly to changes in daylength." *J Pineal Res* 31(4): 294-300.

Thapan, K., J. Arendt, et al. (2001). "An action spectrum for melatonin suppression: evidence for a novel non-rod, non-cone photoreceptor system in humans." *J Physiol* 535(Pt 1): 261-267.

Thomas, K. B., M. Tigges, et al. (1993). "Melatonin synthesis and circadian tryptophan hydroxylase activity in chicken retina following destruction of serotonin immunoreactive amacrine and bipolar cells by kainic acid." *Brain Res* 601(1-2): 303-307.

Torii, M., D. Kojima, et al. (2007). "Two isoforms of chicken melanopsins show blue light sensitivity." *FEBS Lett* 581(27): 5327-5331.

Tosini, G. and J. C. Dirden (2000). "Dopamine inhibits melatonin release in the mammalian retina: in vitro evidence." *Neurosci Lett* 286(2): 119-122.

Tosini, G. and M. Menaker (1996). "Circadian rhythms in cultured mammalian retina." *Science* 272(5260): 419-421.

Tosini, G., N. Pozdeyev, et al. (2008). "The circadian clock system in the mammalian retina." *Bioessays* 30(7): 624-633.

Vannas, A. E., G. S. Ying, et al. (2003). "Myopia and natural lighting extremes: risk factors in Finnish army conscripts." *Acta Ophthalmol Scand* 81(6): 588-595.

Vitale, S., R. D. Sperduto, et al. (2009). "Increased prevalence of myopia in the United States between 1971-1972 and 1999-2004." *Arch Ophthalmol* 127(12): 1632-1639.

Wang, F., J. Zhou, et al. (2011). "Effects of 530 nm Green Light on Refractive Status, Melatonin, MT1 Receptor, and Melanopsin in the Guinea Pig." *Curr Eye Res* 36(2): 103-111.

Weiler, R., W. H. Baldridge, et al. (1997). "Modulation of endogenous dopamine release in the fish retina by light and prolonged darkness." *Vis Neurosci* 14(2): 351-356.

Weiss, S. and F. Schaeffel (1993). "Diurnal growth rhythms in the chicken eye: relation to myopia development and retinal dopamine levels." *J Comp Physiol A Neuroethol Sens Neural Behav Physiol* 172(3): 263-270.

Wiechmann, A. F. and J. G. Hollyfield (1987). "Localization of hydroxyindole-O-methyltransferase-like immunoreactivity in photoreceptors and cone bipolar cells in the human retina: a light and electron microscope study." *J Comp Neurol* 258(2): 253-266.

Wilkinson, M., J. Arendt, et al. (1977). "Determination of a dark-induced increase of pineal N-acetyl transferase activity and simultaneous radioimmunoassay of melatonin in pineal, serum and pituitary tissue of the male rat." *J Endocrinol* 72(2): 243-244.

Witkovsky, P. (2004). "Dopamine and retinal function." *Doc Ophthalmol* 108(1): 17-39.

Zadnik, K., L. A. Jones, et al. (2000). "Myopia and ambient night-time lighting. CLEERE Study Group. Collaborative Longitudinal Evaluation of Ethnicity and Refractive Error." *Nature* 404(6774): 143-144.

Zawilska, J. B., D. J. Skene, et al. (2009). "Physiology and pharmacology of melatonin in relation to biological rhythms." *Pharmacol Rep* 61(3): 383-410.

Zeitzer, J. M., D. J. Dijk, et al. (2000). "Sensitivity of the human circadian pacemaker to nocturnal light: melatonin phase resetting and suppression." *J Physiol* 526 Pt 3: 695-702.

Zmijewski, M. A., T. W. Sweatman, et al. (2009). "The melatonin-producing system is fully functional in retinal pigment epithelium (ARPE-19)." *Mol Cell Endocrinol* 307(1-2): 211-216.

10

Etiology and Clinical Presentation of Astigmatism

Sanja Masnec Olujić
Ghethaldus Ophthalmology Policlinics, Zagreb
Croatia

1. Introduction

A perfect point image of an object point is called a stigmatic image. The term „stigmatic"is derived from the Greek word stigma, which refers to a sharply pointed stylus (Liesegang et al., 2002). Thus, a stigmatic optical system is one able to focus all the light rays from a point source onto a single point. However, in most cases, images are not stigmatic.

In paraxial optics, the focus is stigmatic, and all paraxial rays (those extremely close to the optical axis) focus onto a point. With nonparaxial rays, the focus is generally not stigmatic. Deviations from stigmatic imaging are called aberrations, and, one of a number of ways to classify such aberrations is clinically: into spherical aberrations, regular astigmatism and irregular astigmatism.

Astigmatism is the unequal refraction of the same eye in two different meridians. Unlike the basic types of refraction- emetropia, myopia and hyperopia- where all the light rays enter one focus (on the retina, behind it, or in front of it), in astigmatism there is no a single focus. In basic types of refraction, the cornea is spherical and it refracts equally in all the meridians.

In astigmatism variations in the curvature of the cornea or lens along different meridians prevent the light rays from focusing onto a single point. Corneal refraction depends on the corneal curvature. If the cornea is more curved, the power of refraction is higher and vice versa. Corneal and lenticular astigmatism can complement or cancel each other. Their summation represents the so called "total astigmatism".

Due to the lack of a single focus, an astigmatic eye is not able to see clearly without correction. Astigmatic patients complain of visual disturbances in both far (in myopia) and near vision (in hyperopia), which causes astenopic problems (headache, dizziness, fatigue etc). Additionally, regular, symmetric objects might seem to them irregular, and /or elongated.

2. Astigmatism types

Astigmatism can be regular or irregular. It can also be divided into myopic, hyperopic and mixed/compound astigmatism (where one of the main meridians is hyperopic and the other one myopic).

2.1 Regular astigmatism

In regular astigmatism each meridian refracts regularly and equally, but differently from the other meridians. One of the meridians refracts the most and another one the least. Those two meridians are called the main meridians, and they are perpendicular to each other.

In most cases, one of the main meridians is located vertically and the other one horizontally, but there can also be oblique, still maintaining the 90° angle to each other.

In the remaining meridians, located between the both two main meridians, refraction changes gradually –increases or decreases (Fig 1).

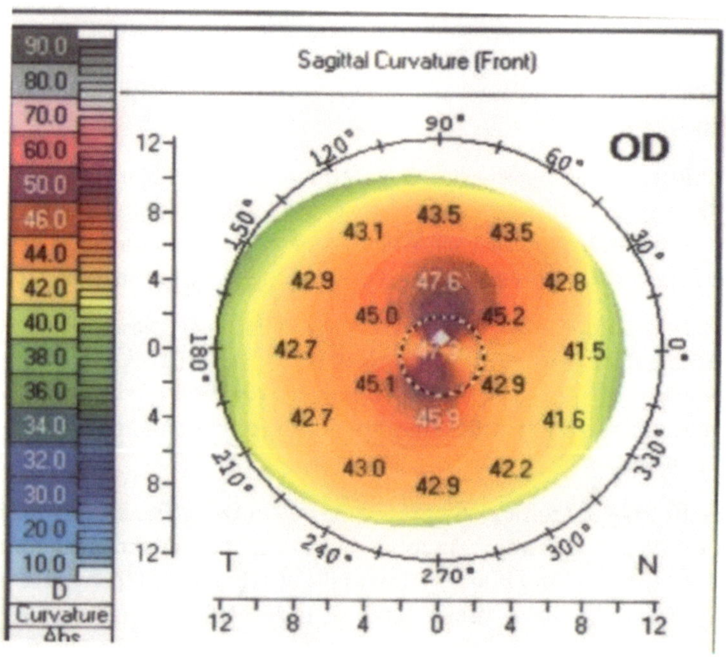

Fig. 1. With-the-rule astigmatism of 5.4 D shown on the topographical map of the anterior corneal surface , with quantitative information on the corneal curvature, astigmatism and its meridians.

Vertical meridian, in most of cases, refracts more then the horizontal, most likely due to the pressure of eyelids onto the cornea. This type of astigmatism is called *with- the- rule* astigmatism and is more common in children (Mohindra et al., 1978).

If the horizontal meridian refracts more, this is called *against- the- rule* astigmatism and is more common in older adults.

The difference in refraction of the two main meridians represents the amount of astigmatism and is represented in diopters (D).

When that difference is no more than 1/2 -3/4 diopters it is a so-called physiological astigmatism and a correction is usually not needed, as it does not lead to visual deterioration or subjective symptoms. Mostly, it is neutralized by the lenticular astigmatism (Parunovic et al., 1995).

Astigmatism over ¾ D can lead to visual disturbances and other subjective symptoms, because the lenticular astigmatism, which rarely exceeds 1-1.5 D, is not able to compensate for the corneal astigmatism.

Regular type astigmatism is rarely greater than 6-7 D.

For a better understanding of astigmatism and its correction, the most important optical concept is the **conoid of Sturm.**

The refractive power, as mentioned above, changes from one meridian to the next, and an astigmatic surface cannot bring a pencil of light rays to a point focus. Two focal lines instead of a single focus are formed. This complex geometrical envelope of a pencil of light rays refracted by a circular spherocylindrical lens is called the **conoid of Sturm.**

The conoid of Sturm has two focal lines, each parallel to one of the main meridians of the spherocylindrical lens. All the light rays in the pencil pass through each of the focal lines. The cross sections of the conoid of Sturm at various points along its length are mostly elliptical, including the portion of the conoid external to the two focal lines. At the dioptric mean of the two focal lines there is a circular cross section of the conoid of Sturm. This circular patch of light rays is called the *circle of least confusion,* and represents the best overall focus for the spherocylindrical lens. The circle of least confusion is the position where all the rays would be brought to focus if the lens had a spherical power equal to the average spherical power of all the meridians of the spherocylindrical lens (Michaels, 1980).

This average spherical power of a spherocylindrical lens represents the spherical equivalent of the lens, and can be calculated by the following equation:

$$\text{Spherical equivalent} = \text{sphere} + \text{cylinder}/2.$$

About 50% of infants in their first years of life show astigmatism of over 1D (Bennet et al., 1989; Mohindra et al., 1978).

Some authors have suggested that this high astigmatism helps the infant to bracket the position of best focus while it learns to accommodate (Howland et al., 1978).

In adults, this high incidence of astigmatism is much smaller. Different studies show that about 15 % of adults have astigmatism greater than 1D, and only 2 % of more then 3D (Yanoff & Duker, 2004).

In the leater group, it is most likely that much of the high astigmatism is due to some form of intraocular surgery, such as cataract surgery (particularly when extracapsular cataract extraction is performed), corneal transplants, corneal lacerations repair, …etc.

Regular astigmatism can be congenital and acquired. Congenital astigmatism is usually inherited. Acquired astigmatism is mostly against-the rule and as mentioned above, can result from various intraocular surgeries.

Most oftenly, astigmatism is static, but it can also change during the life time. With -the - rule astigmatism tends to lessen over the years, and the position of the main meridians can also slightly change during the lifetime.

Regular astigmatism is correctable by cylindrical spectacle lenses and contact lenses.

In with-the rule astigmatism, a correcting plus cylinder lens should be used at or near the 90° axis. In against-the rule astigmatism, a correcting plus cylinder lens should be used at or near the 180° axis.

2.2 Irregular astigmatism

Irregular astigmatism appears when the refraction of light is unequal and irregular in the same meridian of the eye.

That is usually a consequence of pathological changes especially to the cornea (maculae centrales corneae, ulcus, pannus, keratoconus etc) or lens (cataract, posterior capsular opacification, lens subluxation etc).

The visual acuity of such an eye is deteriorated and sometimes monocular diplopia or poliopia occurs. All eyes have at least a small amount of irregular astigmatism, but the term is used clinically only for the stronger irregularities, such as those mentioned above, or occurring with keratoconus.

In the past, irregular astigmatism was not a field of strong interest by clinicians, as it was not very common, and was not treatable. It could not be corrected with spectacles, and rigid contact lenses could alleviate the problem to some extent only if the irregular astigmatism was corneal in origin.

With the development of keratorefractive surgical procedures, it became increasingly of interest, as keratorefractive surgeries may produce visually significant irregular astigmatism, or be used to treat it.

2.2.1 Keratoconus

Keratoconus (conical cornea) is a condition characterized by a progressive corneal steepening, usually inferior to the center of the cornea (Fig. 2.). As a result of a noninflammatory thinning of the corneal stroma eventually myopia is induced, together with irregular astigmatism, leading to an impairment in the quality of vision.

Keratoconus is a bilateral, usually asymmetric, noninflammatory corneal ectasia, which belongs to a group of corneal shape disorders, together with pellucid marginal corneal degeneration and keratoglobus.

By keratometry keratoconus is classified as:

1. mild (< 48 D)
2. moderate (48-54 D)
3. severe (> 54 D).

Epidemiology and pathogenesis

Keratoconus occurs in all ethnic groups with no male or female preponderance.

Rarely, it can be congenital (Smolin, 1987).

In majority of the cases, its onset is at puberty and then progresses until the third to fourth decade of life, with an incidence of approximately 1 per 2000 in the general population, and a prevalence of 54.5 per 100,000 (Hofstetter, 1959; Kennedy et al., 1986).

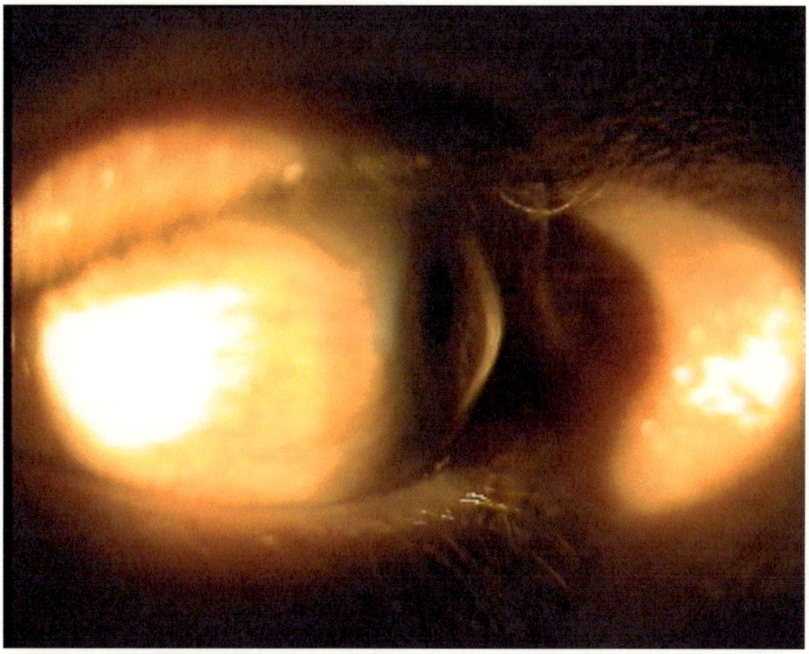

Fig. 2. Keratoconus (conical cornea)

In some cases it may also start later in life and progress at any age.

The etiology of the disease can be divided into three groups:

1. inherited
2. sporadic
3. acquired (secondary or in association to / with other diseases).

The inheritance of keratoconus is still not defined completely. Before the presence of videokeratography it was believed that more than 90 % of cases were sporadic, but recent studies revealed evidence that suggests an autosomal dominant pattern of inheritance (Gonzales & McDonnell, 1992).

Corneal thinning appears to result from a loss of structural components in the cornea, but why this happens is still not clear.

Recent biochemical studies of cornea with keratoconus suggest that enzyme abnormalities in the corneal epithelium, such as increased expression of proteases and other catabolic enzymes (Sawagamuchi et al., 1989) and decreased levels of inhibitors of proteolytic enzymes, may play a role in corneal stromal digestion and degradation (Fukuchi et al., 1994).

Investigations of corneal α1 proteinase inhibitor and α2 macroglobulin (also proteinase inhibitor) support the hypothesis that the degradation process may be aberrant in keratoconus (Sawagamuchi et al., 1994)

Evidence has been provided regarding abnormalities in gene promoters involved in these enzyme activities (Maruyama et al., 2001).

Other studies have reported abnormalities in corneal collagen and its cross-linking, as a potential cause of keratoconus (Bron, 1988).

Some authors have proposed a role for an IL-1 system in the cornea in the pathogenesis of keratoconus. It is suggested that the increased expression of the IL-1 receptor sensitizes the keratocytes to IL-1 released from the epithelium or endothelium, causing a loss of keratocytes through apoptosis and a decrease in stromal mass over time (Wilson et al., 1996).

It is most commonly a single disorder, although much evidence exists that it could be a phenotypic expression of many causes, or part of other multisystem or systemic disorders, as well as ocular non-corneal disorders (Rabinowitz, 1998, table 1).

Multisystem Disorders	Ocular Disorders
Alagille' s syndrome	Aniridia
Albers-Schonberg disease	Anetoderma and bilateral subcapsular cataracts
Angelman syndrome	Ankyloblepharon
Apert' s syndrome	Bilateral macular coloboma
Autographism	Blue sclerae
Anetoderma	Congenital cataracts
Bardet-Biedl syndrome	Ectodermal and mesodermal anomalities
Crouzon' s syndrome	Floppy eyelid syndrome
Down syndrome	Gyrate atrophy
Ehlers-Danlos syndrome	Iridoschisis
Goltz-Gorlin syndrome	Lebers congenital amaurosis
Hyperornithemia	Persistent pupilarry membrane
Icthyosis	Posterior lenticonus
Kurz syndrome	Retinitis pigmentosa
Laurence-Moon-Bardet-Biedl syndrome	Retinal disinsection syndrome
Marphan' s syndrome	Retrolental fibroplasia
Mulvihil-Smith syndrome	Vernal conjunctivitis
Nail patella syndrome	Atopic keratoconjunctivitis
Neurocutaneous angiomatosis	Axenfeld' s anomaly
Neurofibromatosis	Avellino' s dystrophy
Noonan' s syndrome	Chandler' s syndrome
Osteogenesis imperfecta	Corneal amyloidosis
Oculodentodigital syndrome	Deep filiform corneal dystrophy
Pseudoxanthoma elasticum	Essential iris atrophy
Rieger' s syndrome	Fleck corneal dystrophy
Rothmund s syndrome	Fuchs corneal dystrophy
Tourette' s disease	Iridocorneal dystrophy
Turner' s syndrome	Lattice dystrophy
Xeroderma pigmentosum	Microcornea
Congenital hip dysplasia	Pellucid marginal degeneration
False chordae tendineae of left ventricle	Posterior polymorphous dystrophy
Joint hypermobility	Terriens marginal degeneration
Mitral valve prolapse	
Measles retinopathy	
Ocular hypertension	
Thalesselis syndrome	

Table 1. Diseases associated with keratoconus, as reported by different authors

The most common association is with Down syndrome, connective tissue disorders, and Leber's congenital amaurosis (Cullen & Butler, 1963; Iwaszkiewicz, 1989).

Acquired etiologies can be divided into those which are attributed to inflammatory conditions, such as vernal conjunctivitis and those secondary to eye rubbing which can also release inflammatory mediators, such as Leber's congenital amaurosis and Down syndrome.

Many authors report a high incidence of mitral valve prolapse (58%) in patients with advanced keratoconus, while others report of eye rubbing in systemic atopy and cytokine interleukin-1, as a mediator of stromal degradation. Other factors, such as contact lens wear, may play a role in the development of the cone (Krachmer et al.,1984; Sharif et al., 1992).

Also, some studies report 6-8% of cases with positive family history or evidence of familiar transmission (Hallerman & Wilson, 1977; Krachmer et al., 1984).

Ocular manifestations

Early stages of the disorder may not present any symptoms. Cornea may appear normal on slit-lamp examination and there may be no symptoms of the disease. It maya be suspected by an ophthalmologist because the patient cannot be refracted to a 20/20 corrected vision. There might only be a mild steepening of keratometry mires, inferiorly or centrally. In such cases, anterior topography of the central and paracentral cornea will confirm the suspected diagnosis (Krachmer et al, 1984). In advanced cases, there can be a significant visual disturbance followed by a significant visual loss, but, fortunately, patients with keratoconus never become totally blind. Symptoms, as well as clinical signs, are variable and depend on the stage of the progression and on the severity of the disease.

The corneal manifestations include steepening (centrally or paracentrally, most commonly inferiorly or inferotemporally), thinning of the corneal apex, conical protrusion, a ring of iron deposits partially or completely accumulating in the epithelium surrounding the cone *(Fleischer's ring)*, anterior scars at the level of Bowman's membrane, enlarged corneal nerves, increased intensity of the corneal endothelial reflex, and deep vertical lines in stroma and Descemet' s membrane, that disappear momentally under digital pressure during slit-lamp examination *(Vogt' s striae)*.

The steeping of the cornea leads to clinical signs, which include the V-shaped protrusion of the lower eyelid on downgaze due to the ectatic cornea (*Munson's sign*, Fig. 3.), sharply focused light beam at the nasal limbus, produced by lateral illumination *(Rizzuti's sign)*, and a dark reflex using the retroillumination techniques in the area of the cone, when observing the cornea with the pupil dilatation *(Charleaux' s sign)*, and an irregular "scissor" reflex on retinoscopy.

Some patients with advanced keratoconus may occasionally experience sudden visual loss and pain due to the acute rupture of Descemet's membrane (acute hydrops). In such cases the conjunctive may be injected, and diffuse stromal edema appears. These breaks in Descemet's membrane result in acute overhydration and a stromal imbibing of aqueous. The overlying corneal epithelium may become edematous. The edema may last for months and, after the resolution of redness and relief of pain over time, can be replaced by scarring (and the corneal steepness may be reduced).

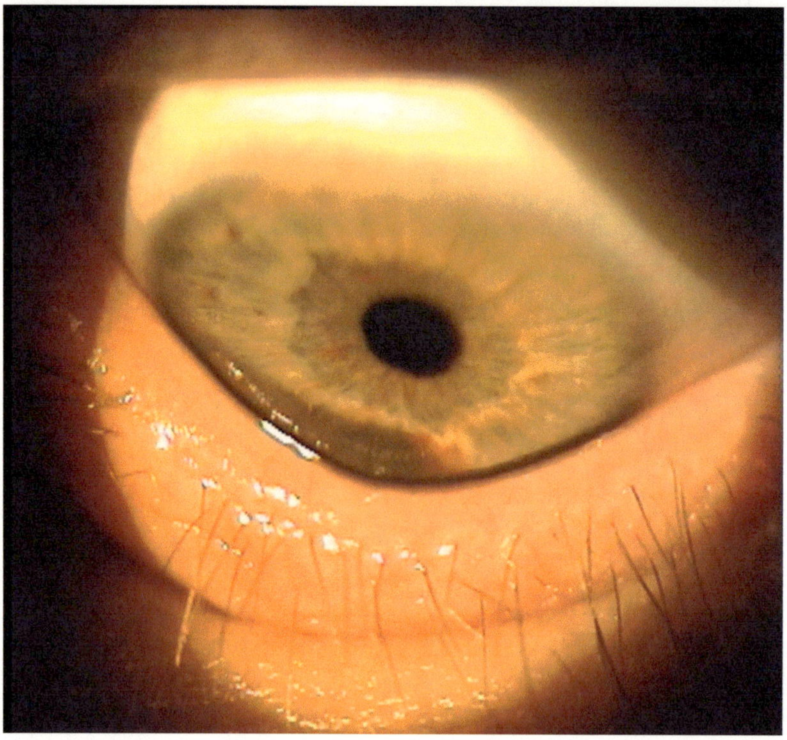

Fig. 3. V-shaped protrusion of the lower eyelid on downgaze due to the ectatic cornea (Munson' s sign)

Histopathology

The classic histopathological triad in keratoconus includes the thinning of the corneal stroma, breaks in Bowman' s layer and iron deposits in the basal layers of the corneal epithelium. Also, every other layer of the cornea can be pathologically affected, depending on the stage of the keratoconus. The endothelium is usually not affected, and the Descemet's membrane is rarely affected, other than in cases of acute hydrops.

Two types of cone morphology may be present. The first one is a „nipple" type cone, located centrally, characterized by small size (5 mm) and steep curvature; the second one is an „oval" type cone, located inferiorly or inferotemporally, characterized by larger size (5-6 mm), and an ellipsoid shape (Perry et al., 1980).

These can be distinguished in most cases on slit-lamp examination, or in the anterior corneal topography.

Diagnosis

To confirm the diagnosis several devices are available from handheld keratoscopes (placido disks), computer-assisted videokeratoscopes to (more recently) computerized videokeratography (Fig.4).

Computer-assisted topographic modeling systems allow the clinicians to detect subtle and minor variations in power distribution of the anterior and posterior corneal surface. The *forme fruste*, or subclinical keratoconus, recognized by Placido disk-based topography, requires caution and is considered a contraindication to refractive surgery. With regard to the identification of forme fruste keratoconus, classification programs on corneal topographers may assist in differentiating between keratoconus suspects, corneal distortion, and even patients having undergone refractive surgery, and normal variations of corneal topography.

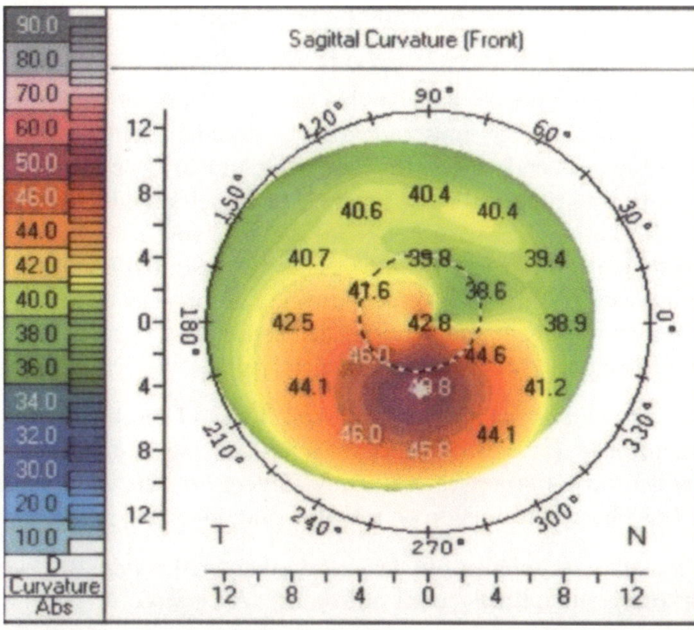

Fig. 4. Color-coded map of peripheral keratoconus. Note the inferior steepening

Rabinowitz has suggested that the diagnosis of keratoconus can be made when keratometry is greater than 47.20 D, the steepening of the inferior cornea compared with the superior cornea is more than 1.2 D, and the skewing of the radial axis of astigmatism is greater then 21° (Rabinowitz YS, 1995).

Differential diagnosis

The differential diagnosis of keratoconus includes other corneal ectasia disorders, such as pellucid marginal corneal degeneration and keratoglobus, and the posttraumatic or post-surgical (after refractive or cataract surgery) corneal ectasia or protrusion of the cornea after corneal ulceration thinning.

Treatment

Treatment of keratoconus starts with spectacles in very early stages, for astigmatism and myopia, and rigid gas permeable contact lenses in cases of inadequate visual acuity correction with spectacles. Contact lenses represent the treatment of choice in 90% of patients (Buxton et al., 1984).

In case of contact lens failure due to a lack of adequate visual acuity, or induced corneal abrasion, apical scarring, neovascularization due to hypoxia, poor lens tolerability and discomfort and lens displacement, surgical procedure is indicated. The most frequent surgical procedure is penetrating keratoplasty, which refers to the full-thickness replacement of diseased corneal tissue with a healthy donor. The main difficulty during surgery is suturing to the thin corneal bed.

Lamellar keratoplasty is also effective, but is not as frequently used as the penetrating keratoplasty, due to technical challenges and it being more time consuming. It is a procedure in which a partial-thickness graft of donor tissue (donor stroma or sclera) is used to provide tectonic stability and /or optical improvement.

There are generally two types of lamellar keratoplasty: anterior and posterior. In the anterior lamellar keratoplasty, the transplanted tissue does not include corneal endothelium and this procedure avoids endothelial rejection. The aim in deep lamellar and posterior lamellar keratoplasty is to replace diseased corneal endothelium while keeping the anterior corneal surface intact, as well as reducing refractive error and irregular astigmatism. In a short amount of time, deep lamellar endothelial keratoplasty (DLEK), Descemet-stripping endothelial keratoplasty (DSEK), Descemet-stripping automated endothelial keratoplasty (DSAEK) and Descemet' s membrane endothelial keratoplasty (DMEK) have become the techniques of choice for partial corneal transplant surgeries.

Descemet's membrane endothelial keratoplasty (DMEK) and Descemet-stripping automated endothelial keratoplasty (DSAEK) are new types of partial-thickness corneal graft operations, in which only the innermost corneal layers are replaced. Visual recovery is quicker, there is less physical restriction on activities and no related suture problems.

The results of lamellar techniques are far better than epikeratoplasty which has been abandoned due to the suboptimal visual outcomes. A keratoconic patient has a 10-20% chance, over her/his lifetime, of needing a corneal transplant (Smiddy et al., 1988; Tuft et al.,1994).

Intracorneal ring segments Intacts can be also used in cases without corneal scarring to reduce myopia and astigmatism. The purpose of Intacts segment implantation is to defer the need for corneal transplantation and restore contact lens tolerance. The placement of Intacts generates the response that interrupts the biomechanical disease progression, and a biomechanical response that allows visual improvement over six months. The improvement in visual acuity and refraction is accomplished by shortening the path length of the portion of the collagen lamellae that are central to the segments. The redistribution of corneal curvature leads to a redistribution of corneal stress, interrupting the biomechanical cycle of the keratoconus progression.

A relatively new method of treating progressive corneal ectasia is **corneal collagen crosslinking (CXL).** Its clinical use has been rapidly increasing since it was originally introduced in 1997 as the first treatment that could improve the biomechanical stability of the weakened cornea. This method is based on combined action of the photo-sensitizer riboflavin (vitamin B2) and ultraviolet A light, which induce the formation of new covalent bonds between the collagen fibers.

This method has been widely accepted since the first introduction by Spoerl and his co-workers at Dresden University in Germany, in 1997 (Spörl et al., 1997).

The recent advances in diagnostic devices resulted in the detection of more subtle corneal changes, suggesting that the sublinical forms are more common than fully developed keratoconus. The iatrogenic post-LASIK ectasia is the second most common corneal ectasia. It usually appears as a result of refractive surgery performed in predisposed individuals or in patients with an undetected early form of keratoconus. Before the introduction of corneal collagen crosslinking, the only treatment that could halt the progression of keratoconus in most cases was the penetrating keratoplasty.

Studies which have been conducted so far demonstrated the beneficial effect in halting the progression of the diseases, with a very low complication rate (Koller et al., 2009; Tomkins & Garzozi, 2008).

The term „crosslinking"refers to the formation of bonds between natural polymer molecules.

The original crosslinking technique described by Wollensak and co-workers is still being used today, with the minor modifications. (Wollensak et al., 2003).

The photopolymerizing effect is induced by the combined action of riboflavin as a photo-sensitizer, and long wavelength ultraviolet (UVA) light of 370 nm. This particular wavelength was chosen so that riboflavin can achieve a maximal absorption while still remaining bellow harmful radiation levels. During the exposure, riboflavin is excited into a triplet state, generating the so-called reactive oxygen species which, in turn, induce the formation of new covalent bonds (disulphide / s-s) between the amino acids of neighboring collagen fibers.

After the application of a local anesthetic, a lid speculum is inserted and central corneal abrasion up to 9.0 mm in diameter is made. According to the protocol of the Institute for Refractive and Ophthalmic Surgery in Zürich, Switzerland, 0.1% riboflavin solution containing 10 mg of riboflavin-5-phosphate diluted in 10 ml of a 20% dextran solution is instilled every 3 minutes, for 30 minutes. After that, central corneal thickness (CCT) is measured. For safety reasons, additional riboflavin 0.1% hypoosmotic drops without dextran should be applied in corneas whose thickness is less than 400 μm. Otherwise, UVA light should not be applied. The cornea is then irradiated for 30 minutes with an UVA illumination device. The device must provide a homogenous UV radiation with irradiance of 3 mW/ cm^2 at the working distance of 5 cm. During irradiation, the cornea is moistened every 3 minutes with the riboflavin 0.1% drops. The total dosage delivered to the cornea in that way is 5.4 J/cm^2. At the end, antibiotic ointment is applied and bandage lens inserted to facilitate the epithelial healing.

Beside the standard CXL, as described above (with removal of the epithelium), the treatment can also be the transepithelial CXL (without removal of the epithelium). The later has less complications, such as death of keratocytes. Not being invasive, it is very well tolerated.

Indications for cross-linking today are clinical and instrumental progression (refractive, topographic, pachimetric, aberrometric) of corneal ectasia disorders such as keratoconus and pellucid marginal degeneration in the last 6-12 months, iatrogenic keratectasia after refractive lamellar surgery and corneal melting not responding to conventional therapy.

Contraindications include corneal thickness of less than 400 μm, central corneal opacity, epithelial healing disorders, such as map dot dystrophy and rheumatic disorders, refractive keratotomy, previous herpes simplex virus keratitis (UV-A may induce herpes reactivation), corneal melting disorders, concurrent infection, severe ocular surface disease, and pregnancy.

In recent years, corneal collagen crosslinking has become a standard treatment for the progressive corneal ectasia in numerous centers throughout the world. Additional basic and clinical research is necessary in order to establish more precise indications and to demonstrate the permanence of the treatment. Despite the evidence in support of the safety of new procedure, future studies are necessary to define its limitations and its long-term efficacy. It has the potential to reduce corneal curvature by approximately 1.0-1.5 D.

Despite the fact that no sight-threatening complications were recorded in the large prospective studies, there are some sporadic reports of stromal haze resistant to topical steroid treatment (Mazzota et al., 2007), diffuse lamellar keratitis in post-LASIK ectasia, herpetic keratitis and iritis (Kymionis et al., 2007), Acanthamoeba keratitis with corneal perforation (Rama et al., 2009), and microbial keratitis (Pollhammer & Cursiefen, 2009; Zamora & Males, 2009). Other potential complications include delay in reepithelization, sterile infiltrates, potential for induction of herpes simples virus and dendritic ulcer, and ocular surface disorders and tear dysfunction (Corkin, 2009).

The reliable data on the turnover rate of the collagen fibers are still insufficient due to the almost complete absence of corneal remodeling (Wollensak & Iomdina., 2009).

However, data such as the increased resistance to the enzymatic degradation in the crosslinked corneas support the theory of the long –lasting effect of the treatment (Spoerl et al., 2004).

2.3 Other corneal ectasias

Pellucid marginal corneal degeneration

Pellucid marginal corneal degeneration is a variant of keratoconus, characterized by a peripheral band of thinning of the inferior cornea and protrusion from the 4 to 8 o'clock position but a 2 mm uninvolved surface of the cornea between the thinning and the limbus.

It has also been described in scleroderma (Sii et al., 2004) and in Sjögren syndrome (Fernández-Barboza et al., 2009).

The thickness of the central cornea is usually normal but with marked against-the-rule astigmatism. It can nicely be recognized by videokeratography due to the typical „butterfly"appearance that represents a large degree of against-the-rule astigmatism (Maguire et al., 1987).

Treatment includes spectacles or contact lenses. Due to the extensive against-the-rule astigmatism, the success rate for fitting those patients with the hard contact lens is lesser than in patients with keratoconus. In case of inadequately vision corrected patients or in case of lens intolerability, large, eccentric penetrating keratoplasty may be considered.

Keratoglobus

In keratoglobus, in contrast to the localized thinning centrally or paracentrally in keratoconus, the entire cornea is thinned out, especially near the limbus, and has a globular protrusion (Krachmer et al., 1984).

It comes in two forms: a congenital or juvenile form and an acquired, adult form. The congenital form can be part of Ehlers-Danlos syndrome type VI, or part of the corneal syndrome associated with blue sclera and red hair (Royce et al., 1990).

The adult form can be associated with blepharitis, vernal keratoconjunctivitis, and orbital diseases than cause proptosis (Cameron, 1993).

It has a recessive pattern of inheritance and is often associated with blue sclerae and other systemic features, such as Ehlers-Danlos syndrome and other systemic connective tissue abnormalities. These kinds of corneas can be so thinned that they are prone to corneal rupture from a minimal trauma.

It was also described in thyroid orbitopathy (Jacobs et al., 1974), and was acquired in pellucid marginal degeneration after extracapsular cataract extraction (Rumelt & Rehany, 1998).

Treatment includes protection from trauma, and protective spectacles are strongly recommended. Hard contact lenses are contraindicated. Lamellar epikeratoplasty should be considered to reinforce thin corneas, and in case of acquired keratoglobus, central penetrating keratoplasty may be successful.

Terrien's marginal corneal degeneration

Terrien's marginal degeneration is a bilateral, slowly- progressive condition with marginal corneal ectasia associated with corneal neovascularisation, lipid deposition along the central edge, thinning and opacification. The cause is unknown, but it is likely to be different from the causes of most degenerations that occurs with age. It can occur at any age, but most frequently in men, 20-40 years old. Two types have been described. First one is slowly-progressive and mostly asymptomatic, and occurs in older population. The second one occurs in younger patients, it is more inflammatory in type and may be associated with episcleritis and scleritis (Iwamoto et al., 1972).

Terrien's marginal degeneration initially starts superiorly with peripheral corneal haze, gradually vascularizes, and is followed by corneal thinning that starts between the limbus and line of lipid deposition. Characteristically, a steeper sloping of the cornea occurs at the advancing edge, without the overlying edge like as in Mooren's ulcer (see below).

The thinning progresses circumferentially, but the overlying epithelium is intact.

Unlike the Mooren's ulcer, usually there is no pain or inflammation, but occasionally, it may present with recurrent painful episodes of inflammation. Perforation may occur, but is rare.

A pseudopterygium may occur in an oblique axis in some patients.

Irregular astigmatism is characteristic in the progressive flattening of vertical meridian, and the high degree of against-the rule astigmatism.

Treatment includes the use of rigid gas-permeable contact lenses. More severe thinning may require crescentic, full-thickness or lamellar keratoplasty (Hahn & Kim, 1993).

Mooren's ulcer

Mooren's ulcer is a progressive, crescentic, peripheral corneal ulceration. Two clinical types have been documented. One type occurs primarily in the older population, it is typically unilateral and more responsive to local therapy. The other is bilateral, painful, progressive corneal destruction, mostly in younger individuals, more resistant to systemic immunosuppression. The pathogenesis of Mooren's ulcer is unknown but appears to involve an autoimmune reaction against a specific target molecule in the stroma, which may occur in genetically susceptible individuals (Gottsch et al., 1999).

It has a characteristic extensive, "overhanging" edge which is absent in Terrien's disease, and progresses with a stromal, yellowish infiltrate at the advancing margin. Over time, overlying epithelial defect develops, followed by stromal melting. In the second type, the inflammation may affect all the layers of cornea and perilimbal tissue, and perforation can occur.

Patients complain of severe pain, photophobia and tearing.

In chronic cases, topographical maps show severe irregular astigmatism and peripheral steepening as a result of peripheral corneal thinning and scarring. Unlike the other forms of peripheral ulcerative keratitis, no clear zone between the ulcer and limbus can be seen.

Treatment includes local, systemic, and surgical therapy. Local therapy includes topical corticosteroids, followed by conjunctival resection if inflammation is not controlled, as well as topical cyclosporine drops. Systemic immunosuppressive treatment of the more aggressive bilateral disease has included corticosteroids, cyclosporine and methotrexate (Brown & Mondino, 1984; Foster, 1985).

Other surgical procedures include epikeratoplasty, lamellar keratoplasty, delimiting keratotomy, conjunctival flap and patch grafts of periostium.

2.4 Residual astigmatism (non-corneal astigmatism)

Corneal astigmatism of more than 2D is present in 5% of general population, while at least 93% of the population has at least 0.5D of corneal astigmatism. The percentage of residual astigmatism is between 10% and 80% (Parunovic et al., 1995).

Spherical rigid contact lens can correct total astigmatism if the correction of cylinder with the spectacles is the same value as the value of corneal astigmatism. In some cases there is a difference in value between astigmatism corrected with the spectacles and corneal astigmatism. Astigmatism that rises from this difference is called residual astigmatism, and does not correlate with the anterior surface of the cornea. Residual astigmatism is in most cases lenticular, but can also be derived from a badly fitted contact lens (a decentrated or deformed contact lens).

Lenticular astigmatism may also be caused by lens subluxation, like in Marfan's syndrome (Konradsen et al., 2010; Yeung & Weissman, 1997), changes in lens contour, like in anterior and posterior lenticonus in Alport' s syndrome (Al-Mahmood et al., 2010; Blaise et al., 2003; Hentati et al., 2008; Kim et al., 2010), lenticular trauma etc.

Residual, lenticular astigmatism is most always against-the-rule astigmatism, rarely more than 1D, and usually is masked by correction of total refractive astigmatism. Residual astigmatism (RA) is calculated by subtracting the value of corneal astigmatism (CA) from the value of astigmatism corrected by the spectacles (SC), according the formula: RA = SC - CA.

Example:
Keratometry: 43.00 / 43.50 x 90
Spectacle correction: -2.00 / -1.50 x 180
Residual astigmatism = (- 1.00 x 180) - (- 0.50 x 180) = - 0.50 x 180

2.5 Surgically induced astigmatism

One of the possible complications of cataract surgery (especially extracapsular and intracapsular cataract extraction), as well as penetrating keratoplasty, is induced astigmatism, which is a major cause of functional disturbance and insufficient uncorrected visual acuity.

The aim of cataract surgery today is rapid visual rehabilitation, the best possible uncorrected visual acuity, and minimal postoperative astigmatism.

The phacoemulsification procedure results in less surgically induced astigmatism than extracapsular cataract extraction, in which the incision is much larger.

Clear corneal incision (CCI) is the most used type of incision in phacoemulsification surgery, because it is less time-consuming and doesn't require cauterization or wound suturing. The location of the CCI affects the degree of postoperative astigmatism.

CCI is made deliberately in the steepest meridian if astigmatism is addressed. It can be made at superior, oblique or temporal locations.

Temporal CCI induces regular astigmatism 90 degrees away from the incision (with-the-rule astigmatism) thus minimizing the postoperative astigmatism (Cilino et al., 1997; Cravy, 1991; Hayashi et al., 1994). It is known to induce the least postoperative astigmatism. Also, the smaller the CCI, the lesser the induced astigmatism.

Oblique scleral tunnel incision predictably reduces astigmatism by simultaneously producing corneal flattening and steepening (Simsek et al., 1998).

Some studies have shown that a small superior CCI induces greater postoperative astigmatism than a small supero-oblique CCI, and a small supero-oblique CCI induces higher postoperative astigmatism than a small temporal CCI (Mendivil, 1996; Reiner et al., 1999; Wirbelauer et al.,1997).

Some authors reported that, although temporal CCI is reported to result in the least induced astigmatism, locating the incision superotemporally or superonasally may ease surgical manipulations during the phacoemulsification cataract surgery for a right-handed surgeon who works from the 12 o' clock position relative to the patient (Ermis et al., 2004).

Performing the procedure from the patient's temporal side may not be possible with the most operating tables, and locating the CCI temporally in left eye may be difficult for a right-handed surgeon who sits at the 12 o' clock position.

Several groups of authors analyzed refractive astigmatism in patients who have had phacoemulsification cataract surgery performed by the oblique clear corneal incision. They provided evidence that the supero-oblique clear corneal incision does not induce the clinically significant amount of oblique astigmatism (Jacobs et al., 1999; Brian et al., 2001; Masnec et al., 2007).

Also, evidence is provided that the superotemporal or superonasal CCI has minimal effect on corneal astigmatism (Masnec et al., 2007).

Further studies on more patients should provide definitive conclusions about the influence of the superotemporal or superonasal clear corneal incision on postoperative astigmatism.

Many studies investigated the influence of different factors, such as the type of a surgery, length of incision and its type (curved, straight, frown), location and width of incision (central vs. peripheral-limbal or scleral), presence or absence of a suture and the suturing method, on postoperative astigmatism (Azar et al., 1997; Roman et al., 1998; Simsek et al.,1998; Wirbelauer et al.,1997)..

Any incisions that are made in the cornea have the potential to change the curvature and therefore the dioptric power of the cornea in that meridian.

The location as well as the width of the incision affects the degree of postoperative astigmatism.

Typically, corneal incisions cause flattening at the axis where they are made. The basic concepts are:

- The larger the incisions, the greater the flattening

The larger the arc length of the corneal incisions, the more effect it has in flattening the cornea at that meridian. Due to the coupling effect, arc lengths of more than 90° are ineffective.

- The more central the incisions, the greater the flattening

Most surgeons prefer performing limbal relaxing incisions (LRIs) at the periphery of the clear cornea. Due to this location, they tend to be more forgiving, heal better, and are less likely to cause irregular astigmatism. But, due to the distance from the central cornea and increased thickness of the cornea at the periphery, these incisions have less effect than astigmatic keratotomy (AK) incisions, which are more centrally placed.

- For penetrating incisions, the shorter the tunnel length, the greater the flattening

Creating an "astigmatically neutral" clear corneal incision during cataract surgery requires the incision to have a sufficient tunnel length. This reduces the compromise of the corneal structure at the incision site and induces little change in the corneal astigmatism. For increasing the astigmatic effect of the corneal incisions, the surgeon can make the tunnel length shorter; however, this results in an incision that may be more prone to leaking during the postoperative period. Surgeon can also vary the position of the corneal incision so that it is placed on the steep axis and, therefore, any induced flattening will help the patient by reducing astigmatism.

- For nonpenetrating incisions, the deeper the incision, the greater the flattening

Most nomograms for LRIs call for nonpenetrating incisions that are placed perpendicularly to corneal tissue. With incisions that are made at 80% or 90% of the corneal thickness, as measured by pachymetry, there is a significant flattening of the corneal astigmatism. As the incisions become more shallow, their effect is lesser, and incisions at less than half corneal depth have little effect on the corneal curvature and power (Budak et al., 1998; Gills et al., 2003; Nichamin, 2006; Thornton, 1994; Wang et al., 2003).

3. Conclusion

Beside the congenital astigmatism which is usually inherited, acquired form of astigmatism can be a result of various intraocular surgeries.

Regular astigmatism is correctable by cylindrical spectacle lenses and contact lenses. In case of irregular astigmatism, cylindrical lenses usually do not help and rigid contact lenses may be useful.

That is usually a consequence of pathological changes of cornea, such as keratoconus, or the lens.

In the past, irregular astigmatism was not very interesting for clinicians because it was not very common and not treatable. However, with the development of keratorefractive surgical procedures, it became increasingly of interest as, in many cases, keratorefractive surgeries produce visually significant irregular astigmatism and, at the same time, may also be able to treat it.

Special focus still remains on keratoconus, a disorder characterized by progressive corneal steepening due to the loss of structural components in the cornea, but its cause is still unclear. It is difficult to treat, and a keratoconic patient has a 10-20% chance, over their lifetime, of needing a corneal transplant. Still, in 90 % of patients contact lenses represent the treatment of choice.

In recent years, corneal collagen crosslinking has become a standard treatment for the progressive corneal ectasia in numerous centers throughout the world, because much evidence has been provided that it can improve biomechanical stability of the weakened cornea.

Additional basic and clinical research is necessary in order to establish more precise indications and to demonstrate the permanence of the treatment. Despite the evidence in support of the safety of this new procedure, future studies are necessary to define its limitations and its long-term efficacy.

4. References

Al-Mahmood, AM., Al-Swailem, SA., Al-Khalaf A., Al-Binali GY. (2010). Progressive Posterior Lenticonus In a Patient with Alport Syndrome. *Middle East Afr J Ophthalmol,* Vol. 17, No. 4 (2010), pp. 379-381

Azar, DT., Stark, WJ., Dodick, J., Khoury, JM., Vitale, S., Enger, C., & Reed, C. (1997). Prospective, randomized vector analysis of astigmatism after three-, one-, and no-suture phacoemulsification. *J Cataract Refract Surg,* Vol. 23, (1997), pp. 1164-73

Bennet, AG., & Rabbits, RB. (1989) *Clinical Visual Optics,* (2nd ed.) , Butterworths, London

Blaise, P., Delanaye, P., Martalo, O., Pierard, GE., Rorive, G., Galand, A. (2003). Anterior lenticonus: diagnostic aid in Alport syndrome. J Fr Ophthalmol, Vol. 26, No.10. (Dec 2003), pp. 1075-82

Brian, J., Jacobs, BS., Bruce, I., Gaynes, OD., Phar, MD., Thomas, A., & Deutch, MD. *J Cataract Refractive Surg,* Vol. 27, (2001), pp. 1176-9

Bron, AJ. (1988). Keratoconus. *Cornea,* Vol. 7, (1988), pp. 163-9

Brown, SI., Mondino BJ. (1984). Therapy of Mooren s ulcer. *Am J Ophthalmol.* Vol. 98. (1984), pp. 1-6

Budak, K., Friedman, NK., Koch, DD. (1998). Limbal relaxing incisions with cataract surgery.. *J Cataract Refract Surg,* Vol. 24, (1998), pp. 503-508

Buxton, JN. (1978) .Contact lenses in keratoconus. *Contact Intraocular Lans Med J,* Vol. 4. (1978), pp. 74

Buxton, JN., Keates, RH., & Hoefle FB. (1984). The contact lens correction of keratoconus. *The CLAO Guide to Basic Science and Clinical Practice : Contact lenses,* (ed), Grune and Stratton, Orlando

Cameron, JA., Cotter, JB., Risco, JM., & Alvarez, H. (1991). Epikeratoplasty for keratoglobus associated with blue sclera. *Ophthalmology,* Vol. 98, (1991), pp. 446-52

Cameron, JA. (1993). Keratoglobus. *Cornea,* Vol. 12, (1993), pp. 124-30

Cameron, JA. (1993). Corneal abnormalities in Ehlers-Danlos syndrome type VI. *Cornea,* Vol. 12, (1993), pp. 54-9

Caporossi, A., Mazzotta, C., Baiocchi, S., & Caporossi, T. (2010). Long-term results of riboflavin ultraviolet a corneal collagen cross-linking for keratoconus in Italy: The Siena eye cross study. *Am J Ophthalmol,* (Feb 2010)

Chan, CC., Sharma, M & Wachler, BS. (2007). Effect of inferior-segment Intacts with and without C3-R on keratoconus. *J Cataract Refract Surg,* Vol. 33, No. 1. (Januar 2007), pp. 75-80

Chang, DF.(2008). Mastering refractive IOLs-the art and science, Slack, ISBN 978-1-55642-859-3

Cillino, S., Morreale, D., Mauceri, A., Ajovalasit, C., & Ponte, F. (1997). Temporal versus superior approach phacoemulsification: short-term postoperative astigmatism. *J Cataract Refract Surg,* Vol. 23, (1997), pp. 267-71

Collin, J., Cochenee, B., & Savary, G. (2001). Intacts inserts for treating keratoconus: one - year results. *Ophthalmology,* Vol. 108, (2001), pp. 1409-14

Corkin, R. (2009). CXL Indications and Patient Selection. *Cataract & Refract Surg Today,* (April 2009), pp.33-35

Cravy, TV. (1991). Routine use of a lateral approach to cataract extraction to achive rapid and sustained stabilisation of postoperative astigmatism. *J Cataract Refract Surg,* Vol. 17, (1991), pp. 415-23

Cullen, JF., & Butler, HG. (1963). Mongolism (Down s syndrome) and keratoconus. *Br J Ophthalmol*, Vol .47, (1963), pp. 321-30

Cupak, K. (2004). *Oftalmologija* (2nd ed), Naknadni zavod globus, ISBN 953-167-163-x, Zagreb

Dana , MR., Putz, JS., & Viana, MAG. (1992). Contact lens failure in keratoconus menagement. *Ophthalmology*, Vol. 99, (1992), pp. 1187-92

Ermis, SS., Inan, UU., & Ozturk, F. (2004). *J Cataract Refract Surg*, Vol. 30, (2004), pp. 1316-19

Ernest, PH., Lavery, KT., & Kiessling, LA. (1994). Relative strenght of scleral corneal and clear corneal incisions constructed in cadaver eyes. *J Cataract Refract Surg*, Vol. 20, (1994), pp. 626-9

Ernest, PH., Fenzl, R., Lavery, KT., & Sensoli, A. (1995) Relative stability of clear corneal incisions in a cadaver eye model. *J Cataract Refract Surg*, Vol. 21, (1995), pp. 39-42

Fernández-Barboza, F., Verdiguel-Sotelo K., Hernández-Löpez, A. (2009). Pellucid marginal degeneration and corneal ulceration, associated with Sjögren syndrome. *Rev Med Inst Mex Seguro Soc*, Vol. 47.(2009), pp. 77-82

Filip, O., Golu, T., & Filip I. (1994). Keratoconus in Albers-Schonberd diases. *Ophthalmologia*, Vol 38. (1994), pp. 247-251

Foote, CS. (1968). Mechanisms of photosensitized oxidation. There are several different types of photosensitized oxidation which may be important in biological systems. *Science*, Vol. 162, No. 857 (November, 1968), pp. 963-70

Foster, CS. (1985). Systemic immunosuppressive therapy for progressive bilateral Mooren' s ulcer. *Ophthalmology*, Vol. 92, (1985), pp. 1436-9

Fukuchi , T., Yue, B., Sugar, J.,S.(1994). Lysosomal enzyme activities in conjunctival tissues of patients with keratoconus. *Arch Ophthalmol*, Vol. 112, (1994), pp: 1368-1374

Gills, JP., Rowsey, JJ. (2003). Managing coupling in secondary astigmatism keratotomy. In: Fine, IH., Packer, M., Hoffman, RS. Eds. *A Complete Surgical Guide for Correcting Astigmatism*. (2003). Thorofare, Slack Incorporated, Nj pp. 131-140

Gills, JP., Wallace, RB., Miller, K. (2003). Reducing pre-existing astigmatism with limbal relaxing incisions. In: Gills, J, ed. *A Complete Surgical Guide for Correcting Astigmatism*. (2003). Thorofare, Slack Incorporated, Nj pp. 99-119

Gonzales, V., & McDonell PJ. (1992). Computer-assisted corneal topography in parents of patients with keratoconus. *Arch Ophthalmol*, Vol. 110, (1992), pp. 1412-4

Gottsch, JD., Li, Q., Ashraf, F. (1999) Cytokine-induced calgranulin C expression in keratocytes. *Clin immunol*, Vol. 91 (1999), pp: 34-40

Grewal, DS., Brar, GS., Jain, R., Sood, V., Singla, M., & Grewal, SP. (2009). Corneal collagen crosslinking using riboflavin and ultraviolet-A light for keratoconus: one year analysis using Scheimpflug imaging. *J Cataract Refract Surg*, Vol. 35, No. 3 (March 2009), pp. 425-32

Hafezi, F., Kanellopoulos, J., Wiltfang, R., & Seiler, T. (2007). Corneal collagen crosslinking with riboflavin and ultraviolet A to treat induced keratectasia after laser in situ keratomileusis. *J Cataract Refract Surg*, Vol. 33, No. 12 (December 2007), pp. 2035-40

Hahn, TW., Kim, JH. (1993). Two step annular tectonic lamellar keratoplasty in severe Terrien s marginal degeneration. *Ophthalmic Surg*. Vol. 24, (1993), pp. 831-4

Hallerman , W . & Wilson, EJ. (1977). Genetische Betractungen uber den Keratoconus. *Klin Monatsb Augenheilk, Vol.* 170, (1977), pp. 906-908

Hayashi, K., Nakao, F., & Hayashi, F. (1994). Corneal topographic analysis of superolateral incision cataract surgery. *Cataract Refract Surg,* Vol. 20, (1994), pp. 392-9

Hentati, N., Sellami, D., Makni, K., Kharrat, M., Hachicha, J., Hammadi, A., Feki, J. (2008). Ocular findings in Alport syndrome: 32 case studies. *J Fr Ophthalmol,* Vol. 31, No. 6. (Jun 2008), pp. 597-604

Hofstetter, H. (1959). A keratoscopic survey of 13,395 eyes. *Am J Optom Acad Optom,* Vol. 36. (1959), pp. 3-11

Howland, HC., Atkinson, J., Braddick, O., & French, J. (1978). Astigmatism measured by Photorefraction. *Science,* Vol. 202, (1978), pp. 331-3

Iwamoto, T., DeVoe AG., Farris RL. (1972). Electron microscopy in cases of marginal degenerations of cornea. *Invest Ophthalmol Vis Sci.,* Vol 11, (1972), pp. 241-57

Iwaszkiewicz, E. (1989). Keratoconus II. Coexisting diseases and theories on its etiology and pathogenesis. *Klin Oczna,* Vol. 91, (1989), pp. 210-211

Jacobs, BJ., Gaynes, BI., & Deutch, TA. (1999). Refractive astigmatism after oblique clear corneal phacoemulsification cataract incision. *J Cataract Refract Surg,* Vol. 25. (1999), pp. 949-52

Jacobs, DS., Green WR., Maumenee, AE. (1974). Acquired keratoglobus. *AJO,* Vol.77, (1974), pp.393-9

Karseras, AG. , & Ruben, M. (1976). Aetiology of keratoconus. *Br J Ophthalmol,* Vol. 60, (1976), pp. 522-5

Kennedy, RH., Bourne, WM., & Dyer JA. (1986). A 48-year clinical and epidemiology study of keratoconus. *Am J Ophthalmol,* Vol. 101, (1986), pp. 267-73

Kim, KS., Kim, MS., Kim JM., Choi, CY. (2010). Evaluation of anterior lenticonus in alport syndrome using tracy wavefront aberrometry and transmission electron microscopy. *Ophthalmic Surg Lasers Imaging,* Vol. 41, No.3 (May-Jun 2010), pp.330-6

Koller, T., Mrochen, M., & Seiler, T. (2009). Complications and failure rates after corneal crosslinking. *J Cataract Refract Surg,* Vol. 35, No. 8 (August 2009), pp. 1358-62.

Konradsen, TR., Koivula, A., Kugelberg, M., Zetterström, C. (2010). Corneal curvature, pachymetry, and endothelial cell density in Marfan syndrome. Acta Ophthalmol (September 2010)

Krachmer, JH., Feder, RS., & Belin, MW. (1984). Keratoconus and related noninflammatory corneal thinning disorders. *Surv Ophthalmol,* Vol. 28, (1984), pp. 293-322

Kymionis, GD., Bouzoukis, DI., Diakonis, VF. (2007). Diffuse lamellar keratitis after corneal crosslinking in patient with post-laser in situ keratomileusis corneal ectasia. *J Cataract Refract Surg,* Vol. 33, (2007), pp. 2135-7

Kymionis, GD., Portaliou, DM., Bouzoukis, DI.(2007). Herpetic keratitis with iritis after corneal crosslinking with riboflavin and ultraviolet A for keratoconus. *J Cataract Refract Surg,* Vol. 33, (2007), pp. 1982-4

Liesegang, TJ., Deutch, TA., & Gilbert Grand, M. (2002-2003). *Optics, Refraction, and Contact lenses, Basic and Clinical Science Course, American Academy of Ophthalmology,* United states of America, ISSN

Maguire, LJ., Klyce, SD., McDonald ME., & Kaufmann HE. (1987). Corneal topography of pellucid marginal degeneration . *Ophthalmology,* Vol. 94, (1987), pp. 519-524

Mandic, Z., Petric ,I., Bencic, G., Vatavuk, Z., & Bojic, L. (2005). Postoperative outcomes after implantation of intraocular lenses in eyes with cataract and uveitis. *Coll Antropol.* Vol .29, No. 1, (March 2005), pp. 9-12, ISSN 03506134

Marcsai, MS., Varley, GA:, & Krachmer, JH. (1990). Development of keratoconus after contact lens wear: patient characteristics. *Arch Ophthalmol,* Vol. 108, (1990), pp. 534-8

Maruyama, Y., Wang, X., & Li, Y. (2001). Involment of sp 1 elements in the promoter activity of genes affected in keratoconus. *Invest Ophthalmol Vis Sci,* Vol. 42, (2001), pp. 1980-5

Masket, S. (1991). Horizontal anchor suture closure method for small incision cataract surgery. *J Cataract Refract Surg,* Vol. 17, (1991), pp. 689-95

Masnec-Paškvalin, S., Čima, I., Iveković, R., Matejčić, A., Novak-Lauš, K., & Mandić, Z. (2007). Comparison of Preoperative and Postoperative Astigmatism after Superotemporal or Superonasal Clear Corneal Incision in Phacoemulsiphication. Coll *Antropol* , Vol. 31, No. (2007), pp. 199-202

Mazzota, C., Balestrazzi, A., Baiocchi, S. (2007). Stromal haze after combined riboflavin-UVa corneal cross-linking in keratoconus: in vivo confocal microscopic evaluation. *Clin Exper Ophthalmol,* Vol. 35, (2007), pp. 580-2

Mendivil, A. (1996). Comparative study of astigmatism through superior and lateral small incisions. *Eur J Ophthalmol,* Vol. 6, (1996), pp. 389-92

Michaels, DD. (1980). A clinical aprprouch. *Visual optics and refraction,* (2nd ed.), Mosby, St Louis

Mohindra, I., Held, R., Gwiazda, J., & Brill, S. (1978) . Astigmatism in Infants. *Science,* Vol. 202, (1978), pp. 329-31

Morlet, N., Minassian, D., & Dart, J. (2001). Astigmatism and the analysis of its surgical correction. *Br J Ophthalmol,* Vol. 85, (2001), pp. 1127-38

Nesburn, AB., Bahri, S., & Salz, J. (1995). Keratoconus detected by videokeratography in candidates for photorefractive keratectomy. *J Refractive Surg,* Vol. 11, (1995), pp. 194-201

Nichamin, LD. (2006). Astigmatism control. *Ophthalmol Clin North Am,* Vol. 19, (2006), pp. 485-493

Oshika, T., Tsuboi, S., & Yaguchi, S. (1994). Comparative study of intraocular lens implantation through 3.2 and 5.5 mm incisions. *Ophthalmology,* Vol. 101, (1994), pp. 1183-90

Oshima, Y., Tsujikawa, K., Oh, A., & Harino, S. (1997). Comparative study of intraocular lens implantation through 3.0 mm temporal clear corneal and superior scleral tunnel self-sealing incisions. *J Cataract Refract Surg,* Vol. 23, (1997), pp. 347-53

Parunovic, A. (1995). *Korekcija refrakcionih anomalija oka,* Bjeletic, ISSN 86-17-04525-6, Beograd

Perry, HD., Buxton, JN., & Fine BS. (1980). Round and oval cones in keratoconus. *Ophthalmology,* Vol. 87, (1980), pp. 905-909

Pollhammer, M., Cursiefen, C. (2009). Bacterial keratitis early after corneal crosslinking with riboflavin and ultraviolet-A. . *J Cataract Refract Surg,* Vol. 3, No.35, (2009), pp.588-9

Pouliquen, Y., Dhermy, P., & Espinasse, MA: (1985). Keratoglobus. *J Fr Ophthalmol,* Vol. 8, (1985), pp. 43-54

Pramanik, S., Musch, DC., Sutphin, JE., & Farjo, AA. (2006). Extended long term outcomes of penetrating keratoplasty for keratoconus. *Ophthalmology,* Vol. 9, No. 113 (September 2006), pp. 1633-8

Rabinowitz, YS. (1995). Videokeratographic indices to aid in screening for keratoconus. *J Refrac Surg* , Vol. 11, (1995), pp. 371-9

Rabinowitz, YS. (1998). Keratoconus. *Surv Ophthalmol,* Vol. 42,No. 4 (Januar 1998), pp. 297-319

Rahi, A., Davies, P., & Ruben, M. (1977). Kratoconus and coexisting atopic disease. *Br J Ophthalmol,* Vol. 61,(1977), pp. 761-4

Rainer, G., Menapace, R., & Vass, C. (1999). Corneal shape changes after temporal and superolateral 3.0 mm clear corneal incisions. *J Cataract Refract Surg,* Vol. 25, (1999), pp. 1121-26

Rama, P., Di Matteo, F., Matuska, S., Paganoni, G., Spinelli, A. (2009). Acanthamoeba keratitis with perforation after corneal crosslinking and bandage contact lens use. . *J Cataract Refract Surg,* Vol. 35, No. 4, (2009), pp. 788-91

Ricchi, B., Lepore, D., & Iossa, M. (1991). Ocular anomalies in Alagille s syndrome, *J Fr Ophthalmol* , Vol 14 (1991), pp. 481-485

Roman, SJ., Auclin, FX., Chong-Sit, DA., & Ullern, MM. (1998). Surgically induced astigmatism with superior and temporal incisions in cases of with-the-rule preoperative astigmatism. *J Cataract Refract Surg,* Vol. 24, (1998), pp. 1636-41

Royce ,PM., Steinmann, B., & Vogel, A. (1990). Brittle cornea syndroma: an haritable connective tissue disorder distinct from Ehlers-Danlos syndrome type VI and fragilitas oculi, with spontaneous perforation of the eye, blue sclerae, red hair, and normal collagen lysyl hydroxylation. *Eur J Pediatr,* Vol. 149, (1990), pp. 465-9

Rumelt, S., & Rehany, U. (1998). Surgically induced keratoglobus in pellucid marginal degeneration. *Eye,* Vol.12, (1998), pp.156-158

Sawagamuchi, S., Yue ,BYT., Sugar J, Ciljoy, JE. (1989). Lysosomal abnormalities in keratoconus. *Arch Ophthalmol,* Vol 108, (1989), pp. 1507-10

Sawagamuchi, S., Twinning, SS., & Yue, BYT. (1994). Alpha 2 macroglobulin levels in normal human and keratoconus corneas. *Invest Ophthalmol Vis Sci,* Vol. 35, (1994), pp. 4008-4014

Sharif, KW., Casey, TA., & Colart, J. (1992). Prevalence of mitral valve prolapse in keratoconus patients. *J R Soc Med,* Vol. 85, (1992), pp. 446-448

Seiler, T., Huhle, S., Spoerl, E., & Kunath, H. (2000). Manifest diabetes and keratoconus : a retrospective case control study. *Graefes Arch Clin Exp Ophthalmol, Vol.* 10, No. 238 (Oct ober 2000), pp. 822-5

Seiler, T., & Hafezi, F. (2006). Corneal cross- linking-induced stromal demarcation line. *Cornea,* Vol. 25, (2006), pp. 1057-9

Sii, F., Lee, GA., Sanfilippo, P., Stephensen, DC. (2004). Pellucid marginal degeneration and scleroderma. *Clin Exp Optom,* Vol 87, (2004), pp. 180-4

Simsek, S., Yasar, T., & Demirok, A. (1998). Effect of superior and temporal clear corneal incisions on astigmatism after sutureless phacoemulsification. *J Cataract Refract Surg,* Vol. 24, (1998), pp. 515-18

Smiddy, WE., Hamburg, TR., Kracher, GP & Stark WJ. (1988). Keratoconus. Contact lens or keratoplasty?. *Ophthalmology,* Vol. 95, (1988), pp. 487-92

Smolin, G. (1987). Dystrophies and degenerations, *The Cornea,* (2nd ed), Little, Brown, Boston

Spörl, E., Huhle, M., Kasper, M., & Seiler, T. (1997). Erhöhung der Festigkeit der Hornhaut durch Vernetzung. *Ophthalmologe,* Vol. 94, No. 12 (December 1997), pp. 902-6

Spörl, E., Huhle, M., & Seiler, T. (1998). Induction of cross-links in corneal tissue. *Exp Eye Res.* Vol. 66, No. 1 (Januar 1998), pp. 97-103

Spoerl, E., Wollensak, G., & Seiler, T. (2004). Increased resistance of crosslinked cornea against enzymatic digestion. *Curr Eye Res,* Vol. 29 (December 2004), pp. 35-40

Spoerl, E., Mrochen, M., & Sliney, D. (2007). Safety of UVA-riboflavin cross-linking of the cornea. *Cornea,* Vol. 26, (2007), pp. 385-9

Thornton, SP. (1994). *Radial and Astigmatic Keratotomy: The American System of Precise, Predictable Refractive Surgery,* Thorofare, Slack Incorporated, NJ

Tomkins, O., & Garzozi, HJ. (2008). Collagen cross-linking: Strengthening the unstable cornea. *Clin Ophthalmol,* Vol. 4,No. 2 (December 2008), pp. 863-7

Tuft, SJ., Moodaley, LC., & Gregory, WM. (1994). Prognostic factors of progression to keratoconus. *Ophthalmology,* Vol. 101, (1994), pp. 439-447

Waller, SG., Steinert, RE., & Wagoner, MD. (1995). Long term results of epikeratoplasty for keratoconus. *Cornea,* Vol. 14, (1995), pp. 84-8

Wang, L., Misra, M., Koch, DD. (2003). Peripheral corneal relaxing incisions combined with cataract surgery. *J Cataract Refract Surg,* Vol. 29, (2003), pp. 712-722

Wilson, SE., Guang, HE., & Weng, J. (1996). Epithelial injury induces keratocyte apoptosis: hypothesized reole of the interleukin-1 system in the modulation of corneal tissue organisation and wound healing. *Exp Eye Res,* Vol. 62, (1996), pp. 325-7

Wirbelauer, C., Anders, N., Pham, DT., & Wollensak, J. (1997). Effect of incision location on preoperative oblique astigmatism after scleral tunnel incision. *Cataract Refract Surg,* Vol. 23, (1997), pp. 365-71

Wollensak, G., Spoerl, E., & Seiler, T. (2003). Riboflavin /ultraviolet-a-induced collagen crosslinking for the treatment of keratoconus. *Am J Ophthalmol,* Vol. 135 (December 2003), pp. 620-7

Wollensak, G., & Iomdina, E. (2008). Long- term biomechanical properties after collagen crosslinking of sclera using glyceraldehyde. *Acta Ophthalmol,* Vol.86 ,No. 8, (December 2008), pp. 887-93

Wollensak, G., & Iomdina, E. (2009). Long term biomechanical properties of rabbit cornea after photodynamic collagen crosslinking. *Acta Ophthalmol,* Vol. 87, No.1, (Februar 2009), pp. 48-51

Yanoff, M., Duker, JS. (2004). *Ophthalmology,* (2nd ed.), Mosby, ISSN 0-323-01634-0, Philadelphia

Yeung, KK., Weissman, BA. (1997). Contact lens correction of patients with Marfan syndrome. *J Am Optom Assoc,* Vol. 68, No. 6, (Jun 1997), pp.367-72

Zamora, KV., Males, JJ. (2009). Polymicrobial keratitis after a collagen cross-linking procedure with postoperative use of a contact lens: a case report. *Cornea*, Vol. 28, No.4, (May 2009), pp. 474-6

11

Wavefront Aberrations

Mirko Resan, Miroslav Vukosavljević and Milorad Milivojević
Eye Clinic, Military Medical Academy, Belgrade, Serbia

1. Introduction

The eye is an optical system having several optical elements that focus light rays representing images onto the retina. Imperfections in the components and materials in the eye may cause light rays to deviate from the desired path. These deviations, referred to as optical or wavefront aberrations, result in blurred images and decreased visual performance (1).

Wavefront aberrations are optical imperfections of the eye that prevent light from focusing perfectly on the retina, resulting in defects in the visual image. There are two kinds of aberrations:

1. Lower order aberrations (0, 1st and 2nd order)
2. Higher order aberrations (3rd, 4th, ... order)

Lower order aberrations are another way to describe refractive errors: myopia, hyperopia and astigmatism, correctible with glasses, contact lenses or refractive surgery. Lower order aberrations is a term used in wavefront technology to describe second-order Zernike polynomials. Second-order Zernike terms represent the conventional aberrations defocus (myopia, hyperopia and astigmatism). Lower order aberrations make up about 85 per cent of all aberrations in the eye.

Higher order aberrations are optical imperfections which cannot be corrected by any reliable means of present technology. All eyes have at least some degree of higher order aberrations. These aberrations are now more recognized because technology has been developed to diagnose them properly. Wavefront aberrometer is actually used to diagnose and measure higher order aberrations. Higher order aberrations is a term used to describe Zernike aberrations above second-order. Third-order Zernike terms are coma and trefoil. Fourth-order Zernike terms include spherical aberration, and so on. Higher order aberrations make up about 15 percent of the overall number of aberrations in an eye.

2. Myopia

Myopia (nearsightedness, shortsightedness) is a refractive error where parallel light rays coming from a distance after refraction through the cornea and lens focus before the retina in the vitreous body and mature behind the focus in the state of divergence generate on retina wasteful circles (Fig. 1 and 3). Because of this, the image that one sees is out of focus when looking at a distant object but comes into focus when looking at a close object. Therefore, shortsighted people cannot see clearly at a distance (2).

Myopia can be classified by cause, degree, clinical features and age of onset. By cause myopia can be: *axial myopia,* attributed to an increase in eyes axial length (more than 24 mm), and *refractive myopia,* attributed to the condition of refractive elements of the eye, like curvature myopia (increased curvature of cornea) or index myopia (variation in the index of refraction of one or more ocular media, like in nuclear cataract). By degree myopia can be: *low myopia* (−3.0 diopters or less), *medium myopia* (between −3.0 and −6.0 diopters), and *high myopia* (−6.0 diopters or more). By clinical features myopia can be: *simple myopia,* characterized by the eye being too long for its optical power or optically too powerful for its axial length, and *degenerative* (*malignant, pathological, progressive*) *myopia* characterized by expressed fundus changes (conus myopicus, staphyloma posticum, degeneratio chorioretinae peripherica, maculopathia) and associated with a high refractive error and subnormal visual acuity after correction. This form of myopia worsen progressively over time and can become complicated with retinal tear and retinal detachment. By age of onset myopia can be: *congenital myopia,* present at birth and persisting through infancy, *youth-onset myopia* (*school myopia*) with onset between around 5 years of age and physical maturity, *early adult-onset myopia* with onset after physical maturity and up to about 40 years of age, and *late adult-onset myopia* with onset after around 55 years of age due to changes in the nucleus of the crystalline lens (2,3,4,5,6).

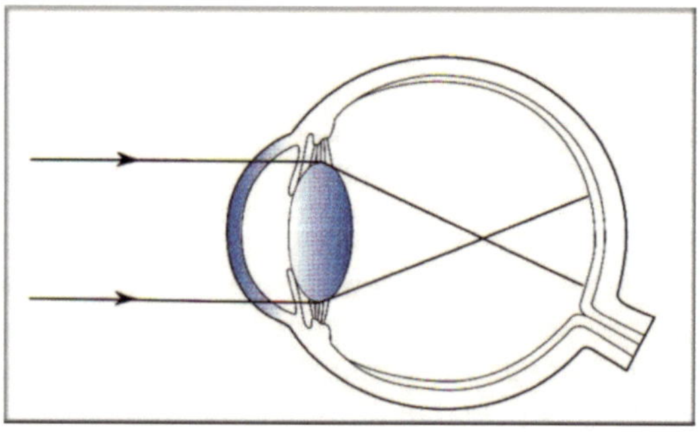

Fig. 1. Myopia with accommodation relaxed. Parallel light rays from infinity focus to a point anterior to the retina, forming a blurred image on the retina (6).

3. Hyperopia

Hyperopia (farsightedness, longsightedness) is a refractive error where parallel light rays coming from a distance after refraction through the cornea and lens focus behind the retina without participation of accommodation (Figs. 2 and 3). Causes of hyperopia are typically genetic and involve an eye that is too short or a cornea that is too flat, so that images focus at a point behind the retina (2).

Hyperopia can be classified by: cause, clinical features and accommodative status. By cause hyperopia can be: *axial hyperopia,* attributed to a decrease in eyes axial length (less than 24 mm), and *refractive hyperopia,* attributed to the condition of refractive elements of the eye like decreased curvature of cornea (cornea plana). By clinical features hyperopia can be: *simple, pathological* (resulting in amblyopia or strabismus), and *functional.* By accommodative status hyperopia can be: *total, latent,* and *manifest.* Total hyperopia occurs in state of full paralysis of accommodation (after application of cycloplegics) and represents the amount of entire refractive error. Latent hyperopia is that part of the refractive error being corrected with accommodation. Manifest hyperopia is the accommodation uncorrected part of hyperopia and becoming closer to the total one with age (2,3,4,5,6).

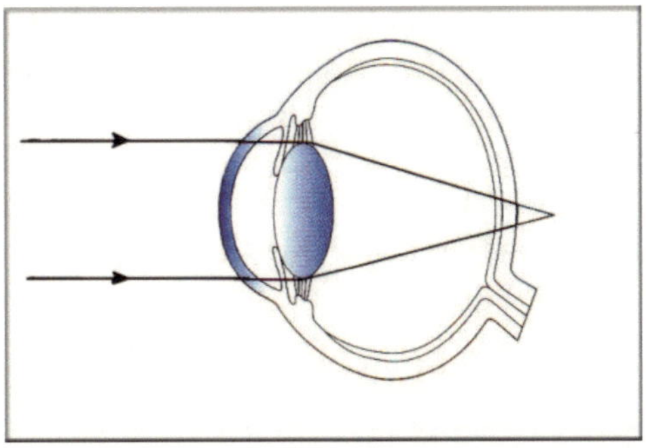

Fig. 2. Hyperopia with accommodation relaxed. Parallel light rays from infinity focus to a point posterior to the retina, forming a blurred image on the retina (6).

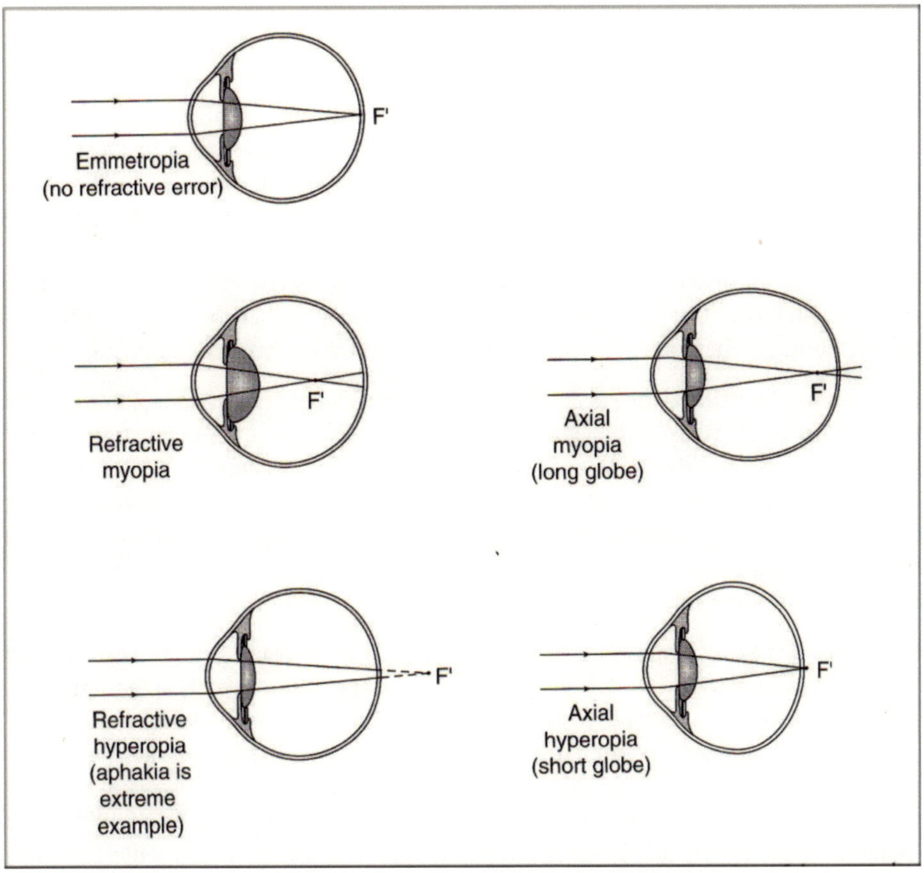

Fig. 3. Refractive errors (myopia and hyperopia) defined by the position of the secondary focal point with respect to the retina, with accommodation fully relaxed. The secondary focal point of a myopic eye is the front of the retina inside the vitreous, whereas the focal point of a hyperopic eye is behind the retina (7).

4. Astigmatism

Astigmatism is a refractive condition in which the eye optical system is incapable of forming a point image for a point object. This is because the refracting power of the optical system varies from one meridian to another. There are complex optical relationships in astigmatism: no focus (as in myopia and hyperopia), but the two focal lines corresponding to main meridians. The meridians of greatest and least refraction are defined as main (principal) meridians. Astigmatism is caused by the cornea or the crystalline lens. Clinically, most astigmatisms are corneal in origin and mainly related to the change in curvature of the cornea (3,4).

There are different types of astigmatism, according to the method of classification (2,3,4,5,6).

Astigmatism is *regular* when two main meridians are 90° to each other; it is correctable with cylindrical or spherocylindrical lenses. Otherwise, the astigmatism is *irregular*. Regular astigmatism is *with-the-rule (direct)* when the steepest corneal meridian is close to 90° (±20°) and *against-the-rule (indirect)* when the steepest meridian is close to 180° (±20°). When the astigmatism is regular but the main meridians do not lie close to 90° or 180°, it is *oblique*.

Astigmatic errors are also described by the location of secondary focal lines relative to the retina (with accommodation relaxed). *Compound myopic* astigmatism occurs when both of the main meridians are myopic, pulling the focal lines off the retina into the vitreous. In *simple myopic* astigmatism, one meridian is emmetropic and the other is myopic, one focal line is on the retina and the other is pulled into the vitreous. *Compound hyperopic* astigmatism occurs when both of the main meridians are hyperopic, pulling the focal lines behind the retina. In *simple hyperopic* astigmatism, one meridian is emmetropic and the other is hyperopic, one focal line is on the retina and the other is pulled behind the retina. *Mixed* astigmatism occurs when one meridian is hyperopic and the other is myopic (Fig. 4).

Astigmatism can be natural or surgically induced. *Natural* astigmatism is common, that is, around 15% of adult population have astigmatism > 1D and 2% have astigmatism > D. Special group of astigmatisms are those surgically induced, *postoperative* astigmatisms. Any surgical intervention in the fibrous mantle of the eye (cornea, sclera) may result in major or minor postoperatively acquired astigmatisms. Classic and most common postoperative astigmatism occurs after cataract surgery, especially after extra- and intracapsular cataract extraction. It is very minimal after phacoemulsification (2).

As noted, the cornea is usually the source of clinically significant amounts of astigmatism. The amount of *corneal* astigmatism, along with the location of meridians of least and greatest refraction, can be easily determined with a keratometer. The vast majority of corneas have with-the-rule astigmatism; a small minority of corneas have against-the-rule or oblique astigmatism, and a small minority have no astigmatism. As compared to corneal astigmatism, *internal* astigmatism is relatively small in amount, tending to slightly vary from one person to another, and is almost always against-the-rule. Main causes of internal astigmatism are the toricity of the back surface of the cornea and the tilting of the crystalline lens. There is no clinical method of measuring internal astigmatism. *Refractive (total)* astigmatism includes both corneal and internal astigmatism and can be determined with refractometry (total determination of refraction) (3).

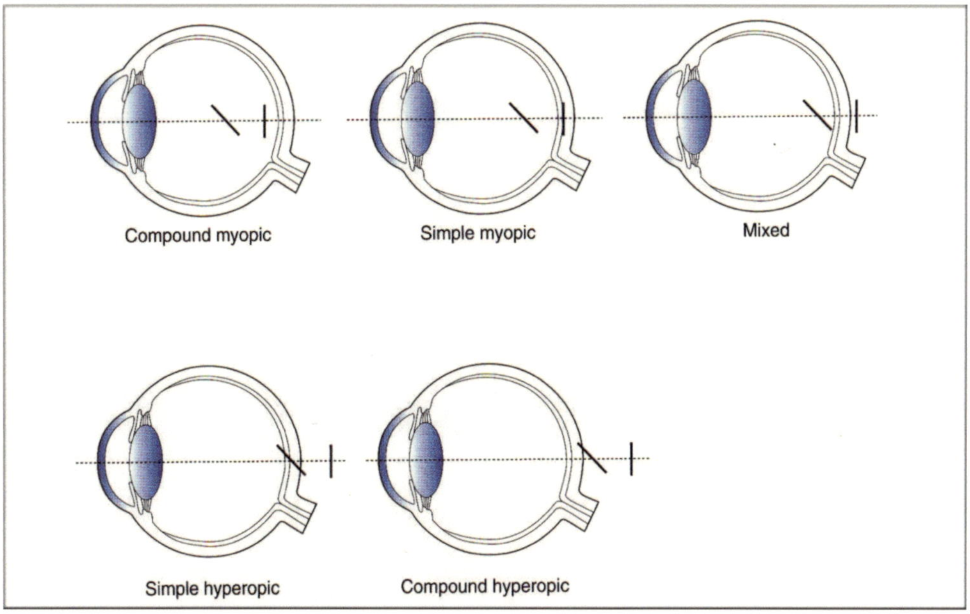

Fig. 4. The locations of focal lines with respect to the retina define the type of astigmatism (6).

5. Higher order aberrations (HOAs)

Within the past decade, rapid improvement in wavefront-related technologies, including the development of sensors for measuring optical properties of the eye in a clinical environment, allowed the ophthalmic community to move the wavefront theory of light transmission from an academic concept to one being central for better understanding of the effect of aberrations on visual performance and the corresponding image-forming properties of the eye. Imperfections in the optics of the eye are now measured and expressed as wave aberration errors. The wave aberration defines how the phase of light is affected as it passes through the eye's optical system, and is usually defined mathematically by a series of Zernike polynomials. Zernike polynomials are used to classify and represent optical aberrations because they consist of terms of same form as the types of aberrations observed when describing the optical properties of the eye, and can be used reciprocally with no misunderstanding. Moreover, the advantage of describing ocular aberrations using the normalized Zernike expansion, generally depicted as a pyramid (Figs. 5 and 6), is that the value of each mode represents the root mean square (RMS) wavefront error attributable to that mode. Coefficients with a higher value identify the modes (aberrations) that have the greatest impact on the overall RMS wavefront error in the eye and thus in reducing the optical performance of the eye (8).

The two most important HOAs are coma and spherical aberration. Coma is the distortion in image formation occurring when a bundle of light rays enters an optical system not parallel to the optic axis. Coma results in off-axis point sources such as stars appearing distorted, with a comet-like tail. Spherical aberration is the blurring of an image, occurring when light from the margin of a lens or mirror with spherical surface comes to a focus shorter than light from the central portion. The changing focal length is caused by deviations in lens or mirror surface from a true sphere.

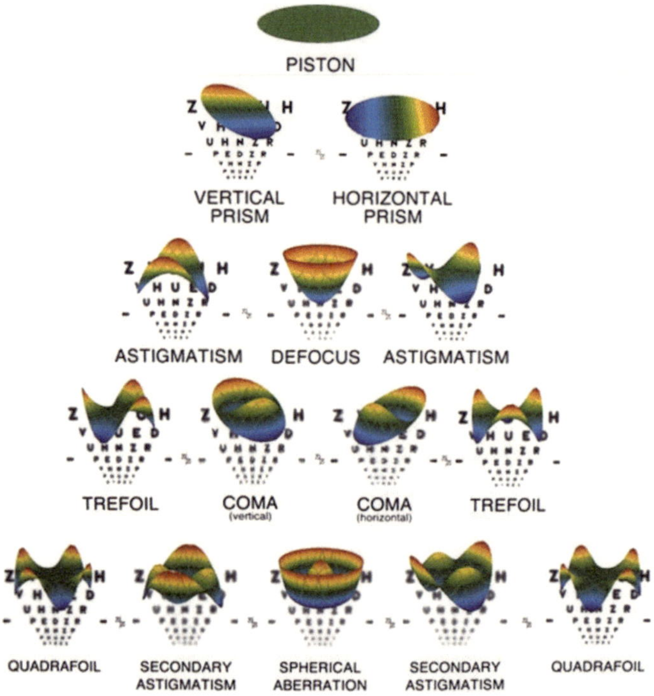

Fig. 5. This chart reveals more common shapes of aberrations created when a wavefront of light passes through eyes with imperfect vision. A theoretically perfect eye (top) is represented by an aberration-free flat plane known, for reference, as piston. (Image: Alcon Inc.)

HOAs are vision errors more complex than lower-order aberrations. HOAs have relatively unfamiliar names such as coma, spherical aberration and trefoil. These types of aberrations can produce vision errors such as difficulty seeing at night, glare, halos, blurring, starburst patterns or double vision (diplopia). No eye is perfect, which means that all eyes have at least some degree of HOAs. These aberrations are now more recognized because technology has been developed to diagnose them properly.

HOAs are measured by aberrometer (wavefront sensor). Aberrometers measure the distortion of a light wave as it is altered by passing through the optics of the eye. A plane wave of monochromatic light will be distorted by optical imperfections. Wavefront sensors do not measure light scatter (from stromal haze or corneal scars), chromatic aberrations or diffraction phenomena. Their effects on vision should be assessed by other means. A useful way to think of distortions in a wavefront is to think of the path length of parallel rays entering the pupil and projecting toward the retina. As light enters the eye from the air, its speed is retarded according to the refractive index of the material along its path to the retina. Arrival time is also influenced by the traveling distance. These two factors, refractive index and linear path variations, are measured with a wavefront sensor. A map can be made to show relevant retardation that a plane wave undergoes as it traverses the optics of the eye. Clinicians are now used to see this information displayed as Zernike polynomial expansion. In order to parcel the wavefront error into individual building blocks, a set of normalized Zernike polynomials is best fit to the measured wavefront error. The coefficient of each Zernike term reveals that term's relative contribution to the total root mean square (RMS) error (Fig. 7) (9).

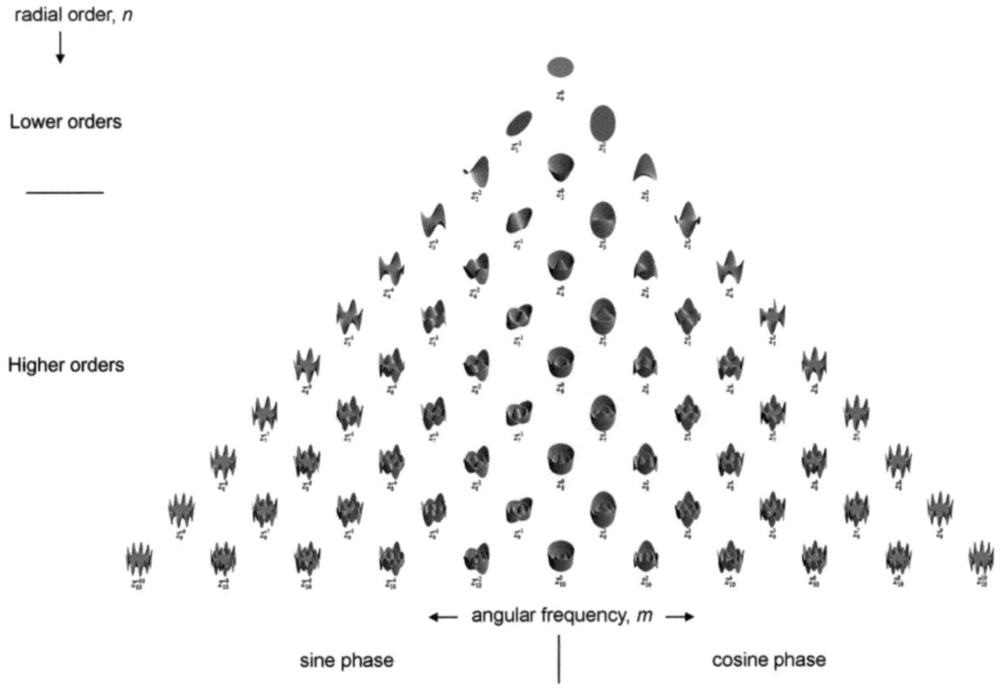

Fig. 6. The Zernike pyramid showing polynomials up to the 10th orders. The 0- to 2nd-order terms represent low optical aberrations in the eye, with 2nd-order terms (i.e. defocus and astigmatism) having the highest contribution to the overall wavefront aberration in the eye. Terms of the 3rd order and higher represent the HOAs. The 3rd- and 4th-order terms are the most prevalent HOA in the human eye (8).

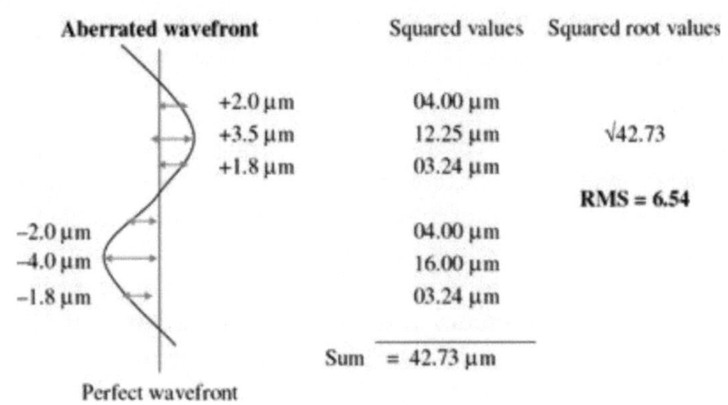

Fig. 7. Graphical representation of root mean squared wavefront error (9).

In the ametropic eye, defocus (i.e. myopia or hyperopia) is by far the largest aberration, followed by astigmatism. These are low order terms. The Zernike pyramid is useful (Table 1). As we follow down the rows from the top, we go from low order to high order. Low order encompasses the top three rows' piston, tilt, tip, and sphere and astigmatism. Row three (i.e. sphere and astigmatism) is what we normally measure and prescribe in spectacles. The fourth row is called third order aberrations, and it continues from there. Anything beyond lower order is lumped under the term of higher order aberrations (HOAs). As observed from the diagram, they have individual names such as coma, and spherical aberration. When interpreting data, we need to know whether the wavefront refers to total aberrations (9).

Plot index	Term	Binomial representation	Polynomial (ρ,θ)
1	Tip	(1,1)	$2\rho\sin(\theta)$
2	Tilt	(1,1)	$2\rho\cos(\theta)$
3	Defocus	(2,0)	$\sqrt{3}\,(2\rho^2 \angle 1)$
4	Astigmatism	(2,2)	$\sqrt{6}\,\rho^2\sin(2\theta)$
5	Astigmatism	(2,2)	$\sqrt{6}\,\rho^2\cos(2\theta)$
6	Vertical coma	(3,1)	$\sqrt{8}\,(3\rho^3 \angle 2\rho)\sin(\theta)$
7	Horizontal coma	(3,1)	$\sqrt{8}\,(3\rho^3 \angle 2\rho)\cos(\theta)$
8	Trefoil	(3,3)	$\sqrt{8}\,\rho^3\sin(3\theta)$
9	Trefoil	(3,3)	$\sqrt{8}\,\rho^3\cos(3\theta)$
10	Spherical aberration	(4,0)	$\sqrt{5}(6\rho^4 \angle 6\rho^2 + 1)$
11	Secondary astigmatism	(4,2)	$\sqrt{10}\,(4\rho^4 \angle 3\rho^2)\sin(2\theta)$
12	Secondary astigmatism	(4,2)	$\sqrt{10}\,(4\rho^4 \angle 3\rho^2)\cos(2\theta)$
13	Tetrafoil	(4,4)	$\sqrt{10}\,\rho^4\sin(4\theta)$
14	Tetrafoil	(4,4)	$\sqrt{10}\,\rho^4\cos(4\theta)$

Table 1. Zernicke pyramid (9).

In the normal ametropic eye, HOAs are a relatively small component, comprising about 10% of eye's overall aberrations. This varies between individuals. Figure 8a shows a 2-D wavefront of a normal ametropic eye with a low amount of HOAs (0.14µm), and Figure 8b shows a subtle form fruste keratoconic eye with a larger amount (0.42µm) of HOAs. Both images are for data at a 6 mm pupil size. It is important to know what the pupil size was when aberrometry was performed, and at what pupil size data was presented, as HOAs increase with increased pupil size (9).

Three different wavefront measuring principles are available to measure aberrations: (1) Hartmann-Shack, (2) Tscherning or ray tracing, and (3) automated retinoscopy. A Hartmann-Shack aberrometer is an outgoing wavefront aberrometer. It measures the shape of the wavefront that is reflected out of the eye from a point source on the fovea. An array of microlenslets is used to subdivide the outgoing wavefront into multiple beams which produce spot images on a video sensor. The displacement of each spot from the corresponding nonaberrated reference position is used to determine the shape of the wavefront. A Tscherning, or ray-tracing, aberrometer is an ingoing instrument. It projects a thin laser beam into the eye, parallel to the visual axis, and determines the location of the beam on the retina by using a photodetector. Once the position of the first light spot on the retina is determined, the laser beam is moved to a new position, and the location of the second light spot on the retina is determined. Aberrations in the optical system cause a shift in the location of the light spot on the retina. The third type, automated retinoscopy, is based on dynamic skiascopy. The retina is scanned with a slit-shaped light beam, and the reflected light is captured by an array of rotating photodetectors over a 360° area. The time difference of the reflected light is used to determine the aberrations. Visser et al. compared total ocular aberrations and corneal aberrations identified with four different aberrometers and determined the repeatability and interobserver variability. In this prospective comparative study, 23 healthy subjects underwent bilateral examination with four aberrometers: the Irx3 (Hartmann-Shack; Imagine Eyes, Orsay, France), Keratron (Hartmann-Shack; Optikon, Rome, Italy), iTrace (raytracing; Tracey Technologies, Houston, TX), and OPD-Scan (Automated Retinoscopy; Nidek, Gamagori, Japan). Six images per eye were obtained. Second-, third- and fourth-order spherical aberrations were exported for 5.0-mm pupils. Results demonstrate that significant differences in measurements were found for several total ocular aberrations (defocus [2,0], astigmatism [2,2], trefoil [3,-3], trefoil [3,3], and spherical aberration [4,0]) and corneal aberrations (defocus [2,0] and astigmatism [2,2]).

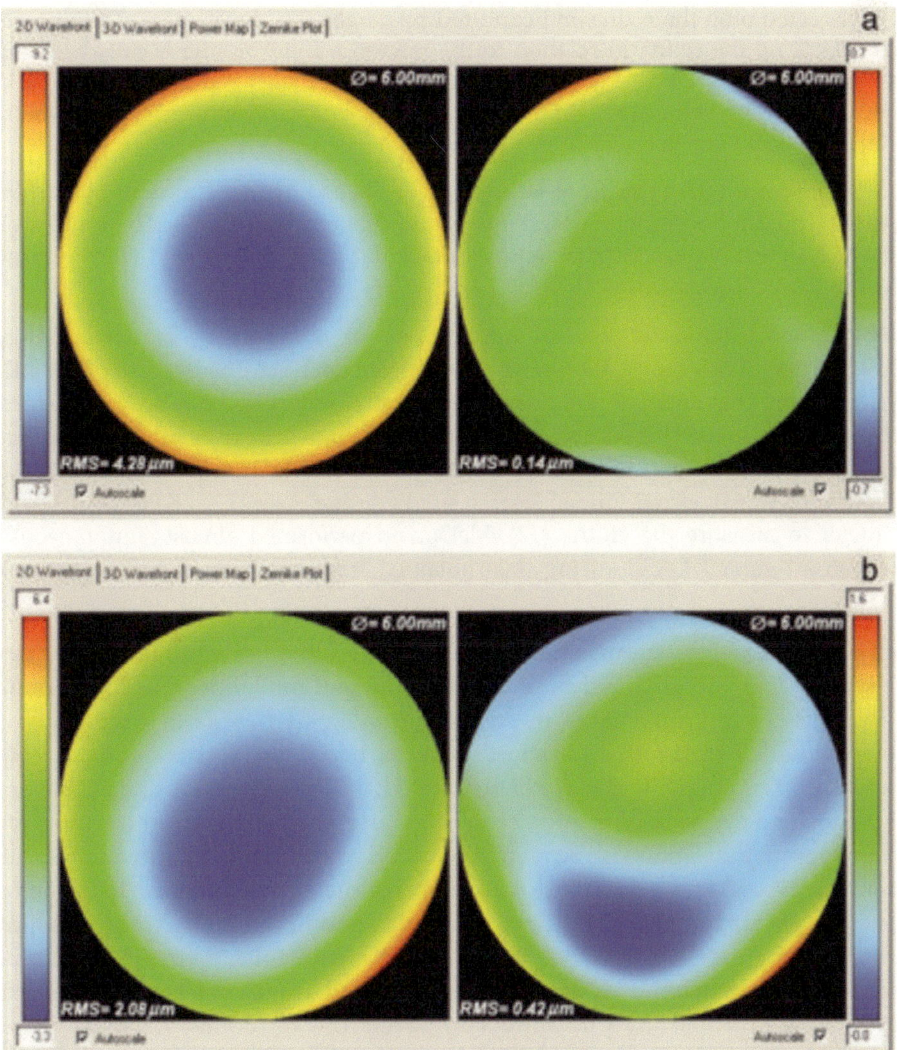

Fig. 8. HOAs represented by 2-D image: (a) eye with low degree, and (b) eye with high degree of HOAs (HOAs measured by Alcon LADARWave) (9).

The Irx3 showed the highest repeatability in measuring total ocular aberrations, followed by the Keratron, OPD-Scan, and iTrace. The repeatability of corneal aberration measurements was highest for the iTrace, followed by the Keratron and OPD-Scan. The OPD-Scan showed a lower interobserver variability, compared with the Irx3, Keratron, and iTrace. In conclusion, total ocular and corneal aberrations are not comparable when measured with different aberrometers. Hartmann-Shack aberrometers showed the best repeatability for total ocular aberrations, and iTrace for corneal aberrations (10).

In our clinic we use WaveLight Analyzer (WaveLight Germany) as aberrometer. Working in the same visible spectrum as the human eye, the WaveLight Analyzer is designed for wavefront measurements on the basis of the Tscherning principle. In order to perform measurements according to the Tscherning principle, an image of regular measurement spots is projected onto the retina and captured by a lightsensitive camera. The distortion of the light spots on the retina in relation to the reference light bundle is calculated and the wavefront error is displayed. Figure 9 shows HOAs in a male aged 32 with myopia on his left eye. Wavefront refraction: -6.54/-1.14 ax 72°, coma: 0.16μm, spherical aberration: 0.02 μm, and pupil diameter: 6.59 mm.

Can HOAs be corrected? Wavefront technology has been advanced enough only in the last few years to produce accurate measurements and diagnoses of HOAs. Some types of new wavefront designed glasses, contact lenses, intraocular lens implants and wavefront-guided laser vision correction can correct HOAs.

One of the most powerful clinical applications of aberrometry is wavefront-guided refractive surgery. With the development of wavefront analyses, the increase of the HOAs of the eye following conventional photorefractive keratectomy (PRK) has been confirmed (11). Wavefront-guided refractive surgery is a technique using excimer or other lasers to correct not only spherical and cylindrical refractive errors but also HOAs. Seiler et al. reported the first application of wavefront-guided laser *in situ* keratomileusis (LASIK) using a Tscherning aberrometer to measure the HOAs (12). McDonald performed almost simultaneously the first wavefront-guided LASIK using data obtained from the Hartmann–Shack wavefront sensor (13).

Several excimer laser platforms are available today. Although various terminology has been used to label, identify, and differentiate treatment modalities, the most commonly used include conventional laser in situ keratomileusis (LASIK); wavefront-guided treatments, which customize ablation patterns based on higher- and lower-order aberration profiles unique to the eye being treated; and wavefront-optimized treatments, which take some eye variables into account but use pre-programmed ablation profiles based on population analysis. Wavefront-guided treatments are intended to reduce preoperative HOAs, and wavefront-optimized treatments are intended to minimize the induction of postoperative HOAs; both modalities minimize significantly postoperative HOA changes compared with conventional LASIK treatments. There are some reported differences in the outcomes of wavefront-guided and wavefront-optimized platforms; however, few studies have directly compared the outcomes of these different technologies. The results in these studies are inconsistent, some indicating an advantage for wavefront-guided treatments and others finding no significant differences between the 2 treatment algorithms for patients without significant preoperative HOAs (14).

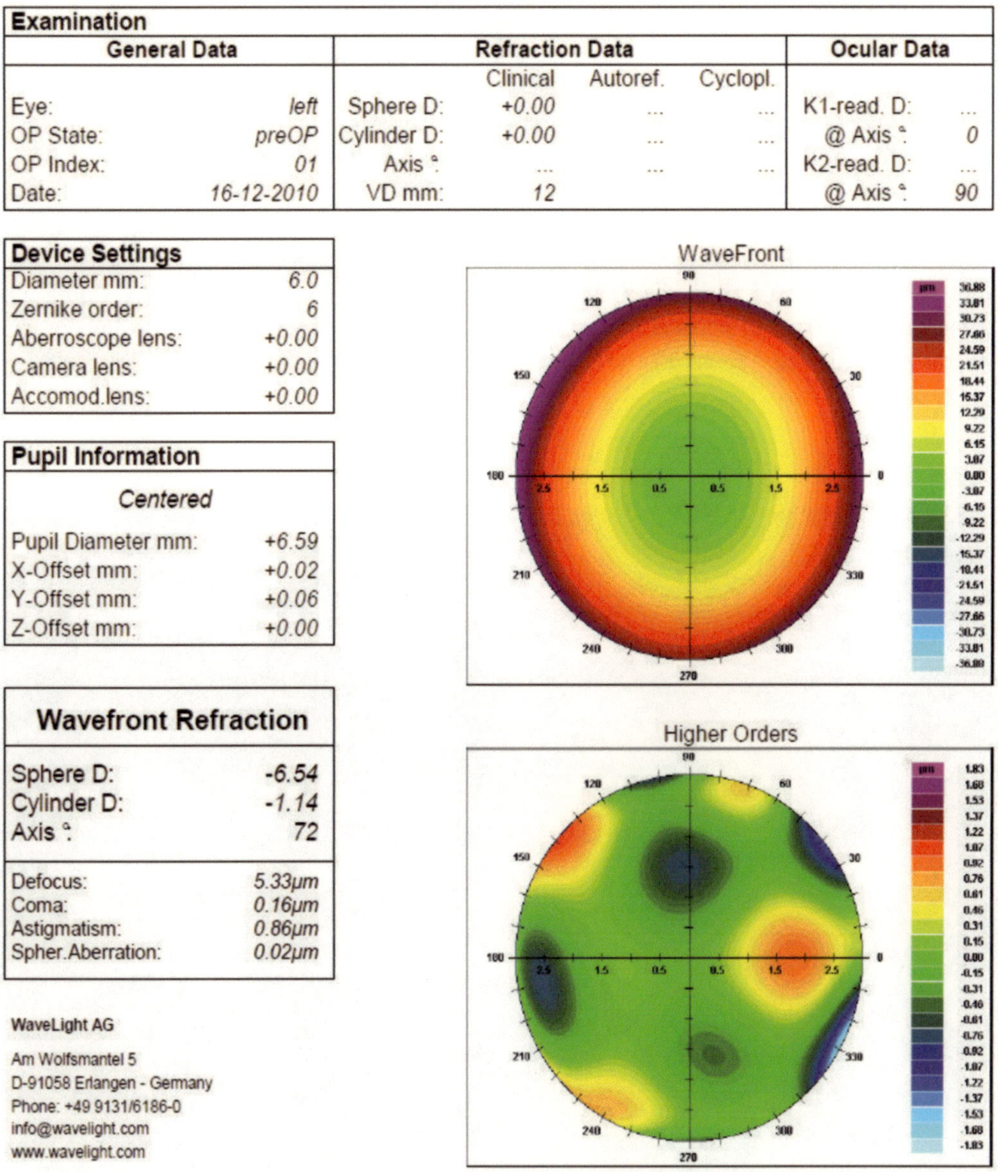

Examination

General Data		Refraction Data	Clinical	Autoref.	Cyclopl.	Ocular Data	
Eye:	left	Sphere D:	+0.00	...	...	K1-read. D:	...
OP State:	preOP	Cylinder D:	+0.00	...	...	@ Axis °:	0
OP Index:	01	Axis °:	...	...	...	K2-read. D:	...
Date:	16-12-2010	VD mm:	12			@ Axis °:	90

Device Settings

Diameter mm:	6.0
Zernike order:	6
Aberroscope lens:	+0.00
Camera lens:	+0.00
Accomod.lens:	+0.00

Pupil Information

Centered

Pupil Diameter mm:	+6.59
X-Offset mm:	+0.02
Y-Offset mm:	+0.06
Z-Offset mm:	+0.00

Wavefront Refraction

Sphere D:	-6.54
Cylinder D:	-1.14
Axis °:	72
Defocus:	5.33µm
Coma:	0.16µm
Astigmatism:	0.86µm
Spher.Aberration:	0.02µm

WaveLight AG
Am Wolfsmantel 5
D-91058 Erlangen - Germany
Phone: +49 9131/6186-0
info@wavelight.com
www.wavelight.com

Fig. 9. Wavefront aberrations recorded on WaveLight Analyzer (WaveLight Germany).

Fares et al. compared the efficiency, predictability, safety, and induced HOAs between wavefront-guided and non-wavefront-guided ablations. Their meta-analysis showed that the increase in HOAs in patients who had wavefront-guided LASIK was lesser than in those who had non-wavefront-guided LASIK (15).

We experienced in our clinic that refractive surgical procedures (LASIK and PRK) induce HOAs and usually do not reduce visual acuity. Here is a brief overview of a case of increasing coma after successful correction of mild myopia using PRK: the patient was a male aged 27, and a PRK method was performed on his right eye with myopia. WaveLight Allegretto (400 Hz) excimer laser was used. HOAs were measured preoperatively and postoperatively on WaveLight Analyzer. Preoperative best spectacle corrected visual acuity of the right eye was with - 0.75/-0.25 ax 134° = 1.0, and postoperative uncorrected visual acuity was 1.0. Optical zone of 6.5 mm and ablated zone of 9.0 mm were used. Coma was increased from 0.02 μm preoperatively to 0.15 μm postoperatively, and sperical aberration was the same (0.08 μm) (Figs. 10 and 11).

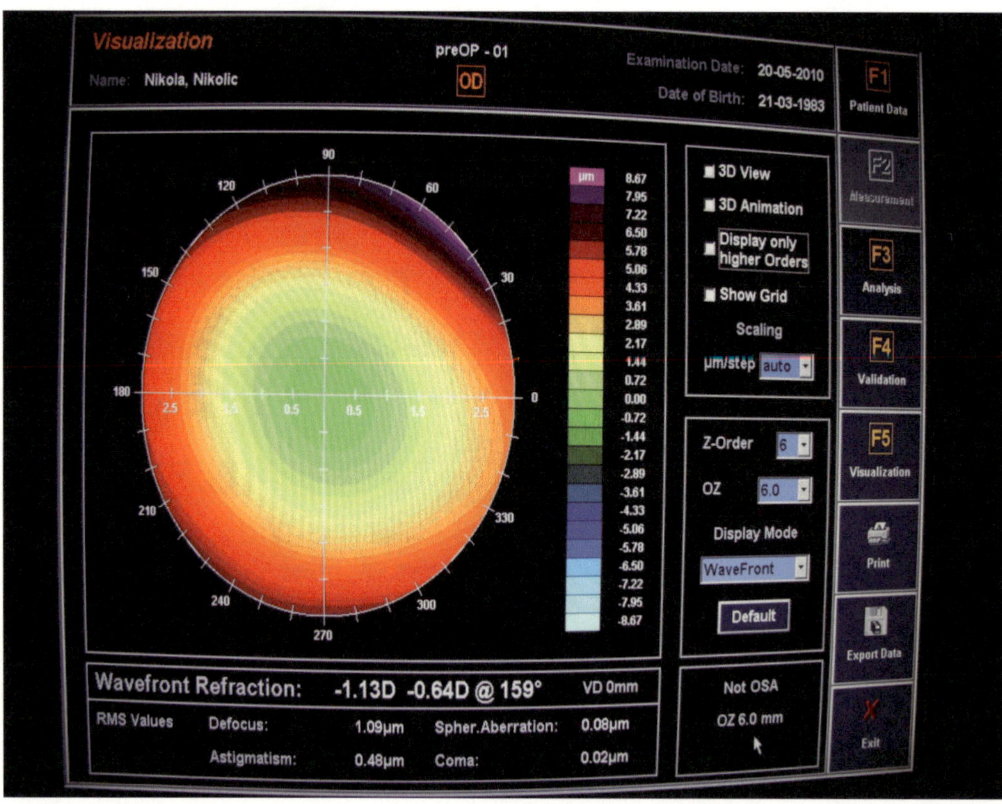

Fig. 10. Picture of wavefront aberrations preoperatively.

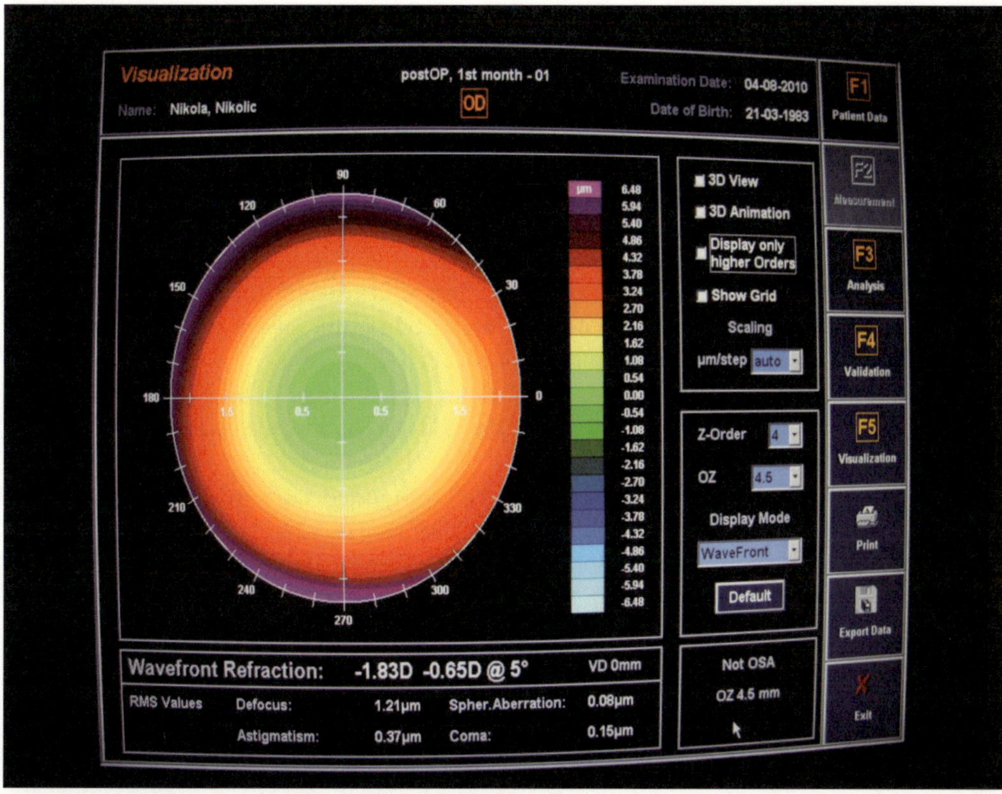

Fig. 11. Picture of wavefront aberrations postoperatively.

6. References

[1] Schwiegerling J. Theoretical limits to visual performance. Surv Ophthalmol 2000; 45:139–146.

[2] Cvetkovic D. Refraction clinic. In: Parunovic A, Cvetkovic D et al, Ed. Correction of refractive errors of the eye. Belgrade: Zavod za udzbenike i nastavna sredstva; 1995. p. 15-44.

[3] Grosvenor T. Anomalies of refraction. In: Grosvenor T, Ed. Primary care optometry. Woburn, MA: Butterworth-Heinemann; 2002. p. 3-26.

[4] Smith ME, Kincaid MC, West CE. Astigmatic lenses. In: Smith ME, Kincaid MC, West CE, Ed. Basic science, refraction, and pathology. St. Louis, Missouri: Mosby; 2002. p. 104-110.

[5] Goss DA, West RW. Optics of refractive error management. In: Goss DA, West RW, Ed. Introduction to the optics of the eye. Woburn, MA: Butterworth-Heinemann; 2002. p. 137-153.

[6] American Academy of Ophthalmology. Optics of the human eye. In: American Academy of Ophthalmology. Clinical optics. San Francisco, CA: American Academy of Ophthalmology; 2007. p. 105-123.

[7] Smith ME, Kincaid MC, West CE. The ametropias. In: Smith ME, Kincaid MC, West CE, Ed. Basic science, refraction, and pathology. St. Louis, Missouri: Mosby; 2002. p. 99-103.

[8] Lombardo M, Lombardo G. Wave aberration of human eyes and new descriptors of image optical quality and visual performance. J Cataract Refract Surg 2010; 36: 313–331.

[9] Lawless MA, Hodge C. Wavefront's role in corneal refractive surgery. Clin Experiment Ophthalmol 2005; 33: 199–209.

[10] Visser N, Berendschot TTJM, Verbakel F, Tan AN, De Brabander J, Nuijts RMMA. Evaluation of the comparability and repeatability of four wavefront aberrometers. Invest Ophthalmol Vis Sci 2011; 52:1302–1311.

[11] Seiler T, Kaemmerer M, Mierdel P, Krinke HE. Ocular optical aberrations after photorefractive keratectomy for myopia and myopic astigmatism. Arch Ophthalmol 2000; 118: 17–21.

[12] Mrochen M, Kaemmerer M, Seiler T. Wavefront-guided laser in situ keratomileusis: early results in three eyes. J Refract Surg 2000; 16: 116–121.

[13] McDonald MB. Summit-Autonomous CustomCornea laser in situ keratomileusis outcomes. J Refract Surg 2000; 16: S617–618.

[14] Perez-Straziota CE, Randleman JB, Stulting RD. Visual acuity and higher-order aberrations with wavefront-guided and wavefront-optimized laser in situ keratomileusis J Cataract Refract Surg 2010; 36: 437–441.

[15] Fares U, Suleman H, Al-Aqaba MA, Otri AM, Said DG, Dua HS. Efficacy, predictability, and safety of wavefront-guided refractive laser treatment: Metaanalysis. J Cataract Refract Surg 2011; 37:1465–1475.

12

Non-Surgical Treatment of Astigmatism

Luciane B. Moreira
Ophthalmology Department, Federal University of Paraná, Curitiba
Brazil

1. Introduction

People with astigmatism have several options available to regain clear vision. They include eyeglasses, contact lenses, orthokeratology and refractive surgery procedures. In this chapter, we will talk about non-surgical treatment only.

2. Eyeglasses

Eyeglasses are a choice for correction for people with regular astigmatism and it doesn't improve vision for irregular astigmatism. They will contain a cylindrical lens prescription for the astigmatism in a specific meridian of the lens which designates the axis of the lens power. Myopia or hyperopia can be associated to astigmatism. Generally, a single vision lens is prescribed so as to provide clear vision at all distances. However, for patients over the age of 40 who have presbyopia, a bifocal or progressive addition lens may be needed in order to focus effectively for near vision work.

A wide variety of lens-types and frame designs are now available for patients of all ages. Eyeglasses are no longer just a medical device that provides needed vision correction, but also a means of enhancing appearance. However, any astigmatism correction numerically higher than a cylinder +1.50 or -2.50 should warrant special consideration of lenses and frames.(1)

Some consideration must be made with the intention of obtaining the best adaptation of the patient to their eyeglasses. A good frame should be lightweight, strong, fit comfortably and suit the wearer's sense of style. Over-sized lenses or much curved frames need to be avoided because they can induce distortion in the periphery of the lens. Eyeglasses with small scaffoldings have a minor possibility of producing alterations in the periphery of the lens. The lesser the distance-vertex, the less will be the disparity in the magnification of the image as it enters the meridians of the astigmatism. The use of negative cylindrical lenses for this sends information to locate the correction of the astigmatism in the posterior part of the lens and consequently next to the ocular globe.(2)

The design of the lens influences the adaptation of the eyeglasses. The lenses of spectacles for correcting astigmatism should have a toric or cylindrical surface in order to give a single focal point in the retina. The thickness of the lens is not the same across its surface. This difference in thickness is increased due to the strength of the astigmatism.(3)

Aspheric lenses are not like conventional lenses in that they do not have a spherical front curvature but instead have differing degrees of curvature. This allows wearers to see clearly whether they are looking directly ahead or to either side. Aspheric lenses can also be combined with a high index material so as to produce extremely thin lenses which provide the same great vision improvement.(1)

Lens material is also important. In general, lenses are made from three materials: plastic, glass, and polycarbonate.(3) Glass is still used for lenses and it is scratch resistant, but it is also heavy and breakable. Polycarbonate and Trivex lenses are designed for high impact resistance and are ideal for occupational hazards, children and athletes. They provide the best eye protection. Plastic is the most used material for lenses. The ones made of high index resin are thin, lightweight, provide good optical quality and do not magnify the eyes as with the others. The term 'Index of refraction' is used to describe the speed at which light travels through a material: a higher index results in thinner lenses.

The lenses of eye glasses can also be upgraded with scratch protectant, anti-reflective, UV-protectants, colour tints, or photochromics. A scratch protectant coating helps the lenses become more resistant against most abrasions. A UV coating helps to reduce the amount of UV rays that enter the eyes by blocking it through the lens. Anti-reflective lenses diminish glare and reflections, and allow people to see your eyes without any problem. They are designed to lighten up the tint when in the shade and darken the tint when in direct sunlight. Polarised lenses are like sunglasses in that they are tinted with a polarisation filter and they block vertical light from placing stress on the eyes. They are good for outdoor activities where the sun will be glaring down.(3)

Doctors should instruct patients about the best glasses for their needs, checking the history and the eye exam of each one. The ideal method is to prescribe the spectacles after eyeglass trials, giving the patients the opportunity to see how they feel in the situations that are common in their everyday life. Often, the physician will try to give the best monocular correction at the refractor to their patients; however, when the patient uses the eyeglasses, with both eyes open, they will not obtain much comfort and will sometimes feel dizzy and get a headache. Ultimately, one needs to take into consideration the binocular vision, the differences between the eyes, the interpupillary distance and the pantoscopic angle of the scaffolding.(4) (figure 1).

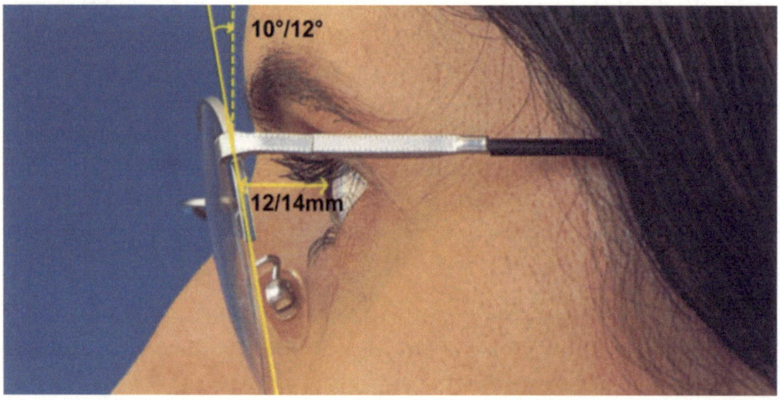

Fig. 1. Pantoscopic angle of glasses.(4)

3. Contact lenses

For some individuals, contact lenses can offer better vision than eyeglasses. They can be used for people with regular and irregular astigmatism, such as keratoconus. They may provide clearer vision and a wider field of view. However, since contact lenses are worn directly on the eyes, they require regular cleaning and care to safeguard eye health(5)

Contact lenses are the first choice for difficult cases such as corneal ecstasies (e.g. keratoconus, keratoglobus and pellucid marginal degeneration). For these cases, there are special lenses with a variety of designs. In this current chapter we will focus only on regular astigmatisms, since to address this kind of adaptation would require a whole chapter to itself.

Almost everybody has the option of using contact lenses. Before initiating any contact lens fitting, it is important to evaluate the patient's motivation, ocular needs, and ocular and medical history. There are four principal indications for contact lens fitting: 1) optical indications (myopia, hyperopia, astigmatism and presbyopia); 2) medical indications (keratoconus, irregular astigmatism, corneal opacification, anisometropia, unilateral aphakia, nystagmus, after refractive surgery or keratoplasty); 3) cosmetic or prosthetic indication to hide imperfections of the eye; 4) therapeutic indications for corneal abrasion.(4)

The contraindications are generally relative, and they will depend upon the criteria of the ophthalmologist's evaluation. Unmotivated patient; poor personal hygiene; inability to follow directions of lens maintenance and handling; inability to understand the risks associated with contact lens use; allergies that affect the eye; immunosuppressed patients, diabetic patients, and alcoholics have a large risk of complications; any effective eye disease affecting the cornea, the conjunctiva and lids as, for example, with inflammations, infections, dry eye, lagophthalmos and glaucoma; moreover, psychological intolerance can be a contraindication for contact lenses use.(4)

Contact lens can be classified by the nature of the material, by their design or by their wearing and replacement schedule, as will seen. A well-made clinical history, along with a complete ophthalmological examination and the patient's needs, determines whether contact lenses are appropriate for each patient(5)

As to the nature of the material of the lens, it can be hard, soft or hybrid. Hard lenses can be non-gas permeable or gas permeable. Polymethylmethacrylate (PMMA) is the polymer from which hard non-gas permeables are made. The disadvantage with this is a lack of gas permeability. The rigid gas permeable lenses (RGP) permit the passage of oxygen and carbon dioxide gas but they contain no water. The general categories of gas permeable polymers are: cellulose acetate butyrate, pure silicone, silicone acrylate and fluorocarbonate. The soft lenses can be hydrogel or silicone hydrogel, both of which have a low water-content (less than 50% water) or high water-content (greater than 50% water). The oxygen transmissibility of a hydrogel lens is directly related to its water-content. For the silicone hydrogel, a higher water-content gives more comfort because it diminishes the roughness of the lens.(6)

There are many designs of lenses. In this chapter, the three basic designs that exist will be addressed: spherical (having anterior and posterior spherical surfaces); aspheric (different radii of curvature in the centre and periphery, simulating the structure of the cornea); and toric (two principal meridians having different radii of curvature; this may be the anterior or posterior surfaces of the lenses or both).[6] Other designs, such as multi-curvature, reverse curve, progressive and bifocal, are related to other refractive errors besides astigmatism and will not be considered here.

The wearing schedule can be: 1) continuous wear (overnight lenses - utilised both during waking and sleeping hours); 2) daily wear (removed daily and not utilised during sleep); 3) flexible wear (removed daily with sporadic sleepers wearing lenses); 4) occasional wear (utilises glasses most of the time and lenses only sometimes, in social activities or sports).[5]

The replacement schedule can be done in three ways: 1) a traditional or conventional way is used when the lens must be replaced annually; 2) the planned replacement way which is nowadays the most used and where the lens needs to be replaced every 15, 30 or 60 days (as defined by the manufacturer's guidelines); 3) disposable lenses, which are probably are the easiest way, because they are immediately discarded after use and do not need maintenance.[5]

Many people ask whether or not RGP lenses are better than hydrogel lenses. The answer to this question depends upon vision accuracy, the comfort and satisfaction of the patient and corneal health. The adaptation of contact lens is different for each person. Generally, to get used to them, the patients need between 1 and 15 days and seem to be easier for those wearing hydrogel lenses than for the ones who wear RGP lenses.

There are many pamphlets to help and teach users how to put on and take off contact lenses, as well as how to store them and keep them clean. However, it is necessary to review these steps at every follow-up visit to the ophthalmologist. The control of contact lens use needs to be done with a specialist every year or else every 6 months, depending on the lens fitting and eye condition.

3.1 Soft contact lenses

Soft contact lenses conform to the shape of the eye. Spherical soft lenses may not be effective in correcting astigmatism;[7] however, toric soft contact lenses can provide a correction for regular astigmatism similar to that of eyeglasses.

A strategy for correcting low degrees of astigmatism with spherical soft lenses is to increase the thickness of the lens. Considering that a thicker or stiffer lens may drape less on the cornea and mask more astigmatism, thicker lenses associated with a special design can give good vision even for irregular astigmatism, such as keratoconus.[5] Another strategy that has been described is the use of lenses with low water-content, since it is not so malleable. However, a low water-content spherical silicone hydrogel material has been shown to have no significant impact on the amount of astigmatism masked.[8]

Visual acuity with a spherical equivalent refraction remained at tolerable limits with the use of spherical contact lenses. Spherical lenses failed to mask corneal toricity during topography, while toric lenses caused central neutralisation and a decrease in corneal cylinder in low and moderate astigmatic eyes.[9]

Soft aspheric contact lenses have been recommended for low astigmatic patients because its design could decrease the level of spherical aberration that is a distortion in image formation. However, clinical studies have reported that non-toric aspheric soft contact lenses did not improve visual acuity significantly when compared to spherical lenses on low astigmats. One reason for why these non-toric lenses do not improve visual acuity is that aspheric soft contact lenses do not correct astigmatism. Additionally, decentration of spherical aberration correction has been shown to induce a coma-like aberration that is another distortion in image formation.(9)

Visual acuity with toric lenses is better than with spherical or aspheric lenses, but initially lens quality and stability was a problem. Nowadays, improved lens designs and the availability of disposable toric contact lenses have resulted in improved health benefits and adaptation(10) Well-fitted hydrogel toric lenses can provide visual acuity and visual performance equivalent to that of spherical RGP lenses.(9)

All the literature agrees that the best way to fit a soft lens is by considering the response to the trial lens fitting. By slit lamp, the physician observes centralisation, the movement of the lens and the lens-cornea relationship. After this, over-refraction has to be done.(5) However, the fitting without trial lens has proven to be an efficient way to prescribe it. 50% to 80% of patients are being fitted successfully with this method for soft toric contact lenses.(11) To fit a soft contact lens, keratometry needs to be done. The base curve of the lens should be approximately 0.6 to 0.8 mm flatter than the average corneal curvature measurement. The lens diameter should be approximately 2.0 mm larger than the horizontal visible iris diameter. The dioptric power of the contact lens should consider the total eye refraction and, if it is greater than 4.00 D, a table for the correction of the vertex distance should be used.(6) It can also be calculated using the following formula:(5)

$$DL = \frac{DA}{1 - d \cdot DA}$$

DL= dioptric power of contact lens.
DA= dioptric power of glasses.
d= vertex distance (which has an average of 12mm).

There remains some disagreement as to when to fit soft toric lenses or else spherical lenses. In practice, high myopia associated with low astigmatism has good acuity with spherical contact lenses; however, low myopes with higher astigmatism had significantly better acuity with toric lenses than with the spherical equivalent.(5)

3.2 Rigid gas permeable lenses

Rigid gas permeable contact lenses maintain their regular shape while on the cornea, and they offer an effective way to compensate for the cornea's irregular shape and improve the vision of persons with astigmatism and other refractive errors.

Gas permeable (GP) lenses could be very acceptable as a viable option for the correction of moderate to severe astigmatism. Patients preferred RGP lenses for visual acuity, especially at near and intermediate distances.(12)

Spherical lenses can compensate for corneal astigmatism up to 3.00 D, although it is known that using them on corneas showing more than 2.00 D of toricity may be inappropriate. Because of this, it is recommended that spherical fittings should be done where the base curve of the lens is equal to the cornea's flattest meridian. The limits of this approach are reached on highly toric corneas where the lens may alter the tear film flow, leading to peripheral desiccation of the cornea (known as 3-9 o'clock staining). This is why a spherical GP lens should be used with extreme caution on a cornea presenting toricity greater than 2.00 D. At present, it is recommended that reliance should be placed on a topographic map of the cornea so as to determine the optimal parameters.(13)

Many methods can be used to find the base curve. That most frequently used by practitioners involves adding 1/3 to 1/4 of the astigmatism measure to K (the flattest meridian of the topographic corneal map).(12) The diameter of the lenses is dependent to the base curve. A great diameter needs a flatter adaptation (table 1). Another tip is to remember is that steeper corneas require lenses with a smaller diameter, and that flatter corneas require lenses with a greater diameter (table 2).(5)

The selected trial lens is placed on the cornea and then, for the evaluation, it is necessary to take into account its comfort, position, movement and stability. The slit lamp evaluates the relationship between the lens and cornea with fluorescein. After the fitting is complete, the over-refraction should be done.

Corneal cylinder	8.6 mm diameter lens	9.2 mm diameter lens	10.2 mm diameter lens
0,00 to 0,50 D	0.25 D STK	On K	0.25 D FTK
0,75 to 1,25 D	0.50 D STK	0,25 D STK	On K
1,50 to 2,00 D	0.75 D STK	0.50 D STK	0.25 D STK
2,25 to 2,75 D	1.00 D STK	0.75 D STK	0.50 D STK
3,00 to 3,50 D	1.25 D STK	1.00 D STK	0.75 D STK

STK = steeper than K / FTK = flatter then K.

Table 1. Base curve lens determination in dependence of lens diameter and topographic corneal cylinder.

Corneal curvature (K)	Lens diameter
38.00 to 42.00 D	9.8 mm or bigger
42.25 to 44.25 D	9.1 to 9.7 mm
44.50 to 50.00 D	9.0 mm or smaller

Table 2. Correlation between corneal curvature flattest meridian of the topographic corneal map (K) and contact lens diameter

Aspheric lenses will always move in the direction of least resistance: this implies that a lens that is restricted along the vertical meridian and which is free along the horizontal meridian will move freely up and down. Conversely, if there is a restriction along the horizontal meridian, the lens will decentre on the nasal or temporal side.(13)

For those wearing RGP contact lenses, only 18% to 22% wear toric correction, suggesting that many practitioners tend to mask astigmatism using spherical equivalence with contact lenses. One reason for this behaviour is that toric gas permeable lenses are more complex to fit and have variable results.[13] Some practitioners will consider toric lenses only if the patient reports unsatisfactory vision in spherical contact lenses or else when the corneal toricity is too great and the fitting has become unstable. Toric lens designs can have different radii of curvature on the front surface, back surface or both of what are known as bitoric lenses.

Back-toric design implies that the back surface of the lens is toric and that its front surface is spherical. This design is most successful when the corneal toricity represents more than two thirds of the refractive astigmatism. Back-toric gas permeable lenses are not designed with prism ballasts; their stabilisation is mainly achieved by the correspondence between the back curves and the corneal toricity. This type of lens is designed with only 66% corneal toricity so as to provide more comfort. However, because of this, the lens will quite certainly rotate in the eye. Clinically, this translates as induced astigmatism that can disturb the visual outcome where it exceeds 0.75 D.[5]

Front-toric designs are designed with the astigmatic correction on the front surface of the lens, leaving the back surface spherical. They are stabilised with a base-down prism and represent the best choice for correcting residual astigmatism, in which the cornea is spherical.[5] Residual astigmatism results from causes other than the shape of the anterior corneal surface and can refer to astigmatism of the posterior cornea surface, lens, and retina.

A bitoric lens offers both surfaces as toric. The back toric surface curves are designed to be aligned with the corneal toricity. Optically speaking, this generates an over-correction of the refractive astigmatism. This is why a front toric surface is needed to compensate the power of the lens. Bi-toric designs are the most popular toric design in RGP contact lens practice, and represent the best choice if corneal toricity is less than or exceeds refractive astigmatism.[5]

For RGP toric lenses, I believe that the most appropriate fitting method is a 4-step approach, known as the two-thirds rule, as seen below.[14]

Step 1. Calculation of corneal toricity: calculate the difference between the two principal meridians of the cornea.

Step 2. Calculation of Base curve 1 (BC-1): the base curve 1 of the lens is determined by dividing the corneal toricity (found in Step 1) into two-thirds and then adding it to the flattest meridian of the cornea.

Step 3. Calculation of base curve 2 (BC-2): the base curve 2 of the lens is determined by flattening the steepest meridian of the cornea according to Remba's rule (Table 3).

Step 4. Calculation of lachrymal lens power and induced astigmatism: this type of astigmatism is induced by the relationship of the back surface of the lens to the cornea, and can be seen doing the over-refraction. If this value is less than 1.00 D, a back-toric design should be ordered because the induced astigmatism is not considered to be a contributing factor affecting visual acuity. At this point, a spherical equivalence is made in order to determine the final power of the back-toric lens. However, if the induced astigmatism value exceeds 1.00 D, a bitoric design should then be selected because the induced astigmatism should be corrected by the addition of the cylinder power to the front-surface of the lens.

Cornea toricity	Flattening of the steepest meridian
2.0 D	0.25 D
3.0 D	0.50 D
4.0 D or more	0.75 D

Table 3. Usable values according to Remba's rule

3.3 Orthokeratology

Orthokeratology (ortho-k) involves the fitting of specially designed rigid contact lenses to reshape the cornea so as to temporarily reduce or eliminate refractive error. The contact lenses are worn for limited periods, such as overnight, and then removed. Persons with mild to moderate myopia and mild astigmatism may be able to temporarily obtain clear vision without lenses for most of their daily activities. Ortho-k does not permanently improve vision, and if the person stops wearing the retainer lenses, the cornea may return to its original condition and vision will be bad again. Ortho-k is a good option for people who need RGP contact lenses to improve vision but who cannot wear common lenses for many reasons.(5) The main reasons for using this kind of lens are: workers in polluted environments or who use chemical products; boxers or water-sports athletes; people who feel discomfort with regular lenses and cannot have refractive surgery; people who have problems with blinking, dry eye, giant papillary conjunctivitis or nystagmus.

Ortho-k makes many changes to the shape of the cornea, as can be seen by topography maps, wave front measurements and pachymetry. The corneal changes induced by reverse-geometry - because of the relatively flat-fitting base curve - create a central flattened zone called the treatment zone, corresponding approximately to the lens back optic zone. Successful ortho-k treatment produces a well-centred regular treatment zone which encompasses the pupil diameter, as revealed by inspection of the difference map on the corneal topographer's data display (figure 2).(15)

The induction of higher-order aberrations with the use of reverse-geometry lenses for overnight ortho-k has been reported.(16) The significant increase in spherical aberrations is seen by the annular zone of mid-peripheral corneal steepening induced by the reverse-geometry lens, and the consequent change in corneal shape from prolate[1] towards oblate[2] asphericity.(16) However, the patients do not complain about these kinds of visual problems. A higher-order aberration is a distortion acquired when light passes through an eye with irregularities. Everyone's eyes have it, but the quantity of it is what determines whether it will affect quality of vision, by giving symptoms as glare, halos, starburst effects and ghost images.

Most of the studies concern ortho-k for myopia of 4.0D and with-the-rule corneal astigmatism of less than 1.50D showing rapid results, with most change after the first night of lens wear and most stability in refractive change after 4 weeks.(17) However, a few studies show good results for irregular astigmatism, such as keratoconus.(15)

Spherical reverse-geometry lenses can be used on toric corneas in order to reduce astigmatism. In a retrospective analysis, Mountford and Pesudovs(18) demonstrated that up

---

[1] The normal cornea is a prolate surface - steeper in the centre and flatter in the periphery.
[2] The oblate surface is a surface after myopic laser photorefractive keratectomy – flatter in the centre and steeper in the periphery.

to 50% of corneal astigmatism could be reduced with standard reverse-geometry ortho-k lenses, provided that the toricity was with-the-rule and restricted to the central region of the cornea. Corneal toricity reaching from limbus to limbus on the topographic map was less amenable to modification by ortho-k lenses.

Toric ortho-k lenses were created for an oval treatment zone and different meridional topographic changes, with more corneal flattening in the meridian requiring more myopic refractive error correction. Details of corneal topographic changes induced by these different ortho-k lens designs over longer periods of wear are yet to be published.[19]

There is slight regression of effect (about 0.25 to 0.75 D) during the day, and lenses must be periodically worn overnight (from every night to every three to four nights) to retain the effect. No serious adverse events have been reported from published clinical studies, although overnight lens adherence and clinically significant corneal staining in the morning after lens removal appear to be relatively common and have caused some clinical concerns in some studies.[20]

Patient satisfaction with overnight ortho-k has been reported as similar to or better than other popular modalities of contact lens wear. Unlike refractive surgery, if patients fail to achieve a subjectively successful outcome, they can cease lens wear and return to other corrective options, such as spectacles or conventional contact lenses. The corneal changes induced by overnight ortho-k are fully reversible on cessation of lens wear.[20]

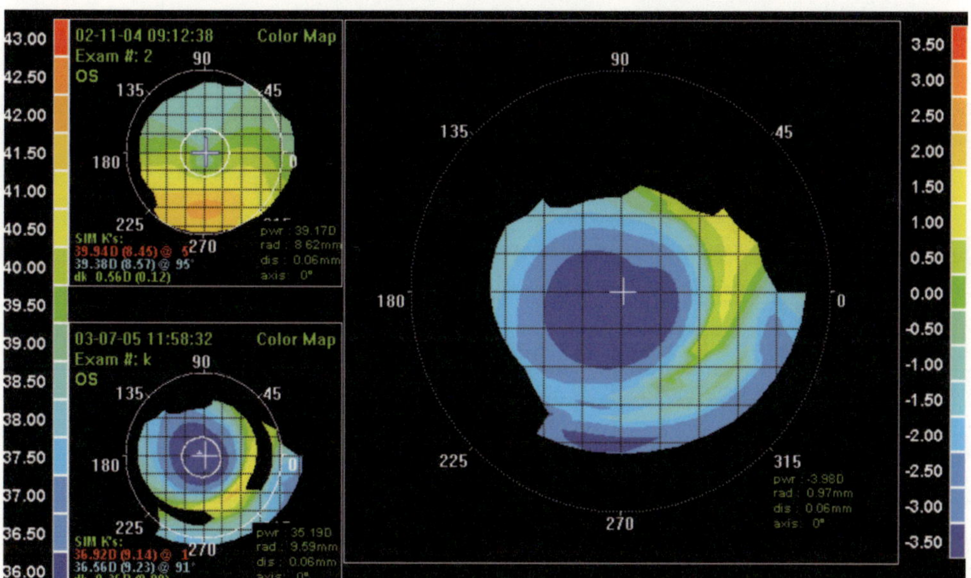

Fig. 2. Topography before and after orthokeratology in a case of irregular astigmatism (keratoconus).[15]

4. Visual stimulation

Brain plasticity in the visual functions of adults has been shown to improve with repetitive practice on specific controlled visual tasks. Through these repetitive practices are initiated neural modifications that lead to an improvement in neuronal efficiency. These neural modifications can enhance image quality by compensating for blurred retinal images due to optical defocus for all the refract errors.(21) It is indicated by those who have good Snellen visual acuity but still have symptoms of ghost images. This commonly happens to people with low astigmatism.

RevitalVision by NeuroVision (NeuroVision Inc., Singapore), based on visual stimulation, have developed a computer programme for amblyopia, post lasik (laser assisted in situ keratomileusis) and post cataract. However, it can be extended for others refractive errors. During training sessions, the user is presented with a series of precise visual tasks consisting of Gabor patches with subtle differences in orientation, size and contrast. Through repetitive practice, the brain is trained to be more efficient and to improve visual processing by improving contrast sensitivity and visual acuity.(22)

Studies showed mean improvements of visual acuity of about 2.0 LogMar, and the contrast sensitivity function also improved at all spatial frequencies. However, the mean refractive error remained unchanged after treatment. Follow-up data for up to 12 months post-treatment showed that the gains were retained.(23) This method has never been proven. The effect is probably related to the memory of the patients, and this would be the reason that the refractive error remains unchanged.

Besides this, it requires more evaluation to see the real value of this kind of stimulation for the treatment of astigmatism.(21-23)

5. Advantages and disadvantages for each correcting method

There are many differences between contact lens and glasses, as can be seen in the chart below, but both need an eye doctor's prescription and periodic evaluation.

Eyeglasses	Contact Lenses
The distance between your eye and the lens sometimes creates distortion.	When worn right on the eye it sometimes can blur because of tears.
Glasses correct only regular astigmatism.	Contact lenses can also correct irregular cornea shape that distorts vision.
Glasses can be inconvenient during games and sports.	Contact lenses are a favourite among athletes.
Poor peripheral vision (visual field) because of the frame.	Your entire field of view is in focus.
Eyeglasses can get dirty and decrease vision.	Contact lenses can form deposits on the lens and blur the vision acuity.
Glasses must be sprayed and wiped several times a day.	Contact lenses should be cleaned, disinfected and stored properly after each use.
Periodic need for tightening or other adjustment.	Maintenance and handling of the lens every day.
Sometimes an uncomfortable weight on your face and ears.	Sometimes uncomfortable in the eye as a strange body, dry eye or allergy.
Glasses are fashionable, functional and complement your outfit.	Cosmetic lens may alter the colour of the eye.

Also, there are advantages and disadvantages associated with various types of contact lens, as seen below. All of the contact lenses require visits to the ophthalmologist for follow-up care.

Lens Types	Advantages	Disadvantages
Soft lenses	Very short adaptation period. More comfortable and more difficult to dislodge than RGP lenses.	Maintenance and handling every day. Do not last long comparing to RGP lenses. Vision may not be as sharp as RGP lenses.
Daily wear disposable lenses	Thinner lenses. Require no cleaning. Minimal risk of eye infection if the wearing instructions are followed.	Do not correct all vision problems.
Extended ware disposable lenses	Can usually be worn up to several days without removal (the wearing period is defined by the manufacturer's guidelines). Require no cleaning.	Do not correct all vision problems. Increases risk of complication with night and day wear. Requires regular monitoring and professional care.
Planned replacement lenses	Require simplified cleaning and disinfection. Good for eye health. Available in most prescriptions.	Vision may not be as sharp as RGP lenses. Maintenance and handling every day.
Rigid gas permeable lenses (RGP)	Excellent vision. Easier than the soft lens for maintenance and handling. Correct most vision problems. Durable, with a relatively long life.	Require consistent wear to maintain good vision. Can slip off the centre of the eye more easily than other types. Debris can easily get under the lenses. Longer period to get used to compared to soft lenses.
Ortoceratologia	Worn only at times of sleeping. Eliminates the use of the lens on walking hour. Short adaptation period. Comfortable to wear. Less friction with the lid. Durable, with a long life.	Correct only low astigmatism and low to moderate myopia. Vision may not be as sharp as with other lenses.

6. Conclusion

Individuals with astigmatism have a wide range of options to correct their vision problems and, together with an eye exam, the selection of the best treatment that meets vision and lifestyle needs must be done.

7. References

[1] Guyton DL. Prescribing cylinders: the problem of distortion. Surv Ophthalmol. 1977 Nov-Dec; 22(3): 177-88.

[2] Moreira ATR. Astigmatismo: atualização continuada - Sociedade Brasileira de Oftalmopediatria. Arq. Bras. Oftalmol. 2001; 64(3): 2712-272.

[3] Stein HA, Freeman MJ, Stenson SM, Kara José N, Coral-Ghanem C, Oliveira PR. Guia CLAO para refração e óculos: um manual para oftalmologistas. Contact Lens Association of Ophthalmologists Inc. (CLAO). Copyright 1999.

[4] Uras R. Optica e refração ocular - coleção de manuais básicos cbo. Cultura Medica, Rio de Janeiro, 2008.

[5] Moreira SB, Moreira H, Moreira LB. Lente de contato. 3° Ed, cultura médica, Rio de Janeiro, 2004.

[6] Mannis MJ, Zadnik K, Coral-Ghanem C, Kara-Jose N. Contact Lens in Ophthalmic Practice. Springer-Verlag, New York, 2004.

[7] Kurna SA, Şengör T, Ün M, Aqui S. Success rates in the correction of astigmatism with toric and spherical soft contact lens fittings clinical ophthalmology 2010: 4 p959-966.

[8] Edmondson L, Edmondson W, Prince R. Masking astigmatism: Ciba focus night and day vs focus monthly. Optom Vis Sci 2003; 80(12): 184.

[9] Berntsen DA, Merchea MM, Richdale K, Mack CJ, Barr JT. FAAO Higher-Order Aberrations when wearing Sphere and Toric Soft Contact Lenses. Optom Vis Sci. 2009 February; 86(2): 115-122.

[10] Morgan PB, Efron SE, Efron N, Hill EA. Inefficacy of aspheric soft contact lenses for the correction of low levels of astigmatism. Optom Vis Sci. 2005; 82(9): 823-828.

[11] Richdale K, Bernsten DA, Mack CJ. Visual acuity with spherical and toric soft lenses in low- to moderate- astigmatic eyes. Optom Vis Sci 2007; 84(10): 969-75.

[12] Giovedi Filho R. Correção do astigmatismo com lentes de contato rígidas: atualização continuada - Sociedade Brasileira de Lentes de contato e córnea - SOBLEC. 2001; 64(5): 485-487.

[13] Michaud, L, Barriault, C, Dionne, A, Karwatsky, P Empirical fitting of soft or rigid gas-permeable contact lenses for the correction of moderate to severe refractive astigmatism: A comparative study Optometry (2009) 80, 375-383.

[14] Michaud L. Understanding and designing toric gas permeable contact lenses: As easy as 1-2-3. Can J Optom 2007; 69(5): 171-81.

[15] Moreira LB. Ortoceratologia nos casos com contra-indicação de cirurgia refrativa por ceratocone incipiente. Universo visual, November 2006.

[16] Hiraoka,T, Matsumoto, Y, Okamoto, F, Yamagushi, T, Hirohara, Y, Mihashi, T, Oshika, T. Corneal higher-order aberrations induced by overnight orthokeratology. *Am J Ophthalmol* 2005; 139: 429–436.

[17] Kang SY, Kim BK, Byun YJ. Sustainability of orthokeratology as demonstrated by corneal topography. Korean Journal of ophthalmology 2007; 21(2): 74-78.

[18] Mountford, J, Pesudovs, K. An analysis of the astigmatic changes induced by accelerated orthokeratology. *Clin Exp Optom* 2002; 85: 284–293.

[19] Baertschi M. Correction of high astigmatism with orthokeratology. Paper presented at the Global Orthokeratology Symposium, Chicago, July 2005.103.

[20] Swarbrick , HA. Orthokeratology review and update *Clin Exp Optom* 2006; 89: 3: 124-43.

[21] Durrie. D. McMinn, P. Computer-based primary visual cortex training for treatment of low myopia and early presbyopia. Trans Am Ophthalmol Soc 2007; 105: 132-140.

[22] http://www.revitalvision.com/doctors/scientificbackground/

[23] Tan, DT and Fong, A. Efficacy of neural vision therapy to enhance contrast sensitivity function and visual acuity in low myopia. J Cataract Refract Surg, 2008. Apr 34(4): 570-7.

13

Treatment Strategies and Clinical Outcomes of Aspheric Surgery for Astigmatism Using the SCHWIND Amaris Platform

Maria C. Arbelaez[1] and Samuel Arba-Mosquera[2,3]

[1]*Muscat Eye Laser Centre,*

[2]*Grupo de Investigación de Cirugía Refractiva y Calidad de Visión, Instituto de Oftalmobiología Aplicada, University of Valladolid, Valladolid,*

[3]*SCHWIND Eye-Tech-Solutions, Kleinostheim,*

[1]*Oman*

[2]*Spain*

[3]*Germany*

1. Introduction

An optical system with astigmatism is one where rays that propagate in two perpendicular planes have different foci. If an optical system with astigmatism is used to form an image of a cross, the vertical and horizontal lines will be in sharp focus at two different distances. The term comes from the Greek α- (a-) meaning "without" and στίγμα (stigma), "a mark, spot, puncture".

There are two distinct forms of astigmatism. The first is a third-order aberration, which occurs for objects (or parts of objects) away from the optical axis. This form of aberration occurs even when the optical system is perfectly symmetrical.

The second form of astigmatism occurs when the optical system is not symmetric about the optical axis. This form of astigmatism is extremely important in vision science and eye care, since the human eye often exhibits this aberration due to imperfections in the shape of the cornea or the lens.

If an optical system is not axisymmetric, either due to an error in the shape of the optical surfaces or due to misalignment of the components, astigmatism can occur even for on-axis object points. Ophthalmic astigmatism is a refraction error of the eye in which there is a difference in degree of refraction in different meridians. It is typically characterized by an aspherical, non-figure of revolution cornea in which the corneal profile slope and refractive power in one meridian is less than that of the perpendicular axis.

Astigmatism causes difficulties in seeing fine detail. In some cases vertical lines and objects such as walls may appear to the patient to be leaning over like the Tower of Pisa. Astigmatism can be often corrected by glasses with a lens that has different radii of curvature in different planes (a cylindrical lens), contact lenses, or refractive surgery.

Astigmatism is quite common. Studies have shown that about one in three people suffers from it. The prevalence of astigmatism increases with age. Although a person may not notice mild astigmatism, higher amounts of astigmatism may cause blurry vision, squinting, asthenopia, fatigue, or headaches.

Astigmatism is an optical defect in which vision is blurred due to the inability of the optics of the eye to focus a point object into a sharp focused image on the retina. This may be due to an irregular or toric curvature of the cornea or lens. The most of the astigmatism is corneal. Astigmatism may also be caused by crystalline lens subluxation, coloboma or lenticonus. There are two types of astigmatism: regular and irregular. Irregular astigmatism is often caused by a corneal scar or scattering in the crystalline lens. Regular astigmatism arising from either the cornea or crystalline lens can be easily corrected.

The refractive error of the astigmatic eye stems from a difference in degree of curvature refraction of the two different meridians (i.e., the eye has different focal points in different planes.) For example, the image may be clearly focused on the retina in the horizontal (sagittal) plane, but not in the vertical (tangential) plane. Astigmatism causes difficulties in seeing fine detail, and in some cases vertical lines (e.g., walls) may appear to the patient to be tilted.

In With-the-rule astigmatism, the eye sees vertical lines more sharply than horizontal lines. Against-the-rule astigmatism reverses the situation. Children tend to have With-the-rule astigmatism and elderly people tend to have Against-the-rule astigmatism. The prevalence of astigmatism increases with age.

Astigmatism may be corrected with eyeglasses, contact lenses, or refractive surgery. Various considerations involving ocular health, refractive status, and lifestyle frequently determine whether one option may be better than another. In those with keratoconus, toric contact lenses often enable patients to achieve better visual acuities than eyeglasses. Once only available in a rigid gas-permeable form, toric lenses are now available also as soft lenses.

2. Aspheric ablation strategies

An aspheric lens or asphere is a lens whose surfaces have a profile that is rotationally symmetric, but is not a portion of a sphere. The asphere's more complex surface profile can reduce or eliminate spherical aberration and also reduce other optical aberrations compared to spheric lenses. Aspheric elements are used to reduce aberrations.

In prescriptions for both farsightedness and nearsightedness, the lens curve flattens toward the edge of the asphere. Aspheric ablation strategies for spherical correction are modified by means of spherical aberration compensations, whereas aspheric ablation strategies for astigmatic correction are modified by means of high-order-asitmgatism aberration compensations.

3. Ocular wavefront (OW) customized ablation strategies

The treatment plan is developed using OW customised aspheric profiles based on Hartmann-Shack sensing[1]. The high-resolution Hartmann-Shack measurements (>800 points for a 7.0-mm pupil) referred to the entire eye. Optical errors centered on the line-of-sight are described by the Zernike polynomials[2] and the coefficients of the Optical Society of America (OSA) standard[3].

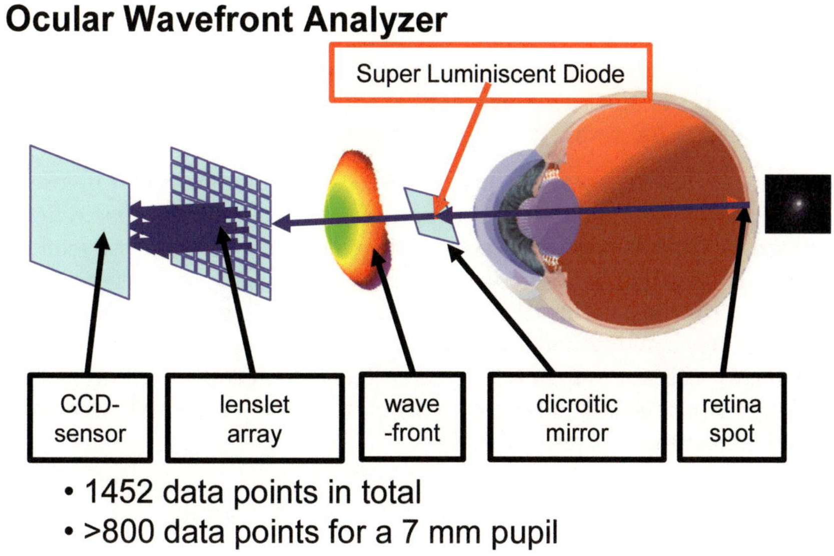

Fig. 1. Principle of the OW measurement.

3.1 Treatment modality

Preoperative topography and aberrometry measurements are taken, and visual acuity, and mesopic pupil size are measured. To determine the ablation profile of the Custom Ablation Manager (CAM), manifest refraction is measured in each eye and crosschecked with objective refraction from the SCHWIND Ocular Wavefront Analyzer[4]. Each eye is planned according to the manifest refraction using the CAM Wavefront customised treatments.

The CAM aspherical profiles were developed with the aim to compensate for the induction of aberrations (especially but not only spherical aberration) observed with other types of profile definitions[5], some of these sources of aberrations are those related to the loss of efficiency of the laser ablation for non-normal incidence[6,7]. Optimization is realized by taking into account the loss of efficiency at the periphery of the cornea in relation to the center, as there is a tangential effect of the spot in relation to the corneal curvature (K (Keratometry) -reading). The software provides K-reading compensation, which considers the change in spot geometry and reflection losses of ablation efficiency.

The base-line for correcting refraction (sphere and cylinder) is aspheric, whereas the high order aberrations measured based on Hartmann-Shack sensing of the entire eye are combined with manifest refraction.

Real ablative spot shape (volume) is considered through a self-constructing algorithm. In addition, there are a randomized flying-spot ablation pattern, and controls for the local repetition rates to minimize the thermal load of the treatment[8].

A central fully corrected ablation zone is used in all eyes with a variable transition size automatically provided by the laser related to the planned refractive correction. Immediately before the ablation, the laser is calibrated per manufacturer's instructions and the calibration settings are recorded.

The CAM software is able to import, visualize, and combine diagnostic data of the eye (manifest refraction and ocular wavefront data in this case) into a customised aspherical ablation profile to optimize the corneal shape. OW based ablations attempt to reduce the wavefront aberration of the entire eye (within Optical Zone, OZ) close to a zero level, compensating, as well, for the aberration induction observed with other types of profiles.

It should be noted that opposing the preoperative wavefront aberration in laser refractive surgery constituted only a first approximation of a perfect refractive correction, as tissue removal occurs. Considerations such as treatment duration or tissue removal make even more difficult to establish a universal optimal profile. Our data suggest that Ocular wavefront customized treatments can only be successful, if the pre-existing aberrations are greater than the repeatability and the biological noise. In particular, the OW customized approach is highly efficient in eyes with greater than 0.25 microns root-mean-square (RMS) ocular HOAb, or where individual components of the OW such as coma, trefoil or spherical aberration are greater than 0.2 microns RMS.

4. Corneal wavefront (CW) customized ablation strategies

The treatment plan is developed using CW customized aspheric profiles based on corneal ray tracing (Salmon 1999[9]). Using the Keratron Scout videokeratoscope (Mattioli & Tripoli 1997[10]) (Optikon 2000 S.p.A, Rome, Italy), the topographical surface and corneal wavefront are analyzed (up to the 7th order). Considering a balanced-eye model (Q-Val -0.25) the departure of the measured corneal topography from the theoretically optimal corneal surface is calculated. Optical errors centered on the line of sight are described by the Zernike polynomials (Zernike 1934[11]) and the coefficients of the Optical Society of America (OSA) standard (Thibos et al. 2002[12]).

Ray tracing is a procedure classically performed by applying Snell's law to the corneal surface. However, it is much simpler to understand corneal wavefront in terms of optical path difference and calculate it by Huygens-Fresnel or "least time" Fermat principles (Salmon 1999[9]; Guirao & Artal 2000[13]).

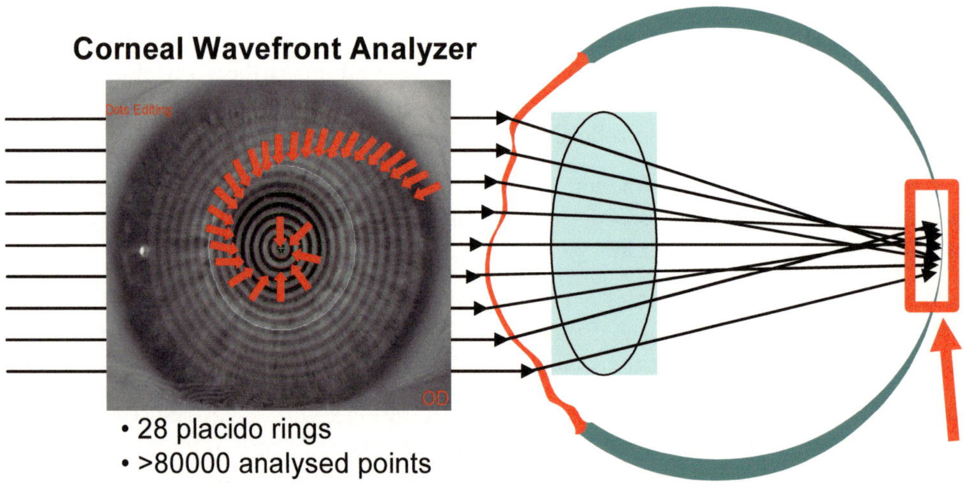

Fig. 2. Principle of the dderivation of the CW.

In corneal wavefront analysis, the type and size of any optical error on the anterior corneal surface are registered, thus allowing a very selective correction. The defects are corrected exactly at their origin - the anterior corneal surface. In this context, the precise localization of defects is crucial to successfully achieving optimal results in laser surgery. The corneal wavefront allows for a very precise diagnosis, thus providing an individual ablation of the cornea in order to obtain perfect results.

Applying this treatment strategy, measurement does not require pupil dilation of the eye, so that the treatment zone is not limited by the pupil and accomodation does not influence the measuring results. Mention is made that in this way forcing a fixed asphericity quotient (Q) on the eyes through the treatment is avoided. Instead, this strategy employs a dynamic postoperative expected asphericity quotient (de Ortueta & Arba-Mosquera 2008[14]), being expressed as:

$$Q_{\exp} = \frac{\frac{1}{n^2} - \frac{1}{4}}{\left(1 + \frac{R \cdot SEq_{cp}}{n-1}\right)^3} - \frac{1}{n^2} \quad (1)$$

where Q_{exp} is the expected/predicted corneal asphericity quotient; R the apical radius of curvature of the preoperative cornea; SEq_{cp} the spherical equivalent to be corrected at the corneal plane; and n the refractive index of the cornea.

The expected quotient of asphericity does not incorporate any compensation for the effect of postop corneal biomechanics / healing response, and it is rather derived from a pure optical model of the cornea.

Preoperative topography and corneal aberrometry measurements are taken, and visual acuity, and mesopic pupil size are measured. Each eye is planned according to the manifest refraction using the CAM wavefront customized treatments. Immediately before ablation, the laser is calibrated according to the manufacturer's instructions and the calibration settings are recorded.

When evaluating the outcomes of wavefront customization strategies, wavefront aberration analysis is mandatory to be able to determine whether the customization aims could be achieved. It has been suggested, as well, that the surface ablation procedures are better suited for the wavefront guided ablation as they would avoid the induction of aberrations due to flap and interface (Chun et al. 2006[15]; Buzzonetti et al. 2004[16]). Now with the introduction of thin and ultrathin planar flaps with femtosecond laser and the newer microkeratomes such as the pendular microkeratome, this aspect of the debate will require further research.

Topography is measured under bright light conditions which might cause pupil constriction and also pupil center shift relative to normal photopic levels. Corneal wavefront customized treatments can only be successful, if the pre-existing aberrations are greater than the repeatability and the biological noise. Considerations such as treatment duration or tissue removal make it more difficult to establish a universal optimal profile.

Furthermore, coupling effects between different high order aberration terms, and between HOAs and manifest refraction is still one of the major sources of residual aberrations after refractive surgery. This topic has been discussed from a theoretical perspective by Bará et al. 2006 [17] and from a clinical perspective by MacRae 2007[18] or Buehren et al. 2007[19]. They all found mutually affecting interactions, for example, between defocus and spherical aberration, or between 3 order aberrations and low order terms, between spherical aberration and coma, or between secondary and primary astigmatisms.

The accuracy, predictability, and stability of the refractive power change, together with the minimal external impact of the CAM ablation profiles on the HOAs, leads to very good results in terms of visual quality. In summary, aspheric CW ablation profiles, designed with CAM software for the AMARIs laser platform, yield visual, optical, and refractive results comparable to those of other wavefront-guided customized techniques for correction of myopia and myopic astigmatism. The CW customized approach shows its strength in cases where abnormal optical systems are expected. Apart from the risk of minimal additional ablation of corneal tissue, systematical wavefront-customized corneal ablation can be considered as a safe and beneficial method.

5. Decision Assistant Wizard

Our definition of "Customisation" is conceptually different and can be stated as: "The planning of the optimum ablation pattern specifically for each individual eye based on its diagnosis and visual demands." It is often the case, that the best approach for planning an ablation is a sophisticated pattern, which can still be simply described in terms of sphere, cylinder, and orientation (axis). The Decision Assistant Wizard, which we present here, is based on our experience with the SCHWIND AMARIS laser. While the general principles of this Decision-Tree based planning (Fig. 3) can basically be applied to any other laser platform offering aspheric and wavefront-guided profiles, some specific aspects concerning both diagnosis and treatments may depend on other manufacturers' specifications.

We begin by acquiring four corneal topographies (Corneal Wavefront Analyzer, SCHWIND eye-tech-solutions GmbH & Co.KG, based on Keratron-Scout, OPTIKON2000, Rome, Italy) and derived CW analyses centred on the line-of-sight for each eye of the patient. We extract the mean, and discard the less representative one (the one with the poorest similarity to the mean). From those remaining three maps, we calculate the mean, and select the most representative one (the one with the highest similarity to the mean).

We continue acquiring, under non pharmacologically dilated pupils, non-cycloplegic conditions, and natural dim light conditions (to avoid pharmacologically induced pupil shifts[20,21]), 3 aberrometries (Ocular Wavefront Analyzer, SCHWIND eye-tech-solutions GmbH & Co.KG, based on irx3, Imagine Eyes, Orsay, France) and objective refractions for each eye of the patient. To minimize the potential accommodative response of the patients, we ask them to "see-through-the-target" instead of "looking at the target." In this way, patients do not try to get a sharp image from the +1.5 D fogged target, since they were instructed to see-through-the-target. From those aberrometries, we calculate the mean, and select the most representative one (the aberrometry map with the highest similarity to the mean).

We continue assessing subjective refraction based upon non-pharmacologic and non-cycloplegic conditions, under natural photopic illumination. We use the objective refraction analyzed for a sub-pupil of 4 mm diameter, as starting refraction for this step. This is particularly useful for determining the magnitude and orientation of the astigmatism. We measure manifest refraction, uncorrected and best spectacle-corrected Snellen visual acuity[22] (UCVA and BSCVA, respectively). Further rules that we impose for accurately determining the manifest subjective refractions among equal levels of BSCVA are: taking the measurement with the least negative (the most positive) spherical equivalent (unmasking latent hyperopia), if several of them are equal in terms of spherical equivalent, we choose the measurement with the least amount of astigmatism (reducing the risk of postoperative shifts in the axis of astigmatism). This is particularly useful for determining the magnitude and orientation of the internal astigmatism as a difference between the topographic astigmatism and the astigmatism of the corneal wavefront analyses compared to the subjective astigmatism the astigmatism of the ocular wavefront analyses.

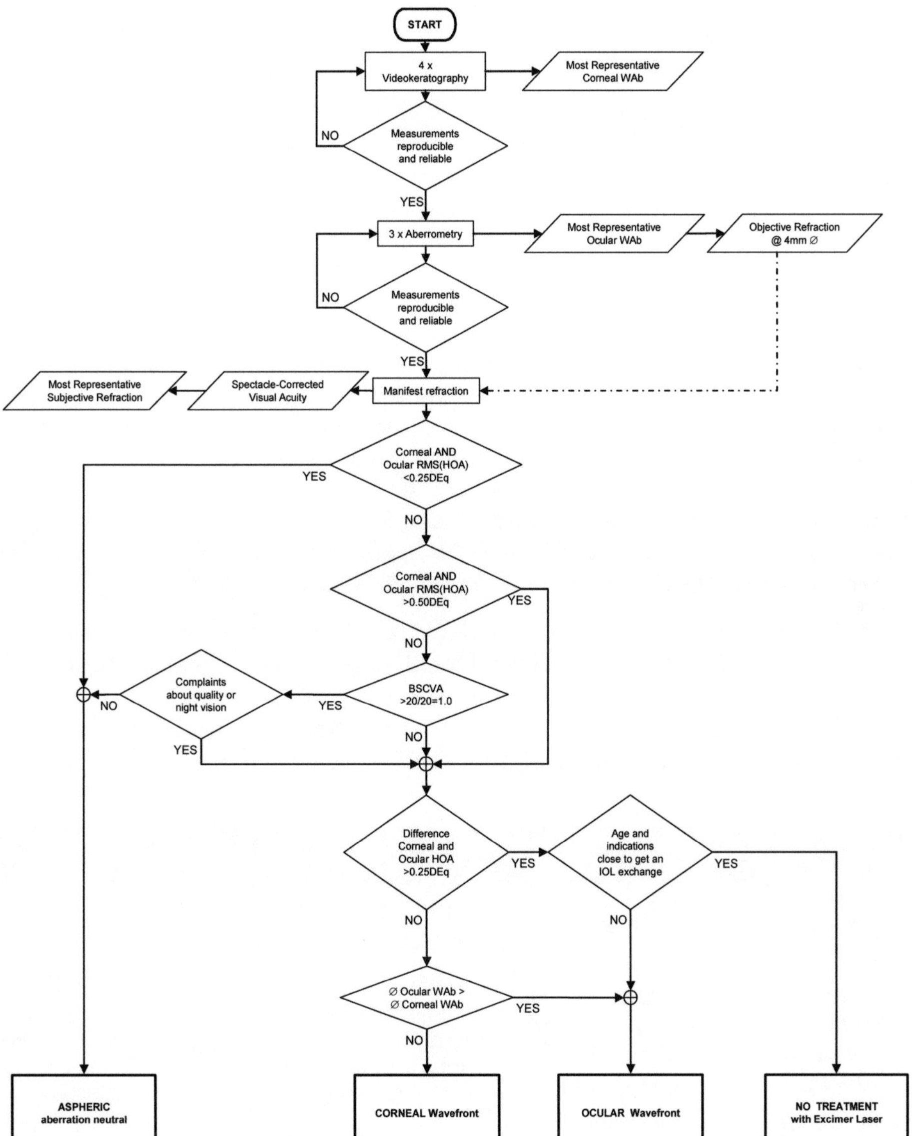

Fig. 3. Decision-Tree applied for selecting the treatment mode (Aspheric aberration neutral, Corneal-Wavefront-Guided, or Ocular-Wavefront-Guided).

The decision process starts by estimating the global optical impairment resulting from the measured wave aberrations. This is done by objectively determining the actual clinical relevance of single terms in a Zernike expansion of the wave aberration. In general, for the same magnitude of aberration, the optical blur produced by high order aberrations increases with increasing radial order and decreases with increasing angular frequencies. Based on this, the dioptric equivalent (DEq) was used.

If the global optical blur for both corneal and ocular wave-aberrations (CWAb and OWAb, respectively) are below 0.25 DEq for both eyes, then the treatment to be applied is Aspheric aberration neutral. If the global optical blur for any corneal or ocular wave-aberrations is between 0.25 DEq and 0.50 DEq for any eye, then we check the BSCVA achieved during the manifest refraction. If the BSCVA is better than 20/20 for both eyes, then we ask the patient about complaints regarding night vision or, in general, quality of vision. If the patient does not report complaints, then the treatment to be applied is Aspheric aberration neutral.

If the patient reports complaints regarding quality of vision, the BSCVA is worse than 20/20 for any eye, or the global optical blur for both corneal and ocular wave-aberrations are above 0.50 DEq for both eyes, then we compare corneal and ocular wave-aberrations. For this, we calculate the differential aberration (CWAb − OWAb, both centred at the line-of-sight) in terms of the Zernike expansion, and estimate the global optical difference. If this global optical difference between corneal and ocular wave-aberrations is below 0.25 DEq for both eyes, we consider both corneal and ocular wave-aberrations as equivalent. In this case, the treatment to be applied depends on the available diameter of the wavefront maps and the scotopic pupil size. If the diameter of the Ocular- or Corneal-WAb map (the one providing the largest diameter) is at least as large as the scotopic pupil size (in natural dark conditions) reduced in 0.25 mm, then Ocular- or Corneal-Wavefront-guided ablation is performed (the one providing the largest diameter), or Aspheric aberration neutral otherwise. Usually the size of the Ocular WAb maps is similar to the size of the scotopic pupils, whereas Corneal WAb maps are wider (up to 10 mm in diameter).

If the global optical difference between corneal and ocular wave-aberrations is above 0.25 DEq for any eye, we consider internal wave-aberration (IWAb) is relevant, then the treatment to be applied is Ocular-Wavefront-guided if the patient is neither in age nor in ophthalmic indications close to get an IOL exchange (due to e.g. lenticular opacities), otherwise no laser corneal refractive treatment is recommended (since IOL exchange is preferred).

Level of aberration	Aspheric aberration neutral	CW-guided	OW-guided
Corneal AND Ocular Wavefronts < 0.25Deq	**Always**	**No**	**No**
Corneal OR Ocular Wavefront between 0.25DEq and 0.50Deq	**If BSCVA > 20/20 AND no complaints about quality or night vision**	**If (BSCVA < 20/20 OR complaints about quality or night vision) AND Internal Wavefront < 0.25DEq**	**If (BSCVA < 20/20 OR complaints about quality or night vision) AND no lenticular problems**
Corneal AND Ocular Wavefronts > 0.50Deq	**If wavefront maps smaller than scotopic pupil**	**If Internal Wavefront < 0.25DEq**	**If no lenticular problems**

Table 1. Indications chart.

There are basically three types of approaches for planning a corneal refractive treatment. The first are those that have as their objective the elimination or reduction of the total aberrations of the eye. The main criticism to this approach argues that the goal "zero aberration" is inconsistent throughout the day due to accommodation, and little lasting, since aberrations change with age[23,24,25]. The second approach is intended to correct all corneal aberrations, since corneal aberrations do not change with age[26,27]. However, this concept might also be wrong considering corneal aberrations interact with internal aberrations, some of them being cancelled, and producing an aberration pattern of the total eye in general different from the aberration pattern of the cornea alone. Therefore, by only removing corneal aberration we might worsen the overall aberrations, since the internal aberration might not find a corneal aberration for compensation. In case that the corneal aberration is of the same sign as the internal aberration, the correction of the corneal aberration would be useful, as it would reduce the total aberration of the eye. A third approach tries not to induce aberrations. This type of treatment is not as ambitious, but much more simple to operate. The goal of the Aberration-Free™ ablation profile is to provide a neutral high-order-aberrations (HOAb) ablation, ie to maintain the same HOAb profile both preoperatively with best spectacle correction and postoperatively without correction.

There is evidence of neural adaptation to the baseline wavefront profile. The interaction between high-order-aberrations can be beneficial to visual quality regardless of the magnitude HOAb. Based on the random nature of the HOAb induction and current research, it may be beneficial to maintain the preoperative wavefront profile for a significant number of refractive surgery candidates.

We are not postulating that customized ablation algorithms in any form (ocular-wavefront-guided, corneal-wavefront-guided, topography-guided) are not be useful. Rather, that specific populations with specific demands deserve specific treatment solutions. Aspheric treatments aimed at preservation of the preoperative HOAb show their strengths in patients with preoperative BSCVA 20/20 or better or in patients where the visual degradation cannot be attributable to the presence of clinically relevant HOAb (e.g. lens opacities).

The corneal wavefront customized approach shows its strength in cases where abnormal corneal surfaces are expected. Apart from the risk of additional ablation of corneal tissue, wavefront customized corneal ablation can be considered a safe and beneficial method. Our experience suggests that wavefront customized treatments can only be successful, if pre-existing aberrations are greater than repeatability (e.g. repeatability of diagnostic[28] and treatment devices) and biological noise (e.g. day-to-day variabilities in visual acuity, refraction, or aberration in the same subject).

Furthermore, coupling effects between different high order aberration terms, and between HOAb and manifest refraction have been found[29,30] for example, between defocus and spherical aberration, or between 3rd order aberrations and low order terms, between spherical aberration and coma, or between secondary and primary astigmatisms. These interactions may provide some relative visual benefits[31], but may as well contribute as sources of uncertainty in the conversion of wavefront aberration maps to refractive prescriptions. Notice that for comparing OWAb and CWAb, the analysis of the IWAb as CWAb - OWAb is mandatory since RMS(IWAb) accounts for any deviation (i.e. inductions and reductions of the wave-aberration both contribute positively to increase the RMS value).

The Decision Assistant Wizard presented here may theoretically be applied to any other laser platform offering aspheric, topography-guided, and wavefront-guided profiles, if appropriate analysis functions for CWAb, OWAb, and IWAb are available. Simplified versions with limited functionalities are also possible, if, for example, neither CW-analyses (i.e. no IWAb) nor topography-guided profiles are available. The desired outcome of non-wavefront-driven refractive surgery is to balance the effects on the wave-aberration, and, to provide normal eyes with perhaps the most natural unaltered quality of vision. While Ocular Wavefront treatments have the advantage of being based on Objective Refraction of the complete human eye system, whereas Corneal Wavefront treatments have the advantage of being independent from accommodation effects or light/pupil conditions; Aspheric treatments have the advantage of saving tissue, time and due to their simplicity offer better predictability.

In highly aberrated eyes, manifest refraction may become an art, a sort of guessing around the least blurred image. In further studies, systematic deviations from the measured manifest refractions, as well as other foreseeable couplings among Zernike coefficients will be evaluated.

6. Minimization of depth and time in laser corneal refractive surgery

In laser corneal refractive surgery, one always aims to reduce the ablated tissue thickness (and, to a minor degree, to reduce the intervention time) because an ectasia of the cornea may result from excessive tissue removal. Customized laser corneal refractive surgery on aberrated eyes may yield better results than the standard procedure[18–21] but generally results in higher ablation depth, volume, and time. Therefore, optimizing the customized treatment to reduce the ablated thickness while retaining the positive aspects is pertinent.[22]

The development of new algorithms or ablation strategies for performing laser corneal refractive surgery in a customized form, minimizing the amount of ablated tissue without compromising the visual quality, and potentially maximizing visual performance without increasing risk factors would be of great value for the refractive surgery community and ultimately for the health and safety of patients. The real impact of tissue-saving algorithms in customized treatments is controversial. Minimizing the amount of tissue must be done in a way that does not compromise the refractive correction or visual performance, and it must be safe, reliable, and reproducible.

In general, for the same amount of equivalent defocus, the optical blur produced by HOAs increases with increasing radial order and decreases with increasing angular frequencies. Based on this blur effect of the single Zernike terms, we have defined a dioptric equivalent:

$$\mathrm{DEq}_n^m = \frac{8\sqrt{2(n+1)(1+\delta_{m0})}\left|C_n^m\right|}{\mathrm{PD}^2} \tag{2}$$

where DEq_n^m is the dioptric equivalent of the optical blur; n, the radial order of the considered Zernike term; m, the angular frequency of the considered Zernike term; δ_{m0}, the Kronecker delta function of the angular frequency and zero (1 for radially symmetric Zernike terms and 0 otherwise); C_n^m, the weight coefficient of the considered Zernike term; and PD, the analysis diameter for the optical blur.

In such a way, the dioptric equivalent produced by HOAs increases with increasing radial order and partly decreases with increasing angular frequencies. This dioptric equivalent metric is identical to the power vector notation for the low orders and allows defining a general optical blur as a general expression for the one proposed by Thibos et al[36]:

$$U_G = \sqrt{\sum \left(\mathrm{DEq}_n^m\right)^2} \tag{3}$$

where U_G is the general optical blur.

We have expressed each of the Zernike terms as a dioptric equivalent in familiar units to help judge the order of magnitude of the effect. Using common clinical limits, the following classification is proposed:

$$\mathrm{DEq}_n^m < 0.50\ \mathrm{D} \Rightarrow \text{might be clinically relevant} \tag{4}$$

$$\mathrm{DEq}_n^m \geq 0.50\ \mathrm{D} \Rightarrow \text{clinically relevant} \tag{5}$$

This represents the proposed objective determination of the actual clinical relevance of the single terms in a Zernike expansion of the wavefront aberration.[22]

6.1 Objective minimization of the maximum depth of a customized ablation based on the Zernike expansion of the wavefront aberration

One of the minimization approaches consists of simplifying the profile by selecting a subset of Zernike terms that minimizes the necessary ablation depth while respecting the Zernike terms considered clinically relevant. The minimize depth (MD+) function analyzes the Zernike pyramid as described in the previous section and evaluates the ablation depth of all possible free combinations of subsets of Zernike terms while fulfilling several conditions:

- Only terms of third or higher order can be disabled.
- Only terms with optical blur dioptric equivalent less than 0.5 D can be disabled.
- For each subset combination of Zernike terms, the low-order terms are recalculated using the automatic refraction balance method.

From this evaluation, the function selects the subset of Zernike terms that needs the minimum amount of maximum depth.

6.2 Objective minimization of the ablation volume of a customized ablation based on the Zernike expansion of the wavefront aberration

The other minimization approach consists of simplifying the profile by selecting a subset of Zernike terms that minimizes the necessary ablation volume while respecting the Zernike terms considered clinically relevant. The minimize volume (MV+) function analyzes the Zernike pyramid as described in the previous section and evaluates the ablation depth of all possible free combinations of subsets of Zernike terms fulfilling several conditions:

- Only terms of third or higher order can be disabled.
- Only terms with optical blur dioptric equivalent less than 0.5 D can be disabled.
- For each subset combination of Zernike terms, the low-order terms are recalculated using the automatic refraction balance method.

From this evaluation, the function selects the subset of Zernike terms that needs the minimum amount of volume for the ablation. Reduced ablation volumes lead to shorter treatment times.

One could use the equivalent defocus applied to each individual Zernike mode to compute its clinical relevance. The basis of the equivalent defocus concept is the notion that the imaging quality of an eye is determined primarily by wavefront variance, and it does not matter which Zernike mode produces that variance. This is only true when the wavefront variance is really small and the image quality is measured by the Strehl ratio. Otherwise, the relationship between wavefront variance and image quality becomes much more complex. It is important to bear in mind that 1 D of ordinary defocus does not necessarily have the same effect as 1 D of equivalent defocus because different types of aberrations affect the retinal image in different ways. Nevertheless, by expressing RMS error in terms of equivalent defocus, the data are put into familiar units that help us judge the order of magnitude of the effect.

Strictly speaking, one cannot consider the clinical relevance of every Zernike term independently without demonstrating whether a single Zernike term is alone responsible for the loss of visual quality. The visual effect of an aberration does not only depend on that specific aberration but also on other possibly present aberrations; for example, the sum of small aberrations, previously considered clinically irrelevant, could lead to a clear loss of overall optical quality. The idea of approximating a distorted wavefront by means of an equivalent dioptric error is much too controversial to be accepted without caution.

Coupling effects between different HOA terms and between HOAs and manifest refraction have been found,[44–46] for example, between defocus and spherical aberration, third-order aberrations and low-order terms, spherical aberration and coma, or secondary and primary astigmatisms. These interactions may provide some relative visual benefits[47] but may also contribute uncertainty in the conversion of wavefront aberration maps to refractive prescriptions.[48,49] One could use more sophisticated equations to model the equivalences between the optical blur produced by the different Zernike terms, but we have used a relatively simple approach driven primarily by the radial order. Different approaches for minimizing tissue ablation in refractive surgery have been proposed and extensively discussed.[22] When to use customized strategies in refractive surgery has been discussed previously as well.[18–21]

Considering that Zernike terms are either planned to be corrected or left uncorrected, visual performance is not compromised because all remaining uncorrected terms are below clinical relevance. The proposed approaches are safe, reliable, and reproducible because of the objective foundation upon which they are based. It is important to note that the selection of the Zernike terms to be included in the correction is not trivial. As mentioned, only Zernike terms considered not clinically relevant or of minor clinical relevance can be excluded from the correction, but they must not necessarily be excluded.

Actually, single Zernike terms considered not clinically relevant will only be disabled when they represent additional tissue for ablation and will be enabled when they help to save tissue. This way, particular cases are represented by the full wavefront correction by disabling all nonclinically relevant terms or by disabling all high-order terms. As per design, the MD group actually optimizes for minimum ablation depth and shows the largest savings for this aim (−8 ± 4 µm, from −20 to −1 µm), whereas the MV group actually optimizes for minimum ablation volume (time) and shows the largest savings for this aim (−8 ± 2 seconds, from -26 to -22 seconds). In this context, and as a rule of thumb, MD minimization could be used in customized myopic treatments when reducing ablation depth is directly related to decreasing the risk of keratectasia, whereas MV minimization could be used in long customized treatments when reducing ablation time is directly related to better maintenance of homogeneous corneal conditions.

7. Surgical technique selection

Excimer laser refractive surgery has evolved full circle. Surface ablations in the form of photorefractive keratectomy (PRK) swiftly evolved into intra-stromal procedure of laser in-situ keratomileusis (LASIK) due to its rapid visual recovery and minimal postoperative discomfort. However, with increasing adoption of LASIK grew the concern for post-LASIK keratectasia. The last few years have therefore, witnessed a renewed interest in alcohol assisted surface ablation procedures to avoid complications of LASIK primarily corneal ectasia and flap and interface related problems.

The decision to perform alcohol assisted LASEK or LASIK is based on preoperative central corneal thickness (measured by ultrasonic pachymetry (DGH-550 Pachette 2, DGH Technologies, USA)) and calculated depth of ablation. LASEK is performed on all patients with central pachymetry less than 500 µm. Eyes with central pachymetry above 500 µm are assigned to either LASEK or LASIK techniques, depending on the central pachymetry and the depth of ablation. The decision is based on the target of limiting the ablation to the anterior one third of the cornea (so as to achieve a residual stromal bed thickness of at least 2/3rd of pre-operative pachymetry). Patients were tested for LASIK in case they do not meet the "2/3" condition they were assigned to the LASEK group.

For corneal and conjunctival anesthesia, two drops of proparacaine HCl 0.5% (Aurocaine®, Aurolab, Madurai, India) are instilled three times before shifting the patient to the operation theatre (OT).

LASIK - Pachymetry is performed before and after flap creation (stromal bed thickness) with both the integrated online coherence pachymeter (Heidelberg, Germany) and ultrasonic pachymeter. Flap is made using LDV femtosecond laser. Contact lens is applied at the end of surgery (Biomedics 55 evolution, Ocular Sciences, Cooper Vision, Hamble, UK) in eyes with 'achieved' flap thickness less than 110 microns to avoid flap displacements, dislocations or striae.

LASEK - 17% alcohol applied for 30 seconds is used for the creation of epithelial flap. Eight or 9 mm diameter epithelial flap is made after incising the corneal epithelium with a trephine. Contact lens is applied at the end of surgery in all LASEK patients.

Postoperative Treatment – For LASIK patients, eye drop Tobradex (Alcon Inc, USA) 3 times a day is used for 1 week along with Oasis soft plugs extended duration (6404 Glendora CA) and preservative free artificial tear drops during the first three months. A bandage contact lens is used during the first night in LASIK patients with flap thickness less than 110µm. For LASEK patients, prior to epithelial healing, eye drops lomefloxacin 0.3 % (Okacin) and pranoprofen (Ofralar, Alcon Inc, USA) are used along with Oasis soft plugs extended duration. Bandage contact lens is applied in all LASEK patients for 5-7 days until complete healing of the epithelial defect. After epithelial healing, preservative free artificial tear eye drops are given along with efemoline eye drops (Fluoromethalone, Novartis Ophthalmics, Switzerland) 3 times a day for 3 months. The steroids are gradually tapered every month to once a day in the last month.

Postoperative follow-up - LASIK patients are followed on first postoperative day, at 1 month, 3 months, and 1 year. LASEK patients are examined on first postoperative day, at 1 week, 1 month, 3 months, and 1 year.

There has been a renewed interest in surface ablation modalities with epithelial repositioning like LASEK to overcome some of the flap and ectasia related complications of LASIK. Though the rate of visual recovery may be slower in surface ablation thus lacking the LASIK 'wow' effect, studies have shown that LASEK is an effective modality for surgical correction of low to moderate myopia.[8-10] However, its utility for correction of high myopia is limited.[11-13] With introduction of thin and ultrathin flaps using femtosecond laser and newer microkeratomes such as the pendular microkeratome, the indications for the 2 surgical modalities are getting indistinct. Introduction of newer ablation profiles such as customized and aspheric ablations has added another aspect to be evaluated.

It has been suggested that surface ablative procedures may be better suited for customized correction though it has not been proven clinically.[1,2,14] It has been suggested that the creation of corneal flap in LASIK patients can induce further higher order aberrations especially coma like aberrations.[15] This may be particularly relevant to thinner flaps which may have a higher incidence of flap striae. The clinical relevance of these flap induced higher order aberrations especially in relation to newer microkeratomes and femtosecond laser and the effect of flap thickness require further investigation.

The aspheric ablation profile is equally successful with both surface ablation as well as intrastromal excimer ablation minimizing the change in higher order aberrations. The latest development in excimer laser refractive is the thin and the ultrathin flap LASIK. It attempts to find the best of both worlds of standard LASIK and surface ablation. Besides pre-existing risk factors, low residual stromal bed thickness is the single most important modifiable factor that increases the risk of iatrogenic post-LASIK ectasia.[38] Thin and ultrathin flap LASIK achieves a thicker residual stromal bed and therefore is believed to decrease the risk of post-LASIK ectasia. Current study indicates that thin and ultrathin LASIK is safe, efficacious, and predictable after short term follow up of 6 months. However, future investigations with long-term follow-up are likely to prove if LASIK utilizing thin and ultrathin flaps translate into the anticipated decreased risk of post-LASIK ectasia.

8. 6D Eye-Tracker

Human eyes have six degrees of freedom to move: X/Y lateral shifts, Z levelling, horizontal/vertical rotations, and cyclotorsion (rotations around the optical axis). The analysis of these movements has been made since the middle of the 20th century. Schwiegerling and Snyder[32] measured eye motion in patients having laser in situ keratomileusis (LASIK) using a video technique and determine centration and variance of the eye position during surgery. They found a standard deviation in the eye movements in all eyes larger than 100 μm. Taylor et al.[33] determined the accuracy of an eye tracking system designed for laser refractive surgery. The system demonstrated an accuracy of 60 μm for an intact cornea and 100 μm for a cornea with a thin flap removed.

Bueeler et al.[34] investigated the lateral alignment accuracy needed in wavefront-guided refractive surgery to improve the ocular optics to a desired level in a percentage of normally aberrated eyes. To achieve the diffraction limit in 95% of the normal eyes with a 7.0 mm pupil, a lateral alignment accuracy of 70 μm or better was required. An accuracy of 200 μm was sufficient to reach the same goal with a 3.0 mm pupil. Bueeler and Mrochen[35] quantified the parallax error associated with localizing corneal positions by tracking the subjacent entrance pupil center by means of optical ray-tracing in a schematic model eye. They found tracking error can amount to 30% (or more for eye trackers mounted closer than 500 mm to the eye) of the detected lateral shift. Thus, if the eye tracker registers a lateral shift of the entrance pupil of 200 μm away from the tracking reference axis, the point of interest located on the cornea would essentially be 260 μm away from this reference axis. A laser pulse fired at that moment would be systematically displaced by 60 μm.

Measuring rotation when the patient is upright[36] to when the refractive treatments are performed with the patient supine may lead to ocular cyclotorsion,[37,38] resulting in mismatching of the applied versus the intended profiles[39,40]. Recently, some equipment can facilitate measurement of and potential compensation for static cyclotorsion occurring when the patient moves from upright to the supine position during the procedure[41], quantifying the cyclorotation occurring between wavefront measurement and laser refractive surgery[42] and compensating for it[43,44,45]. Further measuring and compensating ocular cyclotorsion during refractive treatments with the patient supine may reduce optical "noise" of the applied versus the intended profiles[46,47,48].

In recent times, many studies have discussed the methodologies and implications of ocular cyclotorsion, but not many papers pay attention to the rolling and axial movements of the eye. The more irregular a cornea is, the more important proper eye-tracking. Astigmatism is the most common aberration with a vector nature, so usually are the astigmatic problems the ones more affected or the ones which benefit the most from advanced eye tracking.

8.1 Lateral movements during ablation (1st and 2nd dimension)

AMARIS system includes a pupil-registration module for the eye-tracker subsystem, in which, the first pupil image under the AMARIS system obtained with starting the ablation is taken as reference and its location referred to the limbus is used for any further eye-tracker image in order to determine the pupil centre shift compensation (PCSC).

8.2 Eye rolling during ablation (3rd and 4th dimension)

AMARIS system includes a scleral-registration module for the eye-tracker subsystem, in which, the first few scleral-tracker images under the AMARIS system obtained with starting the ablation are taken as reference (natural rolling) and compared to any further scleral-tracker image in order to determine the eye rolling (ER).

8.3 Static cyclotorsion between upright and supine positions (5th dimension)

AMARIS system includes an eye-registration module for the eye-tracker subsystem, in which, the diagnosis image is taken as reference and compared to an eye-tracker image under the AMARIS system obtained prior to starting the ablation in order to determine the static cyclotorsion component (SCC).

8.4 Dynamic cyclotorsion during ablation (5th dimension)

AMARIS system includes an eye-registration module for the eye-tracker subsystem, in which, the first eye-tracker image under the AMARIS system obtained with starting the ablation is taken as reference and compared to any further eye-tracker image in order to determine the dynamic cyclotorsion component (DCC).

8.5 Axial displacements during ablation (6th dimension)

AMARIS system includes an scleral-registration module for the eye-tracker subsystem, in which, the first few scleral-tracker images under the AMARIS system obtained with starting the ablation are taken as reference (natural level) and compared to any further scleral-tracker image in order to determine the axial displacements (AD).

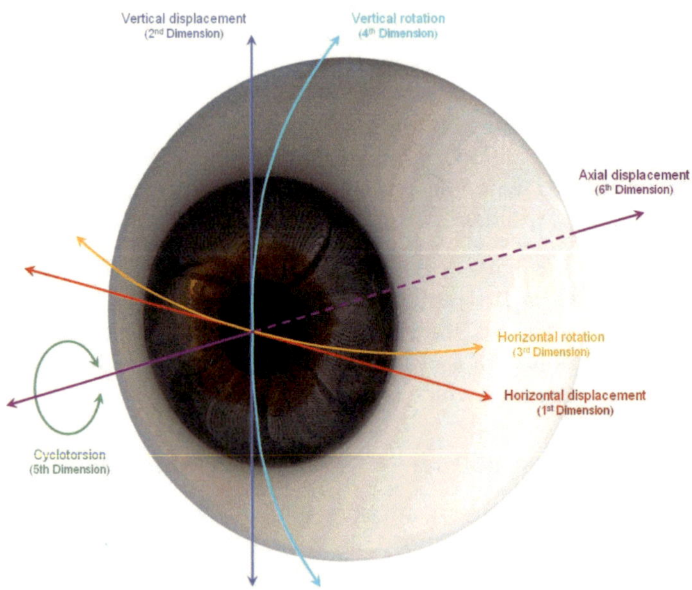

Fig. 4. Lateral movements (vertical and horizontal displacements) 1st and 2nd dimensions, Rolling movements - caused by a tilting of the head or of the eye 3rd and 4th dimensions, Rotations around the visual axis - This happens mostly when changing from upright to supine position, but also during the treatment 5th dimension, cyclotorsion, Movements along the z-axis 6th dimension. All dimensions measured and compensated for static and dynamic movements in an active/passive manner.

The AMARIS TotalTech laser includes compensation for the ocular cyclotorsions occurring from upright to supine position (static cyclotorsion from diagnosis to treatment), as well as the lateral movements, eye rollings, dynamic cyclotorsions, and displacements along the propagation axis occurring during the laser treatment. Further, the differences in pupil size and centre for and during the treatment compared to that during diagnosis[49] are also compensated for, since the theoretical impact of cyclotorted ablations is smaller than decentred ablations or edge effects[50] (coma and spherical aberration[51]). In this way, additional lateral displacements[52] due to cyclotorsions occurring around any position other than the ablation centre are avoided (induced aberrations emanating from lateral displacements always increase with decentration[53]).

A six dimensional eye-tracker is important since uncompensated pupil movements (lateral movements) induce decentrations[32] which can be visually manifested as comatic aberrations[52]. Uncompensated rolling movements induce decentrations as well[35], which can be visually manifested as comatic aberrations[52]. Uncompensated cyclotorsional movements induce aberrations[40], whereas uncompensated axial movements induce undercorrections in an asymmetrical way. Axial movements produce that the laser spots are no longer in focus when they reach the cornea, i.e. ignoring absorption processes in air, for the same energy spot diameter is larger reducing the radiant exposure and the ablation depth of the spot. Axial movements produce as well that off axis pulses hit the cornea more centrally than planned if the eye moves towards the laser system and further peripherally if the eyes moves far from the laser.

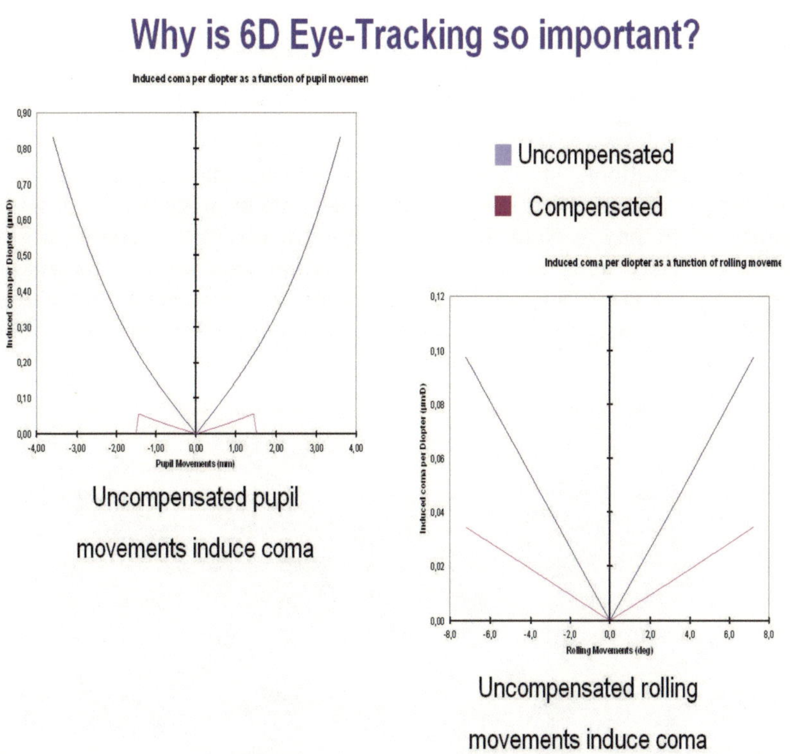

Fig. 5. A six dimensional eye-tracker is important since uncompensated pupil movements (lateral movements) induce decentrations which can be visually manifested as comatic aberrations. Uncompensated rolling movements induce decentrations as well, which can be visually manifested as comatic aberrations.

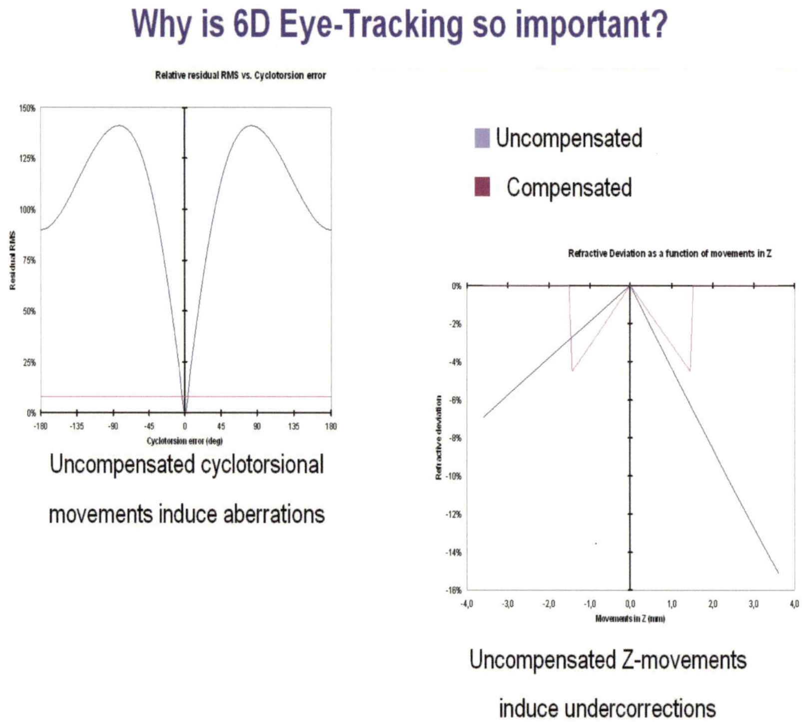

Fig. 6. A six dimensional eye-tracker is important since uncompensated cyclotorsional movements induce aberrations, whereas uncompensated axial movements induce undercorrections in an asymmetrical way. Axial movements produce that the laser spots are no longer in focus when they reach the cornea, i.e. ignoring absorption processes in air, for the same energy spot diameter is larger reducing the radiant exposure and the ablation depth of the spot. Axial movements produce as well that off axis pulses hit the cornea more centrally than planned if the eye moves towards the laser system and further peripherally if the eyes moves far from the laser.

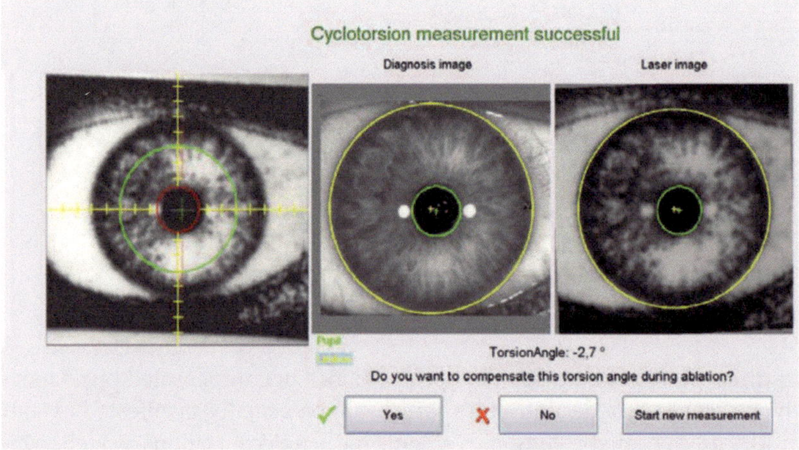

Fig. 7. Static cyclotorsion compensation.

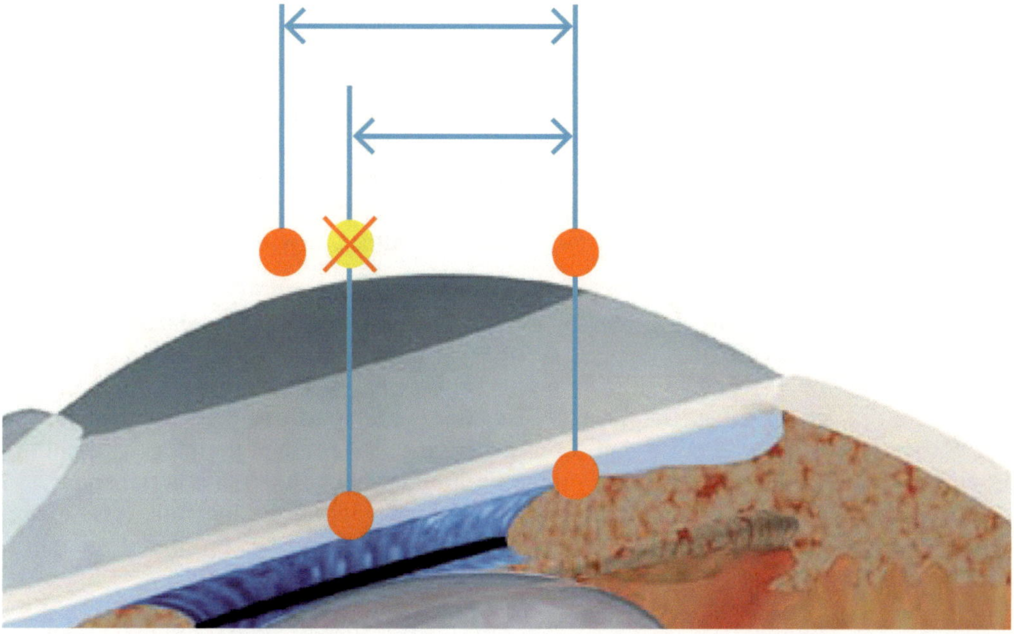

Fig. 8. Rolling compensation.

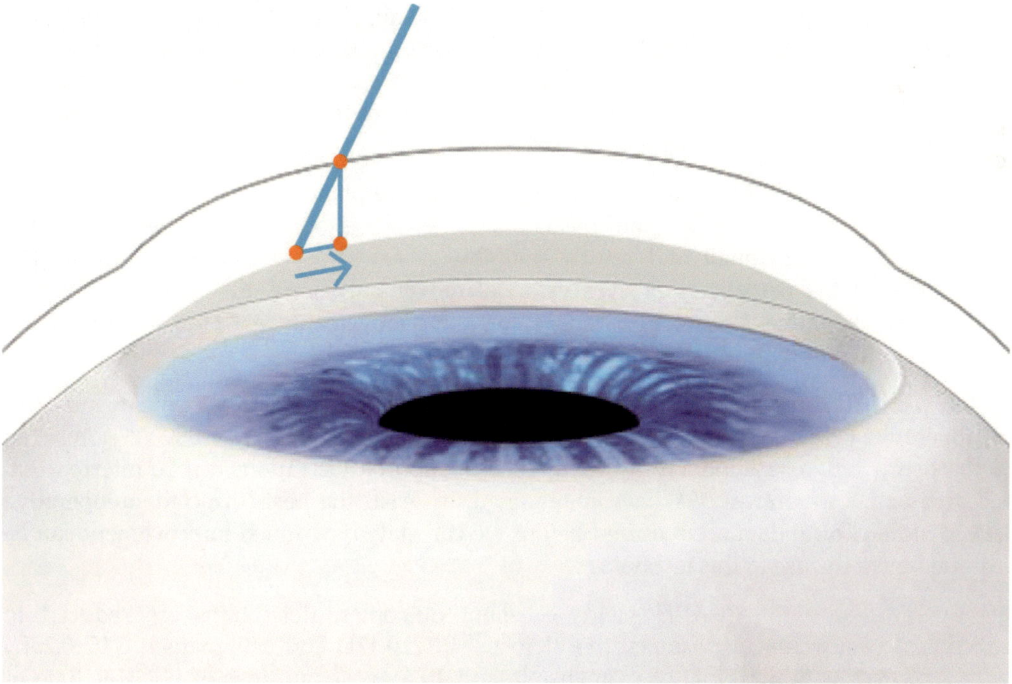

Fig. 9. Axial movements compensation.

In our experience with AMARIS system measuring the pupil displacements, we obtained an average of 150 µm. The distribution of the percentage of eyes vs. pupil displacement showed 3% of eyes had pupil displacements exceeding 1 mm. The ranges for pupil displacements over the treatment are relatively mild, but with peaks of up to about 1.5 mm.

With our system for measuring the rolling movements, we obtained an average value 5°. This value is actually the most commonly accepted value for "natural rolling" measured as angle alpha[54], lambda[55], or kappa[56]. The distribution of the percentage of eyes vs. rolling movements showes 3% of eyes had rolling exceeding 8 deg. The ranges for the rolling movements over the treatment are relatively mild, but with peaks of up to about 10 deg.

With our system for measuring the static cyclotorsional error, we obtained an average cyclotorsion of 1°, lower than the observations of Ciccio et al.,[57] who reported 4°. The distribution of the percentage of eyes vs. cyclotorsional error shows 3% of eyes had cyclotorsion exceeding 8 deg. The mean DCC values over the treatment are relatively small, but with peaks of up to about 5 deg. Considering that the average cyclotorsion resulting from the shift from the upright to the supine position is about ±4 deg,[57] it is not enough to compensate only for the static cyclotorsion without considering the dynamic cyclotorsion during the laser procedure. Finally, the effects of the DCC can be considered as optical "noise" of the applied versus the intended profiles.[58]

Without eye registration technologies,[59,60] considering that maximum cyclotorsion measured from the shift from the upright to the supine position does not exceed ±14 deg,[57] explains why "classical" spherocylindrical corrections in refractive surgery succeed without major cyclotorsional considerations. However, only limited amounts of astigmatism can effectively be corrected for this cyclotorsional error[40]. Currently available eye registration technologies, providing an accuracy of about 1 deg and measuring static and dynamic cyclotorsion components, open a new era in corneal laser refractive surgery, because patients may be treated for a wider range of refractive problems with enhanced success ratios. This requires high-resolution ablation systems as well.[61,62]

With our system for measuring the axial movements, we obtained an average of -300 µm. This negative value is fairly low, but means the patients use to push their head back at the beginning of the treatment and return smoothly closer to level during treatment. The distribution of the percentage of eyes vs. axial movement shows 10% of eyes had axial movements exceeding 1 mm. The ranges for axial movements over the treatment are relatively mild, but with peaks exceeding 1 mm.

In our AMARIS experience of over 8000 treated eyes, 91% of treatments result in a postoperative cylinder within 0.5 D, and 19% of treatments gain lines of BSCVA compared to the preoperative baseline. From the minor induction of aberrations can be inferred that mesopic and low-contrast VA have maintained, at least, the best-corrected preoperative levels. More clinical data are required before we can state how much improvement can be expected from the use of this technology.

6D Eye-Tracker with AMARIS yields excellent outcomes. Refractions are reduced to subclinical values: (mean postoperative defocus -0.12±0.17D and astigmatism 0.15±0.25D) with 70% eyes within ±0.25D of emmetropia and 19% eyes gain lines of BSCVA. Rate of registration is >90% for Cyclotorsion and >80% for Rolling and Axial movements. Mean

Rolling was within ±5° in 52% of the cases, Dynamic Rolling was within ±5° in 66% of the cases, Static Cyclotorsion was within ±4° in 69% of the cases, Dynamic Cyclotorsion was within ±2° in 72% of the cases, and Z-movement was within ±0.5mm in 69% of the cases.

6D Eye-Tracker Controls with the SCHWIND AMARIS are safe and very predictable. In summary, using SCHWIND AMARIS, six-dimensional movements of the eye can be effectively measured and compensated for both static and dynamic conditions during laser corneal ablation.

9. High speed refractive surgery

The range of repetition rates of the laser systems for refractive surgery currently available in the market runs from about 10 Hz to about 1000 Hz (median 250 Hz), with spot size diameters ranging from 6.5 mm to about 0.3 mm (median 1 mm), corresponding to treatment velocities from about 9 s/D to about 1.7 s/D (mean 5 s/D). If we compare these values to the situation at the beginning of the 21st century, a technological quantum leap is observed. In 2001, repetition rates of the laser systems for refractive surgery in the market ranged from about 10 Hz to about 300 Hz (median 50 Hz), with spot size diameters ranging from 6.5 mm to about 0.8 mm (median 2-6 mm), corresponding to treatment velocities from about 19 s/D to about 6 s/D (mean 12 s/D).

To foresee the future trends for these essential values when defining the technological capabilities of a system, four driving forces shall be considered:

- The technological progress of the last 10 years indicating an exponential improvement of the technology
- The non-linear cost-to-benefit ratio for new developments indicating a continued improvement of the technology at a slower rate
- The actual clinical needs for faster or more precise systems indicating a slow-down improvement of the technology achieving maturity and stability
- The limitations imposed by the biological tissue response to the laser interaction (e.g. thermal issues, haze development[63])

Considering these effects, we can hypothesize a scenario with repetition rates of the laser systems for refractive surgery ranging from about 300 Hz to about 1500 Hz, with spot size diameters ranging from 1.5 mm to about 0.2 mm, corresponding to treatment velocities from about 4 s/D to about 1.3 s/D.

However, due to the presence of local frequency controls, the duration of the treatments is no longer inversely proportional to the repetition rate. The duration of the treatments is inversely proportional to the repetition rate only for slow repetition rates (<180 Hz), and stabilizes asymptotically for high repetition rates (>1500 Hz).

10. Bilateral symmetry

Human vision is a binocular process. Having two eyes gives binocular summation in which the ability to detect faint objects is enhanced. It can give stereopsis in which parallax provided by the two eyes' different positions on the head give precise depth perception. Such binocular vision is usually accompanied by binocular fusion, in which a single image is seen despite each eye is having its own image of any object.

Literature suggests that marked anisometropia is uncommon, either in the magnitude of sphere or astigmatism, with few notable exceptions concluding that the axis of astigmatism does not follow any particular rule (mirror or direct symmetry) across right and left eyes.

Porter et al.[64] confirmed in a large population that although the pattern of aberrations varies from subject to subject, aberrations, including irregular ones, are correlated in left and right eyes of the same subject, indicating that they are not random defects. The Indiana Aberration Study by Thibos et al. characterized the aberration structure, and the effects of these aberrations on vision, for a reasonably large population of normal, healthy eyes in young adults, and verified the hypothesis of bilateral symmetry.

Wang et al.[65] found that anterior corneal wave aberrations varied greatly among subjects, but a moderate to high degree of mirror symmetry existed between right and left eyes. To our knowledge, very few studies in the literature have addressed the issue of symmetry of aberrations between eyes after corneal laser refractive surgery[66,67]. Jiménez et al.[66] found that binocular function deteriorates more than monocular function after LASIK, and that this deterioration increases as the interocular differences in aberrations and corneal shape increase. They found that interocular differences above 0.4 μm RMS for 5-mm analysis diameter, lead to a decrease of more than 20% in binocular summation.

If binocular symmetry is manifested on virgin human eyes and it is important for binocular vision, it shall be interesting to assess whether existing symmetry is maintained after treating the cornea for correcting the ametropias using corneal laser refractive surgery. Further analysis of bilateral symmetry according to analysis diameter is also of interest. The analysis of bilateral symmetry should be related to binocular vision status of patients.

Cuesta et al.[68] found that even differences in corneal asphericity might affect the binocular visual function by diminishing the binocular contrast-sensitivity function. Arbelaez et al.[67] found that only four of 25 patients showed preoperatively clinically relevant differences OS vs. OD larger than 0.25 D, whereas 6-month postoperatively only 2 of 25 patients showed clinically relevant differences OS vs. OD larger than 0.25 D. 6-month postoperatively three Zernike terms lost significant correlation symmetry OS vs. OD and 4 Zernike terms gained significant correlation symmetry. However, two of them showed borderline correlations. 6-month postoperatively 6 Zernike terms significantly increased differences in symmetry OS vs. OD and 4 Zernike terms significantly decreased differences in symmetry. However, six of them showed borderline significances of the difference. 6-month postoperatively three patients lost significant correlation symmetry OS vs. OD and one patient gained significant correlation symmetry. However, two of them showed borderline significances of the difference. All these borderline situations actually shall be seen as "almost preserved" bilateral symmetry.

The presented results cannot be extrapolated to patients with symptoms of amblyopia[69], anisometropia, nystagmus, or aniseikonia[70] without further studies. Bilateral symmetry in corneal aberrations does not mean any "good or bad" point for binocular vision. We cannot evaluate exactly the role of aberrations monocularly (patients with high level of aberrations can have an excellent visual acuity and vice-versa); therefore it is more difficult binocularly.

The important question in binocular vision is "the role of interocular-differences," and if they can influence significantly binocular performance. Interocular-differences can be minor but significant for visual performance. Further studies shall help to determine the impact of this on binocular visual performance.

The more irregular a cornea is, the more important proper bilateral symmetry for adequate binocular summation. Astigmatism is the most common aberration with a vector nature, so usually are the astigmatic problems the ones more affected or the ones which benefit the most from losing or preserving bilateral symmetry.

11. Correction of high astigmatism

Because the corneal ablations for refractive surgery treatments induce aberrations (one of the most significant side-effects in myopic LASIK is the induction of spherical aberration[71], which causes halos and reduced contrast sensitivity[72]), special ablation patterns were designed to preserve the preoperative level of high order aberrations[73,74,75]. For the correction of astigmatism many different approaches have been tested, with different degrees of success, through the years[76,77,78,79,80,81].

LASIK has been successfully used for low to moderate myopic astigmatism, whether LASIK is acceptably efficacious, predictable, and safe in correcting higher myopic astigmatism is less documented, specially with regard to the effects of astigmatic corrections in HOA's[82].

The advantage of the Aberration-Free™ ablation profile is that aims being neutral for HOA, leaving the visual print of the patient as it was preoperatively with the best spectacle correction. The correction of astigmatism has been approached using several techniques and ablation profiles. There are several reports showing good results for compound myopic astigmatism using photorefractive keratectomy (PRK) and LASIK, but ablation profiles usually cause a hyperopic shift because of a coupling effect in the flattest corneal meridian. A likely mechanism of this coupling effect is probably due to epithelial remodeling and other effects such as smoothing by the LASIK flap[83]. In cases of large amounts of preoperative astigmatism, deviations from the target refractive outcome are usually attribute to "coupling factors". But, the investigation of the coupling factor remains a rather difficult task, because it seems to be dependent on various factors. Individual Excimer laser systems may have different coupling factors, cutting the flap could alter the initial prescription and also different preoperative corneal curvature (K-reading) may have an influence on the coupling factor.

The most dominant correlations of induced HOAb occurr for C[4,0], and C[6,0] versus defocus correction, for C[4,+2] versus cardinal astigmatism correction, and C[4,-2] versus oblique astigmatism correction. We evaluated the postoperative clinical outcomes and high order aberrations among eyes with astigmatism higher than 2 D that have underwent refractive surgery using the SCHWIND AMARIS laser system. SCHWIND CAM Aberration-Free Aspheric astigmatic treatments have been performed in all cases.

At six-month follow-up, 50 eyes with preoperative astigmatism higher than 2 D were retrospectively analysed. Ablations performed using the SCHWIND AMARIS flying-spot excimer laser system. LASIK flaps were created using Ziemer LDV Femtosecond laser system in all cases.

Inclusion criteria comprised:

- preoperative astigmatism higher than 2 D targeted for emmetropia
- BSCVA ≥ 20/25 (logMAR ≤ +0.1)
- <0.75 μm RMS-HO for 6-mm diameter
- successful completion of 6-month follow-up

We performed following analyses:

- UCVA
- BSCVA
- manifest subjective refraction (SR)
- corneal wavefront up to 7th order at 6-mm diameter without cycloplegia

50 eyes (100%) completed the 6M follow-up, with an average age at the time of the surgery of 28 years (from 17 to 46). 28 eyes were female, and 22 eyes male. 25 patients treated bilaterally. Mean preoperative defocus averaged -3.08 D ± 2.32 D (from -7.13 to -1.00), with mean astigmatism 3.54 D ± 0.85 D (from 2.00 to 4.75). Mean postoperative defocus averaged -0.06 D ± 0.25 D (from -0.75 to +0.75), with mean astigmatism 0.25 D ± 0.26 D (from 0.00 to 1.25). 92% of the eyes ended up in UCVA 20/20 or better. 38% of the eyes gained at least one line of BSCVA (p<.01*). >75% of the eyes within 0.50 D of astigmatism and U-vector, and >90% of the eyes within 1.00 D of astigmatism and U-vector.

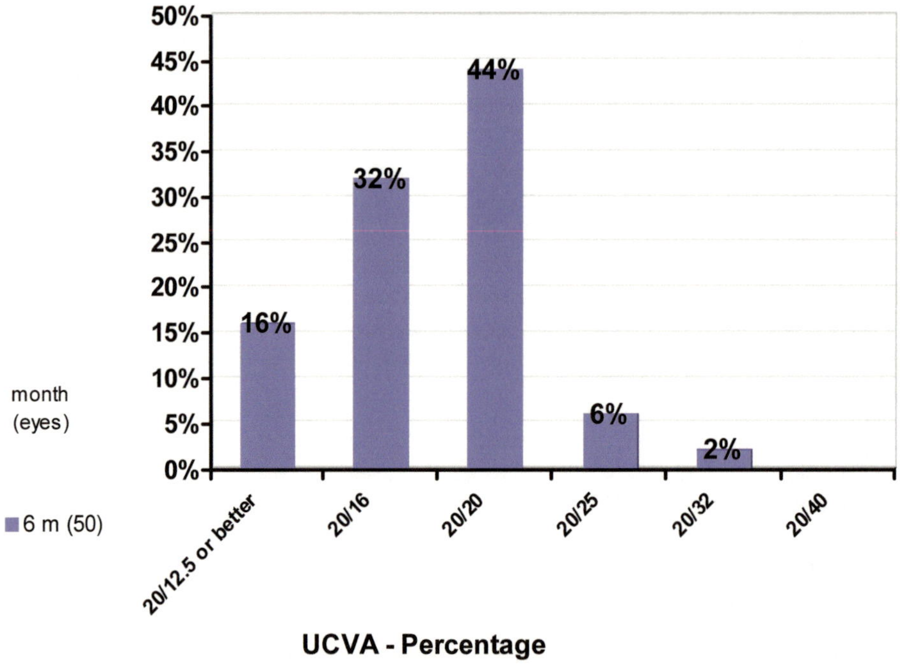

Fig. 10. Efficacy of the correction of moderate to high astigmatism in an aspheric astigmatic setting.

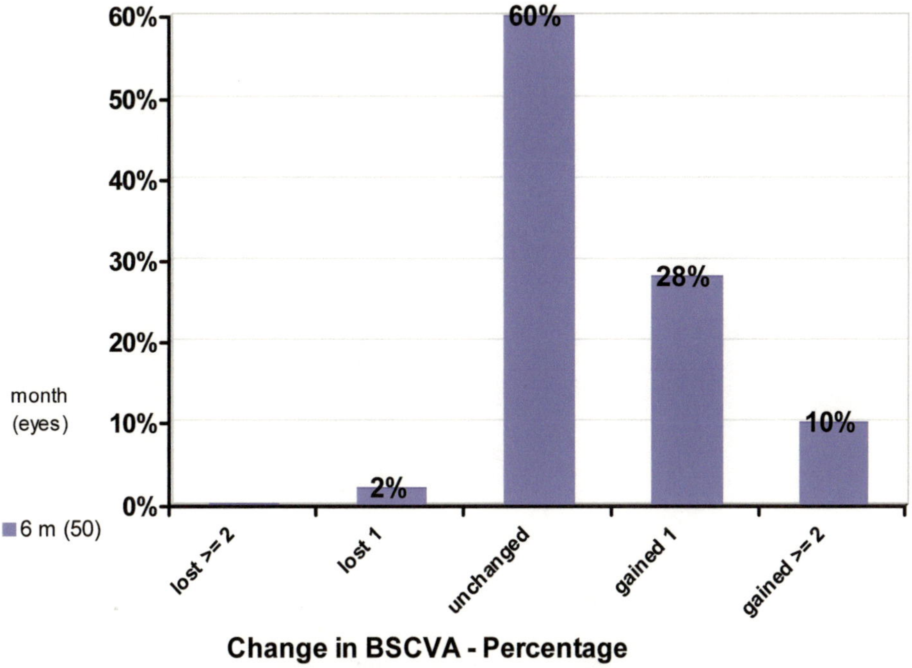

Fig. 11. Safety of the correction of moderate to high astigmatism in an aspheric astigmatic setting.

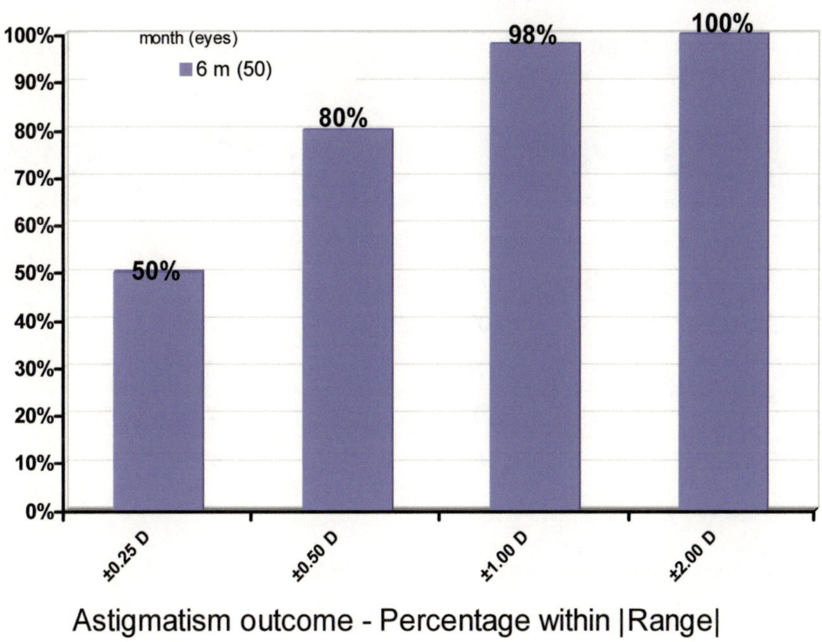

Fig. 12. Refractive astigmatic outcome of the correction of moderate to high astigmatism in an aspheric astigmatic setting.

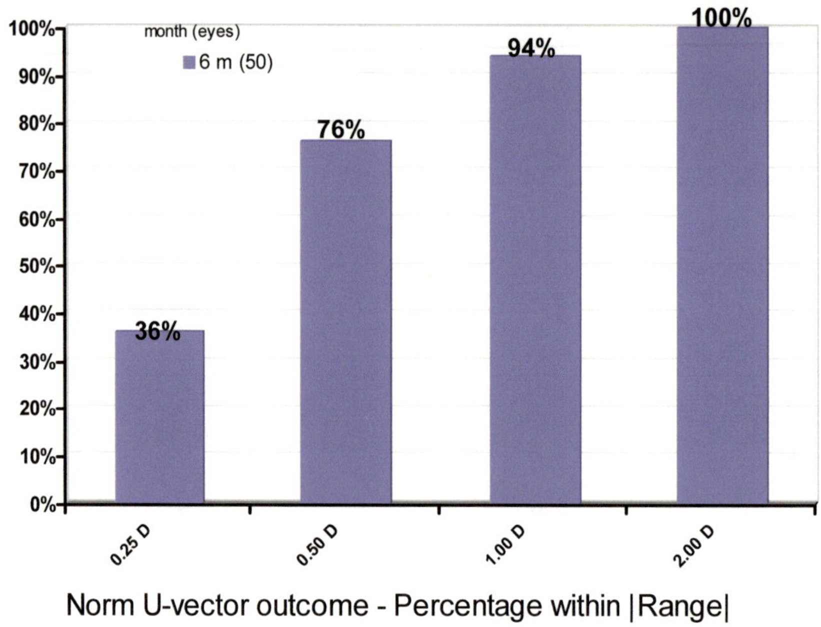

Fig. 13. Residual blur of the correction of moderate to high astigmatism in an aspheric astigmatic setting.

A very slight undercorrection in astigmatism was observed (both cardinal and oblique).

Only 5 HO Zernike terms (out of 30) changed significantly after treatment, whereas 25 HO Zernike terms (out of 30) did not change after treatment.

Zernike term at 6-mm Ø	Preoperative (µm)	Postoperative (µm)	p-value
C[3,-3]	-0.14	-0.02	**<.0001**
C[4,+2]	-0.08	-0.10	**<.05**
C[4,+4]	+0.03	+0.01	**<.05**
C[5,-3]	+0.01	-0.01	**<.0001**
C[6,0]	0.00	+0.03	**<.0001**
HO-RMS	**+0.47**	**+0.57**	**<.0005**

Table 2. Statistically induced Zernike terms.

For all of them, the variation was well below the clinical relevance.

50 high-astigmatism treatments were analysed at 6M follow-up. Results were achieved without applying additional nomograms (residual sphere about 0 D, residual cyl about -0.25 D) (>75% within 0.50 D, >90% within 1.0 D). 6-months follow-up time shows the excellent performance of the system (48% eyes 20/16 or better UCVA, 98% eyes 20/25 or better

UCVA). Aberration-Free astigmatic treatments with SCHWIND AMARIS are safe and very predictable (no eye lost >1 line BSCVA, 5 eyes gained >=2 lines BSCVA).

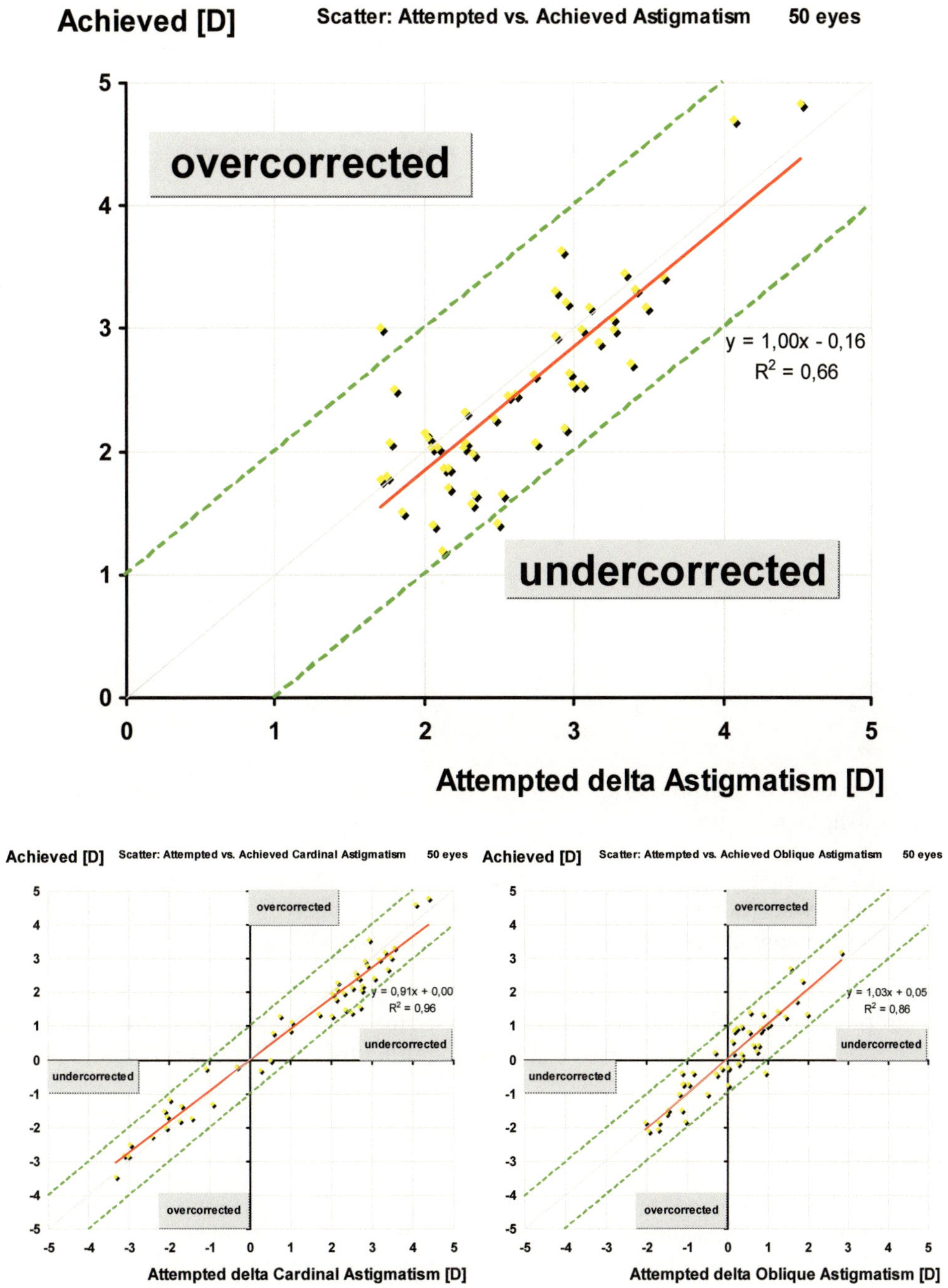

Fig. 14. Scattergram of the correction of moderate to high astigmatism in an aspheric astigmatic setting.

From VA, 92% eyes UCVA 20/20 or better and 38% eyes improved their pre-op BSCVA, due to the minimum aberrations induction by the AMARIS-CAM profile. Despite large defocus and astigmatism magnitudes, minor significant induction of some aberration terms, well below clinically relevant magnitudes. The most dominant correlations of induced HOAb occurred for: C[4,0] vs. Defocus correction, C[4,+2] vs. Cardinal Astigmatism correction, and C[4,-2] vs. Oblique Astigmatism correction.

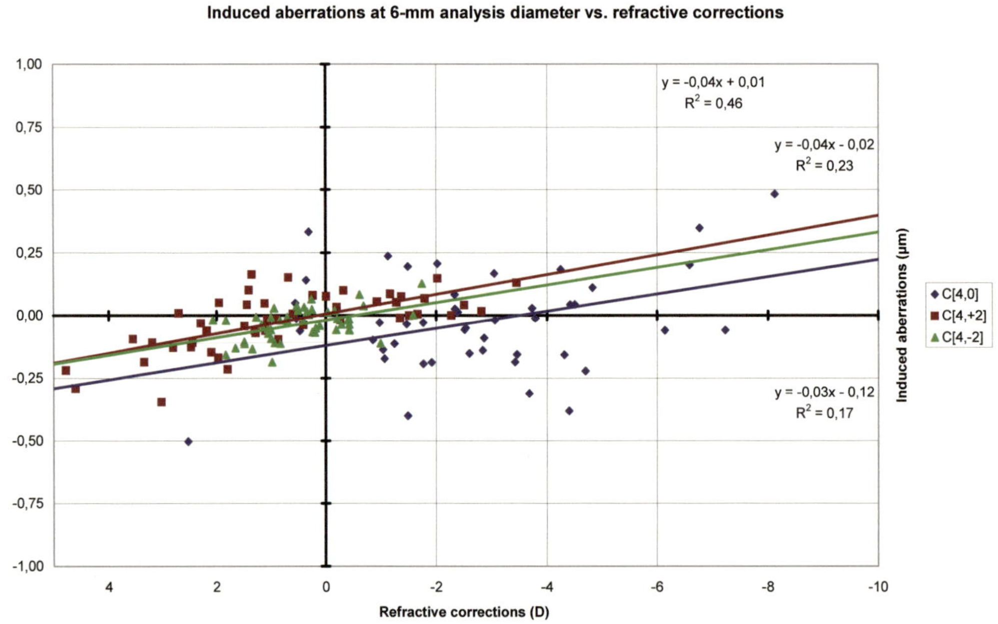

Fig. 15. Induction of aberrations after the correction of moderate to high astigmatism in an aspheric astigmatic setting.

All ablations were non-wavefront-guided treatments. Despite low aberrations, some astigmatisms were not regular. Treatments were centred at the corneal vertex. Despite myopic corrections, 40% of the treatments needed an offset >150 µm.

Laser settings were planned with the manifest astigmatism (magnitude and axis). Topographic astigmatism was not considered for the calculations. No nomogram compensations were applied. With a slight nomogram, further refinements could have been achieved.

12. References

[1] Salmon T. Measurement of Refractive Errors in Young Myopes using the COAS Shack-Hartmann Aberrometer. *Optometry and Vision Science;*2003;Vol 80

[2] Zernike F. Diffraction theory of the knife-edge test and its improved form, the phase-contrast method. *Physica I;* 1934;689-704

[3] Thibos LN, Applegate RA, Schwiegerling JT, Webb R, VSIA Standards Taskforce Members. Standards for reporting the optical aberrations of eyes. *J Refract Surg;* 2002;18:S652-S660

[4] Thibos L, Bradley A, Applegate R. Accuracy and precision of objective refraction from wavefront aberrations. *ISSN 1534-7362* , 2003 ARVO

[5] Marcos S, Cano D, Barbero S. Increase in corneal asphericity after standard laser in situ keratomileusis for myopia is not inherent to the Munnerlyn algorithm. *J Refract Surg;* 2003; 19: S592-6

[6] Dorronsoro C, Cano D, Merayo-Lloves J, Marcos S. Experiments on PMMA models to predict the impact of corneal refractive surgery on corneal shape. *Opt. Express;* 2006; 14: 6142-6156

[7] Arba Mosquera S, de Ortueta D. Geometrical analysis of the loss of ablation efficiency at non-normal incidence. *Opt. Express;* 2008; 16: 3877-3895

[8] Bende T, Seiler T, Wollensak J. Side effects in excimer corneal surgery. Corneal thermal gradients. *Graefes Arch Clin Exp Ophthalmol;* 1988; 226: 277-80

[9] Salmon TO. Corneal contribution to the Wavefront aberration of the eye. *PhD Dissertation;* 1999: 70

[10] Mattioli R, Tripoli NK. Corneal Geometry Reconstruction with the Keratron Videokeratographer. *Optometry and Vision Science* 1997; 74: 881-94

[11] Zernike F. Diffraction theory of the knife-edge test and its improved form, the phase-contrast method. *Monthly Notices of the Royal Astronomical Society;* 1934; 94: 377-384

[12] Thibos LN, Applegate RA, Schwiegerling JT, Webb R, VSIA Standards Taskforce Members. Standards for reporting the optical aberrations of eyes. *J Refract Surg;* 2002;18:S652-S660

[13] Guirao A, Artal P. Corneal wave aberration from videokeratography: accuracy and limitations of the procedure. *J Opt Soc Am A Opt Image Sci Vis.* 2000; 17: 955-65

[14] de Ortueta D, Arba Mosquera S. Mathematical properties of Asphericity: A Method to calculate with asphericities. *J Refract Surg;* 2008; 24: 119-121

[15] Chung SH, Lee IS, Lee YG, Lee HK, Kim EK, Yoon G, Seo KY. Comparison of higher-order aberrations after wavefront-guided laser in situ keratomileusis and laser-assisted subepithelial keratectomy. *J Cataract Refract Surg* 2006; 32:779-84.

[16] Buzzonetti L, Iarossi G, Valente P, Volpi M, Petrocelli G, Scullica L. Comparison of wavefront aberration changes in the anterior corneal surface after laser-assisted subepithelial keratectomy and laser in situ keratomileusis: preliminary study. *J Cataract Refract Surg* 2004; 30: 1929-33.

[17] Bará S, Arines J, Ares J, Prado P. Direct transformation of Zernike eye aberration coefficients between scaled, rotated, and/or displaced pupils. *J Opt Soc Am A.* 2006; 23: 2061-2066.

[18] MacRae S. Aberration Interaction In Aberration Interaction In Wavefront Guided Custom Wavefront Guided Custom Ablation. Wavefront Congress 2007.

[19] Bühren J, Yoon GY, Kenner S, Artrip S, MacRae S, Huxlin K. The effect of decentration on lower- and higher-order aberrations after myopic photorefractive keratectomy (PRK) in a cat model. Wavefront Congress 2007.

[20] Yang Y, Wu F. Technical note: Comparison of the wavefront aberrations between natural and pharmacological pupil dilations. *Ophthalmic Physiol Opt;* 2007; 27: 220-223

[21] Erdem U, Muftuoglu O, Gundogan FC, Sobaci G, Bayer A. Pupil center shift relative to the coaxially sighted corneal light reflex under natural and pharmacologically dilated conditions. *J Refract Surg;* 2008; 24: 530-538

[22] Snellen H. Letterproeven tot Bepaling der Gezichtsscherpte. Utrecht, Weyers, 1862

[23] Radhakrishnan H, Charman WN. Age-related changes in ocular aberrations with accommodation. *J Vis*. 2007; 7: 11.1-21

[24] López-Gil N, Fernández-Sánchez V, Legras R, Montés-Micó R, Lara F, Nguyen-Khoa JL. Accommodation-related changes in monochromatic aberrations of the human eye as a function of age. *Invest Ophthalmol Vis Sci*. 2008; 49: 1736-43

[25] Iida Y, Shimizu K, Ito M, Suzuki M. Influence of age on ocular wavefront aberration changes with accommodation. *J Refract Surg*. 2008; 24: 696-701

[26] He JC, Gwiazda J, Thorn F, Held R, Huang W. Change in corneal shape and corneal wave-front aberrations with accommodation. *J Vis*. 2003; 3:456-63

[27] Atchison DA, Markwell EL, Kasthurirangan S, Pope JM, Smith G, Swann PG. Age-related changes in optical and biometric characteristics of emmetropic eyes. *J Vis*. 2008; 8: 29.1-20

[28] Holzer MP, Sassenroth M, Auffarth GU. Reliability of corneal and total wavefront aberration measurements with the SCHWIND Corneal and Ocular Wavefront Analyzers. *J Refract Surg*; 2006; 22: 917-920.

[29] MacRae S. Aberration Interaction In Wavefront Guided Custom Wavefront Guided Custom Ablation. Wavefront Congress 2007.

[30] Bühren J, Yoon GY, Kenner S, Artrip S, MacRae S, Huxlin K. The effect of decentration on lower- and higher-order aberrations after myopic photorefractive keratectomy (PRK) in a cat model. Wavefront Congress 2007.

[31] McLellan JS, Prieto PM, Marcos S, Burns SA. Effects of interactions among wave aberrations on optical image quality. *Vision Res*; 2006; 46: 3009-3016.

[32] Schwiegerling J, Snyder RW. Eye movement during laser in situ keratomileusis. J Cataract Refract Surg. 2000 Mar;26(3):345-51.

[33] Taylor NM, Eikelboom RH, van Sarloos PP, Reid PG. Determining the accuracy of an eye tracking system for laser refractive surgery. J Refract Surg. 2000 Sep-Oct;16(5):S643-6.

[34] Bueeler M, Mrochen M, Seiler T. Maximum permissible lateral decentration in aberration-sensing and wavefront-guided corneal ablation. J Cataract Refract Surg. 2003 Feb;29(2):257-63.

[35] Bueeler M, Mrochen M. Limitations of pupil tracking in refractive surgery: systematic error in determination of corneal locations. J Refract Surg. 2004 Jul-Aug;20(4):371-8.

[36] Buehren T, Lee BJ, Collins MJ, Iskander DR. Ocular microfluctuations and videokeratoscopy. *Cornea*. 2002; 21: 346-51.

[37] Smith EM Jr, Talamo JH, Assil KK, Petashnick DE. Comparison of astigmatic axis in the seated and supine positions. *J Refract Corneal Surg*. 1994; 10: 615-20.

[38] Smith EM Jr, Talamo JH. Cyclotorsion in the seated and the supine patient. *J Cataract Refract Surg*. 1995; 21: 402-403.

[39] Bueeler M, Mrochen M, Seiler T. Maximum permissible torsional misalignment in aberration-sensing and wavefront-guided corneal ablation. J Cataract Refract Surg. 2004 Jan;30(1):17-25.

[40] Arba-Mosquera S, Merayo-Lloves J, de Ortueta D Clinical effects of pure cyclotorsional errors during refractive surgery. *Invest Ophthalmol Vis Sci*. 2008; 49: 4828-36.

[41] Chernyak DA. From wavefront device to laser: an alignment method for complete registration of the ablation to the cornea. *J Refract Surg*. 2005; 21: 463-8.

[42] Chernyak DA. Cyclotorsional eye motion occurring between wavefront measurement and refractive surgery. *J Cataract Refract Surg*. 2004; 30: 633-8.

[43] Bharti S, Bains HS. Active cyclotorsion error correction during LASIK for myopia and myopic astigmatism with the NIDEK EC-5000 CX III laser. *J Refract Surg*. 2007; 23: S1041-5.

[44] Kim H, Joo CK. Ocular cyclotorsion according to body position and flap creation before laser in situ keratomileusis. *J Cataract Refract Surg*. 2008; 34: 557-61.

[45] Park SH, Kim M, Joo CK. Measurement of pupil centroid shift and cyclotorsional displacement using iris registration. *Ophthalmologica*. 2009; 223: 166-71.

[46] Porter J, Yoon G, MacRae S, Pan G, Twietmeyer T, Cox IG, Williams DR. Surgeon offsets and dynamic eye movements in laser refractive surgery. *J Cataract Refract Surg*. 2005; 31: 2058-66.

[47] Hori-Komai Y, Sakai C, Toda I, Ito M, Yamamoto T, Tsubota K. Detection of cyclotorsional rotation during excimer laser ablation in LASIK. *J Refract Surg*. 2007; 23: 911-5.

[48] Chang J. Cyclotorsion during laser in situ keratomileusis. *J Cataract Refract Surg*. 2008; 34: 1720-6.

[49] Yang Y, Thompson K, Burns S. Pupil location under mesopic, photopic and pharmacologically dilated conditions. *Invest Ophthalmol Vis Sci*. 2002; 43: 2508-2512.

[50] Marcos S, Barbero S, Llorente L, Merayo-Lloves J. Optical response to LASIK surgery for myopia from Total and Corneal Aberration Measurements. *Invest Ophthalmol Vis Sci*. 2001; 42: 3349-3356.

[51] Marcos S. Aberrations and visual performance following standard Laser vision correction. *J Refract Surg*. 2001; 17: S596-S601.

[52] Guirao A, Williams D, Cox I. Effect of rotation and translation on the expected benefit of an ideal method to correct the eyes higher-order aberrations. *J Opt Soc Am A*. 2001; 18: 1003-1015.

[53] Uozato H, Guyton DL. Centering corneal surgical procedures. *Am J Ophthalmol*. 1987; 103: 264-275.

[54] Dunne MC, Misson GP, White EK, Barnes DA. Peripheral astigmatic asymmetry and angle alpha. Ophthalmic Physiol Opt. 1993 Jul;13(3):303-5.

[55] Salmon TO, Thibos LN. Videokeratoscope-line-of-sight misalignment and its effect on measurements of corneal and internal ocular aberrations. *J Opt Soc Am A Opt Image Sci Vis*. 2002 Apr;19(4):657-69.

[56] Hashemi H, Khabazkhoob M, Yazdani K, Mehravaran S, Jafarzadehpur E, Fotouhi A. Distribution of Angle Kappa Measurements with Orbscan II in a Population-Based Survey. *J Refract Surg*. 2010 Jan 28:1-6. doi: 10.3928/1081597X-20100114-06. [Epub ahead of print]

[57] Ciccio AE, Durrie DS, Stahl JE, Schwendeman F. Ocular cyclotorsion during customized laser ablation. *J Refract Surg*. 2005; 21: S772-S774.

[58] Bueeler M, Mrochen M. Simulation of eye-tracker latency, spot size, and ablation pulse depth on the correction of higher order wavefront aberrations with scanning spot laser systems. *J Refract Surg*. 2005; 21: 28-36.

[59] Chernyak DA. Iris-based cyclotorsional image alignment method for wavefront registration. *IEEE Transactions on Biomedical Engineering*. 2005; 52: 2032-2040.

[60] Schruender S, Fuchs H, Spasovski S, Dankert A. Intraoperative corneal topography for image registration. *J Refract Surg*. 2002; 18: S624-S629.

[61] Huang D, Arif M. Spot size and quality of scanning laser correction of higher-order wavefront aberrations. *J Cataract Refract Surg*. 2002; 28: 407-416.

[62] Guirao A,Williams D, MacRae S. Effect of beam size on the expected benefit of customized laser refractive surgery. *J Refract Surg*. 2003; 19: 15-23.

[63] Lohmann CP, Gartry DS, Muir MK, Timberlake GT, Fitzke FW, Marshall J. Corneal haze after excimer laser refractive surgery: objective measurements and functional implications. *Eur J Ophthalmol;* 1991; 1: 173-180.

[64] Porter J, Guirao A, Cox IG, Williams DR. Monochromatic aberrations of the human eye in a large population. *J. Opt. Soc. Am. A* 2001; 18: 1793-1803

[65] Wang L, Dai E, Koch DD, Nathoo A. Optical aberrations of the human anterior cornea. *J Cataract Refract Surg*. 2003; 29: 1514-21

[66] Jiménez JR, Villa C, Anera RG, Gutiérrez R, del Barco LJ. Binocular visual performance after LASIK. *J Refract Surg*. 2006; 22: 679-88

[67] Arbelaez MC, Vidal C, Arba Mosquera S. Bilateral Symmetry before and six-month after Aberration-FreeTM correction with the SCHWIND AMARIS TotalTech laser: Clinical outcomes. *J Optom;*. 2009; in press

[68] Cuesta JR, Anera RG, Jiménez R, Salas C. Impact of interocular differences in corneal asphericity on binocular summation. *Am J Ophthalmol*. 2003; 135: 279-84

[69] Mansouri B, Thompson B, Hess RF. Measurement of suprathreshold binocular interactions in amblyopia. *Vision Res*. 2008 Oct 31. [Epub ahead of print]

[70] Jiménez JR, Ponce A, Anera RG. Induced aniseikonia diminishes binocular contrast sensitivity and binocular summation. *Optom Vis Sci*. 2004; 81: 559-62

[71] Moreno-Barriuso E, Lloves JM, Marcos S. Ocular Aberrations before and after myopic corneal refractive surgery: LASIK-induced changes measured with LASER ray tracing. *Invest Ophthalmol Vis Sci* 2001; 42:1396-1403

[72] Mastropasqua L, Toto L, Zuppardi E, Nubile M, Carpineto P, Di Nicola M, Ballone E. Photorefractive keratectomy with aspheric profile of ablation versus conventional photorefractive keratectomy for myopia correction: six-month controlled clinical trial. *J Cataract Refract Surg;* 2006;32:109-16

[73] Mrochen M, Donetzky C,Wüllner C, Löffler J. Wavefront-optimized ablation profiles: Theoretical background. *J Cataract Refract Surg;* 2004;30:775-785

[74] Koller T, Iseli HP, Hafezi F, Mrochen M, Seiler T. Q-factor customized ablation profile for the correction of myopic astigmatism. *J Cataract Refract Surg;* 2006; 32:584-589

[75] Mastropasqua L, Nubile M, Ciancaglini M, Toto L, Ballone E. Prospective randomized comparison of wavefront-guided and conventional photorefractive keratectomy for myopia with the meditec MEL 70 laser. *J Refract Surg*. 2004; 20: 422-31

[76] McDonnell PJ, Moreira H, Garbus J. Photorefractive keratectomy to create toric ablations for correction of astigmatism. *Arch Ophthalmol* 1991; 109: 710-713.

[77] Argento CJ, Consentino MJ, Biondini A. Treatment of hyperopic astigmatism. *J Cataract Refract Surg* 1997; 23: 1480-1490.

[78] Barraquer C, Gutierrez AM. Results of laser in situ keratomileusis in hyperopic compound astigmatism. *J Cataract Refract Surg* 1999; 25: 1198-1204.

[79] Chayet AS, Montes M, Gómez L, Rodríguez X, Robledo N, MacRae S. Bitoric laser in situ keratomileusis for correcction of simple myopic and mixed astigmatism. *Ophthalmology* 2001; 108: 303-308.

[80] Arbelaez MC, Knorz MC. Laser in situ keramileusis for hyperopia and hyperopic astigmatism. *J Refract Surg* 1999; 15: 406–14.

[81] Vinciguerra P, Sborgi M, Epstein D, et al. Photorefractive keratectomy to correct myopic or hyperopic astigmatism with a cross-cylinder ablation. *J Refract Surg* 1999; 15: S183–5.

[82] Seiler T, Kaemmerer M, Mierdel P, Krinke H-E. Ocular optical aberrations after PRK for myopia and myopic astigmatism. *Arch Ophthalmol* 2000; 118: 17–21

[83] Huang D, Stulting RD, Carr JD, Thompson KP, Waring GO. Multiple regression and vector analysis of LASIK for myopia and astigmatism. *J Refract Surg* 1999; 15: 538-549.

14

Comparing Nomograms of Two Symmetric and Two Asymmetric Intacs® Segments Implantation for Treatment of Pellucid Marginal Degeneration

Luis A. Rodriguez and Anny E. Villegas*
Corneal Clinic, Centro Medico Docente La Trinidad (CMDLT), Caracas Venezuela

1. Introduction

Non-inflammatory progressive corneal ectasia and thinning disease are among the most common abnormalities that refractive surgeons diagnose. Pellucid Marginal Degeneration (PMD) is another ectatic pathology that is rarely detected. PMD is a bilateral, non-inflammatory, progressive peripheral inferior corneal thinning disorder (1,2). Diagnosis is based on the presence of corneal thinning with ectasia characterized by a peripheral band of thinning of the inferior cornea with 1 to 2 mm of normal cornea between this area and the limbus (2,3). The area of thinning typically is epithelialized, clear, avascular, and without lipid deposit. Like keratoconus, PMD is a bilateral progressive disorder although eyes may be asymmetrically affected. Topographic examination is very useful to differentiate this ectatic disorder. The topographic appearance shows a classical "butterfly" pattern that demonstrates large amounts of against-the-rule astigmatism as measured by simulated keratometry and inferior thinning. PMD can also be diagnosed by performing a pachymetric map of the entire cornea, as well as by elevation corneal maps using placido-ring-based videokeratoscopy technology (1).

The etiology of PMD is not clear, and it is not known whether PMD, keratoconus and keratoglobus are distinct diseases or phenotypic variations of the same disorder (4). PMD is usually asymptomatic except for progressive deterioration in uncorrected visual acuity caused by irregular astigmatism (5). Slit-lamp examination shows a peripheral band of thinning with a protrusion ("beer-belly" contour) of the inferior cornea (6,7,8). Topographically, this protrusion in the peripheral inferior cornea has high keratometry powers, radiating toward the center from the inferior oblique meridians, typically in the inferior peripheral cornea. There is an area of flattening in the center of the cornea (5). In transmission electron microscopy of the cornea, abnormal fibrous long-spacing (FSL) collagen with a periodicity of 100 to 110 nm in PMD is revealed, which contrasts with 60 to 64 nm found in normal corneas (9). A study reported in 2002 describes associations with

---

* None of the authors has a financial or proprietary interest in any material or method mentioned in this article.

vernal keratoconjunctivitis, Marfan's syndrome, ocular hypertension, keratoconus, keratoglobus and hydrops (23).

In the early stages, spectacles and contact lenses are the usual treatment approaches; however, in patients who cannot be rehabilitated with these options, a surgical procedure is necessary (10). Different surgical options include crescentic wedge resection, crescentic lamellar keratoplasty, penetrating keratoplasty, epikeratophakia and thermokeratoplasty. However, all these techniques have disadvantages: unpredictability, irreversibility, long period of rehabilitation and significant complication rates (11-16). Authors suggest the use of intracorneal rings (ICR) in glasses/contact lens-intolerant patients affected by early and moderate PMD with against-the-rule astigmatism and inferior peripheral corneal thickness of >450 μm (10). Since ICR mechanically lifts the inferior ectasia of PMD, flattens the soft ectatic corneal tissue, and decreases asymmetrical astigmatism, visual acuity is expected to improve following this procedure (17). Intacs® works on the principle of tissue addition. Peripheral distention is directly proportional to the degree of central corneal flattening, and by an arc-shortening effect it manages to change the shape and power of the central cornea in ectatic eyes without weakening the central or the paracentral cornea (17,18). The aspheric shape of the natural cornea reduces aberrations and minimizes refractive error fluctuations as the pupil changes its size, and therefore reduces visual disturbances such as glare and halos. It is important to observe that Intacs® maintains an aspheric cornea. After placement of ring segments, central cornea has been shown to maintain a prolate shape because Intacs® flattens the peripheral cornea more than the central cornea (19). The major objective of corneal ring segment inserts is to reshape the abnormality by neither removing corneal tissue nor touching the central cornea (20). Various reports have been published illustrating either the symmetrical (inserting two same-size segments) or the asymmetrical (inserting two different size segments) Intacs® implantation techniques for the management of PMD. Both these techniques have been independently shown to improve UCVA, BSCVA and topographic findings (9,10).

Intacs® are polymethylmethacrylate crescent-shaped segments with arc length of 150° and inner and outer diameters of 6.8 mm and 8.1 mm respectively. The ring segments are available in sizes ranging in thickness from 0.25 to 0.45 mm (Table 3).

2. Patients and methods

Symmetric ring segments were implanted in ten (10) eyes and asymmetric ring segments were implanted in nine (9) eyes. Swanson nomogram was used to calculate segment thickness in each eye.

De-Centered Cones (Posterior Float 50% outside the 3 mm optical zone)**		
Spherical Equiv	**Inferior Intacs®**	**Superior Intacs®**
+1.00 to -2.00	.250 mm	.300 mm
-2.00 to -3.00	.250 mm	.350 mm
-3.00 to -4.00	.300 mm	.400 mm*
-4.00 and -5.00	.300 mm	.450 mm*
-5.00 and higher	.350 mm	.450 mm*

**Keratoconus, Pellucid Marginal Degeneration or "Pellucid Like" Nomogram (24)

The election of using asymmetric and symmetric ring segments was based on spherical equivalent and was randomly chosen.

Besides the demographic details, key parameters evaluated during the preoperative and postoperative examination included: slitlamp microscopy, manifest refraction, spherical equivalent (SE), uncorrected visual acuity (UCVA), corneal pachymetry, tonometry, flat and steep keratometry readings and topography (Orbscan II). Postoperatively patients were evaluated at one month, three months, six months and one year.

3. Surgical procedure

Intacs® implantation was performed under topical anesthesia. After the patients were prepared through corneal hydration with balanced saline solution and sterile fields, the geometric center of the cornea was measured and marked. A radial 2 mm incision was performed in the steep corneal meridian with a diamond knife that was calibrated to 85% corneal depth. A vacuum centering guide - sloped shelf ring connected to a KV2000 vacuum system (Addition Technology® 155 Moffett Park Drive, Suite B-1 Sunnyvale, CA 94089-1330 U.S.A.) was positioned to stabilize the globe. Clockwise and counterclockwise stromal dissectors were introduced into the base of the incision to create stromal tunnels. Intacs® of selected thicknesses were placed in the stromal tunnels from each side of the incision. The incision site was closed with one interrupted 10-0 nylon suture. Post-operative medication included an antibiotic/steroid combination taken every six (6) hours for two (2) weeks. All procedures were uneventful and performed by the same surgeon, (LAR).

4. Statistical analysis

The two groups were analyzed for any bias with respect to age, size of segments, initial values of visual acuity, astigmatism, spherical equivalent, flat and steep keratometry readings. Both groups were found to be comparable.

Our study was descriptive and results were represented as averages and percentages (±standard deviations). Confidence intervals were set at 95%.

Paired t test was used to compare the two groups with respect to changes in the following parameters: visual acuity, astigmatism, spherical equivalent, keratometries (flat and steep readings). Visual acuity was expressed in log mar (Snellen equivalent). One-way Anova test was applied to compare the changes in values throughout time in both the symmetric and asymmetric groups. Bonferroni post test was applied in cases where the values were statistically significant. Any value of P less than or equal to 0.05 ($P > 0.05$) was considered statistically significant.

5. Results

Preoperative values in asymmetric group: UCVA 1.00 (log mar); astigmatism: -4.00D; SE: -2.90D, K (flat) 43.09 D; K (steep) 47.02D. (Table 1) UCVA 0.85 (log mar); astigmatism: -4,50D; SE: -2.74D; K (flat) 43.03 D; K (steep) 47.05D. (Table 2)

Tables 1 and 2 show an improvement in visual acuity, reduction in astigmatism, spherical equivalent and decrease in steep and flat keratometry post-op.

Parameter	Initial			Final		
	Mean	SE	CI 95%	Mean	SE	95% CI
Visual Acuity (LogMAR)	1.00	0.14	0.67 – 1.33	0.22	0.04	0.13 – 0.30
Astigmatism	-4.00	0.49	-5.13 - -2.88	-2.11	0.39	-5.25 - -0.55
Spherical Equivalent	-2.90	1.02	-3.08 - -0.06	-1.57	0.62	-3.08 - -0.06
Keratometry Flat	43.09	0.49	41.95 – 44.23	40.79	0.63	39.33 – 42.25
Keratometry Steep	47.02	0.6	45.63 – 48.40	44.51	1.06	42.07 – 46.96

SE: Standard Error; 95% CI: Confidence Interval of mean 95% (Lower – Upper)

Table 1. Initial and Final Values for Visual Acuity (LogMAR), Astigmatism, Spherical Equivalent and Keratometry (Flat and Steep) in Patients with Diagnosis of Pellucid Marginal Degeneration with Insertion Asymmetrical Intacs ® Segments

Parameter	Initial			Final		
	Mean	SE	CI 95%	Mean	SE	95% CI
Visual Acuity (LogMAR)	0.85	0.19	0.42 – 1.28	0.28	0.09	0.09 – 0.48
Astigmatism	-4.50	0.44	-5.5 - -3.5	-3.30	0.54	-4.53 - -2.07
Spherical Equivalent	-2.74	1.08	-5.17 - -0.3	-0.58	0.40	-1.49 – 0.33
Keratometry Flat	43.03	0.27	42.41 – 43.65	42.12	0.50	40.98 – 43.25
Keratometry Steep	47.05	0.79	45.27 – 48.84	45.07	0.48	43.98 – 46.15

SE: Standard Error; 95% CI: Confidence Interval of mean 95% (Lower – Upper)

Table 2. Initial and Final Values for Visual Acuity (LogMAR), Astigmatism, Spherical Equivalent and Keratometry (Flat and Steep) in Patients with Diagnosis of Pellucid Marginal Degeneration with Insertion Symmetrical Intacs ® Segments

The characteristics of the implanted segments were the following:

Asymmetric segments implanted: 300/250 (3), 450/300 (2), 350/250 (2), 450/250 (2).

Symmetric segments implanted: 450 (1), 400 (1), 350 (1), 300 (4), 250 (3).

The asymmetric group had an average age of 29.67 ± 3.42 years, and the symmetric group had an average age of 34.5 ± 3.42 years. The study showed a non-significant statistical difference between the groups (p=0.357).

Visual Acuity in the symmetric group was better than the asymmetric group. In order to compare the two groups and showed a non-significant statistical difference between the two groups (p=0.550). Figure 1

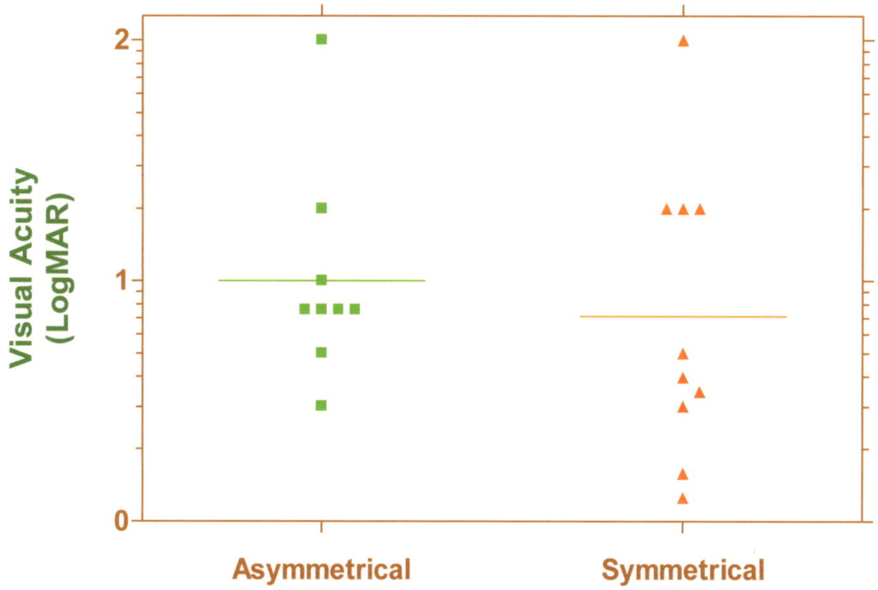

Fig. 1. Initial Values of Visual Acuity in Patients with Diagnosis of Pellucid Marginal Degeneration with Insertion of Symmetrical or Asymmetrical Intacs ® Segments

Spherical equivalent and steep keratometry showed no significant statistical difference in astigmatism between the two groups (p=0.456; p=0.914; p=0.647 respectively). Figure 2, 3 and 4

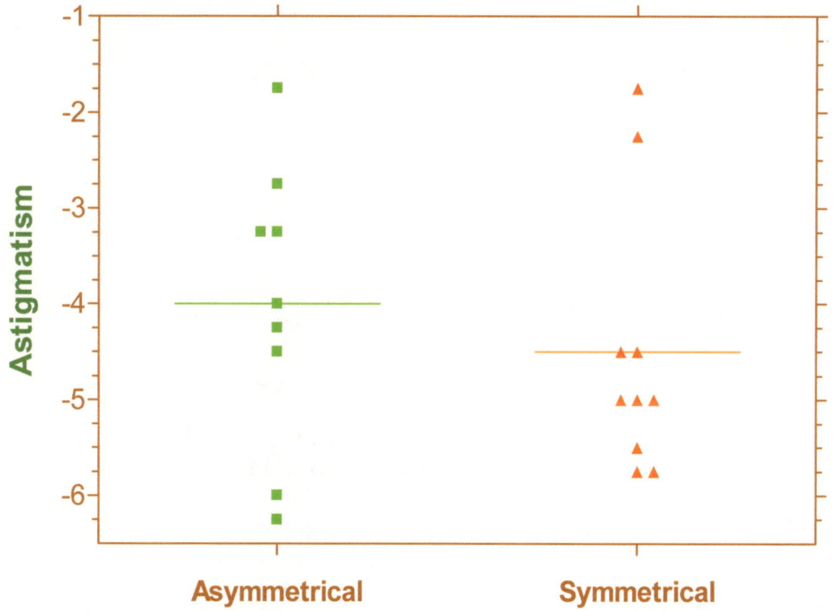

Fig. 2. Initial Values of Astigmatism in Patients with Diagnosis of Pellucid Marginal Degeneration with Insertion of Symmetrical or Asymmetrical Intacs ® Segments

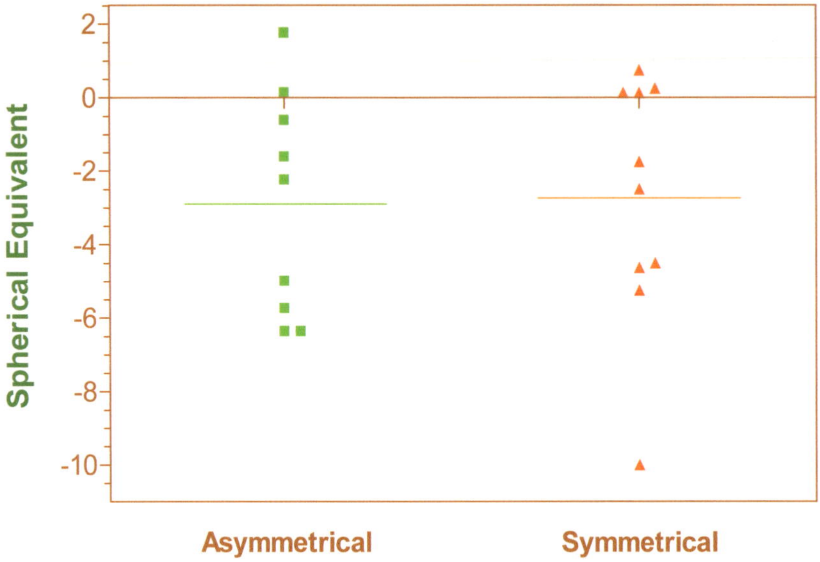

Fig. 3. Initial Values of Spherical Equivalent in Patients with Diagnosis of Pellucid Marginal Degeneration with Insertion of Symmetrical or Asymmetrical Intacs ® Segments

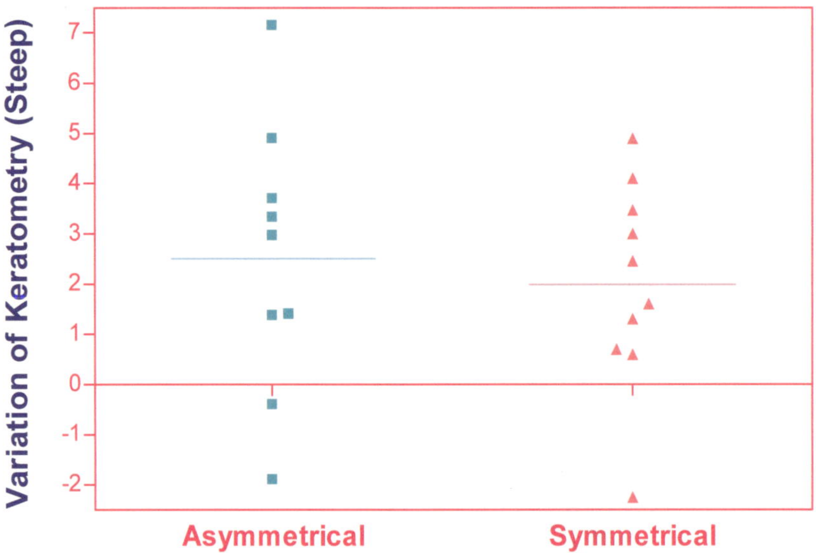

Fig. 4. Variation of Keratometry (Steep) in Patients with Diagnosis of Pellucid Marginal Degeneration with Insertion of Symmetrical or Asymmetrical Intacs ® Segments

After comparing the groups with flat keratometry, a significant statistical difference was found ($p=0.025$). This variation was greater in the asymmetric group. Figure 5

In Figure 6 and 7 the evolution of visual acuity for the asymmetric and symmetric group can be seen. After applying one-way Anova, a significant statistical difference was evidenced ($p<0.0001$ and $p=0.0003$). We subsequently applied the Bonferroni multiple comparison test

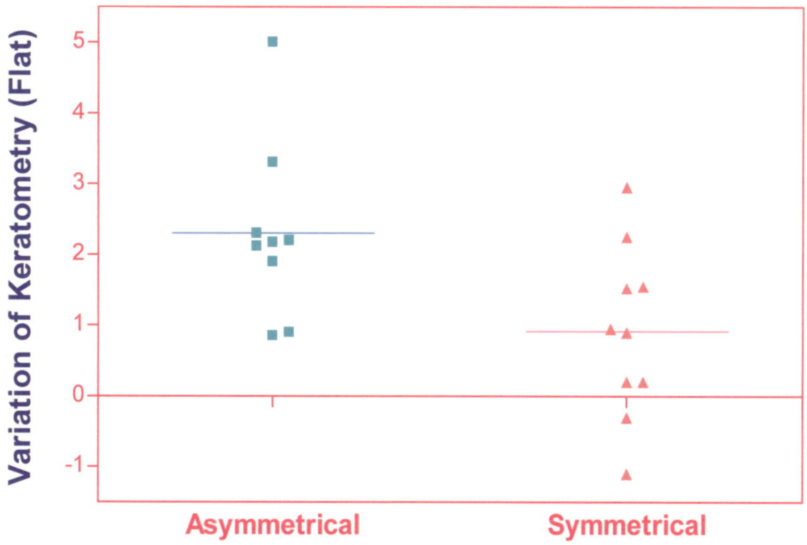

Fig. 5. Variation of Keratometry (Flat) in Patients with Diagnosis of Pellucid Marginal Degeneration with Insertion of Symmetrical or Asymmetrical Intacs ® Segments

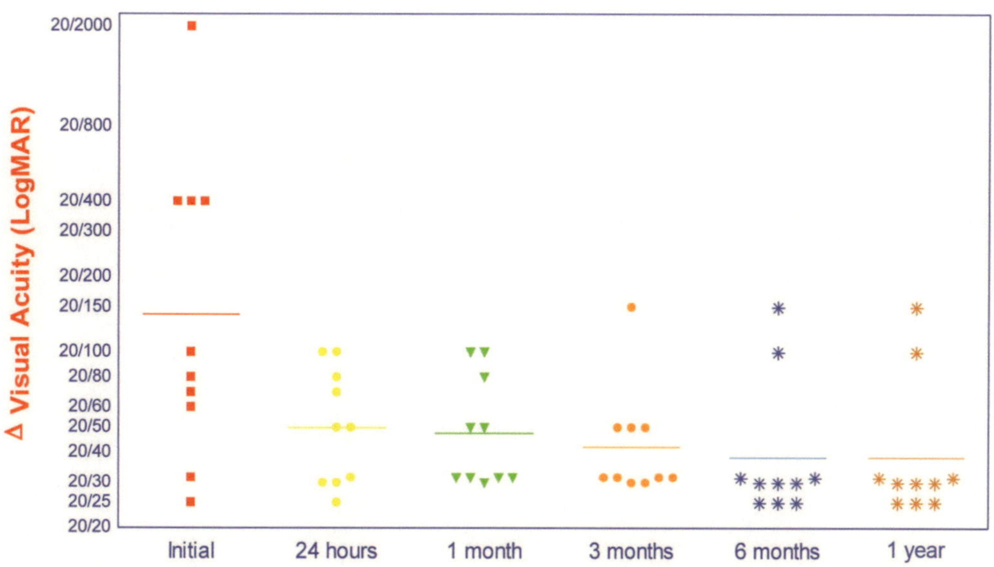

Fig. 6. Time Course of Visual Acuity (LogMAR) in Patients with Diagnosis of Pellucid Marginal Degeneration with Insertion of Asymmetrical Intacs ®

in order to compare each post-operatory time period. No significant statistical differences were seen.

In Figure 8 and 9 the evolution of astigmatism for the asymmetric and symmetric group was shown. With the application of one-way Anova, a significant statistical difference was observed in asymmetric group (p=0.031) while no significant statistical difference was found postoperatively (p =0.074) in symmetric group. The Bonferroni multiple comparison test

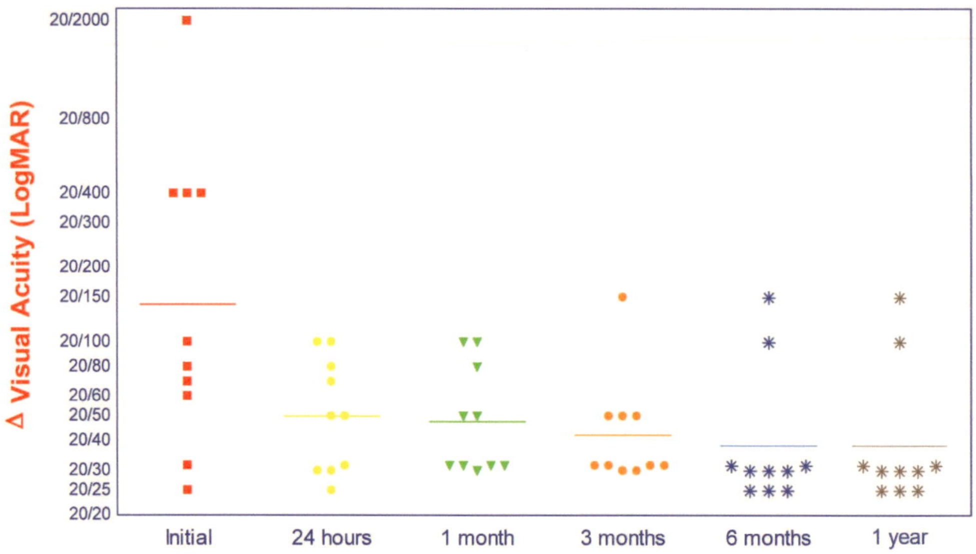

Fig. 7. Time Course of Visual Acuity (LogMAR) in Patients with Diagnosis of Pellucid Marginal Degeneration with Insertion of Symmetrical Intacs ®

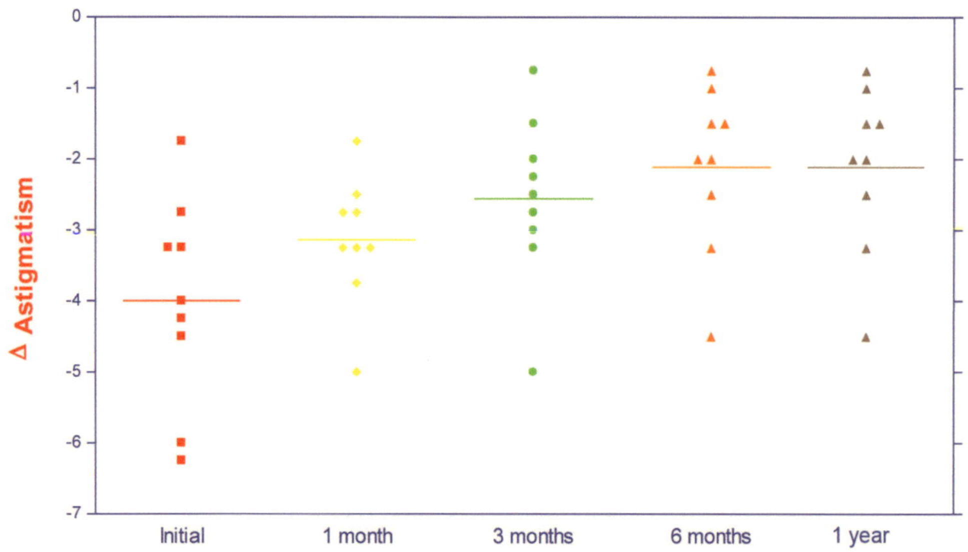

Fig. 8. Time Course of Astigmatism in Patients with Diagnosis of Pellucid Marginal Degeneration with Insertion of Asymmetrical Intacs ®

showed no significant statistical difference between initial and one month, and significant statistical differences between initial and three months and between initial, six months and one year respectively.

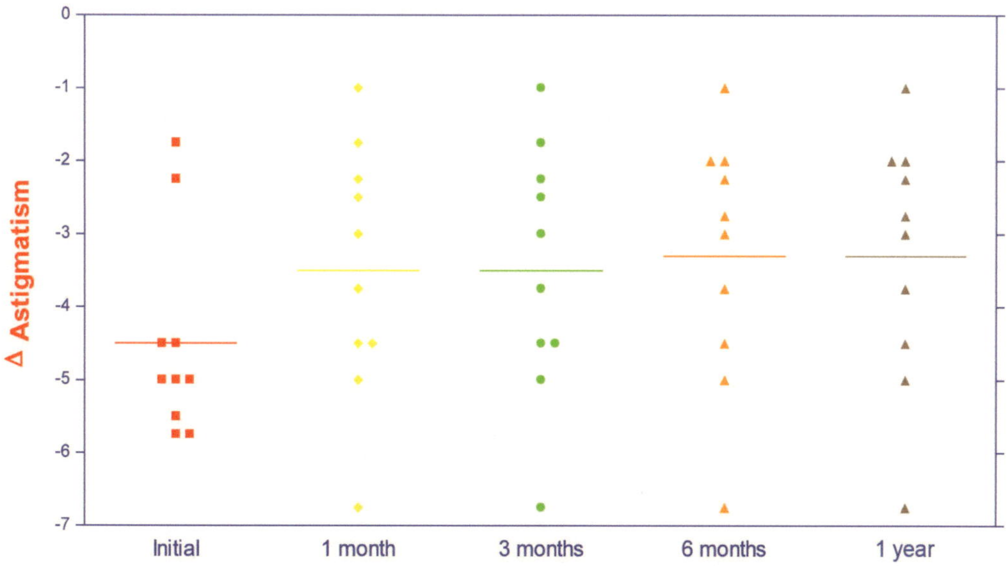

Fig. 9. Time Course of Astigmatism in Patients with Diagnosis of Pellucid Marginal Degeneration with Insertion of Symmetrical Intacs ®

Figures 10 and 11 analyzed the variation of spherical equivalent for the asymmetric and symmetric group. After applying one-way Anova, a significant statistical difference was observed in both groups (p=0.030; p=0.020). In addition we used the Bonferroni multiple comparison test in order to compare each time period and thereby established that the only difference was between initial and first month postoperatively in asymmetric group and initial with six month and first year in symmetric group.

In Figure 12 the evolution of flat keratometry in the asymmetric group is graphed. After the application of one-way Anova, a significant statistical difference was evidenced (p=0.005). We then applied the Bonferroni multiple comparison test in order to compare all the postoperative time periods. The difference found was observed in the comparison between the initial with three months and the initial with six months. No difference was found upon comparing initial with one month, nor when comparing the various time periods after initial (one month, three months, and six months) respectively. No significant statistical difference was observed in symmetric group (p=0.543) figure 13.

In Figure 14 the variation in steep keratometry in the asymmetric group was observed. After applying one-way Anova, a significant statistical difference was observed (p=0.003). In addition we applied the Bonferroni multiple comparison test in order to compare each time period, and the only difference found was when comparing initial with one month.

In Figure 15 we observed the evolution of steep keratometry in the symmetric group. No significant statistical difference was found when one-way Anova was applied (p=0.080).

With respect to the variation in visual acuity (log mar), astigmastism and spherical equivcalent, when both groups were compared with the student's t test, no significant statistical difference was found between them (p=0.366; p=0.412; p=0.344 respectively). Figure 16, 17 and 18.

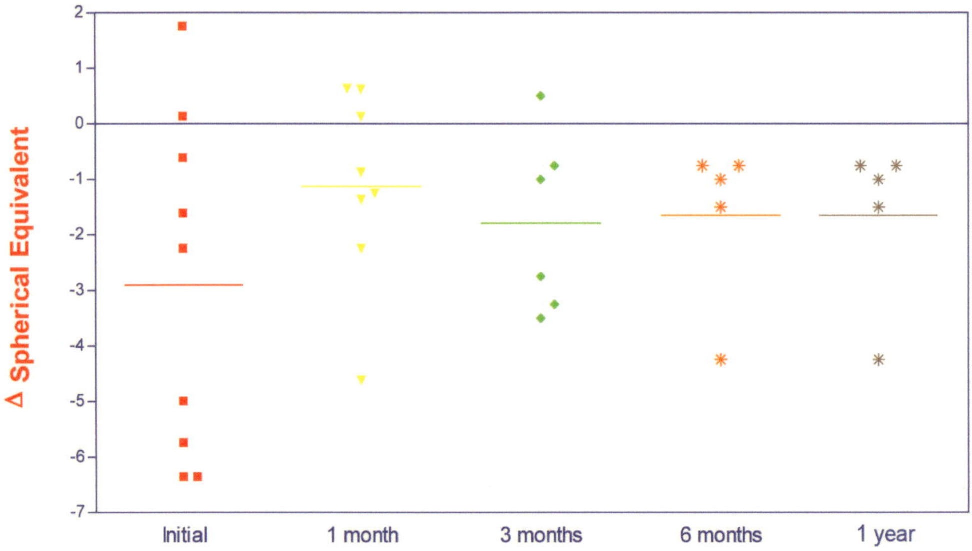

Fig. 10. Time Course of Spherical Equivalent in Patients with Diagnosis of Pellucid Marginal Degeneration with Insertion of Asymmetrical Intacs ®

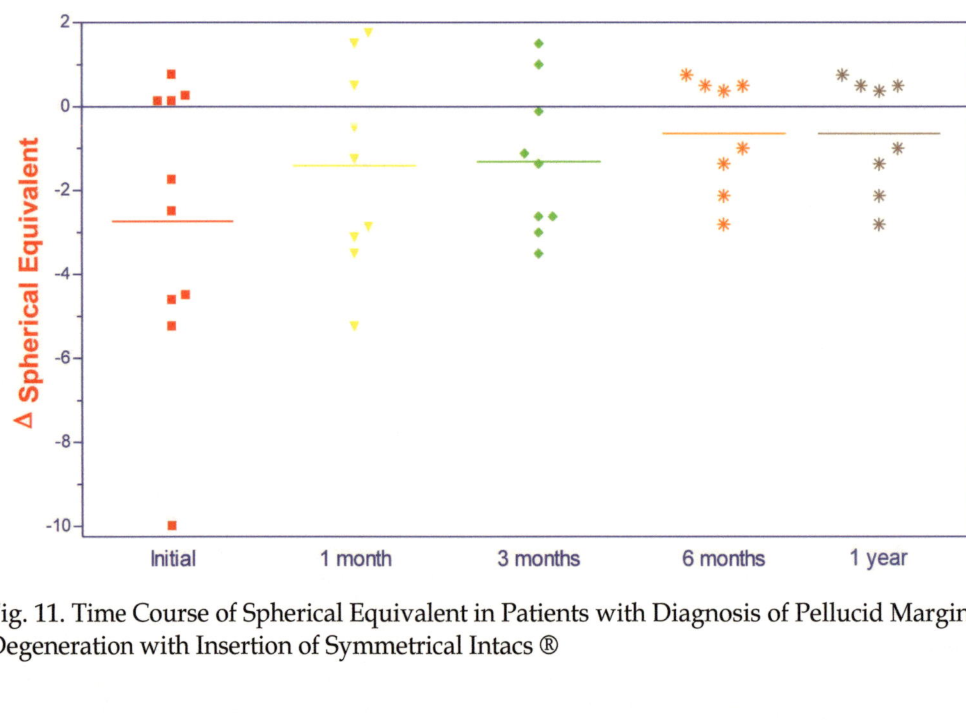

Fig. 11. Time Course of Spherical Equivalent in Patients with Diagnosis of Pellucid Marginal Degeneration with Insertion of Symmetrical Intacs ®

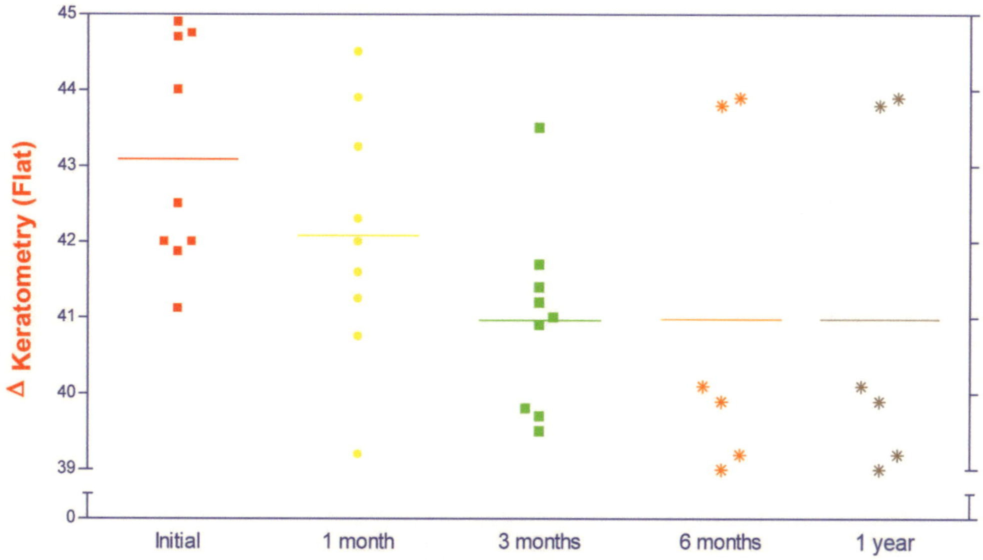

Fig. 12. Time Course of Keratometry (Flat) in Patients with Diagnosis of Pellucid Marginal Degeneration with Insertion of Asymmetrical Intacs ®

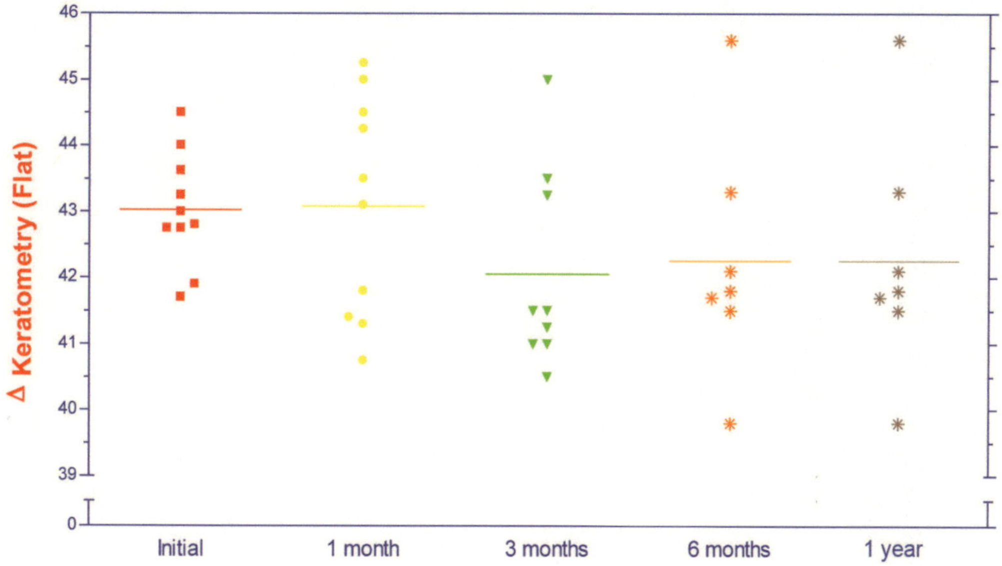

Fig. 13. Time Course of Keratometry (Flat) in Patients with Diagnosis of Pellucid Marginal Degeneration with Insertion of Symmetrical Intacs ®

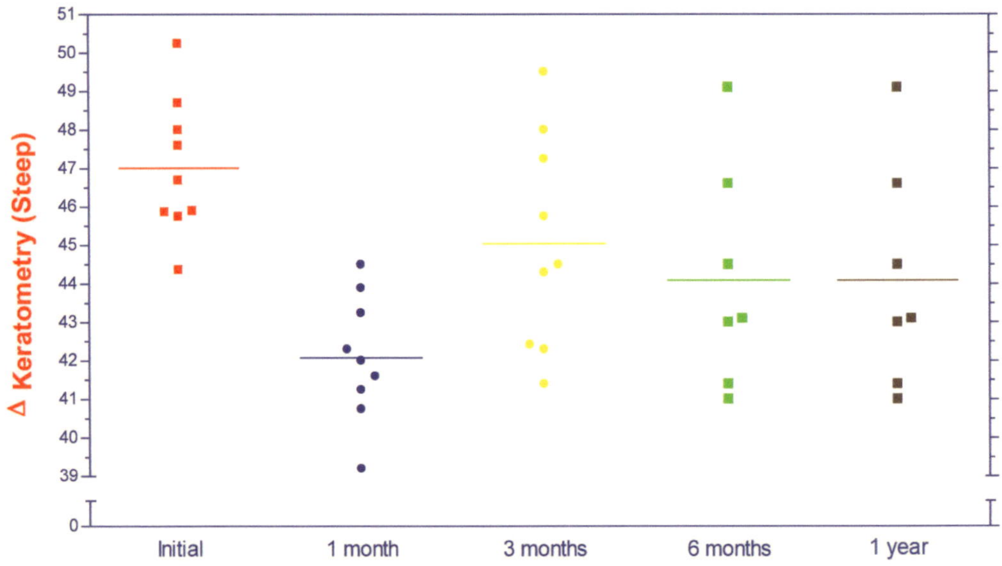

Fig. 14. Time Course of Keratometry (Steep) in Patients with Diagnosis of Pellucid Marginal Degeneration with Insertion of Asymmetrical Intacs ®

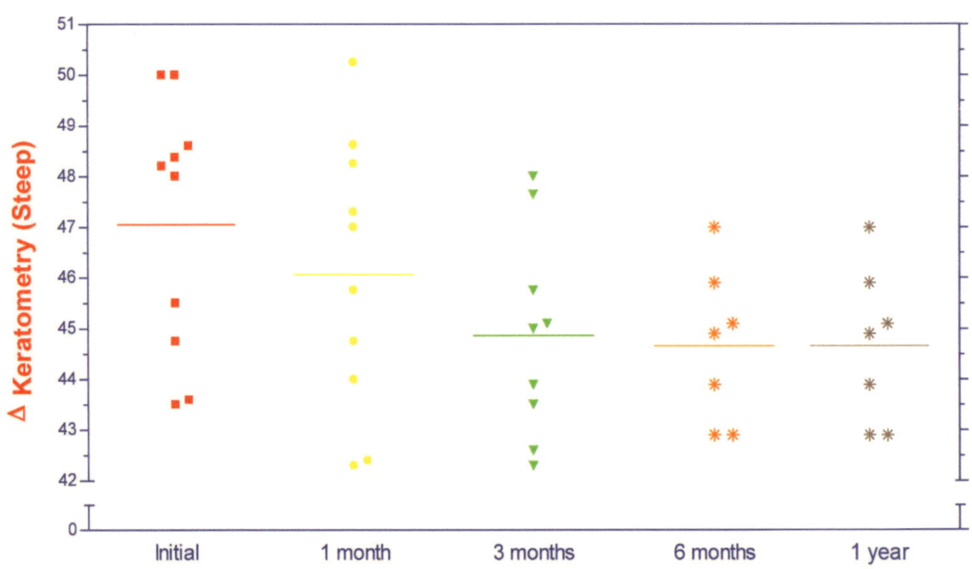

Fig. 15. Time Course of Keratometry (Steep) in Patients with Diagnosis of Pellucid Marginal Degeneration with Insertion of Symmetrical Intacs ®

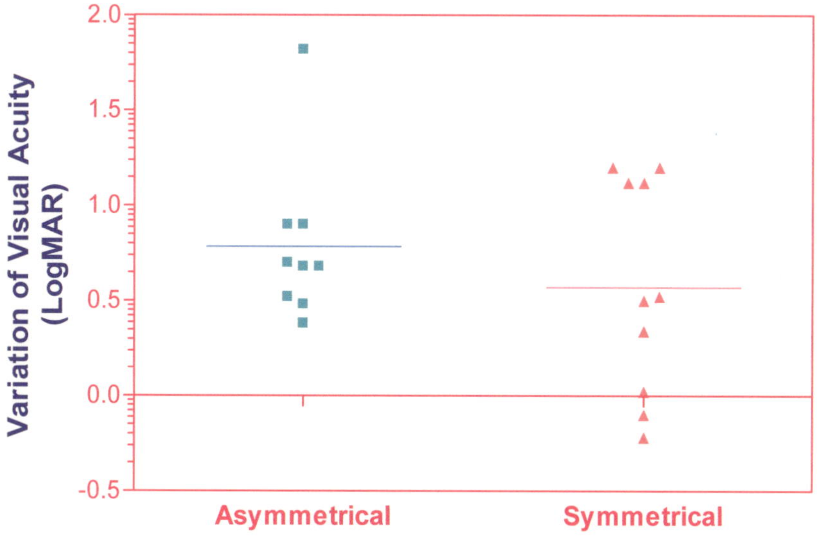

Fig. 16. Variation of Visual Acuity (LogMAR) in Patients with Diagnosis of Pellucid Marginal Degeneration with Insertion of Symmetrical or Asymmetrical Intacs ® Segments

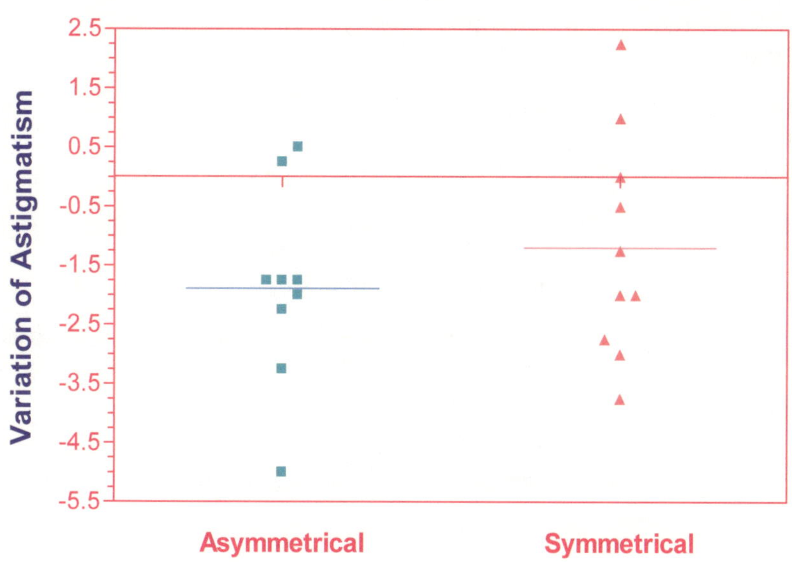

Fig. 17. Variation of Astigmatism in Patients with Diagnosis of Pellucid Marginal Degeneration with Insertion of Symmetrical or Asymmetrical Intacs ® Segments

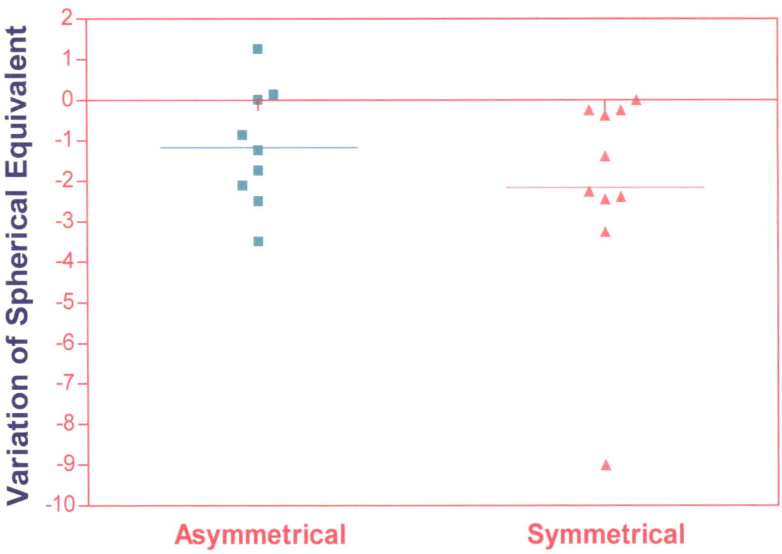

Fig. 18. Variation of Spherical Equivalent in Patients with Diagnosis of Pellucid Marginal Degeneration with Insertion of Symmetrical or Asymmetrical Intacs ® Segments

5.1 Results in asymmetric group

At the end of follow-up period (one year), mean UCVA was 0.22 log mar, ±0,04 (20/30) (95% IC=0.13-0.30). Statistically significant differences were noted throughout the follow-up period ($p < 0.0001$)

Astigmatism value at final follow-up was -2.11D ±0.39 (95% IC= -5.25 – 0.55). P values at all of the postoperative follow-up periods were statistically significant (p=0.001). The maximum improvement in astigmatism was at three months postoperative.

Spherical equivalent mean value was -1.57D ± 0.62 (95% IC=-3.08- 0.06). The changes in mean spherical equivalent during the follow-up period were statistically significant (p=0.030) with maximum improvement at one month postoperative.

Keratometry flat meridian was 40.79D±0.63 (95% IC= 39.33- 42.25). All the changes in mean readings in flat keratometry were statistically significant (p=0.005). Maximum improvement was between three and six months postoperative.

Keratometry steep meridian was 44.51D±1.06 (95% IC= 42.07 – 46.96). The changes in mean readings in steep keratometry were statistically significant (p=0.003) with maximum improvement at first month.

5.2 Results in symmetric group

Mean UCVA was 0.28 log mar, ±0.09 (20/40) (95% IC=0.09-0.48). Statistically significant differences were noted throughout the follow-up period ($p < 0.0003$)

Astigmatism value at final follow-up was -3.30D ±0.54 (95% IC= -4.53 - 2.07). At first year, the difference was not statistically significant (p=0.074).

Spherical equivalent mean values were -0.58D ± 0.40 (95% IC=-1.49 - 0.33). The difference was statistically significant (p=0.020) with maximum improvement at six months postoperative.

Keratometry flat meridian value was 42.12D±0.50 (95% IC= 40.98- 43.25). At first year, the difference was not statistically significant (p=0.543).

Keratometry steep meridian was 45.07D±0.48 (95% IC= 43.98 - 46.15). At first year postoperative the difference was not statistically significant (p= 0.080).

5.3 Comparing results of both groups

Initial visual acuity values were not statistically different between both groups (p=0.550).

Astigmatism initial values were not statistically significant between both groups. (p=0.456). Spherical equivalent values were not statistically significant between both groups (p=0.914). Keratometries (flat and steep) meridian initial values were not statistically significant between both groups (p=0.905 symmetric group), (p=0.972 asymmetric group).

UCVA was not statistically significant between the groups (p=0.366). The difference of final post-op values in astigmatism for the groups was not statistically significant. (p=0.412). The difference of spherical equivalent values at six months post-op between the groups was not statistically significant (p=0.344). The difference of keratometry flat values at six months post-op between the groups was significant (p=0.025) with a better result in the asymmetric group. Keratometry steep values at one year postoperatively in both groups were not statistically significant. (p=0.647).

6. Discussion

Pellucid marginal degeneration (PMD) is a disease with a complicated prognosis in patients who are intolerant to contact lenses (10). Different procedures have been used to treat PMD with unpredictable results. Symmetric and asymmetric Intacs® segments are relatively new devices that reinforce the cornea through the arc-shortening effect of the corneal lamellae that produces flattening of the central cornea. The goal of using Intacs® for PMD is to reshape the cornea without removing tissue by lifting the inferior ectasia, flattening the soft ectatic corneal tissue and decreasing astigmatism. With this treatment, tissue and endothelium is maintained with the benefit that an additive surgical approach is used that adds rigidity and reinforces the ectatic cornea, flattening the central area, and positioning the optical zone in the center of the pupil. This procedure is also reversible. Mularoni et al. proposed a treatment with two asymmetric intracorneal segments in patients with intolerance to contact lenses and early and moderate PMD. Results were great improvement in UCVA, BSCVA and topographical findings (10). Colin J. and Malet F. implanted two symmetric Intacs® segments and followed the progress for two years post operatively obtaining favorable results. The findings in this study indicated that Intacs® segments are an effective long-term treatment for keratoconus and associated ectasia (21). Kymionis et al. reported a case of PMD treated with Intacs® symmetric segments which reported an improvement in corneal topographic pattern. ICR insertion can reduce the corneal steepening and astigmatism associated with PMD (9). Rodriguez Prats et al. reported a reduction of steepening and astigmatism associated with PMD by implanting one inferior segment (17). Sharma M. and Boxer Wachler noted that placement of inferior segment Intacs® alone was more suitable than double segments Intacs® insertion for peripherally located cones (22). Alió et al found that by implanting either one or two segments produced a similar effect in the reduction of the refractive cylinder and the keratometric readings (19). Both methods have similar results especially when concerning the visual acuity.

In our study, we compared implanting two segments in an asymmetric group to implanting two segments in a symmetric group, with a slightly better result in UCVA in the asymmetric group. When we evaluated BCVA, UCVA, spherical equivalent, astigmatism and keratometric readings, the differences between preop and postop values in all parameters were significantly reduced in both groups with statistically significant differences.

We noted that when analyzing nomograms of the symmetric and asymmetric groups, there were no statistically significant differences when comparing the results of both procedures. This is mainly due to similar spherical equivalent and showed that both nomograms were effective. Both groups tolerated spectacles and contact lenses well after the procedures.

In the asymmetric group we implanted intracorneal segments that were thicker in the protrusion area and thinner in the flatter area, taking spherical equivalent into account. This could possibly have led to an overcorrection with the implantation of the thicker segment. When implanting thicker segments in the thinner protrusion area, great skill was used so as not to perforate the cornea or extrude the segment. In the symmetric group we implanted two same thickness segments, also dependent on spherical equivalent. In symmetric implantations there are more articles available that reported success in keratoconus and other ectasias. By implanting thinner segments in the protrusion area, undercorrection was a possibility. The advantage of implanting two segments was that corneal prolate is maintained.

7. References

[1] Sridhar MS, Mahesh S, Bansal AK, Nutheti R, Rao GN Pellucid marginal corneal degeneration. Ophthalmology 2004; 1102-7

[2] Rabinowitz YS, Keratoconus. Surv Ophthalmology 1998; 297-319

[3] Karim Rasheed, Yaron Rabinowitz, MD, Pellucid Marginal Degeneration. Emecine

[4] Santos RM, Bechara SJ, Kara-Jose N. Corneal topography in asymptomatic family members of a patient with pellucid marginal degeneration. Am J Ophthalmology 1999; 205-207.

[5] Kymionis GD, Aslanides IM, Siganos CS, Pallikaris IG. Intacs® for early pellucid marginal degeneration. J Cataract Refract Surg 2004; 230-233

[6] Schlaeppi V., La dystrophie marginale inferieure pellucid de la cornee. Mod Probl Ophthalmology 1957; 672-677

[7] Maguire LJ, Klyce SD, McDonald ME, Kauffmann HE, Corneal topography of pellucid marginal degeneration. Ophthalmology 1987; 519-24

[8] Maeda N, Klyce SD, Tano Y. Detection and classification of mild irregular astigmatism in patients with good visual acuity. Surv Ophthalmology 1998; 53-8

[9] Rodriguez MM, Newsome DA, Krachmer JH.Pellucid marginal cornea degeneration: a clinical pathologic study of two cases. Exp Eye Res 1981; 277-288

[10] Mularoni A, Torreggiani A, Di Biase A, Laffi GL, Tassinari G, Conservative Treatment of Early and Moderate Pellucid Marginal Degeneration. Ophthalmology 2005; 660-666

[11] Rodriguez-Gonzales-Herrero ME, Gutierrez Ortega AR, De Imperial Mora-Figueroa Jm, Surgical treatment of pellucid marginal degeneration associated with cataract [letter]. J Cataract Refract Surg 2000; 309-11

[12] Cameron JA, results of lamellar crescentic resection for pellucid marginal degeneration. IS J Ophthalmology 1992; 296-302

[13] Kremer I, Sperber LT, Laibson PR. Pellucid marginal degeneration treated by lamellar and penetrating keratoplasty [letter]. Arch Ophthalmology 1993; 169-70

[14] Colin J, Cochener B, Savary G, Malet f. Correcting keratoconus with intracorneal rings. J Cataract Refract Surg 2000; 1117-22

[15] Holmes-Higgins DK, Burris TE, INTACS® Study Group. Corneal surface topography and associated visual performance with INTACS® for myopia. Phase III clinical trial results. Ophthalmology 2000; 2061-71

[16] Kymionis GD, Siganos CS, Kounis G, et al. Management of post-LASIK corneal ectasia with Intacs® insert: one year results. Arch Ophthalmology 2003; 332-6.

[17] Rodriguez-Prats J, Galal Ahmed, Garcia-Lledo Magdalena, et al. Intracorneal rings for the correction of pellucid marginal degeneration Cataract Refract Surg 2003; 1421-1424

[18] Burris TE, Baker PC, Ayer CT, et al. Flattening of central corneal curvature with intrastromal corneal rings of increasing thickness: an eye-bank eye study. J Cataract Refract Surg 1993; 182-7.

[19] J.L. Alió, A Artola, A. Hassanein, H Haroun, A Galal, One or two Intacs® segments for the correction of keratoconus. J Cataract Refract Surg 2005; 943-953

[20] Colin J, Velou S, Implantation of Intacs® and a refractive intraocular lens to correct keratoconus. J Cataract Refract Surg 2003; 832-834

[21] Colin J, Cochener B, Savary G, et al. Intacs® inserts for treating keratoconus: one-year results. Ophthalmology 2001; 1409-1414

[22] Sharma M, Boxer Wachler BS. Comparison of single-segment and Double-segment Intacs® for keratoconus and post-LASIK ectasia. Am J Ophthalmology 2006; 891-895

[23] M.S Sridhar, S Mahesh, A.K Bansal, Rishita Nutheti, G.N. Pellucid marginal corneal degeneration. International Center for Advancement of Rural Eye Care, L.V. Prasad Eye Institute, Hyderabad, India. Presented as a poster at: American Academy of Ophthalmology and Pan-American Association of Ophthalmology Joint Meeting, October 20–23, 2002; Orlando.

[24] Swanson M. Developing Solutions for the Ectatic Cornea. Uploaded 2010. Available on web site: http://www.swannkeratoconus.com/main/mnoms.html

15

Toric Intraocular Lenses for the Correction of Astigmatism

Milorad Milivojević,
Miroslav Vukosavljević and Mirko Resan
Eye Clinic, Military Medical Academy, Belgrade, Serbia

1. Introduction

Astigmatism can be corrected with:

1. Glasses and contact lenses
2. Excimer laser refractive procedures (LASIK, PRK)
3. Astigmatic keratotomy
4. Limbal or corneal relaxing and clear corneal incisions
5. Toric intraocular lens

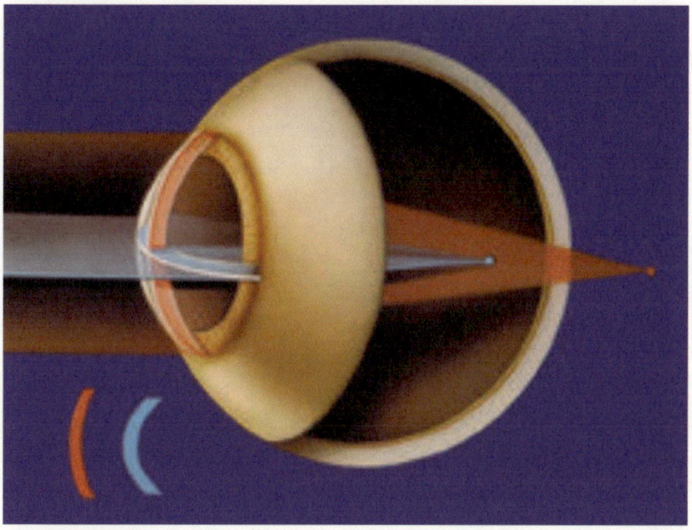

Fig. 1. Eye with astigmatism.

The ideal procedure for the correction of astigmatism should provide: precise and accurate adjustment, safety, predictable outcome, lasting effect and simplicity with an acceptable price. Conventional methods for solving problems such as glasses and/or contact lenses at the present time often do not meet the needs of patients. Whether it is the objective or subjective reasons for a large number of patients tend to avoid wearing glasses or contact lenses.

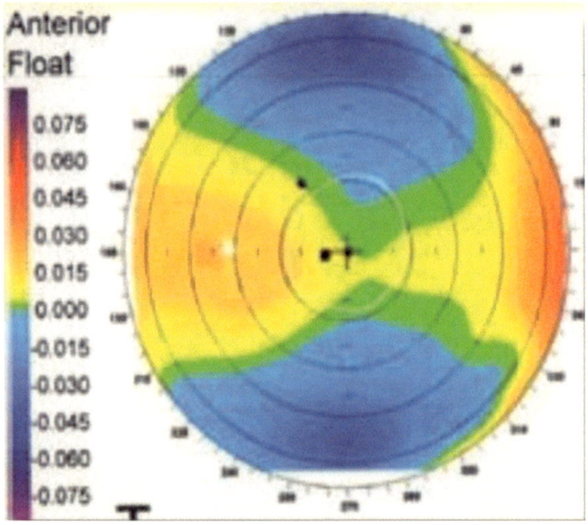

Fig. 2. The topography of corneal astigmatism.

Correcting corneal astigmatism during cataract surgery can increase spectacle independence. For the patient, this has economic benefits as well as desirable cosmetic and practical advantages. Spectacle correction of astigmatism creates meridional magnification, which when coupled with the associated back vertex distance produces retinal images that are asymmetrically magnified and distorted (1).

Company	Intraocular Lens	Range of Spherical IOL Power	Range of Cylindrical IOL Power	Range of Corneal Astigmatism Able to Correct	Percentage of Eyes Susceptible to Correction
Alcon	AcriSof Toric SN60T3/T4/T5 T6/T7T8/T9	+10.0 to +30.0(0.5)	11.5 to 6.0 (1.0)	1.0 to 4.2	34.2
STAAR	AA4203TF AA4203TL	+24.0to+28.5(0.5) +9.5 to 23.5(0.5)	2 and 3.5 2 and 3.5	1.4 and 2.4 1.4 and 2.4	17.1 17.1
Human Optics	Torica-5	-3.0 to +14.0(1.0) +15.0to+25.0(0.5) +26.0to+31.0(1.0)	2.0 to 12.0(0.5)	1.4 to 8.4	22.3
Rayner	T- flex 573T/623T	+6.0 to +26.0(0.5) -10.0 to +35.0(0.5)	1.0 to 6.0(1.0) 1.0 to11.0(0.25)	0.7 to 4.2 0.7 to 7.7	40.5 41.2
Zeiss	Acri.Comfort643TLC Acri.Comfort646TLC	0 to +40.0 -10.0 to +32.0	1.0 to 12.0(0.5) 1.0 to 12.0(0.5)	0.7 to 8.4 0.7 to 8.4	41.2 41.2

Table 1. Range of spherical and cylindrical powers and corneal astigmatism capable of correcting for the toric IOL on the market (1).

According to the literature, it is estimated that 15 to 22.2% of patients who are candidates for cataract surgery have astigmatism greater than 1.50 D. This indicates that a large number of patients still has blurred vision after cataract surgery due to residual astigmatism and require operative correction of distance vision glasses or lenses. (2,3). Since the corneal limbal relaxing incision often have an unpredictable effect on the postoperative visual acuity, and the use of Excimer laser refractive surgery is often not feasible because of it is often contraindicated in elderly people, expensive procedure, requires high technological equipment and expertise of medical personnel. Toric intraocular lenses are the correction of choice for high levels of astigmatism. They promise a predictable method of astigmatic correction with minimal impact to the cornea. However, the effectiveness of a toric IOL is dependent on its orientation. (1,4)

2. Surgical aspects of implantation of toric intraocular lenses

Cataract surgery with implantation of toric intraocular lenses is identical to the normal procedure and requires no special training (4). The difference is reflected in the preoperative treatment, and in celebration of the cylinder axis, which is adjusted to the patient's eye. Toric IOLs need precise positioning to achieve optimal visual results. In accordance with the corneal measurements, reference markers on opposite sides of the pupil need to be established to demarcate the correct axis for IOL orientation. Eye rotation occurs in a supine position and so these markers need to be established pre-operatively. The slit lamp beam axis graticule can be dialed to the correct axis or a bespoke eyepiece graticule can be used to determine where to place the markers, which can be applied to the cornea or conjunctiva using ink or with scratches. Ink should be applied at the last possible minute as it can diffuse by 10° or disappear before implantation is complete. As an alternative, a Neodymium:Yttrium-Aluminum-Garnet (Nd:YAG) laser can be used to mark the cornea. It has been suggested that this improves the accuracy and definition of the markers. Specific toric axis marking instruments exist. One step methods, such as the Devgan Axis Marker (Accutome, Pennsylvania, USA) and the Gerten Pendulum Marker (Geuder, Heidelberg, Germany) are used pre-operatively to determine the required axis. They are dependent on a vertical head position when applied to the cornea. Two-step methods require marking the cornea at the zero and 180 degree positions pre-operatively and then aligning a degree gauge with these markings intra-operatively to establish the correct position (1). The iris architecture is intricate and full marking is done manually or by using the instrument in a sitting position (1,5). Another difference lies in the fact that the shaft of toric IOL to coincide with the axis of the cylinder, marked preoperatively. This is achieved by the end of the operation during the removal of viscoelastic. There are two main surgical factors that can influence IOL rotation. In the early post-operative period careful wound construction is essential. Following surgery, the IOP can fluctuate and in 6.3 per cent of patients, it drops to below 5 mmHg. It is important to emphasize that it is necessary to remove viscoelastic a rotation for maximum stability. Viscoelastic lag could lead to undesirable postoperative implant rotation, and therefore should be brought into question and the desired outcome (1).

Consideration of IOL haptic design is very important when trying to prevent postoperative lens rotation. Over time, the capsular bag contracts to enclose and secure the IOL, however, before this contraction occurs there is potentfor rotation (6). To prevent rotation immediately after implantation, it is important to maximize the contact between the IOL haptic and the capsular bag. A polymethyl methacrylate (PMMA) IOL creates the most friction with the bag, followed by acrylic, with silicon causing the least (7). It is believed that if the implant rotates by more than 30 degrees postoperatively, the effect of cylindrical lenses is lost. The third difference relates to the calculation of the refractive lens, the strength and axis cylinder. As a rule, keratometry very carefully set manually, not automatic keratometer. Must also be taken into account and astigmatism, which will occur as a consequence of the main corneal incision. IOL manufacturers have developed calculators to determine the refractive power lens (as spherical and cylindrical components), and determine the shaft in which the implant should be placed. The data are entered to the calculator are manually specified value keratometry, spherical components required strength, where you are planning a major incision. These calculators are easily and freely available for use on the Internet (8).

3. The outcome of intraocular implantation of toric IOL

When it comes to the outcome of implantation of toric intraocular lenses, it is essential to assess the following parameters:

3.1 Rotational stability in capsular bag

3.1.1 Plate haptic IOLs

Plate haptic IOLs demonstrate excellent long-term stability. In comparison with open-loop haptics, plate haptic IOLs are not as susceptible to the effects of compression from the capsular bag.

The first commercially available toric IOL was the STAAR 4203TF (STAAR Surgical, Company, California, USA), which achieved FDA approval in 1998. It is a biconvex, silicone, plate haptic toric IOL, 10.8 mm in length, with two 1.15-mm positioning holes. The lens is available with a torus of either 2.00 or 3.50 D, which corrects levels of corneal astigmatism between 1.50 and 3.50 D. The lens demonstrates excellent long-term stability once fixation within the capsular bag has been established, 30 however, in the early postoperative period, the lens demonstrates a relatively high incidence of rotation. In its FDA trial, 24 per cent of the lenses rotated more than 10°, 12 per cent more than 20° and 8 per cent more than 30° (9).

The AT-TORBI (Carl Zeiss Meditec, Berlin, Germany) (previously the ACri comfort toric IOL) is an acrylic, bi-toric, plate haptic IOL, 11 mm in length, possessing two positioning holes on the haptic. It is a microincisional lens, and it can be inserted through a 1.5-mm incision. The AT-TORBI has a 6.0-mm optic, and can correct high levels of astigmatism, as it is available with a torus of 1.00 to 12.00 D in 0.50-D steps. Large-scale studies are required to demonstrate the effectiveness of this lens but early results are very promising. In a pilot study involving 21 eyes with 2.00 to 9.00 D of corneal astigmatism, only one lens rotated more than 5° between day one and six months post-operatively, with 76.1 per cent of these subjects achieving a postoperative uncorrected vision of 20/40 or better (10).

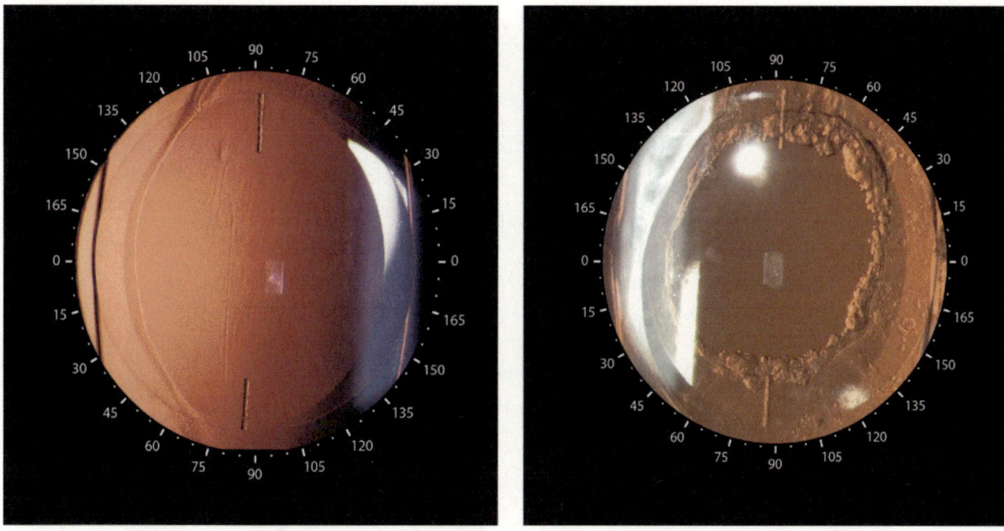

Fig. 3. Slit-lamp retroillumination photographs of a Staar toric intraocular lens with a superimposed digital protractor before (left) and after (right) a circular neodymium-yttrium-aluminum-garnet posterior capsulotomy (9).

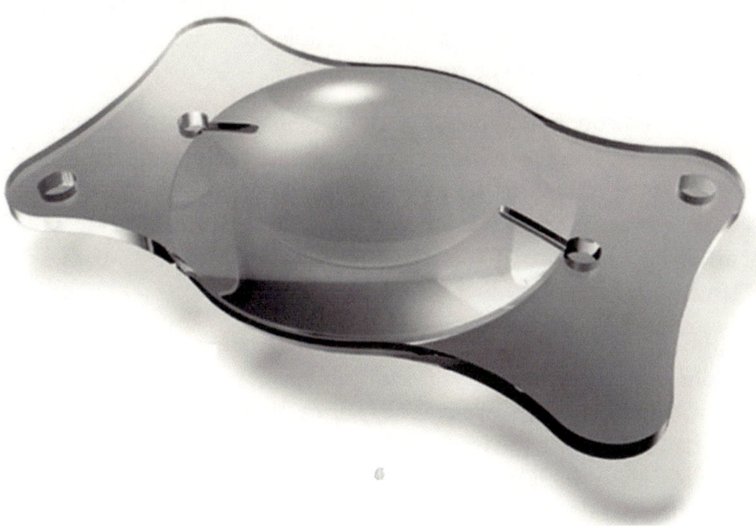

Fig. 4. The ACri comfort toric IOL (10).

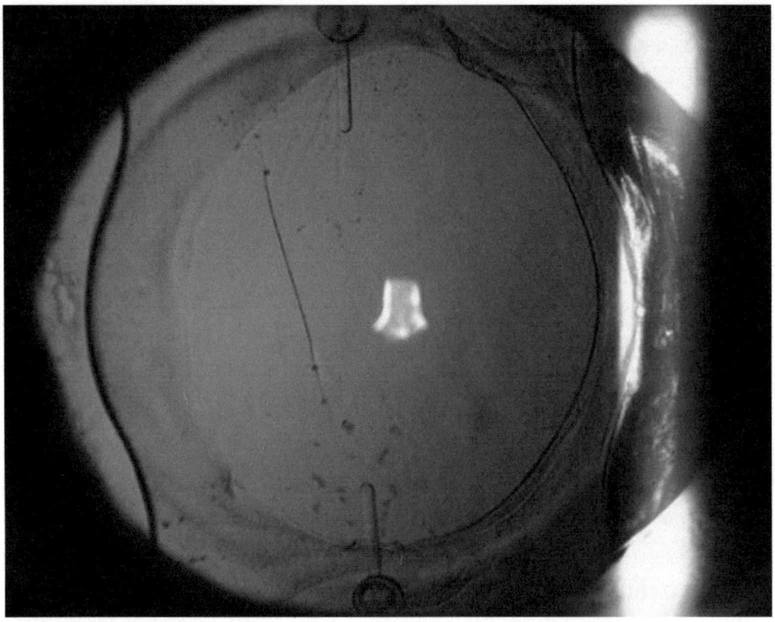

Fig. 5. The ACri comfort toric IOL in situ 3 months postoperatively (10).

3.1.2 Open loop haptic lenses

Open loop haptic lenses compared with previous models (plate haptic IOLs) demonstrate excellent early rotational stability in comparison to plate haptics. The longer loop haptics ensure immediate contact between haptic and capsular bag, maximizing friction in the early postoperative period, however, they are susceptible to late rotation caused by the compression of the capsular bag (11).

The AcrySof toric IOL (Alcon, Fort Worth, USA) is a single-piece acrylic toric IOL with open loop L-shaped haptics. It has a posterior toric surface with three available toric powers 1.50, 2.25 and 3.00 D. It is a 13mm in length with a 6.0mm optic. The AcrySof toric has demonstrated excellent rotational stability results. During its FDA trial, 81.9% of lenses rotated less than 5° and only 2.9% rotated over 10° and only 0.8% of these lenses were repositioned (2,8).

The Torica S (Human Optics, Erlangen, Germany) otherwise known as the Microcyl Toric 6116 (Human Optics), is a three-piece, silicon, Z-shaped open loop haptic toric IOL. It is 11.6mm in length with a 6.0mm optic. The Torica S has a novel haptic design with undulations designed to increase the friction between lens and bag. It has been reported that these undulations maintain the IOLs position but make it difficult to rotate the lens within the bag. To prevent the haptic undulations from causing trauma when rotating the lens, it is recommended that they are compressed against the optic and held away from the capsular bag until the lens is in the required position. In a study of 21 eyes (14 subjects) no lens rotated more than 5°(12).

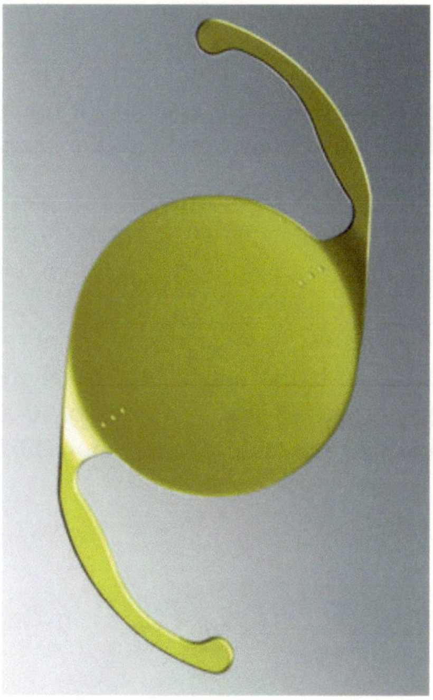

Fig. 6. AcrySof toric IOL.

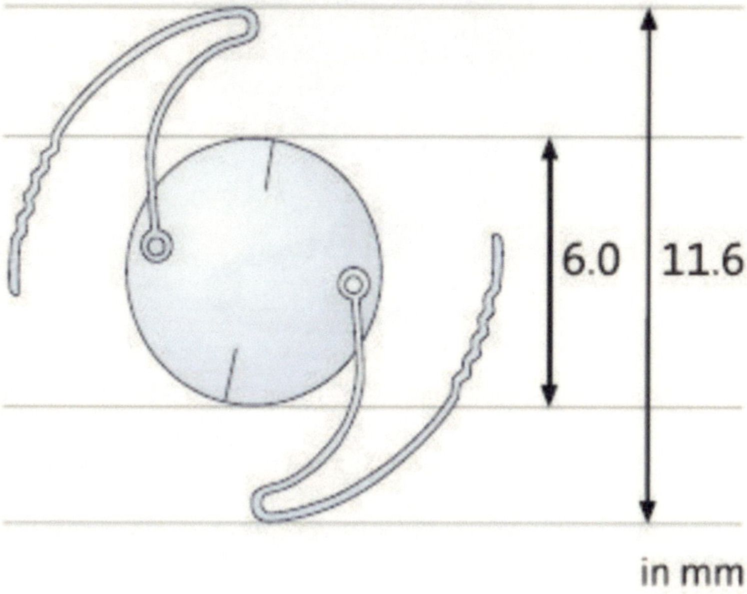

Fig. 7. The Torica-S IOL.

3.1.3 Closed loop haptics IOLs

Closed-loop haptics are a relatively new addition to the toric IOL market. These lenses are typically longer than the plate haptics, which should give good initial contact. The loops have a second insertion on the IOL that may resist capsular compression.

The T-flex toric (Rayner, Hove, UK) is a single-piece, acrylic, closed-loop haptic with anti-vaulting haptic technology. It is available in two sizes; the 573T has a 5.75-mm optic and 12 mm haptics, and the 623T has a 6.25-mm optic and 12.5 mm haptic. The anterior surface of the optic houses the toric surface, which is available with a torus of one to 11 D. The anti-vaulting haptic technology is designed to reduce the effect of compression using a lock and key system. Compression will push the outside of the haptic against the inner haptic, locking it into place. It has been reported that in a group of 10 subjects no lens rotated more than 5° between one week and two years after implantation (13).

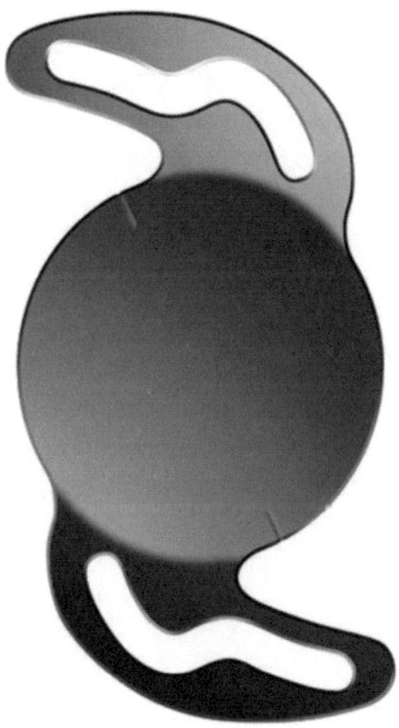

Fig. 8. Rayner T-*flex*® Aspheric Toric IOL.

The Akreos (Bausch & Lomb, Rochester, USA) aspheric platform is a single piece acrylic, closed loop haptic IOL. It has a 6.0-mm optic and is 11 mm in length with a 360° square edge. The IOL is currently being assessed for its viability as a platform for housing a toric surface. A multicenter study has examined the rotational stability of the Akreos haptic housing from one day to six months post-operatively in 97 eyes. This lens was shown to be stable, as 96 per cent of the IOLs rotated no more than 5° and 99% no more than 10° (14).

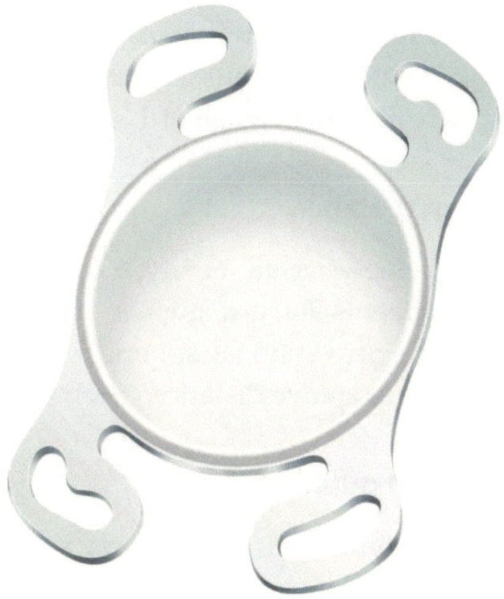

Fig. 9. Akreos™ aspheric IOL.

Tsinopoulos and colleagues (15) reported a new procedure for intra-operative toric intraocular lens (IOL) axis assessment in order to achieve optimal implantation. IOL implantation procedure was directly recorded. An assessor estimated the angle formed by the marked 0–180 axis and the toric IOL axis after implantation with the use of the appropriate software. If IOL implantation was assessed to be inaccurate, the surgeon was advised to correct IOL positioning by rotating the IOL clockwise. The assessment procedure was repeated until accurate IOL positioning was achieved.

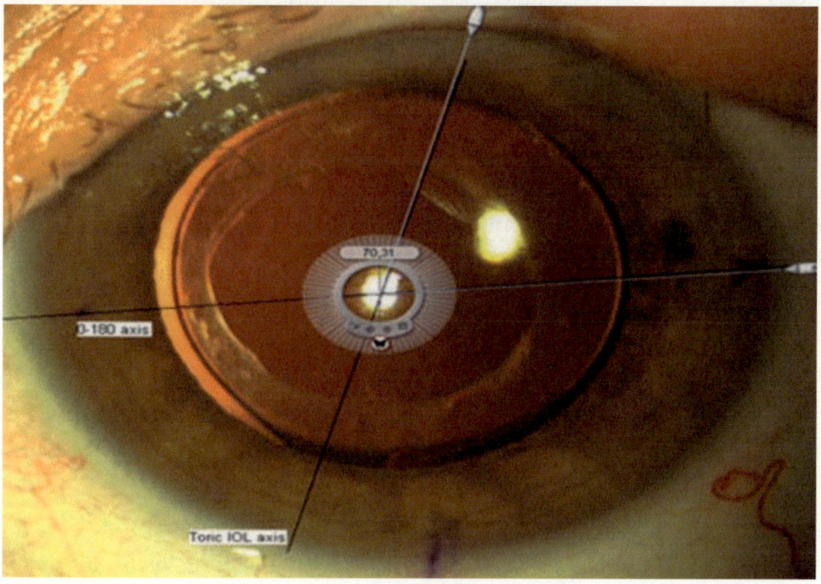

Fig. 10. Intra-operative toric implantation assessment with the use of the appropriate software (15).

3.2 The reduction of absolute residual astigmatism

The average absolute residual astigmatism after implantation of toric intraocular lenses is less than 0.55D. In patients who have significant astigmatism, and implanted them classic spherical lenses residual astigmatism is an average of 1.22D (1).

3.3 Uncorrected visual acuity at distance

Ninety-four percent of patients achieve visual acuity ≥ 0.5 with no correction, which is a remarkable result. Also, these patients have a greater vision improvement at all levels compared with patients who have conventional spherical lens. In 97% of patients whose toric lenses implanted in both eyes maximize distance vision without correction (1,2).

3.3.1 Stability and predictability of outcome

Patients who have significant astigmatism after cataract surgery have the option for correcting glasses or contact lenses. However, for many patients who expect excellent postoperative vision this is unacceptable solution.

Relaxing incisions that had previously been strongly represented in the correction of astigmatism now use fewer surgeons (40%) for the following reasons:

- Unpredictable results in a significant number of cases
- The problem of regression, astigmatism, especially in patients with severe preoperative astigmatism
- Inability to correct high astigmatism
- Paracentral incisions can correct high astigmatism, but more complications
- Healing of incisions can be problematic, since it is predominantly an elderly patient
- Patients with steep corneas and asymmetriastigmatism are not good candidates (1,16).

When speaking of the Excimer laser for the correction of astigmatism, the method is effective and safe, but laser is expensive and this way the correction is often unavailable for most patients (17).

3.3.2 Economic evaluation of toric intraocular lens

Pineda and colleagues (18) assessed the economic value of improved uncorrected visual acuity among patients with cataract and preexisting astigmatism treated with toric intraocular lenses (IOLs) compared with conventional monofocal IOLs. They concluded that toric IOLs reduce lifetime economic costs by reducing the need for glasses or contact lenses following cataract removal. These results can inform physicians and patients regarding the value of toric IOLs in the treatment of cataract and preexisting astigmatism.

Laurendeau and collegues (19) in their study concluded that bilateral toric IOL implants in astigmatic patients decreased spectacle dependence for distance vision and the need for complex spectacles. The economic consequences for patients depended on the national spectacle costs usually incurred after cataract surgery.

4. Conclusion

Toric intraocular lenses are accurate, reliable, predictable, permanently correcting astigmatism in cataract patients who are operated, while the flow of the operation is not extended, or require special training for surgeons already trained. Rotational stability of an IOL is the primary determinant of the refractive outcome. The surgeon should also keep in mind that the final outcome is very important and proper selection of patients, including patients with irregular astigmatism due to the scar tissue forming of the cornea, keratoconus, pellucid marginal degeneration, etc,. New available aspheric toric lens offer a better quality of vision postoperatively (reduction of spherical aberration, further improving contrast sensitivity, and uncorrected visual acuity at a distance). Toric IOLs reduce lifetime economic costs by reducing the need for glasses or contact lenses following cataract removal.

5. References

[1] Buckhurst PJ. Wolffsohn JS. Davies LN, Naroo SA. Surgical correction of astigmatism during cataract surgery. Clin Exp Optom 2010; 93: 409–418.

[2] Bauer NJC, De Vries NE, Webers CAB, Hendrikse F, Nuijts RMMA. Astigmatism management in cataract surgery with the AcrySof toric intraocular lens. J Cataract Refract Surg 2008; 34:1483–1488.

[3] Masket S, Wang L, Belani S. Induced astigmatism with 2.2- and 3.0-mm coaxial phacoemulsification incisions. J Refract Surg 2009; 25: 21–24.

[4] Amesbury EC, Miller KM. Correction of astigmatism at the time of cataract surgery. Curr Opin Ophthalmol 2009; 20: 19–24.

[5] Graether JM. Simplified system of marking the cornea for a toric intraocular lens. J Cataract Refract Surg 2009; 35: 1498–1500.

[6] Patel CK, Ormonde S, Rosen PH, Bron AJ. Postoperative intraocular lens rotation: a randomized comparison of plate and loop haptic implants. Ophthalmology 1999; 106: 2190–2195.

[7] Oshika T, Nagata T, Ishii Y. Adhesion of lens capsule to intraocular lenses of polymethylmethacrylate, silicone and acrylic foldable materials: an experimental study. Br J Ophthalmol 1998; 82: 549–553.

[8] AcrySof Toric Single-Piece Natural IOL Product Information. Fort Worth, TX: Alcon Laboratories, Inc.; 2005.

[9] Jampaulo M, Olson MD, Miller KM. Long-term Staar toric intraocular lens rotational stability. Am J Ophthalmol 2008; 146: 550–553.

[10] Alio JL, Agdeppa MCC, Pongo VC, Kady BE. Microincision cataract surgery with toric intraocular lens implantation for correcting moderate and high astigmatism: pilot study. J Cataract Refract Surg 2010; 36: 44–52.

[11] Chang DF. Comparative rotational stability of single-piece open-loop acrylic and plate-haptic silicone toric intraocular lenses. J Cataract Refract Surg 2008; 34: 1842– 1847.

[12] De Silva DJ, Ramkissoon YD, Bloom PA. Evaluation of a toric intraocular lens with a Z-haptic. J Cataract Refract Surg 2006; 32: 1492–1498.

[13] Narendran R, Vyas A, Bacon P. Centration, rotational stability and outcomes of Rayner T-flexTM toric lens implantation: 2 year results. Proceedings of the XXVII congress of the ESCRS, Barcelona, 2009.

[14] Buckhurst PJ, Wolffsohn JS, Naroo SA, Davies LN. Rotational and centration stability of an aspheric intraocular lens with a simulated toric design. J Cataract Refract Surg 2010; 36: 1523-1528.
[15] Tsinopoulos IT, Symeonidis C, Tsaousis KT, Tsakpinis D, Ziakas NG, Dimitrakos SA. Intra-operative assessment of toric intra-ocular lens implantation. Indian J Ophthalmol 2011; 59: 60-62.
[16] Kaufmann C, Peter J, Ooi K, Phipps S, Cooper P, Goggin M. Limbal relaxing incisions versus on-axis incisions to reduce corneal astigmatism at the time of cataract surgery. J Cataract Refract Surg 2005; 31: 2261–2265.
[17] Sanders DR, Sanders ML. Comparison of the toric implantable collamer lens and custom ablation LASIK for myopic astigmatism. J Refract Surg 2008; 24: 773–778.
[18] Pineda R, Denevich S, Lee WC, Waycaster C, Pashos CL. Economic evaluation of toric intraocular lens. Arch Ophthalmol. 2010; 128: 834-840.
[19] Laurendeau C, Lafuma A, Berdeaux G. Modelling lifetime cost consequences of toric compared with standard IOLs in cataract surgery of astigmatic patients in four Europian countries. Journal of Medical Economics 2009; 12: 230–237.

16

Amblyopia and Foveal Thickness

Elina Landa[1], Shimon Rumelt[1],
Claudia Yahalom[2], Elaine Wong[3] and Lionel Kowal[3]
[1]*Department of Ophthalmology, Western Galilee – Nahariya Medical Center, Nahariya,*
[2]*Department of Ophthalmology, Hadassah University Hospital, Jerusalem,*
[3]*Department of Ophthalmology, Eye and Ear Institute, The University of Melbourne, Melbourne,*
[1,2]*Israel*
[3]*Australia*

1. Introduction

1.1 Definition

Amblyopia in Greek is dullness of vision. It is defined as poor unilateral or bilateral visual acuity due to poor perception in the presence of normal appearing globe.[1] It is caused by poor visual perception during the critical postnatal period required for maturation of the visual pathways and cortex. Clear and corresponding image is required for visual system development in animals including primates.

1.2 Epidemiology

The prevalence of amblyopia in the general population is probably between 2 and 2.5%. The wider range of 1-4% reflects differences in the degree of amblyopia, the studied population and the location. These figures represent the average of the prevalence in the different studies. The frequency of disorder has a socioeconomic impact. These patients have a greater risk for legal blindness if the fellow eye develops a blinding condition or sustain trauma. Indeed, patients with amblyopia as monocular patients are at a greater risk for trauma in the fellow eye although their visual field may be full.

1.3 Development of the visual system

The postnatal visual system development differs in different animals. In humans, the visual acuity improves usually until the age of 5 and this reflects the maturation of both the retina and the visual pathways.[2] The most critical period for amblyopia is the first 2 to 3 years of life.[1] The sensitivity of the visual system to abnormal perception is decreasing gradually afterwards. One should distinguish between the period when amblyopia may develop, which is until 9 years of age (although in most patients, it appears by the age of 5) and the period in which it is treatable, probably until the age of 17.[3]

1.4 Classification

Amblyopia is a result of three mechanisms: deprivation (obscuration of the image on its way to the retina (i.e., ptosis and media opacities), strabismus and refractive (anisometropic or isoamteropic) all causing blurred or non-corresponding images on the fovea.[1] The pathophysiology common to all of these is abnormal binocular interaction and/ or vision deprivation. Strabismic amblyopia occurs in the non-fixating eye and is always unilateral. It occurs in tropia and is more common in esotropia than in exotropia and indeed esotropia is neonatal while exotropia may be neonatal or acquired later in life. It is caused by signaling inhibition of the deviating eye to avoid confusion because of different foveal images between the eyes. Strabismic amblyopia is applied only to cases where the amblyopia is a result of strabismus and not vice versa. In refractive amblyopia, signaling inhibition of the blurred image occurs and in deprivation, there is usually no image. Anisometropia of +2.00, -3.00 and astigmatism of 1.5D or more are associated with amblyopia. The presence of astigmatism causes amblyopia in the astigmatic meridian called meridional amblyopia. Isoametropia of +4.00, -8.00 and astigmatism of 2D or more are associated with bilateral amblyopia. Lesser amount of hypermetropia than myopia is associated with amblyopia because the inability to focus images on the fovea at any distance. While strabismic amblyopia and most of the anisometropic amblyopia are unilateral, isoametropic and some of the deprivative amblyopia are bilateral. Deprivative amblyopia is usually the most profound and most resistant to treatment of all three forms of amblyopia. If it is present in the first 3 months, irreversible nystagmus develops. The unilateral cases are usually the worst.

2. Clinical manifestations

The visual acuity is poorer in the amblyopic eye than in the fellow eye or than in normal eyes and cannot be corrected to full with spectacles or contact lenses. A poorer visual acuity is considered if the visual acuity is less in two Snellen lines or more. Differences in one line may just be fluctuation and within the normal deviation and this is true not only for amblyopia but for all other instances as well. The subject uses the fellow better eye for fixation. The patient sees single signs on the Snellen chart better than several signs in a row (crowding phenomenon or abnormal contour interaction). This is caused by larger receptive fields (larger group of photoreceptors working as a single unit) and lateral inhibition by adjacent fields on the fixating field. Under dim light, the visual acuity decreases in both eyes but the visual acuity of amblyopic eye becomes similar to the normal eye. Thus the decrease in visual acuity is slower in the amblyopic eye than in a normal eye. The use of neutral density filters decreases the visual acuity in the amblyopic eye in much lesser extent compared with eyes with other diseases. In addition, amblyopic eyes have decreased contrast sensitivity, perception of brightness and have longer reaction time.

Other parameters are normal and similar to normal eyes including light perception (visual threshold) and visual field. An afferent pupillary defect is not supposed to occur but is a variable finding.

3. Treatment

Bilateral amblyopia is treated by eliminating the cause of blurred image (removal of the deprivation cause, strabismus surgery or refractive error correction). Unilateral amblyopia is treated similarly along with periodical patching or other penalization of the fellow sound eye. Penalization of the sound eye is usually performed by instilling once drop of atropine sulfate 1% one a day at bedtime. This causes cycloplegia and blurred image in the sound eye and forces the visual system of the amblyopic eye to act. Treatment should be initiated immediately when the condition is diagnosed. The elimination of the deprivative obstacle should be performed as early as possible (usually 2-3 weeks after birth). In strabismic amblyopia, anti-amblyopic treatment is initiated when the condition is diagnosed long before the surgery for strabismus. The reasons for this are improving the possibility to gain binocular vision if visual acuity is improved, easiness to determine the fixation patters, and the strabismus serves as a reminder to the parents on the importance of treatment. Surgery is performed only after achieving alternating fixation and equal visual acuity.

The length of patching or other penalization depends on the severity of the amblyopia. It is increased in direct proportion with the degree of the amblyopia. The follow-up frequency is also increased as the length of patching increases. Amblyopia is more easily reversible if it occurs later (ages 6-9) than earlier in life. Improvement of visual acuity should be both in single and multiple signs on Snellen chart and should be permanent. However, regression may occur and requires re-treatment.

Occlusion may be for full-time (all the day) for several days with one day off, or part time (several hours per day). Full-time occlusion is preserved for severe amblyopia with no binocular vision such as deprivative amblyopia. Full-time occlusion should not exceed one week per one year of age. Part-time treatment is preferred according to the Pediatric Eye Disease Investigator Group (PEDIG) studies because it has a similar outcome as full-time occlusion with less risk for development of amblyopia in the normal fellow eye, especially in the presence of binocular vision and mild amblyopia. Six hours per day of occlusion are sufficient for severe amblyopia of less than 20/100 and 2-3 hours per day for moderate one (better than 20/100). Contact lenses may be employed in anisometropia of more than 3.00D to prevent aniseikonia. However, this is more demanding treatment. Bilateral amblyopia in isoammteropia is usually not treated with occlusion and improves slowly spontaneously once refractive correction has been applied. In all cases, it is essential to rule out the development of amblyopia in the sound eye during treatment.

Obtaining compliance is difficult especially at the beginning of the treatment. The compliance becomes better as visual acuity of the amblyopic eye improves. Children try to remove or pick through the occluder. Therefore, it is better to use eye drops as penalization or a skin sticker rather than a sticker to the eyeglass. A full cooperation is required from the parents. They should be insisting on meticulous treatment for the full period. It is best to occlude when the child is at home under supervision of the parents and to occlude when the child is performing near tasks such as reading or doing homework. A close follow-up is required to ascertain improvement in visual acuity of the amblyopic eye and prevention of developing amblyopia in the fellow eye. In general, the follow-up intervals are one week per each year of life (e.g., a 2-year-old child is followed every 2 weeks). The follow-up includes visual acuity in each eye with full cycloplegic correction after refraction. If the visual acuity decreases, the reason for it should be disclosed. If the correction is not sufficient, it should be adjusted accordingly. If it is sufficient, an adjustment of the anti-amblyopic treatment should be performed. The length of occlusion is gradually decreased if the visual acuity improves to the desired level and no regression is observed in follow-up visits. Occlusion is gradually tapered according to the patient's response. Gradual decrease in occlusion time has been demonstrated to be associated with less recurrence rate than abrupt determination. If regression is noted, the treatment is re-initiated and continued over the vulnerable period (up to the age of 17). Follow-up until the age of 17 is necessary even if the optimal results have been achieved. Recurrence occurs in up to 75% of the patients usually within the first 13 months.[4] If treatment has not been successful after several (usually 6) months, it may be abandoned and visual function will not improve thereafter.

In animal models, L-dopa and bicuculline have been demonstrated to reverse amblyopia.

However, they have not been used in humans because the first one showed only a temporary effect and the second can cause seizures.

4. Prevention

Prevention of amblyopia is of outmost importance. Screening of red reflex at birth should be done to all neonates. Screening programs at preschool and school children are also important.

5. Background

To date, no changes in gross anatomy of the eye were found in the human amblyopic eye. When optical coherence tomography (OCT) was employed to evaluate the overall macular thickness, volume and the retinal nerve fiber layer (RNFL) thickness, it was found that all were similar in one study between strabismic amblyopic and the fellow eyes in 14 patients.[5] Another study did report thicker RNFL in amblyopic eyes than in normal fellow eyes.[6] When the differences in RNFL thickness were compared between amblyopic eyes and normal eyes of other subjects, they were found to be statistically insignificant.[7] In this study, the foveal thickness in the amblyopic eyes was similar to normal control eyes ($p=0.551$), but the authors did not compare it with the normal fellow eye. It would be expected that any differences in the anatomy in vivo between amblyopic and normal eyes would be microscopic. One should also consider the reproducibility of the OCT and the normal variations between normal eyes at different ages. Therefore, to show differences, a comparison should be made first with the fellow normal eye in unilateral amblyopia.

We compared the foveal thickness of amblyopic eyes with the fellow normal eye by OCT. Furthermore, we compared the foveal thickness of amblyopic eyes that underwent successful occlusion therapy with amblyopic eyes refractory to treatment. Such a study has not been previously reported according to Medline® search. The rationale for the current study was that even if the gross anatomy is normal, subtle structural variations such as foveal hypoplasia might exist.

6. Methods

In a prospective study, we compared the foveal thickness of amblyopic eyes with the fellow normal eyes in unilateral strabismic and anisometropic amblyopia by OCT (spectral OCT/SLO, OTI, Ophthalmic Technologies, Toronto, Canada). The inclusion criteria included best-corrected visual acuity (BCVA) of 20/80 or less in the involved eye, BCVA of 20/25 or better of the fellow eye, normal eye exam of each eye and no explanation for the low visual acuity except for amblyopia, presence of one of the causes for amblyopia (anisometropia of more than -3.00D or more than +1.00D, or strabismus), no other ocular, neurologic or systemic disorders, and children between 4 and 10 years of age who can undergo OCT and be treated for amblyopia and that followed the treatment orders. All other patients were excluded from the study. Ocular and general medical history were obtained and the patients underwent a complete ophthalmic examination of each eye including visual acuity by Snellen charts, pupil reactions, slit lamp examination, dilated funduscopic examination with a slit lamp biomicroscopy and indirect ophthalmoscopy.

All eyes were analyzed by OCT. Measurement was performed at the thinnest point of the macular center, representing the fovea. Several topographic 3D, linear and radial scans were obtained. The acceptance criteria of OCT included a central reflex, signal strength of at least 4 and standard deviation of the foveal thickness of less than 10% of the mean for each individual.

Amblyopic patients with refractive errors were treated by refractive full cycloplegic correction. Amblyopic patients with strabismus underwent strabismus surgery. All patients underwent occlusion (patching) therapy of the sound eye at least 6 for months and were followed according to previous recommendations.[3,8-10] Successful treatment was defined as an improvement in visual acuity in the amblyopic eye in at least 2 Snellen lines. The follow-up time ranged between 12 and 54 months.

Statistical analysis was performed with SPSS version 11.5 program (SPSS Inc., Chicago, IL, USA). Paired sample T-test was used for samples larger than 15 and Wilcoxon signed rank test was employed for smaller samples. Two-tailed $p<0.05$ was considered as statistically significant. Approval by the IRB/Ethics Committee was obtained and the patients' parents received a full explanation about the exam.

7. Patients

Nineteen children aged 4-10 with unilateral amblyopia were included. Ten patients had anisometropic (refractive) and 9 had strabismic amblyopia. Eight patients had successful occlusion therapy, while the other 11 had unsuccessful treatment.

8. Results

The foveal thickness in amblyopic eyes was 201±42 μm (average±SD) and in the normal fellow eyes 174±27 μm. The fovea was statistically thicker in the amblyopic eyes of whatever cause than in the normal fellow eye (p=0.011, paired sample T-test). The foveal thickness in eyes with anisometropic amblyopia (n=10) was 194±45 μm and in the fellow eyes of the same patients 167±23 μm (p=0.059, Wilcoxon signed rank test). The foveal thickness in eyes with strabismic amblyopia (n=9) was 210±39 μm and in the fellow eyes of the same patients 181± 30 μm (p=0.070, Wilcoxon signed rank test).

Eight (42%) of the 19 patients experienced improvement in BCVA after occlusion therapy. Six of the 8 had anisometropic and 2 had strabismic amblyopia. From the group of 11 (58%) patients that did not show improvement in BCVA, 4 had anisometropic and 7 had strabismic amblyopia (p=1.000). The foveal thickness in the patients who showed no improvement in BCVA after treatment was 216±41 μm and in their fellow eyes 176±31 μm (p=0.016, Wilcoxon signed rank test) (Table 1). In those who showed improvement, the foveal thickness in the amblyopic eyes was 181±36 μm and in their fellow eyes 171±21 μm (p=0.297, Wilcoxon signed rank test). Examples of the topographic 3-dimensional OCT maps of an amblyopic and normal fellow eye are seen in figures 1 and 2.

Parameter	Amblyopic eye	Fellow eye	P-value
Total (n=19)	201±42	174±27	0.011
Refractive (n=10)	194±45	167±23	0.059
Strabismic (n=9)	210±39	181±30	0.070
VA improvement (n=8)	216±41	176±31	0.016
No VA improvement (n=11)	181±36	171±21	0.297

Mean±SD in μm

Table 1. The foveal thickness in μm as measured by optical coherence tomography in amblyopic versus the normal fellow eye.

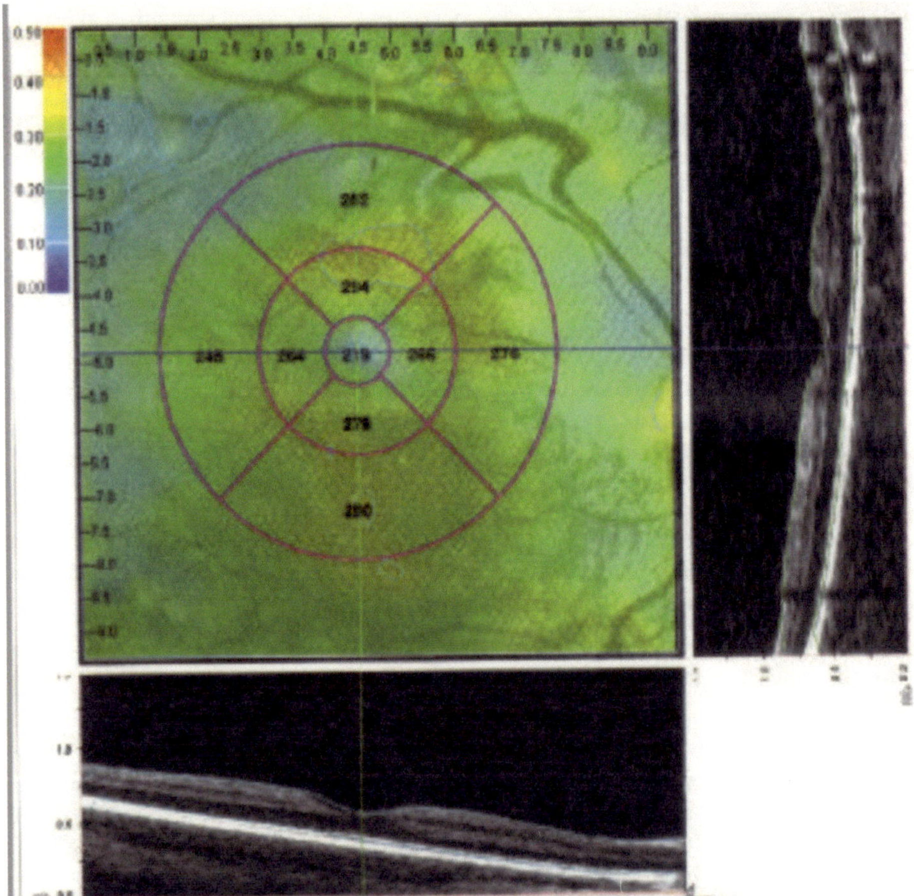

	Avg thick µ	Volume µL
Center	195	
Center circle	219	0.161
Superior inner	294	0.451
Temporal inner	264	0.411
Inferior inner	279	0.428
Nasal inner	266	0.414
Superior outer	252	1.327
Temporal outer	245	1.3
Inferior outer	280	1.474
Nasal outer	276	1.459
Totals	265	7.426

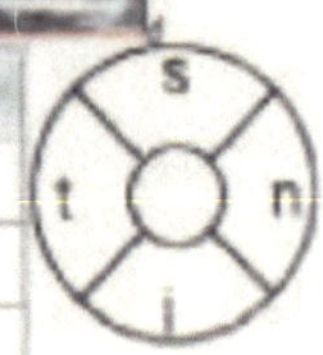

Fig. 1. A topographic 3-dimensional OCT image of the right amblyopic eye of a 10-year-old boy that was refractory to treatment measured a foveal thickness of 195 µm.

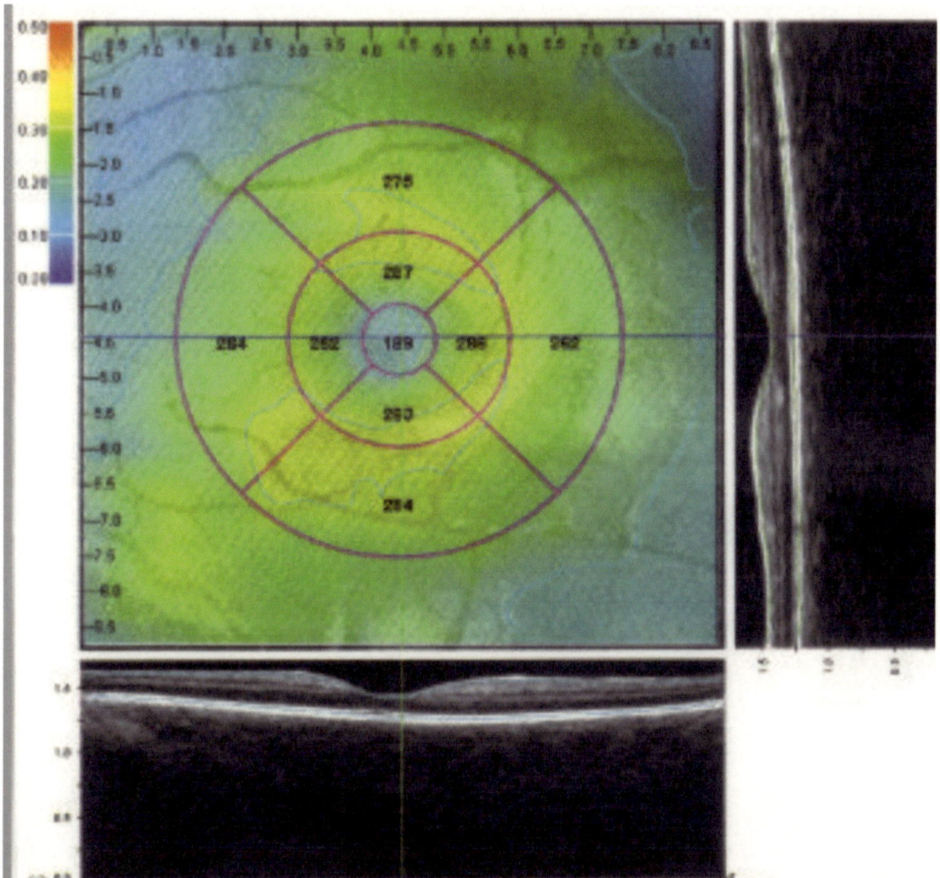

	Avg thick µ	Volume µL
Center	167	
Center circle	189	0.142
Superior inner	287	0.444
Temporal inner	286	0.449
Inferior inner	283	0.437
Nasal inner	262	0.411
Superior outer	275	1.459
Temporal outer	262	1.397
Inferior outer	284	1.504
Nasal outer	264	1.408
Totals	271	7.65

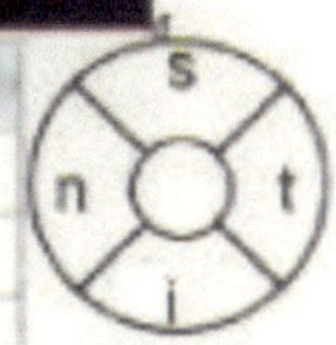

Fig. 2. A topographic 3-dimensional OCT image of the left normal eye of the same patient as in figure 1 measured a foveal thickness of 167 µm. The fovea was thinner in this normal eye than the amblyopic eye.

9. Discussion

Amblyopic eyes are classically considered as having a normal structure.[1] The only changes that have been found were smaller parvocellular cells in layers II, III and V in the ipsilateral lateral geniculate body, layers I, IV and VI of the contralateral lateral geniculate body and reduction in the number of cells in the primary (striate) visual cortex V1 receiving input from the affected eye.[11,12] Reduction was noted in the number of cells receiving binocular input. An increase in the number of cortical cells responding to a contour orientation also occurs. Positron emission tomography demonstrated a reduced cortical activity under visual stimulation of the amblyopic eye.[13]

We found that in the amblyopic eyes the fovea was thicker than in the normal fellow eyes. This was common both for anisometropic and strabismic eyes. Our finding is supported by a recent study in 3,529 children aged 6-12 years that found thicker fovea in amblyopic eyes than in the normal fellow eyes by 5μm.[14] These and our results differ from a recent evaluation of the foveal thickness that did not show statistically significant differences ($p=0.551$) of the foveae in patients with unilateral anisometropic and strabismic amblyopia compared with normal subjects.[7] Nonetheless, the authors did not compare the amblyopic eye with the normal fellow eyes and therefore, did not have an internal control. The differences between our study and the previous one probably relate to variability of foveal thickness in different individuals and indeed such differences were found between different individuals in our study and therefore the standard deviation between different individual was quite high.

Careful review of the OCT images indicated that the foveal thickening was due to either thicker outer retinal layers or immature retinal tissue. The structural feature of the foveae in amblyopic eyes is hypoplasia similar to albinotic and nanophthalmic eyes.[15-18] The fovea is thicker and flatter in these eyes. Since there are no histologic preparations of the retina in amblyopic eyes, it is impossible to determine the exact composition of the foveal area. However, in oculocutaneous albinism the retinal tissue was intact and the Bruch's layer was thickened in one specimen.[19]

We found that amblyopic eyes refractory to occlusion therapy had thicker fovea than those of the normal fellow eyes, while the differences in thickness between amblyopic eyes that responded to treatment and the fellow eyes were insignificant. This finding could have been different if patients and their parents would not be cooperative. No previous study addressed this issue and therefore we cannot compare our data with previous ones.

In our study, patients with anisometropic amblyopia had not statistical significant success of the occlusion therapy compared with patients with strabismic amblyopia. The differences in foveal thickness in the amblyopic and the sound fellow eyes in each group were not statistically significant although they were marginal in the amblyopic eyes of the anisometropic group. The higher number of anisometropic patients that underwent successful occlusion therapy might explain this tendency. A larger population will be required to confirm if the foveal thickness differs in these two groups and if the type of the amblyopia is the cause for different foveal thickness rather than treatment success. The higher success of occlusion therapy in anisometropic amblyopia than in strabismic amblyopia might be related to the thinner foveae in anisometropic patients. Thicker foveae were found in strabismic than in anisometropic amblyopia in another study as well ($p=0.046$).[7]

In our sample, the foveae of the amblyopic eyes were thicker than in the fellow normal eyes except for one in which the thickness was the same and another 3 with thicker normal fovea. Two of these patients experienced an improvement in BCVA after occlusion therapy. If in all future patients, the fovea of the amblyopic eye will be thicker than in the fellow normal eye, the foveal thickness may serve as a prognostic factor for improvement after proper therapy. To validate this, more patients should be recruited and a scale should be established for the measures that may predict improvement or non-improvement. It is possible that there will be patients in whom the fovea in the amblyopic eye would be thinner than in the normal fellow eye and would not experience an improvement in BCVA after treatment. In such event, it may not be possible to predict the success of a treatment based on the foveal thickness at least in those patients.

In patients with bilateral amblyopia, measurements of each fovea and a comparison with normal foveae will be needed. In such cases, the differences might be subtle as after comparing unilateral amblyopic eyes with normal controls and prediction of successful treatment may be difficult. According to our findings, it might be worthwhile to create a database for foveal thickness in the normal population according to age, since the foveal thickness may change with age.[20] In addition, a correlation between BCVA and foveal thickness might be established as well.

OCT measurements in children are demanding because of inattention, especially in children under age 4. In addition, amblyopic eyes tend to fixate less and if nystagmus is present, clear images may not be possible to obtain, unless the eye is mechanically fixated. We should also consider the accuracy and reproducibility of the OCT. When assessing thin layers as in the fovea, if the accuracy and reproducibility are not perfect, subtle differences may not be measured accurately, even if the image resolution is of 2μm. For macular thickness, OCT was found accurate and reproducible[21] and it is expected that with better technologies including high-resolution Fourier-domain OCT, this problem will be solved.

It will be interesting to verify our results in amblyopic adults and to find what is the foveal thickness in children that had regression after treatment. The last and the most intriguing issue is whether treatment influences the foveal thickness. Since the fovea, as well as other structures such as the lateral geniculate body and visual cortex, continue to develop after birth (the "critical" period), it is tempting to hypothesize that in successful treatment, the foveal thickness might also change.

10. Acknowledgments

We thank Orly Yakir, MA for the statistical analysis.

11. References

[1] von Noorden GK. Binocular Vision and Ocular Motility: Theory and Management. 5th Ed. St. Louis: Mosby-Year book Inc. 1996;216-54.
[2] Daw NW. Critical periods and amblyopia. Arch Opthalmol 1998;116:502-5.
[3] Scheiman MN, Hertle RW, Beck RW et at. Randomized trial of treatment of amblyopia in children aged 7 to 17 years. Arch Ophthalmol 2005;123:437-47.

[4] Levartovsky S, Oliver M, Gottesman N, Shimshoni M. Factors affecting long term results of successfully treated amblyopia: initial visual acuity and type of amblyopia. Br J Ophthalmol 1995;79:225-8.
[5] Altintas O, Yüksel N, Ozkan B, Caglar Y. Thickness of the retinal nerve fiber layer, macular thickness, and macular volume in patients with strabismic amblyopia. J Pediatr Ophthalmol Strabismus 2005;42:216-21.
[6] Yen M, Cheng C, Wang A. Retinal nerve fiber layer thickness in unilateral amblyopia. Invest Ophthalmol Vis Sci 2004;45:2224-30.
[7] Kee SY, Lee SY, Lee YC. Thicknesses of the fovea and retinal nerve fiber layer in amblyopic and normal eyes in children. Korean J Ophthalmol 2006;20:177-81.
[8] Park KH, Hwang JM, Ahn JK. Efficacy of amblyopia therapy initiated after 9 years of age. Eye 2004;18:571-4.
[9] Repka MX, Wallace DK, Beck RW et al. Two-year follow-up of a 6-month randomized trial of atropine vs patching for treatment of moderate amblyopia in children. Arch Ophthalmol 2005;123:149-57.
[10] Scheiman MN, Hertle RW, Kraker RT et at. Patching vs atropine to treat amblyopia in children aged 7 to 12 years: a randomiz. Arch Ophthalmol 126;1634-42.
[11] von Noorden GK, Crawford ML, Levacy RA. The lateral geniculate nucleus in human anisometropic amblyopia. Invest Ophthalmol Vis Sci 1983;24:788-90.
[12] Grigg J, Thomas R, Billson F. Neuronal basis of amblyopia: a review. Indian J Ophthalmol 1996;44:69-76.
[13] Demer JL, von Noorden GK, Volkow ND, Gould KL. Imaging of cerebral blood flow and metabolism in amblyopia by positron emission tomography. Am J Ophthalmol 1988;105:337-347.
[14] Huynh SC, Samarawichkama C, Wang XY et al. Macular and nerve fiber layer thickness in amblyopia. The Sydney Childhood Eye Study. Ophthalmology 2009;116:1604-9.
[15] Meyer CH, Lapolice DJ, Freedman SF. Foveal hypoplasia in oculocutaneous albinism demonstrated by optical coherence tomography. Am J Ophthalmol 2002;133:409-10.
[16] Harvey PS, King RA, SummeCG. Spectrum of foveal development in albinism detected with optical coherence tomography. J AAPOS 2006;10:237-42.
[17] Izquierdo NJ, Emanuelli A, Izquierdo JC et al. Foveal thickness and macular volume in patients with oculocutaneous albinism. Retina 2007;27:1227-30.
[18] Bijlsma WR, van Schooneveld MJ, Van der Lelij A. Optical coherence tomography findings for nanophthalmic eyes. Retina 2008;28:1002-7.
[19] Mietz H, Green WR, Wolff SM, Abundo GP. Foveal hypoplasia in complete oculocutaneous albinism. A histopathologic study. Retina 1992;12:254-60.
[20] Neuville JM, Bronson-Castain K, Bears MA Jr et al. OCT reveals regional differences in macular thickness with age. Optom Vis Sci 2009;86:E810-6.
[21] Muscat S, Parks S, Kemp E, Keating D. Repeatability and reproducibility of macular thickness measurements with the Humphrey OCT system. Invest Ophthalmol Vis Sci 2002;43:490-5.

Part 4

Glaucoma

17

Trabecular Surgery

Antonio Fea, Giulia Consolandi, Giulia Pignata, Davide Turco, Paola Cannizzo, Elena Bartoli, Teresa Rolle and Federico M. Grignolo
Clinica Oculistica, Universita' degli Studi di Torino
Italy

1. Introduction

In glaucoma, the most commonly used surgical options attempt to establish communication between the anterior chamber and the subconjunctival space, either by removing part of the trabecular meshwork and thus decreasing resistance to the passage of the aqueous humour or by means of drainage tubes that conduct the aqueous humour toward extraocular subconjunctival reservoirs. Trabeculectomy is still the most widely performed glaucoma procedure worldwide. Nevertheless, it creates an artificial pathway for drainage of aqueous that is less optimal than physiologic outflow and is associated with numerous short and long-term serious complications. Surgical alternatives, such as deep sclerectomy, are more demanding, longer and seem to be surgeon-dependent. Although they achieve a high level of hypotensive effect, these forms of surgery are not exempt from potential complications and are highly dependent on the inflammatory and healing response of the patient.[1] The use of antimetabolites to regulate this healing response is also linked to a higher rate of complications.[2,3,4,5,6]

The interest in new and possibly less invasive surgical techniques to lower intraocular pressure is growing. In particular, to avoid the eventual problems linked to surgical trauma to the conjunctiva and the ensuing inflammatory response, several new *ab interno* methods that attempt to achieve intraocular pressure control have been developed. Some of these methods are aimed at obtaining flow through Schlemm's canal, whereas others point to the possibility of obtaining flow from the anterior chamber to the suprachoroidal space. Gonioscopy is used in these *ab interno* procedures in order to visualize the site of implantation.

2. Visualizing the trabecular meshwork

Trabecular bypass surgery can be performed through the same incision used for phacoemulsification in cases of combined surgery, or by means of a paracentesis, when it is performed as a sole procedure. A temporal incision is warranted because of ease of patient's head positioning. Visualization of the angle using the goniolens should be practiced in cases prior to performing surgery, in order to learn the correct techniques.

In the case of phakic patients, the instillation of a miotic is recommended to minimize the risk of lens injury. If the procedure is carried out under topical anaesthesia it is advisable to introduce lidocaine 1% into the anterior chamber, because some of the surgical manoeuvres can be uncomfortable for the patient. It is perfectly possible to carry out the surgery under topical anaesthesia with intracameral lidocaine; however, when performing the operation for the first few times, it may be advisable to use some form of locoregional anaesthetic (retrobulbar, peribulbar or sub-Tenon).

Once the incision has been made in the temporal cornea, the anterior chamber must be filled with a cohesive viscoelastic that makes it possible to enlarge the region of the angle where surgery is planned.

A perfect view of the trabecular meshwork and of the angle must be achieved. The most common error is failure to position the microscope and/or the patient adequately in order to obtain an adequate view of the trabeculum. The patient's head must be turned approximately 45° away from the surgeon. The microscope should be tilted approximately 30º towards the operating surgeon.

3. Specific devices and surgical techniques

3.1 iStent®

The iStent® trabecular micro-bypass (Glaukos Corporation, Laguna Hills, CA) is made of titanium and coated with heparin (Duraflo® powder). It is L-shaped and measures 1 mm x 0.33 mm, with a nominal snorkel bore diameter of 120 microns (fig.1). The iStent is designed to fit into Schlemm´s canal. The distal portion of the stent is bevelled and sharpened to facilitate penetration into the tissue of the trabecular meshwork. The external surface features three retention arches that impede the movement of the stent once it has been implanted. The implant weighs approximately 0.1 mg. It is delivered preloaded on an insertion device (fig.2) and it is implanted at the level of the trabecular meshwork with the aid of a Swan-Jacob type goniolens (fig.3). Two versions of the iStent are available; one for the right eye and one for the left eye. The difference lies in the orientation of the rails, designed to facilitate the penetration of the implant into the trabecular meshwork. The distal tip of the implant should point towards the patient's feet at all times.

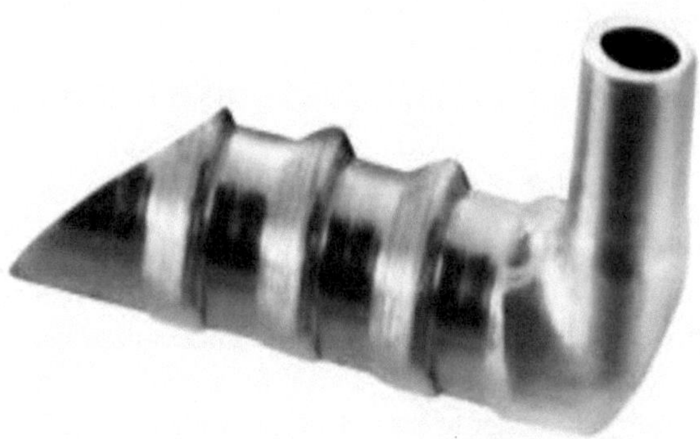

Fig. 1. iStent® trabecular bypass

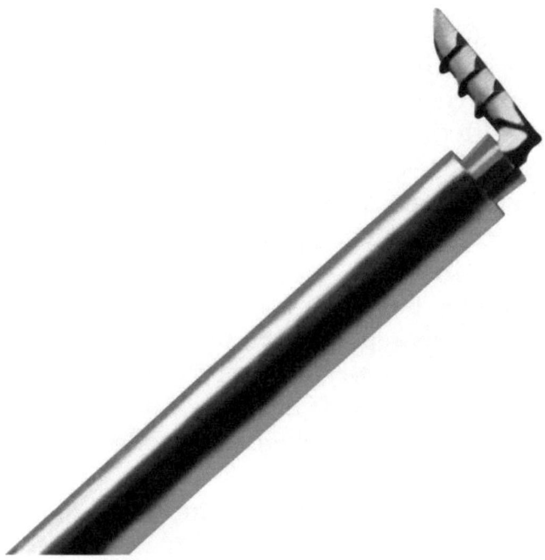

Fig. 2. iStent® trabecular bypass in iStent inserter

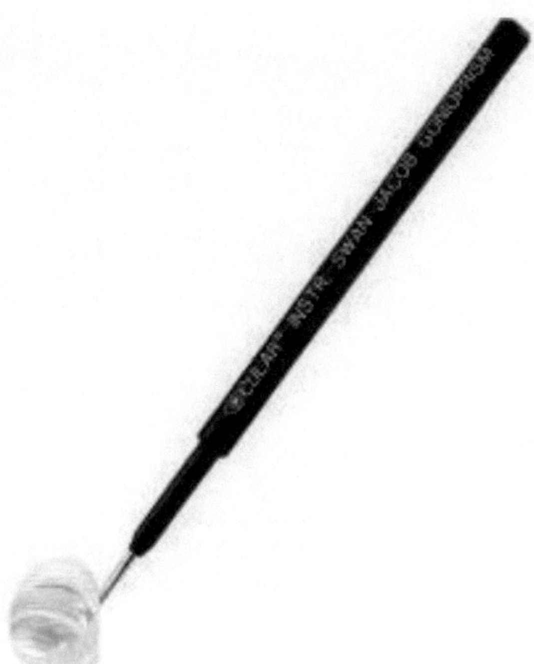

Fig. 3. Swan-Jacob goniolens

In all these techniques the patient is draped as for cataract surgery. Myosis is warranted if the surgery is not combined with phaco. Surgical steps are as follows:

1. A paracentesis is made generally using a 15 degree blade (fig.4).
2. If needed, the pupil is constricted with intracameral miotics and a cohesive viscoelastic is injected in the anterior chamber.
3. The tip of the stent, with the distal part parallel to the trabecular meshwork, should approach the trabecular meshwork at an angle of 15° to facilitate penetration of the tissue (fig.5). The stent should be placed parallel to the plane of the iris with the inner part covered by the meshwork and the lumen away from the iris. Excessive resistance indicates a path that is too perpendicular to the trabeculum or a wrong implantation site. Once the trabecular meshwork covers all of the implant, it should be released by pressing the applicator button. Only the proximal end of the stent should remain visible in the anterior chamber. The stent can be seated in its final position by gently tapping the side of the snorkel with the inserter tip. A small reflux of blood from Schlemm´s canal is common and reflects adequate positioning of the stent.
4. At the end of surgery, blood and viscoelastic are removed(Fig.6). The corneal incision can be hydrated if the paracentesis is not watertight.

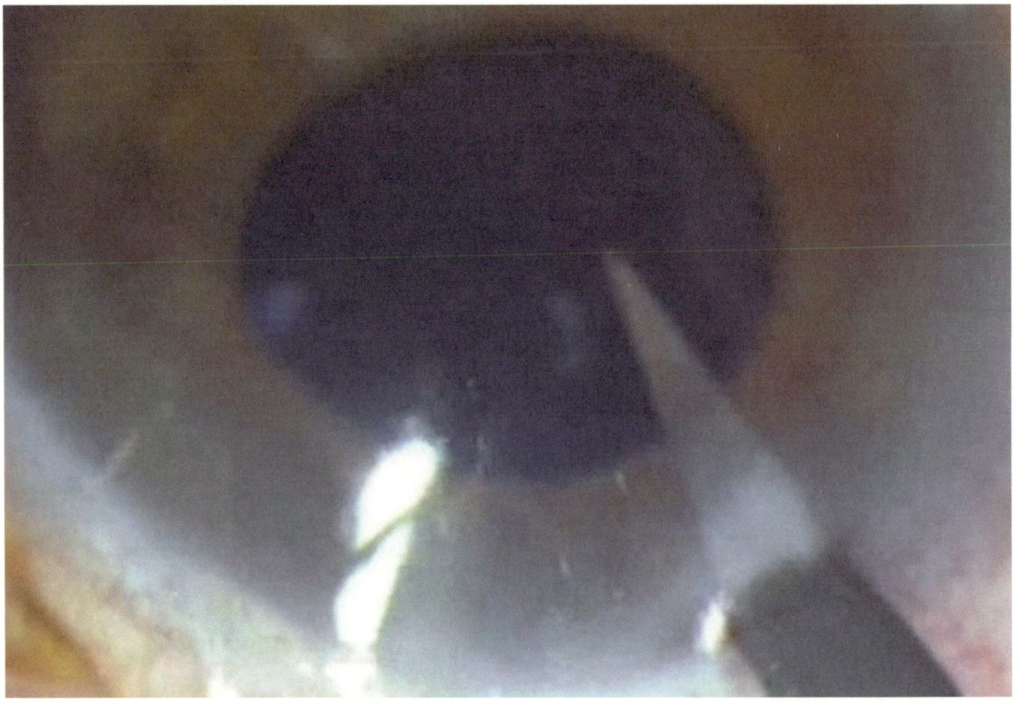

Fig. 4. A paracentesis is performed temporally.

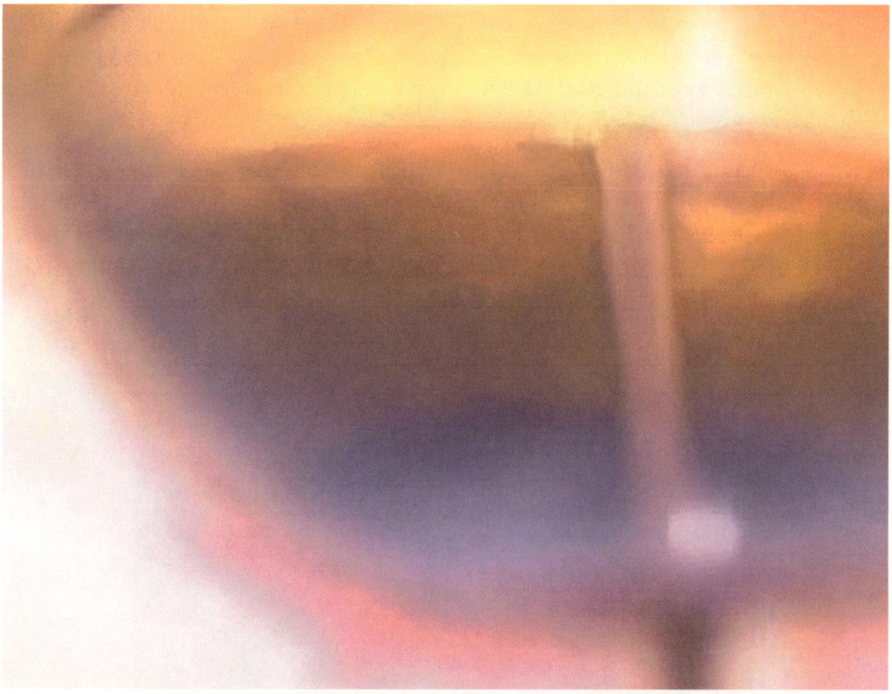

Fig. 5. The iStent is already half way within the trabecular meshwork.

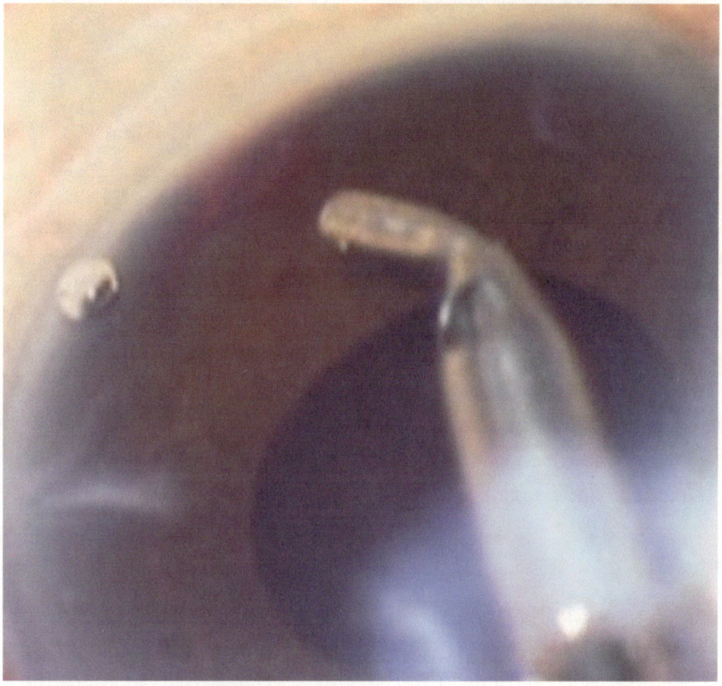

Fig. 6. Residual blood and viscoelastic are washed and aspirated by the anterior chamber with a coaxial I/A tip - the same can be done using a bimanual technique.

The post-operative suggested treatment should be similar to what is commonly used by each surgeon for an uncomplicated phacoemulsification procedure. Generally anti-glaucoma drugs are discontinued post-operatively and reintroduced if the patient does not achieve the target pressure.

iStent *inject is a* second generation trabecular bypass device that is also designed to restore conventional outflow (fig. 7). Two stents come preloaded in a sterile disposable injector that is placed on the meshwork. A stent release button on the injector is used to release the stents one at a time into the proper position (approximately 2-3 clock hours apart (fig. 8).

This new mechanism of implantation allows for implantation of two stents without exiting the inserter from the eye.

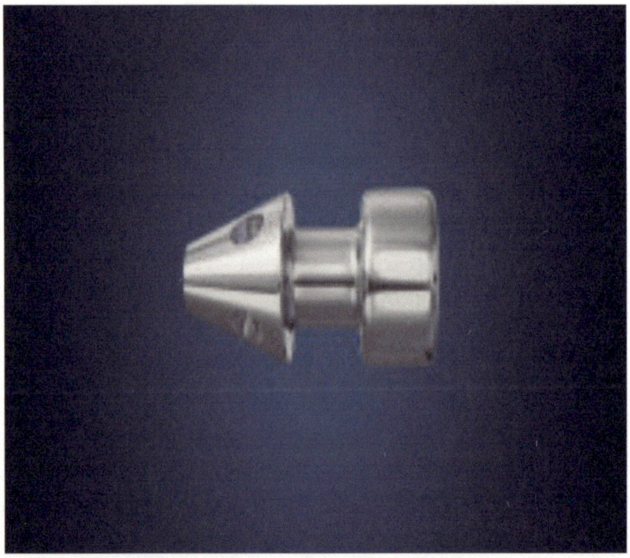

Fig. 7. iStent® inject (image provided by Glaukos)

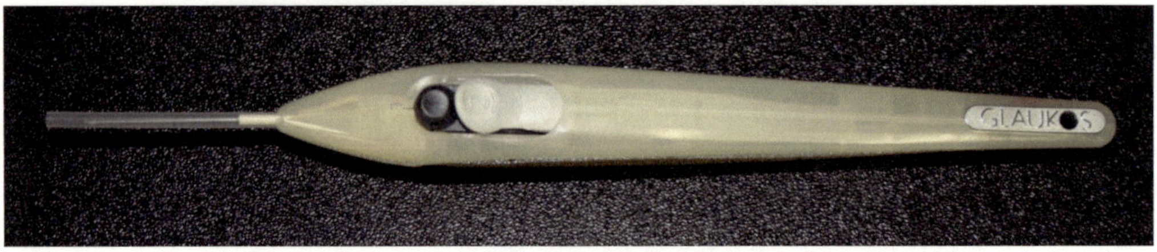

Fig. 8. iStent® inject inserter (image provided by Glaukos)

3.2 Trabectome

The Trabectome™ (NeoMedix Inc., Tustin, CA, USA) device consists of a disposable handpiece tip (19.5-gauge) that will fit through a 1.6mm corneal incision. The handpiece is connected to a console with irrigation and aspiration, and also to a simple electrocautery generator. The foot pedal controls the irrigation, aspiration and electrocautery ablation via a stepwise foot control similar to a phacoemulsification system (fig. 9).

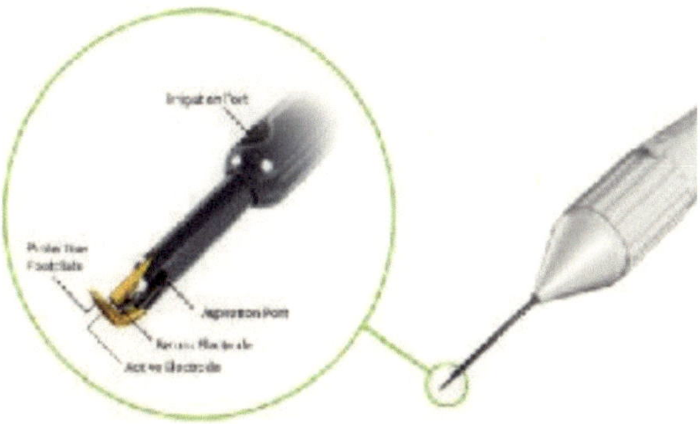

Fig. 9. Trabectome probe and tip

The tip of the handpiece is specially designed with an insulated footplate and is pointed for ease of insertion through the trabecular meshwork into Schlemm´s canal. The footplate is coated with proprietary multilayered polymer, which provides thermal stability, mechanical strength, biocompatibility and chemical resistance in laboratory testing. The aspiration port is in close proximity (approximately 0.3 mm) to the cautery electrode and serves to remove debris during ablation. The irrigation is 3 mm from the surgical site and serves the dual purpose of keeping the eye pressurized and further dissipating heat energy. Although the irrigation and aspiration system role is important, the high-frequency electrocautery generator system is the pivotal point of this technology. The generator is a modified 800 EU unit from Aaron/Bovie (St. Petersburg, FL, USA) and operates at a frequency of 550 kHz with adjustable power setting in 0.1-W increment up to 10 W (recommended range 0.5–1.5 W). The target tissue is disrupted and disintegrated by applying heat energy in bursts with a high-peak power and low duty cycle. This ablation approach equates to high-energy bursts, which are bunched into small increments with comparably long time intervals in between. As a result, disruption and disintegration of tissue is achieved rather than a thermal-cooking effect such as that seen in traditional cautery of blood vessels.[7,8]

Surgical steps: steps 1 and 2 are equal to the previous procedure, although a specially designed blade is provided by the manufacturer to obtain a water-tight paracentesis. A small paracentesis is more important with this procedure because during surgery the viscoelastic material is washed out by the water flowing through the tip of the instrument. 2) The tip of the footplate is inserted through the paracentesis aiming at the trabecular meshwork and then it is inserted through the trabecular meshwork into Schlemm´s canal . A foot switch activates the aspiration and electro-surgical elements that ablate and remove the strip of trabecular meshwork and Schlemm´s canal as the surgeon slowly advances the instrument along the meshwork in a clockwise and then counter clockwise direction using the insertion site as a fulcrum. A strip of trabecular meshwork and Schlemm´s canal spanning 80°–100° is ablated and removed under direct gonioscopic visualization. Intraoperative reflux of blood through the resulting cleft is desirable in this procedure and confirms appropriate ab interno "unroofing" of Schlemm's canal. 4) At the end of surgery any residual viscoelastic or blood present in the anterior chamber is removed. It is generally not necessary to hydrate the paracentesis.

The post-operative suggested treatment includes: antibiotics used for prophylaxis. Pilocarpine 2% qid should be used starting on the first post-operative medication and continued for a month. Lotemax is advised for three weeks and then tapered. Directly post-operative it is advised to continue the previous pre-operative anti-glaucomatous therapy, although prostaglandins should possibly be avoided. .Prof. Baerveldt recommends the eventual use of Latanoprost rather than other prostaglandins if they are absolutely necessary. Iopidine and Brimonidine can be used and are generally suggested. Anti-glaucoma medications can be reduced a month after surgery if target pressure is achieved.

3.3 Other procedures

Other approaches of gonioscopic surgery include the Ivantis method which simulates a short canaloplasty.

Two additional devices are aimed at improving flow of the aqueous humor from the anterior chamber to the suprachoroidal space. These are the Glaukos iStent *supra* and the Transcend Cypass. These devices will not be discussed, because the current data are less than one year post-operative.

4. Results

4.1 iStent

Numerous *in vitro* and *in vivo* studies support the stability, the effectiveness and the safety of the trabecular bypass iStent.

In 2004, Bahler demonstrated *in vitro* that the intraocular pressure was lowered after placement of a single stent, from 21.4 +/- 3.8 mm Hg to 12.4 +/- 4.2 mm Hg ($P < .001$).[9] This corresponded to an 84% increase in facility of outflow. Eyes receiving more than one stent had final IOP of 11.9 +/- 3.7 mm Hg. Nine eyes underwent sequential implantation of additional stents and seven of these had a further decrease of IOP (13.6 +/- 4.1 to 10.0 +/- 4.3; $P = .02$). This work suggested that bypass of the trabecular meshwork lowers IOP in cultured human anterior segments. One stent produced the greatest change in pressure. The sequential addition of more stents further lowered pressure in seven of nine eyes. Parallel to this study the founders/manufacturers of the iStent evaluated the stability of the implant on *ex vivo* eyes confirming that the L shape of the stent could not be moved even with strong traction on the stent itself.

A small clinical case series (n=6) reaffirmed the potential clinical utility of the current titanium version inserted *ab interno* and provided additional confirmation that the device stayed in place and continued to function to lower IOP with fewer medications through follow-up of one year.[10] All patients were seen day one, week one and at 1, 2, 6 and 12 months post-operatively. The mean pre-operative IOP of 20.2 ±6.3 decreased and stabilized at 14 to15 mm Hg with reduced medications out to one year. All devices remained in place and no complications were noted.

A larger prospective, 24-month, uncontrolled, multicenter, multicountry evaluation of 58 patients with uncontrolled primary open-angle glaucoma (including pseudoexfoliation and pigmentary) evaluated the effectiveness of the concurrent phacoemulsification and stent implantation.[11] Of the 48 patients in the per protocol population, 42 completed the 12 months follow-up. At baseline, mean (+/-SD) intraocular pressure (IOP) was 21.7+/-3.98 mmHg. At 12 months, mean IOP was reduced to 17.4+/-2.99 mmHg, a mean IOP reduction of 4.4+/-4.54 mmHg (p<0.001, 18.3%). At baseline, patients were taking a mean 1.6+/-0.8 medications. By 12 months, the mean number of medications was reduced to 0.4+/-0.62 (p<0.001). Half the patients achieved an IOP ≤ 18 mmHg and were able to discontinue hypotensive medication by the 12 month visit. The most commonly reported device-related adverse events were the appearance of stent lumen obstruction (seven eyes) and stent malposition (six eyes). None of the adverse events were deemed serious.

In 2010 Fea compared in a randomized study the results of phacoemulsification alone vs combined surgery (i.e. phacoemulsification and stent implantation).[12] The baseline IOP was similar in the two groups (combined group: 17.9 +/-2.6; control group: 17.3 +/-3.0 mm Hg) with a similar number of medications (2.,0 +/- 0.9 in the combined group and 1.9 +/-0.7 in the control group). Post-operative mean IOP at 15 months was 14.8 +/-1.2 and 15.7 +/- 1.1 respectively in the combined and in the control group (p=0.031). The author demonstrated that at 15 months the mean number of ocular hypotensive medications was significantly lower in the combined group (0.4 +/- 0.7 and 1.3 +/- 1.0, respectively; P = .007). Furthermore, after wash-out of ocular hypotensive medications, IOP was significantly lower in the combined group (16.6 +/- 3.1 mm Hg and 19.2 +/- 3.5 mm Hg). These results confirm the previous observation that IOP reduction could only partially be attributed to phacoemulsification and was in fact enhanced further by implantation of the iStent. The same author previously published a case report demonstrating the effectiveness of the procedure in one pseudophakic patient.[13]

More recently the effect of the iStent on flow was further elucidated by a fluorophotometic study by Fernandez-Barrientos et al.[14] Thirty-three eyes of 33 patients were randomized to either two stents and cataract surgery (n = 17, Group 1) or cataract surgery alone (n = 16, Group 2). Before surgery, flow and outflow facility were similar between Groups 1 and 2 (1.78 +/- 0.44 and 1.74 +/- 0.82 microL/min; P = 0.18; 0.12 +/- 0.03 and 0.13 +/- 0.06 microL/min/mm H; P = 0.71, respectively). At one year, outflow facility was significantly higher in the group with two stents (0.45 +/- 0.27 microL/min/mm Hg in Group 1 and 0.19 +/- 0.05 microL/min/mm Hg in Group 2; P = 0.02).

A larger prospective, randomized, open-label, controlled, multicenter clinical trial with a total of 240 eyes with mild to moderate open-angle glaucoma with intraocular pressure (IOP) ≤ 24 mmHg controlled on one to three medications compared the results of the patients who were randomized to undergo cataract surgery with iStent implantation (treatment group) or cataract surgery only (control).[15] The primary efficacy measure was unmedicated IOP ≤ 21 mmHg at one year. A secondary measure was unmedicated IOP reduction ≥ 20% at one year. Safety measures included best-corrected visual acuity (BCVA), slit-lamp observations, complications and adverse events. The study met the primary efficacy endpoint, with 72% of treatment eyes versus 50% of control eyes achieving the criterion (P<0.001). At one year, IOP in both treatment groups was statistically lower from baseline values. Sixty-six percent of treatment eyes versus 48% of control eyes achieved ≥ 20% IOP reduction without medication (P = 0.003). The overall incidence of adverse events was similar between groups with no unanticipated adverse device effects. This larger series not only further demonstrates the efficacy of the iStent in further lowering the intraocular pressure in patients undergoing cataract surgery, but also points out the safety of the procedure. A longer post-operative follow-up through two years was reported more recently.[16] Best-corrected visual acuity of 20/40 or better was reported in 93% of treatment vs. 91% of control eyes at two years. Over the two year period, post-operative adverse events occurring at a level of 5% or greater included posterior capsular opacification (6% treatment vs. 10% control), elevated IOP (4% vs. 7%, respectively), visual disturbance (3% vs. 7%, respectively) and iritis (1% vs. 5%, respectively). Furthermore, in the treatment group, stent obstruction and malposition occurred in a small percentage of eyes (4% and 3%, respectively) and resolved shortly after occurrence (with or without treatment). The authors concluded that the overall long-term safety of iStents implanted during cataract surgery was similar to that of cataract surgery alone and that the adverse event/complication rate was low through the two year post-operative period.

4.2 Trabectome

The results obtained by the Trabectome can be summarized by a single paper which reports the experience of the Trabectome group. In this retrospective case series the authors reported their experience on follow-up through one year on 143 of 1127 Trabectome surgical procedures, including 102 through one year from 738 Trabectome-only and 41 through one year from 366 Trabectome-phacoemulsification surgeries[17]. It should be pointed out that many eyes at relatively high risk for filtering surgery failure were included after prior failed trabeculectomy or other previous surgeries were included in the study. Considering glaucoma surgery only: 273 underwent SLT, 170 ALT, 20 aqueous shunt surgery, 104 trabeculectomy, five prior Trabectome and five laser iridectomy.

Considering all cases, mean pre-operative IOP of 23.8 +/- 7.7 mm Hg decreased by 39% to 16.5 +/- 4.0 mm Hg at 24 months (n = 50). Intra-operative reflux bleeding occurred in 77.6%. Medications decreased from 2.8 to 1.2 by 24 months. Sixty-five patients (5.8%) had IOP elevation > 10 mm Hg above baseline on day one. Failure led to trabeculectomy in 5.9% (n = 67) and shunt installation in 1.6% (n = 18). Kaplan-Meier failure was defined across groups with at least two weeks follow-up as IOP > 21 mm Hg with or without medications and not reduced by 20% below baseline on two consecutive visits or repeat surgery. For Trabectome-only cases, mean preoperative IOP of 25.7 +/- 7.7 mm Hg was reduced by 40% to 16.6 +/- 4.0 mm Hg at 24 months (n = 46). No prolonged hypotony, choroidal effusion, choroidal haemorrhage or infections occurred. Failure led to trabeculectomy in 8.1% (n = 60) and shunt installation in 1.9% (n = 14). Medications decreased from 2.93 to 1.2 by 24 months. For Trabectome-phacoemulsification cases, baseline IOP of 20.0 +/- 6.2 mm Hg decreased at 12 months to 15.9 +/- 3.3 mm Hg (18%) (n = 45) and medications decreased from 2.63 +/- 1.12 to 1.50 +/- 1.36. Sixteen (4.4%) of 365 had prior failed trabeculectomy and 139 of 365 (38%) had prior laser trabeculoplasty.

Although the the large number of patients who underwent surgery of the study are very impressive, there are major limitations, including the retrospective nature and the fact that a very small number of procedures reported had been followed up postoperatively. Of the 738 patients who underwent only the Trabectome procedure, only 102 had a one year follow-up and of the 366 with combined surgery only 41 were followed up to one year. Furthermore, it is not clear if the patients with a longer follow-up and with available data include those high risk patients who were originally included in the study. If this is the case it would have been very important to analyse if there was any difference in terms of efficacy in the high versus low risk patients.

Recently, Knape and Smith[18] presented the case of a patient who had intra-operative blood reflux onto peripheral iris during trabeculectomy 11 months after Trabectome surgery. After having left the eye firm after surgery, the author did not report any other episode of hyphema during the following period. He hypothesizes that the absence of overlying angle structures, including the roof of Schlemm's canal, may have allowed blood to reflux into the angle and onto peripheral iris during a sudden decrease in intraocular pressure in trabeculectomy surgery. This self-limited episode suggests that the trabeculotomy remained patent, although the patient was not compensated and points out that further studies to assess the consequences of permanent trabecular meshwork tissue removal may be warranted.

More recently, Jea[19] reported on a cohort of patients and showed that a previously failed Trabectome surgery does not seem to impact the effect of subsequent trabeculectomy.

5. Complications prevention and treatment

Bleeding: bleeding with iStent, Trabectome or other trabecular bypass procedures is generally minimal, although aspiration of the blood in phakic eyes is suggested in order to allow proper visualization.. A very rare occurrence of more significant bleeding in the anterior chamber is generally due to damage of the iris either because the surgeon did not aim at the correct site or because involuntary movements occurred during surgery. The use of air or viscoelastics can stop the haemorrhage. It is generally advisable to postpone the trabecular bypass procedure if massive bleeding occurred previously because angle visualization can be difficult and because the source of bleeding and the effect on the angle structures are easier to visualize after the hyphema has cleared.

Malposition: the iStent may at times appear malpositioned. This does not preclude the implantation of another one provided the angle can be visualized. It is advisable to move at least two or three clock hours away from the previous implant to better visualize the meshwork.

Occlusion: occlusion of the Stent by a seemingly fibrinous plug can sometimes be seen during the postoperative follow-up. This may sometimes be eliminated by a single YAG laser spot.

Endothelial damage: although possible, it has never been reported with any of the procedures described.

6. Conclusions

The idea of approaching the surgery site *ab interno* is certainly appealing. The opportunity to perform a more standardized procedure and the opportunity to preserve the conjunctiva and the sites of eventual subsequent surgery are attractive. Furthermore, creating a direct communication between Schlemm's canal and the anterior chamber is a more physiological approach to IOP reduction with a lower rate of complications and a faster surgery compared to any other available approach.

Several studies pointed out the efficacy of the iStent in the reduction of IOP, although these studies were mainly performed in conjunction with cataract surgery. Nevertheless, there is strong evidence both *in vitro* and *in vivo* that the stent insertion actually facilitates outflow independent of the concurrent phacoemulsification. The procedure is safe and complications are mainly limited to a small (and transient) blood reflux into the anterior chamber immediately upon insertion into Schlemm's canal. It should be noted, however, that all studies were performed in eyes with relatively low pre-operative IOP. At present there is no published evidence of the efficacy in patients with severe glaucoma nor what would be the impact in patients with higher baseline IOP.

Upon casual review of the number of cases reported by the papers on the Trabectome and the length of the follow-up, it may appear that the evidence of efficacy of this surgical method is more stringent. The net IOP reduction seems higher with the Trabectome compared to the iStent and patients at higher risk had been treated with this method. However, a more accurate analysis of the literature reveals that a very small number of patients have been followed for a reasonable amount of time. Futhermore, the ablation of part of the trabecular meshwork is certainly a more destructive procedure, although it seems that this fact does not impact upon the results of conventional surgery in the limited series followed for an adequate postoperative timeframe.

IOP outcomes with both approaches are usually in the mid-teens. Although mid-teens IOP might be adequate for initial and moderate patients, traditional filtering surgery with anti-fibrotic enhancement and bleb formation will probably remain the principal surgical approach to eyes with advanced glaucomatous optic neuropathy. Eventually more advanced patients may benefit from trabecular bypass surgery combined with hypotensive medications, but too little data are available at present to sustain this approach. Assuming ongoing clinical studies continue to be favourable, a strong argument can be made for use of these minimally invasive procedures which do not lead to bleb formation nor require anti-fibrotics, early in the glaucoma injury process, especially considering the difficulties of compliance with medical therapy. Neither of these procedures damages the conjunctiva superiorly, leaving surgical alternatives where necessary open. Furthermore, continued development of suprachoroidal stents (such as the iStent supra and the newer Transcend Cypass) may offer additional IOP lowering and thus serve a broader population of patients with more advanced disease.

Given that glaucoma is typically a chronic disease and that the introduction of these methods is relatively new, follow-up of the patients at the moment is limited to two years at maximum.

Trabecular surgery requires some learning curve to visualize the angle using a hand-held gonioprims and the diffuse illumination of the microscope gives a different appearance of the angle's structures as compared with slit lamp gonioscopy. Furthermore, the need for using a hand to hold the gonioprism makes any trabecular surgery strictly bimanual. During surgery, the implantation of the iStent is relatively easier compared with the Trabectome, because it does not need a continuous circumferential movement and because the chamber is well formed with viscoelastics. After the implantation of the device, the blood reflux in the anterior chamber is generally minimal with the iStent.

On the other hand, the Trabectome allows a visual feeling that the trabecular meshwork is ablated, whereas it is sometimes difficult to be sure of the correct iStent placement, especially when blood cannot be completely washed from the angle. Compared to trabeculectomy, additional costs with any device should also be considered. Furthermore at present only the Trabectome has been cleared by the FDA, although U.S. FDA approval of the iStent is expected in the near future.

7. References

[1] Janz NK, Wren PA, Lichter PR, et al. The Collaborative Initial Glaucoma Treatment Study: interim quality of life findings after initial medical or surgical treatment of glaucoma. Ophthalmology 2001;108:1954 -1965

[2] Higginbotham EJ, Stevens RK, Musch DC, et al. Bleb related endophthalmitis after trabeculectomy with mitomycin C. Ophthalmology 1996;103:650–656.

[3] Soltau JB, Rothman RF, Budenz DL, et al. Risk factors for glaucoma filtering bleb infections. Arch Ophthalmol 2000; 118:338 -342.

[4] Greenfield DS, Suner IJ, Miller MP, Kangas TA, Palmberg PF, Flynn HW. Endophthalmitis after filtering surgery with mitomycin. Arch Ophthalmol 1996;114:943–949.

[5] Fontana H, Nouri-Mahdavi K, Lumba J, Ralli M, Caprioli J. Trabeculectomy with mitomycin C: outcomes and risk factors for failure in phakic open-angle glaucoma. Ophthalmology 2006;113:930-6

[6] Anand N, Arora S, Clowes M. Mitomycin C augmented glaucoma surgery: evolution of filtering bleb avascularity, transconjunctival oozing, and leaks. Br J Ophthalmol 2006;90:175-80.

[7] Trabectome description at http://www.ncbi.nlm.nih.gov.proxy-medicina.unito.it/pubmed/16378021.

[8] Trabectome description at http://www.ncbi.nlm.nih.gov.proxy-medicina.unito.it/pubmed/18936637.

[9] Bahler C, Smedley G, Zhou J, Johnson D. Trabecular bypass stents decrease intraocular pressure in cultured human anterior segments. Am J Ophthal 2004; 138:988-994.

[10] Spiegel D, Wetzel W. Haffner DS, Hill RA. Initial clinical experience with the trabecular micro-bypass stent in patients with glaucoma. Adv Ther 2007;24:161-170.

[11] Spiegel D, Wetzel W, Neuhann T, Sturmer J, Hoh H, Garcia-Feijoo J, Martinez de la casa JM, Garcia-Sanchez J. Coexistent primary open-angle glaucoma and cataract: interim analysis of a trabecular micro-bypass stent and concurrent cataract surgery. Eur J Ophthalmol 2009; 19:393-399.

[12] Fea AM. Phacoemulsification versus phacoemulsification with micro-bypass stent implantation in primary open-angle glaucoma. J Cataract Refract Surg 2010;36:407-412.

[13] Fea A, Dogliani M, Macetta F et al. Case report: The trabecular bypass stent in a pseudophakic glaucoma patient: A 1-year follow-up. Clinical Ophthalmology 2008;2:931-934.

[14] Fernández-Barrientos Y, Garcia-Feijoó J, Martínez de la Casa JM, et al. Fluorophotometric study of the effect of the Glaukos trabecular micro-bypass stent on aqueous humor dynamics. Invest Ophthalmol Vis Sci 2010;51:3327-3332.

[15] Samuelson TW, Katz LJ, Wells JM, et al. Randomized evaluation of the trabecular micro-bypass stent with phacoemulsification in patients with glaucoma and cataract. Ophthalmology 2011;118:459-467.

[16] Craven ER. Prospective, Randomized Controlled Trial of Cataract Surgery with Trabecular Micro-Bypass Stent in Mild-Moderate Open Angle Glaucoma: Safety in Two Year Follow-up. Paper presented at 2011 American Society of Cataract and Refractive Surgeons, April, 2011; San Diego, CA.

[17] Minckler D,* Mosaed S, Dustin L, Francis B, AND the Trabectome Study Group†. Trabectome (trabeculectomy-internal approach): additional experience and extended follow-up. Trans Am Ophthalmol Soc 2008;106:149-160
[18] Knape RM and Smith MF. Anterior chamber blood reflux during trabeculectomy in an eye with previous Trabectome surgery. J Glaucoma 2010;19:499–500
[19] Jea SY, Mosaed S, Vold SD, Rhee DJ. Effect of a Failed Trabectome on Subsequent Trabeculectomy. J Glaucoma. 2011 Feb 17. [Epub ahead of print]

Part 5

Retina and Vitreous

18

A Novel Artificial Vitreous Substitute – Foldable Capsular Vitreous Body

Qianying Gao
State Key Laboratory of Ophthalmology, Zhongshan Ophthalmic Center, Sun Yat-sen University, Guangzhou, China

1. Introduction

The natural vitreous is a transparent, gelatinoid structure occupying four-fifths of the volume of the eye. It has a thin, membrane-like structure corresponding to the vitreous cortex that extends from the ora serrata to the posterior pole.[1] It is somewhat spherical but slightly flattened meridionally, and it has a cup-shaped depression in its anterior side. It consists of about 99% water by weight, collagen fibers (types II, V/XI, VI, and IX), hyaluronic acid, opticin, fibrillin, and hyaluronan, which can maintain a certain spatial relationship with dipolar water molecules.[1,2] However, very few cells are found in the vitreous body. These cells are mostly phagocytes that clear useless cellular debris and hyalocytes mainly found at the periphery and that produce hyaluronic acid and collagen. In human adults, the vitreous body has an approximate weight of 4 g, a density of 1.0053-1.0089g cm^{-3}, a refractive index of 1.3345–1.3348, and a PH range of 7.0–7.4. [3-5]

The physiological function of the vitreous body involves supporting adjacent posterior segment structures, providing an ocular refractive medium, and acting as a cell barrier to inhibit cell migration from the retina to the vitreous cavity.[6] With age, the natural vitreous body gradually shrinks and collapses during the course of syneresis. This phenomenon may eventually lead to posterior vitreous detachment and can play a crucial role in the formation of retinal breaks which result in rhegmatogenous retinal detachment if untreated.[7,8]

The removal of diseased vitreous bodies using pars plana vitrectomy combined with artificial vitreous substitutes can restore vision in many patients. These individuals include those affected by proliferative diabetic retinopathy, proliferative vitreoretinopathy, and endophthalmitis or patients otherwise regarded as hopeless.[9-11]

The vitreous body cannot regenerate, so the vitreous cavity must be filled with suitable artificial vitreous substitutes that will keep the retina in place and prevent phthisis bulbi. Artificial vitreous substitutes are one of the most interesting and challenging topics of research in ophthalmology.[2] A number of artificial vitreous substitutes, such as gas, silicone oil, heavy silicone oil, and hydrogels, have been used.[2,12]

There are three major categories of currently available gas vitreous substitutes: air substitutes, expansile gas substitutes, and Xenon. Gases are used for pneumatic retinopexy and post-operative endotamponade. However, they are suitable only as short-term vitreous substitutes (Table 1).[13]

G	Molecular Weight	Purity (mol%)	Expansion Coefficient	Duration* (day)	Expansion Concentration (%)
Air	29	--	0	5-7	-
Xenon	131	99.995	0	1	-
SF6	146	99.9	1.9-2.0	10-14	18
C2F6	88	99.7	1.9	10-14	-
C4F8	138	99.9	3.3	30-35	16+
C3F8	188	99.7	4	55-65	14

Table 1. Physical characteristics of gases as vitreous substitutes

In 1969, Norton et al. highlighted the advantages of clinical management with intravitreal air for the treatment of giant retinal tears.[14] However, the intravitreal longevity of air is only a few days[15] due to diffusion across the retina. The refractive index of the air (1.0008) is also incompatible with optically important tissues. Therefore, these issues limit the use of air. To date, air is mainly used in liquid–air exchanges during vitrectomy procedures.[16]

In 1973, Norton first experimented with sulphur hexafluoride (SF6) and found that the persistence of the gas and its expansile characteristics are superior to air. SF6 expands to twice its volume by dissolving nitrogen, oxygen, and carbon dioxide from the blood. It also stays in the vitreous cavity for about two weeks.[17] In 1980, Lincoff et al. proposed the use of perfluorocarbon gases[18]. These gases expand after intravitreal injection because of the diffusion of other gases from the blood stream. Perfluoropropane expands to four times its original volume by the fourth day after injection. It is also absorbed at a much slower rate than air or sulphur hexafluoride. To date, C3F8 is the agent of choice. Expansile gases last longer in the vitreous chamber than air, but they are spontaneously absorbed in 6 to 80 days and replaced by aqueous humor. Therefore, postsurgical removal is avoided if they cause certain concomitant complications.[19] However, they may induce lens opacification and usually result in a high intraocular pressure (IOP).[20,21] As with air, the refractive indices of gases are also lower (w1.17).[22]

Xenon was tested in rabbit eyes to evaluate its longevity in the vitreous cavity.[23] It is considered as the most promising gas with successful retinal reattachment in all cases. However, the major drawback is its rapid disappearance; almost 90% of Xenon disappears 3 h after introduction.[24]

Silicone oil is hydrophobic, viscous, transparent, and stable. It has a specific gravity of 0.97 g/mL and a refractive index of 1.4. Its viscosity is measured in centistokes and linearly varies with chain lengths and molecular weight. The 1,000 and 5,000 centistoke varieties are commonly used in clinics. The surface tension is approximately 40 mN/m. Introduced by Cibis in 1962,[25] silicone oil has been the most important adjunct for internal tamponade in the treatment of complicated retinal or choroidal detachment for the past five decades. It is commonly applied for the treatment of superior retinal detachment through buoyancy force and high interfacial tension. It is the only substance currently accepted as a long-term vitreous substitute and is the preferred choice in complex retinal detachments, such as long-standing rhegmatogenous retinal detachment, traction retinal detachment, giant retinal tears, proliferative diabetic retinopathy, and severe endoophthalmitis involving the posterior segment.

However, the use of silicone oil has not always been successful. An anatomic success rate of around 70% has been reported,[19] with complications including cataract, keratopathy, anterior chamber oil emulsification, and glaucoma.[26] Several reports have demonstrated the migration of silicone oil droplets into the retina and the optic nerve. Others have shown the widespread loss of myelinated optic nerve fibers due to the oil's free-fluid characteristics within the eye.[27, 28]

Heavy oil, a solution of perfluorohexyloctane and silicone oil prepared as internal tamponade, has recently been used in retinal detachment surgery. However, it causes complications, such as emulsification and inflammatory reaction.[29] Some very recent results are encouraging,[30] but most clinicians are awaiting results from ongoing heavy silicone oil trials.[12]

Hydrogels and smart hydrogels seem to remain as the best candidates as long-term vitreous substitutes because they show excellent transparency and good biocompatibility. They can act as viscoelastic shock-absorbing materials, thereby closely mimicking the behavior of natural vitreous bodies. Hydrogels are networks of polymer chains that can contain over 99.9% water so they are hydrophilic and not flowable. Currently, a number of cross-linked polymeric hydrogels have been proposed, such as poly (vinyl alcohol) (PVA), poly poly (1-vinyl-2-pyrrolidone), poly (acrylamide) (PAA), and poly (ethylene glycol) (PEG).[2,12,31-34] Among these, the PVA and PAA hydrogels are the most promising candidates for long-term vitreous body replacement and are highly recommended for use. They show excellent biocompatibility, are biodegradable, and can closely mimic the physico-mechanical properties of natural vitreous bodies.[2] PEG is a synthetic water-soluble polymer that has been approved by the Food and Drug Administration (FDA) for use in a wide range of biomedical applications, including injectable hydrogels.[35] However, issues such as retinal toxicity, increased IOP, and formation of opacities still need to be addressed.[36] Fragmentation and changes in viscoelastic properties and resiliency after injection through a small-gauge needle have also been found in some types of hydrogels.[36, 37]

Smart hydrogels are a relatively new class of stimuli-sensitive hydrogels. They possess the common properties of conventional hydrogels, and they can respond to a variety of signals, including PH, temperature, light, pressure, electric fields, or chemicals.[38] Temperature-sensitive hydrogels, such as poly(N-isopropylacrylamide), the most extensively studied one, undergo sharp hydrophilic-hydrophobic transition in aqueous media at a lower critical solution temperature of 32 °C, which is close to the body temperature.[39] Generally, smart hydrogels appear promising, but they are still at an early experimental stage, and their long-term toxicity is unknown.[12] Therefore, despite half a century of research efforts to replace the vitreous body of the eye, an ideal and permanent vitreous body replacement has yet to be found.[40,41]

Current research on artificial vitreous bodies aims to determine ideal materials that are nontoxic and inert, thin and transparent, and have good water and oxygen permeability, high compatibility, and good elasticity[46] in order to mimic the natural vitreous perfectly. The materials must be hydrophilic and can form a gel within the vitreous cavity.[35] However, directly injected vitreous substitutes, like silicon oil and heavy silicon oil, often result in severe complications, such as intraocular toxicity, retinal cell proliferation, leakage into the anterior chamber, and difficulty of complete removal if emulsified with time, among others.

Inspired by the structure of the natural vitreous, we postulated a novel foldable capsular vitreous body (FCVB) to restore the shape and function of the natural vitreous body. The FCVB consisted of a capsule, drain tube, and valve. The capsule exactly mimicked the vitreous body using a computer. The intra-capsule pressure can be adjusted from the valve with a syringe, and there is a slice of anti-penetrating metal in the valve. Figure 1 and Table 2 show the images and parameters of the FCVB, respectively.[50] Silicone rubber elastomer has been used for tissue augmentation for many years, [43-45] so it was utilized to manufacture the capsule of FCVB. It showed good oxygen permeability, good mechanical and optical properties (Shore A hardness: 37.4˚, tensile intensity: >5.86 MPa, elongation ratio: >1200%, tear intensity: 34KN/m, transmittance: 93%, Hazes<1%),[46] and good biocompatibility as shown in stable extracts experiment (no significant fever, good genetic safety, and no structural abnormality or apoptosis in the cornea, ciliary body, and retina over a six-month observation period).[50] After pars plana vitrectomy, the seamlessly connected FCVB was triple-folded and inserted into the vitreous cavity through a 3 mm × 1 mm scleral incision without air fluid exchange. Then an injectable medium, such as balanced salt solution (BSS) or silicone oil, can be injected into the capsule and inflated to support the retina. Through the tube–valve system, IOP can be adjusted by the volume of the injected medium. Similar to the glaucoma valve, the valve can be fixed onto the sclera surface. [46]

Component parts		Dimension (mm)	Permissible deviation (mm)
Capsule	Diameter	20.00	±2.00
	Rise of arch	2.00	±0.20
	Radius of curvature of fovea lentis	6.00	±0.50
	Chord length of fovea lentis	9.50	±0.50
	Optic part thickness	0.06	±0.02
Drain tube	Outside diameter	1.50	±0.20
	Inner diameter	1.20	±0.20
	Tube length	4.00	±0.50
	Vertical distance from the open end to the principal axis	7.99	±0.20
Drain valve	Top diameter	4.00	±0.20
	Bottom diameter	6.00	±0.20
	Total thickness	3.50	±0.20
	Puncture part thickness	2.00	±0.20
	Location hole diameter	0.50	±0.05

FCVB, foldable capsular vitreous body; BSS, balanced salt solution.
Note: The FCVB consisted of capsule, drain tube, and valve.The capsule was mimicking the vitreous body exactly by computer, and BSS was injected through the tube-valve system to inflate the capsule.

Table 2. Standard dimensions of the components of the human FCVB

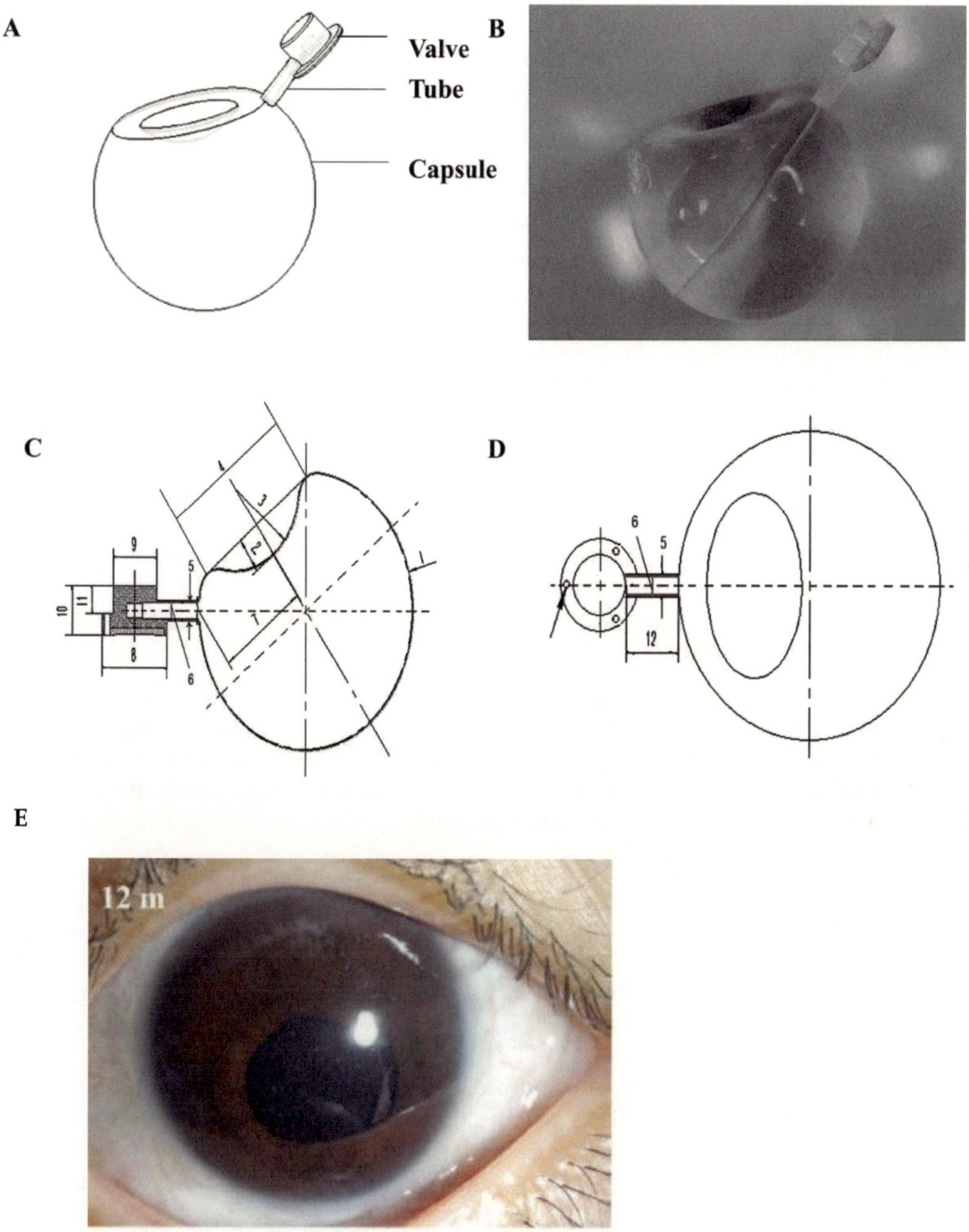

Fig. 1. The human foldable capsular vitreous body (FCVB) consists of vitreous-shape high molecular capsule, tube, and valve. The intra-capsule pressure can be adjusted from the valve with a syringe and there is a slice of anti-penetrating metal in the valve; the designed parameters finely mimic the vitreous shape of a human. (A) Illustration of FCVB. (B) Final sample of the FCVB (Outside the eye). (C) Side view of varied parameters. (D) Vertical view of varied parameters. (E) FCVB inside the eye (Twelve months after implantation).

Theoretically, a new artificial vitreous has the following advantages. First, it does not flow into the anterior chamber and subretinal regions or other sites. Second, it does not emulsify or damage the media over time nor cause it to be isolated in the capsule. Third, it has the capability to support discretionary retina using a 360-degree solid arc.

Developing an irregular vitreous-shaped thin capsule and smoothly connecting it to a very thin diameter tube and a pressure-control valve are very difficult. According to this hypothesis, a mirror steel mold is specially designed to fabricate FCVB using an injection-forming technology that would make the capsule, drainage tube, and valve of the FCVB seamlessly connected. The mold consists of an upper composite die, a lower composite die, and a core.[47] The core shape can be manipulated using a computer to match the human vitreous parameters. The capsular film is 60 μm thick, only one-third the thickness of the retina. In its natural shape, the human FCVB is somewhat spherical, but it is slightly flattened meridionally and has a cup-shaped depression anteriorly.

In the rabbit model of severe retinal detachment, the BSS-filled FCVB was found to mimick the morphology of the natural vitreous very closely and to restore its physiological functions, such as support, refraction, and cellular barriers, during a three-month observation period and without obvious complications. By contrast, the silicone oil control group showed obvious lens opacity, significant hyperopic shift, recurrent retinal detachment, preretinal membrane formation, and vitreoretinal traction.[48] The FCVB capsule can provide the detached retina with a platform to form a flat scar and a barrier to block cell migration from the retina to the vitreous cavity.

Interestingly, the BSS-filled FCVB very slightly changes the refraction compared with silicone oil and heavy silicone oil based on Gullstrand–Emsley and Liou–Brennan schematic eyes.[49] Reports from the State FDA in China show that FCVB has suitably mechanical, optical, and biocompatibility properties.[50] Its optical characteristics indicate that FCVB has high light transmission and laser irradiation stability.

In the early development of breast implants in plastic surgery, similar to current clinical vitreous substitutes, directly injectable materials were used. In fact, hydrophilic polyacrylamide gel (PAAG) was directly injected into the breast. This procedure was practiced widely in China and Eastern Europe in the 1990s. The breast implantation procedure was analogous to the use of silicone oil to replace the vitreous body. However, the injected PAAG was gradually found to induce severe complications, such as inflammation and infection, multiple indurations, hematoma, painful masses, and mastalagia. Currently, the direct injection of PAAG is prohibited, and it has been replaced with the use of capsule-like implants whose fluid substitute is contained in a thin, elastic capsule. This approach to implantation has shown clinical success.[51] In case of severe complications, as mentioned above, the implant can be completely removed without leaving behind residual fluid substitute. Apparently, the development of both artificial vitreous and breast substitutes shared a similar path, and both have suffered setbacks from the direct injection of the fluid substitute into the organ. Therefore, similar lessons can be learned, and the use of a capsule-type implant may be a good replacement for the use of the vitreous body.[46]

The use of FCVBs in the eyes is not yet a common practice worldwide. Therefore, an exploratory study of our new treatment for severe retinal detachment was conducted. The detachment cannot be easily reattached with silicone oil tamponade, such as posterior scleral ruptures with large disruptions of the retina or severe scleral ruptures with retinal and choroidal detachments. It may also have rigid retinal redetachments or inferior holes occurring after silicone or heavy oil tamponade had been attempted. At Zhongshan Ophthalmic Center, 11 patients were implanted with FCVBs filled with BSS,[52] whereas 3 patients were implanted with FCVBs filled with silicone oil.[53] Patients with serious eye inflammation, with only one eye remaining, with silicone oil-filled eyes, with serious heart, lung, liver, or kidney dysfunctions, or have other diseases that make them unsuitable for inclusion were excluded from the research. Retinal reattachments were found by B-scan in 8 (73%) of the 11 eyes at the end of the three-month treatment time; leakage of FCVB caused failure in three eyes. The production method of FCVB was correspondingly revised, and this addressed the problem. No obvious inflammation was observed in any eye after FCVB implantation, and UBM showed that the FCVB did not crush the ciliary body. There was no obvious difference between the FCVB's spectral transmittance before implantation and after removal.[52] Overall, the results showed that FCVB is an effective and safe artificial vitreous body for severe retinal detachments. It can help avoid the complications induced by silicone oil, such as glaucoma, corneal keratopathy, and silicone oil emulsification during a 12-month implantation time.[53]

Current data have demonstrated the theoretical advantages of using FCVBs, as mentioned above. Even if an ideal injectable material can be found, the use of FCVB is necessary to the artificial vitreous body. It acts as a transporter that can be injected with media, such as BSS, silicone oil, heavy oil, and hydrogels. In the present research, BSS was injected into the capsule of FCVB after PPV, and it was demonstrated as a flexible, effective, and safe vitreous substitute over a three-month implantation period.[52] Further multiple-central clinical trials are in progress in China, and the encapsulation of silicone oil, heavy oil, or hydrogels in PPV eyes will be attempted. Some common substances are active, such as collagen, hyaloronic acid, water, and the natural vitreous that consists of approximately 99% water and 1.0% inorganic salts, organic lipids, and hyaluronan[1], so these are not recommended as encapsulated tamponades in PPV eyes.

In addition, tiny (300 nm) apertures (Fig.2)[54] exist in the capsule, so the FCVB can release dexamethasone sodium phosphate and Protein kinase Cα. It can also be used as an intravitreal drug delivery system in addition to serving as a vitreous substitute.[54,55] Therefore, without the need to change its chemical properties, FCVB may provide a common vehicle for different drug releases, including antibiotics, anti-proliferative agents, and vascular endothelial growth factor antagonists.

The present exploratory clinical study was not large enough to provide a definitive conclusion. Further, the effects of FCVB on the lens should be further evaluated because 10 of 11 eyes were aphakic, and only one eye was phakic.[52] Based on this trial, a nine-hospital clinical trial is currently in progress in China to ascertain FCVBs' safety and efficacy as a vitreous substitute. The FCVB produced by Guangzhou Vesber Co. Ltd. is still in the stage of clinical trial, so it is not commercially available.

FCVBs have some similarities to thin elastic capsule breast implants and tissue expander systems used in plastic surgery. However, they also have differences, which are as follows. (1) Production methods: FCVBs are formed by injection forming technology and have a US patent, whereas capsule breast implants and tissue expander systems are made by dip forming for large balloons. (2) Sample size: Producing an irregular vitreous-shaped thin capsule and smoothly connecting it to a 1.2 mm diameter tube and a pressure-control valve are major challenges. However, capsule breast implants and tissue expander systems are large and easily made. (3) Implantation site: FCVBs are implanted into the vitreous cavity and come into contact with very tender tissues, such as the retina, ciliary body, lens, and anterior chamber. However, capsule breast implants and tissue expander systems directly come into contact with adipose tissues. Therefore, there are a number of safety issues in the use of FCVBs, which have to be addressed.

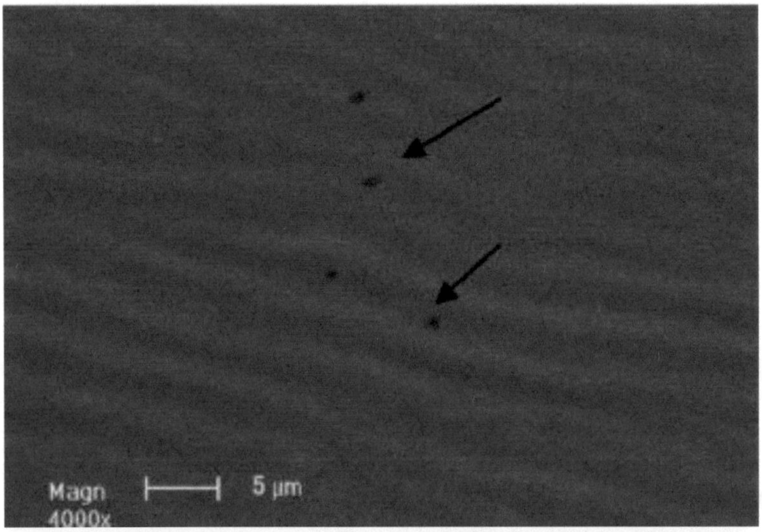

(A)

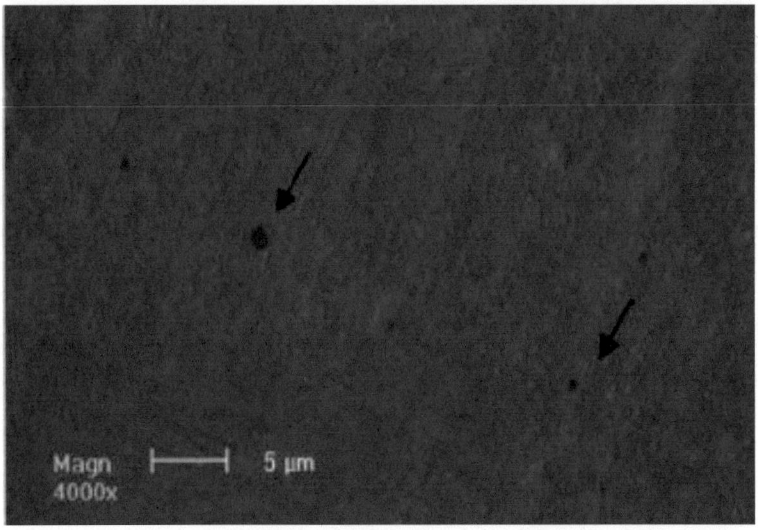

(B)

Fig. 2. Scanning electron microscope images of the capsule of the FCVB. Before implantation (**A**) and at the end of the observation time (**B**) 300-nm-mili apertures in the capsule were observed (*arrows*).

In conclusion, a new paradigm for the fabrication of a vitreous body substitute using FCVB was proposed in the current work. FCVB was established as an acceptable replacement as it closely mimics the morphology and restores the physiological function of the vitreous body. This idea provided us with a novel approach in researching on a new therapy strategy mimicking the natural vitreous that has been used for nearly half a century.

2. Acknowledgments

This study was supported by the National Nature Science Foundation of China (30973258) and National High-tech R&D Program of China (863 Program, 2009AA2Z404). I would like to thank my postgraduates, Shuyi Mai, Peijuan Wang, Ting Wang, Xuyuan Sun and Zhen Huang, for collecting the data.

3. References

[1] Green WR, Sebag J. Vitreoretinal interface. In: Ryan SJ, eds. Retina. 4th ed. Philadelphia, USA: Elsevier Mosby, 2006:1921-1989.

[2] Baino F. Towards an ideal biomaterial for vitreous replacement: Historical overview and future trends. Acta Biomater 2011; 7: 921-935.

[3] Gloor BP. The vitreous. In: Moses RA, Hart WM, editors. Adler's physiology of the eye. St. Louis: CV Mosby Co.; 1987: 246–267.

[4] Sebag J. Macromolecular structure of the corpus vitreus. Prog Polym Sci 1998; 23: 415-446.

[5] Chirila TV, Hong Y. The vitreous humour. In: Black J, Hastings GW, editors. Handbook of biomaterial properties. London: Chapman & Hall; 1998: 125–31.

[6] Goff MM Le, Bishop PN. Adult vitreous structure and postnatal changes. Eye. 2008; 22: 1214-1222.

[7] Byer NE. Natural history of posterior vitreous detachment with early management as the premier line of defense against retinal detachment. Ophthalmology. 1994;101:1503-1514.

[8] Los LI, Van Der Vorp RJ, Van Luyn MJA, Hooymans JMM. Age-related liquefaction of vitreous body: LM and TEM evaluation of the role of proteoglycans and collagen. Invest Ophthalmol Vis Sci 2003; 44: 2828–2833.

[9] Castellarin A, Grigorian R, Bhagat N, Del Priore L, Zarbin MA. Vitrectomy with silicone oil infusion in severe diabetic retinopathy. Br J Ophthalmol 2003; 87: 318-321.

[10] Quiram PA, Gonzales CR, Hu W, et al. Outcomes of vitrectomy with inferior retinectomy in patients with recurrent rhegmatogenous retinal detachments and proliferative vitreoretinopathy. Ophthalmology 2006; 113: 2041-2047.

[11] Yoon YH, Lee SU, Sohn JH, Lee SE. Result of early vitrectomy for endogenous Klebsiella pneumoniae endophthalmitis. Retina 2003; 23: 366-370.

[12] Kleinberg TT, Tzekov RT, Stein L, Ravi N, Kaushal S. Vitreous substitutes: a comprehensive review. Surv Ophthalmol. 2011; 56: 300-323

[13] 13. Ryan SJ, 4th edition, Retina, London, England: Elsevier/Mosby 127: 2137-2149.

[14] 14. Norton EWD, Aaberg T, Fung W and Curtin VT. Giant retinal tears. I. Clinical management with intravitreal air. Trans Am Ophthalmol Soc. 1969; 67: 374–393.

[15] 15. Marcus DM, D'Amico DJ, Mukai S. Pneumatic retinopexy versus scleral buckling forrepair of primary rhegmatogenous retinal detachment. Int Ophthalmol Clin. 1994; 34: 97-108.

[16] 16. Brinton DA, Wilkinson CP. Retinal detachment-principles and practice. Oxford, UK: Oxford University Press; 2009.

[17] 17. Norton EWD. Intraocular gas in the management of selected retinal detachments. Trans Am Acad Ophthalmol Otolaryngol. 1973; 77: 85-98.

[18] 18. Lincoff HA, Mardirossian J, Lincoff A, Ligget P, Iwamoto T, Jakobiec F. Intravitreal longevity of three perfluorocarbon gases. Arch Ophthalmol. 1980; 98:1610-1611.

[19] 19. Azen SP, ScottIU, Flynn HW Jr, et al.Silicone oil in the repair of complex retinal detachments. A prospective observational multicenter study. Ophthalmology. 1998;105(9):1587-1597.

[20] 20. Lee DA, Wilson MR, Yoshizumi MO,et al. The ocular effects of gases when injected into the anterior chamber of rabbit eyes. Arch Ophthalmol.1991;109(4):571-575.

[21] 21. Wilkinson C, Rice T. Instrumentation, materials, and treatment alternatives,in Craven L (ed) Michels Retinal Detachment.St.Louis, MO, Mosby,ed 21996,pp 391--461.

[22] 22. Yaws CL, Braker W. Matheson Gas Data Book. Appendix18, Refractive index, dipole moment and radius of gyration. New York, McGraw--Hill Professional, 2001, ed7, p919.

[23] 23. Lincoff A, Lincoff H, Solorzano C, Iwamoto T. Selection of Xenon gas for rapidly disappearing retinal tamponade. Arch Opthalmol. 1982; 100: 996-997.

[24] 24. Lincoff H, Kreissig I. Applications of Xenon gas to clinical retinal detachment. Arch Ophthalmol. 1982; 100:1083-1085.

[25] 25. Cibis PA, Becker B, Okun E, Canaan S. The use of liquid silicone in retinal detachment surgery. Arch Ophthalmol. 1962; 68: 590–599.

[26] 26. Soman N, Banerjee R. Artificial vitreous replacements. Biomed Mater Eng. 2003; 13: 59-74.

[27] 27. Ichhpujani P, Jindal A, Jay Katz L. Silicone oil induced glaucoma: a review. Graefe's Arch Clin Exp Ophthalmol. 2009; 247:1585-1593.

[28] La Cour M, Lux A, Heegaard S. Visual loss under silicone oil. Klin Monbl Augenheilkd. 2010; 227: 181-184.

[29] Bhisitkul RB, Gonzalez VH. "Heavy oil" for intraocular tamponade in retinal detachment surgery. Br J Ophthalmol. 2005; 89: 649-650.

[30] Rizzo S, Genovesi-Ebert F, Vento A, et al. Heavy silicone oil(densiron-68) for the treatment of persistent macular holes: densiron-68 endotamponade for persistent macular holes. Graefes Arch Clin Exp Ophthalmol. 2009;247:1471-1476

[31] Maruoka S, Matsuura T, Kawasaki K, et al. Biocompatibility of polyvinylalcohol gel as a vitreous substitute. Curr Eye Res. 2006; 31: 599-606.

[32] Hong Y, Chirila TV, Vijayasekaran S, Dalton PD, Tahija SG, Cuypers MH, et al. Crosslinked poly(1-vinyl-2-pyrrolidinone) as a vitreous substitute. J Biomed Mater Res 1996;30: 441–448.

[33] Hamilton PD, Aliyar HA, Ravi N. Biocompatibility of thiol-containing polyacrylamide polymers suitable for ophthalmic applications. Polym Prep 2004;45: 495–496.

[34] Pritchard CD, Crafoord S, Andréasson S, Arnér KM, O'Shea TM, Langer R, Ghosh FK. Evaluation of viscoelastic poly(ethylene glycol) sols as vitreous substitutes in an experimental vitrectomy model in rabbits. Acta Biomater. 2011;7: 936-943.

[35] Sawhney AS, Pathak CP, Hubbell JA. Bioerodible hydrogels based on photopolymerized poly(ethylene glycol)-co-poly(alpha-hydroxy acid) diacrylate macromers. Macromolecules 1993; 26: 581-587.

[36] Chirila TV, Hong Y, Dalton PD, Constable IJ, Refojo MF. The use of hydrophilic polymers as artificial vitreous. Prog Polym Sci. 1998; 23 (3): 475–508.

[37] Chirila TV, Hong Y. Poly (1-vinyl-2-pyrrolidinone) hydrogels as vitreous substitutes: a rheological study. Polym Int. 1998;46:183–195.

[38] Chaterji S, Kwon IK, Park K. Smart polymeric gels: redefining the limits of biomedical devices. Prog Polym Sci. 2007;32: 1083-122.

[39] Tanaka T, Fillmore D, Sun ST, Nishio I, Swislow G, Shah A. Phase transitions in ionic gels. Phys Rev Lett 1980; 45: 1636-9.

[40] Steijns D, Stilma JS. Vitrectomy: in search of the ideal vitreous replacement. Ned Tijdschr Geneeskd. 2009;153: A 433.

[41] Soman N, Banerjee R. Artificial vitreous replacements. Biomed Mater Eng. 2003; 13: 59-74.

[42] Colthurst MJ, Williams RL, Hiscott PS, Grierson I. Biomaterials used in the posterior segment of the eye. Biomaterials. 2000; 21: 649-665.

[43] Berry MG, Davies DM. Breast augmentation: Part I--A review of the silicone prosthesis. J Plast Reconstr Aesthet Surg. 2010; 63 (11):1761-8.

[44] Stavrou D, Weissman O, Winkler E, Yankelson L, Millet E, Mushin OP, Liran A, Haik J. Silicone-based scar therapy: a review of the literature. Aesthetic Plast Surg. 2010;34 (5):646-51.

[45] Prather CL, Jones DH. Liquid injectable silicone for soft tissue augmentation. Dermatol Ther. 2006; 19 (3):159-68

[46] 46. Gao Q, Mou S, Ge J, et al. A new strategy to replace the natural vitreous by a novel capsular artificial vitreous body with pressure-control valve. Eye. 2008; 22: 461-468.

[47] Gao Q. A novel method and mould for foldable capsular vitreous body, China patent (200810199177.3)(2008).

[48] Chen J, Gao Q, Liu Y, et al. Evaluation of morphology and functions of a foldable capsular vitreous body in rabbit eye. Journal of Biomedical Materials Research: Part B, 2011;97: 396-404.

[49] Gao Q, Chen X, Ge J, et al. Refractive shifts in four selected artificial vitreous substitutes based on Gullstrand-Emsley and Liou-Brennan schematic eyes. Invest Ophthalmol Vis Sci 2009; 50: 3529-3534.

[50] Liu Y, Jiang Z, Gao Q, et al. Technical standards of foldable capsular vitreous body regarding mechanical, optical and biocompatible properties. Artif Organs. 2010; 34: 836-845.

[51] Gampper TJ, Khoury H, Gottlieb W, Morgan RF. Silicone gel implants in breast augmentation and reconstruction. Ann Plast Surg 2007;59: 581–590.

[52] Lin X, Ge J, Gao Q, et al. Evaluation of the flexibility, efficacy, and safety of a foldable capsular vitreous body in the treatment of severe retinal detachment. Invest Ophthalmol Vis Sci. 2011; 52(1):374-381.

[53] Lin X, Wang Z, Gao Q, et al. Preliminary efficacy and safety of a silicone oil-filled foldable capsular vitreous body in the treatment of severe retinal detachment. Retina. 2011, Proof.

[54] Liu Y, Ke Q, Chen J, et al. Dexamethasone sodium phosphate sustained mechanical release in the foldable capsular vitreous body. Invest Ophthalmol Vis Sci. 2010; 51: 1636-1642.

[55] Chen X, Liu Y, Gao Q, et al. Protein kinase Cα downregulation via siRNA-PKCα released from foldable capsular vitreous body in cultured human retinal pigment epithelium cells. Int J Nanomed. 2011; 6: 1303-1311.

19

Endophthalmitis

Phillip S. Coburn and Michelle C. Callegan
University of Oklahoma Health Sciences Center, Dean McGee Eye Institute, Oklahoma City, Oklahoma, USA

1. Introduction

Endophthalmitis is an infection of the anterior and posterior segments of the eye resulting from the introduction of microorganisms following a surgical procedure (postoperative), traumatic penetrating injury (posttraumatic), or metastasis from an infection of a distant site in the body (endogenous). Endophthalmitis can develop into panophthalmitis if the infectious agent invades the cornea and sclera. The vast majority of cases of endophthalmitis result from intraocular surgical procedures, in particular cataract surgery (West et al., 2005). Over the past several decades, the number of postoperative endophthalmitis cases has risen steadily, owing to the increase in the number of invasive ocular surgeries performed (West et al., 2005). The etiological agents responsible for endophthalmitis include both Gram-positive and Gram-negative bacteria and fungi. Cases of post-surgical endophthalmitis are usually a result of the introduction of members of the normal microbiota of the eyelid and skin surrounding the eye, the most common cause being coagulase-negative staphylococci (CNS) (West et al., 2005). Cases of posttraumatic endophthalmitis are more frequently caused by environmental bacteria, the most common being *Staphylococcus aureus* and *Bacillus cereus* (Jonas et al., 2000; Meredith, 1999; O'Brien & Choic, 1995; Thompson et al., 1993). Frequent causes of endogenous endophthalmitis (EE) include *S. aureus*, streptococcal species, *B. cereus*, and Gram-negative bacteria including *Klebsiella pneumoniae*, *Escherichia coli*, and fungal agents such as *Candida albicans* (Greenwald et al., 1986; Jackson et al., 2003; Okada et al., 1994; Romero et al., 1999; Shammas, 1977; Shrader et al., 1990).

The clinical hallmarks of endophthalmitis are acute vision loss, severe ocular pain, periorbital swelling, hypopyon, proptosis, and the presence of white cells and flare in the anterior chamber and vitreous (Lemley and Han, 2007). The visual prognosis can vary widely depending on the infectious agent, ranging from mild inflammation and full resolution to devastating blindness and loss of the eye. Therapy for endophthalmitis caused by avirulent skin microbiota typically results in complete resolution and full vision recovery. However, posttraumatic or endogenous endophthalmitis caused by virulent pathogens may not respond to therapeutic intervention and result in partial to complete vision loss, and in some instances, evisceration or enucleation of the infected eye.

This chapter will present a summation of the latest findings of epidemiological studies and discuss current therapeutic modalities. Moreover, the bacteriology and the current state of knowledge regarding the pathogenesis and host/pathogen interactions will be explored.

Given that a number of detailed and authoritative reviews of endophthalmitis in general have been published in the last ten years, and given the paucity of reviews on endogenous bacterial endophthalmitis, this chapter will primarily focus on this route of endophthalmitis.

2. Endogenous endophthalmitis

2.1 Historical perspective

Endogenous or metastatic endophthalmitis results from microorganisms seeding the bloodstream from a distant focus of infection and invading the posterior segment of the eye via a compromised blood retinal barrier (BRB) (Arevalo et al., 2010; Greenwald et al., 1986; Jackson et al., 2003; Okada et al., 1994; Romero et al., 1999; Shammas, 1977; Shrader et al., 1990). While this form of endophthalmitis is rare, the potential for blindness in one or both eyes is high. To date, almost nothing is known about the pathogenesis of endogenous endophthalmitis (EE), even though this disease ranks as one of the most devastating infections of the eye. In the pre-antibiotic era, the majority of cases of endophthalmitis resulted in poor visual outcome. From 1944 to 1966, approximately 73% of endophthalmitis cases resulted in a final visual acuity of hand motion vision or worse. The clinical outcome of endophthalmitis improved somewhat upon the introduction of intravitreal antibiotics and vitrectomy (Neveu and Elliot, 1959; Peyman et al., 1978). Even after the introduction of intravitreal antibiotic therapy and vitrectomy, the visual outcome of EE has not improved significantly in over 50 years (Jackson et al., 2003). Morever, there is a paucity of information on the pathogenic mechanisms of this disease from both the causative agent and host perspectives. The majority of patients have an underlying condition and are immunocompromised (Jackson et al., 2003). The leading predisposing condition of EE is diabetes mellitus type 2, but intravenous drug abuse, immunosuppressive agents, malignancies, and AIDS are also underlying conditions (Arevalo et al., 2010). Symptoms of EE typically include ocular pain, blurring or loss of vision, purulent discharge, and photophobia. EE may present as focal white nodules on the lens capsule, iris, retina, or choroid, or as a ubiquitous inflammation of multiple ocular tissues resulting in purulent exudate throughout the globe. In addition, inflammation can spread to involve the orbital soft tissue (Arevalo et al., 2010).

EE was first identified and described by the German pathologist Rudolf Ludwig Karl Virchow in 1856 (Virchow, 1856). While the causative agent was not identified, it may have been bacterial. In 1894, German ophthalmologist Theodor Axenfeld reported in a treatise on endogenous endophthalmitis that the majority of cases involved only one eye and were a result of the deposition of septic emboli in the uvea (Axenfeld, 1894). However, in one-third of cases, both eyes were affected and infection was selectively localized to the retina. Axenfeld postulated that although bacteria were found in all branches of the carotid and ophthalmic arteries, the predilection for the retina was probably due to the smaller size of the retinal capillaries and „the presence of areas of disease in the capillary walls favoring the lodgment there of micro-organisms" (Tooker, 1938). Collins and Mayou (1925) further speculated that „the retina becomes infiltrated with polymorphonuclear leukocyes, which make their way inward, collecting in large numbers between the retina and the hyaloid membrane and in the neighboring vitreous". Axenfeld noted in his writings that approximately one-third of patients with EE also had endocarditis, and that the vegetations were the likely source of bacteria infecting the eye. In 1916, a case of unilateral EE in a 19 year-old soldier with cerebrospinal meningitis was described (Weakley, 1916). Gram-negative diplococci, presumably *Neisseria meningitidis,* was cultured from both the cerebrospinal fluid and from the anterior chamber of the left eye. The patient was treated with repeated injections of antimeningococcus serum into the spinal column, which resulted in complete resolution of the meningitis. Interestingly, infection and inflammation of the affected eye was also resolved, leading the case author to speculate that the antiserum therapy may have contributed to the rapid clearance of the infection. Regardless of whether the antiserum had any effect on clearing the infection, the patient retained only perception of light visual acuity (Weakley, 1916). In 1938, Tooker described a case of unilateral EE in a patient that was readmitted to the hospital after having undergone ear surgery (Tooker, 1938). The left eye was severely inflammed and visual acuity was perception of light only. Blood cultures were positive for staphylococci and the patient expired from septicemia three days following readmission. An autopsy revealed bronchial pneumonia, vegetative endocarditis, and abscesses in the kidneys, spleen, and liver. Examination of the left eyeball revealed two primary foci in the retina and ciliary body. Tooker concluded that staphylococcal emboli lodged in the retinal and ciliary capillaries, entered the vitreous chamber, and induced a robust inflammatory response. Tooker reported that the patient had been in excellent condition prior to the ear surgery, blood glucose levels were normal, and no other underlying condition was present. It is therefore possible that a systemic inflammatory response induced a breakdown in the blood retinal barrier allowing staphylococci to invade the vitreous humor.

Even after the introduction of antibiotic therapy, visual outcomes following EE remained poor. Walker and Fenwick (1962) reported a case of fulminate bilateral endophthalmitis following streptococcal septicemia. In spite of aggressive treatment with systemic steroids, hydrocortisone ointment, and local and systemic antibiotics, vision in the right eye was perception of light, and in the left was count fingers. More recently, Jackson et al. (2003) reviewed 267 cases of EE and found that the visual prognosis was uniformly poor. These authors offered a number of possible explanations for the poor visual outcome of EE, including misdiagnosis owing to the fact that EE may mimic other ocular conditions, the rapid progression of the disease, and the failure to recognize the overlap between ocular and systemic infection (Jackson et al., 2003). Since the earliest reports of EE, little progress has been achieved in improving the visual prognosis of this disease. This highlights the necessity for studies to characterize the factors that contribute to the pathogenesis of EE, both from the host and the bacterial perspectives.

2.2 Epidemiology and bacteriology

Current epidemiological studies indicate that EE accounts for approximately 2 to 15% of all cases of infectious endophthalmitis (Arevalo et al., 2010; Puliafito et al., 1982). The often poor visual outcome and potential for bilateral blindness make EE one of the most destructive and devastating ocular infections. In recent reviews of cases of bacterial EE, 41% of cases resulted in a final visual acuity of count fingers or better, 26% of infected eyes lost all useful vision, and 29% required enucleation or evisceration (Greenwald et al., 1986; Jackson et al., 2003; Shammas, 1977). The vast majority of infections are unilateral, with disagreement among studies as to whether there is a predilection for the right or left eye (Arevalo et al., 2010; Greenwald et al., 1986; Jackson et al., 2003; Okada et al., 1994). Bilateral infections occur in approximately 25% of patients with EE (Arevalo et al., 2010). As stated earlier, over 50% of EE patients have an underlying medical condition, with diabetes being the most prevalent. Additional populations at risk include immunocompromised patients, patients with prolonged indwelling devices, and intravenous drug abusers. Sources of infection include suppurative liver disease, endocarditis, urinary tract infection, and meningitis (Jackson et al., 2003). Virtually any organism that can infect the bloodstream has the capability to cause EE, but frequent causes include opportunistic and environmental pathogens such as *Staphylococcus aureus*, *Streptococcus sp.*, *Clostridium septicum*, coagulase-negative *Staphylococcus*, *Bacillus cereus*, *Listeria monogocytogenes*, *Escherichia coli*, *Klebsiella pneumoniae*, *Serratia marcescens*, *Pseudomonas aeruginosa*, and *Neisseria meningitidis* (Arevalo et al., 2010). However, *S. aureus* and *K. pneumoniae* dominate as bacterial causes of Gram-positive and Gram-negative cases of EE, respectively.

S. aureus is a Gram-positive bacterium found as a member of the normal microbiota of skin and mucosa, but can cause a variety of systemic, skin, and deep tissue infections and is a leading cause of contact lens-associated corneal infections (Callegan et al., 1994; Callegan et al., 2002b). The association between *S. aureus* EE and the prolonged use of indwelling prosthetics has been reported in diabetics and patients with other underlying immunocompromise with increasing frequency (Jackson et al., 2003; Major et al., 2010; Ness and Schneider, 2009; Nixdorff et al., 2009; Okada et al., 1994). *S. aureus* causes the majority of the cases of EE in Western countries and Europe (Ho et al., 2011). The emergence of lineages resistant to methicillin in the 1960s has prompted a public health crisis due to the difficulty in treating methicillin-resistant *S. aureus* (MRSA) infections and the increasing trend of infection among individuals with fully competent immune systems. MRSA infections may be community acquired (CA) or healthcare-associated (HA), with CA-MRSA being easier to treat but considerably more virulent. Coinciding with an increase in the prevalence of MRSA strains is an increase in MRSA ocular infections (Blomquist, 2006; Major et al., 2010). Recently, Ho et al. (2011) described a series of 7 patients (8 eyes) from a single institution that were diagnosed with EE caused by MRSA. Treatment of these cases consisted of intravitreal tap and injection of vancomycin and ceftazidime, as well as intravenous vancomycin. While retinal detachment occurred in 6 of 8 eyes, most of the patients experienced improved visual acuity from initial presentation, and only one eye lost all vision and required enucleation. Previous reports found that only 23.5% of cases of MRSA EE resulted in a visual acuity better than 20/200, whereas these authors found that 37.5% of eyes showed a final visual acuity of better than 20/200 (Ho et al., 2011). The authors contend that the higher than usual retinal detachment rate observered in their study might have been due to the higher than normal time between onset of EE and presentation, generally a mean time of 3.5 to 7.1 days versus a mean time of 17 days in their study (Ho et al., 2011).

K. pneumoniae is responsible for the majority of cases of EE due to Gram-negative bacteria and is the leading cause of EE throughout East Asia (Arevalo et al., 2010). Similar to MRSA, *K. pneumoniae* represents a therapeutic challenge due to increasing rates of acquisition of antibiotic resistance determinants. Although *K. pneumoniae* is found in the environment and as a commensal member of the gastrointestinal tract microbiota, it is also a frequent cause of healthcare-associated infections such as pneumonia, bacteremia, and urinary tract infections (Chang et al., 2002; Chuang et al., 2006; Fang et al., 2004; Fung et al., 2002;). *K. pneumoniae* has become the leading cause of pyogenic liver abscess in patients in Taiwan and other countries in the Far East (Chang et al., 2000; Wang et al., 1998), and reports of *K. pneumoniae* EE resulting from septicemia following pyogenic liver abscesses in diabetics are increasing (Chang et al., 2002; Chen et al., 2004; Chuang et al., 2006; Fang et al., 2004; Fung et al., 2002;).

In a case review of 18 patients with EE in Korea, Chung et al. (2011) also reported a close association between diabetes and infection with *K. pneumoniae*, and these factors were linked to a poor visual prognosis. These findings highlight the necessity for increased scrutiny of diabetic patients that present with ocular symptoms.

2.3 Diagnosis and therapeutic modalities

Early diagnosis and the initiation of treatment are critical to controlling infection and improving the visual prognosis of EE. Diagnosis of EE is difficult to establish based on clinical presentation alone because of the nonspecific nature of the symptomology. Diagnosis is usually based on clinical presentation and additional methods such as fundoscopy, ultrasonography, optical coherence tomography, and magnetic resonance imaging (Jackson et al., 2003). When EE is suspected, cultures of blood, vitreous and aqueous humor, and Gram stains are criticial for confirmation (Arevalo et al., 2010). Symptoms of systemic disease may also be useful in diagnosis, however only 57% of patients with EE manifested systemic signs of infection (Okada et al., 1994). Moreover, EE might be missed in patients with systemic infection until ocular pain and vision loss are experienced. Therapy for diagnosed bacterial EE consists of administration of systemic antibiotics such as third generation cephalosporins, vancomycin, and aminoglycosides (Lemley and Han, 2007). Fourth generation fluoroquinolones are also used at the discretion of the physician (Lemley and Han, 2007). Therapy also consists of intravitreal injection of 1 mg vancomyin per 0.1 ml for Gram-positive and 2.25 mg ceftazidime per 0.1 ml for Gram-negative pathogens and/or the aminoglycoside amikacin (0.4 mg). Jackson et al. (2003) reported in a literature review that vitrectomy is beneficial in cases of severe EE caused by highly virulent organisms and increases the likelihood of a better visual outcome by threefold. Vitrectomy is also indicated for cases of EE complicated by retinal detachment (Arevalo et al., 2010). As stated earlier, however, the visual outcome of EE has not improved in over 50 years. The lack of clinical improvements in EE is likely due to the lack of a reproducible animal model in which to study this disease; a disease model would be beneficial in terms of therapeutic testing and analysis of pathogenesis.

2.4 Pathogenesis

EE is one of the most frequently blinding intraocular infections, however little is known about the interplay of host and bacterial factors that contribute to the development of this disease. Moreover, the pathogenic mechanisms underlying the migration of bacteria toward and into the eye, inflammation, and vision loss have not been addressed. It is also unknown as to why diabetes is a common predisposing condition, although there are a number of possible explanations. Diabetes compromises the eye both immunologically and architecturally, resulting in changes that may weaken the ability of the eye to exclude organisms during systemic infection. One of the most serious and common complications among diabetics, specifically those with type 2 diabetes, is diabetic retinopathy (Aiello et al., 1998; Engler et al., 1991). During the progression of diabetic retinopathy, the vasculature, glia, and neurons of the retina are affected. The initial changes that occur within the retinal vasculature are the death of pericytes and thickening of the basement membrane, which lead to capillary leakage and occlusion. These changes ultimately result in macular edema, formation of new vessels, and neuroretinal degeneration (Asnaghi et al., 2003; Fong et al., 2003; Martin et al., 2004; Neely and Gardner, 1998; Qaum et al., 2001; Takeda et al., 2001).

Increases in vascular endothelial growth factor (VEGF) and the cytokines interleukin (IL)-1β, IL-6, IL-8, and tumor necrosis factor alpha (TNFα) in diabetic retinas contribute to angiogenesis and to breakdown in the BRB, implying an association with inflammation in the disease process (Jo et al., 2010). Intercellular adhesion molecule 1 (ICAM-1) and CD18 are upregulated and contribute to increased leukocyte adhesion to the endothelial wall. This is turn results in endothelial cell injury and death (Funatsu et al., 2005; Miyamoto et al., 1998; Miyamoto et al., 1999; Schroder et al., 1991). Elevated expression of matrix metalloproteases in the retina may also facilitate increases in vascular permeability and degradation of tight junction complexes, leading to BRB dysfunction (Giebel et al., 2005). Retinal pigment epithelia (RPE) and vascular endothelium, barrier cells of the BRB, also undergo changes in hyperglycemic environments *in vitro* and *in vivo*, including increases in VEGF that may contribute to vascular permeability (Amrite et al., 2006; Losso et al., 2010). The deterioration of the BRB during the development of diabetic retinopathy may allow pathogens to more readily invade the interior of the eye and might partially explain the link between diabetes and an increased risk of acquiring EE. Unfortunately, a clinical link between patients with diabetic retinopathy and EE has not been reported, only speculated. Retinal vascular permeability is not the only change occurring in a diabetic individual. Diabetes also compromises the innate immune response and depresses the ability to clear infections in general. Polymorphonuclear leukocytes (PMN) are of critical importance in clearing pathogens from the bloodstream and in the eye during acute bacterial endophthalmitis (Callegan et al., 1999; Ramadan et al., 2006; Ramadan et al., 2008; Wiskur et al., 2008). These important cells are impaired in diabetics. PMN defects in chemotaxis, phagocytosis, and bactericidal activity have been reported in the context of diabetes (Delamaire et al., 1997; Walrand et al., 2004) and PMN from diabetic mice and humans are incapable of phagocytizing and killing both *S. aureus* and *K. pneumoniae* (Lin et al., 2006; Park et al., 2009). These defects in the ability of PMNs to clear bacteria that are destined to cross a compromised blood retinal barrier may also contribute to the development and pathogenesis of EE, but this has not been scientifically analyzed.

Virtually nothing is known about the bacterial factors that contribute to the pathogenesis of EE. *S. aureus* and *K. pneumoniae* possess a repertoire of factors with demonstrable roles in the virulence of these species in a number of animal models of infection, however it is currently unknown if they contribute to the pathogenesis of EE. *S. aureus* expresses a number of adhesins, including the fibronectin binding proteins FnbpA and FnbpB (Green et al., 1995), the fibrinogen-binding proteins ClfA and ClfB (McDevitt et al., 1994), and the collagen binding protein Cna (Patti et al., 1992) that have been shown to mediate attachment to extracellular matrix and plasma proteins, a crucial first step in initiating infections. *S. aureus* synthesizes alpha-toxin, a cytolysin shown to be important in corneal infections (Callegan et al., 1994) and endophthalmitis (Booth et al., 1998; Callegan et al., 2002b). *S. aureus* also secretes a host of other secreted cytolytic toxins including the beta-, gamma- and delta-toxins, and Panton-Valentine leukocidin (Plata et al., 2009) that may contribute to structural damage within the eye, or in the case of Panton-Valentine leukocidin (PVL) have either anti- or pro-inflammatory effects. PVL lyses neutrophils at higher concentrations but is a potent stimulator of the release of proinflammatory cytokines such as IL-8 at lower concentrations (Otto, 2010). Some strains of *S. aureus* are also encapsulated, rendering them resistant to phagocytosis and more virulent in animal models of sepsis (Luong and Lee, 2002; Thakker et al., 1998). Most clinical isolates of *S. aureus* produce either Type 5 or Type 8 capsular polysaccharide (Roghmann et al., 2005). The capsule of *S. aureus* may afford a survival advantage and prevent clearance from the bloodstream as well as the vitreous humor, especially in diabetics with impaired clearance mechanisms.

K. pneumoniae produces at least five major virulence factors that contribute to the pathogenesis of infection and include capsular serotype, hypermucoviscosity phenotype (HMV), lipopolysaccharide (LPS), siderophores, and pili. However, nothing is known about their potential contribution to EE pathogenesis. There are 77 capsular serotypes, however serotype K1 predominates among bacteremia, liver abscess, and EE isolates in Taiwan (Fung et al., 2002). Capsule production is likely to impede clearance of *K. pneumoniae* from the bloodstream and from the eye. The HMV phenotype is enriched among highly virulent, invasive strains of *K. pneumoniae*, especially those causing EE (Fang et al., 2004; Fang et al., 2007; Fung et al., 2002; Karama et al., 2008; Keynan and Rubinstein, 2008; Lee et al., 2006). Strains that express this phenotype possess a thick, viscous capsule-associated mucopolysaccharide web (Wiskur et al., 2008). Two commonly studied genes are associated with HMV: *magA* (mucoviscosity-associated gene A), which encodes a 43 kd outer membrane protein that has not been characterized (Fang et al., 2004), and *rmpA* (regulator of the mucoid phenotype A), a regulatory gene that controls the synthesis of the extracapsular mucopolysaccharide (Nassif et al., 1989). It has been shown that HMV confers resistance to serum killing and phagocytosis, and contributes to virulence in mice (Fang et al., 2004). *magA*- transposon mutants, which lost the HMV phenotype displayed serum sensitivity, became phagocytosis susceptible, and were avirulent in a mouse model (Fang et al., 2004). *magA* was located within a 35-kb locus containing 24 open reading frames (ORFs) with homologies to genes involved in exopolysaccharide biosynthesis or export and glycosylation (Chuang et al., 2006). This locus may represent a novel pathogenicity island responsible for the hypervirulence seen with certain *K. pneumoniae* pathogenic strains (Chuang et al., 2006). HMV+ *K. pneumoniae* are the most common cause of EE in Southeast Asia, with cases of EE caused by HMV+ *K. pneumoniae* on the rise in Western countries (Keynan and Rubinstein, 2008; Lederman and Crum, 2005). Our laboratory has previously shown that the HMV phenotype contributes to the pathogenesis of experimental *K. pneumoniae* endophthalmitis. In this model, an HMV+ strain caused significantly greater inflammation and greater loss of visual function than an HMV- strain following direct injection of bacteria into the vitreous (Wiskur et al., 2008). Further, the HMV+ strain was not readily cleared from the eye in this model (Wiskur et al., 2008). More recently, the *magA* gene was directly linked to the pathogenesis of EE in experimental *K. pneumoniae* endophthalmitis. Hunt et al. compared a wildtype HMV+ *K. pneumoniae* strain with an isogenic mutant defective in the *magA* gene, and found that mice infected with the *magA*- strain showed a significantly improved visual outcome relative to mice infected with the wildtype strain (Hunt et al., 2011). These results clearly demonstrate a role for the HMV phenotype in *K. pneumoniae* endophthalmitis. As this direct injection model circumvents systemic infection, it remains to be seen whether the HMV phenotype is important for crossing the BRB and establishing EBE.

The lipopolysaccharide O side chain has been shown to confer serum resistance to *K. pneumoniae* by preventing the deposition of complement components on the bacterial cell membrane and the ensuing complement-mediated cell lysis (Tomas et al., 1986). It is therefore possible that *K. pneumoniae* LPS from cells migrating near the BRB might elicit increases in permeability in the retinal vasculature that result in leakiness, facilitating entry into the eye. Metrickin et al. (1995), demonstrated that *E. coli* LPS induced a dose-dependent breakdown of the BRB. The siderophores enterobactin and aerobactin could also potentially be involved. While enterobactin is synthesized by nearly all isolates of *K. pneumoniae*, aerobactin is less frequently detected (Podschun et al., 1993). However, only *K. pneumoniae* isolates with capsular serotype K1 or K2 that produced aerobactin were more virulent (LD_{50} $<10^3$ cfu), and transfer of the genes necessary for synthesis of aerobactin into an avirulent strain increased the virulence by 100-fold (Nassif and Sansonetti, 1986). *K. pneumoniae* produce two types of pili or fimbriae, type 1 and type 3, that mediate attachment to epithelial cells. The type 1 fimbrial adhesion gene *fimH* was shown to be enriched among blood isolates (Yu et al., 2006), and the type 3 fimbrial adhesion protein MrkD has been demonstrated to contribute to virulence by binding to epithelial cells of the urogenital, repiratory, and gastrointestinal tracts (Sebghati et al., 1998), and the type 3 fimbrial shaft protein MrkA is required for biofilm formation on intravenous and urinary catheters and human extracellular matrix (Jagnow and Clegg, 2003; Langstraat et al., 2001). It is conceivable that these pili mediate adherence to structures in the eye and aid in the establishment of EE. However, as for all of the above discussed factors, no studies have been conducted evaluating the importance of these virulence traits to EE pathogenesis due to the lack of a well-characterized animal model of this disease.

3. Postoperative endophthalmitis

Postoperative endophthalmitis is the most common type of endophthalmitis and most frequently occurs following cataract surgery, with 90% of cases occuring following this procedure (Lemley and Han, 2007). The rates of postoperative endophthalmitis have been increasing over the past several years, owing to increases in the number of cataract surgeries and other types of intraocular surgeries performed. This raises concerns due to the ever-growing population of the elderly that require cataract surgery. Millions of cataract surgeries are performed each year. Fortunately, the rate of occurrence of post-cataract endophthalmitis remains low, ranging between 0.06% and 0.25% (O'Brien et al., 2007; West et al., 2005). Among the types of cataract surgeries performed, phacoemulsification accounted for approximately 48% of the postoperative endophthalmitis cases, while 38.5% and 6.6% of cases followed extracapsular or intracapsular extraction, respectively (Ng et al., 2005). Postoperative endophthalmitis can occur after other types of surgery such as secondary intraocular lens placement, pars plana vitrectomy, penetrating keratoplasty, and even after corneal suture removal (Lemley and Han, 2007).

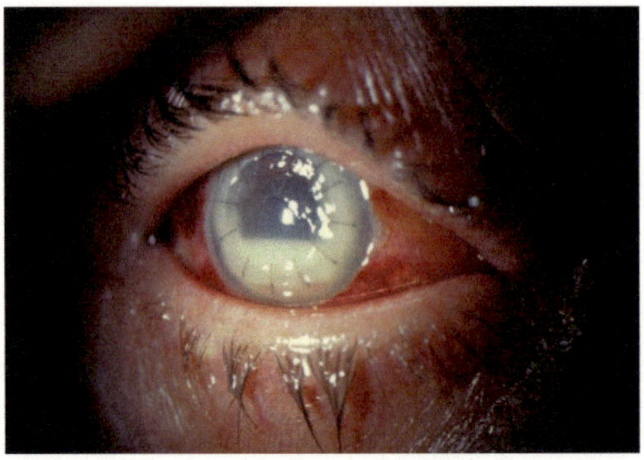

Fig. 1. Acute endophthalmitis caused by *Staphylococcus aureus* in a 43-year-old patient 3 days following a triple surgical procedure (penetrating keratoplasty, cataract extraction, and posterior chamber intraocular lens). Note the hypopion in the anterior chamber. The vitreous was also involved. Reproduced with kind permission from Dr. Rumelt

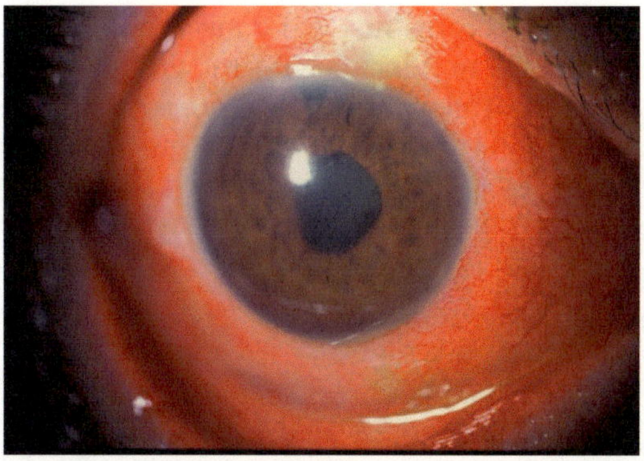

Fig. 2. Bleb-associated endophthalmitis due to *Streptococcus pneumoniae* in the right eye of a 63-year-old patient, 2 weeks after trabeculectomy. Note the whitening of the filtering bleb due to inflammatory infiltrate. There was also inflammation of the anterior and posterior segment. The earliest sign of endophthalmitis is infiltration of the bleb by inflammatory cells, and when the anterior and posterior segments are still normal, this is defined as "blebitis". Reproduced with kind permission from Dr. Rumelt

Preventative measures consist of prophylactic intracameral antibiotics or prophylactic subconjunctival antibiotic injection following cataract surgery (Kelkar et al., 2008). Patients with acute postoperative endophthalmitis generally present between 1 to 2 weeks following surgery. Endophthalmitis has also been reported to occur after intravitreal injection of anti-VEGF agents for the treatment of age-related macular degeneration (AMD). While the rate of endophthalmitis following intravitreal injection of these agents is equivalent to that of postoperative endophthalmitis following cataract surgery, approximately 0.16%, the increasing number of elderly patients requiring this type of therapy is a significant cause for alarm (Gragoudas et al., 2004).

Endophthalmitis must be distinguished from sterile inflammation following surgery. Diagnosis is established by visual acuity measurements, fundoscopy, and ERG, followed by microbiological evaluation of aqueous and vitreous samples (Lemley and Han, 2007). Gram-positive bacteria are the leading cause of postoperative endophthalmitis cases, with coagulase-negative staphylococcal (CNS) isolates being the most common, causing 47–70% of all postoperative endophthalmitis cases (Han et al., 1996). *S. aureus* account for approximately 10%, *Streptococcus* species for 9%, *Enterococcus* species for 2.2%, and Gram-negative bacteria for approximately 6% (Han et al., 1996). Fortunately, postoperative endophthalmitis caused by CNS is relatively mild and is more easily resolved with antibiotic and anti-inflammatory therapy (Josephberg, 2006). The visual prognosis is generally favorable, with 84% of cases resulting in at least 20/100 visual acuity, and 50% of these cases resulted in 20/40 visual acuity (Josephberg, 2006). Less virulent bacteria such as *Propionibacterium acnes* and CNS, and the fungal organism *Candida parapsilosis* are the most common causative agents of chronic endophthalmitis (Lemley and Han, 2007). Patients with this form of endophthalmitis typically present several months following surgery (Lemley and Han, 2007). Postoperative endophthalmitis caused by *S. aureus*, species of streptococci, enterococci, *Bacillus*, and Gram-negative bacteria can cause a more explosive and fulminant infection. The visual outcome of severe infections is uniformly poor, with only 30% of eyes attaining 20/100 visual acuity (Josephberg, 2006). The primary treatment is typically a single intravitreal injection of antibiotics consisting of 1.0 mg vancomycin per 0.1 ml, and 2.25 mg ceftazidime per 0.1 ml or 400 µg amikacin per 0.1 ml. Fourth generation fluoroquinolones can also be employed because of their broad spectrum of activity and usefulness against Gram-negative bacteria. Vitrectomy and corticosteriod therapy are are often advocated as adjunct treatment modalities (Lemley and Han, 2007), however corticosteriod treatment is still considered controversial.

4. Posttraumatic endophthalmitis

Posttraumatic endophthalmitis is a complication of a penetrating injury to the eye and is not as frequent as postoperative endophthalmitis. However, the rate of infection is higher and the visual prognosis is poorer following penetrating injury to the globe than following surgical procedures. The infection rates following traumatic injury to the globe range from 3% to 17% (Meredith, 1999; O'Brien and Choi, 1995; Thompson et al., 1993). The rates increase substantially when a foreign body remains in the globe and range from 11 to 30% (Boldt et al., 1989; Brinton et al., 1984; Thompson et al., 1993). Other risk factors include age greater than 50 and a more than 24 hour delay prior to presentation (Thompson et al., 1993). Those patients who presented for intraocular foregin body removal greater than 24 hours following injury were approximately 4-fold more likely to acquire endophthalmitis (Thompson et al, 1993), highlighting the necessity of seeking immediate medical attention following penetrating injury. Staphylocci and *B. cereus* rank as the number one and two causes, respectively, and together account for 95% of cases (Das et al., 2005; Lemley and Han, 2007).

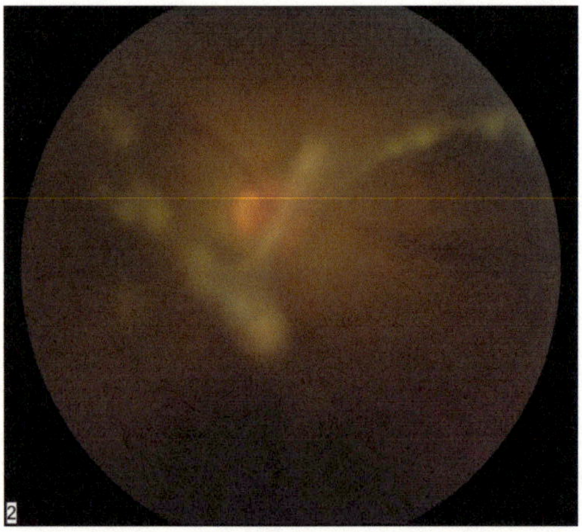

Fig. 3. Fundoscopic exam of a patient with *Staphylococcus aureus* endophthalmitis after a penetrating ocular injury. The findings of endophthalmitis in the vitreous may include not only flare and cells, but also fibrin in various degrees of organization. Organization to fibrotic bands may results in traction retinal detachment due to contraction of such bands. Reproduced with kind permission from Dr. Rumelt

B. cereus is ten times more likely to be the causative agent of posttraumatic than postoperative endophthalmitis, especially in cases involving organic or soil-contaminated intraocular foreign bodies (Das et al., 2005). Other causative agents include CNS, streptococcal species, clostridial species, fungi, and protozoa such as acanthamoeba (Lemley and Han, 2007; Rumelt et al., 2001).

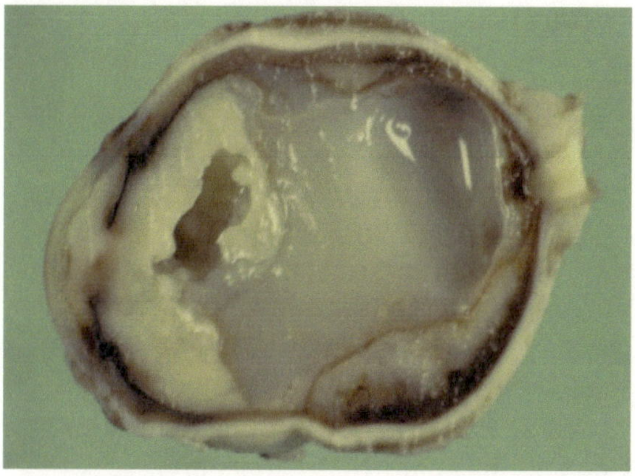

Fig. 4. Gross pathologic specimen of the globe affected by *Pseudomonas aeruginosa* endophthalmitis. The patient lost his vision in the eye and it became a blind, painful eye that underwent enucleation. Note the massive necrosis of the ocular tissues. Reproduced with kind permission from Dr. Rumelt

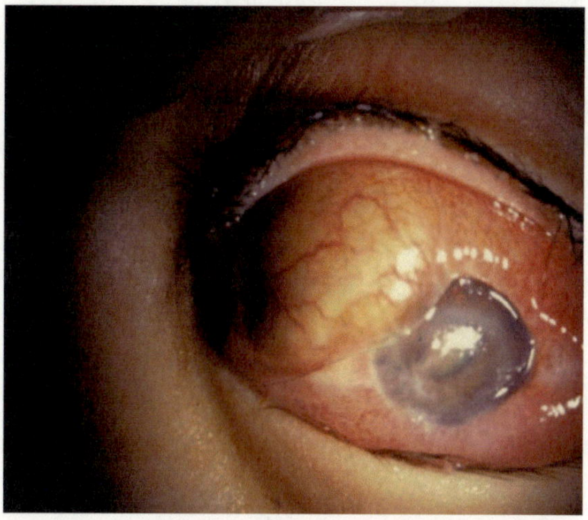

Fig. 5A. Endophthalmitis caused by the gas-forming bacterium *Clostridium bifermentans*. The endophthalmitis was caused following ocular penetrating injury be a soiled-contaminated foreign body. Note the brownish discoloration of the conjunctiva and a subconjunctival gas bubble. The patient was treated with intravenous and intravitreal panicillin and clyndamycin, but lost his vision despite the treatment. Reproduced with kind permission from Elsevier, Inc., in Rehany U, Dorenboim Y, Lefler E, Schirer E. Ophthalmology. 1994;101:839-42.

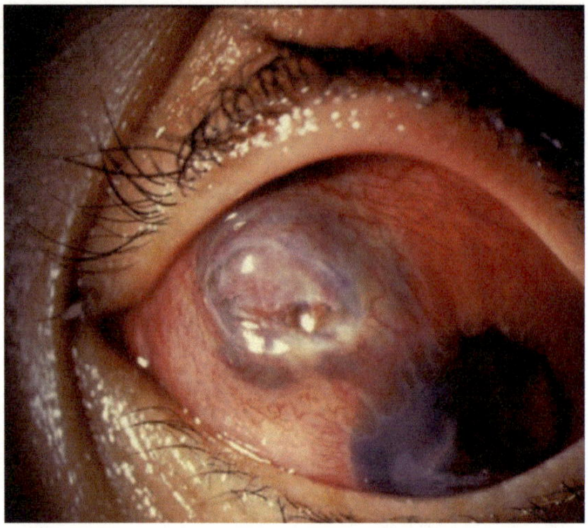

Fig. 5B. The same patient as in 5A a few days later. Note that the conjunctiva has become necrotic, the color became purple, and the gas bubble ruptured. Reproduced with kind permission from Elsevier, Inc., in Rehany U, Dorenboim Y, Lefler E, Schirer E. Ophthalmology. 1994;101:839-42.

When penetrating injury occurs, the foreign body should be removed as soon as possible, especially when the material is organic or soil contaminated due to the potential for *B. cereus* contamination (Lemley and Han, 2007). In some cases, for example where the foreign body is inert glass and is located in a sensitive position such as the retina, it may not be desirable to remove the object. Even relatively minor injuries to the eye can result in severe endophthalmitis with devastating outcomes. Cases have been described following penetrating injury to the eye due to orthodontic headgear (Blum-Hareuveni et al., 2006). Diagnosis of posttraumatic endophthalmitis is established by visual acuity tests, slit-lamp examination, and ophthalmoscopy, as well as computed tomography and ultrasound (Lemley and Han, 2007). For posttraumatic endopthalmitis, treatment consists of administration of intravitreal 1 mg vancomycin per 0.1 ml, 2.25 mg ceftazidime per 0.1 ml or 400 μg amikacin per 0.1 ml (Lemley and Han, 2007). Even with early therapy, the outcomes are often poor due to the potential virulence of the infecting bacterium and the explosive inflammatory response.

5. Experimental endophthalmitis and the roles of bacterial and host factors

A rabbit model of experimental endophthalmitis has been used to assess the contribution of both bacterial and host factors to the development of endophthalmitis. This model mimics the infection course after introduction of bacteria directly into the posterior segment of the eye that would occur following a surgical procedure or penetrating injury, but does not allow for the analysis of host immunological status and bacterial factors that contribute to the development of EE. This model system allows intravitreal injection across the pars plana of low inocula that allow the bacterium under study to adapt to the intraocular environment of the eye and replicate (Booth et al., 1995; Booth et al., 1997; Callegan et al., 1999a; Jett et al., 1992; Sanders et al., 2010; Sanders et al., 2011). Depending on the infecting organisms, infection symptoms in the rabbit model develop over a period ranging from 6 hours to 3 days, and a number of infection parameters can be repeatedly monitored and quantitative data obtained. Parameters that can be monitored include ocular inflammation, fibrin deposition, electrophysiologic measurement of retinal function, and bacterial growth and distribution. Infiltration of inflammatory cells can be quantified by slit lamp biomicroscopy in which progressive inflammation is scored in different anatomical locations within the eye (Callegan et al., 1999a). Inflammation and fibrin deposition can be qualitatively assessed by analysis of thin-section histopathology. Retinal damage as a result of the production of toxin by the bacterium under study or by bystander damage due to PMN activity in the eye can be measured by electroretinography (ERG). Using the rabbit model, Callegan et al. (1999a) found that supernatants from from *B. cereus* and *S. aureus* caused retinal damage and were highly inflammogenic, suggesting that secreted toxins are of primary importance to the pathogenesis of endophthalmitis. Callegan and colleagues did not find individual roles for the *B. cereus* membrane damaging toxins hemolysin BL, phosphatidylinositol-specific phopholipase C, and phosphatidylcholine-specific phospholipase C in this model, however, other toxins controlled by the global regulator *plcR* were found to contribute to pathogenesis of experimental *B. cereus* endophthalmitis (Callegan et al., 1999b; Callegan et al., 2002a; Callegan et al., 2003). The *S. aureus* alpha- and beta-toxins, but not the gamma-toxin, were shown to make an important contribution to endophthalmitis (Booth et al., 1998; Callegan et al., 2002b). Isogenic mutants deficient in each of the toxin-encoding genes were compared in this model. Injection of rabbit eyes with the gamma-toxin deficient mutant had no impact on retinal function when compared with the wildtype strain. However, the alpha- and beta-toxin deficient mutants were attenuated when compared with the wildtype. After 2 days, rabbit eyes infected with the alpha- or beta-toxin deficient mutant showed 40% and 60% retinal function retained, respectively, as compared with 20% retained in rabbits infected with the wildtype strain. Moreover, a cumulative effect was observed as a result of inactivation of all three toxin loci on retention of retinal function (Callegan et al., 2002b). This model has also been used as a sensitive measure of the contribution of enterococcal virulence factors to pathogenesis. Jett et al. (1992) demonstrated that the course and severity of disease was significantly determined by the *E. faecalis* biocomponent cytolysin. The cytolysin destroyed the neural tissue of the retina and its architecture over a period of 24 - 72 hours. The toxicity to retinal tissue was not attenuated by either antibiotic and/or anti-inflammatory therapy when infection involved a cytolytic strain, although an isogenic, non-cytolytic infection completely resolved when both of these treatments were provided 24 h postinfection. These studies showed not only the contribution of the cytolysin to the pathogenesis of enterococcal endophthalmitis, but also the importance of inflammatory sequelae. Engelbert et al. (2004) demonstrated that the *E. faecalis* gelatinase and serine protease in concert contributed to pathogenesis in this model as double mutants in these genes were significantly attenuated when compared to the single mutants. Callegan et al. (1999a) also utilized this model to implicate the contribution of bacterial cell wall components in inciting an inflammatory response during endophthalmitis. Injection of metabolically inactive bacteria or cell wall sacculi elicited significant intraocular inflammation. The rabbit model has also been used to implicate the *Streptococcus pneumoniae* capsule in the pathogenesis of endopthalmitis (Sanders et al., 2011). Infection with an isogenic unencapsulated *S. pneumoniae* mutant strain resulted in significantly lower slit lamp examination scores, significantly greater retinal function, and significantly less neutrophil infiltration into the eye compared with the wildtype parental strain in this model. Moreover, they demonstrated the efficacy of immunizing with the *S. pneumoniae* pneumolysin in protecting the eye from retinal damage during *S. pneumoniae* endophthalmitis (Sanders et al., 2010). In summary, the rabbit model of experimental endophthalmitis has proven invaluable in assessing the role of bacterial virulence factors and identifiying potentially new therapeutic targets.

More recently, a mouse model of experimentally induced endophthalmitis has been employed to explore various aspects of disease development, course, and outcome. As with the rabbit model, infection parameters can be qualitatively and quantitatively measured including bacterial growth, ocular inflammation, and retinal function. Ocular inflammation can be qualitatively assessed via thin-section histopathology as well as quantified by slit-lamp biomicrosopy and indirect measurements of PMN influx by a myeloperoxidase ELISA (Ramadan et al., 2006). As stated earlier, Wiskur et al. (2008) implicated the HMV phenotype in the persistence of *K. pneumoniae* in the eye by comparing the bacterial growth of an HMV+ to that of an HMV- strain after intravitreal injection of 100 CFU. The HMV- strain did not grow to the same level as the HMV+ strain and were cleared with 27 hours. HMV+ infected eyes underwent phthisis within 24 hours. This study provided evidence that the HMV phenotype makes an important contribution to *K. pneumoniae* endophthalmitis pathogenesis. As discussed above, Hunt et al. (2011) confirmed these findings using a *magA*-mutant of *K. pneumoniae* in the mouse endophthalmitis model. *S. aureus* cell wall teichoic acids have also been shown to contribute to the pathogenesis of endophthalmitis and that inhibitors of cell wall teichoic acid synthesis might serve as candidates for therapy of *S. aureus* endophthalmitis in this model (Suzuki et al., 2011).

An important aspect of the murine model of experimental endophthalmitis is that factors of the host immune system can be assessed by comparison of the infection course in genetic knockout mouse strains with that in wildtype strains of the same genetic background. Ramadan and colleagues (2006) showed that as early as 4 hours post-injection with *B. cereus*, significant decline in retinal function and PMN infiltration were observed, which coincided with an increase in the proinflammatory cytokine TNF-α. In TNF-α knockout mice, *B. cereus* replicated more rapidly, retinal function declined more sharply, and fewer PMN infiltrated the eye. These findings illustrate the power of this model in allowing the repeated measurement of multiple infection parameters and showed that damage to the retina occurred earlier than was previously thought. Furthermore, the necessity of TNF-α in PMN recruitment and control of *B. cereus* replication was established. Engelbert and Gilmore (2005) used C3 and FasL knockout out mice to dissect components of the innate immune and ocular immune privilege systems in controlling *S. aureus* endophthalmitis. The infection course in C3 knockout eyes followed a similar course to their wildtype counterparts, suggesting that complement does not play a significant role in ocular defense against *S. aureus* infection. On the other hand, the membrane-bound Fas ligand (FasL), which functions to maintain the immune privilege status of the eye by inducing apoptosis in infiltrating inflammatory cells, was found to be criticial in bacterial clearance. Mice deficient in FasL were unable to control *S. aureus* infection after injection of an inoculum that is cleared in wildtype mice (Engelbert and Gilmore, 2005). The host heat shock protein alphaB-crystallin was shown to be upregulated in the retina and prevent apoptosis and retinal damage during murine *S. aureus* endopthalmitis (Whiston et al., 2008). These authors found that mice deficient in the production of this molecular chaperone displayed increased retinal apoptosis and damage, and that *S. aureus* produced a protease capable of cleaving this protective protein. Finally, Kumar et al. (2010) suggested that the host toll-like receptor (TLR) 2 is involved in controlling infection by *S. aureus* in this model by showing that pretreatment of mice with intravitreal injections of the TLR2 ligand Pam3Cys reduced bacterial load when compared with mock-injected animals. In summary, the murine model of experimental endopthalmitis has proven to be invaluable in analyzing both host and bacterial factors that contribute to this disease. The growing number of available genetic knockouts in components of the innate and adaptive immune systems and the relative ease of use will continue to make the murine model key to understanding the complex interplay between host and bacterial factors during the initiation, course, and resolution of endophthalmitis.

6. Conclusions

Endophthalmitis remains a relatively rare infection, but the potential for vision loss and/or blindness is significant. The potential for poor prognosis, which depends on the causative organism and the immune status of the patient, remains high despite antibiotic and surgical intervention. Research on the contribution of bacterial virulence factors has implicated both secreted toxins and proteases, capsules, and the intraocular host response to bacterial cell wall components in the pathogenesis of experimental *B. cereus, S. aureus, E. faecalis, S. pneumoniae,* and *K. pneumoniae* endophthalmitis. Moreover, components of the host inflammatory response and mediators of ocular immune privilege have been shown to play critical roles in controlling experimental *B. cereus* and *S. aureus* endophthalmitis. Virtually nothing is known about the contribution of bacterial or host virulence factors to the development of EE. The fact that visual prognosis of EE and other types of bacterial endophthalmitis caused by pathogenic organisms remains uniformly poor highlights the need for continuing research on the interactions between the offending pathogen, the internal structures of the eye, underlying disease state and the immune response.

7. Acknowledgments

Portions of the work presented in this review were supported by the National Institutes of Health Grant R01EY012985 (to MCC), a Lew R. Wasserman Award from Research to Prevent Blindness (to MCC), a National Institutes of Health CORE Grant P30EY012190 (to Robert E. Anderson, OUHSC), and an unrestricted grant to the Dean A. McGee Eye Institute from Research to Prevent Blindness.

8. References

Aiello, L., Gardner, T., King, G., Blankenship, G., Cavallerano, J., Ferris, F., Klein, R. (1998). Diabetic retinopathy. *Diabetes Care,* Vol.21, pp. 143-156.

Amrite, A., Ayalasomayajula, S., Cheruvu, N., Kompella, U. (2006). Single periocular injection of celecoxib-PLGA microparticles inhibits diabetes-induced elevations in retinal PGE2, VEGF, and vascular leakage. *Invest. Ophthalmol. Vis. Sci.,* Vol.47, pp. 1149-1160.

Arevalo, J., Jap, A., Chee, S., Zeballos, D. (2010). Endogenous endophthalmitis in the developing world. *Int. Ophthalmol. Clin.,* Vol.50, pp. 173-187.

Asnaghi, V., Gerhardinger, C., Hoehn, T., Adeboje, A., Lorenzi, M. (2003). A role for the polyol pathway in the early neuroretinal apoptosis and glial changes induced by diabetes in the rat. *Diabetes*, Vol.52, pp. 506-511.

Axenfeld, T. (1894). *Arch. F. Ophth.*, pp. 103.

Blomquist, P. (2006). Methicillin-resistant *Staphylococcus aureus* infections of the eye and orbit (an American Ophthalmological Society thesis). *Trans. Am. Ophthalmol. Soc.*, Vol.104, pp. 322–345.

Blum-Hareuveni, T., Rehany, U., Rumelt, S. (2006). Devastating endophthalmitis following penetrating ocular injury during night sleep from orthodontic headgear: case report and literature review. *Graefes Arch. Clin. Exp. Ophthalmol.*, Vol.244, pp. 253-258.

Boldt, H., Pulido, J., Blodi, C., Folk, J., Weingeist, T. (1989). Rural endophthalmitis. *Ophthalmology*, Vol.96, pp. 1722-1726.

Booth, M., Atkuri, R., Nanda, S., Iandolo, J., Gilmore, M. (1995). Accessory gene regulator controls *Staphylococcus aureus* virulence in endophthalmitis. *Invest. Ophthalmol. Vis. Sci.*, Vol.36, pp. 1828-1836.

Booth, M., Cheung, A., Hatter, K., Jett, B., Callegan, M., Gilmore, M. (1997). Staphylococcal accessory regulator (*sar*) in conjunction with *agr* contributes to *Staphylococcus aureus* virulence in endophthalmitis. *Infect. Immun.*, Vol.65, pp. 1550-1556.

Booth, M., Hatter, K., Miller, D., Davis, J., Kowalski, R., Parke, D., Chodosh, J., Jett, B., Callegan, M., Penland, R., Gilmore, M. (1998). Molecular epidemiology of *Staphylococcus aureus* and *Enterococcus faecalis* in endophthalmitis. *Infect. Immun.*, Vol.66, pp. 356-360.

Brinton, G., Topping, T., Hyndiuk, R., Aaberg, T., Reeser, F., Abrams, G. (1984). Posttraumatic endophthalmitis. *Arch. Ophthalmol.*, Vol.102, pp. 547-550.

Callegan, M., Booth, M., Jett, B., Gilmore, M. (1999a). Pathogenesis of gram-positive bacterial endophthalmitis. Infect. Immun., Vol.67, pp. 3348-3356.

Callegan, M., Cochran, D., Kane, S., Gilmore, M., Gominet, M., Lereclus, D. (2002a). Contribution of membrane-damaging toxins to *Bacillus* endophthalmitis pathogenesis. *Infect.Immun.*, Vol.70, pp. 5381–5389.

Callegan, M., Engelbert, M., Parke, D., Jett, B., Gilmore, M. (2002b). Bacterial endophthalmitis: epidemiology, therapeutics, and bacterium-host interactions. *Clin. Microbiol. Rev.*, Vol.15, pp. 111-124.

Callegan, M., Engel, L., Hill, J., O'Callaghan, R. (1994). Corneal virulence of *Staphylococcus aureus*: roles of alpha-toxin and protein A in pathogenesis. *Infect. Immun.*, Vol.62, pp. 2478-2482.

Callegan, M., Jett, B., Hancock, L., Gilmore, M. (1999b). Role of hemolysin BL in the pathogenesis of extraintestinal *Bacillus cereus* infection assessed in an endophthalmitis model. *Infect. Immun.*, Vol. 67, pp. 3357-3366.

Callegan, M., Kane, S., Cochran, D., Gilmore, M., Gominet, M., Lereclus, D. (2003). Relationship of *plcR*-regulated factors to *Bacillus* endophthalmitis virulence. *Infect. Immun.*, Vol.71, pp. 3116–3124.

Chang, S., Fang, C., Hsueh, P., Chen, Y., Luh, K. (2000). *Klebsiella pneumoniae* isolates causing liver abscess in Taiwan. *Diagn. Microbiol. Infect. Dis.*, Vol.37, pp. 279-284.

Chen, Y., Kuo, H., Wu, P., Kuo, M., Tsai, H., Liu, C., Chen, C. (2004). A 10-year comparison of endogenous endophthalmitis outcomes: an east Asian experience with *Klebsiella pneumoniae* infection. *Retina*, Vol.24, pp. 383-390.

Chuang, Y., Fang, C., Lai, S., Chang, S., Wang, J. (2006). Genetic determinants of capsular serotype K1 of *Klebsiella pneumoniae* causing primary pyogenic liver abscess. *J. Infect. Dis.*, Vol.193, pp. 645-654.

Chung, K., Kim, Y., Song, Y., Kim, C., Han, S., Chin, B., Gu, N., Jeong, S., Baek, J., Choi, J., Kim, H,, Kim, J. (2011). Clinical review of endogenous endophthalmitis in Korea: a 14-year review of culture positive cases of two large hospitals. *Yonsei Med. J.*, Vol.52, pp. 630-634.

Collins, E., and Mayou, M. (1925). In: *Pathology and Bacteriology of the Eye*, P. Blakiston's Son & Co., Philadelphia.

Das, T., Kunimoto, D., Sharma, S., Jalali, S., Majji, A., Nagaraja, R., Gopinathan, U., Athmanathan, S. (2005). Relationship between clinical presentation and visual outcome in postoperative and posttraumatic endophthalmitis in south central India. *Indian J. Ophthalmol.*, Vol.53, pp. 5-16.

Delamaire, M., Maugendre, D., Moreno, M., Le Goff, M., Allannic, H., Genetet, B. (1997). Impaired leucocyte functions in diabetic patients. *Diabet. Med.*, Vol.14, pp. 29-34.

Engelbert, M., Gilmore, M. (2005). Fas ligand but not complement is critical for control of experimental *Staphylococcus aureus* endophthalmitis. *Invest. Ophthalmol. Vis. Sci.*, Vol.46, pp. 2479-2486.

Engelbert, M., Mylonakis, E., Ausubel, F., Calderwood, S., Gilmore, M. (2004). Contribution of gelatinase, serine protease, and fsr to the pathogenesis of *Enterococcus faecalis* endophthalmitis. *Infect. Immun.*, Vol.72, pp. 3628-3633.

Engler, C., Krogsaa, B., Lund-Andersen, H. (1991). Blood-retina barrier permeability and its relation to the progression of diabetic retinopathy in type 1 diabetics. An 8-year follow-up study. *Graefes Arch. Clin. Exp. Ophthalmol.*, Vol.229, pp. 442-446.

Fang, C., Chuang, Y., Shun, C., Chang, S., Wang, J. (2004). A novel virulence gene in *Klebsiella pneumoniae* strains causing primary liver abscess and septic metastatic complications. *J. Exp. Med.*, Vol.199, pp. 697-705.

Fang, C., Lai, S., Yi, W., Hsueh, P., Liu, K., Chang, S. (2007). *Klebsiella pneumoniae* genotype K1: an emerging pathogen that causes septic ocular or central nervous system complications from pyogenic liver abscess. *Clin. Infect. Dis.*, Vol.45, pp. 284-293.

Fong, D., Aiello, L., Gardner, T., King, G., Blankenship, G., Cavallerano, J., Ferris, F., Klein, R. (2003). American Diabetes Association: Diabetic retinopathy. *Diabetes Care*, Vol.26, pp. 226-229.

Funatsu, H., Yamashita, H., Sakata, K., Noma, H., Mimura, T., Suzuki, M., Eguchi, S., Hori, S. (2005). Vitreous levels of vascular endothelial growth factor and intercellular adhesion molecule 1 are related to diabetic macular edema. *Ophthalmology*, Vol.112, pp. 806-16.

Fung, C., Chang, F., Lee, S., Hu, B., Kuo, B., Liu, C., Ho, M., Siu, L. (2002). A global emerging disease of *Klebsiella pneumoniae* liver abscess: is serotype K1 an important factor for complicated endophthalmitis? *Gut*, Vol.50, pp. 420-424.

Giebel, S., Menicucci, G., McGuire, P., Das, A. (2005). Matrix metalloproteinases in early diabetic retinopathy and their role in alteration of the blood-retinal barrier. *Lab. Invest.*, Vol.85, pp. 597-607.

Gragoudas, E., Adamis, A., Cunningham, E., Feinsod, M., Guyer, D. (2004). Pegaptanib for neovascular age-related macular degeneration. *N. Engl. J. Med.*, Vol.351, pp. 2805-2816.

Greene, C., McDevitt, D., François, P., Vaudaux, P., Lew, D., Foster, T. (1995). Adhesion properties of mutants of *Staphylococcus aureus* defective in fibronectin binding proteins and studies on the expression of the *fnb* genes. *Mol. Microbiol.,* Vol.17, pp. 1143–1152.

Greenwald, M., Wohl, L., Sell, C. (1986). Metastatic bacterial endophthalmitis: a contemporary reappraisal. *Surv Ophthalmol.*, Vol.31, pp. 81-101.

Han, D., Wisniewski, S., Wilson, L., Barza, M., Vine, A., Doft, B., Kelsey, S. (1996). Spectrum and susceptibilities of microbiologic isolates in the Endophthalmitis Vitrectomy Study. *Am. J. Ophthalmol.*, Vol.122, pp. 1-17. Erratum in: *Am. J. Ophthalmol.*, Vol.122, pp. 920.

Ho, V., Ho, L., Ranchod, T., Drenser, K., Williams, G., Garretson, B. (2011). Endogenous methicillin-resistant *Staphylococcus aureus* endophthalmitis. *Retina*, Vol.31, pp. 596-601.

Hunt, J., Wang, J., Callegan, M. (2011). Contribution of mucoviscosity associated gene A (*magA*) to virulence in experimental *Klebsiella pneumoniae* endophthalmitis. *Invest. Opthalmol. Vis. Sci.*, Vol. 52, pp. 6860-6866.

Jackson, T., Eykyn, S., Graham, E., Stanford, M. (2003). Endogenous bacterial endophthalmitis: a 17-year prospective series and review of 267 reported cases. *Surv Ophthalmol.*, Vol.48, pp. 403-423.

Jagnow, J., Clegg, S. (2003). *Klebsiella pneumoniae* MrkD-mediated biofilm formation on extracellular matrix- and collagen-coated surfaces. *Microbiology*, Vol.149, pp. 2397-2405.

Jett, B., Jensen, H., Nordquist, R., Gilmore, M. (1992). Contribution of the pAD1-encoded cytolysin to the severity of experimental *Enterococcus faecalis* endophthalmitis. *Infect. Immun.*, Vol.60, pp. 2445-2452.

Jo, D., Kim, J., Kim, J. (2010). How to overcome retinal neuropathy: the fight against angiogenesis-related blindness. *Arch. Pharm. Res.*, Vol.33, pp. 1557-65.

Jonas, J., Knorr, H., Budde, W. (2000). Prognostic factors in ocular injuries caused by intraocular or retrobulbar foreign bodies. *Ophthalmology, Vol.*107, pp. 823–828.

Josephberg, R. (2006). Endophthalmitis: the latest in current management. *Retina*, Vol.26, pp. S47-S50.

Karama, E., Willermain, F., Janssens, X., Claus, M., Van den Wijngaert, S., Wang, J., Verougstraete, C., Caspers, L. (2008). Endogenous endophthalmitis complicating *Klebsiella pneumoniae* liver abscess in Europe: case report. *Int. Ophthalmol.*, Vol.28, pp. 111-113.

Kelkar, A., Kelkar, J., Amuaku, W., Kelkar, U., Shaikh, A. (2008). How to prevent endophthalmitis in cataract surgeries? *Indian J. Ophthalmol.*, Vol.56, pp. 403–407.

Keynan, Y., Rubinstein, E. (2008). Endogenous endophthalmitis caused by hypermucoviscous *Klebsiella pneumoniae*: an emerging disease in Southeast Asia and beyond. *Curr. Infect. Dis. Rep.*, Vol.10, pp. 343-345.

Kumar, A., Singh, C., Glybina, I., Mahmoud, T., Yu, F. (2010). Toll-like receptor 2 ligand-induced protection against bacterial endophthalmitis. *J. Infect. Dis.*, Vol.201, pp. 255-263.

Langstraat, J., Bohse, M., Clegg, S. (2001). Type 3 fimbrial shaft (MrkA) of *Klebsiella pneumoniae*, but not the fimbrial adhesin (MrkD), facilitates biofilm formation. *Infect. Immun.*, Vol.69, pp. 5805-5812.

Lederman, E., Crum, N. (2005). Pyogenic liver abscess with a focus on *Klebsiella pneumoniae* as a primary pathogen: an emerging disease with unique clinical characteristics. *Am. J. Gastroenterol.*, Vol.100, pp. 322-331.

Lee, H., Chuang, Y., Yu, W., Lee, N., Chang, C., Ko, N., Wang, L., Ko, W. (2006). Clinical implications of hypermucoviscosity phenotype in *Klebsiella pneumoniae* isolates: association with invasive syndrome in patients with community-acquired bacteraemia. *J. Intern. Med.*, Vol.259, pp. 606-614.

Lemley, C., Han, D. (2007). Endophthalmitis: a review of current evaluation and management. *Retina*, Vol.27, pp. 662-680.

Lin, J., Siu, L., Fung, C., Tsou, H., Wang, J., Chen, C., Wang, S., Chang, F. (2006). Impaired phagocytosis of capsular serotypes K1 or K2 *Klebsiella pneumoniae* in type 2 diabetes mellitus patients with poor glycemic control. *J. Clin. Endocrinol. Metab.*, Vol.91, pp. 3084-3087.

Losso, J., Truax, R., Richard, G. (2010). Trans-resveratrol inhibits hyperglycemia-induced inflammation and connexin downregulation in retinal pigment epithelial cells. *J. Agric. Food Chem.* Vol.58, pp. 8246-8252.

Luong, T., Lee, C. (2002). Overproduction of type 8 capsular polysaccharide augments *Staphylococcus aureus* virulence. *Infect. Immun.*, Vol.70, pp. 3389-3395.

Major, J., Engelbert, M., Flynn, H., Miller, D., Smiddy, W., Davis, J. (2010). *Staphylococcus aureus* endophthalmitis: antibiotic susceptibilities, methicillin resistance, and clinical outcomes. *Am. J. Ophthalmol.*, Vol.149, pp. 278-283.

Martin, P., Roon, P., Van Ells, T., Ganapathy, V., Smith, S. (2004). Death of retinal neurons in streptozotocin induced diabetic mice. *Invest. Ophthalmol. Vis. Sci.*, Vol.45, pp. 3330-3336.

McDevitt, D., François, P., Vaudaux, P., Foster, T. (1994). Molecular characterization of the fibrinogen receptor (clumping factor) of *Staphylococcus aureus*. *Mol. Microbiol.*, Vol.11, pp. 237–248.

Meredith, T. (1999). Posttraumatic endophthalmitis. *Arch. Ophthalmol., Vol.*117, pp. 520–521.

Metrickin, D., Wilson, C., Berkowitz, B., Lam, M., Wood, G., Peshock, R. (1995). Measurement of blood-retinal barrier breakdown in endotoxin-induced endophthalmitis. *Invest. Ophthalmol. Vis. Sci.*, Vol. 36, pp. 1361–1370.

Miyamoto, K., Hiroshiba, N., Tsujikawa, A., Ogura, Y. (1998). In vivo demonstration of increased leukocyte entrapment in retinal microcirculation of diabetic rats. *Invest. Opthalmol. Vis. Sci.*, Vol.39, pp. 2190-2194.

Miyamoto, K., Khosrof, S., Bursell, S–E., et al. (1999). Prevention of leukostasis and vascular leakage in streptozotocin-induced diabetic retinopathy via intercellular adhesion molecule-1 inhibition. *Proc. Natl. Acad. Sci. USA.*, Vol.96, pp. 10836-10841.

Nassif, X., Honoré, N., Vasselon, T., Cole, S., Sansonetti, P. (1989). Positive control of colanic acid synthesis in *Escherichia coli* by *rmpA* and *rmpB,* two virulence-plasmid genes of *Klebsiella pneumoniae. Mol. Microbiol.*, Vol.3, pp. 1349-1359.

Nassif, X., Sansonetti, P. (1986). Correlation of the virulence of *Klebsiella pneumoniae* K1 and K2 with the presence of a plasmid encoding aerobactin. *Infect. Immun.*, Vol.54, pp. 603-608.

Neely, K., Gardner T. (1998). Ocular neovascularization: clarifying complex interactions. *Am. J. Pathol.*, Vol.153, pp. 665-670.

Ness, T., Schneider, C. (2009). Endogenous endophthalmitis caused by methicillin-resistant *Staphylococcus aureus* (MRSA). *Retina*, Vol.29, pp. 831-834.

Neveu, M., Elliot, A. (1959). Prophylaxis and treatment of endophthalmitis. *Am. J. Ophthalmol.*, Vol.48, pp. 368-373.

Ng, J., Morlet, N., Pearman, J., Constable, I., McAllister, I., Kennedy, C., Isaacs, T., Semmens, J., Team EPSWA. (2005). Management and outcomes of postoperative endophthalmitis since the endophthalmitis vitrectomy study: the Endophthalmitis Population Study of Western Australia (EPSWA)'s fifth report. *Ophthamology,* Vol.112, pp. 1199–1206.

Nixdorff, N., Tang, J., Mourad, R., Skalweit, M. (2009). SAME is different: a case report and literature review of *Staphylococcus aureus* metastatic endophthalmitis. *South Med. J.*, Vol.102, pp. 952-956.

O'Brien, T., Arshinoff, S., Mah, F. (2007). Perspectives on antibiotics for postoperative endophthalmitis prophylaxis: potential role of moxifloxacin. *J. Cataract Refract. Surg.*, Vol.33, pp. 1790-1800.

O'Brien, T., Choi, S. (1995). Trauma-related ocular infections. *Int. Ophthalmol. Clin. N. Am., Vol.*8, pp. 667–679.

Okada, A., Johnson, R., Liles, W., D'Amico, D., Baker, A. (1994). Endogenous bacterial endophthalmitis. Report of a ten-year retrospective study. *Ophthalmology,* Vol.101, pp. 832-838.

Otto, M. (2010). Basis of virulence in community-associated methicillin-resistant Staphylococcus aureus. *Annu. Rev. Microbiol.*, Vol.64, pp. 143-16.

Park, S., Rich, J., Hanses, F., Lee, J. (2009). Defects in innate immunity predispose C57BL/6J-Leprdb/Leprdb mice to infection by *Staphylococcus aureus*. *Infect. Immun.*, Vol.77, pp. 1008-1014.

Patti, J., Jonsson, H., Guss, B., Switalski, L., Wiberg, K., Lindberg, M., Höök, M. (1992). Molecular characterization and expression of a gene encoding a *Staphylococcus aureus* collagen adhesion. *J. Biol. Chem.,* Vol.267, pp. 4766–4772.

Peyman, G., Vastine, D., Raichard, M. (1978). Postoperative endophthalmitis: experimental aspects and their clinical application. *Ophthalmology,* Vol.85, pp. 374-385.

Plata, K., Rosato, A., Wegrzyn, G. (2009). *Staphylococcus aureus* as an infectious agent: overview of biochemistry and molecular genetics of its pathogenicity. *Acta. Biochim. Pol.*, Vol.56, pp. 597-612.

Podschun, R., Sievers, D., Fischer, A., Ullmann, U. (1993). Serotypes, hemagglutinins, siderophore synthesis, and serum resistance of *Klebsiella* isolates causing human urinary tract infections. *J. Infect. Dis.*, Vol.168, pp. 1415-1421.

Puliafito, C., Baker, A., Haaf, J., Foster, C. (1982). Infectious endophthalmitis. Review of 36 cases. *Ophthalmology.*, Vol.89, pp. 921-929.

Qaum, T., Xu, Q., Joussen, A., Clemens, M., Qin, W., Miyamoto, K., Hassessian, H., Wiegand, S., Rudge, J., Yancopoulos, G., Adamis, A. (2001). VEGF-initiated blood-retinal barrier breakdown in early diabetes. *Invest. Ophthalmol. Vis. Sci.,* Vol.42, pp. 2408-2413.

Ramadan, R., Moyer, A., Callegan, M. (2008). A role for tumor necrosis factor-alpha in experimental *Bacillus cereus* endophthalmitis pathogenesis. *Invest. Ophthalmol. Vis. Sci.*, Vol.49, pp. 4482-4489.

Ramadan, R., Ramirez, R., Novosad, B., Callegan, M. (2006). Acute inflammation and loss of retinal architecture and function during experimental *Bacillus* endophthalmitis. *Curr. Eye Res.*, Vol.31, pp. 955-965.

Roghmann, M., Taylor, K., Gupte, A., Zhan, M., Johnson, J., Cross, A., Edelman, R., Fattom, A. (2005). Epidemiology of capsular and surface polysaccharide in *Staphylococcus aureus* infections complicated by bacteraemia. *J. Hosp. Infect.*, Vol.59, pp. 27-32.

Romero, C., Rai, M., Lowder, C., Adal, K. (1999). Endogenous endophthalmitis: case report and brief review. *Am Fam Physician*, Vol.60, pp. 510-514.

Rumelt, S., Cohen, I., Lefler, E., Rehany, U. (2001). Corneal co-infection with *Scedosporium apiospermum* and *Acanthamoeba* after sewage-contaminated ocular injury. *Cornea*, Vol.20, pp. 112-116.

Sanders, M., Norcross, E., Moore, Q., Fratkin, J., Thompson, H., Marquart, M. (2010). Immunization with pneumolysin protects against both retinal and global damage caused by *Streptococcus pneumoniae* endophthalmitis. *J. Ocul. Pharmacol. Ther.*, Vol.26, pp. 571-577.

Sanders, M., Norcross, E., Robertson, Z., Moore, Q., Fratkin, J., Marquart, M. (2011). The *Streptococcus pneumoniae* capsule is required for full virulence in pneumococcal endophthalmitis. *Invest.Ophthalmol. Vis. Sci.*, Vol.52, pp. 865-872.

Schroder, S., Palinski, W., Schmid-Schonbein, G. (1991). Activated monocytes and granulocytes, capillary nonperfusion, and neovascularization in diabetic retinopathy. *Am. J. Pathol.*, Vol.139, pp. 81-100.

Sebghati, T., Korhonen, T., Hornick, D., Clegg, S. (1998). Characterization of the type 3 fimbrial adhesins of *Klebsiella* strains. *Infect. Immun.*, Vol.66, pp. 2887-2894.

Shammas, H. (1977). Endogenous *E. coli* endophthalmitis. *Surv Ophthalmol.*, Vol.21, pp. 429-435.

Shrader, S., Band, J., Lauter, C., Murphy, P. (1990). The clinical spectrum of endophthalmitis: incidence, predisposing factors, and features influencing outcome. *J Infect Dis.*, Vol.162, pp. 115-120.

Suzuki, T., Campbell, J., Swoboda, J., Walker, S., Gilmore, M. (2011). Role of wall teichoic acids in *Staphylococcus aureus* endophthalmitis. *Invest. Ophthalmol. Vis. Sci.*, Vol.52, pp. 3187-3192.

Takeda, M., Mori, F., Yoshida, A., Takamiya, A., Nakagomi, S., Sato, E., Kiyama, H. (2001). Constitutive nitric oxide synthase is associated with retinal vascular permeability in early diabetic rats. *Diabetologia*, Vol.44, pp. 1043-1050.

Thakker, M., Park, J., Carey, V., Lee, J. (1998). *Staphylococcus aureus* serotype 5 capsular polysaccharide is antiphagocytic and enhances bacterial virulence in a murine bacteremia model. *Infect. Immun.* Vol.66, pp. 5183-5189.

Thompson, S., Parver, L., Enger, C., Meiler, W., Liggett, P. (1993). Infectious endophthalmitis after penetrating injuries with retained intraocular foreign bodies. *Ophthalmology, Vol.*100, pp. 1468–1474.

Tomás, J., Benedí, V., Ciurana, B., Jofre, J. (1986). Role of capsule and O antigen in resistance of *Klebsiella pneumoniae* to serum bactericidal activity. *Infect. Immun.*, Vol.54, pp. 85-89.

Tooker, C. (1938). Metastatic septic endophthalmitis with ring abscess of the cornea-case report, clinical history, and pathologic anatomy. *Trans. Am. Ophthalmol. Soc.*, Vol.36, pp. 77-88.

Virchow, R. (1856). Uber capillare embolie. *Virchow Arch. Pathol. Anato.*, Vol.9, pp. 307-308.

Walker, C., Fenwick, P. (1962). Bilateral fulminating endophthalmitis with streptocococcal septicaemia. *Br. J. Ophthalmol.*, Vol.46, pp. 281-284.

Walrand, S., Guillet, C., Boirie, Y., Vasson, M. (2004). *In vivo* evidences that insulin regulates human polymorphonuclear neutrophil functions. *J. Leukoc. Biol.*, Vol.76, pp. 1104-1110.

Wang, J., Liu, Y., Lee, S., Yen, M., Chen, Y., Wang, J., Wann, S., Lin, H. (1998). Primary liver abscess due to *Klebsiella pneumoniae* in Taiwan. *Clin. Infect. Dis.*, Vol.26, pp. 1434-1438.

Weakley, A. (1916). Metastatic endophthalmitis in a case of cerebro-spinal meningitis. *Br. Med. J.*, Vol.1, pp. 47-48.

West, E., Behrens, A., McDonnell, P., Tielsch, J., Schein, O. (2005). The incidence of endophthalmitis after cataract surgery among the US Medicare population increased between 1994 and 2001. *Ophthalmology, Vol.*112, pp. 1388–1394.

Whiston, E., Sugi, N., Kamradt, M., Sack, C., Heimer, S., Engelbert, M., Wawrousek, E., Gilmore, M., Ksander, B., Gregory, M. (2008). alphaB-crystallin protects retinal tissue during *Staphylococcus aureus*-induced endophthalmitis. *Infect. Immun.*, Vol.76, pp. 1781-1790.

Wiskur, B., Hunt, J., Callegan, M. (2008). Hypermucoviscosity as a virulence factor in experimental *Klebsiella pneumoniae* endophthalmitis. *Invest. Ophthalmol. Vis. Sci.*, Vol.49, pp. 4931-4938.

Yu, W., Ko, W., Cheng, K., Lee, H., Ke, D., Lee, C., Fung, C., Chuang, Y. (2006). Association between *rmpA* and *magA* genes and clinical syndromes caused by *Klebsiella pneumoniae* in Taiwan. *Clin. Infect. Dis.*, Vol.42, pp. 1351-1358.

20

Retinal Detachment – An Update of the Disease and Its Epidemiology – A Discussion Based on Research and Clinical Experience at the Prince Charles Eye Unit, Windsor, England

Irina Gout, Faye Mellington, Vikas Tah,
Mahmoud Sarhan, Sofia Rokerya, Michael Goldacre and Ahmed El-Amir
Oxford University
England

1. Introduction

Retinal detachment is a potentially blinding condition. It is caused by separation of neurosensory retina from the underlying retinal pigment epithelium. Despite treatment advances, functional results remain poor (with only 42% achieving 6/12 vision and only 28% if the macula is involved). There are three distinct types of retinal detachment: rhegmatogenous (RRD), tractional and exudative. For the purpose of this chapter we will focus on RRD.

RRD demonstrates wide geographical variation with incidence reported between 6.3 and 17.9 per 100, 000[1] with 7300 new cases estimated annually in the UK[29]. Risk factors include myopia, increasing age and certain vitreoretinal conditions. Horseshoe tears, giant tears and round holes have been shown the most common along with lattice degeneration[7].

Vitreoretinal traction is responsible for most RRD. As the vitreous becomes syneretic (liquefied) with age, a posterior vitreous detachment (PVD) occurs. In most cases, the vitreous separates from the retina without any sequelae. However, in certain eyes, strong vitreoretinal adhesions are present and the occurrence of a PVD can lead to a retinal tear; then, fluid from the liquefied vitreous can enter the sub-retinal space through the tear, leading to a retinal detachment.

Several studies have investigated the epidemiology and risk factors associated with RRD. These differ in their methodology making comparison of data difficult [1,2,4,6,11,29]. RRD incidence varies with ethnicity and is strongly associated with increasing age, myopia and certain vitreoretinal degenerations including lattice degeneration and round holes. Abnormal vitreoretinal adhesions, which may be visible or invisible, are present in many eyes. Among the visible ones are lattice degeneration and cystic retinal tufts. When a PVD occurs and encounters such an area, a retinal tear may form. Due to changes in cataract surgery trends, the proportion of pseudophakic retinal detachment presenting to specialised centres appears to be increasing. The incidence is lower in phacoemulsification than extra and intracapsular cataract extraction.

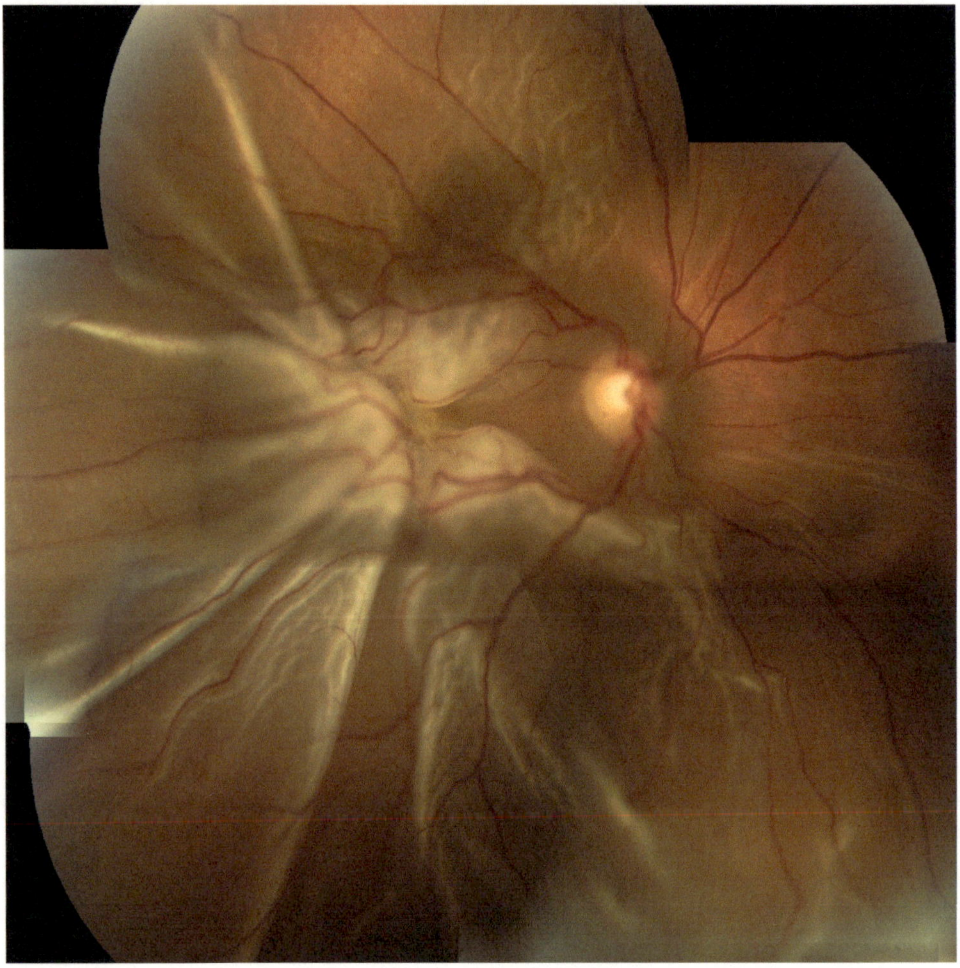

Fig. 1. Retinal detachment

Obtaining an accurate estimate of rhegmatogenous retinal detachment incidence in England and associated risk factors is essential in understanding the healthcare burden related to this disorder. We investigated the epidemiology of rhegmatogenous retinal detachment and associated clinical features by analysing routinely collected hospital statistics for England, using the Hospital In-patient Enquiry (HIPE) and Hospital Episode Statistics (HES) from 1968 to 2004, and for the Oxford National Health Service Region using the Oxford Record Linkage Study (ORLS) from 1963 to 2004. A literature review is also presented.

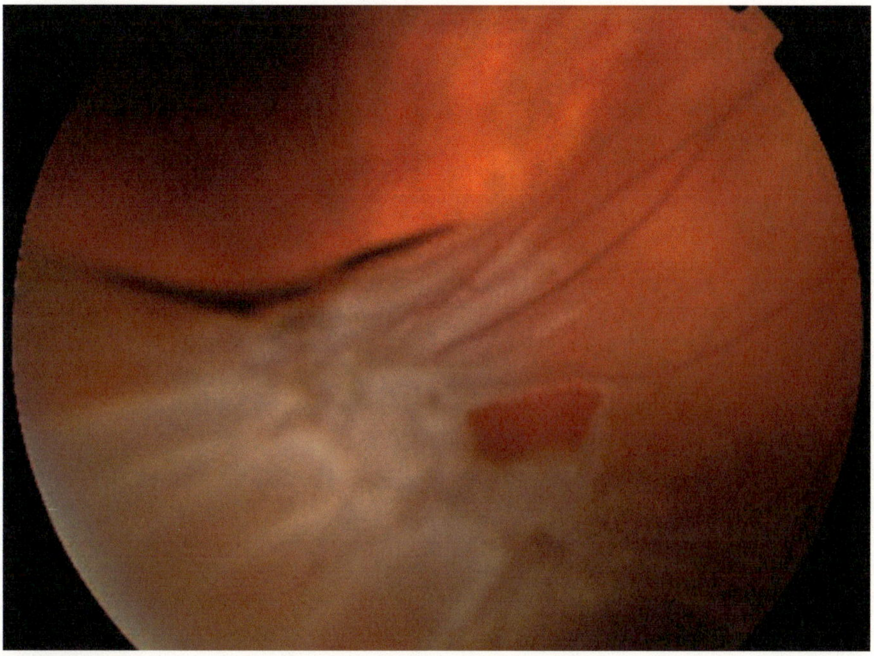

Fig. 2. Retinal break

2. Methods

At the start date for our national analysis, 1968, national hospital statistics for England were collected as the HIPE. This system ceased in 1985 and was replaced, though not until 1989 by HES. Both HIPE and HES are statistical databases of demographic, medical and administrative information about each episode of hospital care. HES include data on all "day cases" or office procedures, as well as patients admitted for overnight stay, whereas the HIPE did not include day cases.. The Oxford Record Linkage Study (ORLS) was also used for all patients treated in the Oxford Regional Health Authority area.

The International Classification for Disease (ICD) by the World Health Organisation was used to identify rhegmatogenous retinal detachment. The codes included ICD-7 (1955) code 386, ICD-8 (1965) code 376, ICD-9 (1977) codes 361.0, 361.1, 361.8 and 361.9, ICD-10 (1992) codes H33.0, H33.2, H33.4 and H33.5.

National HES for England were analysed to produce a geographical profile of hospital admission for retinal detachment by the Local Authority (LA) between 1998 and 2005. The data were used to construct a map showing the person-based admission rate per 100 000 resident population for each LA, expressed as an average annual rate. The LAs were arranged into quintiles: the fifth of LAs with the lowest rates are shown with the lightest colour, and the fifth of LAs with the highest rates are shown with the darkest colour.

The association with affluence was studied using the Index of Multiple Deprivation score for 1998-2005 (n= 57,949) as a measure of deprivation levels. The study population was split into quintiles from least deprived to the most deprived. Standardised admission ratios and 95% confidence intervals were calculated to evaluate statistical significance. Seasonal variation by monthly analysis was studied for detachment surgery from 1989-2006 (n=169,417).

The datasets were anonymised; approval to analyse them in a programme of research undertaken by the Unit and affiliated University, was obtained through the NHS Central Office for Research Ethics Committees (reference 04/Q2006/176).

3. Incidence

The English National and ORLS admission rates for retinal detachment surgery were just over 10 episodes per 100 000 population in the late 1960s. They rose nationally steadily, but gradually, to around 22 episodes per 100 000 population by 2004.

The ORLS data show rates based on the number of people admitted to hospital for retinal detachment surgery as well as the number of episodes of care for surgery (episodes of separate admission or transfers within an admission, or both). The scale of multiple admissions per person was small, although an increase in multiple recording is evident in recent years as seen in the recent divergence between the rates for episodes and people (figure 3). The figure confirms that the increase in hospital episodes in the 1990s represents an increase in the number of people treated (all RRD admissions were operated). It also shows more accurately than the English figures (which omit data for 1986–8) that the start of rapid increase in surgery was about 1989–90.

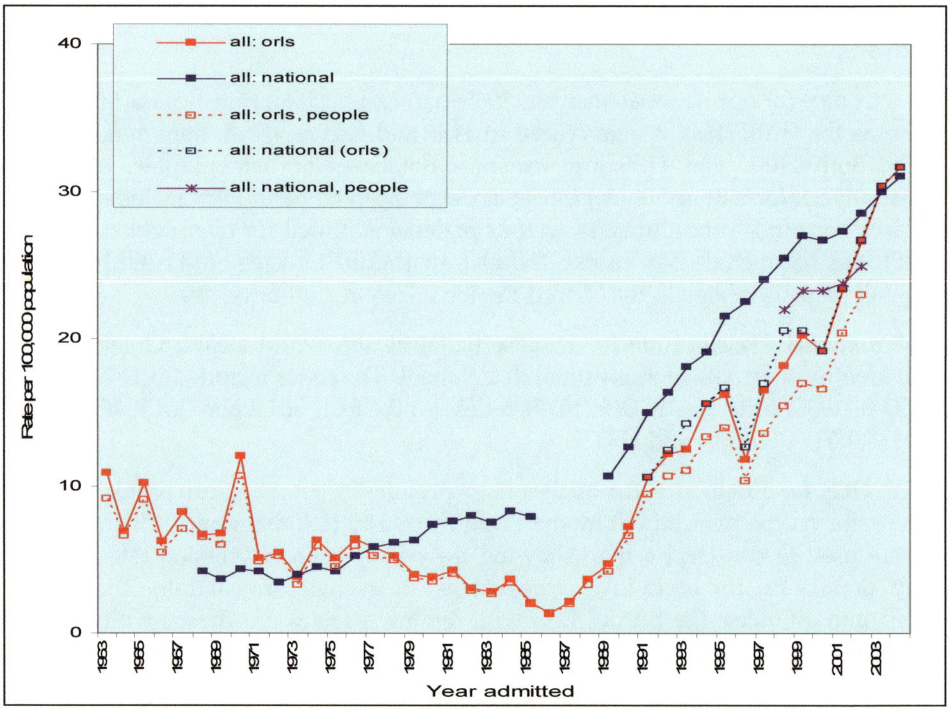

Fig. 3. Hospital admission rates 1963-2004 for Retinal surgery for ORLS and National data measured as episodes and people per year, male and female, all ages, all sources of admission, any mention

The reported annual incidence of rhegamatogenous retinal detachment in other studies around the world varies from 4-17.9 per 100 000 population [1,2,4,8,10,12,13,32,38]. Studies with small sample size, potential for sampling error and varied methodologies underlie these different results.

4. Geographic variation

The people rate for the national data is at its peak at 16 per 100,000 in 2004. There is a suggestion that the rate has reached its peak as the rate fluctuated between15-16 per 100,000 from 1998 to 2004. The people rate for the Oxford data continues to show a rise to 20 per 100,000 in 2004. This can be explained by the fact that Oxford remains a tertiary referral centre for retinal detachment and serves patients from outside the region and so the service throughput may not represent the local population. Bilaterality was not investigated but most series support a bilateral rate of retinal detachment of between 5-15%.

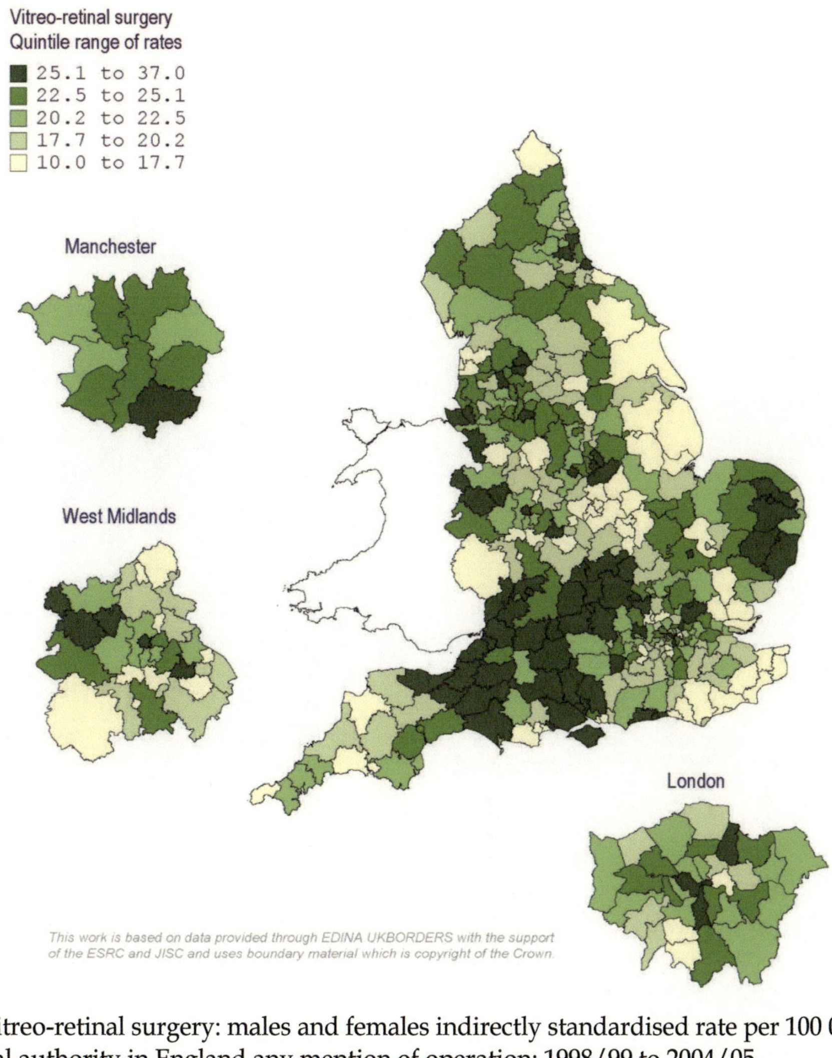

Fig. 4. Vitreo-retinal surgery: males and females indirectly standardised rate per 100 000: each local authority in England any mention of operation: 1998/99 to 2004/05

Figure 4 shows a geographical profile of the annual rate of retinal detachment surgery by LA. LAs showed a wide variation in rates of retinal detachment surgery, ranging from 7 to 23 people per 100 000 population. This reflects the relative infancy of retinal surgery service provision in comparison to cataract surgery for example and highlights the need for more service provision for patients in England.

5. Age distribution

The prevalence of PVD increases with age; occurring in 11% of 60-69 year olds, 46% of 80-89 year olds and occurring earlier in myopes. The highest incidence rate of detachment was found in the 70-74 age group with rates of 60 per 100,000. The incidence rate in under 20 year old females was the lowest noted; <3 per 100,000. The bimodal distribution with a secondary peak in younger ages (24-30 years) reflects the highly myopic group.

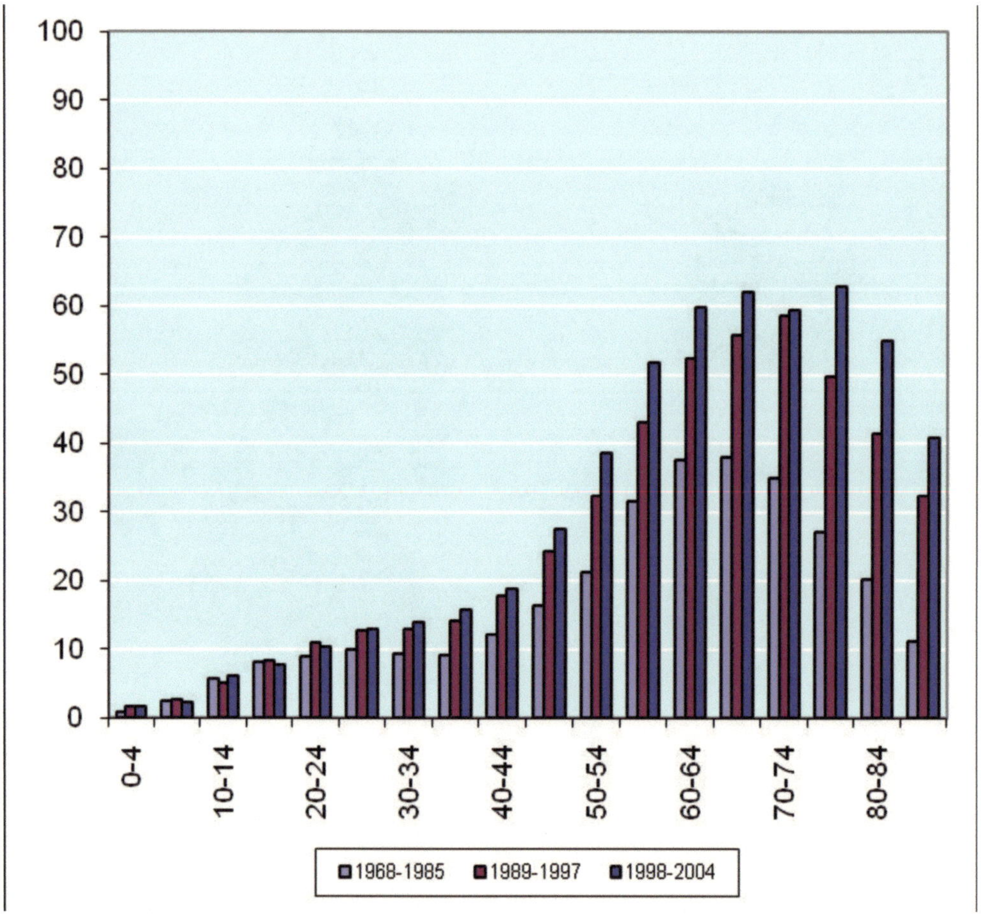

Fig. 5. Admission rates for retinal detachment per 100,000 population: all sources, males, National data

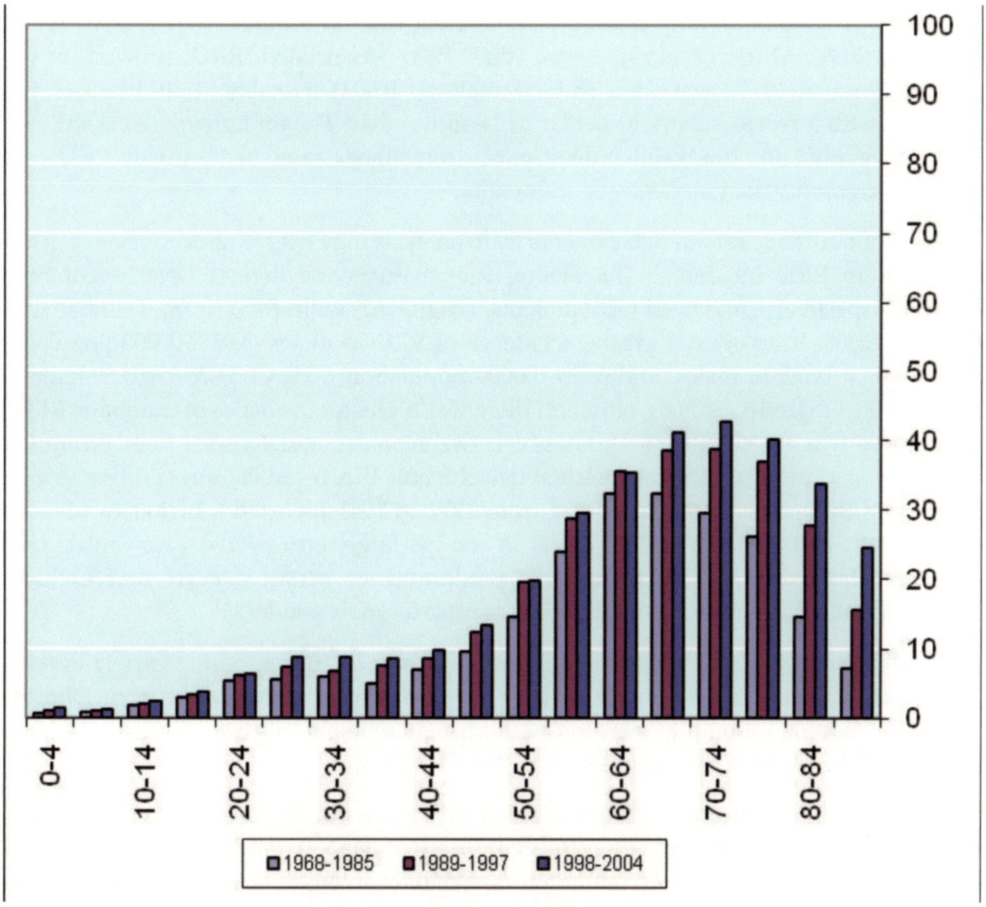

Fig. 6. Admission rates for retinal detachment per 100,000 population: all sources, females, National data

6. Gender

Figures 5 and 6 presents national and ORLS admission rates for retinal detachment surgery analysed by age and sex, and over three time periods (1968–1985, 1989–1997 and 1998–2004) for men and women separately. Three contrasting time periods were selected: one relatively long historical period, when rises in rates were fairly modest, and two more recent periods, when rises were more evident. Over these time periods, the rate of retinal detachment surgery shows a bi-modal distribution with peaks at the 24-30 and 70-74 age groups for both men and women. There was a 6 times higher risk in the 70-74 age group for both males and females. The rate of retinal detachment surgery for all age groups shows a 1.5 times male preponderance.

While some reports indicate a sex distribution corresponding with that of the general population, most indicate a male preponderance[2-6]. This may be related to an inherent gender risk, though an increased rate of ocular trauma may be contributory. Furthermore, the higher proportion of myopia in young males may partly explain this.

In a prospective study which involved 1130 cases of RRD in Scotland over a 2-year period from 2007-2009, Mitry *et al.*, reported that PVD -associated RRD showed a male preponderance of 61.7% male vs. 38.2% female (P<0.001). Notably, 1 in 10 cases were associated with a recent history of ocular or head trauma.[7] The underlying sex distribution could not account for this gender discrepancy but higher rates of traumatic RRD or an inherent increased risk in men may be influential.[8]

Exclusion of traumatic retinal detachments from analysis may negate or even reverse gender differences in RRD incidence. The Beijing Rhegmatogenous Retinal Detachment Study Group prospectively reviewed 528 patients diagnosed with RRD from October 1999-September 2000. It reported a greater incidence of RRD in males (8.98/100000 population; 95% CI 8.07 - 10.13 in males, and 6.78/100000 population; 95% CI 5.97 - 7.76 in females). However, on subgroup analysis, although there was a greater incidence of traumatic RRD in males, there was no significant difference between males and females in nontraumatic, phakic, aphakic and pseudophakic retinal detachments.[11] A Swedish retrospective study of 590 cases of RRD over a 10-year period from 1971 to 1981 reported a higher incidence of non-traumatic RRD in females.[12] However in another large retrospective case-control study (1032 cases from 1995 to 2001), the male predominance persisted even after excluding trauma-related RRD, with a reported 2.15 odds ratio for male gender.[13]

The sex difference, that is a higher incidence of RRD in men, also appears to apply to retinal detachment incidence after cataract surgery. A small retrospective study from Olmstead County, Minnesota, found that men were 2.9 times more likely to have a retinal detachment after cataract surgery than women (P<0.001; 95%CI 1,8-4.4).[14]

Other possible explanations include increased myopia and axial length in men, as well as gender differences in the anatomy of the vitreoretinal base. [15, 16] Myopia is a well-known risk factor for retinal detachment and an increase in axial length is significantly associated with an increased risk of RRD.[17-19] Axial length is related to height and men tend to be taller than women.[20] Anatomical differences in the vitreoretinal base (with males having larger eyes hence longer vitreous chambers as described in 1912 by Salzmann's Anatomy and Histology of the Human Eyeball) can be in the form of greater migration of the posterior vitreous base towards the retina in males as reported by Wang et al, in their study of donor eyes.[21] This may predispose males to retinal breaks after PVD, either from greater dynamic vitreoretinal traction and/or an increase in vitreoretinal irregularities of the posterior border.

7. Cataract extraction and other ophthalmic operations

Cataract operation is the most common ophthalmic surgical procedure worldwide. Even with the best technique and in healthy eyes this procedure is associated with an increased risk of retinal detachment. There is a higher rate of PVD after cataract extraction and a lower hyaluronic acid concentration causing vitreous collapse **5**. Increased rates of cataract surgery (phacoemulsification, internal and external capsular cataract extraction) and higher life expectancy may also contribute to retinal detachment. The cumulated six year risk of detachment after cataract surgery is increased by a factor of 6 to 8, increasing linearly for 20 years[22].

The risk is increased if there are complications during cataract surgery. There is a statistically significant higher incidence of RRD after posterior capsule rupture and anterior vitrectomy than after uncomplicated phacoemulsification, 16% versus 0.75% according to one study[23].The estimated risk of retinal detachment after cataract surgery is 5 to 16 per 1000 uncomplicated cataract operations[24].The risk may be much higher in those who are highly myopic, with a frequency of 7% reported in one study[25].Young age at cataract removal further increased risk in this study. A vitreo-retinal centre in London analysed cases of rhegmatogenous retinal detachment in 1980 and again in 1999 finding that pseudophakia rose from 0.8% to 24%. This may explain the steady rise in retinal detachment we found as shown in figure 7 in England over the last 4 decades. Most series report that about 50% of RRD occur during the first year following cataract surgery. Long term risk of retinal detachment after extracapsular and phacoemulsification cataract surgery at 2, 5, and 10 years was estimated in one study to be 0.36%, 0.77%, and 1.29%, respectively[26].

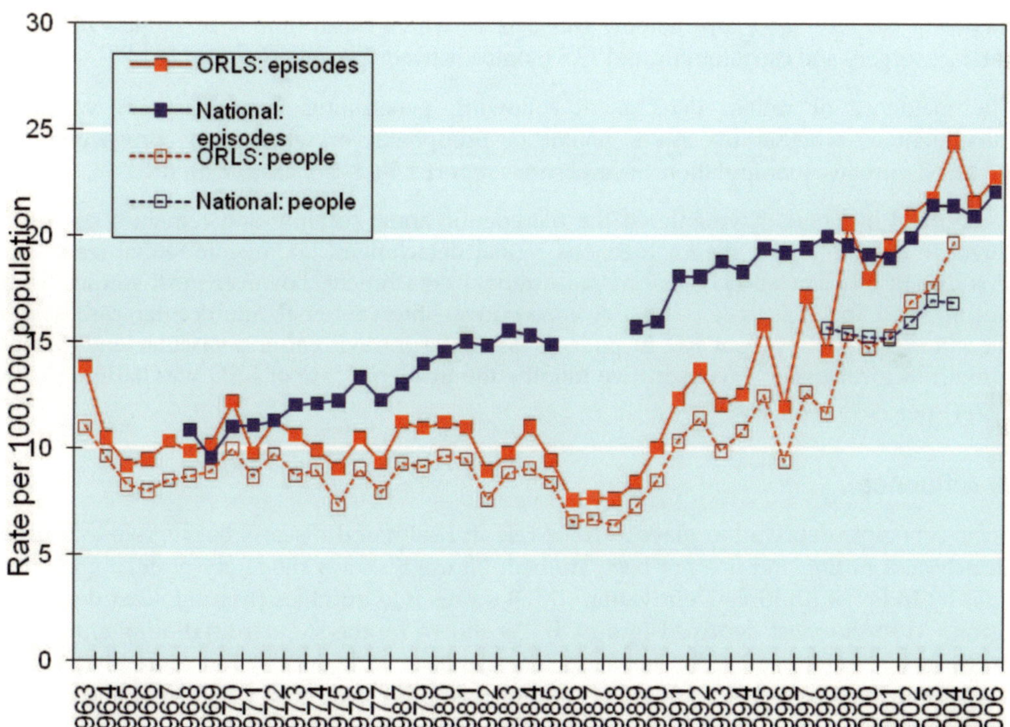

Fig. 7. Hospital admission rates (per 100,000 population) for retinal detachment: National & ORLS data 1963-2004(06) measured as episodes and people per year, all ages, males and females, all sources, any mention

The exact mechanism contributing to retinal detachment related to cataract surgery is not fully known, however several hypothesis have been postulated. It is well known that cataract extraction alters the physiology of the eye. Removal of a larger cataractous lens in aphakia or its replacement with a smaller lens implant in pseudophakia is responsible for the anterior shift of the iris lens diaphragm resulting in a relative increase in volume of the vitreous cavity. The removal of the lens and its anterior capsule also disturbs the diffusion barriers and results in a more liquefied vitreous with a reduced hyaluronic acid content . This is associated with a higher rate of PVD. Direct evidence between cataract surgery and PVD comes from a recently published study from New Zealand [33]. The study showed that among 149 patients aged 50 to 60 years who underwent unilateral cataract surgery, the incidence of PVD after five years was 51 per cent in the treated eyes, compared to only 21 per cent in their unoperated fellow eyes. Other possible mechanisms leading to a retinal detachment have been implicated to be the inflammatory vitreoretinal adhesions and retinal breaks caused by surgical trauma.

ND:Yag capsulotomy following cataract operation carries a potential to induce PVD, and thereby cause a retinal detachment [23]. The risk factors include myopia, lattice degeneration and retinal detachment in the fellow eye. No relationship has been established between energy application and incidence of retinal detachment. According to one study the incidence of RD following Nd:YAG laser capsulotomy was 0.82% , with a mean time of 32 months between cataract surgery and capsulotomy and 13.5 months between capsulotomy and RD.[23]

The incidence of retinal detachment following penetrating keratoplasty is variable, dependent on whether the eye is phakic or pseuphakic or whether the procedure has involved vitreous manipulation. Several series report 2.4-6.8% of cases with RRD[28]

Intravitreal injections have entered the therapeutic arena recently and remain a potential threat to causation of a rhegmatogenous retinal detachment. Iaterogenic retinal tears and rips due to misdirected needles can cause retinal detachment, however most studies have documented that this risk is low. A consecutive, interventional, multicenter case series measured the incidence of RD in patients receiving intravitreal anti-vascular endothelial growth factor. During 36 consecutive months the incidence rate of RRD was 0.013% (5/35 942) (1 per 7188 injections)[29].

8. Affluence

Socio-economic deprivation plays a major role in health and disease, but its role in retinal detachment in England has not been studied. Figure 8 shows the study population being split by Index of Multiple Deprivation (IMD) scores into quintiles from the least deprived (group 1) to the most deprived (group 5). As shown by the standardised admission ratio (with lower and upper 95% CIs) there is a gradient with deprivation score showing a significant relationship, though not strong, between affluence (least deprived) and retinal detachment surgery. There's about a 10% difference between the least deprived quintile and the most deprived (n= 57,949).

The Scottish Retinal Detachment Study Group, based on 12 months prospective research between 1 November 2007 and 31 October 2008, assessed 572 patients diagnosed with primary retinal detachment[29]. They came to the conclusion that retinal detachment is twice as common among the more affluent than those living in areas of deprivation. This might be as those in poorer areas may present later if at all to medical services and the more affluent tend to have greater myopic prevalence.

IMD Group	Index of Multiple Deprivation Score	No. of LA's	Observed	Expected	o/e	SAR	Confidence Interval (Lower)	Confidence Interval (Upper)
1 Least Deprived	8,36	71	9924	9150,1	1,08	108,5	106,3	110,6
2	12,68	70	9807	9615,1	1,02	102,0	100,0	104,0
3	17,13	70	9585	9793,4	0,98	97,9	95,9	99,9
4	22,92	70	11701	11903,7	0,98	98,3	96,5	100,1
5 Most Deprived	33,35	71	16932	17486,6	0,97	96,8	95,4	98,3
Total			57949	57949,0		100,0		

Fig. 8.

High myopia is one of the risk factors in patients with retinal detachment. It was documented that there is an association of short sightedness with intelligence quotient (IQ) and thus higher income and socio-economic status[31,32]. Saw et al. report the association between retinal detachment and educational achievement in a study of 1204 school children aged 10 to 12 in Singapore. Using the nonverbal Raven Standard Progressive Matrix test Intelligence Quotient they concluded that non-verbal IQ is a strong risk factor for myopia[32]. Higher prevalence of myopia in the most affluent quartile could explain the increased incidence in this group.

However, we cannot exclude the possibility that affluence is associated with some other, hitherto undefined, risk factor such as genetic factors. The latest evaluation by the Scottish Retinal Detachment Study Group investigated the influence of genetic predilection on primary RRD in 2011. They show a doubled risk of the condition in those having an affected sibling[33]. Whilst ethnicity could not be studied we know that the incidence of retinal detachment is lower in Asians and in Blacks[34].

As the risk of retinal detachment has direct connection with the most affluent group of population, there are implications for service planning, as there is likely to be a greater need for vitreoretinal services in wealthier areas.

9. Seasonality

Seasonal variation in RRD incidence has been widely reported. Most studies describe a summer peak and winter trough; others vice versa and some no seasonal variation at all[35-39]. This is likely attributed to increased sun exposure and outdoor activities in summer[36].

Figure 9 shows that the rate of retinal detachment surgery is higher in summer peaking in July with the lowest rates being in January-February. This pattern is most striking in males under

40 in whom there is relatively lower presentation in winter (lower incidence in December-February). The association with season was statistically significant at the level of p=0.01.

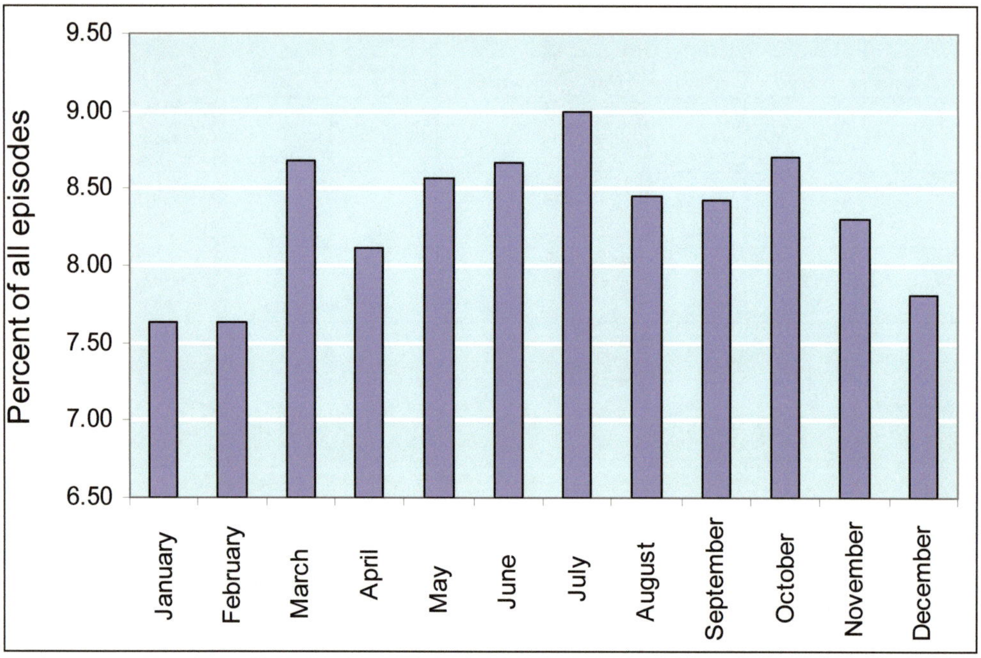

Fig. 9. Retinal detachment: monthly percentages of all FCEs, National data, male and females, any mention 1989-2006

We found a statistically significant summer peak and winter trough at the level of p=0.01 (n=115,450). The effect of light and temperature on the vitreous has been implicated. This study showed that the seasonal variation was most striking in younger males suggesting another association other than the season itself. Could this subgroup of patient be more active during the summer months and be more likely to experience trauma and PVD formation?

In a large retrospective review of 2314 patients with primary RRD in Germany, Thelen *et al.* (1997) reported a significant mid-summer peak incidence (n in July = 228) and winter trough (mean n December to January = 161) with a difference of 36% between the two periods. They noted a close correlation between seasonal incidence of RRD and seasonal incidence of light hours per day and considered a potential role of light-induced changes on vitreoretinal adhesion.[35]

Mansour *et al.* (2009) retrospectively reviewed the charts of 211 patients undergoing idiopathic RRD repair in one referral centre in Lebanon over a 13-year period. They reported a significant (P<0.05) increase in RRD in spring and summer compared to autumn and winter (56% vs. 44%). Interestingly, there was a significantly younger age of onset of RRD in the warmer months (47 vs. 54, P= 0.007).[36]

In contrast, a retrospective evaluation of RRD in Kuwait from 1981 to 1987 reported a peak incidence in winter (with the highest level in November) and a trough in the summer months.[38] These findings have not been replicated elsewhere.

Studies reporting no apparent seasonal variation in RRD incidence include the large prospective population-based study by the Beijing Rhegmatogenous Retinal Detachment Study Group. There were no seasonal differences in incidence even after further classification of retinal detachments into blunt traumatic, aphakic and pseudophakic and non-traumatic phakic.[39]

Possible explanations for seasonal variation in RRD incidence include: variations in light and temperature affecting vitreous structure, and increased outdoor activity and consequent trauma during periods of longer daylight hours and warmer weather [35].

Posterior vitreous detachment (PVD) is widely accepted as a contributory factor in RRD. Mitry *et al.* (2011) found that more than 85% of RRDs are associated with PVD and associated tractional retinal tears.[40] The influence of climatic variables namely seasonality, air temperature, solar radiation and humidity on PVD rates was elegantly evaluated by Rahman *et al.* (2002).[41] They retrospectively reviewed 567 patient records diagnostically coded as PVD in the Oxford Eye Casualty over a 2-year period. They excluded cases with a precipitating cause for PVD such as blunt trauma, retinal vascular disease and diabetes, and looked for a correlation between ambient temperatures, humidity and solar radiance and PVD incidence. Interestingly, they found no statistically significant difference in the total numbers of new patients attending the Eye casualty over the summer months compared to winter (912 from April to September vs. 839 October to March). They did however note a strong association ($P= 0.035$) between weekly average air temperatures and PVD incidence. Air temperatures of the previous week also correlated positively with PVD incidence ($P = 0.028$). The higher the average air temperature the higher the weekly rate of PVD. As such, increased physical activity and dehydration associated with higher ambient temperatures may alter vitreous structure and thereby increase the incidence of PVD and, in turn, RRD. Further investigation into the role of increased temperature on the biochemical structure of the vitreous and retinal detachment rates is needed.

10. Conclusion

The data on overall incidence of RRD worldwide has been inconsistent. The incidence varies with the population studied and is limited by study design and inclusion criteria. Few recent estimates of incidence have used large samples sizes. These studies show national data and provides longitudinal information, a more inclusive estimate of incidence and its' variation over time.

The highest annual incidence of RRD in England is in the 70-74 year age group with a secondary peak in young myopes and a higher overall incidence in males. Retinal detachment is correlated with affluence and season in England and there is geographic variation. This data sheds light into understanding the epidemiology of RRD in England. This would be particularly useful in designing and developing vitreo-retinal services to meet local needs.

11. Clinical features and management summary

Patients perceive flashing lights and floaters acutely. It probably arises from the mechanical stimulation of vitreoretinal traction on the retina. Floaters are opacities in the vitreous cavity that cast a shadow in the patient's visual field. Cobwebs are caused by condensation of the collagen fibers. Floaters can also indicate fresh blood due to the rupture of a retinal vessel during an acute PVD. Patients often describe a black curtain (visual field defect) once the subretinal fluid accumalates. When the macula becomes detached (ie, extension of subretinal fluid into the macula), the patient experiences a drop in central vision.

Cell and flare may be seen in the anterior chamber and the intraocular pressure is usually lower in the affected eye. Pigment in the anterior vitreous ('tobacco dusting' or a Shaffer sign) is usually present and this represents release of retinal pigment epithelium through the retinal break. Once the retina becomes detached, it assumes a slightly opaque color secondary to intraretinal edema. It has a corrugated appearance and undulates freely with eye movements unless severe proliferative vitreoretinopathy is present.

Patients with a RRD should be referred to a vitreoretinal specialist immediately. Regardless of the surgical technique chosen, the surgical goals are to identify and close all the breaks with minimum iatrogenic damage. Closure of the breaks occurs when the edges of the retinal break are brought into contact with the underlying RPE. This is accomplished either by bringing the eye wall closer to the detached retina (using a scleral buckle) or by pushing the detached retina toward the eye wall (intraocular tamponade with a gas bubble or silicone oil). Sealing of the breaks is accomplished by creating a strong chorioretinal adhesion around the breaks; this may be completed with cryotherapy or laser photocoagulation.

Scleral buckles usually are made of solid silicone and silicone sponges. Indirect ophthalmoscopy is used to localize all the breaks. Once the breaks are localized, they are usually treated with cryotherapy. A buckling element is chosen and sutured over the breaks. The drainage of the subretinal fluid is a controversial topic among vitreoretinal specialists. The retina can be reattached by either technique and the technical details are outside the remit of this chapter.

Currently, many surgeons use pars plana vitrectomy surgery (PPV) to treat primary uncomplicated retinal detachments. A central core vitrectomy and removal of the vitreous from the margins of the breaks is the next step. Drainage of subretinal fluid through a break internally is then performed. Intraocular tamponade with either gas or silicone oil is chosen according to the surgeon's preference. The advantages of gas are that it has a higher surface tension than silicone oil and it dissipates on its own. The disadvantage is that it expands with changing atmospheric pressure. Patients with an intraocular gas bubble should not fly. Transconjunctival and suture-less small-gauge vitrectomy has gained popularity in the past few years. 23 and 25 gauge systems have several potential advantages over traditional 20-gauge vitrectomy including improved patient comfort, faster wound healing, decreased inflammation, less conjunctival scarring, and a decrease in surgical time in opening and closing.

More than 90% of RRD cases can expect anatomical success with reattachment following one operation. Further surgery is required in the failed cases.

12. References

[1] Mitry D, Charteris DG, Fleck BW, Campbell H, Singh J. 1The epidemiology of rhegmatogenous retinal detachment: geographical variation and clinical associations. . Br J Ophthalmol. 2010 Jun;94(6):678-84. Epub 2009 Jun 9.

[2] Pollinghorne PJ, Craig JP. Northern New Zealand Rhegmatogenous Retinal Detachment Study: epidemiology and risk factors. *Clin Experiment Ophthalmol.* 2004;32:159-63.

[3] Mowatt L, Shun-Shin G, Price N. Ethnic differences in the demand incidence of retinal detachments in two districts in the West Midlands. *Eye.* 2003;17:63-70.

[4] Limeira-Soares PH, Lira RP, Arieta CE, *et al.* Demand incidence of retinal detachment in Brazil. *Eye.* 2007;21:348-52.

[5] Ivanisevic M, Bojic I, Eterovic D. Epidemiological study of nontraumatic phakic rhegmatogenous retinal detachment. *Ophthalmic Res.* 2000;32:237-9.

[6] Rosman M, Wong TY, Ong SG *et al.* Retinal detachment in Chinese, Malay and Indian residents in Singapore: a comparative study on risk factors, clinical presentation and surgical outcomes. *Int Ophthalmol.* 2001;24:101-6.

[7] Mitry D, Singh J, Yorston D, Siddiqui MA, Wright A, Fleck BW, Campbell H, Charteris DG. The Predisposing Pathology and Clinical Characteristics in the Scottish Retinal Detachment Study. *Ophthalmology.* 2011 May 9. [Epub ahead of print].

[8] Mitry D, Chalmers J, Anderson K, Williams L, Fleck BW, Wright A, Campbell H. Temporal trends in retinal detachment incidence in Scotland between 1987 and 2006. *Br J Ophthalmol.* 2011;95:365-369

[9] Wong TY, Tielsch JM. A population-based study on the incidence of severe ocular trauma in Singapore. *Am J Ophthalmol.* 1999;128(3):345-51.

[10] Wong TY, Tielsch JM, Schein OD. Racial difference in the incidence of retinal detachment in Singapore. *Arch Ophthalmol.* 1999;117(3):379-83.

[11] Li X; Beijing Rhegmatogenous Retinal Detachment Study Group. Incidence and epidemiological characteristics of rhegmatogenous retinal detachment in Beijing, China. *Ophthalmology.* 2003;110(12):2413-7.

[12] Tornquist R, Stenkula S, Tornquist P. retinal detachment. A study of a population-based patient material in Sweden 1971-1981. I. Epidemiology. *Acta Ophthalmol (Copenh).* 1987;65(2):213-22.

[13] Chou SC, Yang CH, Lee CH, Yang CM, Ho TC, Huang JS, Lin CP, Chen MS, Shih YF. Characteristics of primary rhegmatogenous retinal detachment in Taiwan. *Eye.* 2007;21:1056-1061.

[14] Rowe JA, Erie JC, Baratz KH, Hodge DO, Gray DT, Butterfield L, Robertson D. Retinal Detachment in Olmstead County, Minnesota, 1976 Through 1995. *Ophthalmology.* 1999;106(1):154-9.

[15] Bourne RR, Dineen BP. Ali SM, Noorul Huq DM, Johnson GJ. Prevalence of refractive error in Bangladeshi adults: results of the National Blindness and Low Vision Survey of Bangladesh. *Ophthalmology.* 2004;111(8):1150-60.

[16] Dandona R, Dandona L, Srinivas M, Giridhar P, McCarty CA, Rao GN. Population-based assessment of refractive error in India: the Andhra Pradesh eye disease study. *Clin Experiment Ophthalmol.* 2002; 30(2):84-93.

[17] Schepens CLDM. Data on the natural history of retinal detachment. *Arch Ophthalmol.* 1961;66:47-58.

[18] Cambiaggi A. Myopia and Retinal Detachment: statistical study of their relationships. *Am J Ophthalmol.* 1964;58:642-50.

[19] Sheu SJ, Ger LP, Chen JF. Male sex as a risk factor for pseudophakic retinal detachment after cataract extraction in Taiwanese adults. *Ophthalmology.* 114(10):1898-903.

[20] Tan CS, Chan YH, Wong TY, Gazzard G, Niti M, Ng TP, Saw SM. Prevalence and risk factors for refractive errors and ocular biometry parameters in an elderly Asian population: the Singapore Longitudinal Aging Study (SLAS). *Eye.* 2011 July 1 [Epub ahead of print].

[21] Wang J, McLeod D, Henson DB, Bishop PN. Age-dependent changes in the basal retinovitreous adhesion. *Invest Ophthalmol Vis Sci.* 2003;44(5):1793-800.

[22] Lois N, Wong D. Pseudophakic retinal detachment. *Surv Ophthalmol.* Sep-Oct 2003;48(5):467-87.

[23] Powell SK, Olson RJ. Incidence of retinal detachment after cataract surgery and neodymium: YAG laser capsulotomy. *J Cataract Refract Surg.* 1995 Mar;21(2):132-5.

[24] Ramos M, Kruger EF, Lashkari K (2002). "Biostatistical analysis of pseudophakic and aphakic retinal detachments". *Seminars in ophthalmology* 17 (3–4): 206–13.

[25] Hyams SW, Bialik M, Neumann E (1975). "Myopia-aphakia. I. Prevalence of retinal detachment". *The* British journal of *ophthalmology* 59 (9): 480–2.

[26] J.A. Rowe, J.C. Erie, K.H. Baratz et al. (1999). "Retinal detachment in Olmsted County, Minnesota, 1976 through 1995". Ophthalmology 106 (1): 154–159.

[27] Hilford D, Hilford M, Mathew A, Polkinghorne PJ. Posterior vitreous detachment following cataract surgery. *Eye 2009; 23:1388-1392.*

[28] Forstot SL, Binder PS, Fitzgerald C, Kaufman HE. The incidence of retinal detachment after penetrating keratoplasty. *Am J Ophthalmol.* Jul 1975;80(1):102-5.

[29] Meyer CH, Michels S, Rodrigues EB, Hager A, Mennel S, Schmidt JC, Helb HM, Farah ME. Incidence of rhegmatogenous retinal detachments after intravitreal antivascular endothelial factor injections. Acta Ophthalmol. 2011 Feb;89(1):70-5. doi: 10.1111/j.1755-3768.2010.02064.x. Epub 2010 Dec 22.

[30] Mitry D, Charteris DG, Yorston D, Siddiqui MA, Campbell H, Murphy AL, Fleck BW, Wright AF, Singh J; Scottish RD Study Group. The epidemiology and socioeconomic associations of retinal detachment in Scotland: a two-year prospective population-based study. Invest Ophthalmol Vis Sci. 2010 Oct;51(10):4963-8.

[31] Williams C, Miller LL, Gazzard G, Saw SM. A comparison of measures of reading and intelligence as risk factors for the development of myopia in a UK cohort of children. Br J Ophthalmol. 2008 Aug;92(8):1117-21.

[32] Saw SM, Tan SB, Fung D et al. IQ and the association with myopia in children. *Invest Ophthalmol Vis Sci.* 2004;45(9):2943–2948.

[33]Polkinghorne PJ, Craig JP. Northern New Zealand Rhegmatogenous Retinal Detachment Study: epidemiology and risk factors.Clin Experiment Ophthalmol. 2004 Apr;32(2):159-63.

[34] Mitry D, Williams L, Charteris DG, Fleck BW, Wright AF, Campbell H. Population-based estimate of the sibling recurrence risk ratio for rhegmatogenousretinal detachment. Invest Ophthalmol Vis Sci. 2011 Apr 20;52(5):2551-5.

[35] Thelen U, Gerding H, Clemens S. Rhegmatogenous retinal detachments. Seasonal variation and incidence. *Ophthalmologe.* 1997;94(9):638-41.

[36] Mansour AM, Hamam RN, Sibai TA, Farah TI, Mehio-Sibai A, Kanaan M. Seasonal variation of retinal detachment in Lebanon. *Ophthalmic Res.* 2009;41(3):170-4.

[37] Paavola M, Chehova S, Forsius H. Seasonal variations in retinal detachment in Northern Finland and Novosibirsk. *Acta Ophthalmol (Copenh).* 1983;61(5):806-12.

[38] Al Samarrai AR. Seasonal variations of retinal detachment among Arabs in Kuwait. *Ophthalmic Res.* 1990;22(4):220-3.

[39] Li X; Beijing Rhegmatogenous Retinal Detachment Study Group. Incidence and epidemiological characteristics of rhegmatogenous retinal detachment in Beijing, China. *Ophthalmology.* 2003;110(12):2413-7.

[40] Mitry D, Singh J, Yorston D, Siddiqui MA, Wright A, Fleck BW, Campbell H, Charteris DG. The Predisposing Pathology and Clinical Characteristics in the Scottish Retinal Detachment Study. *Ophthalmology.* 2011 May 9. [Epub ahead of print].#

[41] Rahman R, Ikram K, Rosen PH, Cortina-Borja M, Taylor ME. Do climatic variables influence the development of posterior vitreous detachment? *Br J Ophthalmol.* 2002;86(7):829.

21

Retinal Vascular Occlusions

Mario Bradvica, Tvrtka Benašić and Maja Vinković
University of Josip Juraj Strossmayer, Medical School Osijek, University Hospital Osijek
Croatia

1. Introduction

Retinal vascular occlusions are serious diseases and significant causes of blindness that include arterial and venous obstructions. The causes, pathogenesis, clinical characteristics, prognosis, and response to therapy are influenced by the location of the occlusion in the retinal vasculature and by the extent of retinal nonperfusion.

The hallmark of clinical presentation in the retinal occlusive disease is painless loss of vision, which can be asymptomatic, gradual with only mildly reduced visual acuity, or sudden and reduced to counting fingers depending on the extent of the irrigation area of the affected vessel. The clinical presentation aids in distinguishing the type of the occlusion, which may be classified according to the anatomical site of the occlusion.

2. Retinal Artery Occlusion

Retinal artery occlusion (RAO) represents an ophthalmologic emergency. In 1859, von Graefe first described central retinal artery occlusion (von Graefe, 1859). Retinal artery obstruction may be classified as follows: central (CRAO), affecting the retinal vessel at the optic nerve, hemicentral (occasional, only when one of the two trunks of the CRA is occluded) (Akkoyun et al., 2006; Karagoz et al., 2009; Schmidt & Kramer-Zucker, 2011), branch (BRAO), obstruction distally to the lamina cribrosa of the optic nerve, cilioretinal (CLRAO) and central sparing cilioretinal artery (Hayreh, 2011). Obstructions more proximal to the central retinal artery, in the ophthalmic artery, or even in the internal carotid artery, may produce visual loss as well. More proximal obstructions usually cause a more chronic form of visual problem—the ocular ischemic syndrome often associated with occlusive carotid disease (Kearns & Hollenhorst, 1963).

Central retinal artery occlusion results in sudden visual loss and is therefore one of the most important topics in ophthalmology. Branch retinal artery occlusion causes sudden segmental visual loss and may recur to involve other branch retinal arterioles. Amaurosis fugax is a common transient acute retinal ischemic condition. Acute retinal arterial occlusive disorders together comprise one of the major causes of acute visual loss (Hayreh, 2011). Only anecdotal reports have described spontaneous recovery of vision, and case series have shown only up to 14% of spontaneous recovery (Atebara et al., 1995).

The majority of retinal arterial obstructions are either thrombotic or embolic in nature (an embolus is visible only in 20% of the patients with branch or central retinal artery occlusion)

(Rumelt & Brown, 2003). Arterial occlusions in the eye are almost always due to microembolism and the major source of microemboli is the plaque(s), which may be present with or without any significant carotid artery stenosis. Thus, absence of significant stenosis of the carotid artery does not necessarily rule out the carotid artery as the source of microembolism (Hayreh et al., 2009).

Immediate intervention improves chances of visual recovery, but even then, the prognosis is rather poor, with only 21-35% of eyes retaining useful vision (Jain & Juang, 2009), because it dominantly depends on the type of the occlusion (Hayreh & Zimmerman, 2005). Although restoration of vision is of immediate concern, retinal artery occlusion is a forerunner for other systemic diseases that must be evaluated promptly. Establishing of the cause of obstruction is essential. In case of giant cell arteritis causing occlusion immediate treatment is urgent.

2.1 Epidemiology

Central retinal artery obstruction (CRAO) is a rare event – it has been estimated to account for about 0.85 in 100,000 per year (Jain & Juang, 2009). The mean age at onset is about 60 years, with a range from the first to the ninth decade of life (Duker, 2003). Bilateral obstruction occurs in 1-2% of cases (Brown, 1994). CRAOs account for 58% of acute RAOs, BRAOs for 38%, and cilioretinal artery occlusions (CLRAOs) (Jain & Juang, 2009). There are discrepancies among authors regarding the prevalence of men over women. Some advocate the ratio 2:1 (Duker, 2003) whereas the others found slightly more frequent occurrence in men (Hayreh et al., 2009). A large case series documented that approximately one fourth of patients with CRAO had a form with the cilioretinal sparing (Brown & Shields, 1979). The incidence of CLRA occlusion (CLRAO) varies in different studies from none to 32% (Justice & Lehmann 1976), which would be the most acceptable data, because the incidence was calculated by reviewing stereoscopic color fundus photographs as well as FA; the incidence of CLRAO is in direct proportion with the presence of cilioretinal artery in the population. FA is the most reliable way to ascertain the true incidence because the CLRA dyes concurrently with the filling of the choroid and usually before the start of filling of the CRA. The arteries occurred bilaterally in 14.6% (Justice & Lehmann, 1976).

Multiple studies have shown increased mortality in patients with retinal arterial emboli (Bruno et al., 1995; Ho et al., 2008; Lindley et al., 2009). The frequency of retinal emboli increases with age and are more common in men than in women. Bilateral are rare, although multiple emboli in a single eye may be seen in up to one third of cases. They are associated with the presence of carotid artery disease (CAD), hypertension, smoking, and possibly diabetes (Wong & Klein, 2002). The large Beaver Dam Eye Study calculated the prevalence of retinal arteriolar emboli of 1.3% in the population ranged from 43-86 years, and the 5-year incidence of 0.9%, the 10-year incidence of 1.5% for the same population, and also confirmed a significantly higher hazard of dying from a stroke in people with retinal emboli (Klein et al., 1999; Klein et al., 2003).

Debate exists in the literature on the prevalence and etiology of neovascularization (NV) following CRAO. The reported prevalence varies from 2.5% to 31.6%. Studies have reported prevalence of 18.2% of neovascularization and 15.2% of neovascular glaucoma (NVG) (Duker et al., 1991; Rudkin et al., 2010). In branch retinal artery occlusion, the incidence is even rarer. Neovascularization is more likely to occur in persons with concurrent diseases and not CRAO per se, as with diabetes, severe carotid artery disease or generalized atherosclerosis (Hayreh & Podhajsky, 1982). Clinical cases have been reported in which neovascular glaucoma developed after branch retinal artery occlusion (Brown & Reber, 1986); most probably they are a result of later complete CRAO rather than pure BRAO.

2.2 Pathophysiology and histology

Visual loss from retinal arterial occlusion (RAO) occurs from the loss of blood supply to the inner layer of the retina. Blood supply to the retina originates from the central retinal (CRA) and the cilioretinal (CLRA) artery. The primary source of blood supply to both arteries - the ophthalmic artery (OA), usually the first intracranial branch of the internal carotid artery (ICA), does not always originate from the ICA; the most common abnormal origin is the middle meningeal artery (Hayreh, 2011; Morandi et al., 1998). The central retinal artery arises independently in 37.5% from the ophthalmic artery, in 59.5% by a common trunk with one or another posterior ciliary artery (PCA), and extremely rarely with other branches of the OA. Numerous anastomoses are established by the branches of the CRA with other branches of the OA, mostly pial. The study showed that these pial anastomoses were usually large enough to establish a variable amount of collateral circulation in the eye having an occlusion of the CRA. This was also demonstrated by fluorescein fundus angiography (FA) (Hayreh, 2011; Hayreh & Weingeist, 1980). The central retinal artery supplies the retina as it branches into smaller segments upon leaving the optic disc. The so-called "branch retinal arteries" are in fact arterioles after the first branching in the retina which don't have either an internal elastic lamina or a continuous muscular layer (Hayreh, 2011). A retinal vascular bed does not own any anastomoses; it is end-arterial system. The cilioretinal artery belongs to the PCA system; it usually originates from the peripapillary choroid or directly from one of the PCAs and supplies the part of the macular retina. The CLRA has a characteristic hook-like appearance at its site of entry into the retina at the optic disc margin, usually on the temporal side. Branch retinal artery occlusion (BRAO) occurs when the embolus lodges in a more distal branch of the retinal artery. BRAO typically involves the temporal retinal vessels and usually does not require treatment, unless perifoveolar vessels are threatened (Ho et al., 2008).

Acutely, obstruction of the central retinal artery results in inner retinal layer edema and pyknosis of the ganglion cell nuclei. Ischemic necrosis results and the retina become opacified and yellow-white in appearance. The opacity is most dense in the posterior pole as a result of the increased thickness of the nerve fiber layer and ganglion cells in this region. The opacification takes as little as 15 minutes to several hours before becoming evident and resolves in 4-6 weeks. Furthermore, the foveola assumes a cherry-red spot because of a combination of 3 factors: (i) the intact retinal pigment epithelium and choroid underlying the fovea, (ii) the foveolar retina is nourished by the choriocapillaris, and (iii) the thinnest NFL at this location. The late stage shows a homogenous scar replacing the inner layer of the retina. Pigmentary changes are typically absent since the retinal pigment epithelium remains unaffected (Kearns & Hollenhorst, 1963).

It has been shown experimentally on animal studies that the retinal damage is irreversible after 105 minutes of completely occluded circulation, but may recover at 97 minutes (Hayreh et al., 2004), and the treatment instituted at any time beyond 4h after the onset of

CRAO cannot have any scientific rationale for improvement of vision. However, complete occlusion or retinal artery circulation in humans is rare with retinal artery disease; thus, retinal recovery is possible even after days of ischemia (Brown & Magargal, 1988). Controversy exists regarding the optimal window of treatment in humans, but the conservative approach involves treatment up to 24 hours (Kearns & Hollenhorst, 1963).

The retinal artery could be occluded due to embolism, vasoobliteration (atherosclerotic plaques, giant-cell arteritis and other types of vasculitis) and vascular compression (a retrobulbar mass - hematoma, neoplasm, retrobulbar injections may lead to an optic nerve and central retinal artery compression) (Korner-Stiefbold, 2001), angiospasm, hemodynamic or hydrostatic arterial occlusion (Hayreh, 2011). By far the most common cause of nonarteritic RAO is the embolism. Emboli are usually of three types: cholesterol - Hollenhorst plaque, platelet-fibrin, calcified, and occasionally myxomatous, or bacterial. The incidence is 74%, 15.5% and 10.5% for the first 3 types, respectively (Arruga & Sanders, 1982). They are mostly of carotid and/or cardiac origin (Korner-Stiefbold, 2001). The major source of embolism in the carotid arteries is plaque (66%), whereas a significant carotid stenosis (>50%) accounts for only 30% of cases (Hayreh et al., 2009; Korner-Stiefbold, 2001; Younge, 1989). Statistically, Caucasians, when compared to African Americans, have significantly different incidence of ICA stenosis, which is 41% and 3.4% for the each group, respectively (Ahuja et al., 1999). A significant stenosis of the extracranial internal carotid artery is the most common identified condition associated with retinal and ocular ischemia (Biousse, 1997; Mizener et al., 1997; Sharma et al., 1998). It represents the hemodynamic cause, and, especially if associated with nocturnal arterial hypotension, can lead to transient CRAO (Hayreh & Zimmerman, 2005). The sources of emboli in heart are valvular lesions, patent foramen ovale, myxoma and endocarditis (Mangat, 1995; Reese & Shafer, 1978; Schmidt et al., 2005; Sharma et al., 1997). It must be remembered though, that the absence of any abnormality on color Doppler ultrasound or echocardiography does not exclude carotid artery or the heart as the source of microembolism, because of the test-resolution and location of the plaque/stenosis.

Animal studies have shown that, serotonin in atherosclerotic vessels produces vasospasm of the central retinal artery (CRA) and/or posterior ciliary artery (PCA) in various combinations (but not vasospasm of the arterioles in the retina). It is postulated that in some atherosclerotic individuals this mechanism may play an important role in the development of ischemic disorders of the retina and optic nerve head (ONH), including amaurosis fugax, CRA occlusion and anterior ischemic optic neuropathy, and possibly also glaucomatous optic neuropathy, particularly in normal tension glaucoma (Hayreh, 1999).

Central retinal arterial occlusions could be divided into permanent or transient; arteritic (usually gigantocellular arteritis) or nonarteritic occlusion. The transient is the nonarteritic and could occur due to (i) transient impaction of an embolus, (ii) fall of perfusion pressure in the retinal vascular bed below the critical level (night arterial hypotension, hypovolemic shock, hemodialysis, spasm of CRA, marked carotid artery disease, ocular ischemia, or a rise of intraocular pressure because of orbital swelling, acute angle-closure glaucoma, neovascular glaucoma (NVG) with ocular ischemia), and (iii) vasospasm of the atherosclerotic lesions (induced by the platelet-aggregation plaque secreting serotonin) (Hayreh, 2011).

Branch arterial occlusion is usually due to embolism and occasionally vasculitis. It could be recurrent (Barak et al., 1997; Beiran et al., 1995; Beversdorf et al., 1997; Johnson et al., 1994). Most of these cases probably have Susac's syndrome (autoimmune endotheliopathy leading to encephalopathy, BRAO and hearing loss) (Susac et al., 2007). The etiology of this syndrome is still unknown, but the prognosis is good in most cases. Spontaneous resolution usually occurs, but early treatment minimizes the risk of sequelae (Van Winden & Salu, 2010).

2.3 Causes

Embolism of the carotid artery and the heart are the most common causes of retinal artery obstruction. Carotid artery disease causes retinal arterial occlusion by three mechanisms: embolism, hemodynamic changes in significantly stenosed carotid artery, and arterial spasm. The major source of emboli is plaques in the carotid arteries, and much less frequently stenosis. According to some studies, hemodynamically significant carotid artery stenosis was found in about 18%of patients with acute RAO (Sharma et al., 1998) and as previously mentioned, Hayreh et al. suggest that the presence of plaques on Doppler color imaging is of more value in determining the cause of acute occlusive event rather than the embolus itself (Hayreh, 2005). The probable cause is the microembolism, which may not produce hemodynamically significant stenosis recordable on Doppler color imaging but may indeed account for the retinal artery occlusion. As shown in the study, carotid Doppler and/or angiography showed the presence of plaques in 71% in CRAO and 66% in BRAO (Hayreh et al., 2009). The fluctuation of hemodynamic factors, especially drops in blood pressure in nocturnal hypotension along with significant stenosis of the carotid artery may be responsible for transient retinal artery occlusion (Hayreh & Zimmerman, 2005; McCullough et al., 2004). Based on experimental studies on animals, the investigators have introduced the possible role of serotonin, released by platelet aggregation on atherosclerotic plaques in the carotid artery, causing transient vasospasm of the central retinal artery and thus potentially inducing retinal artery occlusion and retinal ischemic disorders.

Systemic cardiovascular diseases have a well known association with retinal arterial occlusive disease in elderly people (Sharma, 1998). Therefore, a careful history should include identifying the possible underlying causes such as arterial hypertension, diabetes mellitus, hyperlipidemia, carotid artery disease, coronary artery disease, cerebrovascular disease and symptoms suggestive of temporal arteritis. Cigarette smoking has been described significantly more common among these patients than in the general population. In patients with no obvious systemic risk factors and especially in subjects under the age of 40, the other causative options should be considered, which include systemic vasculitis, blood dyscrasias, drug abuse, hypercoagulabile states, infective diseases, migraine and prolonged direct pressure to the globe in unconscious patients (Brown et al., 1981; Graham, 1990; Greven et al., 1995).

Coagulopathies from sickle cell anemia or antiphospholipid antibodies are more common etiologies for CRAO in patients younger than 30 years of age and the proposed mechanisms involve increase in coagulation factor or platelet activity, thrombocytosis, interaction of lupus anticoagulant and anticardiolipin antibodies with phospholipids as well as the deficiencies of protein C and S and resistance to activated protein C (Comp & Esmon, 1984; Love & Santoro, 1990; Palmowski-Wolfe et al., 2007; Vignes et al., 1996). Increased levels of homocysteine have been linked with higher incidence of occlusive vascular incidents damaging the vascular endothelium and thus increasing atherosclerotic changes and the formation of blood cloths. Therefore, in cases of suspected homocystinuria or heterozygosity for homocystinuria an oral methionine loading test may be performed since this state may be preventable by taking appropriate vitamin supplements (Boers et al., 1985; Weger et al., 2002; Wenzler et al., 1993). In cases of clinical suspicion, the HIV testing may be indicated since there have been case reports of CRAO or BRAO associated with HIV infection (Conway et al., 1995). A variety of other diseases, including systemic lupus erythematosus, polyarteritis nodosa, dengue fever, West Nile virus, sickle cell disease, Takayasu's arteritis, after smallpox vaccination, Churg-Strauss syndrome, ocular Behçet's disease, Fabry's disease, Susac'c syndrome, and head injury may present with retinal occlusive disorders. It is necessary to exclude these states if there is a young person with sudden loss of vision, fundoscopic findings of arterial occlusion, central or branch, and no obvious identifiable systemic risk factors as above mentioned. In conclusion, arterial occlusive disease of the retina is the result of either arteriosclerotic thrombosis, embolic impaction (predominantly atheromatous plaques of carotid bifurcation, or the internal carotid artery, but also consisting of different material - fat, parasites, talc, air), vasculitis, vasospasm or systemic hypotension. These numerous potential causes mandate often time-consuming and expensive lab tests, and sometimes a causative management of the underlying disease. The possible causes and underlying states associated with retinal arterial occlusion are incorporated in Table 1.

2.4 Clinical presentation

2.4.1 Symptoms

The main presenting symptom of the arterial occlusive disease is loss of vision, usually monocular, which may be sudden (seconds to minutes) blurring, decrease or total loss of vision. The extent of visual loss depends on the type of the occlusion. In central artery occlusions, visual loss is central and dense. In branch artery occlusions, visual loss may go unnoticed if only a section of the peripheral visual field space is affected. Various types of the retinal artery occlusion have different degree of visual acuity (VA) drop; CRAO characterizes severely decreased VA (counting fingers to light perception); BRAO has VA 20/20 to counting fingers; VA in cilioretinal occlusion ranges from 20/30-20/60; CRAO with cilioretinal sparing has VA 20/30 to hand motion, depending on the amount of the papillomacular bundle supplied by the patent vessel; combined CRAO and CRVO have VA counting fingers to light perception (Rumelt S, Brown GC, 2004). The patients with CRAO without cilioretinal sparing rarely regained any useful vision (Brown & Shields, 1979).

Pain accompanying the visual loss is unusual and usually denotes associated ocular ischemic syndrome (Werner et al. 1994). Rarely, in cases associated with arterial spasm, a relapsing and remitting course of visual loss precedes central retinal artery obstruction. Amaurosis fugax precedes visual loss in about 10% of patients involving transient loss of vision lasting seconds to minutes, but which may last up to 2 hours (Brown, 1999). The vision usually returns to baseline after an episode of amaurosis fugax.

2.4.2 Signs

In CRAO, the first signs are afferent pupillary defect on the affected side and segmental arterial blood flow ("box- carring"), which appear immediately at the occlusion and are accompanied by the various degree of diminished visual acuity. Later signs are retinal opacification and cherry-red spot and optic disc pallor, attenuation of the retinal arteries, arterio-arteriolar collaterals or neovascular glaucoma (as a complication). Von Graefe was the first one who described typical fundoscopic findings associated with occlusion of the central retinal artery: whitish, edematous retina attributable to infarction, especially at the posterior pole where the nerve fibre layer and ganglion cell layer are the thickest (Beatty & Au Eong, 2000). As these layers are absent in the fovea, the underlying choroidal vascular bed can be seen in this area, thus giving rise to the classic cherry-red spot (Fig. 1.). In the presence of a patent cilioretinal artery, the retinal region served by the unobstructed vessel is not involved (Fig. 2.). Disc pallor and retinal vascular narrowing are characteristic of the late stage of CRAO. The characteristic of BRAO is retinal edema in the distribution of the affected vessel only (Fig. 3.). Obstruction of a cilioretinal artery, or even a macular branch arteriole, gives cloudy, edematous appearance of the macula and affects central vision. In acute stage, the arteries appear thin and attenuated while cherry red spot and ground glass appearance may take hours to develop. In severe blockages, both veins and arteries may manifest "box-carring" or segmentation of the blood flow.

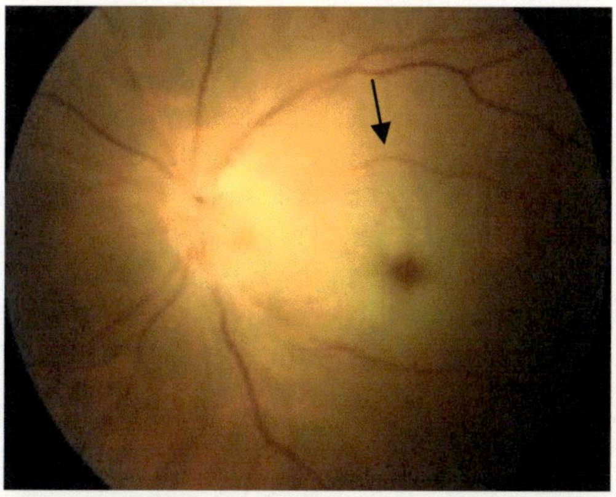

Fig. 1. Central retinal artery occlusion, note foveal cherry red spot and ground glass appearance of the macula (arrow)

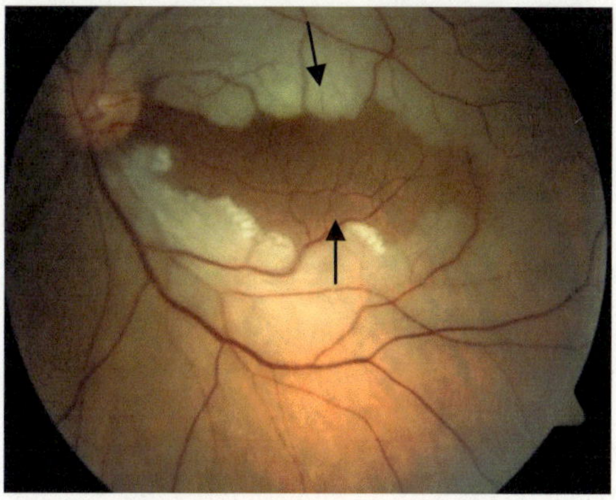

Fig. 2. Cilioretinal sparing central artery occlusion; sparing between the disc and fovea (arrows), representing irrigation area of the cilioretinal artery

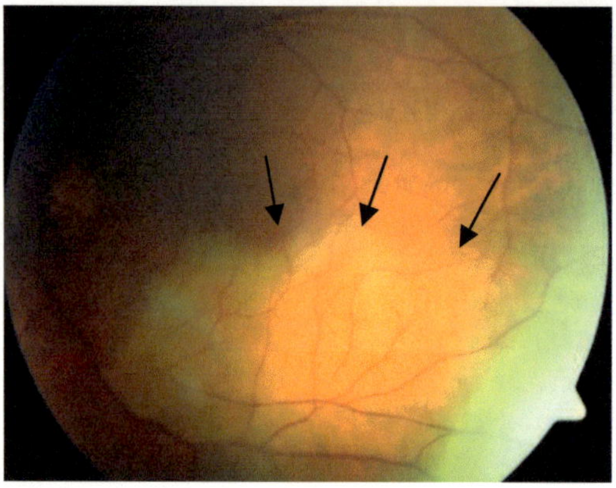

Fig. 3. Branch retinal artery occlusion; note pale, edematous retina in the area of affected vessel (arrows)

Late complication of CRAO is a neovascularization which indicates severe retinal ischemia and is more common at the far periphery and not at the optic disc or the posterior pole, and may complicate with vitreous or preretinal hemorrhage (Duker & Brown, 1989). This is why, in most cases, they are not observed clinically or angiographically with standard angle fundus camera. Only ischemia is usually seen by fluorescein angiography. The typical angiographic finding of neovascularization is the leakage of dye, whereas collateral shunting vessels do not present with such a feature. The fundoscopic findings typically resolve within days to weeks of the acute event, and residual optic atrophy may be the only physical finding. This feature also explains why it is crucial to treat the far periphery of the retina by cryo in addition to treatment by photocoagulation, in cases that the retinal periphery cannot be treated by photocoagulation.

Acute simultaneous obstruction of both the retinal and choroidal circulations is referred to as an ophthalmic artery obstruction. It can be differentiated clinically from central retinal artery obstruction by the following features: severe visual loss—bare or no light perception; intense ischemic retinal whitening that extends beyond the macular area; little to no cherry-red spot; pronounced choroidal perfusion defects on fluorescein angiography; nonrecordable electroretinogram; and late retinal pigment epithelium alterations (Brown et al., 1986). Cases of ophthalmic artery obstruction usually have associated local orbital or systemic diseases: orbital mucormycosis, orbital trauma, retrobulbar anesthesia, depot corticosteroid injection, atrial myxoma, or carotid artery disease (Sullivan et al., 1983). In conjunction with ipsilateral ischemic optic neuropathy, temporal arteritis may produce ophthalmic artery obstruction.

2.5 Evaluation and imaging

To summarize and to choose a rational approach in the workup, it is our opinion that the evaluation should be related to the age group. We recommend the following procedures to be undertaken in the persons over 50 years: the physical examination with complete cardiovascular assessment, ECG, the lab tests including full blood count, erythrocyte sedimentation rate, C reactive protein, fasting blood glucose, lipidogram, urine analysis, Doppler color imaging of the carotid arteries, and transthoracic echocardiography in patients with cardioembolic risk factors.

In the younger patients and those with unidentifiable systemic risk factors these are the proposed investigations: fluorescein angiography, vasculitis screen including anticardiolipin antibodies, antinuclear antibodies, anti-double stranded DNA antibodies, routine coagulation tests (prothrombin time, partial thromboplastin time), specialized clotting factor and platelet activity studies (levels of protein S, protein C, antithrombin III, plasminogen activator, plasminogen activator inhibitor, fibrinogen and resistance to activated protein C) and homocysteine.

Systemic cardiovascular disease	
	Hypertension, Diabetes mellitus, Atheromatous disease, Cardiac-valvular disease, bacterial endocarditis, myxoma, arrhythmias
Coagulopathies	
	Antiphospholipid antibodies, Protein C deficiency, Protein S deficiency, Antithrombin III deficiency, Elevation of platelet factor 4, Sickle cell anemia, Homocysteine
Systemic vasculitis	
	Polyarteritis nodosa, Temporal arteritis, Kawasaki's syndrome, Wegener's granulomatosis, Susac's disease, Systemic lupus erythematosus
Oncologic	
	Metastatic tumors, Leukemia, Lymphoma
Infective diseases	
	Syphilis, HIV
Trauma	
	Direct ocular compression, Penetrating injury, Retrobulbar injection, Orbital trauma, Purtscher's disease
Ocular conditions	
	Preretinal arterial loops, Optic nerve drusen, Necrotizing herpetic retinitis, Toxoplasmosis
Other causes	
	Oral contraceptives, Pregnancy, Drug abuse, Migraine

Table 1. Systemic and ocular conditions related to retinal arterial occlusion

It is important to exclude temporal arteritis in older patients, since it follows different clinical course and mandates the prompt administration of systemic corticosteroids. Giant cell arteritis is concerned as approved clinically if two of the three symptoms or signs exist: headache, tenderness over the temple and high sedimentation rate. Biopsy only approves it and treatment should not be deferred for biopsy result. It should be immediately initiated if two or more of the above are present. The purpose of the treatment is to prevent visual loss of the fellow eye, which usually occurs within 10 days of the event in one eye. Apart from the sudden, painless, nonprogressive vision loss in one eye, the patients may have headaches, jaw claudication, scalp tenderness, proximal muscle and joint aches, anorexia, weight loss, or fever.

All patients with acute retinal arterial occlusion must be evaluated for the source of embolism, which is the commonest cause for its development. The imaging techniques are used to confirm the diagnosis in uncertain cases and these are fluorescein angiography, visual field testing, optical coherence tomography and electroretinography.

2.5.1 Fluorescein angiography

Fluorescein angiography is not routinely indicated in the acute phase of arterial occlusive disease. The angiographic findings in both types, CRAO and BRAO (Fig. 4.), include delayed arm-to-retina time which is over 12 seconds (Richard G. et al., 1998), reduced arterial caliber and "cattle-trucking" of the blood column in the branch arteries. Sometimes, it may be minutes before the retinal arterial tree fills with fluorescein. Arteriovenous transit is also delayed, and late staining of the disc is common.

The CLRA dyes concurrently with the filling of the choroid and usually before the start of filling of the CRA (Justice & Lehmann, 1976).

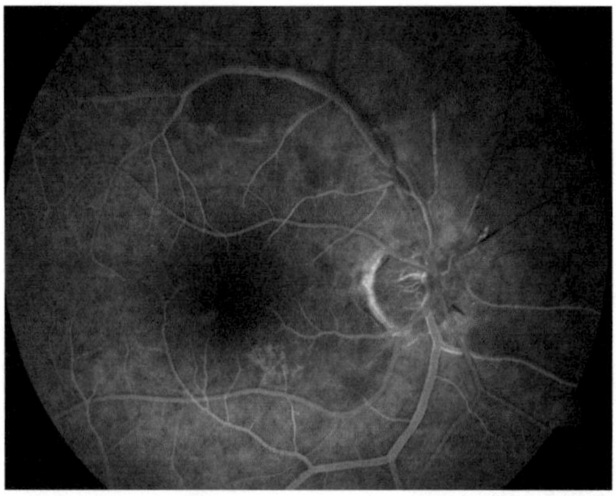

Fig. 4. Superior branch retinal artery occlusion of the right eye. Note the delayed filling of the dye in the superior quadrant of retina

2.5.2 Visual field testing

Visual fields show a remaining temporal island of peripheral vision. In cases of a patent cilioretinal artery, a small intact central island is found as well.

2.5.3 Electroretinography

Electroretinography characteristically shows a decreased to absent b-wave with intact a-wave.

2.5.4 Optical Coherence Tomography (OCT)

Optical coherence findings depend on the duration of the ischemia. Acute stages show increased reflectivity in the inner retinal layers and decreased reflectivity of the photoreceptor layer due to the shadowing effect (Fig. 4.). If involved, the macular region shows cystoid changes with loss of the foveolar contour. Old cases of arterial occlusion are presented with macular thinning with increased reflectivity of the retinal structure denoting ischemia.

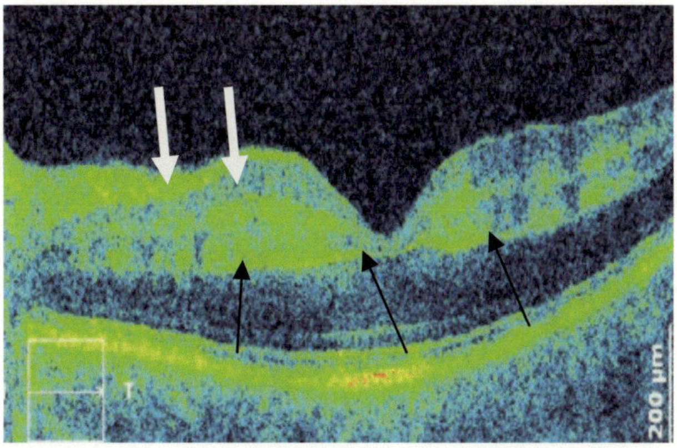

Fig. 5. CRAO - OCT changes, retinal edema in the inner layers (white arrows) denoting ischemia and the shadowing effect in the photoreceptor layer (black arrows)

2.5.5 Color Doppler imaging

Color Doppler imaging is an ultrasonographic evaluation of the blood flow characteristics of the retrobulbar circulation. Color Doppler studies of acute central retinal artery obstruction show diminished to absent blood flow velocity in the central retinal artery, generally with intact flow in the ophthalmic and choroidal branches (Sharma, 1998). Color Doppler imaging can be used to detect calcific emboli at the lamina cribrosa and also may be used to monitor blood flow changes induced by therapy. In addition, carotid artery studies may be carried out concurrently with ocular blood flow determinations to evaluate the possible causes of the central retinal artery obstruction. It is, however, important to determine the presence of plaques in the inspected vessels that are often the source of microemboli responsible for the occlusive event. In doubtful cases, the above-mentioned physical examination and laboratory testing should be carried out, especially in subjects younger than 40 years of age (Table 2).

2.6 Differential diagnosis

Ocular ischemic syndrome

Purtscher's retinopathy

Severe commotio retinae

Inflammatory or infectious retinitis

2.7 Management

Due to the poor prognosis of retinal artery occlusions, several treatment approaches have been attempted. These can be divided into two major categories: (1) conservative treatment, including mechanical (ocular massage and paracentesis), pharmacologic, and other means; and (2) invasive treatment, including catheterization of the proximal ophthalmic artery, usually through the femoral artery with infusion of thrombolytic agents. Any treatment that results in a statistically higher percentage of visual recovery compared with the spontaneous recovery rate and has a low risk for morbidity and mortality could be considered the treatment of choice (Rumelt & Brown, 2003).

2.7.1 Management of central retinal artery occlusion

Conservative treatment

- First step is arterial vasodilatation using sublingval isosorbid dinitrat, or CO_2 rebreathing in the bag;
- Reduction of intraocular pressure (IOP) and improvement of perfusion by means of antiglaucomatous treatment topically (timolol, etc), systemically (manitol), or surgically by paracenthesis;
    - Ocular massage to move embolus further downstream through artery circulation in distant arterioles. Begin ocular massage with 3-mirror contact lens. Press the lens repeatedly for 10 seconds until the appearance of pulsation; or in the absence of pulsation, until collapse of the retinal blood flow. Observation for improvement of retinal blood flow is made through the lens during the ocular massage. If blood supply improves, ocular massage can be stopped and no further steps are required. If the blood flow does not improve, ocular massage should be continued meticulously for approximately 20 minutes. In addition, treatment prior to 24 hours is more highly to be successful and the success depends on the type of the embolus (calcified are the resistant ones). No light perception is also indication to start treatment. Our experience supports the statement of others that even patients with no light perception may recover (this was also seen in cases of orbital compartment syndrome) (Rumelt et al, 1999);
    - During the ocular massage, administer acetazolamide 500 mg IV;
    - During the ocular massage, administer mannitol 20% 1 mg/kg IV or glycerol 1ml/kg PO;
    - Scleral paracenthesis or anterior chamber paracenthesis - anesthetize the limbus with q-tip soaked with lidocaine 4%, and perform anterior chamber paracentesis with 25-G needle withdrawing 0.2 ml of aqueous humor;
- Antiplatelet therapy (streptokinase 750 000 I.U. IV, urokinase), heparin therapy, isovolemic haemodilution, which basically make no sense if there is no circulation in the occluded artery and agents cannot reach the embolus (Hayreh, 2011);
- Pentoxyfilline injection intravenously to reduce red blood cell rigidity;
- Systemic steroids, in case where CRAO is caused by giant cell arteritis;
- yperbaric oxygenation is one of the promising ways of treatment (Weinberger et al., 2002; Bradvica et al., 2009), which can override the time to artery recanalization. However, there is still need for further evaluation because of the lack of greater randomized studies.

Invasive treatment

- Nd:Yag laser arteriotomy and embolectomy (Opremcak et al., 2008), although this rather invasive treatment frequently caused vitreous hemorrhage and need for vitrectomy, so it requires further evaluation;
- Local intraarterial trombolysis, one of the very enthusiastically announced approaches in CRAO therapy, which is suspended due to a high adverse reactions incidence as

reported by the last European Assessment Group for Lysis in the Eye Study (EAGLE) (Schumacher et al., 2010). Probable reason for the high complication rate was the inexperience of some of the participating physicians. The results and complications were much lower when the procedure was performed by one group (Schmidt et al., 1992; Schumacher et al., 1993).

Since the outcome of invasive treatment depends on the experience of the physician and therefore is not applicable to most centers, the best treatment so far is the conservative multi-step treatment that requires the persistence of the physician (Rumelt et al, 1999).

2.7.2 Management of branch retinal artery occlusion

Management of BRAO depends on the type of occlusion; either it is permanent or transient. In permanent BRAO, like in CRAO there are a lot of advocated treatments but none of them has proven efficient. Transient BRAO does not require any treatment at all except a thorough diagnostics to establish the cause of the occlusion and possibly prevent permanent BRAO from occurring. Nonarteritic cilioretinal artery occlusion (CLRAO) can be treated with any of the procedures described in CRAO treatment. Only arteritic CLRAO associated with giant cell arteritis (GCA) has to be treated with a high dose of steroids, i.e. treat GCA to prevent affecting the other eye and total blindness.

It is important that CRAO and BRAO are both emergencies and any procedures leading to recanalization, or improving the outflow, have to be done urgently inside 97 min from the onset of occlusion (Hayreh et al., 2004), and certainly not after 240 min, because after that time the most part of the retinal tissue function is probably destroyed. It has to be emphasized though that these results are valid for experimental models in primates and for complete occlusion and not for humans that usually have partial obstruction. That is probably the reason why the treatment may be successful even more than 24 hours after the occlusion and the onset of symptoms. Therefore, prevention and education of patients to present immediately to an ophthalmologist or emergency care unit may be the one of the measures of improving the chances of treatment in such patients.

3. Retinal Vein Occlusion

Retinal vein occlusion (RVO) has been recognized as an entity since 1855 (Liebreich, 1855) and is one of the most common causes of acquired retinal vascular abnormality in adults as well as the frequent cause of visual loss. However, the pathogenesis and management of this disorder remains somewhat of an enigma. Current treatments for RVO and its sequelae are still evolving.

CRVO and HCRVO are commonly subdivided into nonischemic and ischemic (hemorrhagic) types according to the degree of obstruction. Ischemic type occurs in more severe (complete) obstruction. Such a distinction is relevant to the clinician, since these two types have very different clinical features, visual outcomes, complications, prognosis and management. Nonischemic RVO is a comparatively benign disease, with central scotoma, essentially due to macular edema, as its major complication, with no risk of ocular neovascularization. Ischemic RVO, by contrast, is a seriously blinding disease, since up to two thirds of patients develop the devastating complications of ischemia, and neovascularization that lead to neovascular glaucoma which causes blindness (Hayreh, 1994).

Retinal vein obstruction is divided into central (CRVO), an occlusion of the central retinal vein resulting in four quadrants of retinal involvement; hemi-central retinal vein occlusion (HCRVO) and branch (BRVO) which consists of major BRVO, an occlusion of either a major branch retinal vein draining one quadrant of the retina, macular BRVO (Hayreh, 1994), an occlusion of a macular branch vein draining a portion of the macula, and peripheral BRVO, an occlusion of a branch retinal vein draining a portion of the retinal periphery. According to the most study data, hemicentral (HCRVO) is an anatomic variant of central retinal vein occlusion (CRVO). Thus, HCRVO acts more like CRVO in terms of risk factors, visual outcome, risk of neovascularization, and response to laser treatment (Appiah & Trempe, 1989). CRVO and BRVO have both differences and similarities in pathophysiology, underlying systemic associations, average age of onset, clinical presentation, prognosis (natural history, complication rate) and treatment.

Furthermore, central and hemi-central occlusion are divided into ischemic and nonischemic subtypes each having different clinical implications and ischemic carrying the risk of developing macular edema and devastating consequences regarding the visual function.

3.1 Epidemiology

The worldwide RVO prevalence, according to the meta-analysis which used pooled data from 15 different international studies involving over than 50,000 participants, ranged from 30 to 101 years, has been calculated per 1000 as follows: 5.20 for any RVO, 4.42 for BRVO, and 0.80 for CRVO. On the basis of these rates, projected to the world population, 16.4 million adults are affected by RVO (Rogers et al., 2010). For comparison, more than 171 million adults with diabetes worldwide either have diabetic retinopathy or are at risk of developing this potentially blinding disease, according to a 2005 World Health Organization report (Wild et al., 2004). An estimated 13.9 million people globally are affected by BRVO and 2.5 million by CRVO. Prevalence varied by race/ethnicity and increased with age, but did not have a sex predilection. The age- and sex-standardized prevalence of any RVO was 3.7 per 1000 in whites, 3.9 per 1000 in blacks, 5.7 per 1000 in Asians, and 6.9 per 1000 in Hispanics. Prevalence of CRVO was lower than BRVO in all ethnic populations. Although BRVO prevalence appears to be highest in Asians and Hispanics and lowest in whites, the authors assume this may reflect differences in the prevalence of RVO risk factors, varying methodologies or definitions among reviewed studies (Rogers et al., 2010). Ischemic central retinal vein obstructions account for 20–25% of all central retinal vein obstructions (Klein et al., 2000).

3.2 Pathophysiology

All types of RVO are multifactorial in origin. A whole host of local and systemic factors acting in different combinations and to different extent may produce the vascular occlusion. The role of the various factors may vary, with some as predisposing factors and other as precipitating ones in one group and vice versa in another. Most investigators accept that BRVO and CRVO represent varying degrees of the same underlying disease process. Yet, other clinicians and researchers argue that ischemic and nonischemic types are distinct clinical entities. It is also essential to understand that CRVO and HCRVO are very different from BRVO pathogenetically. In conclusion, it is a mistake to try to explain all types of RVO by one common pathogenetic mechanism (Hayreh, 1994).

3.2.1 Central Retinal Vein Occlusion

The pathogenesis of CRVO is not fully understood and there are marked controversies on the pathogenesis of ischemic and especially nonischemic CRVO. A combination of vascular, anatomic, and inflammatory factors contributes to its pathophysiology.

The occlusive mechanisms in CRVO are mostly these: (i) external mechanical compression of the vein (i.e. by sclerotic adjacent central retinal artery and common adventitia, especially in elderly persons, structural changes in lamina cribrosa, e.g., glaucomatous cupping, inflammatory swelling in optic nerve and orbital disorders) followed by secondary endothelial proliferation; (ii) primary venous wall disease (degenerative or inflammatory); and (iii) hemodynamic disturbances produced by a variety of factors (e.g., hyperdynamic or sluggish circulation, blood dyscrasias, disturbances on the arterial side, etc.). Consequently, a stagnation of the vein flow occurs and a thrombus formation ensues (Hayreh, 1994; Williamson, 1997).

There are multiple anatomic variations of the branching pattern to the central retinal vein. In 20% of eyes there are, as a congenital abnormality, two trunks of the central retinal vein (CRV) in the optic nerve (instead of the usual one), and the merging of the trunks occurs posterior to the lamina cribrosa (Chopdar, 1984; S. S. Hayreh & M. S. Hayreh, 1980). If one of these trunks is occluded, the result is a nonperfusion to superior or inferior retina. Additionally, the venous outflow from the nasal retina may occur via a branch of one of the temporal branches, rather than an independent nasal vein. In an eye with such a branching pattern, an inferior or superior HCRVO may occur if one the venous branches that drain the nasal and temporal retina is occluded (Sanborn & Magargal, 1984). So, considering the various possible scenarios that can result in a HCRVO, a consensus as to whether HCRVO is a variant of BRVO or CRVO still has not been reached.

CRVO is significantly more common in patients with raised intraocular pressure (IOP) and glaucoma (up to 5- to 10-fold increased risk) (Risk factors for central retinal vein occlusion. The Eye Disease Case-Control Study Group, 1996). To maintain the blood flow, the pressure in the CRV at the optic disc has to be higher than the IOP, otherwise a retinal venous stasis and sluggish venous outflow occur (Hayreh, 2005).

There is much more congruence of the data on the pathogenesis of the ischemic CRVO. Most probably ischemic CRVO represents a more extensive (or complete) obstruction while non-ischemic RCVO represents a milder (partial) obstruction. A conception suggests that the vessels are in a tight compartment within limited space for displacement, because of a common adventitial sheath as CRA and CRV exit the optic nerve head and pass through a narrow opening in the lamina cribrosa. This anatomical position *per se* predisposes to thrombus formation in the central retinal vein. But, CRV has multiple tributaries during its course in the optic nerve, pial outside the optic nerve, none in the lamina cribrosa, and only a small one in the prelaminar region. These tributaries establish anastomoses with the surrounding veins. Since the severity of retinal venous stasis depends upon the site of occlusion in the CRV, and the number of available tributaries anterior to it, the site of the occlusion is likely to be much posteriorly to the lamina cribrosa in nonischemic CRVO than in ischemic CRVO (Hayreh, 2005). There is a possibility of changing nonischemic CRVO to ischemic in some patients, probably due to a further precipitous gradual or sudden fall of perfusion pressure (Hayreh, 1994).

Occlusion of the central retinal vein leads to the retention of the blood in the retinal venous system, and increased resistance to venous blood flow subsequently causes a stagnation of the blood and ischemic damage to the retina. It has been postulated that ischemic damage to the retina stimulates increased production of vascular endothelial growth factor (VEGF) in the vitreous cavity. Increased levels of VEGF stimulate neovascularization of the posterior and anterior segment (responsible for secondary complications due to CRVO). Also, it has been shown that VEGF causes capillary leakage leading to macular edema (which is the leading cause of visual loss in both ischemic CRVO and nonischemic CRVO) (Boyd et al., 2002; Noma et al., 2008; Pe'er et al., 1998).

The prognosis of CRVO depends upon the reestablishment of patency of the venous system by recanalization, dissolution of clot, or formation of optociliary shunt vessels.

3.2.2 Combined Retinal Vein and Artery Occlusion

A central retinal artery obstruction combined with central retinal vein obstruction can occur rarely (Richards, 1979), and the mechanism is probably increased pressure on both central retinal artery and vein. The most common cause for combined CRAO and CRVO is retrobulbar anesthetic injection, caused probably by inadvertent injection into the optic nerve sheath (Torres, 2005). If no CRV tributaries are available anterior to the site of occlusion in the CRVO, it converts the circulation into a closed loop and this results in complete hemodynamic block of the retinal circulation, and secondary CRAO. This condition is invariably diagnosed as simultaneous occlusion of CRA and CRV (Hayreh, 2005). Nonischemic CRVO associated with cilioretinal artery occlusion (CLRAO) is usually a result of transient rise i.e. a functional obstruction of the blood pressure in the entire retinal capillary bed due to a sudden blockage of blood flow by a thrombus in the CRV, which, in turn, results in a physiologic block in the CLRA circulation (Theoulakis et al., 2010). Within a day or two, with the development of venous collaterals by the CRV, the blood pressure in the retinal vascular bed falls, and normal cilioretinal filling occurs. However, the severity of retinal ischemia and associated visual loss depends upon the length of time elapsed before the circulation was re-established (Hayreh, 1994).

3.2.3 Branch Retinal Vein Occlusion

Branch retinal vein occlusion is defined as a focal occlusion of a retinal vein at an arterio-venous crossing site. In all but a few rare cases, the BRVO occurs at crossing sites where the artery is passing anteriorly (superficially) to the vein (Duker & Brown, 1989; Weinberg et al., 1990). The upper temporal vascular arcade is more often involved than the lower temporal vascular arcade. Most BRVOs involve the area inside the temporal vascular arcades (macular BRVO), whereas peripheral BRVOs are more rarely seen, partly because they tend to be asymptomatic (Christoffersen & Larsen, 1999).

The arterio-venous crossing plays an important role in the pathogenesis of BRVO, and the anterior position of the arteriole at the crossing somehow renders the underlying vein vulnerable to occlusion. It seems logical to assume that sclerotic retinal arteriole probably compresses the accompanying vein because of a common thickened, adventitial and glial sheath; however, histopathological studies failed to confirm this view. In addition, turbulent flow may injure the vessel wall exposing it for thrombus formation (Hayreh, 1994; Williamson, 1997).

3.3 Causes

Retinal vascular occlusions all have overlapping clinical presentation as well as the similar underlying causes. They are all multifactorial in origin and each patient may have a unique combination of systemic and local factors leading to the occlusive event (Hayreh, 1994). Since the systemic vascular disease is a possible underlying pathophysiological cause, it is important to ask about history of hypertension, diabetes mellitus, any condition predisposing embolic events (endocarditis, atrial fibrillation, atherosclerotic disease, drug and alcohol abuse, hypercoagulabile states) (Klein et al., 2003; Schmidt et al., 2007). Also, the questions regarding possible trauma as well as the undertaken surgical procedures should not be omitted from the medical history since the prolonged pressure to the globe may lead to the ischemic event.

The well-known risk factors contributing to retinal vein occlusions are systemic vascular diseases. The most recognized risk factors for retinal vein occlusion are hypertension, diabetes mellitus, arteriosclerosis and hyperlipidemia. Also, cigarette smoking has been related to increased risk of RVO. They predominately affect the older age group of patients but the younger patients may also develop this type of retinal occlusive disorder and they account for 10-15% of patients with RVO. Mild central retinal vein obstructions in patients younger than 50 years have been referred to as papillophlebitis or optic disc vasculitis. An inflammatory optic neuritis or vasculitis is hypothesized as the cause (Fong, 1992).

According to the recent studies by Hayreh et al. there may be some difference in the risk factors between CRVO and BRVO, with higher prevalence of hypertension, venous disease, peripheral vascular disease and peptic ulcer in the latter (Hayreh et al., 2001). This suggests that it may not be correct to generalize about these underlying causes for the entire group of retinal vein occlusions.

In addition to well-recognized risk factors, new thrombophilic factors have been investigated in these patients. The role of thrombophilic risk factors in RVO is controversial and the studies are showing conflicting results. Hyperhomocysteinemia as well as low levels of vitamin B_6 and folic acid have been identified as independent risk factors (Sofi et al., 2008; Taubert, 2008). Other potential risk factors include elevated factor V Leiden, protein C or S deficiency, anti-cardiolipin antibodies or lupus anticoagulant. Blood dyscrasias and dysproteinemias result in hyperviscosity syndromes, which may appear similar to central retinal vein obstruction but possibly represent curable disease. Hyperviscosity syndromes may produce a bilateral retinopathy similar to central retinal vein obstruction and may, in fact, induce a true central retinal vein obstruction with thrombus formation (Bandello et al., 1994). Simultaneous bilateral disease is an unusual finding in central retinal vein obstructions but occurs more commonly in hypercoagulabile and hyperviscous states. Diseases such as sickle cell disease, polycythemia vera, leukemia, and multiple myeloma are but a few of the possibilities. When there is a patient with bilateral central retinal vein obstructions, especially simultaneous, the medical and laboratory evaluation should include a search for evidence of hyperviscous and hypercoagulabile syndromes (Marcucci et al., 2001) Severe anemia with thrombocytopenia can masquerade as a central retinal vein obstruction, and it is differentiated from a central retinal vein obstruction by a complete blood count with platelets.

In combined central retinal vein occlusion with branch retinal artery occlusion systemic associations other than hypertension and diabetes have not been confirmed. In combination with central retinal artery occlusion associated systemic or local disease is the rule—collagen vascular disorders, leukemia, orbital trauma, retrobulbar injections, and mucormycosis have been implicated (Jorizzo, 1987).

Oral contraceptive use in women may be associated with both thromboembolic disease and central retinal vein obstruction (Stowe et al., 1978). In addition, acute hypertensive retinopathy with disc edema may resemble bilateral central retinal vein obstruction. Obstructive sleep apnea affects more patients with retinal vein obstruction than other disorders and treatment of the sleep apnea may help prevent central vein obstruction (Glacet-Bernard et al., 2010). Other rare associations include closed-head trauma, optic disc drusen, and arteriovenous malformations of retina.

The Eye Disease Case-Control Study Group reported that the risk of CRVO is decreased in men with increased levels of physical activity and increased alcohol consumption (Risk factors for central retinal vein occlusion. The Eye Disease Case-Control Study Group, 1996). The same study group reported a decreased risk of CRVO with the use of postmenopausal estrogens and an increased risk with higher erythrocyte sedimentation rates in women.

An ocular risk factor for the development of central retinal vein occlusion is raised intraocular pressure; the risk of central retinal vein occlusion in glaucoma patients is 5-fold to 10-fold increase (Risk factors for central retinal vein occlusion. The Eye Disease Case-Control Study Group, 1996). Unlike CRVO and HCRVO, glaucoma plays no role in the pathogenesis of BRVO (Hayreh, 1994).

In ischemic CRVO, for example, neovascular glaucoma develops in about 45%. The chronic hypoxia of the retinal tissue induces ocular neovascularization by producing the vasoproliferative factor, which is the proposed mechanism in CRVO whereas in CRAO, there is acute retinal ischemia and infarction responsible for the occlusive event. Also a surprisingly small proportion of patients (2.5%) have the course of illness complicated with neovascular glaucoma (Hayreh, 2011).

3.4 Clinical presentation

3.4.1 Symptoms

Retinal vein occlusion is characterized by painless unilateral loss of vision. It may be subtle in character, with intermittent episodes of blurred vision. In other cases, it may be sudden and dramatic. The nonischemic type is often the more subtle of the two, while the ischemic type is prone to the more acute clinical presentations and may be accompanied by pain.

Ischemic CRVO Acute, markedly decreased visual acuity ranged from 20/200 (6/60) to hand-motion is the usual initial complaint. A prominent afferent pupillary defect is typical. Pain at the time of evaluation may occur if neovascular glaucoma already had developed.

Nonischemic CRVO The majority of patients with central retinal vein obstruction (75–80%) fall into nonischemic form. Patients usually have mild to moderate decreased visual acuity, although this can vary from normal to as poor as the finger counting. Transient visual obscuration may also be a complaint.

Branch retinal vein occlusion is characterized by painless decrease in vision on the affected eye and some patients may have a scotoma.

Combined Retinal Vein and Artery Occlusion Such patients present with acute, severe loss of vision, usually to bare or no light perception. The visual prognosis is generally poor.

3.4.2 Signs

The distinction between the ischemic and nonischemic type is important, because they carry a totally different prognosis regarding visual recovery and potential complication, which may result in permanent visual deterioration.

Both types of central retinal vein obstruction, ischemic and nonischemic, have similar fundoscopic findings—dilated, tortuous retinal veins and retinal hemorrhages in all four quadrants, optic disc swelling, cotton wool spots and macular edema (Fig. 5). Hemorrhages can be superficial, dot and blot, and/or deep. They may vary in severity, covering the whole fundus and sometimes even obscuring retinal and choroidal details, or can be limited to the peripheral fundus only. Vitreous hemorrhage may ensue when bleeding breaks through the internal limiting membrane. The optic disc is usually edematous during the early-stage disease, but the edema may persist in chronic cases (Ehlers & Fekrat, 2011). Many or all of the pathological retinal findings may resolve over the 6-12 months following diagnosis. The resolution of retinal hemorrhages may be complete whereas the optic nerve may appear normal, but optociliary collateral vessels are common finding. In spite the resolution of macular edema, a persistent cystoid macular edema can linger and result in permanent visual loss, often leading to pigmentary changes, epiretinal membrane formation, or subretinal fibrosis.

Ischemic CRVO The presence of cotton-wool spots located around the posterior pole is characteristic of and more common with ischemic CRVO (Fig. 6.). In ischemic CRVO, the ganglion cells in the macular retina are irreversibly damaged by ischemia during the initial stages of the disease; therefore, there is little chance of improvement of visual acuity in such an eye. The distinction between the two types of vein obstructions remains somewhat arbitrary and is based on the total area of nonperfusion on fluorescein angiography. However, dense intraretinal hemorrhage in acute stages may block retinal fluorescence and renders it impossible to determine the extent of retinal nonperfusion. Therefore, it is important to take into account other clinical features such as poor initial visual acuity, the presence of an afferent pupillary defect, neovascularization as well as the functional tests - visual field testing (Goldmann) and electroretinography (ERG) to establish the perfusion status of the retina (Hayreh et al., 2011). In central retinal vein obstruction, perfusion of the inner retina is affected, so that the amplitude of the b-wave is decreased relative to the a-wave; the b-to-a ratio has been shown to be reduced. Some studies indicate that a b-to-a ratio of less than 1 suggests an ischemic central retinal vein obstruction (Matsui et al., 1994). It is only the ischemic CRVO eye which is at risk of developing ocular neovascularization (Hayreh et al., 1983; Natural history and clinical management of central retinal vein occlusion. The Central Vein Occlusion Study Group, 1997). The incidence of anterior segment neovascularization in ischemic central retinal vein obstruction is 60% or higher and has been documented as early as 9 weeks after onset of an occlusive event. The greatest risk of developing anterior segment neovascularization is during the first 7 months, after which the risk of dreaded complication of neovascular glaucoma falls dramatically to minimal. Neovascularization of the optic disc and retinal neovascularization may be seen as well, but they are less common. As with nonischemic central retinal vein obstruction, the findings may decrease or resolve 6–12 months after diagnosis. The anterior segment structures may show signs of ischemia: congestion of the conjunctival and ciliary vessels, corneal edema, iris and anterior chamber angle neovascularization with development of synechial changes predisposing the development of secondary glaucoma.

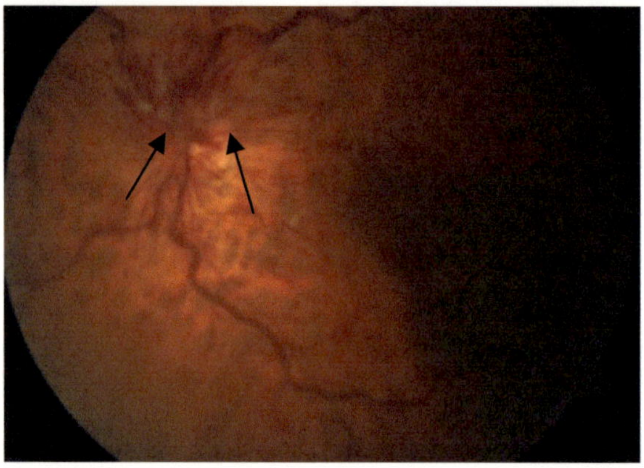

Fig. 6. Central retinal vein occlusion; dilated, tortuous retinal veins and retinal hemorrhages in all four quadrants, optic disc swelling (arrows), cotton wool spots and macular edema

Nonischemic CRVO Neovascularization of either the anterior or posterior segment is rare in a true nonischemic central retinal vein obstruction (less than 2% incidence), although conversion from an initially nonischemic vein obstruction to the ischemic variety is fairly common. The Central Vein Occlusion Study Group noted that 34% of nonischemic central retinal vein occlusions (CRVOs) progressed to become ischemic within 3 years and 15% of the study group converted within the first 4 months (Natural history and clinical management of central retinal vein occlusion. The Central Vein Occlusion Study Group, 1997).

Hemicentral RVO In hemicentral retinal vein obstruction venous outflow from the superior or inferior parts of retina is impaired. Although they involve half of the retina, in terms of visual outcome, the risk of neovascularization, and response to the laser treatment, they resemble the ischemic variant of the disease.

Branch retinal vein occlusion (Fig. 7.) Intraretinal hemorrhages (usually flame shaped), retinal edema, and cotton-wool spots are seen in the distribution of a retinal vessel.

Papillophlebitis The characteristic finding is optic disc edema out of proportion to the retinal findings, cotton-wool spots that ring the optic disc, and occasionally cilioretinal artery obstructions or even partial central retinal artery obstructions. Although spontaneous improvement occurs, the course is not always benign. Approximately 30% of these patients may develop the ischemic type of occlusion, a final visual acuity of 20/200 in nearly 40% of these subjects, and neovascular glaucoma has been reported (Fong, 1992).

Combined Retinal Vein and Artery Occlusion Examination shows a cherry-red spot combined with features of a central retinal vein obstruction, which include dilated, tortuous veins that have retinal hemorrhages in all four quadrants (Fig. 8.). The risk of neovascularization of the iris is about 75%. Exceptionally, a patient may manifest spontaneous improvement (Jorizzo, 1987). Branch retinal artery obstruction combined with simultaneous central retinal vein obstruction has also been reported. This rare entity behaves as a central retinal vein obstruction. Neovascularization of the iris is possible.

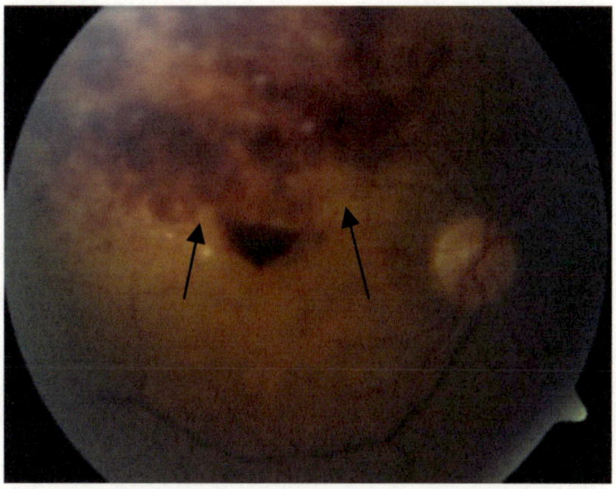

Fig. 7. Branch retinal vein occlusion; note hemorrhages and edema in superior temporal quadrant (arrows)

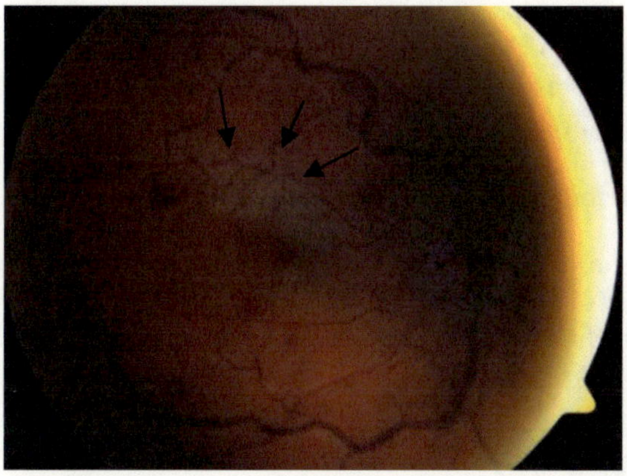

Fig. 8. Combined branch retinal artery occlusion (BRAO) and central retinal vein occlusion (CRVO) of the right eye, ischemia involving superior macular branches (arrows), optic disc swelling, tortuous veins and dot and blot hemorrhages

3.5 Evaluation and imaging

3.5.1 Systemic evaluation

Given the heterogenity of risk factors and their possible interaction in these subjects, the following algorithm of patients with RVO is proposed in the Table 2. As for the arterial occlusive retinal disease, these tests should be performed in younger patients and in doubtful cases.

We feel that, as with the arterial occlusive disease, the stepwise approach to each patient should be tailored, taking into account the age of the patient. Therefore the investigations in the patients older than 50 years of age should consist of: cardiovascular risk assessment, ECG, carotid and vertebral artery Doppler color imaging, echocardiogram; the lab tests including full blood count, erythrocyte sedimentation rate, C reactive protein, fasting blood glucose, lipidogram. The younger patients should be evaluated for thrombophilia, hyperviscosity syndromes, screening for autoimmune diseases and women should be asked about the use of oral contraceptives. Of course, other possible causes of retinal vein occlusions should be considered in cases of normal findings and the investigations should be expanded in stepwise approach, since each case may have a unique combination of risk factors and underlying causes.

Cardiovascular risk factors assessment (diabetes, hypertension, smoking habitus, dyslipidemia, BMI)
ECG
Carotid and vertebral artery Doppler color imaging
Echocardiogram (transthoracic, transesophageal in selected cases)
Lab tests (complete blood count, fasting glucose, lipidogram, autoimmune screen in selected cases: ANA, anti ENA, anti DNA; homocysteine level, folic acid, vitamin B12 and B6, antiphospholipid antibodies)
Thrombophilia assessment in subjects younger than 50 years (factor V Leiden, antithrombin, protein C, protein S)

Table 2. Proposed systemic work-up in RVO patients

Although most cases are diagnosed straightforward from the fundus appearance, the following ancillary tests may be undertaken to distinguish between ischemic or milder, nonischemic form, which is very important in terms of the treatment options as well as the natural course and visual prognosis of the patients.

3.5.2 Fluorescein angiography

Arteriolar filling is usually normal, but venous filling in the affected vessel is usually delayed in the acute phase. Hypofluorescence caused by hemorrhage and capillary nonperfusion are common findings, and dilated, tortuous veins are seen (Fig. 9a.). The retinal vessels, particularly the vein walls, may stain with fluorescein, especially at the site of the occlusion (Fig.10.). The very important distinction should be made between neovascular fronds, which may show profuse leakage of dye, vs. collateral vessels, which do not leak fluorescein. Cystoid macular edema (Fig. 9b.) appears in the late stage of the angoigram shows typically petaloid pattern and may involve the entire fovea or just several clock hours, depending on the distribution of the obstruction. It is, however, important to emphasize that in early stages the retinal angiograms may be misleading because of the masking by abundant hemorrhages and the fact that retinal capillary obliteration is a progressive phenomenon which takes at least 3-4 weeks or even longer to develop after the occurrence of ischemic CRVO (Hayreh, 1994).

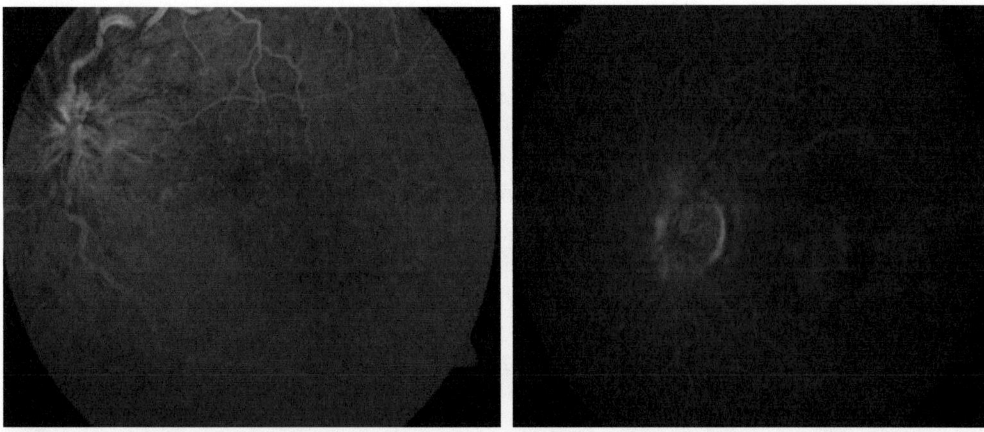

Fig. 9. Fluorescein angiogram of the left eye with central retinal vein occlusion a and b. a) staining of blood vessel walls, disc hyperfluorescence and blockage from intraretinal hemorrhage b) the late stages of angiogram shows leakage of dye in cystoid macular edema, with characteristic "petaloid" appearance.

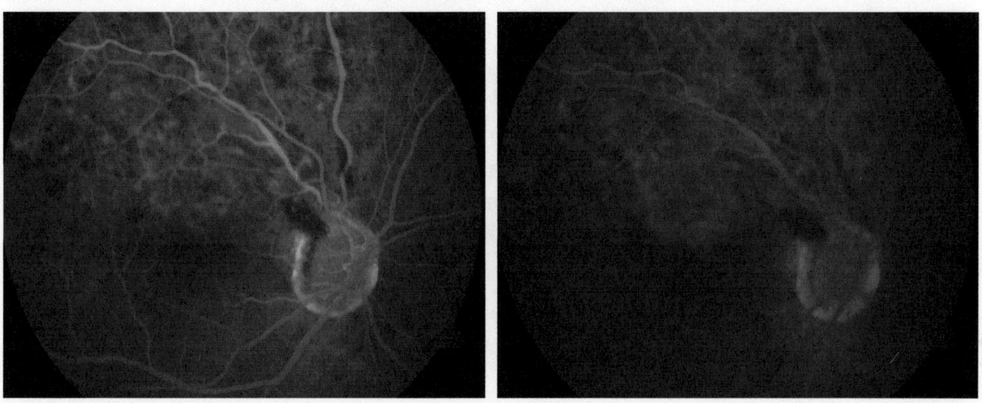

Fig. 10. Fluorescein angiogram of the right eye with superior branch retinal vein occlusion a and b. a) blockage of dye with hemorrhages, mottled areas of intraretinal leakage and microaneurysm formation with vascular teleangiectasia in the upper parts b) the late stages of angiogram shows further diffuse leakage of dye, through all layers of the retina, affecting the macular region as well.

3.5.3 Optical coherence tomography

The optical coherence tomograms show increase in the retinal thickness, which is seen as a loss of macular contour. In the area of edematous retina the presence of cystoids spaces denotes the existence of cystoid macular edema (Fig. 11.). The retinal hemorrhages, subretinal fluid accumulation, cotton wool spots and optic disc edema may also be visualized on OCT. OCT is useful in the management and treatment of the macular edema; it also offers certain advantages over angiograms because it quantifies the macular thickness useful in monitoring the response to treatment and gives valuable data on distribution of the fluid, is not invasive and has no potentially serious side effects. There have been some disputes whether the macular thickness correlates significantly with visual acuity (Nussenblatt et al., 1987). What counts is the improvement in visual functions and not the anatomy. Several factors were predictive of better visual acuity outcomes and more favorable OCT outcomes, including younger age and shorter duration of macular edema, respectively. These factors may assist clinicians in predicting disease course for patients with CRVO and BRVO (Scott et al., 2011). Loss of foveal IS/OS junction line and absence of inner retinal layers in late stage significantly correlated with poorer visual outcome. Macular ischemia by fluorescein angiography shows significant correlation with thinner central subfield thickness, loss of inner retinal layers (Lima, 2011).

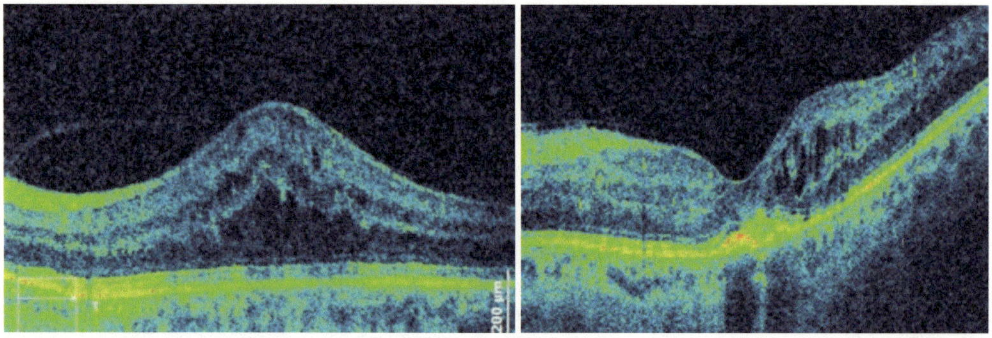

Fig. 11 a and b. Optical coherence tomography (OCT) changes of eye with central retinal vein occlusion a) Cystoid macular edema prior to anti-VEGF injection; b) Cystoid macular edema after anti-VEGF injection treatment Cross-section goes through inferior retina to superior retina, capturing the abnormally thickened retina associated with intracellular edema.

3.6 Differential diagnosis

Hypertensive retinopathy

Diabetic retinopathy

Ocular ischemic syndrome

Juxtafoveal retinal telangiectasia

Radiation retinopathy

Retinal artery occlusion

Retinal detachment

Vitreous hemorrhage

3.7 Management

Some treatments have addressed the venous outflow and the majority the sequelae of the venous occlusion (i.e. cystoid macular edema, neovascularization). In the following text the advocated treatment options are discussed.

3.7.1 Management of branch retinal vein occlusion

Etiology treatment

- Isovolemic hemodilution, used to lower plasma viscosity and to improve retinal perfusion. However, the true benefit of hemodilution has not been established because the published reports have used a combination therapy in the hemodilution groups ;
- Laser chorioretinal venous anastomosis, performed to bypass the occluded site by inducing a communication between the involved branch vein and the choroidal circulation by placing a laser burn directly on the vein and then on the adjacent Bruch's membrane. During the healing process, a chorioretinal anastomosis may form. The technique is studied on CRVO patient, but the small number of BRVO case series were reported (Bavbek et al., 2005; Fekrat et al., 1998);
- Pars plana vitrectomy and arteriovenous sheathotomy. Arteriovenous sheathotomy, in which the retinal vein and artery are surgically separated at the arteriovenous crossing by cutting the common adventitial sheath bare the same idea of improving perfusion. Several small, uncontrolled series have shown good results in improving macular edema and macular perfusion. However, others have reported a lack of efficacy of this procedure (Le Rouic et al., 2001; Cahill et al., 2003).

Sequelae treatment

- Grid laser photocoagulation. The Branch Vein Occlusion Study (BVOS) demonstrated the efficacy of grid laser photocoagulation in the treatment of BRVO-related macular edema. According to the study, grid photocoagulation performed in the first 12 months of onset of the occlusion can, compared to the natural course, improved the response almost twice (Argon laser photocoagulation for macular edema in branch vein occlusion. The Branch Vein Occlusion Study Group, 1984) Argon laser grid or sector treatment result in resolution of the edema but do not improve visual acuity;
- Sector Scatter Retinal Laser Photocoagulation. This treatment was also evaluated during the BVOS study in the ability of preventing the development of neovascularization and vitreous hemorrhage in the BRVO. It is recommended that scatter photocoagulation should be used in BRVO, if and when neovascularization occurs (Argon laser scatter photocoagulation for prevention of neovascularization and vitreous hemorrhage in branch vein occlusion. A randomized clinical trial. Branch Vein Occlusion Study Group, 1986);
- Intravitreal corticosteroids, using a long lasting corticosteroid such as triamcinolone (IVTA), or biodegradable carrier containing dexamethasone to manage macular edema. SCORE study was conducted to compare IVTA versus standard of care, i.e. grid-pattern macular photocoagulation (Scott et al., 2009). The results of this study suggest that both procedures have a similar effect on resolving macular edema and improving visual acuity, but IVTA has more side effects (increasing IOP, cataract progression). In a randomized pilot study of subjects with cystoid macular edema (CME) secondary to BRVO, the increase in visual acuity was significantly greater in those treated with combination of IVTA and grid-pattern laser photocoagulation than in the eyes treated with grid-pattern laser alone, suggesting that IVTA can be effective as an adjunctive treatment to laser (Parodi et al., 2008). Allergan conducted an international study at 167 centers in 24 countries on the effect of intravitreal dexamethasone sustained release delivery system (Ozurdex). The data for the first 6 months was released (Haller et al., 2010). It appears that visual acuity was significantly better in the group of patients who received 0.7 mg dexamethasone implant than in the control group after 60 and 90 days, but is similar 180 days after the treatment. Ozurdex received FDA approval for treatment of macular edema

secondary to BRVO in 2009. An implantable fluocinolone acetonide (Retisert, Bausch and Lomb, Rochester, NY), at present being registered for the intravitreal treatment of chronic non-infectious uveitis, is also being evaluated for the treatment of BRVO and CRVO. The beneficial effect of intravitreal corticosteroids is limited in time and repeated treatment is associated with the accumulation of the complications including steroid-induced glaucoma, cataract, endophthalmitis and retinal detachment. IOP sparing corticosteroids may only prevent glaucoma but not the other side-effects;

- Intravitreal Anti-Vascular Endothelial Growth Factor. It was noticed that VEGF plays a substantial role in the development of CME and neovascular complication in RVO patients. The first intravitreally used drug was bevacizumab, originally developed for the intravenous treatment of colorectal carcinoma metastases, but widely used for treating RVO complications and other retinal disorders (e.g. diabetic macular edema, age related macular degeneration). Several studies have reported a decrease in retinal thickness and improved visual acuity after receiving bevacizumab (Kreutzer et al., 2008; Kriechbaum et al., 2008; Pai et al., 2007). Visual acuity usually increased to maximum in 3-6 weeks after the injections (Stahl et al., 2007). A subsequent decrease in visual acuity appeared to be closely related to an increase in CME. Early recurrence of CME should prompt consideration for retreatment. The most appropriate timing interval between injections is still unclear. The other anti-VEGF agents on the market are pegaptanib, the first FDA approved intravitreal agent (for the treatment of neovascular age-related macular degeneration - ARMD) and ranibizumab, the first FDA approved agent for the treatment of not only ARMD but also macular edema caused by BRVO, based on the results of BRAVO study. Results of phase III BRAVO study show us that after six monthly intravitreal injections of ranibizumab 55% (0.3mg group), and 61% (0.5mg group) gain more than 15 letters, compared to 28.8% in the control group. Also a central foveal thickness decreased by 158 microns in the control group versus 337 microns in the 0.3 mg group and by 345 microns in the 0.5 mg group. Adverse events are rare - one retinal detachment in the 0.3 mg group, one endophthalmitis and one myocardial infarction in 0.5 mg group, and one stroke in the control group. According to our experience as well as numerous other authorities it is doubtfull that myocardial infarction and stroke are caused by the local treatment with anti-VEGF, since they are most prominent in the older population which is prone to these conditions (Rosenfeld, 2006). After six months the control group received intravitreal ranibizumab on as needed basis; i.e. if macular edema occurs. Therefore, the long-term results remain unknown. We can say that, according to this data, the use of anti-VEGF agents become an important option in macular edema treatment secondary to BRVO;
- Pars plana vitrectomy with removal of the posterior hyaloid is effective in resolving CME (only if the traction is the cause of retinal edema and usually if the duration of the edema is less than 6 months) and improving visual acuity (Figueroa et al., 2004). Due to complications associated with these procedures, such as vitreous hemorrhage, intraoperative retinal tears, rhegmatogenous retinal detachment and cataract development, they are not often in use.

3.7.2 Management of central retinal vein occlusion

Etiology treatment

- Isovolemic hemodilution. Several studies have suggested the presence of abnormal blood viscosity in CRVO patients. Based on that assumption, some authors have advocated the use of hemodilution in CRVO, but other (Hayreh, 2003) claim that there is little scientifically valid evidence of beneficial effects of this therapy;

- Anticoagulant and antiplatelet therapy. Although no clear ocular benefit of antithrombotic drugs has been demonstrated, antiplatelet drugs (e.g. aspirin) are prescribed for many patients, including CRVO patients. Hayreh (Hayreh, 2002) claims that this therapy as well as the anticoagulant therapy, such as recombinant tissue plasminogen activator (rt-PA), is contraindicated and even harmful for CRVO patients. Some authors have tried local application of rt-PA into retinal branch vein but the results are controversial and complication rate (haemophtalmus, neovascular glaucoma, retinal detachment, eye phthysis) is unacceptably high; rt-PA should penetrate the retina to exert its activity
- Chorioretinal venous anastomosis. The techniques explained earlier may create an anastomosis, but also carry significant risks. Given the variable success rate, these techniques are rarely employed;
- Surgical decompression of the retinal vein. Proposed procedures can be divided into two mayor types; the first is the vitrectomy with radial optic neurotomy, in which a surgeon's approach is from inside the globe, and the second is optic nerve sheet decompression using orbital "outer" approach. Because of the danger and invasiveness of the procedures and the lack of scientific explanation (Hayreh et al., 2002), there is a need for a larger study to eventually find a place for these procedures in the management of CRVO.

Treatment directed at sequelae

- When speaking of sequelae treatment, we have to add an antiglaucomatous treatment as needed if increase of IOP occurs. Local medical therapy such as, β-blocker (timolol 0,5%), α-2 agonists (brimonidine 0'1-0,2%), carbonic anhydrase inhibitor (acetazolamide, dorzolamide) and panretinal photocoagulation. If failed, the other method of treatment has to be applied such as (i) trabeculectomy with antimetabolites as a first step when there is potential to improve state, (ii) aqueous shunt implants as a second step, and (iii) diode laser cyclophotocoagulation or retinal cryoablation , and in the worst case, with no vision and the patient suffering from great pain, (iv) evisceration or enucleation should be considered (Sivak-Callcott et al., 2001);
- Grid-pattern laser photocoagulation. According to CVOS study, these procedures have no beneficial effect on the visual outcome in macular edema due to CRVO, either ischemic or non-ischemic;
- Scatter panretinal laser photocoagulation. It has been almost universally accepted that prophylactic panretinal photocoagulation (PRP) is the treatment of choice to prevent neovascular glaucoma or treat neovascular glaucoma itself in ischemic CRVO. CVOS study revealed that there is no benefit of the prophylactic PRP in the eyes with ischemic CRVO. These results have led to the recommendation that PRP should be applied promptly after the identification of intraocular neovascularization in eyes with ischemic CRVO to minimize the risk of the development of neovascular glaucoma;
- Corticosteroids. Steroids reduce vascular permeability and stabilize the blood-retina barrier. The mechanism for these effects involves inhibition of the production of inflammatory mediators and vascular permeability factors (e.g. VEGF) as well as the stabilization of the vascular endothelial cell tight junctions. The inhibition of VEGF production may further help prevent neovascular sequelae. Some authors have proposed for some patients the systemic use of corticosteroids (Hayreh, 2010) in high

oral doses of about 80 mg of prednisone to control macular edema, which is the main cause of visual loss. Most of the patients with CRVO according to the SCORE study respond to intravitreal triamcinolone application of either 1 or 4 mg doses compared to the standard care in terms of improving visual acuity of more than 15 letters. As far as the safety is concerned, there are more complications such as cataract formation and IOP elevation in the triamcinolone group. Complications rate is higher in the group with higher dose (4 mg) (Ip et al., 2009). Although triamcinolone is a long lasting corticosteroid, it appears that it is not enough and it leads to the development of sustained corticosteroid delivery devices, which release the drug longer. One of them is Retisert which has good results in chronic refractory CME (Ramchandran et al., 2008), with the best results 12 month after injection. However, the complication rates are very high - all phakic eyes developed visually significant cataracts, and 92% have had an elevation of IOP that needed intervention. Allergan conducted an international study on dexamethasone sustained delivery devices (Ozurdex) and the six month results have been published. In CRVO subgroup of patients a significantly better result in gaining visual acuity (more than 15 letters) has been recorded in the group which received 0.7 mg implant compared with control group at 30 and 60 days control point, and not significantly better at 90 and 180 days point. There were no significant differences in cataract formation between groups and ocular hypertension occurred in only 4% of patients receiving an implant. In 2009 FDA gave approval for the Ozurdex in the treatment of macular edema secondary to CRVO;

- Intravitreal anti vascular endothelial growth factor (anti-VEGF). As VEGF plays a key role in the pathophysiology of CRVO, several anti-VEGF treatments have been developed to decrease VEGF and block vascular permeability and angiogenic activity (bevacizumab, ranibizumab, pegaptanib). According to the results of CRUISE study, FDA released approval of intravitreal ranibizumab for the treatment of CRVO (Brown et al., 2010);
- In cases of refractory CME secondary to CRVO with no resolution after bevacizumab or IVTA individually, a combination treatment with both agents may result in resolution of CME and significant recovery of visual acuity (Ehlers & Fekrat, 2011; Ekdawi & Bakri, 2007). These results suggest that for some patients, the complementary actions of bevacizumab and IVTA on VEGF and inflammation may be more effective than either therapy used alone in the treatment of RVO. Further studies examining multi-modal therapy are needed to answer these questions regarding optimal therapy. Probably a combined treatment or new drugs will have a better efficacy.

4. Ocular Ischemic Syndrome

Obstructions more proximal to the central retinal artery usually cause a more chronic form of visual problem - the ocular ischemic syndrome. Ocular ischemic syndrome (OIS) is a condition that has a variable spectrum of signs and symptoms that result from chronic ocular insufficiency, usually secondary to severe carotid artery disease (CAD). Moreover, they may be the first manifestations of CAD (Dugan & Green, 1991). OIS was firstly described in 1963 and named *venous stasis retinopathy* (Hedges, 1963; Kearns & Hollenhorst, 1963).

4.1 Epidemiology

The OIS occurs at a mean age of 65 years and generally does not develop before 50 years of age. Men outnumber women by a ratio of 2:1, because of the higher incidence of atherosclerosis in men (Brown & Magargal, 1988). No racial predilection exists. Bilaterally OIS occurs up to 22% of cases (Mendrinos et al., 2010). The incidence of OIS is not known precisely, but is estimated at 7.5 cases per million people annually (Sturrock & Mueller, 1984).

Different studies found various incidence of OIS development in patients with hemodynamically significant CAD, which is 4%, 18%, and 1.5% respectively (Kearns & Hollenhorst, 1963; Kearns et al., 1978; Klijn et al., 2002). Ipsilateral transient monocular visual loss is the hallmark of carotid insufficiency and occurs in 30-40% of patients with CAD. CAD on the one common (CCA) or internal carotid artery (ICA) is often accompanied by occlusion or stenosis of the opposite carotid artery (Mendrinos et al., 2010).

4.2 Pathophysiology and causes

Both stenosis and occlusion of the common or internal carotid arteries are responsible for ipsilateral ocular signs and symptoms that may herald a devastating cerebral infarction (Biousse, 1997). The decreased vascular perfusion results in tissue hypoxia and increased ocular ischemia, leading to neovascularization (Leibovitch et al., 2009; Kahn et al., 1986; Takaki et al., 2008).

Patients who develop OIS show decreased blood flow in the retrobulbar vessels and reversal of blood flow in the ophthalmic artery (OA) (Mendrinos et al., 2010). OA shunts blood flow away from the eye to the low-resistance intracranial circuit. This blood steal leads to further reduction of retrobulbar blood flow, hypoperfusion, and subsequently ocular ischemia.

OIS develops especially in patients with poor collateral circulation between the internal and external arterial systems or between the two ICAs. The occurrence of cerebral infarctions and poor neurologic prognosis could also be explained by the insufficient collateral circulation.

4.3 Clinical presentation

Ocular ischemic syndrome encompasses a spectrum of ocular signs and symptoms that are the result of ocular hypoperfusion caused by severe carotid artery obstruction.

4.3.1 Symptoms

The presenting symptom is a variable degree of visual loss often accompanied by pain caused either by ischemia of the globe or elevated intraocular pressure in neovascular glaucoma. The natural course of the ischemic syndrome is generally poor, although there is certain proportion of cases with milder clinical picture retaining the visual function.

4.3.2 Signs

The anterior segment signs are often present: neovascularization of the iris in approximately two thirds of eyes at the time of initial examination; corneal edema and striae usually concurrent with increased pressure from neovascular glaucoma. Although the iris neovascularization is the presenting sign in large percentage of patients with ischemic syndrome, only one third of cases develop secondary neovascular glaucoma. This may be due to a lower arterial supply of the ciliary body causing hypotony or normal pressure in spite neovascular changes in the iridocorneal angle. There may be signs of mild anterior chamber reaction in 20% of these eyes with flare being a more prominent feature than the cellular response (Kahn et al., 1986). Advanced lens opacification may also be present in the late stages of this syndrome. The fundoscopic findings may mimic other vascular retinal disorders and involutive changes seen in elderly population: constriction, straightening and narrowing of the arteries, dilated retinal veins, but without accentuated tortuosity commonly seen in vein occlusions. Venous beading may resemble features of proliferative diabetic retinopathy. In the majority of cases there are dot and blot retinal hemorrhages distributed diffusely around the periphery, but they can spread onto the posterior pole. The other features of retinal ischemia may also be present: cherry red spot appearance, cotton wool exudates, optic atrophy and edema.

4.4 Evaluation and imaging

A careful clinical examination and lab tests (ESR, CRP) must be undertaken to exclude possible temporal arteritis, which may resemble this clinical entity and mandates different diagnostic and therapeutic approach, which may prevent further visual loss and potentially blindness.

4.4.1 Fluorescein and indocyanine green angiography

Besides clinical examination, fluorescein angiography (FA) can help to establish the diagnosis of ocular ischemic syndrome. Prolonged choroidal filling time is the most specific angiographic sign of ocular ischemic syndrome (Mendrinos et al., 2010). Patchy filling of the choroid that lasts more than 5 seconds is seen in about 60% of eyes affected by ocular ischemic syndrome (Brown & Margargal, 1998). Staining of the retinal vessels, both the major vessels and its branches, is another sign seen in 85% of eyes with ocular ischemic syndrome. Demonstration of a well-demarcated leading edge of fluorescein dye within a retinal artery is a typical sign of OIS. Other findings on fluorescein angiography include an increased arteriovenous transit time (over 11 seconds), macular edema, retinal capillary nonperfusion, and evidence of microaneurysms (especially in the periphery) (Richard et al., 1998).

Indocyanine green angiography (ICG) shows signs of choroidal hypoperfusion - occlusion of choriocapillaries with filling defects in the posterior pole or the mid-periphery. There is also prolonged arm to choroid (over 10 seconds) and intrachoroidal circulation time (over 5-6 seconds). Another characteristic finding is slow filling of the watershed zones of the choroids) (Richard et al., 1998).

4.4.2 Electroretinography

Electroretinography demonstrates a decrease in both a and b waves in these eyes, which is in contrast to the sparing of the a wave found in central retinal artery occlusions (Brown et al., 1982).

It is of paramount role to assess the carotid artery function since the endarterectomy procedure reduces the risk of stroke as life threatening consequence and there is some evidence of improvement in retinal function viewed through the improvement of a and b waves in electroretinography, as well as the normalization of preoperative retrograde ophthalmic artery flow shown on Doppler color imaging (Kawaguchi et al., 2001; Story et al., 1995).

4.4.3 Duplex carotid ultrasonography

Duplex carotid ultrasonography combines B-mode ultrasound and Doppler ultrasound providing the morphologic imaging and flow velocity data. It is the most commonly used noninvasive method in evaluation of carotid artery obstruction.

Color Doppler imaging is a noninvasive tool for assessing the velocity of blood flow in the retrobulbar circulation. Diminished velocities of the blood flow in the central retinal artery, choroidal vessels, and ophthalmic artery are typical. There may be a reversal of flow in the ophthalmic artery, as well. Color Doppler imaging may assess the carotid arteries simultaneously.

4.4.4 Invasive diagnostics

If noninvasive carotid artery evaluation is unremarkable in an eye that shows signs suggestive of ocular ischemia, conventional carotid arteriography or digital subtraction angiography may be required to detect possible chronic obstruction of the ophthalmic artery (Wardlaw et al., 2006).

The new minimally invasive methods, magnetic resonance angiography and computed tomographic angiography are evolving and improving as adjunctive diagnostic tests in evaluating the patients with carotid occlusive disease.

4.5 Differential diagnostic

Diabetic retinopathy

Nonischemic central retinal venous occlusions

Giant cell arteritis

Takayasu arteritis

Ischemic optic neuropathy

Retinal artery occlusion

Neovascular glaucoma

4.6 Management

Management of OIS is basically multidisciplinary and the task of the ophthalmologist is to treat ocular condition, recognize the possible cause of OIS and refer the patient to a cardiologist, neurologist or other specialists, where they can get proper treatment of the cause of OIS.

Ophthalmology treatment consists of increased IOP control, management of neovascularization and control of anterior segment inflammation.

- Anterior segment inflammation is usually treated with topical steroids and long acting cycloplegic agents;
- Increased IOP, usually controlled with topical β-adrenergics blockers, ά-agonists and topical or oral carbonic anhydrase inhibitors to reduce aqueous production; prostaglandins (could increase ocular inflammation) and pilocarpin should be avoided;

- Ocular neovascularization following carotid occlusive disease is usually managed with panretinal photocoagulation and can prevent neovascular glaucoma (Carter, 1984; Chen et al., 2001). If PRP is not possible due to media opacities or refractory miosis, other modalities such as transconjunctival cryotherapy of peripheral retina or transscleral diode laser retinopexy should be considered to prevent neovascularization. In any case, PRP works effectively and reduces the iris neovascularization in only 36% of patients with OIS (Sivalingam et al., 1991). In other cases it can even get worse (Turut & Malthieu, 1986), which suggests that uveal ischemia can induce neovascularization, as it is shown on animal model (Hayreh & Baines, 1973). Therefore, in the cases where there is retinal ischemia, prophylactic PRP is advisable. Neovascularization and macular edema caused by OIS can be also treated with intravitreal bevacizumab (Amselem et al., 2007). In this case report neovascularization regressed, but there was no improvement in VA or IOP. Macular edema can also be treated with triamcinolone intravitreally, reducing macular edema and improving visual acuity (Klais & Spaide, 2004). Further investigation with a more reliable sample is needed to establish the role of this therapy in IOS patient. Additionally, we have to mention that when neovascular glaucoma occurs it is usually refractory to medical therapy and if panretinal photocoagulation failed the other method of treatment has to be applied, such as (i) trabeculectomy with antimetabolites as a first step when there is potential to improve state, (ii) aqueous shunt implants as a second step, and (iii) diode laser cyclophotocoagulation or retinal cryoablation, and in the worst case, with no vision and the patient suffering from great pain (iv) evisceration or enucleation should be considered (Sivak-Callcott et al., 2001).

Medical treatment includes conservative treatment by other specialists in order to manage associated systemic diseases or states such as coronary artery disease, hiperlipidemia, hypertension, diabetes mellitus etc.

Some of the surgical treatment is advocated to manage carotid stenosis and to improve ocular ischemia (Costa et al. 1999; Chaer & Makaroun, 2008; Sivalingam et al., 1991), such as carotid artery endarterectomy (CEA), carotid artery stenting (CAS) or extracranial-intracranial arterial bypass surgery (EC-IC), but without sufficient evidence to claim improvement of the ocular state with this treatment, except for CEA, where studies show some beneficial effect on the patient who has mild ocular ischemia and less effect on the patient with a greater degree of ocular ischemia, where retinal damage has probably become irreversible.

In conclusion, we can say that the ocular ischemic syndrome is a rare, vision-threatening condition and since the ophthalmologists may be the first to deal with such patients, they should be aware of the clinical presentation of OIS and recognize it early enough to start treating the condition when visual acuity is preserved enough and when prognosis is better. The continuing improvements in the diagnostic techniques, medical management and surgical treatment of carotid artery occlusive disease make the role of ophthalmologists increasingly important in the early detection and management of the OIS and its comorbidity.

5. Conclusion

Retinal vascular occlusions are an important cause of visual loss, particularly in elderly patients with multifactorial pathophysiological arms uniquely intertwined in each patient. They are often referred to as a „stroke"in the eye due to symptoms and clinical picture, often dramatic in its presentation. It also emphasizes the tremendous influence on patient's quality of life.

Apart from the similar clinical symptoms of visual loss there are some distinctive features that direct the clinician towards the diagnosis of arterial or venous occlusion. A thorough examination should assess the degree of vision loss by testing visual acuity, the presence of afferent pupillary defect, visual field testing, slit lamp examination of both anterior and posterior segments of the eye as well as ERG, which along with afferent pupillary defect and visual field testing provides the most sensitive diagnostic test in distinguishing between ischemic and non ischemic types of the occlusive disease (Hayreh, 2005). Visual acuity alone is not sufficient to validate peripheral retinal function but solely central vision. Therefore, it has been advocated by some authors to combine morphologic and functional tests in order to establish the type of the occlusion which has tremendous impact on the clinical course, prognosis and management of each case. The oxymetry (Gehlert et al., 2010) offers new possible tool in evaluating the perfusion status of the retina as this is extremely important prognostic factor when deciding which diagnostic and therapeutic algorithm should be undertaken in patient with occlusive disorder.

In conclusion we can say that retinal vascular occlusions are very common ocular diseases and the causes of visual loss with poor perspectives in the past, but recent studies on various medications and treatment modalities raise hope between a patient and ophthalmologist for establishing the proper treatment. Although we still cannot foresee, prevent, or causatively and successfully treat occlusive diseases of the retina, there are promising, recently introduced novel options focused on the management of visually deteriorating complications. Intravitreal agents, especially anti-VEGF medications and intravitreal corticosteroid implants have drastically changed the visual outcome for the affected patients. The perspective looks brighter as the development of the most effective treatment regimens and their combinations is evolving. Probably a combined therapy will better act than a single one. Developing new drugs is warranted.

6. Acknowledgement

Authors would like to thank Zoran Pletikosa, MD on providing them with useful medical sources from some databases unavailable to them in a time of writing this chapter.

7. References

Ahuja, R. M., Chaturvedi, S., Eliott, D., Joshi, N., Puklin, J. E., & Abrams, G. W. (1999). Mechanisms of retinal arterial occlusive disease in African American and Caucasian patients. *Stroke, 30*(8), 1506-1509.

Akkoyun, I., Baskin, E., Caner, H., Agildere, M. A., Boyvat, F., & Akova, Y. A. (2006). [Hemicentral retinal artery occlusion associated with moyamoya syndrome]. *Ophthalmologe, 103*(10), 888-891.

Amselem, L., Montero, J., Diaz-Llopis, M., Pulido, J. S., Bakri, S. J., Palomares, P., et al. (2007). Intravitreal bevacizumab (Avastin) injection in ocular ischemic syndrome. *Am J Ophthalmol, 144*(1), 122-124.

Appiah, A. P., & Trempe, C. L. (1989). Differences in contributory factors among hemicentral, central, and branch retinal vein occlusions. *Ophthalmology, 96*(3), 364-366.

Argon laser photocoagulation for macular edema in branch vein occlusion. The Branch Vein Occlusion Study Group. (1984). *Am J Ophthalmol, 98*(3), 271-282.

Argon laser scatter photocoagulation for prevention of neovascularization and vitreous hemorrhage in branch vein occlusion. A randomized clinical trial. Branch Vein Occlusion Study Group. (1986). *Arch Ophthalmol, 104*(1), 34-41.

Arruga, J., & Sanders, M. D. (1982). Ophthalmologic findings in 70 patients with evidence of retinal embolism. *Ophthalmology, 89*(12), 1336-1347.

Atebara N. H., Brown, G. C., & Cater, J. (1995). Efficacy of anterior chamber paracentesis and Carbogen in treating acute nonarteritic central retinal artery occlusion. *Ophthalmology* 102:2029–2034.

Bandello, F., Vigano D'Angelo, S., Parlavecchia, M., Tavola, A., Della Valle, P., Brancato, R., et al. (1994). Hypercoagulability and high lipoprotein(a) levels in patients with central retinal vein occlusion. *Thromb Haemost, 72*(1), 39-43.

Barak, N., Ferencz, J. R., Freund, M., & Mekori, Y. (1997). Urticaria in idiopathic bilateral recurrent branch retinal arterial occlusion. *Acta Ophthalmol Scand, 75*(1), 107-108.

Bavbek, T., Yenice, O., & Toygar, O. (2005). Problems with attempted chorioretinal venous anastomosis by laser for nonischemic CRVO and BRVO. *Ophthalmologica, 219*(5), 267-271.

Beatty, S., & Au Eong, K. G. (2000). Acute occlusion of the retinal arteries: current concepts and recent advances in diagnosis and management. *J Accid Emerg Med, 17*(5), 324-329.

Beiran, I., Dori, D., Pikkel, J., Goldsher, D., & Miller, B. (1995). Recurrent retinal artery obstruction as a presenting symptom of ophthalmic artery aneurysm: a case report. *Graefes Arch Clin Exp Ophthalmol, 233*(7), 444-447.

Beversdorf, D., Stommel, E., Allen, C., Stevens, R., & Lessell, S. (1997). Recurrent branch retinal infarcts in association with migraine. *Headache, 37*(6), 396-399.

Biousse, V. (1997). Carotid disease and the eye. *Curr Opin Ophthalmol, 8*(6), 16-26.

Boers, G. H., Smals, A. G., Trijbels, F. J., Fowler, B., Bakkeren, J. A., Schoonderwaldt, H. C., et al. (1985). Heterozygosity for homocystinuria in premature peripheral and cerebral occlusive arterial disease. *N Engl J Med, 313*(12), 709-715.

Boyd, S. R., Zachary, I., Chakravarthy, U., Allen, G. J., Wisdom, G. B., Cree, I. A., et al. (2002). Correlation of increased vascular endothelial growth factor with neovascularization and permeability in ischemic central vein occlusion. *Arch Ophthalmol, 120*(12), 1644-1650.

Bradvica, M., Barać, J., Benašić, T., Kalajdžić Čandrlić, J., Štenc Bradvica, I., & Biuk, D. (2009). Treatment of occlusion of the central retinal artery with hyperbaric oxygenation - our experience on eight patients. *Medicinski Glasnik, 6*(1), 4.

Brown, D. M., Campochiaro, P. A., Singh, R. P., Li, Z., Gray, S., Saroj, N., et al. (2010). Ranibizumab for macular edema following central retinal vein occlusion: six-month primary end point results of a phase III study. *Ophthalmology, 117*(6), 1124-1133 e1121.

Brown, G. C. (1994). Retinal artery obstructive disease. In S. J. Ryan (Ed.), *Retina* (2 ed., Vol. 2, pp. 1361-1377). St. Louis: Mosby.

Brown, G. (1999). Retinal arterial occlusive disease. In D. Guyer (Ed.), *Retina-Vitreous-Macula* (Vol. 1, pp. 271-285).

Brown, G. C., Magargal, L. E., Shields, J. A., Goldberg, R. E., & Walsh, P. N. (1981). Retinal arterial obstruction in children and young adults. *Ophthalmology, 88*(1), 18-25.

Brown, G. C., Magargal, L. E., & Sergott, R. (1986). Acute obstruction of the retinal and choroidal circulations. *Ophthalmology, 93*(11), 1373-1382.

Brown, G. C., & Magargal, L. E. (1988). The ocular ischemic syndrome. Clinical, fluorescein angiographic and carotid angiographic features. *Int Ophthalmol, 11*(4), 239-251.

Brown, G. C., & Reber, R. (1986). An unusual presentation of branch retinal artery obstruction in association with ocular neovascularization. *Can J Ophthalmol, 21*(3), 103-106.

Brown, G. C., & Shields, J. A. (1979). Cilioretinal arteries and retinal arterial occlusion. *Arch Ophthalmol, 97*(1), 84-92.

Bruno, A., Jones, W. L., Austin, J. K., Carter, S., & Qualls, C. (1995). Vascular outcome in men with asymptomatic retinal cholesterol emboli. A cohort study. *Ann Intern Med, 122*(4), 249-253.

Cahill, M. T., Kaiser, P. K., Sears, J. E., & Fekrat, S. (2003). The effect of arteriovenous sheathotomy on cystoid macular oedema secondary to branch retinal vein occlusion. *Br J Ophthalmol, 87*(11), 1329-1332.

Carter, J. E. (1984). Panretinal photocoagulation for progressive ocular neovascularization secondary to occlusion of the common carotid artery. *Ann Ophthalmol, 16*(6), 572-576.

Chaer, R. A., & Makaroun, M. S. (2008). Evolution of carotid stenting: indications. *Semin Vasc Surg, 21*(2), 59-63.

Chen, K. J., Chen, S. N., Kao, L. Y., Ho, C. L., Chen, T. L., Lai, C. C., et al. (2001). Ocular ischemic syndrome. *Chang Gung Med J, 24*(8), 483-491.

Chopdar, A. (1984). Dual trunk central retinal vein incidence in clinical practice. *Arch Ophthalmol, 102*(1), 85-87.

Christoffersen, N. L., & Larsen, M. (1999). Pathophysiology and hemodynamics of branch retinal vein occlusion. *Ophthalmology, 106*(11), 2054-2062.

Comp, P. C., & Esmon, C. T. (1984). Recurrent venous thromboembolism in patients with a partial deficiency of protein S. *N Engl J Med, 311*(24), 1525-1528.

Conway, M. D., Tong, P., & Olk, R. J. (1995). Branch retinal artery occlusion (BRAO) combined with branch retinal vein occlusion (BRVO) and optic disc neovascularization associated with HIV and CMV retinitis. *Int Ophthalmol, 19*(4), 249-252.

Costa, V. P., Kuzniec, S., Molnar, L. J., Cerri, G. G., Puech-Leao, P., & Carvalho, C. A. (1999). The effects of carotid endarterectomy on the retrobulbar circulation of patients with severe occlusive carotid artery disease. An investigation by color Doppler imaging. *Ophthalmology, 106*(2), 306-310.

Dugan, J. D., Jr., & Green, W. R. (1991). Ophthalmologic manifestations of carotid occlusive disease. *Eye (Lond), 5 (Pt 2)*, 226-238.

Duker, J. S. (2003). Retinal Arterial Obstruction. In M. Yanoff, J. S. Duker & A. J. James (Eds.), *Ophthalmology* (2nd ed.). St. Louis: Mosby.

Duker, J. S., & Brown, G. C. (1989a). Anterior location of the crossing artery in branch retinal vein obstruction. *Arch Ophthalmol, 107*(7), 998-1000.

Duker, J. S., & Brown, G. C. (1989b). Neovascularization of the optic disc associated with obstruction of the central retinal artery. *Ophthalmology, 96*(1), 87-91.

Duker, J. S., Sivalingam, A., Brown, G. C., & Reber, R. (1991). A prospective study of acute central retinal artery obstruction. The incidence of secondary ocular neovascularization. *Arch Ophthalmol, 109*(3), 339-342.

Ehlers, J. P., & Fekrat, S. (2011). Retinal vein occlusion: beyond the acute event. *Surv Ophthalmol, 56*(4), 281-299.

Ekdawi, N. S., & Bakri, S. J. (2007). Intravitreal triamcinolone and bevacizumab combination therapy for macular edema due to central retinal vein occlusion refractory to either treatment alone. *Eye (Lond), 21*(8), 1128-1130.

Fekrat, S., Goldberg, M. F., & Finkelstein, D. (1998). Laser-induced chorioretinal venous anastomosis for nonischemic central or branch retinal vein occlusion. *Arch Ophthalmol, 116*(1), 43-52.

Figueroa, M. S., Torres, R., & Alvarez, M. T. (2004). Comparative study of vitrectomy with and without vein decompression for branch retinal vein occlusion: a pilot study. *Eur J Ophthalmol, 14*(1), 40-47.

Fong, A. C., Schatz, H., McDonald, H. R., Burton, T. C., Maberley, A. L., Joffe, L., et al. (1992). Central retinal vein occlusion in young adults (papillophlebitis). *Retina, 12*(1), 3-11.

Gehlert, S., Dawczynski, J., Hammer, M., & Strobel, J. (2010). Haemoglobin Oxygenation of Retinal Vessels in Branch Retinal Artery Occlusions over Time and Correlation with Clinical Outcome. *Klin Monbl Augenheilkd, 227*(12), 976-980.

Glacet-Bernard, A., Leroux les Jardins, G., Lasry, S., Coscas, G., Soubrane, G., Souied, E., et al. (2010). Obstructive sleep apnea among patients with retinal vein occlusion. *Arch Ophthalmol, 128*(12), 1533-1538.

Graham, E. M. (1990). The investigation of patients with retinal vascular occlusion. *Eye (Lond), 4 (Pt 3)*, 464-468.

Greven, C. M., Slusher, M. M., & Weaver, R. G. (1995). Retinal arterial occlusions in young adults. *Am J Ophthalmol, 120*(6), 776-783.

Haller, J. A., Bandello, F., Belfort, R., Jr., Blumenkranz, M. S., Gillies, M., Heier, J., et al. (2010). Randomized, sham-controlled trial of dexamethasone intravitreal implant in patients with macular edema due to retinal vein occlusion. *Ophthalmology, 117*(6), 1134-1146 e1133.

Hayreh, S. S. (1994). Retinal vein occlusion. *Indian J Ophthalmol, 42*(3), 109-132.

Hayreh, S. S. (1999). Retinal and optic nerve head ischemic disorders and atherosclerosis: role of serotonin. *Prog Retin Eye Res, 18*(2), 191-221.

Hayreh, S. S. (2002). t-PA in CRVO. *Ophthalmology, 109*(10), 1758-1761; author reply 1761-1753.

Hayreh, S. S. (2003). Management of central retinal vein occlusion. *Ophthalmologica, 217*(3), 167-188.

Hayreh, S. S. (2005). Prevalent misconceptions about acute retinal vascular occlusive disorders. *Prog Retin Eye Res, 24*(4), 493-519.

Hayreh, S. S. (2010). Central Retinal Vein Occlusion from webeye.ophth.uiowa.edu/dept/crvo/

Hayreh, S. S. (2011). Acute retinal arterial occlusive disorders. *Prog Retin Eye Res, 30*(5), 359-394.

Hayreh, S. S., & Baines, J. A. (1973). Occlusion of the vortex veins. An experimental study. *Br J Ophthalmol, 57*(4), 217-238.

Hayreh, S. S., & Hayreh, M. S. (1980). Hemi-central retinal vein occulsion. Pathogenesis, clinical features, and natural history. *Arch Ophthalmol, 98*(9), 1600-1609.

Hayreh, S. S., Opremcak, E. M., Bruce, R. A., Lomeo, M. D., Ridenour, C. D., Letson, A. D., et al. (2002). Radial optic neurotomy for central retinal vein obstruction. *Retina, 22*(3), 374-377; author reply 377-379.

Hayreh, S. S., & Podhajsky, P. (1982). Ocular neovascularization with retinal vascular occlusion. II. Occurrence in central and branch retinal artery occlusion. *Arch Ophthalmol, 100*(10), 1585-1596.

Hayreh, S. S., Podhajsky, P. A., & Zimmerman, M. B. (2009). Retinal artery occlusion: associated systemic and ophthalmic abnormalities. *Ophthalmology, 116*(10), 1928-1936.

Hayreh, S. S., Podhajsky, P. A., & Zimmerman, M. B. (2011). Natural history of visual outcome in central retinal vein occlusion. *Ophthalmology, 118*(1), 119-133 e111-112.

Hayreh, S. S., Rojas, P., Podhajsky, P., Montague, P., & Woolson, R. F. (1983). Ocular neovascularization with retinal vascular occlusion-III. Incidence of ocular neovascularization with retinal vein occlusion. *Ophthalmology, 90*(5), 488-506.

Hayreh, S. S., & Weingeist, T. A. (1980). Experimental occlusion of the central artery of the retina. I. Ophthalmoscopic and fluorescein fundus angiographic studies. *Br J Ophthalmol, 64*(12), 896-912.

Hayreh, S. S., Zimmerman, B., McCarthy, M. J., & Podhajsky, P. (2001). Systemic diseases associated with various types of retinal vein occlusion. *Am J Ophthalmol, 131*(1), 61-77.

Hayreh, S. S., & Zimmerman, M. B. (2005). Central retinal artery occlusion: visual outcome. *Am J Ophthalmol, 140*(3), 376-391.

Hayreh, S. S., Zimmerman, M. B., Kimura, A., & Sanon, A. (2004). Central retinal artery occlusion. Retinal survival time. *Exp Eye Res, 78*(3), 723-736.

Hedges, T. R., Jr. (1963). Ophthalmoscopic findings in internal carotid artery occlusion. *Am J Ophthalmol, 55*, 1007-1012.

Ho, T. Y., Lin, P. K., & Huang, C. H. (2008). White-centered retinal hemorrhage in ocular ischemic syndrome resolved after carotid artery stenting. *J Chin Med Assoc, 71*(5), 270-272.

Ip, M. S., Scott, I. U., VanVeldhuisen, P. C., Oden, N. L., Blodi, B. A., Fisher, M., et al. (2009). A randomized trial comparing the efficacy and safety of intravitreal triamcinolone with observation to treat vision loss associated with macular edema secondary to central retinal vein occlusion: the Standard Care vs Corticosteroid for Retinal Vein Occlusion (SCORE) study report 5. *Arch Ophthalmol, 127*(9), 1101-1114.

Jain, N., & Juang, P. S. C. (2009, Jun 30, 2009). Retinal Artery Occlusion. Retrieved Jun 12, 2011, from http://emedicine.medscape.com/article/799119-overview

Johnson, M. W., Thomley, M. L., Huang, S. S., & Gass, J. D. (1994). Idiopathic recurrent branch retinal arterial occlusion. Natural history and laboratory evaluation. *Ophthalmology, 101*(3), 480-489.

Jorizzo PA, K. M., Shults WT, Linn ML. (1987). Visual recovery in combined central retinal artery and central retinal vein occlusion. *Am J Ophthalmol, 104*, 358-363.

Justice, J., Jr., & Lehmann, R. P. (1976). Cilioretinal arteries. A study based on review of stereo fundus photographs and fluorescein angiographic findings. *Arch Ophthalmol, 94*(8), 1355-1358.

Kahn, M., Green, W. R., Knox, D. L., & Miller, N. R. (1986). Ocular features of carotid occlusive disease. *Retina, 6*(4), 239-252.

Karagoz, B., Ayata, A., Bilgi, O., Uzun, G., Unal, M., Kandemir, E. G., et al. (2009). Hemicentral retinal artery occlusion in a breast cancer patient using anastrozole. *Onkologie, 32*(7), 421-423.

Kawaguchi, S., Okuno, S., Sakaki, T., & Nishikawa, N. (2001). Effect of carotid endarterectomy on chronic ocular ischemic syndrome due to internal carotid artery stenosis. *Neurosurgery, 48*(2), 328-332; discussion 322-323.

Kearns, T. P., & Hollenhorst, R. W. (1963). Venous-Stasis Retinopathy of Occlusive Disease of the Carotid Artery. *Proc Staff Meet Mayo Clin, 38*, 304-312.

Kearns, T. P., Siekert, R. G., & Sundt, T. M. (1978). The ocular aspects of carotid artery bypass surgery. *Trans Am Ophthalmol Soc, 76*, 247-265.

Klais, C. M., & Spaide, R. F. (2004). Intravitreal triamcinolone acetonide injection in ocular ischemic syndrome. *Retina, 24*(3), 459-461.

Klein, R., Klein, B. E., Jensen, S. C., Moss, S. E., & Meuer, S. M. (1999). Retinal emboli and stroke: the Beaver Dam Eye Study. *Arch Ophthalmol, 117*(8), 1063-1068.

Klein, R., Klein, B. E., Moss, S. E., & Meuer, S. M. (2000). The epidemiology of retinal vein occlusion: the Beaver Dam Eye Study. *Trans Am Ophthalmol Soc, 98*, 133-141; discussion 141-133.

Klein, R., Klein, B. E., Moss, S. E., & Meuer, S. M. (2003). Retinal emboli and cardiovascular disease: the Beaver Dam Eye Study. *Arch Ophthalmol, 121*(10), 1446-1451.

Klijn, C. J., Kappelle, L. J., van Schooneveld, M. J., Hoppenreijs, V. P., Algra, A., Tulleken, C. A., et al. (2002). Venous stasis retinopathy in symptomatic carotid artery occlusion: prevalence, cause, and outcome. *Stroke, 33*(3), 695-701.

Korner-Stiefbold, U. (2001). [Central retinal artery occlusion--etiology, clinical picture, therapeutic possibilities]. *Ther Umsch, 58*(1), 36-40.

Kreutzer, T. C., Alge, C. S., Wolf, A. H., Kook, D., Burger, J., Strauss, R., et al. (2008). Intravitreal bevacizumab for the treatment of macular oedema secondary to branch retinal vein occlusion. *Br J Ophthalmol, 92*(3), 351-355.

Kriechbaum, K., Michels, S., Prager, F., Georgopoulos, M., Funk, M., Geitzenauer, W., et al. (2008). Intravitreal Avastin for macular oedema secondary to retinal vein occlusion: a prospective study. *Br J Ophthalmol, 92*(4), 518-522.

Le Rouic, J. F., Bejjani, R. A., Rumen, F., Caudron, C., Bettembourg, O., Renard, G., et al. (2001). Adventitial sheathotomy for decompression of recent onset branch retinal vein occlusion. *Graefes Arch Clin Exp Ophthalmol, 239*(10), 747-751.

Leibovitch, I., Calonje, D., & El-Harazi, S. M. (2009, May 13, 2009). Ocular Ischemic Syndrome *The Medscape from WebMD Journal of Medicine* Retrieved June 11, 2011, from http://emedicine.medscape.com/article/1201678-overview

Liebreich, R. (1855). Ophthalmoskopische Notizen: Ueber die Farbe des Augengrundes. *Albrecht Von Graefes Arch Ophthalmol, 1*, 333-343.

Lima, V. C., Yeung, L., Castro, L.C., Landa, G. & Rosen, R. B. (2011). Correlation between spectral domain optical coherence tomography findings and visual outcomes in central retinal vein occlusion. *Clin Ophthalmol,* 5:299-305.

Lindley, R. I., Wang, J. J., Wong, M. C., Mitchell, P., Liew, G., Hand, P., et al. (2009). Retinal microvasculature in acute lacunar stroke: a cross-sectional study. *Lancet Neurol, 8*(7), 628-634.

Love, P. E., & Santoro, S. A. (1990). Antiphospholipid antibodies: anticardiolipin and the lupus anticoagulant in systemic lupus erythematosus (SLE) and in non-SLE disorders. Prevalence and clinical significance. *Ann Intern Med, 112*(9), 682-698.

Mangat, H. S. (1995). Retinal artery occlusion. *Surv Ophthalmol, 40*(2), 145-156.

Marcucci, R., Bertini, L., Giusti, B., Brunelli, T., Fedi, S., Cellai, A. P., et al. (2001). Thrombophilic risk factors in patients with central retinal vein occlusion. *Thromb Haemost, 86*(3), 772-776.

Matsui, Y., Katsumi, O., Sakaue, H., & Hirose, T. (1994). Electroretinogram b/a wave ratio improvement in central retinal vein obstruction. *Br J Ophthalmol, 78*(3), 191-198.

McCullough, H. K., Reinert, C. G., Hynan, L. S., Albiston, C. L., Inman, M. H., Boyd, P. I., et al. (2004). Ocular findings as predictors of carotid artery occlusive disease: is carotid imaging justified? *J Vasc Surg, 40*(2), 279-286.

Mendrinos, E., Machinis, T. G., & Pournaras, C. J. (2010). Ocular ischemic syndrome. *Surv Ophthalmol, 55*(1), 2-34.

Mizener, J. B., Podhajsky, P., & Hayreh, S. S. (1997). Ocular ischemic syndrome. *Ophthalmology, 104*(5), 859-864.

Morandi, X., Le Bourdon, E., Darnault, P., Brassier, G., & Duval, J. M. (1998). Unusual origin of the ophthalmic artery and occlusion of the central retinal artery. *Surg Radiol Anat, 20*(1), 69-71.

Natural history and clinical management of central retinal vein occlusion. The Central Vein Occlusion Study Group. (1997). *Arch Ophthalmol, 115*(4), 486-491.

Noma, H., Funatsu, H., Mimura, T., & Hori, S. (2008). Changes of vascular endothelial growth factor after vitrectomy for macular edema secondary to retinal vein occlusion. *Eur J Ophthalmol, 18*(6), 1017-1019.

Nussenblatt, R. B., Kaufman, S. C., Palestine, A. G., Davis, M. D., & Ferris, F. L., 3rd. (1987). Macular thickening and visual acuity. Measurement in patients with cystoid macular edema. *Ophthalmology, 94*(9), 1134-1139.

Opremcak, E., Rehmar, A. J., Ridenour, C. D., Borkowski, L. M., & Kelley, J. K. (2008). Restoration of retinal blood flow via translumenal Nd:YAG embolysis/embolectomy (TYL/E) for central and branch retinal artery occlusion. *Retina, 28*(2), 226-235.

Pai, S. A., Shetty, R., Vijayan, P. B., Venkatasubramaniam, G., Yadav, N. K., Shetty, B. K., et al. (2007). Clinical, anatomic, and electrophysiologic evaluation following intravitreal bevacizumab for macular edema in retinal vein occlusion. *Am J Ophthalmol, 143*(4), 601-606.

Palmowski-Wolfe, A. M., Denninger, E., Geisel, J., Pindur, G., & Ruprecht, K. W. (2007). Antiphospholipid antibodies in ocular arterial and venous occlusive disease. *Ophthalmologica, 221*(1), 41-46.

Parodi, M. B., Iacono, P., & Ravalico, G. (2008). Intravitreal triamcinolone acetonide combined with subthreshold grid laser treatment for macular oedema in branch retinal vein occlusion: a pilot study. *Br J Ophthalmol, 92*(8), 1046-1050.

Pe'er, J., Folberg, R., Itin, A., Gnessin, H., Hemo, I., & Keshet, E. (1998). Vascular endothelial growth factor upregulation in human central retinal vein occlusion. *Ophthalmology, 105*(3), 412-416.

Ramchandran, R. S., Fekrat, S., Stinnett, S. S., & Jaffe, G. J. (2008). Fluocinolone acetonide sustained drug delivery device for chronic central retinal vein occlusion: 12-month results. *Am J Ophthalmol, 146*(2), 285-291.

Reese, L. T., & Shafer, D. (1978). Retinal embolization from endocarditis. *Ann Ophthalmol, 10*(12), 1655-1657.

Richard, G., Saubrane, G., & Yanuzzi, L. A. (1998). *Fluorescein and ICG Angiography: Textbook and atlas.* (2 Rev Exp ed.). New York, N.Y. U.S.A. : Thieme.

Richards, R. D. (1979). Simulataneous occlusion of the central retinal artery and vein. *Trans Am Ophthalmol Soc, 77,* 191-209.

Risk factors for central retinal vein occlusion. The Eye Disease Case-Control Study Group. (1996). *Arch Ophthalmol, 114*(5), 545-554.

Rogers, S., McIntosh, R. L., Cheung, N., Lim, L., Wang, J. J., Mitchell, P., et al. (2010). The prevalence of retinal vein occlusion: pooled data from population studies from the United States, Europe, Asia, and Australia. *Ophthalmology, 117*(2), 313-319 e311.

Rudkin, A. K., Lee, A. W., & Chen, C. S. (2010). Ocular neovascularization following central retinal artery occlusion: prevalence and timing of onset. *Eur J Ophthalmol, 20*(6), 1042-1046.

Rosenfeld, P. J., Rich, R. M., & Lalwani, G. A. (2006). Ranibizumab: Phase III clinical trial results. *Ophthalmol Clin North Am, 19*(3), 361-372.

Rumelt, S., Dorenboim, Y., & Rehany, U. (1999). Aggressive systematic treatment for central retinal artery occlusion. *Am J Ophthalmol, 128*(6), 733-738.

Rumelt, S., & Brown, G. C. (2003). Update on treatment of retinal arterial occlusions. *Curr Opin Ophthalmol* 14 - (3):139-141.

Rumelt, S., & Brown, G. C. (2004). A systematic approach to evaluate and treat retinal arterial occlusions. Handouts for a course on retinal arterial occlusions for the American Academy of ophthalmology Meetings.

Sanborn, G. E., & Magargal, L. E. (1984). Characteristics of the hemispheric retinal vein occlusion. *Ophthalmology, 91*(12), 1616-1626.

Schmidt, D., Schumacher, M., & Wakhloo, A. K. (1992). Microcatheter urokinase infusion in central retinal artery occlusion. *Am J Ophthalmol, 113*(4), 429-434.

Schmidt, D., Hetzel, A., & Geibel-Zehender, A. (2005). Retinal arterial occlusion due to embolism of suspected cardiac tumors -- report on two patients and review of the topic. *Eur J Med Res, 10*(7), 296-304.

Schmidt, D., Hetzel, A., Geibel-Zehender, A., & Schulte-Monting, J. (2007). Systemic diseases in non-inflammatory branch and central retinal artery occlusion--an overview of 416 patients. *Eur J Med Res, 12*(12), 595-603.

Schmidt, D., & Kramer-Zucker, A. (2011). [Hemicentral Retinal Artery Occlusion due to Oral Contraceptives.]. *Klin Monbl Augenheilkd.*

Schumacher, M., Schmidt, D., & Wakhloo, A. K. (1993). Intra-arterial fibrinolytic therapy in central retinal artery occlusion. *Neuroradiology, 35*(8), 600-605.

Schumacher, M., Schmidt, D., Jurklies, B., Gall, C., Wanke, I., Schmoor, C., et al. (2010). Central retinal artery occlusion: local intra-arterial fibrinolysis versus conservative treatment, a multicenter randomized trial. *Ophthalmology, 117*(7), 1367-1375 e1361.

Scott, I. U., Ip, M. S., VanVeldhuisen, P. C., Oden, N. L., Blodi, B. A., Fisher, M., et al. (2009). A randomized trial comparing the efficacy and safety of intravitreal triamcinolone with standard care to treat vision loss associated with macular Edema secondary to branch retinal vein occlusion: the Standard Care vs Corticosteroid for Retinal Vein Occlusion (SCORE) study report 6. *Arch Ophthalmol, 127*(9), 1115-1128.

Scott, I. U., VanVeldhuisen, P. C., Oden, N. L., Ip, M. S., Blodi, B. A., Hartnett, M. E., & Cohen, G. (2011). Baseline predictors of visual acuity and retinal thickness outcomes in patients with retinal vein occlusion: Standard Care Versus COrticosteroid for REtinal Vein Occlusion Study report 10. *Ophthalmology* 118 (2):345-52.

Sharma, S. (1998). The systemic evaluation of acute retinal artery occlusion. *Curr Opin Ophthalmol, 9*(3), 1-5.

Sharma, S., Pater, J. L., Lam, M., & Cruess, A. F. (1998). Can different types of retinal emboli be reliably differentiated from one another? An inter- and intraobserver agreement study. *Can J Ophthalmol, 33*(3), 144-148.

Sharma, S., Sharma, S. M., Cruess, A. F., & Brown, G. C. (1997). Transthoracic echocardiography in young patients with acute retinal arterial obstruction. RECO Study Group. Retinal Emboli of Cardiac Origin Group. *Can J Ophthalmol, 32*(1), 38-41.

Sivak-Callcott, J. A., O'Day, D. M., Gass, J. D., & Tsai, J. C. (2001). Evidence-based recommendations for the diagnosis and treatment of neovascular glaucoma. *Ophthalmology, 108*(10), 1767-1776; quiz1777, 1800.

Sivalingam, A., Brown, G. C., & Magargal, L. E. (1991). The ocular ischemic syndrome. III. Visual prognosis and the effect of treatment. *Int Ophthalmol, 15*(1), 15-20.

Sofi, F., Marcucci, R., Bolli, P., Giambene, B., Sodi, A., Fedi, S., et al. (2008). Low vitamin B6 and folic acid levels are associated with retinal vein occlusion independently of homocysteine levels. *Atherosclerosis, 198*(1), 223-227.

Stahl, A., Agostini, H., Hansen, L. L., & Feltgen, N. (2007). Bevacizumab in retinal vein occlusion-results of a prospective case series. *Graefes Arch Clin Exp Ophthalmol, 245*(10), 1429-1436.

Story, J. L., Held, K. S., Harrison, J. M., Cleland, T. P., Eubanks, K. D., & Brown, W. E., Jr. (1995). The ocular ischemic syndrome in carotid artery occlusive disease: ophthalmic color Doppler flow velocity and electroretinographic changes following carotid artery reconstruction. *Surg Neurol, 44*(6), 534-535.

Stowe, G. C., 3rd, Zakov, Z. N., & Albert, D. M. (1978). Central retinal vascular occlusion associated with oral contraceptives. *Am J Ophthalmol, 86*(6), 798-801.

Sturrock, G. D., & Mueller, H. R. (1984). Chronic ocular ischaemia. *Br J Ophthalmol, 68*(10), 716-723.

Sullivan, K. L., Brown, G. C., Forman, A. R., Sergott, R. C., & Flanagan, J. C. (1983). Retrobulbar anesthesia and retinal vascular obstruction. *Ophthalmology, 90*(4), 373-377.

Susac, J. O., Egan, R. A., Rennebohm, R. M., & Lubow, M. (2007). Susac's syndrome: 1975-2005 microangiopathy/autoimmune endotheliopathy. *J Neurol Sci, 257*(1-2), 270-272.

Takaki, Y., Nagata, M., Shinoda, K., Tatewaki, S., Yamada, K., Matsumoto, C. S., et al. (2008). Severe acute ocular ischemia associated with spontaneous internal carotid artery dissection. *Int Ophthalmol, 28*(6), 447-449.

Taubert, M., Dowd, T. C., & Wood, A. (2008). Malnutrition and bilateral central retinal vein occlusion in a young woman: a case report. *J Med Case Reports, 2*, 77.

Theoulakis, P. E., Livieratou, A., Petropoulos, I. K., Lepidas, J., Brinkmann, C. K., & Katsimpris, J. M. (2010). Cilioretinal artery occlusion combined with central retinal vein occlusion - a report of two cases and review of the literature. *Klin Monbl Augenheilkd, 227*(4), 302-305.

Torres, R. J., Luchini, A., Weis, W., Frecceiro, P. R., & Casella, M. (2005). Combined central retinal vein and artery occlusion after retrobulbar anesthesia--report of two cases. *Arq Bras Oftalmol,* 68(2):257-61.

Turut, P., & Malthieu, D. (1986). [Failure of laser photocoagulation in ischemic retinopathy associated with carotid occlusion]. *Bull Soc Ophtalmol Fr, 86*(11), 1297-1299.

Van Winden, M., & Salu, P. (2010). Branch retinal artery occlusion with visual field and multifocal erg in Susac syndrome: a case report. *Doc Ophthalmol* 121(3):223-9.

Vignes, S., Wechsler, B., Elmaleh, C., Cassoux, N., Horellou, M. H., & Godeau, P. (1996). Retinal arterial occlusion associated with resistance to activated protein C. *Br J Ophthalmol, 80*(12), 1111.

von Graefe, A. (1859). Ueber Embolie der Arteria centralis retinae als Ursache plotzlicher Erblindung. *Albrecht Von Graefes Arch Ophthalmol, 5,* 136-157.

Wardlaw, J. M., Chappell, F. M., Best, J. J., Wartolowska, K., & Berry, E. (2006). Non-invasive imaging compared with intra-arterial angiography in the diagnosis of symptomatic carotid stenosis: a meta-analysis. *Lancet, 367*(9521), 1503-1512.

Weger, M., Stanger, O., Deutschmann, H., Leitner, F. J., Renner, W., Schmut, O., et al. (2002). The role of hyperhomocysteinemia and methylenetetrahydrofolate reductase (MTHFR) C677T mutation in patients with retinal artery occlusion. *Am J Ophthalmol, 134*(1), 57-61.

Weinberg, D., Dodwell, D. G., & Fern, S. A. (1990). Anatomy of arteriovenous crossings in branch retinal vein occlusion. *Am J Ophthalmol, 109*(3), 298-302.

Weinberger, A. W., Siekmann, U. P., Wolf, S., Rossaint, R., Kirchhof, B., & Schrage, N. F. (2002). [Treatment of Acute Central Retinal Artery Occlusion (CRAO) by Hyperbaric Oxygenation Therapy (HBO)--Pilot study with 21 patients]. *Klin Monbl Augenheilkd, 219*(10), 728-734.

Wenzler, E. M., Rademakers, A. J., Boers, G. H., Cruysberg, J. R., Webers, C. A., & Deutman, A. F. (1993). Hyperhomocysteinemia in retinal artery and retinal vein occlusion. *Am J Ophthalmol, 115*(2), 162-167.

Werner, M. S., Latchaw, R., Baker, L., & Wirtschafter, J. D. (1994). Relapsing and remitting central retinal artery occlusion. *Am J Ophthalmol, 118*(3), 393-395.

Wild, S., Roglic, G., Green, A., Sicree, R., & King, H. (2004). Global prevalence of diabetes: estimates for the year 2000 and projections for 2030. *Diabetes Care, 27*(5), 1047-1053.

Williamson, T. H. (1997). Central retinal vein occlusion: what's the story? *Br J Ophthalmol, 81*(8), 698-704.

Wong, T. Y., & Klein, R. (2002). Retinal arteriolar emboli: epidemiology and risk of stroke. *Curr Opin Ophthalmol, 13*(3), 142-146.

Younge, B. R. (1989). The significance of retinal emboli. *J Clin Neuroophthalmol, 9*(3), 190-194.

22

Induction of Branch Retinal Vein Occlusion by Photodynamic Therapy with Rose Bengal in a Rabbit Model

Xiao-Xu Zhou[1], Yan-Ping Song[2], Yu-Xing Zhao[2] and Jian-Guo Wu[1,2]
[1]*Tianjin Medical University Eye Center, Tianjin,*
[2]*Department of Ophthalmology of PLA Wuhan General Hospital, Wuhan,*
People's Republic of China

1. Introduction

Branch retinal vein occlusion (BRVO) is a common vascular disorder that is frequently associated with severe vision loss due to its complications. There are two forms of BRVO, the ischaemic and the non-ischemic, both leading to loss of visual acuity. About 20-30% of the BRVOS are ischemic and the majority of them develop secondary glaucoma and rubeosis. [1] Although this disorder was first reported by J. von Michel in 1878, its pathogenesis has still not been fully understood, and no effective therapy has been developed for this disorder [1-3]. Comparative research on this disorder is based on clinical models of BRVO.

The pathological features of BRVO can be more accurately reproduced by a photodynamic method to induce thrombosis in retinal vessels[4-14] than by using other methods such as laser coagulation[15-17], electrocoagulation of the retinal vein via the vitreous body[18], intravenous thrombin instillation[19-21] and endothelin-I injection into the posterior vitreous body[22, 23]. In the photodynamic method, a photosensitizing agent, namely, rose Bengal, is injected intravenously. This dye absorbs light maximally at a specific wavelength of 550 nm. Dye activation in the presence of molecular oxygen leads to the generation of singlet oxygen, which in turn acts locally to injure or destroy the vascular endothelium. The altered endothelium provides a surface for platelet aggregation and subsequent thrombosis. By using this method, thrombi can be produced in vessels. Because relatively low light intensities are required to initiate this process, the thermal effects on the surrounding tissues are minimized.

In this investigation, we used a Xenon arc lamp as the light source, and visible light was transmitted through an intraocular fiber to induce BRVO in pigmented rabbits. The characteristics of BRVO were evaluated quantitatively, and histological studies were performed to support the clinical findings. The results provided a framework for future applications of this technique.

2. Materials and methods

2.1 Animals and husbandry

Thirty-two male Standard Chinchilla rabbits were purchased from the Experimental Animal Center of Tianjin Medical University (Tianjin, China) and allowed to acclimate upon arrival for 10 d before the initiation of the experiment. At the beginning of the study, the animals were aged 3–4 months and weighed 2.5–3.5 kg. All experimental animals were housed in individual cages under stable environmental conditions: diet, commercial pellet diet (Lushifu, Beijing, China) and tap water ad libitum; relative humidity, 45–55%; temperature, 18°C; and light-dark cycle, 12/12 h (intensity, 300 lux).

The study was approved by the Ethics Committee of Tianjin medical university. All animal experiments were performed in accordance with the conventions of the Association for Research in Vision and Ophthalmology (ARVO) for ethics in animal experimentation.

2.2 Experimental design

The 32 rabbits (32 eyes, 32 vessels) were randomly divided into 15 treatment groups (n = 2) and 1 control group (n = 2). The treatment groups were administered 5 different rose Bengal doses (3, 6, 9, 12 and 15 mg/kg) and exposed to light of 3 different intensities (600, 1000 and 1400 lux) 1 min later. In the control group rabbits, the vessels were exposed to a light intensity of 1400 lux for 20 min without injection of the rose Bengal dye.

2.3 Experimental procedure

In preparation for the treatment and follow-up examinations, the rabbits were fully anesthetized with an intramuscular injection of 60 mg/kg ketamine (Beijing Shuanghe Pharmaceuticals, Beijing, China) and 8 mg/kg xylazine (Beijing Shuanghe Pharmaceuticals, Beijing, China). The pupils were dilated using 0.5% tropicamide eye drops (Beijing Shuanghe Pharmaceuticals, Beijing, China).

Rose Bengal (tetrachloro-tetraiodo-fluorescein sodium; certified purity, 90%; Sigma, St. Louis, MO) was dissolved in normal saline (30 mg/ml), sterilized by passage through a 0.22-μm filter and injected intravenously in doses of 3, 6, 9, 12 or 15 mg/kg before the light treatment. A Xenon arc lamp (Anshijia Instrument Co. Ltd., Beijing, China) was used as a light source, and light was transmitted by using a 0.2-mm intraocular illumination fiber (Alcon (China) Ophthalmic Product Co. Ltd., Shanghai, China). Light intensity was measured using a digital lux meter (LX-9621; Landtek Instrument Co. Ltd., Guangzhou, China). Average values of 600, 1000 and 1400 lux, for the low, medium and high settings, respectively, were obtained with less than 3% variation in repeated measurements throughout the study.

According to the treatment protocol, the rabbits were placed on a stage under a surgical microscope (OPTON Universal S3; Germany). 2% methylcellulose solution (Zhengda Co. Ltd., Shandong, China) is dropped on the cornea to couple the input light into the 30-degree prism lens (Anshijia Instrument Co. Ltd., Beijing, China). The operations were observed by using a contact lens and a surgical microscope. A 25-gauge trocar (Alcon (China) Ophthalmic Product Co. Ltd., Shanghai, China) was used to make an incisions in the conjunctiva and sclera at the projection holes located supratemporally 3 mm from the corneal limbus, then the needle was removed and the intraocular fiber was inserted through the incision and its direction was toward optic disc, the depth was 10 mm. Rose Bengal was injected intravenously through the marginal ear vein. After 1 min, the trunk vessels adjacent to the optic disc of 1~ 3 mm were exposed to a beam of white light. The duration of continuous exposure to light did not exceed 20 min, and the exposure time was recorded if complete vascular occlusion was observed. The fiber finally was then taken out and the sclera was finally sutured.

Fundus fluorescein angiography (FFA) was performed using a fundus camera (Zeiss FF450IR; Carl Zeiss Far East Co. Ltd., Beijing, China) before the treatment and everyday after the treatment until the occluded vein reopened. The 5 mg aqueous fluorescein sodium (100 mg/ml, Baiyunshan Pharmaceuticals Co. Ltd., Guangzhou, China) was injected into ear veins immediately prior to FFA under anesthesia and pupil dilation those were as same as the prior.

2.4 Experimental observation

The rate and duration of vessel occlusion are confirmed with an ophthalmoscope and by FFA. The blood flow was confirmed by a scleral depressor transiently applied pressure on the equator of the eyeball, thereby the higher intraocular pressure (IOP) reduced the flow rate until freely moving red blood cells were seen. Once the scleral depressor was removed, a rapid uninterrupted column of blood flow passed through without the presence of stagnant red blood cells. [9] These dynamic phenomenons were monitored by an ophthalmoscope and it was the character of reperfused vessels.

When reperfusion was noted on post-treatment day 1, the number of days of occlusion was defined as 0. When the vessel was observed to be occluded on day 1 but not on day 2, the number of days of occlusion was defined as 1 and so on.

Two rabbits in the control group and 1 rabbit in the treatment groups in whom BRVO was confirmed by FFA were euthanized using intravenous overdose of pentobarbital sodium (Beijing Shuanghe Pharmaceuticals, Beijing, China). Their eyes were enucleated and prepared for light microscopic examination by using standard techniques. Sections (5-μm-thick) were stained with haematoxylin/eosin. The remaining rabbits were euthanized by administering an overdose of pentobarbital sodium at the end of the experiment.

2.5 Statistical analysis

A partial correlation coefficient was used to analyze the relationship between the time of thrombosis, the drug dose, and light intensity. A P value of 0.05 or less was considered statistically significant. All data were analysed with the SPSS 11.5 software.

3. Results

3.1 Evaluation of BRVO animal model

BRVO models were developed in 22 of the 30 rabbits in the treatment group. The fundus could be observed in detail by using a surgical microscope (please see supplemental video 1). In the site exposed to light, photodynamic injury resulted in white debris (plaque-like thrombi) and the stagnation of blood flow. FFA showed the engorged distal ends of the venules proximal to the occlusion site and peripheral retinal oedema in the BRVO area (Figure 1).

Histological sections were studied to confirm the presence and extent of the photodynamic lesions. Retinal vein damage was confined to the area of direct light exposure in the treatment groups. Histological examination revealed thrombi consisting of platelet aggregates, stagnant red blood cells and a few white blood cells. Occluded retinal vein histological section indicated that compact thrombus filled the entire vein cavity and occlusion is evident. (Figure 2).

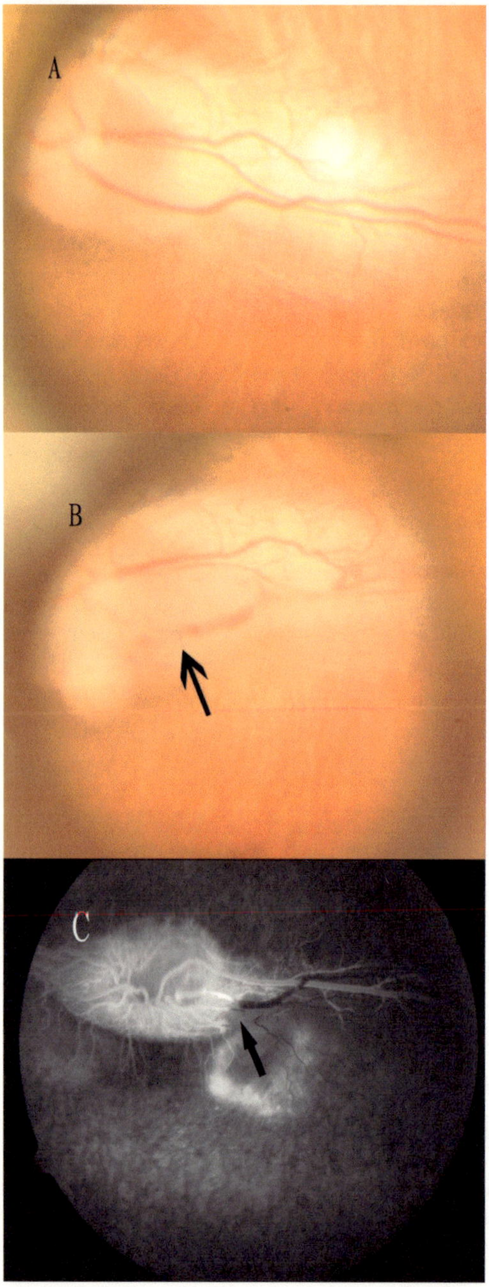

Fig. 1. **Photodynamic thrombosis of a branch retinal vein in a pigmented rabbit eye.** Initial formation of a thrombosis in the target vein (A) and complete obliteration of the vessel lumen (B). FFA showed a delay in the time required for angiosclerosis in the distal end of the vein and discontinuous intravenous blood flow in the vicinity of the optic disc (C). Arrows indicate the occlusion site and peripheral retinal oedema.

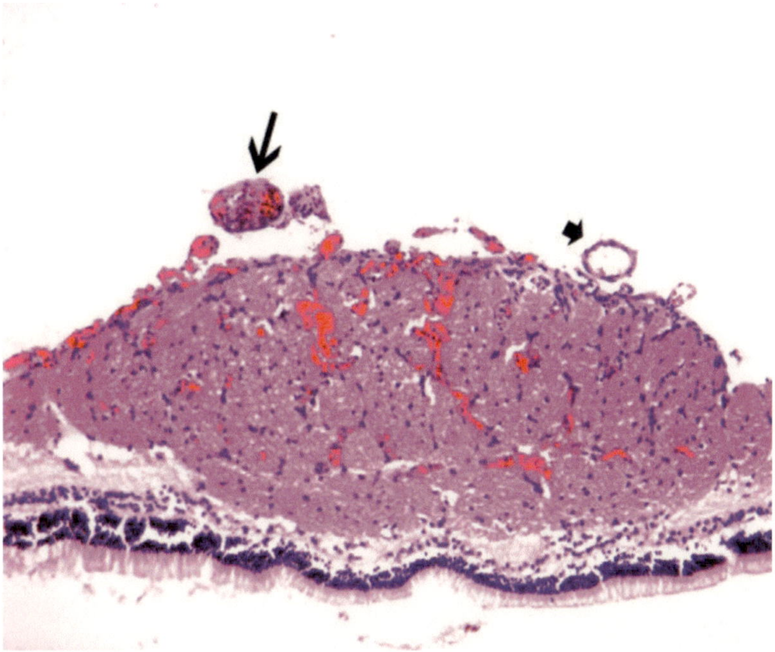

Fig. 2. **Histological findings.** Two hours after thrombosis, the thrombus filled the entire vein cavity (long arrow), and the artery was normal (short arrow). The thrombus consisted of platelet aggregates, stagnant red blood cells and a few white blood cells. Magnification, 200×.

The control vessels and the blood flow through them were as same as those in healthy animals. The histological sections from the rabbits that were not injected with rose Bengal showed no evidence of photochemical or thermal retinal damage in the site that was exposed to a light intensity of 1400 lux (maximum light intensity) for 20 min.

3.2 Dose- and light-response studies

Vein occlusion in the pigmented rabbits was considered as the end point for determining dose- and light-response relationships. In 22 successful BRVO models, the time required to produce an occlusion decreased with an increase in the dose of rose Bengal administered and the light intensity. Rose Bengal at doses of more than 9 mg/kg was effective in producing BRVO; a dose of 6 mg/kg was ineffective in producing BRVO at a light intensity of 600 lux. At a dose of 3 mg/kg, small plaques also developed in the target vessel; however, they did not progress to vascular occlusions in 20 min even if the light intensity was as high as 1400 lux. The total light energy required to produce an occlusion increased from an average of 600 lux with 9 mg/kg of rose Bengal to 1000 lux with 6 mg/kg of rose Bengal. The time of occurrence of thrombosis showed a negative correlation with the drug dose and light intensity. A decrease in the time required for the development of BRVO corresponded to a higher drug dose (partial $r = -0.7895$; $P < 0.001$) and a higher light intensity (partial $r = -0.9060$; $P < 0.001$) (Figure 3).

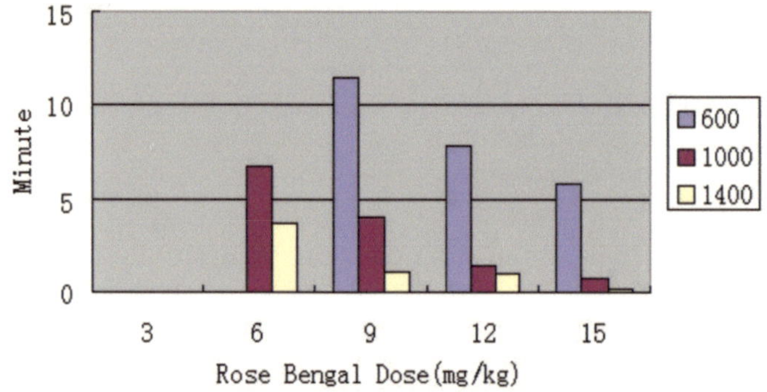

Fig. 3. **The relationship between the time required for thrombosis and the dose of rose Bengal and the light intensity.** The mean value of the time required for thrombosis was determined (n = 2). Complete BRVO formation did not occur when a dose of 3 mg/kg rose Bengal was used, and a dose of 6 mg/kg rose Bengal was ineffective in producing BRVO at a light intensity of 600 lux.

3.3 Duration of occlusion

In the early period of BRVO in the animal models, FFA and fundus photography documented the blood along the circuitous expanded vein, and retinal oedema that was similar to the lesion in humans. The area of the white thrombus gradually decreased with time, and the angiostenosis in the distal end of the retinal vein also gradually decreased. In 21 cases, the minimum duration record for the reopening of an occlusion was 3 d and the maximum, 10 d (Figure 4).

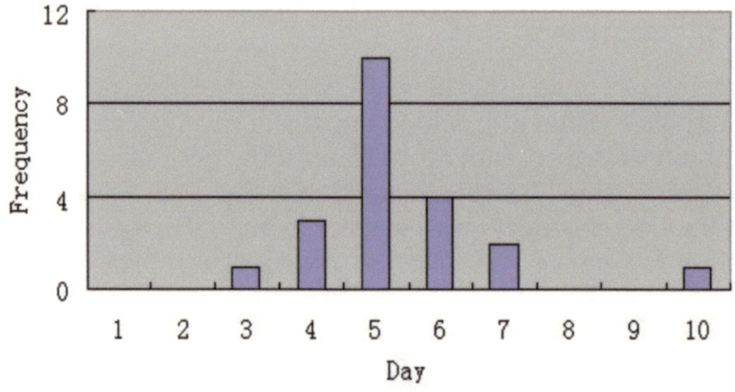

Fig. 4. **The frequency of the duration of vessel occlusion.** The duration of BRVO varied from 3 to 10 d. The data correspond to a Gaussian distribution ($P < 0.01$); the 95% confidence bound was 4.73-6.03 d, and the mean duration of vessel occlusion was 5.38 ± 1.43 d (n = 21).

4. Discussion

While developing an animal model, the following factors should be considered: the animal species used, the ease of development and reproducibility of the model and the degree of similarity of the model with the human disease. In this study, we focus on optimizing the method used to induce experimental thrombosis.

The animal species that are usually selected for the development of BRVO animal models are mouse, rat, rabbit, cat, pig, dog and monkey. Mice[14] and rats[5-7, 9] are suitable for the development of large numbers of RVO models for research because of their low price, easy availability and breeding management. Further, these models enable easy identification of the retinal artery and vein. However, the eye of mice or rats is too small to permit investigative surgical procedures. The structure of the retina in pigs[12, 15], cats[8] or dogs[4] is similar to that in humans except that it does not have a macular region. The retinal blood supply in rhesus monkeys[16, 17] is similar to that in human; however, the sources of these animals are limited, and they are difficult to breed and manage. Compared with the eyeballs of other animal species, the rabbit eyeball is sufficiently large to operate[19-23]. Further, rabbits are inexpensive, can be easily bred and the FFA of the rabbit eye is stable. Therefore, we selected pigmented rabbits for our study.

The combination of intraocular fibre illumination with the administration of rose Bengal should be classified as a photodynamic method of inducing BRVO because the wavelength of visible light include 550 nm. These findings correspond to Virchow's hypothesis of thrombosis in humans. Compared with the photodynamic method, laser coagulation[15-17] requires higher energy and a longer exposure time, which would inevitably result in heat injury and disruption of the vessel wall, and subsequently, frequent bleeding. Electrocoagulation of the retinal vein via the vitreous body[18] utilizes electrothermal energy to destroy the vascular endothelium and block the vessels, which is different from the process of thrombosis. In intravitreous thrombin instillation method[19-21], the location of the retinal thrombus could not be determined; thus, the thrombus may occlude other regions but not the target vessels. The injection of endothelin-I into the posterior vitreous body[22, 23] caused complete occlusion of the temporal retinal vessels, but this vasospastic mechanism is also unsuitable for application in the experimental induction of thrombosis because actual clinical BRVO was occluded at one or some spots in vein.

Presently, an argon (Ar) laser is often used as the excitation light source in the photodynamic method because its wavelength of 514 nm is similar to the light absorption peak of rose Bengal. However, heat injury from laser-coagulation to the retinal tissue and its vessels is observed. Moreover, due to the pulsed excitation of the laser, continuous exposure of the vessel to the laser beam is impossible. Consequently, it is difficult to adjust the level of energy used in this procedure: if the energy level is too low, no thrombus formation occurs and if it is too high, vessel hemorrhage occurs[8]. Some researchers utilize common light sources such as slit lamps and Xenon lamps to develop BRVO animal models. However, the use of these light sources resulted in an extensive arteriovenous obstruction caused due to the exposure of a large area to the light source, therefore, these light sources are not suitable for studying a typical BRVO[9, 10, 13]. In a previous study, we use a microsurgical illumination system, which comprised a 0.9-mm intraocular fibre that served as an endoilluminator to produce RVO in pigs[11]; the intraocular fibre illuminated the nearby retinal vascular target and by localizing energy, it is able to produce a thrombus as effectively as laser irradiation. However, the diameter of the retinal trunk vein in rabbits was only 150–200 μm, and the microsurgical system was too wide to the rabbit. Therefore, in this study, we used a Xenon arc lamp as a light source and designed a 0.2 mm fiber for illumination to ensure that the light beam irradiate the trunk vein and not the accompanying artery. We find that this is a simple and reliable system for developing BRVO models in rabbits.

The process of formation of BRVO in our rabbit model can be visualized and photographed using a surgical microscope. At the site exposed to light, the following course of thrombogenesis is recognized: photodynamic injury resulted in a decrease in the rate of venous blood flow; this is followed by the appearance of stagnant red blood cells in the vessel, the gradual accumulation of white debris (plaque-like thrombi) and the development of a vascular occlusion. The distal ends of the venules are engorged proximal to the occlusion site. The morphological and histopathological changes are similar to Kohner's results[24]. No changes were observe in the light microscopic images of the control vessels; this confirmes that illumination do not produce heat injury in the retinal vessels and tissue.

The dose- and light-response studies show that the time of occurrence of thrombosis correlate negatively with the drug dose and light intensity; further, the basic set of parameters require to produce an occlusion is an average light intensity of 600 lux, a rose Bengal dose of 9 mg/kg and an exposure time of 11.5 min or an average light intensity of 1000 lux, a rose Bengal dose of 6 mg/kg and an exposure time of 6.75 min. Thus, we suggest that the optimum parameters should be 1000 lux, 9 mg/kg of rose Bengal and an exposure time of 3–5 min. This suggestion is based on the following considerations: the experimental dose of rose Bengal in this model is maintained as low as possible to prevent the leakage of rose Bengal into the vitreous humour and the anterior chamber[12]; the energy level of the light used to induce thrombosis is higher than that in the breeding conditions (300 lux); this ensures that thrombosis occur only in the area exposed to the light and not in other vessels. On the other hand, the exposure time of 3–5 min was suitable for operation. The optimization of this method may aid investigators in controlling thrombus formation more precisely.

Clinical BRVO is a disease of long duration and various types [1-3]; however, the experimental occlusion is maintained for 3 to 10 d (average, 5.38 d) in our model. This may be attributed to the use of young and healthy experimental animals, the sudden generation of an obstruction in the normal vascular bed and the activation of an autochthonous repair mechanism; all these factors result in rapid thrombolysis. Therefore, this BRVO model is very suitable for observation of immediate therapy experiment, for example, surgery; and not suitable for long-term drug treatment studies.

5. References

[1] Hayreh SS, Podhajsky PA, Zimmerman MB. Branch retinal artery occlusion: natural history of visual outcome. Ophthalmology. 116:1188-94. e1-4(2009).

[2] Hayreh SS, Zimmerman B, McCarthy MJ, et al. Systemic diseases associated with various types of retinal vein occlusion. Am J Ophthalmol.131:61-77(2001).

[3] Shahid H, Hossain P, Amoaku WM. The management of retinal vein occlusion: is interventional ophthalmology the way forward?. Br J Ophthalmol. 90:627- 39(2006).

[4] Tameesh MK, Lakhanpal RR, Fujii GY, et al. Retinal vein cannulation with prolonged infusion of tissue plasminogen activator (t-PA) for the treatment of experimental retinal vein occlusion in dogs. Am J Ophthalmol. 138:829-39(2004)

[5] Kang SG, Chung H, Hyon JY. Experimental preretinal neovascularization by laser-induced thrombosis in albino rats. Korean J Ophthalmol. 13(2):65-70(1999)

[6] Ham DI, Chang K, Chung H. Preretinal neovascularization induced by experimental retinal vein occlusion in albino rats. Korean J Ophthalmol.11:60-64(1997)

[7] Shen W, He S, Han S, et al. Preretinal neovascularisation induced by photodynamic venous thrombosis in pigmented rat. Aust N Z J Ophthalmol. 24:50-52(1996)

[8] Si BX, Zhang MN, Huang HB, et al. [Experimental retinal vein occlusion in cats]. Chin Inter J Ophthalmol.7:987-989(2007)

[9] Wilson CA, Hatchell DL. Photodynamic retinal vascular thrombosis. Rate and duration of vascular occlusion. Invest Ophthalmol Vis Sci. 32:2357-2365(1991)

[10] Nanda SK, Hatchell DL, Tiedeman JS, et al. A new method for vascular occlusion. Photochemical initiation of thrombosis. Arch Ophthalmol. 105:1121-1124(1987)

[11] Zhang XL, Ma ZZ, Hu YT, et al. Direct tissue plasminogen activator administration through a microinjection device in a pig model of retinal vein thrombosis. Curr Eye Res. 24:263-267(2002)

[12] Zhang XL, Hu YT, Ma ZZ, et al. [Experimental retinal vein occlusion induced by photodynamic approach]. Chin J Ophthalmol. 39:220-223(2003)

[13] Royster AJ, Nanda SK, Hatchell DL, et al. Photochemical initiation of thrombosis. Fluorescein angiographic, histologic, and ultrastructural alterations in the choroid, retinal pigment epithelium, and retina. Arch Ophthalmol. 106:1608-1614(1988)

[14] Zhang H, Sonoda KH, Qiao H, et al. Development of a new mouse model of branch retinal vein occlusion and retinal neovascularization. Jpn J Ophthalmol. 51:251-257(2007)

[15] Pournaras CJ, Tsacopoulos M, Strommer K, et al. Experimental retinal branch vein occlusion in miniature pigs induces local tissue hypoxia and vasoproliferative microangiopathy. Ophthalmol. 97:1321-1328(1990)

[16] Hamilton AM, Kohner EM, Rosen D, et al. Experimental retinal branch vein occlusion in rhesus monkeys. I. Clinical appearances. Br J Ophthalmol. 63:377-387(1979)

[17] Minamikawa M, Yamamoto K, Okuma H, et al. [Experimental retinal branch vein occlusion]. Nippon Ganka Gakkai Zasshi. 93:691-697(1989)

[18] Chan CC, Green WR, Rice TA. Experimental occlusion of the retinal vein. Graefes Arch Clin Exp Ophthalmol. 224:507-512(1986)

[19] Matsumoto M. [Experimental study on earlier thrombogenic process in thrombin induced retinal venous obstruction in rabbit eye]. Nippon Ganka Gakkai Zasshi. 96:1132-1141(1992)

[20] Tamura M. Neovascularization in experimental retinal venous obstruction in rabbits. Jpn J Ophthalmol. 45:144-150(2001)

[21] Sakuraba T. [Experimental retinal vein obstruction induced by transadventitial administration of thrombin in the rabbit]. Nippon Ganka Gakkai Zasshi. 93:978-985(1989)

[22] Takei K, Sato T, Nonoyama T, et al. A new model of transient complete obstruction of retinal vessels induced by endothelin-1 injection into the posterior vitreous body in rabbits. Graefes Arch Clin Exp Ophthalmol. 231:476-481(1993)

[23] Sato T, Takei K, Nonoyama T, et al. [Endothelin-1-induced vasoconstriction in retinal blood vessels in the rabbit]. Nippon Ganka Gakkai Zasshi. 97:683-689(1993)
[24] Kohner EM, Dollery CT, Shakib M. Experimental retinal branch vein occlusion. Am J Ophthalmol. 69:7782−8251(1970)

23

Regulation of Angiogenesis in Choroidal Neovascularization of Age Related Macular Degeneration by Endogenous Angioinhibitors

Venugopal Gunda[1] and Yakkanti A. Sudhakar[1,2]
[1]*Cell Signaling, Retinal and Tumor Angiogenesis Laboratory, Department of Genetics, Boys Town National Research Hospital, Omaha, NE,*
[2]*Department of Biochemistry and Molecular Biology, University of Nebraska Medical Center, Omaha, NE, USA*

1. Introduction

The sense of vision has utmost significance and the loss of vision leads to the impairment of active human behavior as evident in pathological disorders that affect vision. Among different pathological visual disorders, Age Related Macular Degeneration (AMD/ARMD) is of serious concern as a leading cause of blindness, observed with aging globally. The clinical manifestation of AMD includes retinal damage with the degeneration of macula, leading to the partial or complete loss of acuity in vision. One form of pathologic AMD named, "wet form of AMD", involves the growth of new blood vessels from the choroid which lies underneath the retina, leading to the pathological blood vessel growth termed as Choroidal Neovascularization (CNV), with subsequent damage to the retina. Thus, choroidal neovascularization reflects a pathological angiogenic condition, where the loss of regulation over angiogenesis leads to the retinal damage. It also indicates that, the regulation of pathological angiogenesis can be an efficient strategy in preventing CNV of AMD. Though, some genetic disposition and aging factors are identified as peculiar etiological factors causing AMD; recent studies have shown that different cellular mechanisms regulating angiogenesis are common in different angiogenic scenarios including CNV. Further, the role of different endogenous angiogenesis inhibitors/angioinhibitors conferring the tissues with angiogenic regulation has been deciphered, which can be applied for regulation of CNV in AMD through inhibition of angiogenic signaling mechanisms. The present chapter provides an overview of the role of factors leading to choroidal neovascularization, the mechanisms underlying such angiogenesis and also the scope for endogenous angioinhibitors in regulation of CNV of AMD.

1.1 Retina and choroid

Retina is the inner most layer of the eye, which possesses anatomically ten distinct layers that are broadly categorized into two layers. The inner neural layer comprising of extensive nervous tissue towards the vitreous chamber and the outer retinal pigmented epithelium (RPE) adhering to the choroid. Some of the functions of the RPE include the phagocytosis of outer retinal segmental discs, maintenance of chorio-capillaries, fluid and electrolyte balance in subretinal space. Choroid is the highly vascular and pigmented tissue of the eye lying between the retina and the sclera. It consists of lamina suprachoroidea adhering to sclera, followed by lamina vesculosa, chorio-capillaries, stroma and Bruch membrane adhering to the RPE. Choroid is rich in vasculature and the extracellular matrix (ECM) components, including collagen and elastin fibers. It provides nutrient, metabolite and gaseous exchange to the retina by diffusion through chorio-capillaries.

1.2 Choroidal neovascularization in age related macular degeneration

The histological proximity between retinal pigmented epithelium and choroid confers not only physiological but also pathological effect on RPE. The mechanical barrier that separates the RPE from choroid is the Bruch membrane, which in turn consists of basement membrane secreted by RPE, inner collagenous layer, elastic layer, outer collagenous zone and the basement membrane of chorio-capillaries acting as a mechanical barrier for the underlying chorio-capillaries, but facilitating diffusion of metabolites and gaseous exchange for RPE. In cases of CNV the Bruch membrane is distorted with initial deposition of lipid and protienaceous component called 'drusen' followed by the growth and penetration of blood capillaries from choroid into Bruch membrane, finally leading to the leakage of fluid into sub-retinal spaces and retinal or retinal pigmented epithelial damage (Green, 1999; Green and Enger, 1993; Jager et al., 2008).

1.3 Factors for choroidal neovascularization in age related macular degeneration

Pathological neovascularization in CNV of AMD is considered to be contributed by both the angiogenesis and vasculogenesis, which are the processes of *de-novo* blood vessel formation (Chan-Ling et al., 2011; Jager et al., 2008). Angiogenesis is the process of formation of new blood vessels from the pre-existing ones, which involves the role of different cell types and remodeling of ECM. The inception of different cell types involved in the angiogenesis, such as, the endothelial cells (ECs) of RPE and choroid involved in CNV, mural cells and inflammatory cells occurs through vasculogenesis, by the differentiation of endothelial progenitor cells (EPCs). The EPCs found in the normal circulation are recruited into angiogenic sites, where they differentiate into different cell types leading to angiogenesis (Chan-Ling et al., 2011; Jager et al., 2008). However, the salient feature of neovascularization involves the common sequential events of angiogenesis including the proliferation of ECs, degradation of ECM or vascular basement membrane (VBM) by ECs through secretion of proteases, migration and differentiation of ECs into tip and stalk cells, lumen development, ECM reorganization and finally vessel anastomosing into functional capillaries (Carmeliet and Jain, 2000). These sequential steps of angiogenesis are considered to be common for CNV, which are initiated by the release of angiogenic factors by the RPE and other cell types differentiated from EPCs or infiltrating through the leaky capillaries in response to aging evoked stress (Alon et al., 1995; Grossniklaus et al., 2002). The initiating cellular and physiological factors that lead to the secretion of angiogenic factors by ECs and other cell types have been identified in different studies, which can be systematically framed for synergistic interpretation of etiological factors leading to CNV.

The normal function of phagocytosis and degradation of phagocytosed membranes is impaired with aging in RPE, leading to the accumulation of lipofuscin in these cells, with senescence (Marshall, 1987; Young and Bok, 1969). Ischemia and hypoxia evident in the ocular tissues of CNV are identified as factors promoting free radical generation in RPE and also the release of cellular lipids and proteinaceous deposits into the Bruch membrane (Spaide et al., 2003). Thus, impairing Bruch membrane's barrier function and in turn leading to the secretion of different angiogenic factors like vascular endothelial growth factor (VEGF), transforming growth factor-β (TGF- β), basic fibroblast growth factor (bFGF), insulin-like growth factor-1 and platelet derived growth factor (PDGF) by the RPE and the macrophages and stromal cells that are recruited by the differentiation of EPCs (Alon et al., 1995; Grossniklaus et al., 2002; Lu and Adamis, 2006; Penn et al., 2008; Young and Bok, 1969). Damage to the Bruch membrane is considered to enhance the diffusion of the growth factors, which elicit angiogenic signaling in the ECs (Lu and Adamis, 2006; Marshall, 1987; Penn et al., 2008).

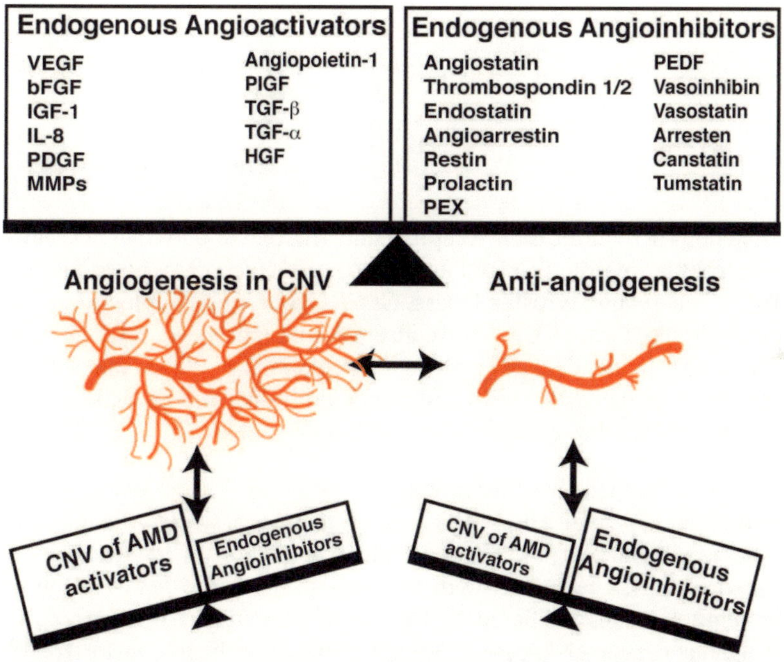

Fig. 1. **The angiogenic balance between endogenous angioactivators and angioinhibitors regulate vascular homeostasis.** Angiogenesis under physiological and pathological conditions is associated with up-regulation of endogenous angioactivators and/or down-regulation of endogenous angioinhibitors. Up-regulation of angioinhibitors and/or down-regulation of angioactivators may be associated with impaired neovascularization capacity in the choroidal neovascularization in age related macular degeneration (CNV of AMD). VEGF, vascular endothelial growth factor; bFGF, basic fibroblast growth factor; IGF-I, insulin-like growth factor-I; IL-8, interleukin-8; PDGF, platelet-derived growth factor; PlGF, placental growth factor; TGF-α and β, transforming growth factor-α and β;
HGF, Hepatocyte growth factor

Endogenous Angioactivators	Potent Receptors	Angiogenic action
Vascular endothelial growth factor (VEGF) & Placental growth factor (PlGF)	VEGFRs (Flt-1, Flk-1, KDR, Flt-4), Neuropilins, HSPG, integrins	Increases EC permeability, proliferation, migration, NO, uPA/PAI-1 & MMP production Inhibiting EC apoptosis, Promotes ECM degradation Monocyte migration
Transforming growth factor-β (TGF-α, −β)	Transforming growth factor receptors	Increased vessel stability and organization, promote secretion of ECM components
basic Fibroblast growth factor (bFGF)	FGFRs, HSPG, integrins	Promotes EC proliferation, migration, tube formation, ECM degradation, vessel maturation
Insulin-like growth factor-1 (IGF-1)	Insulin-like growth factor receptors	Promotes EC migration, proliferation, tube formation
Platelet derived growth factor (PDGF)	PDGF-α, −β, GPCRs, integrins	Increases EC permeability, proliferation, migration
Angiopoietin-1	Tie-2, integrins	EC sprouting, Vessel stabilization
Hepatocyte growth factor (HGF)	Hepatocyte growth factor receptor	Promotes tubulogenesis along with other factors
Interleukin-8 (IL-8)	C-X-C chemokine receptor type (CXCR-1,2)	Activates neovascularization increasing invasiveness of different cell types
Matrix metalloproteinases (MMPs)		Degradation of ECM components promoting EC migration and vessel organization, release of ECM or cell surface bound/sequestred angiogenic fcators

Table 1. Endogenous activators, their receptors and angiogenic activities (EC: endothelial cell, ECM: extracellular matrix, FGFRs: Fibroblast growth factor receptors, Flk-1: Fetal liver kinase-1, Flt-1, 4: fms-related tyrosine kinase, GPCRs: G-protein coupled receptors, HSPG: Heparan sulfate proteoglycan, KDR: kinase insert domain receptor, MMP: matrix metallo proteinase, NO: nitric oxide, Pak: p21 protein activated kinase, PDGF: platelet derived growth factor, Tie: tyrosine kinase with immunoglobulin-like and EGF-like domains, VEGFRs: vascular endothelial growth factor receptors)

The integrins and other ECM binding receptors present on ECs are essential in maintaining the ECM promoted survival and migration in angiogenesis (Avraamides et al., 2008; Mettouchi and Meneguzzi, 2006). The synergistic activation of integrins and other ECM binding receptors on ECs by the growth factors and cytokines leads to the activation of different signaling cascades mediated by the kinases, secondary messengers, transcription factors such as, nuclear factor kappa β (NF-κβ), hypoxia inducible factor-1α (HIF-1α), and other enzymes such as, inducible nitric oxide synthase (iNOS), cyclooxygenase-2 (COX-2) and metalloproteinases (MMPs) (Avraamides et al., 2008; Boosani et al., 2007; Egeblad and Werb, 2002; Mettouchi and Meneguzzi, 2006; Oklu et al., 2010). The transcription factors that are stabilized, up-regulated or expressed under hypoxia also lead to activation of different signaling cascades that promote effective survival and proliferation of ECs. The secretion of proteases such as matrix metallo-proteinases (MMPs) including collagenases and elastases, which degrade the collagen and elastin of vascular basement membrane (VBM) promote the migration of ECs. The urokinase is another proteinase, which binds to its receptors (urikanse binding receptor, uPAR) and activates signaling cascades leading to the secretion of MMPs, which promote migration of ECs and angiogenesis. The organization and differentiation of migrating ECs into tip and stalk cells is further enumerated to be regulated by Wingless type (Wnt)/Frizzled-Notch signaling that provides an insight about formation of functional capillaries in neovascular vessels (Dejana, 2010; Zerlin et al., 2008).

The inflammatory cells that are recruited through the expression of cytokines such as monocyte chemo-attractant protein-1 (Ccl2/MCP-1), Chemokine (C-X-C motif) liagnd 1 (CXCL1), macrophage inflammatory protein-1/-2 (MIP-1, MIP-2) are also considered to play role in CNV progression (Hendricks, 2006). Further, the intriguing stimulative role of Bruch membrane in promoting AMD is also being deciphered by identifying the complement components 3a and 5a (C3a and C5a), which lead to the up-regulation of VEGF-A (Nozaki et al., 2006). Thus, the orchestration of various signaling events at different stages of angiogenesis leads to the neovascularization. The angiogenic ECs lining the neovascular vessels arising due to the above factors in CNV are found to possess fenestrations and also organize into defective capillaries leading to the leakage of macromolecules as well as vascular cells into the Bruch membrane and sub-retinal spaces leading to the degeneration of macula of retina (Dvorak et al., 1995; Roberts and Palade, 1995).

2. Endogenous angioinhibitors

In addition to the angiogenic factors, which activate angiogenesis, tissues and ECM also possess angioinhibitors, which have the potency to inhibit the angiogenesis and thus, regulating the pathological angiogenesis by inhibiting the signaling mechanisms activated by angiogenic factors (Boosani et al., 2010; Sudhakar and Kalluri, 2010, Zhang and Ma, 2007). Nearly, 40 endogenous angioinhibitors have been characterized and some of them are found in the ocular tissues or secreted into vasculature and released into ocular tissues, where they exhibit angio-inhibition and finally regulation of CNV (Boosani et al., 2011; Sudhakar and Kalluri, 2010). The significance of imbalance in the levels of endogenous angioinhibitors and angioactivators in regulation of vascular homeostasis can be summarized as in Figure 1. This significance was also ascertained by the evaluations showing the correlation between the decrease in specific angioinhibitors and the progression of CNV (Bhutto et al., 2008).

2.1 Mechanisms of regulation of CNV by endogenous angioinhibitors

2.1.1 Vasoinhibins

The vasoinhibins (14-18 kDa) are antiangiogenic peptides found in the pituitary, retina and extrapituitary tissues. They constitute the amino terminal regions of three different precursors; prolactin, growth hormone and placental lactogen. Though their precursors do not exhibit angioinhibitory activities; vasoinhibins found in the tissues or those expressed using recombinant methods exhibit antiangiogenic properties (Clapp et al., 2008). The therapeutic potential of vasoinhibins in regulating angiogenesis in CNV and tumor growth was evaluated and studies indicate that adenovirus mediated expression of vasoinhibins inhibits CNV, *in-vivo* and also angiogenesis (Zhou et al., 2010). Mechanisms of regulation of EC survival, proliferation and migration by the vasoinhibins have been deciphered in different studies; nevertheless, the receptors through which the mechanisms are mediated still remain enigmatic. Vasoinhibins regulate the EC migration and survival through inhibition of VEGF and bFGF stimulated MAPK activation (D'Angelo et al., 1995).

Endogenous Angioinhibitor	Parent molecule	Receptors	Mode of action/ Inhibition pathways
Vasoinhibins	Prolactin, growth hormone	Not known	Sos/Ras/MAPK or eNOS /Raf/MAPK, Ca2+/ eNOS/protein phosphatase 2, Ras/Tiam-1/Rac1/Pak1, Bcl-XL, NF-kβ, caspases
PEDF	PEDF	Not known	Possible apoptosis
Arresten	Collagen IV, α1 NC1	α1β1 integrin, HSPG	Raf/MEK/ERK1/2/p38-MAPK, HIF-1α, MMPs
Canstatin	Collagen IV, α2 NC1	αVβ3, αVβ5 integrins, Fas	procaspse-8 and -9, Akt/ FAK/mToR, eIF-4EBP-1, Ribosomal S6-kinase
Tumstatin	Collagen IV, α3NC1	CD47/IAP, αVβ3, α6β1 integrins	FAK/Akt/PI3K/mTOR/ eIF-4EBP1/NFκB, COX-2 signaling
Endostatin	Collagen XVIII-NC1	αVβ1/α5β1 integrins, HSP, glypican, caveolin-1	Ras/Raf/KDR/Flk-1 / ERK/p38-MAPK/p125 FAK/HIF1α/Ephrin/TNFα/NFκB, Wnt signaling
Angiostatin	Plasminogen	ATP synthases, αVβ3 integrin, angiomotin	αVβ3 integrin mediated apoptotis, ATP synthase
Thrombospondins	TSP	CD36, IAP, CD47, HSPG, α3β1 , other integrins	Src-family kinases/ Caspase-3/p38 MAPK, TGF-β signaling
Endorepellin	Perlecan	α2β1 integrins, lipid rafts, caveolin	cAMP-PKA/FAK/p38-MAPK/Hsp27, SHP-1, Ca2+ signaling

Table 2. Endogenous angioinhibitors, their precursors, cell surface receptors and mode of action AMD/ARMD: Age related macular degeneration, Akt: protein kinase B, Bcl-XL: B-cell lymphoma-extra large, bFGF: basic fibroblast growth factor, Ccl2/MCP-1: chemoattractant protein-1, CD(CD47, CD36): cluster of differentiation, CNV: choroidal neovascularization, COX-2: cyclooxygenase-2, eIF-4EBP-1: eukaryotic translation initiation factor-4E binding protein-1, eNOS: endothelial nitric oxide synthase, ECs: endothelial cells, ECM: extracellular matrix, EPCs: endothelail progenitor cells, ERK1/2: extracellular signal-regulated kinase1/2, FAK: focal adhesion kinase, Flk-1: fetal liver kinase-1, HIF-1α: hypoxia inducible factor-1α, Hsp: heat shock protein, HSPG: Heparan sulfate proteoglycan, IAP: integrin associated protein, KDR: kinase insert domain receptor, MAPK: Mitogen activated protein kinase, MEK: MAPK-ERK kinase, MMPs: matrix metallo proteinases, mToR: mammalian target of rapamycin, NF-kβ: nuclear factor kappa β, Pak: p21 protein activated kinase, PDGF: platelet derived growth factor, PEDF: Pigment epithelium derived factor, PEX: noncatalytic Carboxy-terminal hemopexin-like domain of MMP, PI3K: phosphatidyl inositol 3-kinase, Rac: Ras-related C3 botulinin toxin susbtrate 1, Raf: Ras activated factor, Ras: Rat sarcoma, RPE: retinal pigmented epithelium, SHP: Src homology region 2 domain-conatining phopshatase, Sos: Son of sevenless, Src: Schmidt-Ruppin A-2 sarcoma viral oncogene homolog, Tiam: T-lymphoma invasion and metastasis-inducing protein, TGF-β: transforming growth factor β, TNFα: tumor necrosis factorα, TSP: thrombospondin, VBM: vascular basement membrane, VEGF: vascular endothelial growth factor, Wnt: wingless-type

VEGF activated Sos/Ras/MAPK or eNOS/Raf/MAPK-mediated proliferative signaling and Ca2+/eNOS/protein phosphatase-2 mediated vascular permeability and vasodilatation were shown to be inhibited by the vasoinhibins (Gonzalez et al., 2004; Ziche and Morbidelli, 2000). In addition vasoinhibins also inhibit the migration of EC stimulated by IL-1β through Ras/Tiam-1/Rac-1/Pak1 and promote apoptosis through conversion of Bcl-XL to proapoptoctic Bcl-Xs and NF-kβ mediated activation of initiator and effector caspases (Martini et al., 2000; Tabruyn et al., 2003).

2.1.2 Pigment Epithelium Derived Factor (PEDF)

Pigment epithelium derived factor (PEDF) is a 50 kDa, secreted, serpin family glycoprotein, first identified from the cultured fetal RPE conditioned media (Tombran-Tink et al., 1991). PEDF accumulates in the vitreous humor and is also expressed in different adult tissues (Tombran-Tink et al., 1991). Addition of PEDF to the cultured HUVECs increased the number of TUNEL positive cells suggesting apoptotic mode of action of PEDF and thus, possibly preventing EC response to ischemia *in-vivo* (Ho et al., 2007). The levels of PEDF were found to be decreased in Bruch membrane with progression of AMD and concomitant increase in VEGF levels were also identified with decrease in PEDF levels (Bhutto et al., 2008). Different methods of PEDF upregulation have been applied to investigate the effect of PEDF on CNV. Intravitreous injections of adenovirus expressing the PEDF and ultrasound-microbubble technique of noninvasive gene transfer of PEDF gene in rats exhibited significant decrease in the CNV (Gehlbach et al., 2003; Zhou et al., 2009). However, studies also demonstrate that PEDF at lower doses (90µg/ml) has negative effect on CNV whereas; higher doses (2-4 fold) can augment CNV; thus, indicating a strategic approach to be developed during clinical trials for CNV treatment with PEDF (Apte et al., 2004).

2.1.3 Angiostatin

Angiostatins are 38-45 kDa kringle domains derived by the protease activity of parent molecule plasminogen, which itself has significant role in activation of fibrinogen and blood clotting (Hayashi et al., 2008). Some of the angiostatin peptide derivates exhibit anti-angiogenic properties including inhibition of EC proliferation, tube formation and migration. The application of angiostatins in regulating CNV of AMD was evaluated by the expression of the angiostatins *in-vivo*, using viral vectors (Lai et al., 2001). Angiostatins bind to ATP synthases on the surface of ECs leading to their apoptotic death (Burwick et al., 2005; Tarui et al., 2001). Further αVβ3 integrin and angiomotin are also shown to bind angiostatin and induce apoptosis (Burwick et al., 2005; Tarui et al., 2001).

2.1.4 Thrombospondins

Thrombospondins (TSPs) are secreted ECM glycoproteins playing key role in the cellular and ECM interactions (Bornstein, 2001; Lawler, 2000). The NH2-terminal peptides derived from the TSPs, by the action of different proteases are identified to possess angioinhibitory properties. TSP-1 and TSP-2 are trimeric globular domain subunits (145 kDa) categorized into subgroup-A and subgroup-B consists of TSP's 3-5, which are pentameric subunits (110 kDa) (Bornstein, 2009). TSP-1 was the first identified ECM derived endogenous angioinhibitor from many normal tissues and produced by a variety of cells including platelets, megakaryocytes, epithelial, endothelial and stromal cells (Bornstein, 2009). TSP-1 is secreted by the retinal-pigmented epithelium (RPE) and regulates angiogenesis in normal eye (Miyajima-Uchida et al., 2000). Immunolocalization studies showed decrease in the levels of TSP in the chorio-capillaries and the Bruch membrane of AMD samples (Bhutto et al., 2008). Wispostatin-1 (WISP-1) repeat derived peptide from TSP-1 was shown to inhibit the CNV in LASER induced CNV mice models (Cano Mdel et al., 2009). TSP-1 induces apoptosis in ECs through CD36 and integrin associated protein (IAP)/Src-family protein kinases/Caspase-3/p38 MAPK signaling (Dawson et al., 1997). In addition TSP-1 can also bind to different integrins, including CD47 and heparin sulfated proteoglycans (Kaur et al., 2011). Thus the significance of TSPs in regulation of CNV have been evaluated through detection of endogenous levels in pathological tissues and also by evaluating the effects of TSPs both *in vitro* and *in vivo.*

2.1.5 Arresten

Arresten [α1(IV)NC1], is the 26 kDa collagen type IV, α1 chain derived non-collagenous domain, which functions via binding to $\alpha 1\beta 1$ integrin and heparan sulfate proteolgycans, regulating bFGF and VEGF stimulated activation of ECs (Boosani and Sudhakar, 2006; Colorado et al., 2000; Sudhakar et al., 2005). It inhibits the survival of mouse lung endothelial cells through inhibition of FAK phopshorylation in AKT independent manner (Sudhakar et al., 2005). FAK inhibition by arresten via $\alpha 1\beta 1$ integrin leads to inhibition of downstream Raf/MEK/ERK1/2/p38 MAPK signaling and HIF-1α expression **(Figure 2)**. Inhibition of HIF-1α by arresten is critical in preventing hypoxic survival of ECs through VEGF regulation (Sudhakar et al., 2005). Arresten inhibited VEGF-mediated angiogenesis by promoting apoptosis, caspase-3/PARP activation and negatively impacting FAK/p38-MAPK phosphorylation, Bcl-2 and Bcl-x_L expressions leading to mouse retinal endothelial cell (MREC) death (Boosani et al., 2009). In addition angioinhibitory activity of arresten was found to inhibit bFGF induced proliferation of MREC *in-vitro* in a dose dependent manner. It also inhibited the bFGF-induced migration of MREC mediated by MMP-2 activity but not the expression levels of MMP-2 (Boosani et al., 2010). Thus, arresten was shown to effect the proliferation and migration of choroidal endothelial cells and regulate CNV of AMD. The endothelial specific inhibitory actions of arresten may be of benefit in the treatment of a variety of eye diseases with a neovascular component.

2.1.6 Canstatin

It is the 24 kDa collagen type IV, α2 derived non-collagenous domain [α2(IV)NC1], which binds to the $\alpha V\beta 3$ and $\alpha V\beta 5$ integrins and inhibits EC proliferation, migration and tube formation by enhancing apoptosis in these cells (Magnon et al., 2005; Magnon et al., 2007; Petitclerc et al., 2000; Roth et al., 2005). The antiangiogenic efficacy of canstatin in regulating the neovascularization of cornea was also evaluated using the recombinant canstatin in alkali burn induced neovascularization study (Lima et al., 2006; Wang et al., 2011). Cantstain was shown to induce apoptosis through the induction of Fas-ligand, activation of procaspse-8 and -9 cleavage, reduction in membrane potential, inhibition of Akt, FAK, mToR, eIF-4E/4E-BP1 and ribosomal S6-kinase phosphorylations, in cultured HUVECs **(Figure 2)** (Panka and Mier, 2003).

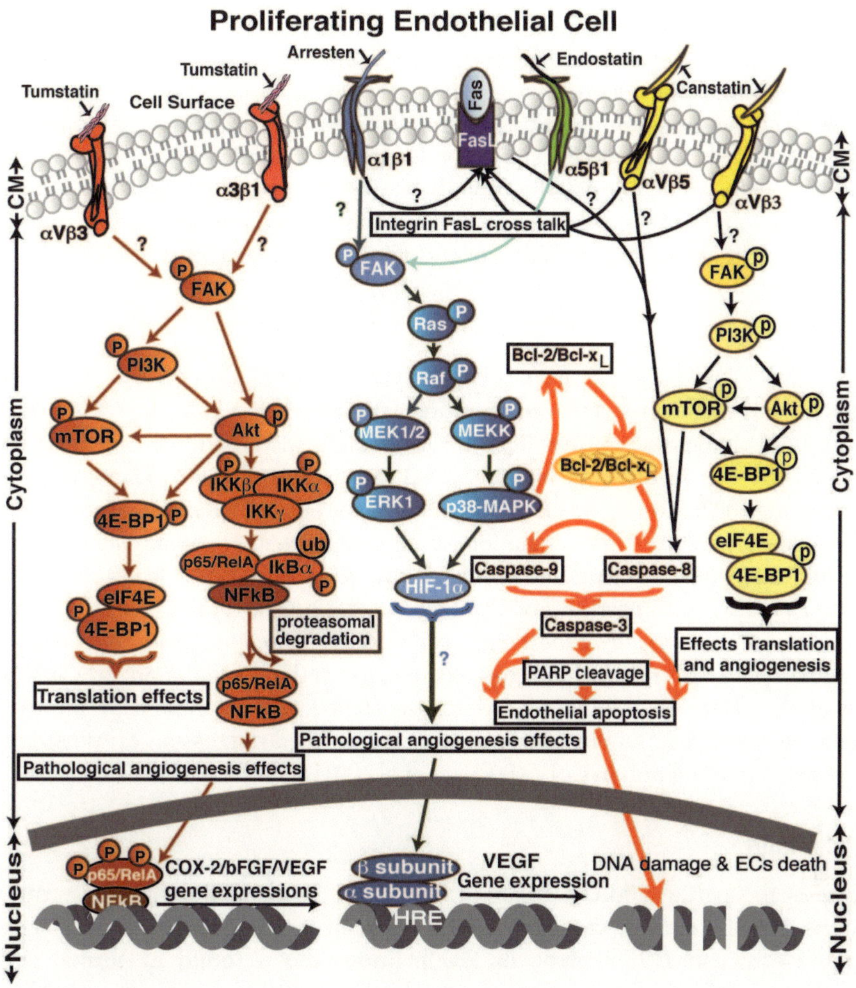

Fig. 2. **Schematic illustration of distinct angioinhibitory signaling mediated by different extracellular matrix (ECM) reloaded molecules.** Tumstatin, arresten, canstatin and endostatin interact with $\alpha V\beta 3/\alpha 3\beta 1$, $\alpha 1\beta 1$, $\alpha V\beta 3/\alpha V\beta 5$ and $\alpha 5\beta 1$ integrins respectively, to inhibit the phosphorylation of focal adhesion kinase (FAK). Tumstatin: It binds to $\alpha V\beta 3$ and $\alpha 3\beta 1$ integrins and inhibits the pathway that includes phosphorylation of FAK, PI3-K, Akt, mTOR, 4E-BP1 and eIF4E to decrease endothelial cell protein synthesis and proliferation. In addition tumstatin also inhibits NFκB mediated signaling in hypoxic conditions leading to the inhibition of COX-2, VEGF and bFGF expressions, resulting in inhibition of hypoxic tumor angiogenesis. Arresten: It binds to $\alpha 1\beta 1$ integrin and inhibit phosphorylation FAK, causes inhibition of Ras, Raf, extra cellular signal related kinase 1 (ERK1) and p38 MAPK pathways that leads to inhibition of HIF-1α and VEGF expression resulting in inhibition of endothelial cell migration, proliferation and tube formation. In addition arresten initiates two apoptotic pathways, involving activation of caspase-9 and -8, leading to activation of caspase-3 and PARP cleavage. (a) Arresten activates caspase-3 directly through inhibition of FAK/p38-MAPK/Bcl-2/Bcl-x_L and activation of caspase-9; (b) Integrin $\alpha 1\beta 1$ cross talk with Fas-L through mitochondrial pathway and leads to activation of caspase-8 and-3 in

proliferating endothelial cells. Canstatin: It binds to αVβ3/αVβ5 integrins and inhibits two apoptotic pathways, involving activation of caspase-8 and casoase-9, leading to activation of caspase-3. Canstatin activates procaspase-9 not only through inhibition of the FAK/PI3K/AKT pathways but also by integrins cross talking mitochondrial pathway through Fas-L dependent caspase-8 activation leads to endothelial cell apoptosis. CM represents cell membrane. Endostatin: It binds to α5β1 integrin and inhibit phosphorylation FAK, causes inhibition of Ras, Raf, extra cellular signal related kinase-1 (ERK1) and p38 MAPK pathways that leads to inhibition of endothelial cell migration and tube formation.

2.1.7 Tumstatin

Tumstatin [α3(IV)NC1], is a 28 kDa collagen type IV, α3 chain derived non-collagenous domain with anti-angiogenic and proapoptotic activities. It binds to the CD47/IAP, αVβ3, α3β1 and α6β1 integrins and inhibits the signaling cascade mediated by FAK, Akt, PI3K/mTOR/eIF-4E/4E-BP1 and NFκB/COX-2 (Boosani et al., 2007; Hamano et al., 2003; Maeshima et al., 2002; Monboisse et al., 1994; Sudhakar et al., 2003). Inhibition of eIF-4E/4E-BP1 by tumstatin leads to the regulation of cap dependent translational level of genes, whereas inhibition of transcriptional factor signaling such as NFκB leads to regulation of genes such as COX-2 at transcriptional level (Figure 2) (Boosani et al., 2007). Thus, tumstatin exhibits gene regulation in endothelail cell-specific and integrin-dependent manner. Angioinhibitory effect of tumstatin has been evaluated in regulation of CNV in mice (Boosani et al., 2011). Recombinant tumstatin regulated tube formation by mouse corneal endothelial cells (MCECs) *in-vitro* and adenoviral mediated expression of tumstatin *in-vivo* in mice has shown reduction in CNV (Boosani et al., 2011; Gunda et al., 2011).

2.1.8 Endostatin

Endostatin is the partial 20-kDa fragment of collagen type XVIII, carboxy terminal non-collagenous domain, derived from the parent collagen by proteolytic cleavage activities of elastase and cathepsin-L (Felbor et al., 2000). Endostatin is found in normal circulation enabling it to be utilized as an effective angioinhibitor without toxic effects (Fukai et al., 2002). Lower levels of endostatin have been recorded in CNV samples compared to the healthy donor eyes and within the tissues of progressive AMD (Bhutto et al., 2008; Fukai et al., 2002). Deletion of endostatin or collagen type XVIII massively up-regulates LASER induced CNV; where as administration of physiological concentrations of endostatin was able to inhibit such CNV in these mice (Marneros et al., 2007). Endostatin also down regulates the expression of VEGF in experimental CNV rat models (Takahashi et al., 2003). These observations along with the evidence of inhibition of CNV with intravenous injection of adenoviral vectors that express secretable endostatin, confirm the significance of endostatin in regulation of CNV (Mori et al., 2001; Wickstrom et al., 2003).

Endostatin elicits the anti-proliferative and anti-migratory effects by binding to different EC surface molecules and regulating the signaling cascades (Faye et al., 2009). Recombinant endostatin binds to αV integrin as shown in human endothelial cells (Rehn et al., 2001). Further studies have also shown localization of endostatin in the lipid rafts and association with caveolae (Wickstrom et al., 2002; Wickstrom et al., 2003). Surface plasmon resonance assays characterized the binding of endostatin to both αVβ1 integrins and the heparin sulfates and also localization to the lipid rafts (Ricard-Blum et al., 2004). *In-vitro* assays using ECs also showed the co-localization of endostatin with $\alpha5\beta1$ integrin, actin stress fibers, membrane anchor protein and caveolin-1, which enumerates the interaction of endostatin with caveolae, inhibiting EC migration through the disassembly of actin stress fibers/focal adhesions, activation of Src and impaired fibronectin deposition by ECs in response to bFGF (Wickstrom et al., 2002; Wickstrom et al., 2003; Sudhakar et al., 2003). Binding of endostatin with integrins also down-regulates the activity of RhoA-GTPase and inhibits signaling pathways mediated by small kinases of the Ras and Raf families (Ricard-Blum et al., 2004). In addition, binding to the KDR/Flk-1, endostatin inhibits the VEGF-induced tyrosine phosphorylation of KDR/Flk-1 and activation of ERK, p38 MAPK, and p125FAK in HUVECs (Kim et al., 2002; Sudhakar et al., 2003). Further signaling cascades regulated by the endostatin are being identified, which are mediated by activator protein 1 (Id), HIF1α, ephrin, tumor necrosis factor-α (TNFα), nuclear factor-κB (NFκB), coagulation cascades, adhesion molecules and Wnt, which indicate the potential role of endostatin as an endogenous angioinhibitor (Nyberg et al., 2005) **(Figure 2).**

2.2 Scope for endogenous angioinhibitors in CNV treatment

Current modalities of treatment for the CNV in AMD include the regulation of angiogenesis as angiogenesis being one of the pathological factors of neovascularization. The therapies such as LASER photocoagulation, photodynamic therapy and anti-VEGF therapies using Macugen or Lucentis, that are currently being applied to regulate the CNV have their own constraints such as development of lesions, loss of acuity in vision and frequent administration, respectively (Gallemore and Boyer, 2006). Alternative strategies for the treatment of CNV in AMD are therefore being developed in which the specific targeting on angiogenesis can be possible. Endogenous angioinhibitors are considered as one of the area to be explored in this arena to include them in regimens of complementary treatments for the regulation of CNV (Chappelow and Kaiser, 2008; Do, 2009). The signaling cascades regulated by some of endogenous angioinhibitors have been identified **(Table 2 and Figure 2),** which enabled the application of those inhibitors in CNV.

3. Conclusions

The cellular, extracellular milieu and genetic factors responsible for the neovascularization arising in AMD are being deciphered with emphasis on identifying those factors that play a key role in the inception and progression of CNV. In this scenario, different etiological factors have been identified which regulate angiogenesis, effecting both extracellular milieu and intracellular angiogenic signaling pathways. Identification of the signaling cascades leading to the pathological angiogenesis in CNV has further lead to the possibility of regulating CNV, by focusing on signaling pathways as one of the targets. Application of endogenous angioinhibitors has proven as a promising strategy in this scenario of inhibiting angiogeneic pathways that are identified in CNV. The inhibitors such as vasoinhibins, PEDF, angiostatin, endostatin, tumstatin, canstatin and arresten that have been so far evaluated for regulation of CNV have not only shown promising evidence of CNV regulation, but also provided new strategies for inhibiting CNV through differential mode of actions. Such variation exhibited by different endogenous angioinhibitors can be beneficial in targeting CNV using different combinations of these inhibitors. It can be realized that these naturally occurring inhibitors can pose low immune reactions and thus, an efficient way of regulating diseases. Further, clinical studies using individual and combinations of endogenous angioinhibitors, included in different regimens along with current therapies of CNV would elaborate the application of endogenous angioinhibitors for regulating CNV of AMD.

4. Acknowledgements

This study was supported by Flight Attendant Medical Research Institute Young Clinical Scientist Award Grant FAMRI-062558, NIH/NCI Grant RO1CA143128, Dobleman Head and Neck Cancer Institute Grant DHNCI-61905 and startup research funds of Cell Signaling, Retinal and Tumor Angiogenesis Laboratory at Boys Town National Research Hospital to YAS.

5. References

Alon, T., Hemo, I., Itin, A., Pe'er, J., Stone, J., and Keshet, E. (1995). Vascular endothelial growth factor acts as a survival factor for newly formed retinal vessels and has implications for retinopathy of prematurity. Nat Med *1*, 1024-1028.

Apte, R. S., Barreiro, R. A., Duh, E., Volpert, O., and Ferguson, T. A. (2004). Stimulation of neovascularization by the anti-angiogenic factor PEDF. Invest Ophthalmol Vis Sci *45*, 4491-4497.

Avraamides, C. J., Garmy-Susini, B., and Varner, J. A. (2008). Integrins in angiogenesis and lymphangiogenesis. Nat Rev Cancer *8*, 604-617.

Bhutto, I. A., Uno, K., Merges, C., Zhang, L., McLeod, D. S., and Lutty, G. A. (2008). Reduction of endogenous angiogenesis inhibitors in Bruch's membrane of the submacular region in eyes with age-related macular degeneration. Arch Ophthalmol *126*, 670-678.

Boosani, C. S., Gunda, V., Wang, S., Sheibani, N., and Sudhakar, A. Y. (2011). Tumstatin inhibits Choroidal Neovascularisation by Inhibiting MMP-2 activation *in-vitro* and *in-vivo.* Mol Vision. (Publication ahead of print).

Boosani, C. S., Mannam, A. P., Cosgrove, D., Silva, R., Hodivala-Dilke, K. M., Keshamouni, V. G., and Sudhakar, A. (2007). Regulation of COX-2 mediated signaling by alpha3 type IV noncollagenous domain in tumor angiogenesis. Blood *110*, 1168-1177.

Boosani, C.S., Nalabothula, N., Munugalvadla, V., Cosgrove, D., Keshamouni, V. G., Sheibani, N., and Sudhakar, A. (2009). FAK and p38-MAP kinase-dependent activation of apoptosis and caspase-3 in retinal endothelial cells by α1(IV)NC1. *Invest. Ophthalmol. Vis. Sci. 50*, 4567-4575.

Boosani, C. S., Nalabothula, N., Sheibani, N., and Sudhakar, A. (2010). Inhibitory effects of arresten on bFGF-induced proliferation, migration, and matrix metalloproteinase-2 activation in mouse retinal endothelial cells. Curr Eye Res *35*, 45-55.

Boosani, C. S., and Sudhakar, A. (2006). Cloning, purification, and characterization of a non-collagenous anti-angiogenic protein domain from human alpha1 type IV collagen expressed in Sf9 cells. Protein Expr Purif *49*, 211-218.

Bornstein, P. (2001). Thrombospondins as matricellular modulators of cell function. J Clin Invest *107*, 929-934.

Bornstein, P. (2009). Thrombospondins function as regulators of angiogenesis. J Cell Commun Signal *3*, 189-200.

Burwick, N. R., Wahl, M. L., Fang, J., Zhong, Z., Moser, T. L., Li, B., Capaldi, R. A., Kenan, D. J., and Pizzo, S. V. (2005). An Inhibitor of the F1 subunit of ATP synthase (IF1) modulates the activity of angiostatin on the endothelial cell surface. J Biol Chem *280*, 1740-1745.

Cano Mdel, V., Karagiannis, E. D., Soliman, M., Bakir, B., Zhuang, W., Popel, A. S., and Gehlbach, P. L. (2009). A peptide derived from type 1 thrombospondin repeat-containing protein WISP-1 inhibits corneal and choroidal neovascularization. Invest Ophthalmol Vis Sci *50*, 3840-3845.

Carmeliet, P., and Jain, R. K. (2000). Angiogenesis in cancer and other diseases. Nature *407*, 249-257.

Chan-Ling, T., Dahlstrom, J. E., Koina, M. E., McColm, J. R., Sterling, R. A., Bean, E. G., Adamson, S., Hughes, S., and Baxter, L. C. (2011). Evidence of hematopoietic differentiation, vasculogenesis and angiogenesis in the formation of human choroidal blood vessels. Exp Eye Res *92*, 361-376.

Chappelow, A. V., and Kaiser, P. K. (2008). Neovascular age-related macular degeneration: potential therapies. Drugs *68*, 1029-1036.

Clapp, C., Thebault, S., Arnold, E., Garcia, C., Rivera, J. C., and de la Escalera, G. M. (2008). Vasoinhibins: novel inhibitors of ocular angiogenesis. Am J Physiol Endocrinol Metab *295*, E772-778.

Colorado, P. C., Torre, A., Kamphaus, G., Maeshima, Y., Hopfer, H., Takahashi, K., Volk, R., Zamborsky, E. D., Herman, S., Sarkar, P. K., Ericksen, M. B., Dhanabal, M., Simons, M., Post, M., Kufe, D. W., Weichselbaum, R. R., Sukhatme, V. P., and Kalluri, R. (2000). Anti-angiogenic cues from vascular basement membrane collagen. Cancer Res *60*, 2520-2526.

D'Angelo, G., Struman, I., Martial, J., and Weiner, R. I. (1995). Activation of mitogen-activated protein kinases by vascular endothelial growth factor and basic fibroblast growth factor in capillary endothelial cells is inhibited by the antiangiogenic factor 16-kDa N-terminal fragment of prolactin. Proc Natl Acad Sci U S A *92*, 6374-6378.

Dawson, D. W., Pearce, S. F., Zhong, R., Silverstein, R. L., Frazier, W. A., and Bouck, N. P. (1997). CD36 mediates the In vitro inhibitory effects of thrombospondin-1 on endothelial cells. J Cell Biol *138*, 707-717.

Dejana, E. (2010). The role of wnt signaling in physiological and pathological angiogenesis. Circ Res *107*, 943-952.

Do, D. V. (2009). Antiangiogenic approaches to age-related macular degeneration in the future. Ophthalmology *116*, S24-26.

Dvorak, H. F., Brown, L. F., Detmar, M., and Dvorak, A. M. (1995). Vascular permeability factor/vascular endothelial growth factor, microvascular hyperpermeability, and angiogenesis. Am J Pathol *146*, 1029-1039.

Egeblad, M., and Werb, Z. (2002). New functions for the matrix metalloproteinases in cancer progression. Nat Rev Cancer *2*, 161-174.

Faye, C., Moreau, C., Chautard, E., Jetne, R., Fukai, N., Ruggiero, F., Humphries, M. J., Olsen, B. R., and Ricard-Blum, S. (2009). Molecular interplay between endostatin, integrins, and heparan sulfate. J Biol Chem *284*, 22029-22040.

Felbor, U., Dreier, L., Bryant, R. A., Ploegh, H. L., Olsen, B. R., and Mothes, W. (2000). Secreted cathepsin L generates endostatin from collagen XVIII. EMBO J *19*, 1187-1194.

Fukai, N., Eklund, L., Marneros, A. G., Oh, S. P., Keene, D. R., Tamarkin, L., Niemela, M., Ilves, M., Li, E., Pihlajaniemi, T., and Olsen, B. R. (2002). Lack of collagen XVIII/endostatin results in eye abnormalities. EMBO J *21*, 1535-1544.

Gallemore, P. R., and Boyer, D. S. (2006). PDT or Anti-VEGF for AMD treatment. Review of Ophthalmology online.

Gehlbach, P., Demetriades, A. M., Yamamoto, S., Deering, T., Duh, E. J., Yang, H. S., Cingolani, C., Lai, H., Wei, L., and Campochiaro, P. A. (2003). Periocular injection of an adenoviral vector encoding pigment epithelium-derived factor inhibits choroidal neovascularization. Gene Ther *10*, 637-646.

Gonzalez, C., Corbacho, A. M., Eiserich, J. P., Garcia, C., Lopez-Barrera, F., Morales-Tlalpan, V., Barajas-Espinosa, A., Diaz-Munoz, M., Rubio, R., Lin, S. H., Martinez de la Escalera, G., and Clapp, C. (2004). 16K-prolactin inhibits activation of endothelial nitric oxide synthase, intracellular calcium mobilization, and endothelium-dependent vasorelaxation. Endocrinology *145*, 5714-5722.

Green, W. R. (1999). Histopathology of age-related macular degeneration. Mol Vis *5*, 27.

Green, W. R., and Enger, C. (1993). Age-related macular degeneration histopathologic studies. The 1992 Lorenz E. Zimmerman Lecture. Ophthalmology *100*, 1519-1535.

Grossniklaus, H. E., Ling, J. X., Wallace, T. M., Dithmar, S., Lawson, D. H., Cohen, C., Elner, V. M., Elner, S. G., and Sternberg, P., Jr. (2002). Macrophage and retinal pigment epithelium expression of angiogenic cytokines in choroidal neovascularization. Mol Vis *8*, 119-126.

Gunda, V., Wang, S., Sheibani, N., and Sudhakar, A. (2011). Inhibitory effect of tumstatin on corneal neovascularization both in-vitro and in-vivo. J Clinic Experment Ophthalmol (publication ahead of time).

Hamano, Y., Zeisberg, M., Sugimoto, H., Lively, J. C., Maeshima, Y., Yang, C., Hynes, R. O., Werb, Z., Sudhakar, A., and Kalluri, R. (2003). Physiological levels of tumstatin, a fragment of collagen IV alpha3 chain, are generated by MMP-9 proteolysis and suppress angiogenesis via alphaV beta3 integrin. Cancer Cell *3*, 589-601.

Hayashi, M., Tamura, Y., Dohmae, N., Kojima, S., and Shimonaka, M. (2008). Plasminogen N-terminal activation peptide modulates the activity of angiostatin-related peptides on endothelial cell proliferation and migration. Biochem Biophys Res Commun *369*, 635-640.

Hendricks, R. L. (2006). Interaction of angiogenic and immune mechanisms in the eye. Semin Ophthalmol *21*, 37-40.

Ho, T. C., Chen, S. L., Yang, Y. C., Liao, C. L., Cheng, H. C., and Tsao, Y. P. (2007). PEDF induces p53-mediated apoptosis through PPAR gamma signaling in human umbilical vein endothelial cells. Cardiovasc Res *76*, 213-223.

Jager, R. D., Mieler, W. F., and Miller, J. W. (2008). Age-related macular degeneration. N Engl J Med *358*, 2606-2617.

Kaur, S., Kuznetsova, S. A., Pendrak, M. L., Sipes, J. M., Romeo, M. J., Li, Z., Zhang, L., and Roberts, D. D. (2011). Heparan sulfate modification of the transmembrane receptor CD47 is necessary for inhibition of T cell receptor signaling by thrombospondin-1. J Biol Chem *286*, 14991-15002.

Kim, Y. M., Hwang, S., Pyun, B. J., Kim, T. Y., Lee, S. T., Gho, Y. S., and Kwon, Y. G. (2002). Endostatin blocks vascular endothelial growth factor-mediated signaling via direct interaction with KDR/Flk-1. J Biol Chem *277*, 27872-27879.

Lai, C. C., Wu, W. C., Chen, S. L., Xiao, X., Tsai, T. C., Huan, S. J., Chen, T. L., Tsai, R. J., and Tsao, Y. P. (2001). Suppression of choroidal neovascularization by adeno-associated virus vector expressing angiostatin. Invest Ophthalmol Vis Sci *42*, 2401-2407.

Lawler, J. (2000). The functions of thrombospondin-1 and-2. Curr Opin Cell Biol *12*, 634-640.

Lima, E. S. R., Kachi, S., Akiyama, H., Shen, J., Aslam, S., Yuan Gong, Y., Khu, N. H., Hatara, M. C., Boutaud, A., Peterson, R., and Campochiaro, P. A. (2006). Recombinant non-collagenous domain of alpha2(IV) collagen causes involution of choroidal neovascularization by inducing apoptosis. J Cell Physiol *208*, 161-166.

Lu, M., and Adamis, A. P. (2006). Molecular biology of choroidal neovascularization. Ophthalmol Clin North Am *19*, 323-334.

Maeshima, Y., Colorado, P. C., Torre, A., Holthaus, K. A., Grunkemeyer, J. A., Ericksen, M. B., Hopfer, H., Xiao, Y., Stillman, I. E., and Kalluri, R. (2000). Distinct antitumor properties of a type IV collagen domain derived from basement membrane. J Biol Chem *275*, 21340-21348.

Maeshima, Y., Sudhakar, A., Lively, J. C., Ueki, K., Kharbanda, S., Kahn, C. R., Sonenberg, N., Hynes, R. O., and Kalluri, R. (2002). Tumstatin, an endothelial cell-specific inhibitor of protein synthesis. Science *295*, 140-143.

Magnon, C., Galaup, A., Mullan, B., Rouffiac, V., Bouquet, C., Bidart, J. M., Griscelli, F., Opolon, P., and Perricaudet, M. (2005). Canstatin acts on endothelial and tumor cells via mitochondrial damage initiated through interaction with alphavbeta3 and alphavbeta5 integrins. Cancer Res *65*, 4353-4361.

Magnon, C., Opolon, P., Ricard, M., Connault, E., Ardouin, P., Galaup, A., Metivier, D., Bidart, J. M., Germain, S., Perricaudet, M., and Schlumberger, M. (2007). Radiation and inhibition of angiogenesis by canstatin synergize to induce HIF-1alpha-mediated tumor apoptotic switch. J Clin Invest *117*, 1844-1855.

Marneros, A. G., She, H., Zambarakji, H., Hashizume, H., Connolly, E. J., Kim, I., Gragoudas, E. S., Miller, J. W., and Olsen, B. R. (2007). Endogenous endostatin inhibits choroidal neovascularization. FASEB J *21*, 3809-3818.

Marshall, J. (1987). The ageing retina: physiology or pathology. Eye (Lond) *1 (Pt 2)*, 282-295.

Martini, J. F., Piot, C., Humeau, L. M., Struman, I., Martial, J. A., and Weiner, R. I. (2000). The antiangiogenic factor 16K PRL induces programmed cell death in endothelial cells by caspase activation. Mol Endocrinol *14*, 1536-1549.

Mettouchi, A., and Meneguzzi, G. (2006). Distinct roles of beta1 integrins during angiogenesis. Eur J Cell Biol *85*, 243-247.

Miyajima-Uchida, H., Hayashi, H., Beppu, R., Kuroki, M., Fukami, M., Arakawa, F., Tomita, Y., and Oshima, K. (2000). Production and accumulation of thrombospondin-1 in human retinal pigment epithelial cells. Invest Ophthalmol Vis Sci *41*, 561-567.

Monboisse, J. C., Garnotel, R., Bellon, G., Ohno, N., Perreau, C., Borel, J. P., and Kefalides, N. A. (1994). The alpha 3 chain of type IV collagen prevents activation of human polymorphonuclear leukocytes. J Biol Chem *269*, 25475-25482.

Mori, K., Ando, A., Gehlbach, P., Nesbitt, D., Takahashi, K., Goldsteen, D., Penn, M., Chen, C. T., Melia, M., Phipps, S., Moffat, D., Brazzell, K., Liau, G., Dixon, K. H., and Campochiaro, P. A. (2001). Inhibition of choroidal neovascularization by intravenous injection of adenoviral vectors expressing secretable endostatin. Am J Pathol *159*, 313-320.

Nozaki, M., Raisler, B. J., Sakurai, E., Sarma, J. V., Barnum, S. R., Lambris, J. D., Chen, Y., Zhang, K., Ambati, B. K., Baffi, J. Z., and Ambati, J. (2006). Drusen complement components C3a and C5a promote choroidal neovascularization. Proc Natl Acad Sci U S A *103*, 2328-2333.

Nyberg, P., Xie, L., and Kalluri, R. (2005). Endogenous inhibitors of angiogenesis. Cancer Res *65*, 3967-3979.

Oklu, R., Walker, T. G., Wicky, S., and Hesketh, R. (2010). Angiogenesis and current antiangiogenic strategies for the treatment of cancer. J Vasc Interv Radiol *21*, 1791-1805; quiz 1806.

Panka, D. J., and Mier, J. W. (2003). Canstatin inhibits Akt activation and induces Fas-dependent apoptosis in endothelial cells. J Biol Chem *278*, 37632-37636.

Penn, J. S., Madan, A., Caldwell, R. B., Bartoli, M., Caldwell, R. W., and Hartnett, M. E. (2008). Vascular endothelial growth factor in eye disease. Prog Retin Eye Res *27*, 331-371.

Petitclerc, E., Boutaud, A., Prestayko, A., Xu, J., Sado, Y., Ninomiya, Y., Sarras, M. P., Jr., Hudson, B. G., and Brooks, P. C. (2000). New Functions for Non-collagenous Domains of Human Collagen Type IV. Novel integrin ligands inhibiting angiogenesis and tumor growth in vivo. J Biol Chem *275*, 8051-8061.

Rehn, M., Veikkola, T., Kukk-Valdre, E., Nakamura, H., Ilmonen, M., Lombardo, C., Pihlajaniemi, T., Alitalo, K., and Vuori, K. (2001). Interaction of endostatin with integrins implicated in angiogenesis. Proc Natl Acad Sci U S A *98*, 1024-1029.

Ricard-Blum, S., Feraud, O., Lortat-Jacob, H., Rencurosi, A., Fukai, N., Dkhissi, F., Vittet, D., Imberty, A., Olsen, B. R., and van der Rest, M. (2004). Characterization of endostatin binding to heparin and heparan sulfate by surface plasmon resonance and molecular modeling: role of divalent cations. J Biol Chem *279*, 2927-2936.

Roberts, W. G., and Palade, G. E. (1995). Increased microvascular permeability and endothelial fenestration induced by vascular endothelial growth factor. J Cell Sci *108 (Pt 6)*, 2369-2379.

Roth, J. M., Akalu, A., Zelmanovich, A., Policarpio, D., Ng, B., MacDonald, S., Formenti, S., Liebes, L., and Brooks, P. C. (2005). Recombinant alpha2(IV)NC1 domain inhibits tumor cell-extracellular matrix interactions, induces cellular senescence, and inhibits tumor growth in vivo. Am J Pathol *166*, 901-911.

Spaide, R. F., Armstrong, D., and Browne, R. (2003). Continuing medical education review: choroidal neovascularization in age-related macular degeneration--what is the cause? Retina *23*, 595-614.

Sudhakar, A., and Boosani, C. S. (2008). Inhibition of tumor angiogenesis by tumstatin: insights into signaling mechanisms and implications in cancer regression. Pharm Res *25*, 2731-2739.

Sudhakar, A., and Kalluri, R. (2010). Molecular mechanisms of angiostatis. Encyclopedia of the eye *3 M-P*, 52-59.

Sudhakar, A., Nyberg, P., Keshamouni, V. G., Mannam, A. P., Li, J., Sugimoto, H., Cosgrove, D., and Kalluri, R. (2005). Human alpha1 type IV collagen NC1 domain exhibits distinct antiangiogenic activity mediated by alpha1beta1 integrin. J Clin Invest *115*, 2801-2810.

Sudhakar, A., Sugimoto, H., Yang, C., Lively, J., Zeisberg, M., and Kalluri, R. (2003). Human tumstatin and human endostatin exhibit distinct antiangiogenic activities mediated by alpha vbeta 3 and alpha 5beta 1 integrins. Proc Natl Acad Sci U S A *100*, 4766-4771.

Tabruyn, S. P., Sorlet, C. M., Rentier-Delrue, F., Bours, V., Weiner, R. I., Martial, J. A., and Struman, I. (2003). The antiangiogenic factor 16K human prolactin induces caspase-dependent apoptosis by a mechanism that requires activation of nuclear factor-kappaB. Mol Endocrinol *17*, 1815-1823.

Takahashi, K., Saishin, Y., Silva, R. L., Oshima, Y., Oshima, S., Melia, M., Paszkiet, B., Zerby, D., Kadan, M. J., Liau, G., Kaleko, M., Connelly, S., Luo, T., and Campochiaro, P. A. (2003). Intraocular expression of endostatin reduces VEGF-induced retinal vascular permeability, neovascularization, and retinal detachment. FASEB J *17*, 896-898.

Tarui, T., Miles, L. A., and Takada, Y. (2001). Specific interaction of angiostatin with integrin alpha(v)beta(3) in endothelial cells. J Biol Chem *276*, 39562-39568.

Tombran-Tink, J., Chader, G. G., and Johnson, L. V. (1991). PEDF: a pigment epithelium-derived factor with potent neuronal differentiative activity. Exp Eye Res *53*, 411-414.

Wang, Y., Yin, H., Chen, P., and Xie, L. (2011). Inhibitory Effect of Canstatin in Alkali Burn-Induced Corneal Neovascularization. Ophthalmic Res *46*, 66-72.

Wickstrom, S. A., Alitalo, K., and Keski-Oja, J. (2002). Endostatin associates with integrin alpha5beta1 and caveolin-1, and activates Src via a tyrosyl phosphatase-dependent pathway in human endothelial cells. Cancer Res *62*, 5580-5589.

Wickstrom, S. A., Alitalo, K., and Keski-Oja, J. (2003). Endostatin associates with lipid rafts and induces reorganization of the actin cytoskeleton via down-regulation of RhoA activity. J Biol Chem *278*, 37895-37901.

Young, R. W., and Bok, D. (1969). Participation of the retinal pigment epithelium in the rod outer segment renewal process. J Cell Biol *42*, 392-403.

Zerlin, M., Julius, M. A., and Kitajewski, J. (2008). Wnt/Frizzled signaling in angiogenesis. Angiogenesis *11*, 63-69.

Zhang, S. X., and Ma, J. X. (2007). Ocular neovascularization: Implication of endogenous angiogenic inhibitors and potential therapy. Prog Retin Eye Res *26*, 1-37.

Zhou, S. Y., Xie, Z. L., Xiao, O., Yang, X. R., Heng, B. C., and Sato, Y. (2010). Inhibition of mouse alkali burn induced-corneal neovascularization by recombinant adenovirus encoding human vasohibin-1. Mol Vis *16*, 1389-1398.

Zhou, X. Y., Liao, Q., Pu, Y. M., Tang, Y. Q., Gong, X., Li, J., Xu, Y., and Wang, Z. G. (2009). Ultrasound-mediated microbubble delivery of pigment epithelium-derived factor gene into retina inhibits choroidal neovascularization. Chin Med J (Engl) *122*, 2711-2717.

Ziche, M., and Morbidelli, L. (2000). Nitric oxide and angiogenesis. J Neurooncol *50*, 139-148.

24

NRF2 and Age-Dependent RPE Degeneration

Yan Chen, Zhenyang Zhao,
Paul Sternberg and Jiyang Cai
Vanderbilt Eye Institute,
Vanderbilt University Medical Center, Nashville, TN,
USA

1. Introduction

Retinal pigment epithelium (RPE) is a single layer of epithelial cells lined between the neurosensory retina and choriocapillaris. It is part of the blood-retinal barrier and is a central component of the visual phototransduction pathway. RPE cells regenerate 11-cis-retinal by RPE65 isomerase and its related enzymes and chaperones (Moiseyev et al., 2006; Xue et al., 2004). They are professional phagocytes and are responsible for the clearance of daily shed photoreceptor outer segments (POS) (Young, 1967; Young & Bok, 1969). The multi-step process of phagocytosis includes receptor-mediated binding of POS to the RPE (Finnemann et al., 1997), internalization (Feng et al., 2002; Finnemann & Silverstein, 2001), transport to lysosome and degradation. The importance of RPE phagocytosis has been clearly illustrated by the Royal College of Surgeons (RCS) rats, which carry a mutation in *Mertk* gene (D'Cruz et al., 2000). MERTK is a membrane-associated receptor tyrosine kinase and is activated upon binding of POS to the RPE (Feng et al. 2002). In RCS rats, loss-of-function mutation of *Mertk* causes defects in phagocytosis and consequently these animals develop inherited retinal dystrophy and photoreceptor apoptosis (Tso et al., 1994). In addition to their roles in the visual cycle, RPE cells provide vital support for the structure and function of the outer retina. They transport ions, water and nutrients between choroidal blood supply and the retina, and synthesize melanin which absorbs light and shields the retina. RPE-produced growth factors, such as vascular endothelial growth factor (VEGF), are indispensable for the choroidal vasculature (Saint-Geniez et al., 2009).

Degeneration of the RPE with aging is an initiating event in age-related macular degeneration (AMD), a major cause of blindness in elderly people. Approximately 11% of persons between ages 65 and 74 have AMD, with prevalence rates rising to 30% in individuals at age 75 or older (Lee et al., 2003). Vision loss in AMD occurs through photoreceptor loss in the macula, the central area of the retina, and results either from a gradual "geographic atrophy" of the RPE (dry or atrophic disease) or from leakage and/or bleeding from choroidal neovascularization (CNV) (wet or neovascular disease). During CNV, blood vessels break through Bruch's membrane, leading to rapid loss of central vision in many cases. In recent years anti-VEGF agents have achieved unprecedented success in preserving visual acuity in patients with CNV (Brown et al., 2006; Rosenfeld et al., 2006; Galbinur et al., 2009). Detailed clinical aspects of wet AMD and anti-VEGF therapy are covered by other chapters of this book.

The genetic and biochemical mechanisms of RPE degeneration in dry AMD, however, remain largely unknown. Several hypothetical models have been proposed, including accumulation of lipofuscin and its bisretinoid fluorophore (Sparrow et al., 2003; Zhou et al., 2006), iron overload (Dunaief, 2006; Hahn et al., 2004), autoimmune response (Hollyfield et al., 2008) and exposure to double strand RNA (Ambati, 2011; Kaneko et al., 2011). All of them have suggested clinical associations with AMD and their causal relationships to the disease have been demonstrated by respective animal models (Ramkumar et al., 2010). Oxidative stress is a common mechanism underlying these diversified pathological processes. Photooxidation of the bisretinoids can produce singlet oxygen and release methylglyoxal to form advanced glycation end product (Wu et al., 2010). Iron overload increased isoprostane, a marker of lipid peroxidation, in the RPE/choroid (Hadziahmetovic et al., 2008). Mice immunized with serum albumin conjugated with carboxyethylpyrrole, an oxidation product of docosahexaenoic acid, developed signs of RPE degeneration and deposition of complement proteins in the Bruch's membrane (Hollyfield et al., 2008). Oxidative stress can downregulate DICER1, a RNA processing enzyme whose deficiency was shown to cause Alu RNA-induced cytotoxicity and RPE apoptosis (Kaneko et al., 2011).

Results from earlier clinical and laboratory studies also support the contributing roles of oxidative stress to AMD. Smoking is the strongest environmental risk factor of AMD (Cano et al., 2010; Smith et al., 2001) and has been clearly associated with oxidative stress (DeBlack, 2003; Mitchell et al., 2002; Pryor et al., 1983; Smith et al., 2001). A number of interventional studies showed that antioxidant supplementation had protective effects against development of AMD or limiting its progression. Experimental animals fed with diets supplemented with antioxidants demonstrated an increased resistance to retinal degeneration (Ham et al., 1984; Organisciak et al., 1985; Tso et al., 1984). Results from the Age-Related Eye Disease Study (AREDS) showed that supplemental antioxidants (vitamin C, vitamin E and beta carotene) and zinc can decrease the risk of progression from intermediate AMD to advanced AMD by 25% (AREDS 2000 & 2001). Taken together, the findings from the research of the past two decades suggest that AMD is a multifactorial disease, with oxidative stress viewed as a common mechanism involved in the gene-environmental interaction of its etiololgy.

Oxidative stress is due to an imbalance between the generation of reactive oxygen species and their clearance by antioxidant systems. The RPE has powerful endogenous antioxidant capacity to overcome the high level of oxidative stress, which is caused by both focal light exposure and high metabolic rate of the retina. In addition to utilizing direct radical scavengers such as β-carotene, ascorbic acid and α-tocopherol, RPE cells have an elaborate enzymatic antioxidant system that can prevent and repair oxidative injury. Nuclear factor erythroid 2-related factor 2 (NRF2) is a master regulator of cellular antioxidant and detoxification responses (Kensler et al., 2007). We and others have shown previously that elevating the transcriptional activity of NRF2 can protect against oxidative injury to the RPE; while mice that are deficient of NRF2 developed pathological features similar to human AMD (Zhao et al., 2011; Cano et al., 2010). Oral zinc supplementation, which was used in the AREDS to slow AMD progression, can activate NRF2-dependent antioxidant system in the RPE (Ha et al., 2006). More recently, a newer class of NRF2 inducers, which are based on synthetic triterpenoid 2-cyano-3,12-dioxooleana-1,9-dien-28-oic acid (CDDO) and its derivatives, have achieved potent protection in various models of retinal damage (Pitha-Rowe et al. 2009). In this chapter we will review past and recent literature reports, based on cell culture, animal models and human clinical studies, to address how NRF2 regulates RPE function both *in vitro* and *in vivo*.

2. NRF2-dependent antioxidant defense

NRF2 is a transcription factor that controls the expression of phase 2 detoxification genes. It heterodimerizes with members of the Maf family of transcription factors and binds to the *cis*-acting antioxidant response element in the promoter regions of various phase 2 genes (Katsuoka et al., 2005; Motohashi et al., 2004). The latter encode a group of enzymes, such as glutamate-cysteine ligase, glutathione S-transferase, glutathione peroxidase, heme oxygenase, NAD(P)H:quinone reductase and glutamate-cysteine exchanger, which are essential for detoxification of xenobiotics and endogenous reactive intermediates (Kensler et al., 2007; Wakabayashi et al. 2010). NRF2-deficient mice showed increased sensitivity to a variety of pharmacological and environmental toxicants (Kensler et al., 2007; Rangasamy et al., 2004). The protective effects of NRF2 inducers have been tested in a number of models of human diseases, including cancer, neurodegeneration, cardiovascular disease, and liver and lung injury (Kensler et al., 2007; Wakabayashi et al., 2010).

Activation of NRF2 is subjected to multiple levels of regulation. Under basal conditions, NRF2 is sequestered by its inhibitor protein, Keap1, and is targeted for Cullin 3/Rbx1-mediated ubiquitination and degradation (Cullinan et al., 2004; Furukawa & Xiong, 2005; Kobayashi et al., 2004). Upon conditions of oxidative stress or exposure to electrophilic compounds, NRF2 protein can be liberated from Keap1 and will translocate into nucleus to mediate gene trasncription. As illustrated in Fig. 1, there are six Neh (NRF2 ECH homology) domains that are responsible for most of the functions of NRF2. The Neh domains show amino acid sequence homology conserved between different species including human, rodents and chicken (McMahon et al., 2004; Zhang et al., 2007).

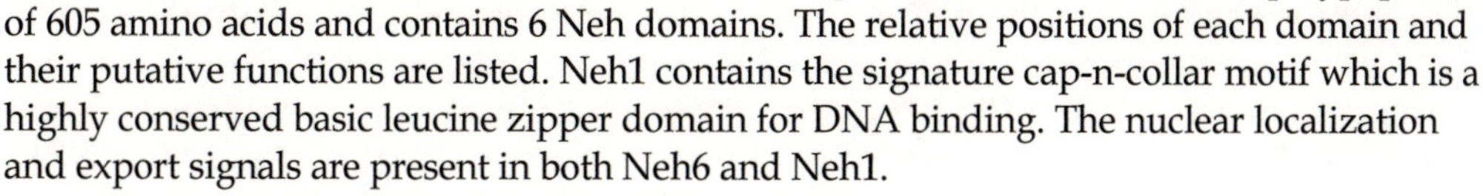

Fig. 1. Illustration of the Neh domains of the NRF2 protein. Human NRF2 is a polypeptide of 605 amino acids and contains 6 Neh domains. The relative positions of each domain and their putative functions are listed. Neh1 contains the signature cap-n-collar motif which is a highly conserved basic leucine zipper domain for DNA binding. The nuclear localization and export signals are present in both Neh6 and Neh1.

3. NRF2-mediated protection in cultured RPE cells

Compounds that promote the nuclear translocation of Nrf2 and elevate its transcriptional activity can protect against oxidative injury in cultured RPE cells. In 2001, Talalay and colleagues first reported that sulforaphane could prevent RPE cell death caused by treatments with menadione, t-butyl hydroperoxide, 4-hydroxynonenal and peroxynitrite (Gao et al., 2001). Since then numerous other studies reported the protective effects of a wide range of structurally-different NRF2 inducers including isothiocyanates (sulforaphane) (Gao & Talalay, 2004), polyphenols (curcumin, resveratrol and flavonoids) (Alex et al., 2010; Johnson et al., 2009; Mandal et al., 2009), 1,2,dithiole-3-thiones (oltipraz) (Nelson et al., 2002), zinc (Ha et al., 2006) or triterpenoids (Pitha-Rowe et al., 2009). Many of them are naturally occurring compounds present in fruits and vegetables, making them ideal for dietary supplementation. Some of the compounds have either gone through human clinical trials or are currently used for other applications. For instances, zinc was used in the AREDS supplementation either alone or with antioxidant vitamins. Oltipraz, a dithiole derivate, is used in treating schistosomiasis and cancer chemoprevention (Jacobson et al., 1997). A common mechanism underlying the antioxidant and detoxification functions of NRF2 is to increase cellular glutathione (GSH) synthesis.

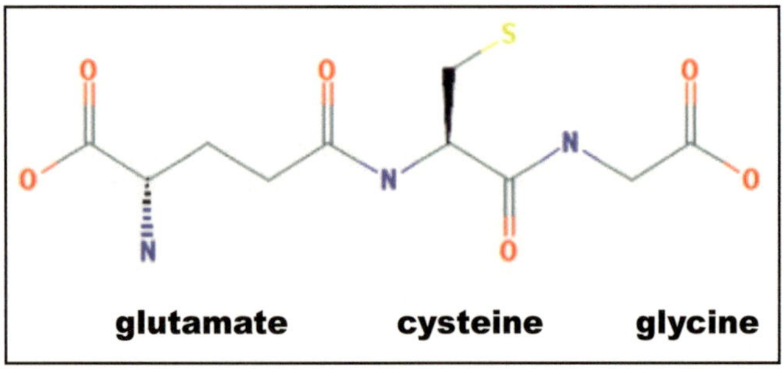

Fig. 2. Structure of glutathione. The γ-glutamylcysteine is formed by a peptide bond between the carboxylate group of glutamate and animo group of cysteine. The sulfhydryl group of cysteine is responsible for the antioxidant function of the tripeptide.

GSH is a tripeptide consisted of glutamate, cysteine and glycine. It contains a unique peptide bond between the amine group of cysteine and the carboxyl group of the glutamate side chain so that it is much more resistant to degradation by peptidase (Fig. 2). The sulfhydryl group of cysteine of GSH can be used by glutathione S-transferase to conjugate electrophilic centers on a wide variety of substrates (Pool-Zobel et al., 2005). GSH is also used by glutathione peroxidase to reduce lipid hydroperoxides and hydrogen peroxide to alcohols and water, respectively. The glutamate cysteine ligase (GCL) is the rate-limiting enzyme of GSH synthesis. It generates γ-glutamylcysteine from glutamate and cysteine. NRF2 inducers can elevate the mRNA levels of the catalytic and modulatory subunits of GCL. Cystine uptake by the RPE is mediated by a sodium independent, cystine/glutamate exchanger (Bridges et al., 2001; Ishii et al., 1992). The transporter is consisted of two subunits, xCT as the light chain and 4F2hc as the heavy chain (Wagner et al., 2001). NRF2 controls the expression of *xCT* gene (Sato et al., 1999). In *xCT* knock out mice, the plasma cystine concentration almost doubled, resulted from decreased tissue uptake (Sasaki et al., 2002). The *xCT-/-* mice showed more several renal injury caused by ischemia-reperfusion (Shibasaki et al., 2009). Thus, NRF2 inducers can increase both the rate of GSH synthesis and cellular concentration of its amino acid precursor.

Monitoring the RPE glutathione content is a reliable assay for initial screening of model compounds designed to activate NRF2. For instance, RPE cells pretreated with oltipraz showed increased total and mitochondrial GSH. At 50 μM, oltipraz increased total cellular GSH by 18% and mitochondrial GSH by 50%, and achieved significant protection against tert-butylhydroperoxide-induced RPE cell death (Nelson et al., 2002). Similar results were obtained from cells pretreated with dimethylfumarate (DMF) for 24 hours (Nelson et al., 1999). However, when the time course of the DMF was evaluated, a transient decrease in GSH levels was found that preceded the increase noted at later time points. Compared to vehicle-treated control cells, cells pretreated with DMF for 3 hours showed a significant reduction in viability when further challenged by peroxide (Nelson et al, 1999). Thus, the initial decrease of GSH after DMF treatment rendered the RPE cells more sensitive to oxidative injury, although it can subsequently lead to a feedback increase of GSH synthesis and a more robust antioxidant response (Nelson et al., 1999). Many of the NRF2 inducers are thiol-reacting compounds and may cause a similar initial depletion of cellular GSH. Therefore, although the *in vitro* culture system does not present the complexity of the retinal microenvironment and cell-cell interaction *in vivo*, it is a valuable tool for assessing both the pharmacological properties of new NRF2 inducers and their potential toxicities. For treatment of a chronic disease like AMD, the RPE cells are already stressed by oxidative burden and may not tolerate transient GSH depletion after repeated administration of agents that react with cellular thiols with low selectivity.

4. Ocular pathology of *Nrf2* knockout mice

Nrf2 knockout mice have normal embryonic development (Chan et al., 1996) and their basal level of antioxidant status in many tissues is not different from age-matched wild type mice. However, the *Nrf2* null mice show increased sensitivity to a variety of pharmacological and environmental toxicants (Cano et al., 2010; Kensler et al., 2007; Osburn & Kensler, 2008). Depending upon the stimuli, injuries occur in different organs and tissues. The phenotypes vary, but commonly involve oxidative and inflammatory stress. For ocular pathology, neonatal *Nrf2* knockout mice develop more severe retinal vaso-obliteration at early phase after hyperoxia exposure (Uno et al., 2010). NRF2 also modulates the innate immune response in the retina and iris-ciliary body in a mouse model of uveitis induced by intraperitoneal injection of lipopolysaccaride (Nagai et al., 2009).

Aging and smoking are the major demographic and environmental risk factor of AMD, respectively. Cano and colleagues (2010) reported that NRF2-deficient mice were more susceptible to smoking-induced retinal injury. At 8 months, *Nrf2* null mice showed a mild degree of ultrastructural change in the RPE. Comparing to age-matched wild type mice, RPE of the knockout mice exposed to cigarette smoking for 6 months (starting at 2 months) displayed markedly increased staining of 8-hydroxydeoxyguanosine, an indicator of accumulated oxidative DNA damage (Cano et al., 2010). On electron microscopy, *Nrf2*$^{-/-}$ smoking mice displayed abnormal RPE basal infoldings and vacuoles, without apparent changes of the choroidal endothelium or sub-RPE deposit formation (Cano et al., 2010). Thickening and deposits in the outer collagenous layer of Bruch's membrane were often observed in smoking mice. The data suggest that NRF2-mediated protection to the RPE is important against chronic environmental toxicities associated with AMD.

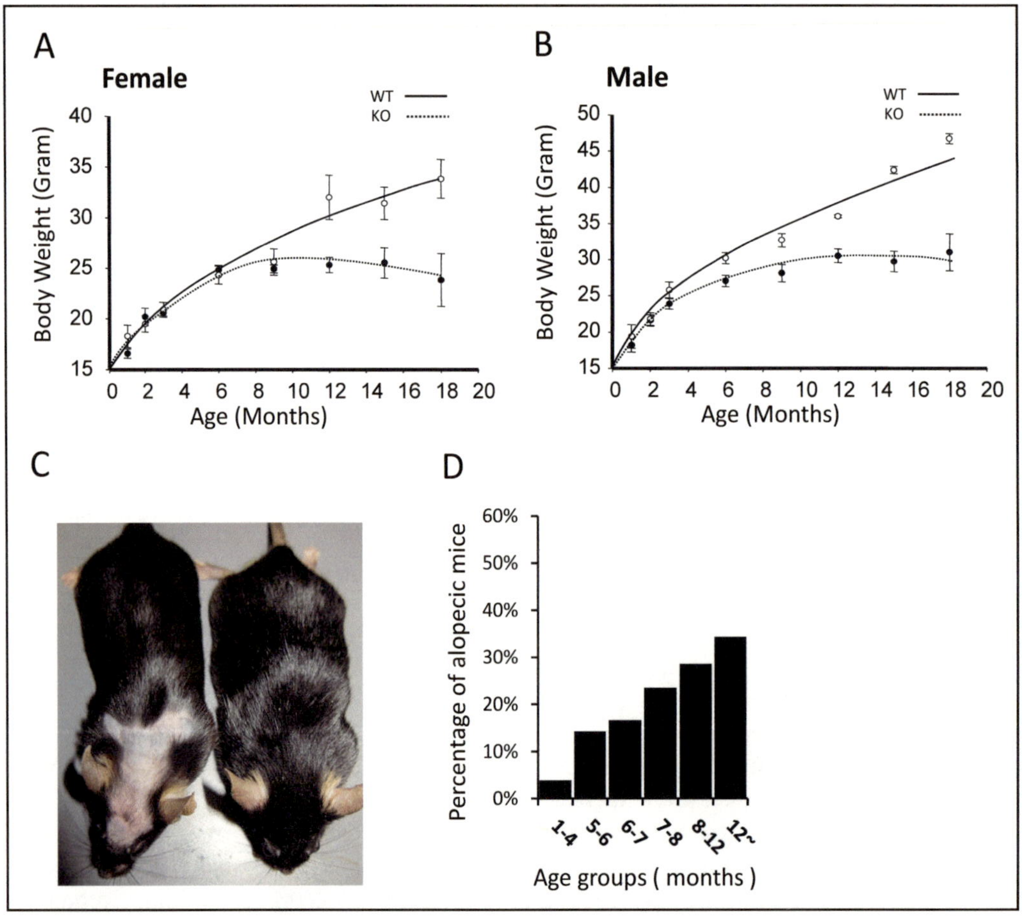

Fig. 3. Accelerated aging in *Nrf2-/-* mice. (A) and (B) Growth curves of male and female *Nrf2-/-* mice and their age-matched littermates. Knockout animals showed a lower body weight after the first year. (C) and (D) Hair loss in *Nrf2-/-* mice. A representative picture of a 12-month-old alopecic *Nrf2-/-* mice is shown in (C). Hair loss was often first observed between 5 to 6 months of age (D).

We recently reported that *Nrf2-/-* mice developed age-related RPE and choroidal degeneration resembling cardinal features of human AMD (Zhao et al., 2011). The *Nrf2-/-* mice have accelerated aging. Some of the animals exhibited extensive hair loss (alopecia), which began as early as 4 months and peaked at 8 months (Fig. 3). Interestingly, more female *Nrf2-/-* mice suffered from hair loss than male ones; this could possibly be attributed to the higher susceptibility of female mice to autoimmune diseases as reported by Takahashi and colleagues (Yoh et al., 2001). After 12 months, the *Nrf2-/-* mice started to show lower body weight than the age-matched wild type littermates (Fig. 3). The life expectancy of *Nrf2-/-* mice is about 20 months which is only 60% of wild type mice with the same genetic background (Pearson et al., 2008).

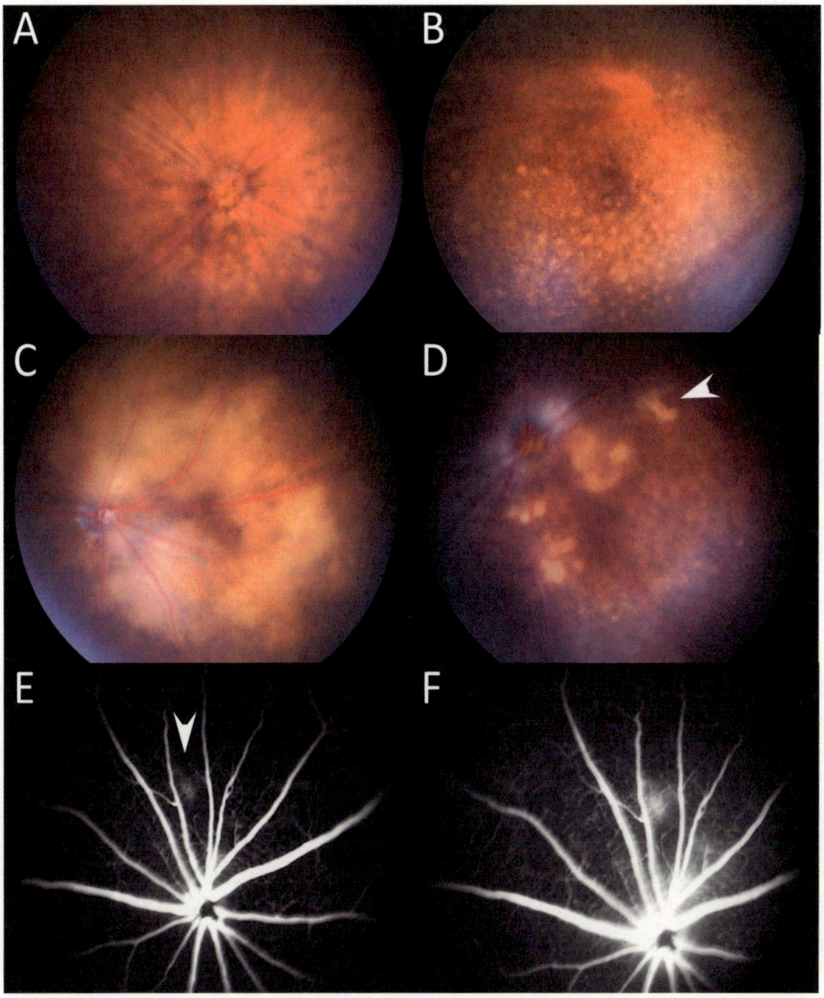

Fig. 4. Fundus examinations of *Nrf2*-/- mice. (A) Normal fundus image taken from a 12-month-old wild type mouse. (B) Drusen like deposits developed in the peripheral retina of an 8-month-old *Nrf2*-/- mouse. (C) Yellowish patchy lesions found in a 14-month-old *Nrf2*-/- mouse. (D-F) A 16-month-old knockout mouse developed extensive RPE lesions (D), one of which showed hyperfluorescence in both early (E) and late (F) phase of fluorescein angiography. Arrowheads in D and E indicate the same lesion.

Drusen-like deposits were noted in around 70% of eyes from *Nrf2*-/- mice, as examined by funduscopy between 8 to 11 months (Fig. 4B). With aging, these small, dome-shaped whitish spots in the fundus tended to become confluent yellowish lesions, gradually increasing in area (Fig. 4C). Atrophic RPE lesions were frequently seen in *Nrf2*-/- mice after the first year (Fig 4C and 4D). Some of these lesions would eventually develop into sites of CNV, which were identified by both fundus fluorescein angiography (Fig 4E and 4F) and histopathology (Zhao et al., 2011). Moderate but statistically significant decreases in both a- and b-wave amplitudes on ERG were observed between the *Nrf2*-/- and wild-type mice at 12 months of age (Zhao et al., 2011), indicating compromised visual function in knockout mice.

The fundus phenotype in aged *Nrf2-/-* mice was further confirmed by histology (Fig. 5 and Zhao et al., 2011), which showed drusen formation, extensive RPE atrophy with numerous vacuoles, increased autofluorescence inside the RPE layer and CNV. Thickening of the Bruch's membrane with age and basal laminar and basal linear deposit were found exclusively in *Nrf2-/-* mice by electron microscopy (Zhao et al., 2011). Immunostaining of eye sections revealed increased deposition of proteins that are related to innate immunity (i.e., C3d, vitronectin and serum amyloid P) and marker of oxidative injury (nitrotyrosine) between the RPE and Bruch's membrane in *Nrf2-/-* mice (Zhao et al., 2011). The same proteins have been found in drusen and Bruch's membrane of human AMD eyes (Crabb et al., 2002; Mullins et al., 2000).

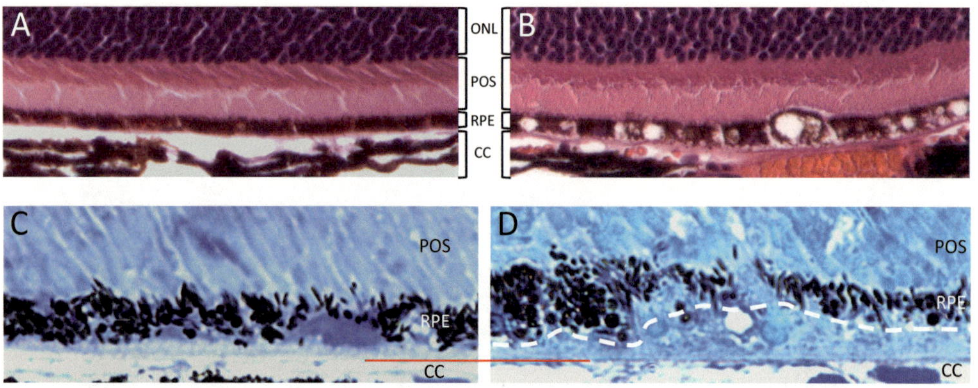

Fig. 5. Histology examination of retina of *Nrf2-/-* mice. (A) A 14-month-old wild type mouse showed normal structure of the outer retina. (B) Representative image of RPE degeneration with big vacuoles, taken from a 14-month-old *Nrf2-/-* mouse. (C-D) Semi-thin sections from a 12-month-old wild-type mouse (C) and an age-matched *Nrf2-/-* mouse (D). Bruch's membranes of the two were aligned at the same level (red line). Note that the RPE layer was elevated due to heterogeneous deposits (under the dotted line) in the sub-RPE space. (A and B: Paraffin section with hematoxylin and eosin staining. C and D: Plastic section with toluidine blue staining. ONL: outer nuclear layer; POS: photoreceptor outer segment; CC: choriocapillaris)

The accelerated degeneration after middle age and the typical pathology of the RPE/choroid indicate that the *Nrf2-/-* model shares many features of human AMD. At advanced age, the retinal pathology progressed from atrophic form to neovascularization and about 15% of the *Nrf2-/-*mice developed spontaneous CNV (Zhao et al., 2011). Photoreceptor degeneration was moderate and was probably secondary to RPE dysfunction. Rodents do not have macula and, therefore, cannot be used to generate ideal models of AMD. On the other hand, mechanistic studies exploring the molecular and biochemical mechanisms of age-related RPE degeneration and CNV can greatly benefit from animal models that at least partially reproduce representative lesions commonly seen in human AMD eyes. Animal models, such as the *Nrf2-/-* mice, will display the dynamic process of the disease and offer windows of intervention that can either slow down or accelerate the progression. Similar experiments will be difficult if not impossible to perform with human eyes mainly at late stages of AMD.

5. Pharmacological interventions that activate NRF2 *in vivo*

A number of *in vivo* studies have investigated the protective roles of NRF2 inducers in models of retinal injury and inflammation. A study by Yodoi and colleagues (Tanito et al., 2005) showed that sulforaphane, a prototypic NRF2 inducer, could upregulate thioredoxin in both the RPE and neural retina, and was effective in protecting photoreceptors from photo-oxidative damage. Compared to vehicle-treated controls, mice received sulforaphane showed fewer apoptotic cells in the outer nuclear layer and RPE, and had moderate but statistically significant improvement of both a- and b-wave amplitudes. At four days after light exposure, the ONL was significantly thicker in sulforaphane-treated mice (Tanito et al., 2005). Sulforaphane also delayed photoreceptor cell death in *tubby* mouse, a model of Usher syndrome (Kong et al., 2007). Homozygous *tubby* mice develop progressive photoreceptor degeneration shortly after birth. Sulforaphane-treated *tub/tub* mice showed significantly increased ONL thickness and b-wave amplitude at P28 and P34, as compared to vehicle-treated animals (Kong et al., 2007).

For human clinical studies, AREDS reported (2001) that supplementation with zinc alone, or antioxidants plus zinc, decreased the risk of progression towards advanced AMD by 20%. We showed that zinc could activate NRF2 both in cultured RPE cells and in RPE of NRF2 reporter mice (Chen et al., data not shown). In an ancillary study of AREDS, we analyzed the effects of long-term zinc supplementation on plasma thiol metabolites and their redox status (Moriarty-Craige et al., 2007). There was a significant decrease in plasma cystine concentration in the zinc-supplemented group. The systemic effects may be due to increased tissue uptake of cystine, as NRF2 regulates the transporter protein xCT (Sasaki et al., 2002). These results prove the concept that long term dietary supplementation of an NRF2 inducer is a feasible approach for treating early stage AMD patients.

A new class of synthetic triterpenoids derivatives of oleanolic acid have been tested both in cultured RPE cells and *in vivo*. These agents exerted highly potent activity at concentration as low as 10 nM. They reacted with a broad range of accessible protein thiols and activate NRF2 about 10 times more potently (by the ARE reporter assay) than previously used compounds (Pitha-Rowe et al., 2009). The *in vivo* protection against light-induced retinal toxicity has been demonstrated. Mice receiving 200 mg/kg CDDO-trifluoroethylamide (-TFEA) showed significantly increased ONL thickness after light-induced retinal degeneration (Pitha-Rowe et al., 2009). CDDO-imidazolide decreased mouse leukocyte adherence to retinal vasculature after lipopolysaccaride treatment, and reduced expression of inflammatory mediators including ICAM-1, IL-6, COX-2, TNF-α and MCP-1 (Nagai et al., 2009; Cano et al., 2010). CDDO-methyl ester inhibited neutrophil infiltration in vitreous and internal limiting membrane after retinal ischemia-reperfusion induced by high intraocular pressure, and inhibited degeneration of retinal capillary (Wei et al., 2011). The CDDO compounds are currently under clinical trials for chronic kidney disease and type 2 diabetes. Their potential applications in treating dry AMD can be explored in human studies in the near future.

6. Signaling pathways that regulate NRF2 activation

The interaction between Keap1 and NRF2 is considered as a major determinant of the stability and function of NRF2 (Dinkova-Kostova et al., 2002; Hong et al., 2005). Electrophilic compounds, such as sulforaphane, can directly react with various cysteine residues of Keap1 and consequently cause dissociation and activation of NRF2 (Eggler et al., 2005). Keap1-

deficient hepatocytes had increased NRF2 activity and were more resistant to acetaminophen (Okawa et al., 2006). In addition to thiol modification and redox regulation, it is well established that there are cross-talk between the protein kinase pathways and NRF2-dependent antioxidant system (Sherratt et al., 2004).

Several phosphorylation sites of NRF2 protein have been mapped out and associated to its activity (Fig. 6). Phosphorylation of NRF2 at Serine 40 by protein kinase C promotes its dissociation from Keap1 and translocation into the nucleus (Bloom and Jaiswal, 2003; Huang et al., 2002). Phosphorylation at Tyrosine 568 by a Src subfamily kinase Fyn controls the export and inactivation of NRF2 at the late phase of induction (Jain and Jaiswal, 2006; Salazar et al., 2006). Other Src subfamily kinases, Src, Yes and Fgr, can also function as negative regulators of NRF2 by phosphorylating the protein at Tyr568 (Niture et al., 2011). A recent study by Rada et al (2011) demonstrated that a serine cluster in the Neh6 domain (Ser335, 338, 342, 347, 351, and 355) (Fig. 1) of NRF2 can be phosphorylated by glycogen synthase kinase-3β (GSK-3β). The phosphorylation enhanced the association between Nrf2 and SCF/β-TrCP, which is an adaptor protein for ubiquitin ligase and targets NRF2 for cullin-1/Rbx1-mediated degradation (Rada et al., 2011). Thus, phosphorylation of NRF2 by GSK-3β will facilitate it proteosomal degradation and inhibit its transactivation function. GSK-3β may also act upstream of Src family kinases (Jain and Jaiswal, 2006; Kaspar and Jaiswal, 2011). It remains elusive whether those two mechanisms work independently or additively. Mitogen-activated protein kinases (MAPKs) have been shown to phosphorylate NRF2 at Ser215, 408, 558, 577 and Tyr559; however, impacts on NRF2 location and activity were marginal after phosphorylation at those residues (Sun et al., 2009).

Results from the functional studies consistently showed that inhibition of the PI3K/Akt pathway decreased NRF2 activation induced by a variety of stimuli in different cell lines, while expression of a constitutive active mutant of Akt increased NRF2 activity, indicating that PI3K/Akt signalling is a positive regulator of NRF2 (Chen et al., 2009; Jain and Jaiswal, 2006; Kang et al., 2000; Lee et al., 2001; Wang et al., 2008). PI3K/Akt controls NRF2 via multiple indirect mechanisms. They can facilitate translocation of NRF2 into the nucleus via rearrangement of cytoskeletal actin (Kang et al., 2002). They are upstream kinases of GSK-3β. Akt phosphorylates GSK-3β at Ser9 and inhibits its kinase activity, which in turn will potentiate NRF2 activation because GSK-3β is its negative regulator (Jain and Jaiswal, 2006; Niture et al., 2011; Rada et al., 2011; Salazar et al., 2006).

There are other kinases that can be positive regulators of NRF2. PKR-like endoplasmic reticulum kinase phosphorylates and activates NRF2 under conditions of ER stress (Cullinan and Diehl, 2004; Cullinan et al., 2003). Casein kinase 2 phosphorylates endogenous NRF2 and regulates its activity and degradation (Pi et al., 2007). MAPK family proteins, extracellular signal-regulated protein kinases (ERKs) and the c-Jun N-terminal kinases (JNK), also play positive roles in NRF2-signaling pathway (Shen et al., 2004; Yu et al., 2000a; Zipper and Mulcahy, 2003). However, the positive regulation by ERKs and JNK may not through direct phosphorylation of NRF2 (Shen et al., 2004; Zipper and Mulcahy, 2003). Instead, they may upregulate NRF2 activity by phosphorylating and activating Nrf2 binding partner, such as the nuclear transcriptional coactivator CBP (Shen et al., 2004; Yu et al., 2000a). The p38 kinase may either stimulate or inhibit NRF2 activity, depending on the different type of cells and the pharmacological agents used for the studies (Yu et al., 2000b; Zipper and Mulcahy, 2000).

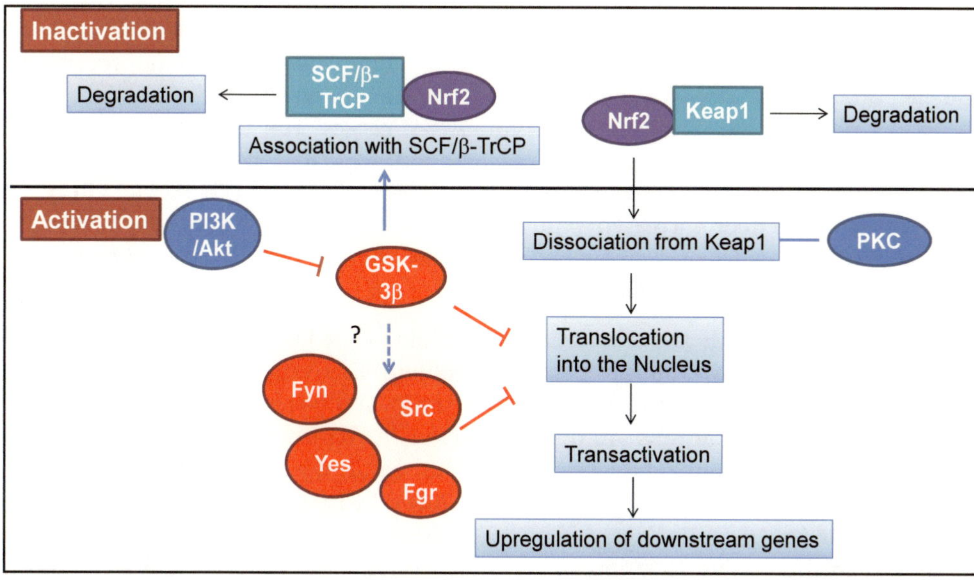

Fig. 6. Regulation of NRF2 activity by protein phosphorylation. There are positive and negative regulators of upstream kinases that function at various steps of the signalling pathway. Phosphorylation can leads to either its activation or degradation/inactivation.

Because of the multiple putative phosphorylation sites of NRF2, and its dual regulation by cellular redox status and protein phosphorylation, it is difficult to clearly define its upstream signalling network both at basal level and in response to oxidative stress. Identification of authentic phosphorylation sites and development of antibodies specific for phosphorylated NRF2 can greatly advance our knowledge in this area. More importantly, most of the works on signal transduction of NRF2 have been performed in transformed cancer cells, which harbour genetic and biochemical variations and function quite differently from the RPE. Future mechanistic studies of NRF2 will be needed to address cell type-specific signalling mechanisms involved in RPE aging and degeneration.

7. Potential mechanisms linking NRF2 to AMD

A unique pathology of AMD is that RPE degeneration occurs before severe loss of photoreceptors, a retinal phenotype also seen in NRF2-deficient mice. In contrast, in model systems of retinal toxicities, animals exposed to excessive levels of oxidative stress often showed much more severe retinal degeneration than the RPE damage. Compared to epithelial cells, neurons are less efficiently protected by the endogenous antioxidant system. The outer segments of rods and cones have very low GSH (Winkler 2008). As shown in both the SOD1- and SOD2-deficient mice, severe loss of neurons occurred before or at the same time of RPE degeneration (Imamura et al. 2006; Justilien et al., 2007). In *Vldlr-/-* mice, antioxidant supplementation protected retinal degeneration and improved the retinal electrophysiology (Dorrell et al., 2009). The fact that *Nrf2-/-* mice showed preferential loss of RPE suggests that NRF2 can have functions other than antioxidant protection.

It is noteworthy that the retinal ultrastructure of aged *Nrf2*$^{-/-}$ mice showed signs of dysregulated autophagy (Zhao et al., 2011). Autophagy is a major self-renewal process which is essential for organelle turnover and removal of aggregated proteins that cannot be processed by proteasome (Klionsky 2007). During autophagy, unwanted proteins and organelles are sorted to double-membrane autophagosomes, which are further delivered to and fused with lysosomes to degrade the sequestered cargos. The accumulation of various intermediate forms of autophagic vacuoles and multivesicular bodies in the RPE and Bruch's membrane was evident on EM images of aged *Nrf2*$^{-/-}$ mice (Zhao et al. 2011). This can be caused by either increased autophagic flux or decreased final degradation by lysosome. Similar findings of dysregulated autophagy were reported in another study using human AMD eyes (Wang et al., 2009).

Autophagy is of particular importance in non-dividing cells like neurons and RPE which, unlike proliferating cells, are incapable of diluting the waste products by mitosis. Dysregulated autophagy is considered as pathogenic in various neurodegenerative diseases; and the underlying mechanisms are disease-specific. In Alzheimer's disease, mutations in presenilin-1 impairs lysosomal targeting of v-ATPase V0a1, which is essential for lysosome acidification and protease activation (Lee et al., 2010). In Parkinson's disease, mutated α-synuclein cannot be efficiently degraded by autophagy (Cuervo et al., 2004). In Huntington's disease, mutant huntingtin may impair the initial cargo assembly of autophagic vesicles (Martinez-Vicente et al., 2010). It has been hypothesized that dysregulated autophagy is also involved in AMD (Wang et al., 2009; Kaarniranta 2010).

NRF2 can be an important regulator of RPE autophagy via multiple mechanisms. In normal RPE cells, autophagy is responsible for the removal of ubiquitinated and/or aggregated proteins. Cargos inside autophagosomes will be delivered to lysosome for degradation and recycled for catabolism. NRF2 is likely involved in autophagosome formation. Several previous studies reported that p62, which is a receptor protein of ubiquitinated proteins and essential for the initial assembly of autophagosome, is transcriptionally regulated by NRF2 (Komatsu et al., 2010). Whether NRF2 controls other specific molecular components of the autophagy pathway remains to be characterized by future studies. Accelerated accumulation of lipofuscin was observed in *Nrf2*$^{-/-}$ RPE (Zhao et al., 2011). Reactive metabolites from bisretinoids inhibit lysosome-mediated autophagic degradation. NRF2-dependent detoxification can be protective in both formation and elimination of lipofuscin-related metabolic waste products. Thus, compromised NRF2 signalling can impact both the early and late stages of RPE autophagy.

NRF2 may also be involved in the innate immune response that amplifies the initial RPE lesions in AMD. As shown in the uveitis model, NRF2-deficient retina had higher number of infiltrated leukocytes and increased production of pro-inflammatory cytokines (Cano et al., 2010). Thioredoxin 1, a downstream protein of NRF2, can interact with complement factor H and regulate its activation (Inomata et al., 2008). Autophagy can be a possible mechanistic link between oxidative stress and inflammation (Levine et al., 2011). Elevated cellular stress will cause increased damage to proteins and organelles and overwhelm the degradation capacity of RPE autophagy. Consequently, the undigested wastes could be exported into Bruch's membrane via exocytosis and deposited in the sub-RPE space (Wang et al., 2009). The exported proteins, possibly in oxidatively modified forms, may further promote drusen formation and cause local inflammation mediated by complement proteins and macrophages. Loss of endothelial fenestration was observed in choriocapillaris of aged *Nrf2-/-* mice (Zhao et al., 2011). In human AMD eyes, choroidal vascular degeneration occurs in areas of geographic atrophy (McLeod et al., 2009; Mullins et al. 2011). Decreased transport function of choroidal vessels can facilitate the accumulation of damaged proteins in the sub-RPE space and Bruch's membrane.

Single nucleotide polymorphisms (SNPs) in the coding region of *NRF2* gene have been detected in human cancerous tissues (Shibata et al. 2008). Functional polymorphisms in the promoter region of *NRF2* have been reported (Marzec et al., 2007). However, according to the GWAS data (Chen et al., 2010), NRF2 is not a major risk allele of AMD and SNPs of *NRF2* are unlikely to be a major genetic factor. A recent study showed that age-dependent decline of NRF2 function could be caused by upstream regulatory mechanisms, such as GSK-3β, that control its localization and activity (Tomobe et al., 2011). Defining these mechanisms will open up new revenues of intervention to prevent oxidative injury and RPE loss during dry AMD. Unlike the inherited genetic variations, the biochemical changes associated with RPE aging are likely treatable.

8. Conclusion

NRF2 is a protein that has been extensively studied in cancer and other chronic human diseases. Accumulating evidence suggests that NRF2-mediated signalling pathways have central roles in protecting the RPE cells from aging and age-related degeneration. The *Nrf2-/-* mice represent a new model for translational and mechanistic studies of AMD. Agents that activate Nrf2 are potential candidates for treating AMD and other retinal diseases involving oxidative and inflammatory stress.

9. Acknowledgment

This work was supported by International Retinal Research Foundation, NIH grants EY019706, EY07892, EY018715, P30 EY08126, and Research to Prevent Blindness, Inc.

10. References

AREDS (2000). The Age-Related Eye Disease Study: a clinical trial of zinc and antioxidants--AREDS Report No. 2. *Journal of Nutrition* Vol.130, No.5S (Suppl), (May 2000), pp. 1516S-1519S, ISSN 0022-3166

AREDS (2001).A randomized, placebo-controlled, clinical trial of high-dose supplementation with vitamins C and E, beta carotene, and zinc for age-related macular degeneration and vision loss: AREDS report no. 8. *Archives of Ophthalmology* Vol.119, No.10, (October 2001), pp. 1417-1436, ISSN 0003-9950

Alex, A.F., Spitznas, M., Tittel, A.P., Kurts, C., & Eter, N. (2010). Inhibitory effect of epigallocatechin gallate (EGCG), resveratrol, and curcumin on proliferation of human retinal pigment epithelial cells in vitro. *Current Eye Resesearch* Vol.35, No.11, (November 2010), pp. 1021-1033, ISSN 1460-2202

Ambati, J. (2011). Age-related macular degeneration and the other double helix. The Cogan Lecture. *Investigative Ophthalmology & Visual Science* Vol.52, No.5, (April 2011), pp. 2165-2169, ISSN 0146-0404

Bloom, D.A., & Jaiswal, A.K. (2003). Phosphorylation of Nrf2 at Ser40 by protein kinase C in response to antioxidants leads to the release of Nrf2 from INrf2, but is not required for Nrf2 stabilization/accumulation in the nucleus and transcriptional activation of antioxidant response element-mediated NAD(P)H:quinone oxidoreductase-1 gene expression. *Journal of Biological Chemistry* Vol.278, No.45, (November 2003), pp. 44675-44682, ISSN 0021-9258

Bridges, C.C., Kekuda, R., Wang, H., Prasad, P.D., Mehta, P., Huang, W., Smith, S.B., & Ganapathy, V. (2001). Structure, function, and regulation of human cystine/glutamate transporter in retinal pigment epithelial cells. *Investigative Ophthalmology & Visual Science* Vol.42, No.1, (January 2001), pp. 47-54, ISSN 0146-0404

Brown, D.M., Kaiser, P.K., Michels, M., Soubrane, G., Heier, J.S., Kim, R.Y., Sy, J.P., & Schneider, S. (2006). Ranibizumab versus verteporfin for neovascular age-related macular degeneration. *New England Journal of Medicine* Vol.355, No.14, (October 2006), pp. 1432-1444, ISSN 0028-4793

Cano, M., Thimmalappula, R., Fujihara, M., Nagai, N., Sporn, M., Wang, A.L., Neufeld, A.H., Biswal, S., & Handa, J.T. (2010). Cigarette smoking, oxidative stress, the anti-oxidant response through Nrf2 signaling, and Age-related Macular Degeneration. *Vision Resesearch* Vol.50, No.7, (March 2010), pp. 652-664, ISSN 0042-6989

Chan, K., Lu, R., Change, J.C. & Kan, Y.W. (1996) NRF2, a member of the NFE2 family of transcription factors, is not essential for murin erythropoiesis, growth, and development. *Proceedings of the National Academy of Sciences of the United States of America* Vol.93, No.24, (November 1996), pp. 13943-13948, ISSN 1091-6490

Chen, J. B., Wang, L., Chen, Y., Sternberg, P., & Cai, J. (2009). Phosphatidylinositol 3 Kinase Pathway and 4-Hydroxy-2-Nonenal-Induced Oxidative Injury in the RPE. *Investigative Ophthalmology & Visual Science* Vol.50, No.2, (February 2009), pp. 936-942, ISSN 0146-0404

Chen, W., Stambolian, D., Edwards, A.O., Branham, K.E., Othman, M., et al. (2010) Genetic variants near TIMP3 and high-density lipoprotein-associated loci influence susceptibility to age-related macular degeneration. *Proceedings of the National Academy of Sciences of the United States of America* Vol.107, No.16, (April 2010), pp. 7401-7406, ISSN 1091-6490

Crabb, J.W., Miyagi, M., Gu, X., Shadrach, K., West, K.A., Sakaguchi, H., Kamei, M., Hasan, A., Yan, L., Rayborn, M.E., et al. (2002). Drusen proteome analysis: an approach to the etiology of age-related macular degeneration. *Proceedings of the National Academy of Sciences of the United States of America* Vol.99, No.23, (November 2002), pp. 14682-14687, ISSN 1091-6490

Cullinan, S.B., & Diehl, J.A. (2004). PERK-dependent activation of Nrf2 contributes to redox homeostasis and cell survival following endoplasmic reticulum stress. *Journal of Biological Chemistry* Vol.279, No.19, (May 2004), pp. 20108-20117, ISSN 0021-9258

Cullinan, S.B., Gordan, J.D., Jin, J., Harper, J.W., & Diehl, J.A. (2004). The Keap1-BTB protein is an adaptor that bridges Nrf2 to a Cul3-based E3 ligase: oxidative stress sensing by a Cul3-Keap1 ligase. *Molecular and Cell Biology* Vol.24, No.19, (October 2004), pp. 8477-8486, ISSN 0270-7306

Cullinan, S. B., Zhang, D., Hannink, M., Arvisais, E., Kaufman, R. J., & Diehl, J. A. (2003). Nrf2 is a direct PERK substrate and effector of PERK-dependent cell survival.

Molecular and Cellular Biology Vol.23, No.20, (October 2003), pp. 7198-7209, ISSN 0270-7306

Cuervo, A.M., Stefanis, L., Fredenburg, R., Lansbury, P.T. & Sulzer, D. (2004) Impaired degradation of mutant α-synuclein by chaperone-mediated autophagy. *Science* Vol.305, No.5688, (August 2004), pp. 1292-1295, ISSN 0036-8075

D'Cruz, P.M., Yasumura, D., Weir, J., Matthes, M.T., Abderrahim, H., LaVail, M.M., & Vollrath, D. (2000). Mutation of the receptor tyrosine kinase gene Mertk in the retinal dystrophic RCS rat. *Human Molecular Genetics* Vol.9, No.4, (March 2000), pp. 645-651, ISSN 0964-6906

DeBlack, S.S. (2003). Cigarette smoking as a risk factor for cataract and age-related macular degeneration: a review of the literature. *Optometry* Vol.74, No.2, (February 2003), pp. 99-110, ISSN 1558-1527

Dinkova-Kostova, A.T., Holtzclaw, W.D., Cole, R.N., Itoh, K., Wakabayashi, N., Katoh, Y., Yamamoto, M., & Talalay, P. (2002). Direct evidence that sulfhydryl groups of Keap1 are the sensors regulating induction of phase 2 enzymes that protect against carcinogens and oxidants. *Proceedings of the National Academy of Sciences of the United States of America* Vol.99, No.18, (September 2002), pp. 11908-11913, ISSN 1091-6490

Dorrell, M.I., Aguilar, E., Jacobson, R., Yanes, O., Gariano, R., Heckenlively, J., Banin, E., Ramirez, G.A., Gasmi, M., Bird, A., Siuzdak G. & Friedlander, M. Antioxidant or neurotrophic factor treatment preserves function in a mouse model of neovascularization-associated oxidative stress. *Journal of Clinical Investigation* Vo.119, No.3, (March 2009), pp. 611-623, ISSN 0021-9738

Dunaief, J.L. (2006). Iron induced oxidative damage as a potential factor in age-related macular degeneration: the Cogan Lecture. *Investigative Ophthalmology & Visual Science* Vol.47, No.11, (November 2006), pp. 4660-4664, ISSN 0146-0404

Eggler, A.L., Liu, G., Pezzuto, J.M., van Breemen, R.B., & Mesecar, A.D. (2005). Modifying specific cysteines of the electrophile-sensing human Keap1 protein is insufficient to disrupt binding to the Nrf2 domain Neh2. *Proceedings of the National Academy of Sciences of the United States of America* Vol.102, No.29, (July 2005), pp. 10070-10075, ISSN 1091-6490

Feng, W., Yasumura, D., Matthes, M.T., LaVail, M.M., and Vollrath, D. (2002). Mertk triggers uptake of photoreceptor outer segments during phagocytosis by cultured retinal pigment epithelial cells. *Journal of Biological Chemistry* Vol.277, No.19, (May 2002), pp. 17016-17022, ISSN 0021-9258

Finnemann, S.C., Bonilha, V.L., Marmorstein, A.D., & Rodriguez-Boulan, E. (1997). Phagocytosis of rod outer segments by retinal pigment epithelial cells requires alpha(v)beta5 integrin for binding but not for internalization. *Proceedings of the National Academy of Sciences of the United States of America* Vol.94, No.24, (November 1997), pp. 12932-12937, ISSN 1091-6490

Finnemann, S.C., & Silverstein, R.L. (2001). Differential roles of CD36 and alphavbeta5 integrin in photoreceptor phagocytosis by the retinal pigment epithelium. *Journal of Experimental Medicine* Vol.194, No.9, (November 2001), pp. 1289-1298, ISSN 0022-1007

Furukawa, M., & Xiong, Y. (2005). BTB protein Keap1 targets antioxidant transcription factor Nrf2 for ubiquitination by the Cullin 3-Roc1 ligase. *Molecular and Cell Biology* Vol.25, No.1, (January 2005), pp. 162-171, ISSN 0270-7306

Galbinur, T., Averbukh, E., Banin, E., Hemo, I., & Chowers, I. (2009). Intravitreal bevacizumab therapy for neovascular age-related macular degeneration associated with poor initial visual acuity. *British Journal of Ophthalmology* Vol.93, No.10, (October 2009), pp. 1351-1352, ISSN 0007-1161

Gao, X., Dinkova-Kostova, A.T., & Talalay, P. (2001). Powerful and prolonged protection of human retinal pigment epithelial cells, keratinocytes, and mouse leukemia cells against oxidative damage: the indirect antioxidant effects of sulforaphane. *Proceedings of the National Academy of Sciences of the United States of America* Vol.98, No.26, (December 2001), pp. 15221-15226, ISSN 0027-8424

Gao, X., & Talalay, P. (2004). Induction of phase 2 genes by sulforaphane protects retinal pigment epithelial cells against photooxidative damage. *Proceedings of the National Academy of Sciences of the United States of America* Vol.101, No.28, (July 2004), pp. 10446-10451, ISSN 0027-8424

Ha, K.N., Chen, Y., Cai, J., & Sternberg, P., Jr. (2006). Increased glutathione synthesis through an ARE-Nrf2-dependent pathway by zinc in the RPE: implication for protection against oxidative stress. *Investigative Ophthalmology & Visual Science* Vol.47, No.6, (June 2006), pp. 2709-2715, ISSN 0146-0404

Hadziahmetovic, M., Dentchev, T., Song, Y., Haddad, N., He, X., Hahn, P., Pratico, D., Wen, R., Harris, Z.L., Lambris, J.D., et al. (2008). Ceruloplasmin/hephaestin knockout mice model morphologic and molecular features of AMD. *Investigative Ophthalmology & Visual Science* Vol.49, No.6, (June 2008), pp. 2728-2736, ISSN 0146-0404

Hahn, P., Qian, Y., Dentchev, T., Chen, L., Beard, J., Harris, Z.L., & Dunaief, J.L. (2004). Disruption of ceruloplasmin and hephaestin in mice causes retinal iron overload and retinal degeneration with features of age-related macular degeneration. *Proceedings of the National Academy of Sciences of the United States of America* Vol.101, No.38, (September 2004), pp. 13850-13855, ISSN 0027-8424

Ham, W.T., Jr., Mueller, H.A., Ruffolo, J.J., Jr., Millen, J.E., Cleary, S.F., Guerry, R.K., and Guerry, D., 3rd (1984). Basic mechanisms underlying the production of photochemical lesions in the mammalian retina. *Current Eye Research* Vol.3, No.1, (January 1984), pp. 165-174, ISSN 0271-3683

Hollyfield, J.G., Bonilha, V.L., Rayborn, M.E., Yang, X., Shadrach, K.G., Lu, L., Ufret, R.L., Salomon, R.G., and Perez, V.L. (2008). Oxidative damage-induced inflammation initiates age-related macular degeneration. *Nature Medicine* Vol.14, No.2, (February 2008), pp. 194-198, ISSN 1078-8956

Hong, F., Sekhar, K.R., Freeman, M.L., & Liebler, D.C. (2005). Specific patterns of electrophile adduction trigger Keap1 ubiquitination and Nrf2 activation. *Journal of Biological Chemistry* Vol.280, No.36, (September 2005), pp. 31768-31775, ISSN 0021-9258

Huang, H.C., Nguyen, T., & Pickett, C.B. (2002). Phosphorylation of Nrf2 at Ser-40 by protein kinase C regulates antioxidant response element-mediated transcription. *Journal of Biological Chemistry* Vol.277, No.45, (November 2002), pp. 42769-42774, ISSN 0021-9258

Imamura, Y., Noda, S.,Hashizume, K., Shinoda, K., Yamaguchi, M., Uchlyama, S., Shimizu, T., Mizushima, Y., Shirasawa, T. & Tsubota, K. Drusen, choroidal neovascularization, and retinal pigment epithelium dysfunction in SOD1-deficient mice: a model of age-related macular degeneration. *Proceedings of the National Academy of Sciences of the United States of America* Vol.103, No.30, (July 2006), pp. 11282-11287, ISSN 0027-8424

Imomata, Y., Tanibara, H., Tanito, M., Okyama, H., Hoshino, Y., Kinumi, T., Kawaji, T., Kondo, N., Yodoi, J & Nakamura H. Suppression of choroidal neovascularization by thioredoxin-1 via interaction with complement factor H. *Investigative Ophthalmology & Visual Science* Vol.49, No.11, (November 2008), pp. 5118-5125, ISSN 0146-0404

Ishii, T., Sato, H., Miura, K., Sagara, J., & Bannai, S. (1992). Induction of cystine transport activity by stress. *Annals of the New York Academy of Sciences* Vol.663, (November 1992), pp. 497-498, ISSN 0077-8923

Jacobson, L.P., Zhang, B.C., Zhu, Y.R., Wang, J.B., Wu, Y., Zhang, Q.N., Yu, L.Y., Qian, G.S., Kuang, S.Y., Li, Y.F., et al. (1997). Oltipraz chemoprevention trial in Qidong, People's Republic of China: study design and clinical outcomes. *Cancer Epidemiology, Biomarkers & Prevention* Vol.6, No.4, (April 1997), pp. 257-265, ISSN 1055-9965

Jain, A. K., & Jaiswal, A.K. (2006). Phosphorylation of tyrosine 568 controls nuclear export of Nrf2. *Journal of Biological Chemistry* Vol.281, No.17, (April 2006), pp. 12132-12142, ISSN 0021-9258

Johnson, J., Maher, P., and Hanneken, A. (2009). The flavonoid, eriodictyol, induces long-term protection in ARPE-19 cells through its effects on Nrf2 activation and phase 2 gene expression. *Investigative Ophthalmology & Visual Science* Vol.50, No.5, (May 2009), pp. 2398-2406, ISSN 0146-0404

Justilien, V., Pang, J.J., Renganathan, K., Zhan, X., Crabb, J.W., Kim, S.R., Sparrow, J.R., Hauswirth, W.W. & Lewin, A.S. SOD2 knockdown mouse model of early AMD. *Investigative Ophthalmology & Visual Science* Vol.48, No.10, (October 2007), pp. 4407-4420, ISSN 0146-0404

Kaarniranta, K. (2010) Autophagy-hot topic in AMD. *Acta Ophthalmologica* Vol.88, No.4, (June 2010), pp. 387-388, ISSN 1755-3768

Kaneko, H., Dridi, S., Tarallo, V., Gelfand, B.D., Fowler, B.J., Cho, W.G., Kleinman, M.E., Ponicsan, S.L., Hauswirth, W.W., Chiodo, V.A., et al. (2011). DICER1 deficit induces Alu RNA toxicity in age-related macular degeneration. *Nature* Vol.471, No.7338, (March 2011), pp. 325-330, ISSN 0028-0836

Kang, K. W., Lee, S. J., Park, J. W., & Kim, S. G. (2002). Phosphatidylinositol 3-kinase regulates nuclear translocation of NF-E2-related factor 2 through actin rearrangement in response to oxidative stress. *Molecular pharmacology* Vol.62, No.5, (November 2002), pp. 1001-1010, ISSN 0026-895X

Kang, K. W., Ryu, J. H., & Kim, S. G. (2000). The essential role of phosphatidylinositol 3-kinase and of p38 mitogen-activated protein kinase activation in the antioxidant response element-mediated rGSTA2 induction by decreased glutathione in H4IIE hepatoma cells. *Molecular pharmacology* Vol.58, No.5, (November 2000), pp. 1017-1025, ISSN 0026-895X

Kaspar, J.W. & Jaiswal, A.K. (2011) Tyrosine phosphorylation control nuclear export of Fyn, allowing Nrf2 activation of cytoprotective gene expression. *FASEB Journal* (March 2011), pp 1076-1087, ISSN 0892-6638.

Katsuoka, F., Motohashi, H., Ishii, T., Aburatani, H., Engel, J.D., & Yamamoto, M. (2005). Genetic evidence that small maf proteins are essential for the activation of antioxidant response element-dependent genes. *Molecular and Cell Biololgy* Vol.25, No.18, (September 2005), pp. 8044-8051, ISSN 0270-7306

Kensler, T.W., Wakabayashi, N., & Biswal, S. (2007). Cell survival responses to environmental stresses via the Keap1-Nrf2-ARE pathway. *Annual Review of Pharmacology and Toxicology* Vol.47, (2007), pp. 89-116, ISSN 0362-1642

Klionsky, D.J. (2007) Autophagy: from phenomenology to molecular understanding in less than a decade. *Nature Review Molecular &Cell Biology* Vol.8, (November 2007), pp. 931-937, ISSN 1471-0072

Kobayashi, A., Kang, M.I., Okawa, H., Ohtsuji, M., Zenke, Y., Chiba, T., Igarashi, K., and Yamamoto, M. (2004). Oxidative stress sensor Keap1 functions as an adaptor for Cul3-based E3 ligase to regulate proteasomal degradation of Nrf2. *Molecular and Cell Biology* Vol.24, No.16, (August 2004), pp. 7130-7139, ISSN 0270-7306

Komatsu, M., Kurokawa, H., Waguri, S., Taguchi, K., Kobayashi, A., et al. (2010) The selective autophagy substrate p62 activates the stress responsive transcription factor Nrf2 through inactivation of Keap1. *Nature Cell Biology* Vol.12, No.3, (March 2010), pp. 213-224, ISSN 1465-7392

Kong, L., Tanito, M., Huang, Z., Li, F., Zhou, X., Zaharia, A., Yodoi, J., McGinnis, J.F., & Cao, W. (2007). Delay of photoreceptor degeneration in tubby mouse by sulforaphane. *Journal of Neurochemistry* Vol.101, No.4, (May 2007), pp. 1041-1052, ISSN 0022-3042

Lee, J. M., Hanson, J. M., Chu, W. A., & Johnson, J. A. (2001). Phosphatidylinositol 3-kinase, not extracellular signal-regulated kinase, regulates activation of the antioxidant-responsive element in IMR-32 human neuroblastoma cells. *Journal of biological chemistry* Vol.276, No.23, (June 2001), pp. 20011-20016, ISSN 0021-9258

Lee, J.-H., Yu, W.H, Kuma A., Lee, S., Mohan, P.S., Peterhoff, C.M., Wolfe, D.M., Martinez-Vicente, M., Massey, A.C., Sovak, G., Uchiyama, Y., Westaway, D., Cuervo, A.M. & Nixon, R.A. (2010) Lysosomal proteolysis and autophagy require presenilin 1 and are disrupted by Alzheimer-related PS1 mutations. *Cell* Vol.141, No.7, (June 2010), pp 1146-1158, ISSN 0092-8674

Lee, P. P., Feldman, Z. W., Ostermann, J., Brown, D. S., & Sloan, F. A. (2003). Longitudinal prevalence of major eye diseases. *Archives of Ophthalmology* Vol.121, No.9, (September 2003), pp. 1303-1310, ISSN 0003-9950

Levine, B., Mizushima, N. & Virgin, H.W. (2011) Autophagy in immunity and inflammation. *Nature* Vol.469, (January 2011), pp. 323-335, ISSN 0028-0836

Mandal, M. N. A., Patlolla, J. M. R., Zheng, L., Agbaga, M. P., Tran, J. T. A., Wicker, L., Asus-Jacobi, A., Elliott, M. H., Rao, C. V., & Anderson, R. E. (2009). Curcumin protects retinal cells from light-and oxidant stress-induced cell death. *Free Radical Biology and Medicine* Vol.46, No.5, (March 2009), pp. 672-679, ISSN 0891-5849

Marzec, J. M., Christie, J. D., Reddy, S. P., Jedlicka, A. E., Vuong, H., Lanken, P. N., Aplenc, R., Yamamoto, T., Yamamoto, M., Cho, H. Y., & Kleeberger, S. R. (2007). Functional polymorphisms in the transcription factor NRF2 in humans increase the risk of acute lung injury. *Faseb Journal* Vol.21, No.9, (July 2007), pp. 2237-2246, ISSN 0892-6638 1546-1726

Martinez-Vicente, M., Talloczy, Z., Wong, E., Tang, G., Koga, H., et al. (2010) Cargo recognition failure is responsible for inefficient autophagy in Huntington's disease. *Nature Neuroscience* Vol.13, (April 2010), pp. 567-576, ISSN

McLeod, D. S., Grebe, R., Bhutto, J., Merges, C., Baba, T., & Lutty, G. A. (2009) Relationship between RPE and choriocapillaris in age-related macular degeneration. *Investigative Ophthalmology & Visual Science* Vol.50, No. 10, (October 2009), pp 4982-4991, ISSN 0146-0404

McMahon, M., Thomas, N., Itoh, K., Yamamoto, M., & Hayes, J. D. (2004). Redox-regulated turnover of Nrf2 is determined by at least two separate protein domains, the redox-sensitive Neh2 degron and the redox-insensitive Neh6 degron. *Journal of Biological Chemistry* Vol.279, No.30, (July 2004), pp. 31556-31567, ISSN 0021-9258

Mitchell, P., Wang, J. J., Smith, W., & Leeder, S. R. (2002). Smoking and the 5-year incidence of age-related maculopathy - The Blue Mountains Eye Study. *Archives of Ophthalmology* Vol.120, No.10, (October 2002), pp. 1357-1363, ISSN 0003-9950

Moiseyev, G., Takahashi, Y., Chen, Y., Gentleman, S., Redmond, T. M., Crouch, R. K., & Ma, J. X. (2006). RPE65 is an iron(II)-dependent isomerohydrolase in the retinoid visual cycle. *Journal of Biological Chemistry* Vol.281, No.5, (February 2006), pp. 2835-2840, ISSN 0021-9258

Moriarty-Craige, S.E., Ha, K.N., Sternberg, P. Jr., Lynn, M., Bressler, S., Gensler, G. & Jones, D.P. (2007) Effects off long-term zinc supplementation on plasma thiol metabolites and redox status in patients with age-related macular degeneration. *American Journal of Ophthalmology* Vo.143, No.2, (February 2007), pp. 206-211, ISSN 0002-9394

Motohashi, H., Katsuoka, F., Engel, J. D., & Yamamoto, M. (2004). Small Maf proteins serve as transcriptional cofactors for keratinocyte differentiation in the Keap1-Nrf2 regulatory pathway. *Proceedings of the National Academy of Sciences of the United States of America* Vol.101, No.17, (April 2004), pp. 6379-6384, ISSN 0027-8424

Mullins, R. F., Johnson, M. N., Faidley, E. A., Skeie, J. M., & Huang, J. (2011) Choriocapillaris vascular dropout related to density of drusen in human eyes with early age-related macular degeneration. *Investigative Ophthalmology & Visual Science* Vol.52, No. 3, (March 2011), pp 1606-1612, ISSN 0146-0404

Mullins, R. F., Russell, S. R., Anderson, D. H., & Hageman, G. S. (2000). Drusen associated with aging and age-related macular degeneration contain proteins common to extracellular deposits associated with atherosclerosis, elastosis, amyloidosis, and dense deposit disease. *Faseb Journal* Vol.14, No.7, (May 2000), pp. 835-846, ISSN 0892-6638

Nagai, N., Thimmulappa, R. K., Cano, M., Fujihara, M., Izumi-Nagai, K., Kong, X. O., Sporn, M. B., Kensler, T. W., Biswal, S., & Handa, J. I. (2009). Nrf2 is a critical modulator of the innate immune response in a model of uveitis. *Free Radical Biology and Medicine* Vol.47, No.3, (August 2009), pp. 300-306, ISSN 0891-5849

Nelson, K. C., Armstrong, J. S., Moriarty, S., Cai, J. Y., Wu, M. W. H., Sternberg, P., & Jones, D. P. (2002). Protection of retinal pigment epithelial cells from oxidative damage by oltipraz, a cancer chemopreventive agent. *Investigative Ophthalmology & Visual Science* Vol.43, No.11, (November 2002), pp. 3550-3554, ISSN 0146-0404

Nelson, K.C., Carlson, J, Newman, M.L., Sternberg, P. Jr., Jones, D.P., Kavanagh, T.J., Diaz, D., Cai, J. & Wu M. (1999) Effect of dietary inducer dimethylfumarate on glutathione in cultured human retinal pigment epithelial cells. *Investigative Ophthalmology & Visual Science* Vol.40, No. 9, (August 1999), pp 1927-1935, ISSN 0146-0404

Niture, S.K., Jain, A.K., Shelton, P.M. & Jaiswal, A.K. (2011) Src subfamily kinases regulate nuclear export and degradation of the transcription factor Nrf2 to switch off Nrf2-mediated antioxidant activation of cytoprotective gene expression. *Journal of Biological Chemistry.* in press, (June 2011), ISSN 0021-9258

Okawa, H., Motohashi, H., Kobayashi, A., Aburatani, H., Kensler, T. W., & Yamamoto, M. (2006). Hepatocyte-specific deletion of the keap1 gene activates Nrf2 and confers potent resistance against acute drug toxicity. *Biochemical and Biophysical Research Communications* Vol.339, No.1, (January 2006), pp. 79-88, ISSN 0006-291X

Organisciak, D. T., Wang, H. M., Li, Z. Y., & Tso, M. O. M. (1985). The Protective Effect of Ascorbate in Retinal Light Damage of Rats. *Investigative Ophthalmology & Visual Science* Vol.26, No.11, (November 1985), pp. 1580-1588, ISSN 0146-0404

Osburn, W. O., & Kensler, T. W. (2008). Nrf2 signaling: An adaptive response pathway for protection against environmental toxic insults. *Mutation Research-Reviews in Mutation Research* Vol.659, No.1-2, (July-August 2008), pp. 31-39, ISSN 1383-5742

Pearson, K.J., Lewis, K.N., Price, N.L., et al. (2008) Nrf2 mediates cancer protection but not prolongevity induced by caloric restriction. *Proceedings of the National Academy of Sciences of the United States of America* Vol.105, No.7, (February 2008), pp. 2325-2330, ISSN 0027-8424

Pi, J., Bai, Y., Reece, J. M., Williams, J., Liu, D., Freeman, M. L., Fahl, W. E., Shugar, D., Liu, J., Qu, W., Collins, S., & Waalkes, M. P. (2007). Molecular mechanism of human Nrf2 activation and degradation: role of sequential phosphorylation by protein kinase CK2. *Free Radical Biology & Medicine* Vol.42, No.12, (June 15 2007), pp. 1797-1806, ISSN 0891-5849

Pitha-Rowe, I., Liby, K., Royce, D., & Sporn, M. (2009). Synthetic Triterpenoids Attenuate Cytotoxic Retinal Injury: Cross-talk between Nrf2 and PI3K/AKT Signaling through Inhibition of the Lipid Phosphatase PTEN. *Investigative Ophthalmology & Visual Science* Vol.50, No.11, (November 2009), pp. 5339-5347, ISSN 0146-0404

Pool-Zobel, B., Veeriah, S., & Bohmer, F. D. (2005). Modulation of xenobiotic metabolising enzymes by anticarcinogens - focus on glutathione S-transferases and their role as targets of dietary chemoprevention in colorectal carcinogenesis. *Mutation Research-Fundamental and Molecular Mechanisms of Mutagenesis* Vol.591, No.1-2, (December 2005), pp. 74-92, ISSN 0027-5107

Pryor, W. A., Prier, D. G., & Church, D. F. (1983). Electron-Spin Resonance Study of Mainstream and Sidestream Cigarette-Smoke - Nature of the Free-Radicals in Gas-Phase Smoke and in Cigarette Tar. *Environmental Health Perspectives* Vol.47, (January 1983), pp. 345-355, ISSN 0091-6765

Rada, P., Rojo, A. I., Chowdhry, S., McMahon, M., Hayes, J. D., & Cuadrado, A. (2011). SCF/{beta}-TrCP promotes glycogen synthase kinase 3-dependent degradation of the Nrf2 transcription factor in a Keap1-independent manner. *Molecular and Cellular Biology* Vol.31, No.6, (March 2011), pp. 1121-1133, ISSN 1098-5549

Ramkumar, H. L., Chan, C. C., & Zhang, J. (2010). Retinal ultrastructure of murine models of dry age-related macular degeneration (AMD). *Progress in Retinal and Eye Research* Vol.29, No.3, (May 2010), pp. 169-190, ISSN 1350-9462

Rangasamy, T., Cho, C. Y., Thimmulappa, R. K., Zhen, L. J., Srisuma, S. S., Kensler, T. W., Yamamoto, M., Petrache, I., Tuder, R. M., & Biswal, S. (2004). Genetic ablation of Nrf2 enhances susceptibility to cigarette smoke-induced emphysema in mice. *Journal of Clinical Investigation* Vol.114, No.9, (November 2004), pp. 1248-1259, ISSN 0021-9738

Rosenfeld, P. J., Brown, D. M., Heier, J. S., Boyer, D. S., Kaiser, P. K., Chung, C. Y., & Kim, R. Y. (2006). Ranibizumab for neovascular age-related macular degeneration. *New England Journal of Medicine* Vol.355, No.14, (October 2006), pp. 1419-1431, ISSN 0028-4793

Saint-Geniez, M., Kurihara, T., Sekiyama, E., Maldonado, A. E., & D'Amore, P. A. (2009). An essential role for RPE-derived soluble VEGF in the maintenance of the choriocapillaris. *Proceedings of the National Academy of Sciences of the United States of America* Vol.106, No.44, (November 2009), pp. 18751-18756, ISSN 0027-8424

Salazar, M., Rojo, A. I., Velasco, D., de Sagarra, R. M., & Cuadrado, A. (2006). Glycogen synthase kinase-3beta inhibits the xenobiotic and antioxidant cell response by direct phosphorylation and nuclear exclusion of the transcription factor Nrf2. *Journal of Biological Chemistry* Vol.281, No.21, (May 2006), pp. 14841-14851, ISSN 0021-9258

Sasaki, H., Sato, H., Kuriyama-Matsumura, K., Sato, K., Maebara, K., Wang, H. Y., Tamba, M., Itoh, K., Yamamoto, M., & Bannai, S. (2002). Electrophile response element-mediated induction of the cystine/glutamate exchange transporter gene expression. *Journal of Biological Chemistry* Vol.277, No.47, (November 2002), pp. 44765-44771, ISSN 0021-9258

Sato, H., Tamba, M., Ishii, T., & Bannai, S. (1999). Cloning and expression of a plasma membrane cystine/glutamate exchange transporter composed of two distinct proteins. *Journal of Biological Chemistry* Vol.274, No.17, (April 1999), pp. 11455-11458, ISSN 0021-9258

Shen, G., Hebbar, V., Nair, S., Xu, C., Li, W., Lin, W., Keum, Y. S., Han, J., Gallo, M. A., & Kong, A. N. (2004). Regulation of Nrf2 transactivation domain activity. The differential effects of mitogen-activated protein kinase cascades and synergistic stimulatory effect of Raf and CREB-binding protein. *Journal of Biological Chemistry* Vol.279, No.22, (May 2004), pp. 23052-23060, ISSN 0021-9258

Sherratt, P. J., Huang, H. C., Nguyen, T., & Pickett, C. B. (2004). Role of protein phosphorylation in the regulation of NF-E2-related factor 2 activity. *Methods in Enzymology* Vol.378, (2004), pp. 286-301, ISSN 0076-6879

Shibata, T., Iuchi, Y., Okada, F., Kuwata, K., Yamanobe, T., Bannai, S., Tomita, Y., Tomita, Y. & Fujii J. (2009) Aggravation of ischemia-reperfusion-triggered acute renal failure in *xCT*-deficient mice. *Archives of Biochemistry and Biophysic* Vol.490, No.1, (October 2009),pp. 63-69, ISSN 0003-9861

Shibata, T., Ohta, T., Tong, K.I., Kokubu, A., Odogawa, R., Tsuta, K., Asamura, H., Yamamoto, M. & Hirohashi S. (2008). Cancer related mutations in *NRF2* impair its recognition by Keap1-Cul3 E3 ligase and promote malignancy. *Proceedings of the*

National Academy of Sciences of the United States of America Vol.105, No.36, (September 2008), pp. 13568-13573, ISSN 0027-8424

Smith, W., Assink, J., Klein, R., Mitchell, P., Klaver, C. C. W., Klein, B. E. K., Hofman, A., Jensen, S., Wang, J. J., & de Jong, P. T. V. M. (2001). Risk factors for age related macular degeneration - Pooled findings from three continents. *Ophthalmology* Vol.108, No.4, (April 2001), pp. 697-704, ISSN 0161-6420

Sparrow, J. R., Fishkin, N., Zhou, J. L., Cai, B. L., Jang, Y. P., Krane, S., Itagaki, Y., & Nakanishi, K. (2003). A2E, a byproduct of the visual cycle. *Vision Research* Vol.43, No.28, (December 2003), pp. 2983-2990, ISSN 0042-6989

Sun, Z., Huang, Z., & Zhang, D. D. (2009). Phosphorylation of Nrf2 at multiple sites by MAP kinases has a limited contribution in modulating the Nrf2-dependent antioxidant response. *PLoS One* Vol.4, No.8, (August 2009), pp. e6588, ISSN 1932-6203

Tanito, M., Masutani, H., Kim, Y. C., Nishikawa, M., Ohira, A., & Yodoi, J. (2005). Sulforaphane induces thioredoxin through the antioxidant-responsive element and attenuates retinal light damage in mice. *Investigative Ophthalmology & Visual Science* Vol.46, No.3, (March 2005), pp. 979-987, ISSN 0146-0404

Tomobe, K., Shinozuka, T., Kuroiwa, M. & Nomura Y. (2011) Age-related changes of Nrf2 and phosphorylated GSH-3β in a mouse model of accelerated aging (SAMP8). *Archives of Gerontology and Geriatrics* Article in Press, ISSN 0167-4943

Tso, M. O. M., Woodford, B. J., & Lam, K. W. (1984). Distribution of Ascorbate in Normal Primate Retina and after Photic Injury - a Biochemical, Morphological Correlated Study. *Current Eye Research* Vol.3, No.1, (January 1984), pp. 181-191, ISSN 0271-3683

Tso, M. O. M., Zhang, C., Abler, A. S., Chang, C. J., Wong, F., Chang, G. Q., & Lam, T. T. (1994). Apoptosis Leads to Photoreceptor Degeneration in Inherited Retinal Dystrophy of Rcs Rats. *Investigative Ophthalmology & Visual Science* Vol.35, No.6, (May 1994), pp. 2693-2699, ISSN 0146-0404

Uno, K., Prow, T. W., Bhutto, I. A., Yerrapureddy, A., McLeod, D. S., Yamamoto, M., Reddy, S. P., & Lutty, G. A. (2010). Role of Nrf2 in retinal vascular development and the vaso-obliterative phase of oxygen-induced retinopathy. *Experimental Eye Research* Vol.90, No.4, (April 2010), pp. 493-500, ISSN 0014-4835

Wagner, C. A., Lang, F., & Broer, S. (2001). Function and structure of heterodimeric amino acid transporters. *American Journal of Physiology-Cell Physiology* Vol.281, No.4, (October 2001), pp. C1077-C1093, ISSN 0363-6143

Wakabayashi, N., Slocum, S. L., Skoko, J. J., Shin, S., & Kensler, T. W. (2010). When NRF2 Talks, Who's Listening? *Antioxidants & Redox Signaling* Vol.13, No.11, (December 2010), pp. 1649-1663, ISSN 1523-0864

Wang, A. L., Lukas, T. J., Yuan, M., Du, N., Tso, M. O., & Neufeld, A. H. (2009). Autophagy and Exosomes in the Aged Retinal Pigment Epithelium: Possible Relevance to Drusen Formation and Age-Related Macular Degeneration. *PLoS One* Vol.4, No.1, (January 8 2009), pp. e4160, ISSN 1932-6203

Wang, L., Chen, Y., Sternberg, P., & Cai, J. (2008). Essential roles of the PI3 kinase/Akt pathway in regulating Nrf2-dependent antioxidant functions in the RPE. *Investigative Ophthalmology & Visual Science* Vol.49, No.4, (April 2008), pp. 1671-1678, ISSN 0146-0404

Wei, Y., Gong, J., Yoshida, T., Eberhart, C.G., Xu, Z., Kombairaju P., Spron, M.B., Handa, J.T. & Duh, E.J. (2011) Nrf2 has a protective role against neuronal and capillary degeneration in retinal ischemia-reperfusion injury. *Free Radical Biology & Medicine* Vol.51, No.1 (July 2011), pp 216-224, ISSN 0891-5849

Winkler, B.S. (2008) An hypothesis to account for the renewal of outer segments in rod and cone photoreceptor cells: renewal as a surrogate antioxidant. *Investigative Ophthalmology & Visual Science* Vol.49, No.8, (August 2008), pp. 3259-3261, ISSN 0146-0404

Wu, Y. L., Yanase, E., Feng, X. D., Siegel, M. M., & Sparrow, J. R. (2010). Structural characterization of bisretinoid A2E photocleavage products and implications for age-related macular degeneration. *Proceedings of the National Academy of Sciences of the United States of America* Vol.107, No.16, (April 20 2010), pp. 7275-7280, ISSN 0027-8424

Xue, L. L., Gollapalli, D. R., Maiti, P., Jahng, W. J., & Rando, R. R. (2004). A palmitoylation switch mechanism in the regulation of the visual cycle. *Cell* Vol.117, No.6, (June 11 2004), pp. 761-771, ISSN 0092-8674

Yoh, K., Itoh, K., Enomoto, A., Hirayama, A., Yamaguchi, N., Kobayashi, M., Morito, N., Koyama, A., Yamamoto, M., & Takahashi, S. (2001). Nrf2-deficient female mice develop lupus-like autoimmune nephritis. *Kidney International* Vol.60, No.4, (October 2001), pp. 1343-1353, ISSN 0085-2538

Young, R. W. (1967). The renewal of photoreceptor cell outer segments. *The Journal of Cell Biology* Vol.33, No.1, (April 1967), pp. 61-72, ISSN 0021-9525

Young, R. W., & Bok, D. (1969). Participation of the retinal pigment epithelium in the rod outer segment renewal process. *The Journal of Cell Biology* V ol.42, No.2, (August 1969), pp. 392-403, ISSN 0021-9525

Yu, R., Chen, C., Mo, Y. Y., Hebbar, V., Owuor, E. D., Tann, T. H., & Kong, A. N. T. (2000). Activation of mitogen-activated protein kinase pathways induces antioxidant response element-mediated gene expression via a Nrf2-dependent mechanism. *Journal of Biological Chemistry* Vol.275, No.51, (December 2000), pp. 39907-39913, ISSN 0021-9258

Yu, R., Mandlekar, S., Lei, W., Fahl, W. E., Tan, T. H., & Kong, A. N. (2000). p38 mitogen-activated protein kinase negatively regulates the induction of phase II drug-metabolizing enzymes that detoxify carcinogens. *Journal of Biological Chemistry* Vol.275, No.4, (January 2000c), pp. 2322-2327, ISSN 0021-9258

Zhang, J., Hosoya, T., Maruyama, A., Nishikawa, K., Maher, J. M., Ohta, T., Motohashi, H., Fukamizu, A., Shibahara, S., Yamamoto, M., & Itoh, K. (2007). Nrf2 Neh5 domain is differentially utilized in the transactivation of cytoprotective genes. *Biochemical Journal* Vol.404, (June 2007), pp. 459-466, ISSN 0264-6021

Zhao, Z. Y., Chen, Y., Wang, J., Sternberg, P., Freeman, M. L., Grossniklaus, H. E., & Cai, J. Y. (2011). Age-Related Retinopathy in NRF2-Deficient Mice. *PLoS One* Vol.6, No.4, (April 2011), pp. e19456 ISSN 1932-6203

Zhou, J. L., Jang, Y. P., Kim, S. R., & Sparrow, J. R. (2006). Complement activation by photooxidation products of A2E, a lipofuscin constituent of the retinal pigment epithelium. *Proceedings of the National Academy of Sciences of the United States of America* Vol.103, No.44, (October 2006), pp. 16182-16187, ISSN 0027-8424

Zipper, L. M., & Mulcahy, R. T. (2000). Inhibition of ERK and p38 MAP kinases inhibits binding of Nrf2 and induction of GCS genes. *Biochemical and Biophysical Research Communications* Vol.278, No.2, (November 2000), pp. 484-492, ISSN 0006-291X

Retinitis Pigmentosa in Northern Sweden – From Gene to Treatment

Irina Golovleva and Marie Burstedt
University Hospital of Umeå, Umeå, Sweden

1. Introduction

Blindness is a loss of vision resulting in the inability to continue with a normal lifestyle. The prevalence of blindness varies from country to country and from region to region within the same country. An average estimate of the number of blind people in industrialized countries is 1–2 per 2000, compared to 5–10 per 1000 in developing countries. According to World Health Organisation estimates, there are between 27 and 35 million blind people in the world today.

Retinal dystrophies and degenerations represent a heterogeneous group of disorders affecting the function of the retina. They are characterized by degeneration of photoreceptors or adjacent cells such as retinal pigment epithelium or Müller cells. Retinitis pigmentosa (RP), hereditary maculopathies, and age-related macular degeneration (AMD) are representative of these diseases. RP as well as macular degeneration can be part of syndromes with symptoms from other organs or organ systems, for example, Usher syndrome with RP and deafness. More than 190 loci for different retinal diseases have been localized, and 140 genes have been identified (http://www.sph.uth.tmc.edu/Retnet/).

In northern Sweden the presence of all hereditary disorders is higher than in the southern part of the country. Explanations offered include a low migration rate in the sixteenth to nineteenth centuries and a certain number of marriages among relatives, which influenced the presence of autosomal recessive disorders. Furthermore, a disposition to a genetic abnormality in a geographically restricted area gave rise to a 'founder' effect, which influenced the presence of autosomal dominant disorders. These factors are taken into consideration in studies of all hereditary disorders, including those affecting vision.

2. Retinitis pigmentosa

Retinitis pigmentosa is a genetically and clinically heterogeneous group of hereditary retinopathies characterized by a degeneration of photoreceptors (rods primary) with a progressive loss of peripheral vision. This leads to night blindness, 'tunnel vision', and eventually, complete blindness. Typical signs of the disease, except for night blindness and progressive loss of the peripheral visual field, are typical pigment deposition in the retina, attenuation of the retinal blood vessels, and optic disc pallor. The diagnosis is confirmed by an abnormal or extinguished electroretinogram (ERG). RP can be nonsyndromic, syndromic, or systemic, when multiple tissues are affected. Nonsyndromic RP can be inherited in autosomal dominant (15–25%), autosomal recessive (5–20%), and X-linked (5–15%) manners (Daiger & Pagon, 2000). However, an inheritance pattern is still unknown in many cases. So-called simplex usually represents an isolated case without any family history. Due to different degrees of penetrance and expressivity of RP genes, the phenotype can vary between families and even within the same family (Shintani et al., 2009).

The prevalence in the United States and Europe is approximately 1/3500 to 1/4000, and the disorder is the most common cause of blindness among young adults. In Denmark the lifetime risk of developing RP is 1/2500 (Haim et al., 2002), and in Sweden it is 1/2000 (Burstedt et al., 1999). Similar frequencies can be expected in other populations, but they have not been well documented. Frequency of RP in certain isolated or consanguineous populations might be higher due to mutations in particular genes (Daiger & Pagon, 2000). Among known loci and genes there are 57 identified for autosomal dominant RP and autosomal recessive RP. Many genes associated with RP encode proteins functioning as photoreceptor transcription factors; others are involved in phototransduction and the visual cycle or photoreceptor structure (Phelan & Bok, 2000; Fig. 1). Despite many retinal diseases having been mapped to specific chromosomal regions, the genes and their functions still have not been identified in all cases.

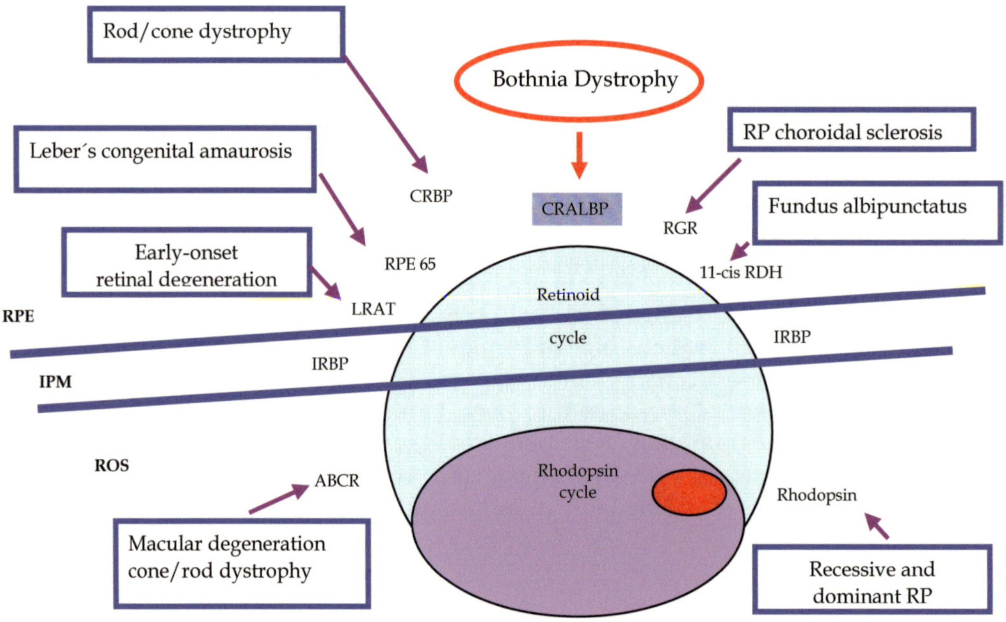

Fig. 1. Visual cycle proteins cause retinal degenerations. CRBP = cellular retinol binding protein, RPE65 = retinal pigment epithelium-specific protein 65kDa, LRAT = lecithin retinol acyltransferase, IRBP = interphotoreceptor retinoid-binding protein, RPE = retinal pigment epithelium, IPM = interphotoreceptor matrix, ROS = rod outer segment, ABCR = retina-specific ATP-binding cassette transporter, CRALBP = retinaldehyde-binding protein 1, RGR = retinal G protein coupled receptor, 11-cis RDH = retinol dehydrogenase 5 (11-cis/9-cis).

In Västerbotten County of northern Sweden 160 RP cases were identified and genetic defects were found in 66%, representing 79 patients with autosomal recessive RP of Bothnia type and 27 patients with autosomal dominant RP. However, genetic mechanisms of RP are still unknown in patients from other counties of northern Sweden. In this chapter we will focus on a disease with characteristic phenotype common in northern Sweden form of autosomal recessive RP, Bothnia dystrophy.

2.1 Autosomal recessive RP, Bothnia Dystrophy (BD)

Examination of medical records for patients with RP in Västerbotten County in northern Sweden has shown an accumulation of cases with a unique phenotype of RP called Bothnia dystrophy. Bothnia is the region in northern Sweden west of the Gulf of Bothnia, historically known as Bothnia Occidentalis (Fig. 2). Affected individuals showed night blindness with onset in early childhood, retinitis punctata albescens (RPA) at some stage of the disease, macular degeneration, and markedly elevated dark adaptation (DA) thresholds.

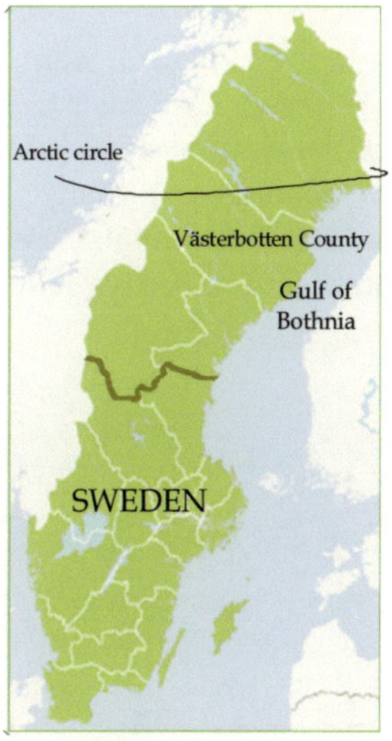

Fig. 2. The map shows the location of Västerbotten County in Scandinavia.

2.1.1 Genetic cause of BD

Initially, twenty patients from seven families originating from the same geographic area were included in the linkage analysis study aimed at identifying a disease-causing gene (Burstedt et al., 1999). All affected individuals had a nonsyndromic type of retinal degeneration inherited in an autosomal recessive way (Fig. 3). By statistical two-point lod (logarithm [base 10] of odds) score analysis, which is used to determine the linkage between trait and a chromosome marker, BD was mapped between the markers D15S526 and FES on chromosome 15q26.1. The D15S116, located near the *RLBP1* gene showed a maximum lod score of 7.79. Since lod score greater than 3 is considered evidence for linkage, the *RLBP1* gene was a strong candidate to cause the BD. Mutation analysis showed that all patients were homozygous for a cytosine (C) to thymine (T) change in exon 7 of the *RLBP1* gene, resulting in a substitution of a conservative arginine to tryptophan at position 234 (c.700C>T, p.R234W) in encoded cellular retinaldehyde-binding protein (Burstedt et al., 1999). No homozygotes for the c.700C>T mutation were found among 33 unaffected control subjects who underwent ophthalmologic examinations or 92 anonymous blood donors.

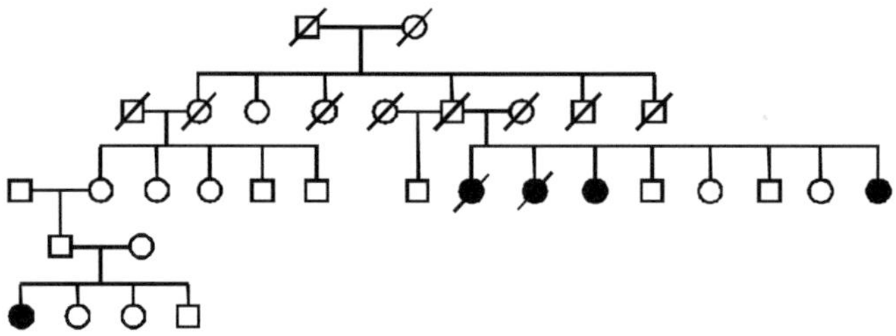

Fig. 3. A pedigree demonstrating autosomal recessive inheritance of BD in one of the families used for linkage analysis study.

2.1.2 Compound heterozygosity in BD

Sixty-nine BD cases homozygous for the c.700C>T were identified amongst patients with retinal dystrophies. In addition, 10 patients with similar to BD phenotype were heterozygous. Further screening for known mutations causing autosomal recessive RP revealed a second *RLBP1* mutation, a thymine (T) to adenine (A) change, resulting in a substitution of a methionine to lysine, c.677 T>A, p.M226K (Köhn et al., 2008). R234W and M226K were shown to be allelic and the patients were compound heterozygotes, c.[677T>A]+[700C>T] (Fig. 4).

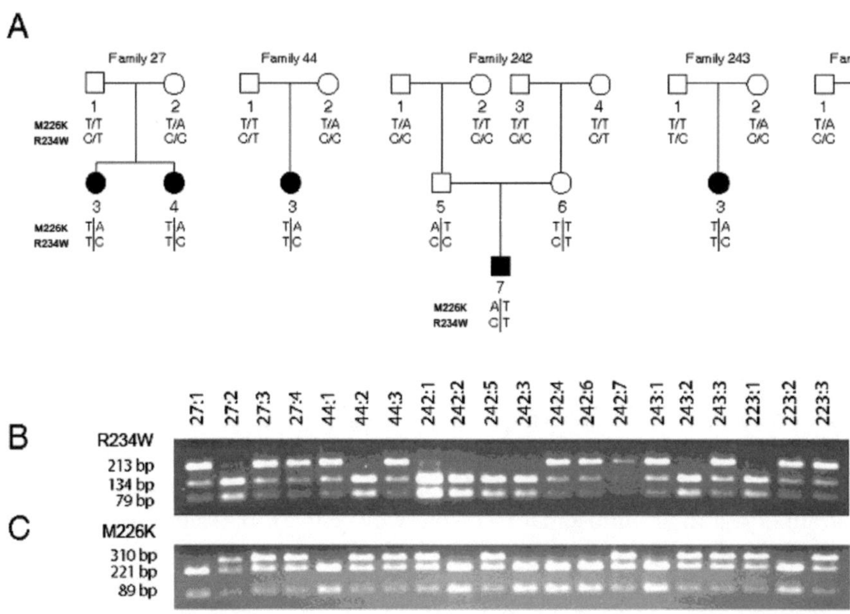

Fig. 4. Pedigrees of compound heterozygotes (A) and segregation analysis of *RLBP1* c.700C>T (B) and c.677T>A (C) performed by polymerase chain reaction and restriction fragment length polymorphism. (Figure published in Invest Ophthal Vis Sci, 2008;49(7):3172–3177).

Frequency of c.677 T>A allele in a matched control population was 0.0021. Among RP patients from northern Sweden two were homozygotes for p.M226K mutation. Based on allele frequency of R234W (3/250) and M226K (1/466), we believe that R234W was the first mutation to appear in northern Sweden, resulting in expected disease incidence of 1.5 per 10,000 in a population of 257,000 inhabitants.

Notably, one *RLBP1* compound heterozygote BD patient tested for 848 mutations in 29 genes causing autosomal dominant RP was shown to be a carrier of a mutation in carbonic anhydrase IV (CAIV), known to be associated with autosomal dominant retinitis pigmentosa RP17 (Rebello et al., 2004; Yang et al., 2005). Presence of this sequence variant in 6 out of 143 blood donors from a control Swedish population (4%) and phenotype undistinguishable from the other BD patients casts doubt on the pathogenic role of the CAIV (Köhn et al., 2008), though modifier genes switching off the mutant CAIV protein or other factors resisting its function in carriers of Swedish origin remain to be investigated.

2.1.3 *RLBP1* mutations in RP

To date, at least 12 mutations representing single nucleotide changes, in addition to small and one gross deletion have been reported (http://www.hgmd.cf.ac.uk). First homozygous *RLBP1* mutation was found in a consanguineous family of Indian origin and in one of consanguineous kindred from Saudi Arabia, both diagnosed with retinitis punctata albescens (Maw et al., 1997; Katsanis et al., 2001). Three additional mutations in the *RLBP1* gene were identified in the patients of European ancestry with recessively inherited RPA (Morimura et al., 1999), and in patients of Newfoundland origin with a severe rod cone dystrophy two splice junction mutations were detected (Eichers et al., 2002). The reported cases of retinal degeneration associated with *RLBP1* mutations were either homozygous or compound heterozygous (Demirci et al., 2004; Eichers et al., 2002; Fishman et al., 2004; Morimura et al., 1999; Nakamura et al., 2005). One of the compound heterozygotes, a Japanese patient with RPA, carried the c.700C>T mutation on one allele (Nakamura et al., 2005). Finally, changes involving single nucleotides are not the only type of mutation that affects the *RLBP1* gene. A large homozygous deletion was described in a RPA patient (Humbert et al., 2006).

2.1.4 Cellular retinaldehyde-binding protein (CRALBP)

RLBP1 gene mapped to chromosome 15q26 (Rosenfeld & Dryja, 1995) encodes the human cellular retinaldehyde-binding protein (CRALBP) expressing in outer epithelium of the iris, ciliary body pigment epithelium, cornea, optic nerve, pineal gland, Müller cells of the retina, and retinal pigment epithelium (RPE) (Bridges et al., 1987; Bunt-Milan & Saari, 1983; Eisenfeldt et al., 1985; Futterman & Saari, 1977; Saari et al., 1997; Sarthy, 1996). In the RPE, CRALBP functions as a carrier protein for endogenous retinoids, such as 11-cis-retinol, participating in the visual cycle. 11-cis-retinol can either be stored as an ester in the RPE or become oxidized to 11-cis-retinal by 11-cis-retinol dehydrogenase for visual pigment regeneration, and consecutively recycled back to the outer segment of photoreceptor cells of the retina (Saari, 1990). In vitro studies indicate that the presence of CRALBP diminishes the esterification and enhances oxidation of 11-cis-retinol (Saari et al., 1994).

A missense mutation of a conserved residue arginine at position 150 of CRALBP abolished binding to 11-cis-retinaldehyde. The mutation was shown to be associated with an atypical form of autosomal recessive RP in a small consanguineous Indian family (Maw et al., 1997).

We evaluated binding activities for two recombinant mutant proteins causing BD (Golovleva et al., 2003). M226K mutation completely abolished binding of the recombinant protein with 11-cis retinaldehyde, while the R234W, in contrast, increased binding activity of the recombinant CRALBP (Fig. 5). Double mutant M226K + R234W showed less solubility than the wild type rCRALBP (Köhn et al., 2008).

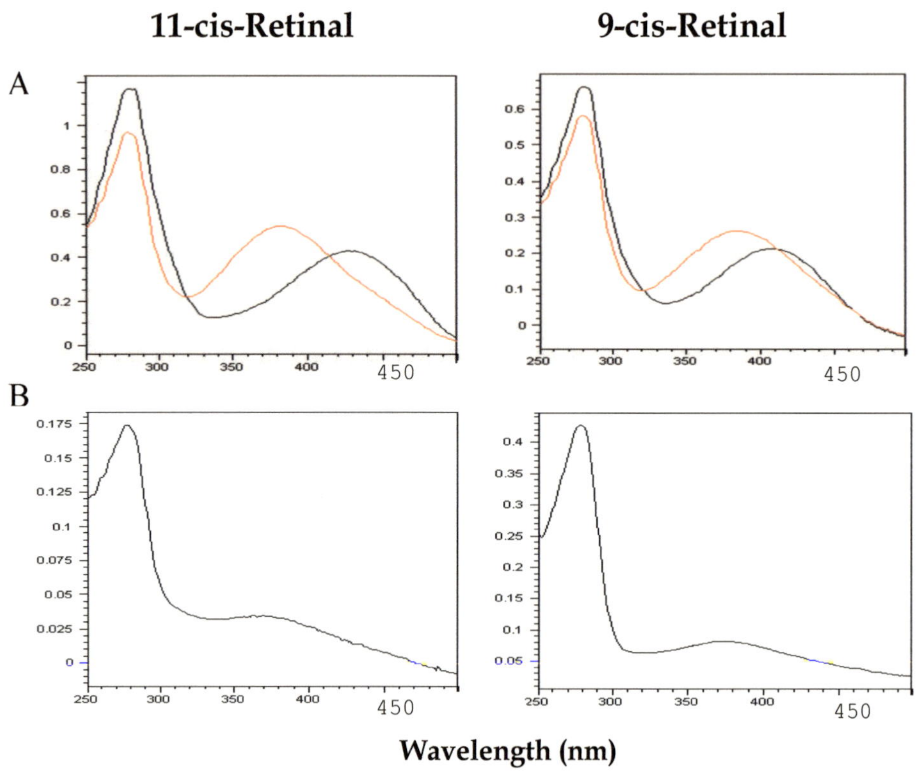

Fig. 5. Retinoid binding analysis of CRALBP mutants R234W (A) and M226K (B). UV-visible absorption spectra are shown before and after exposure to bleaching illumination following retinoid labelling with either 11-cis- or 9-cis-retinal. Spectra from wild-type rCRALBP (black line) and mutant R234W (red line) are indistinguishable and reflect stoichiometric binding of 11-cis- and 9-cis-retinal. The absorption spectra from mutant M226K show no chromophore absorbance at 425 nm or 400 nm, indicating no bound retinoid (Figure published in J Biol Chem, 2001;278:14,12397–12402).

We also analysed *RLBP1* promoter by sequencing 4kb in the upstream region in two BD compound heterozygotes. Seven single nucleotide polymorphisms (SNP) were identified; six had been reported previously and one was unique (cytosine to thymine change at position 2614, C2614T). Haplotype was constructed for BD patients. R234W and C2614T were both associated with BD phenotype. In experiments with reporter gene expression, decrease of expression level was shown when using either the entire 'affected' promoter haplotype or only C2614T (Golovleva, personal communication).

Thus, M226K mutation resulted in loss of functional CRALBP, which is true even for R234W mutant, since gene expression was decreased due to sequence variant in promoter.

2.2 Phenotype of retinitis pigmentosa of Bothnia type

All 79 patients originating from Västerbotten County, with a population of 257,000 inhabitants, present the phenotype caused by loss of CRALBP function.

2.2.1 Clinical findings and effects of age

The BD phenotype is characterized by central and peripheral degeneration of the retina with a unique expression of retinitis pigmentosa. All BD patients from the north of Sweden being homozygous for either the c.700C>T (p.R234W) (n = 67) or for the c.677T>A (p.M226K) (n = 2), and compound heterozygous [c.677T>A]+[c.700C>T] (p.M226K+p.R234W) (n = 10), have a clinical expression of the disease with a progression of retinal degeneration. The progressive maculopathy in BD presents an overall decrease of the visual acuity (VA) with age, leading to legal blindness in early adulthood (Fig. 6; Burstedt et al., 2001).

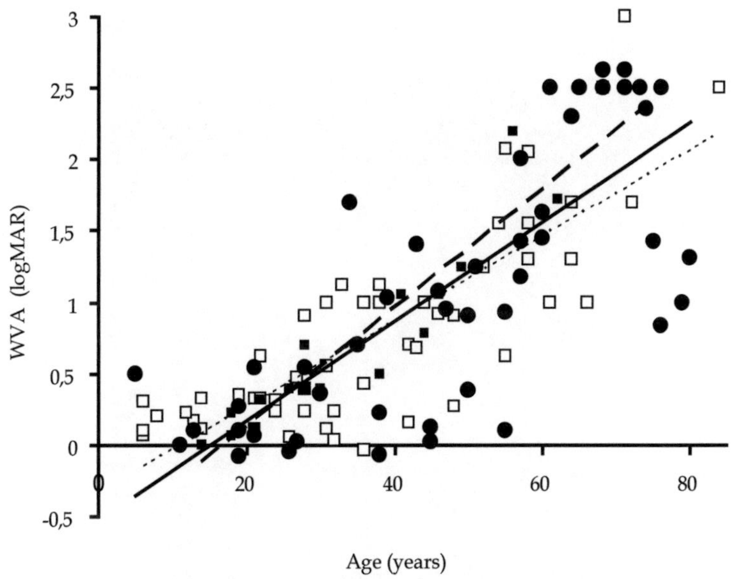

Fig. 6. Scatterplot of BD patients showing the relation of weighted distance logMAR visual acuity (WVA) with age. (•) Single observations of WVA vs. age in homozygotes c.700C>T (p.R234W); n = 49, (y = 0.035 × -0.53). (□) Retrospective recordings of WVA vs. age in compound heterozygotes [c.677T>A] + [c.700C>T] (p.M226K + p.R234W); n = 10 (y = 0.04 × −0.7), and homozygotes c.677T>A (p.M226K) (■); n = 2 (y = 0.03 × -0.32). Trendlines are drawn.

Notably, testing of monocular low-contrast VA using Sloan letter logarithmic translucent contrast charts (10% and 2.5%, Precision Vision®) allowed recording of measurable results, predominantly in the younger patients (Burstedt et al., 2005).

The retinal findings in BD patients show distinct maculopathy with central pigment deposits in the teens, and areolar maculopathy is observed in the younger adults (Burstedt et al., 1999, 2001, 2010). In the peripheral retina the pigmentations are similar to a 'salt and pepper' pattern and round retinal atrophies develop paracentrally and/or peripherally with age. The areolar atrophies are the most common peripheral findings in BD fundus as the degeneration progresses, though discrete pigmentations with an appearance similar to bone spicules may occasionally be found. No premature cataract of significance is observed in BD, and in advanced cases narrowing of the retinal vessels and pale optic disc are not typical findings (Fig. 7).

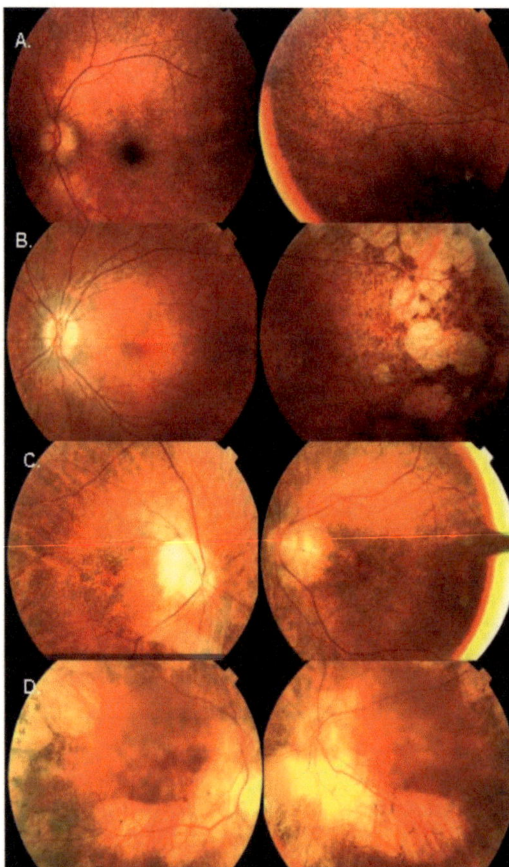

Fig. 7. Fundus photography. (A) 16-year-old girl, discrete central maculopathy and peripheral mottling, (WVA, weighted visual acuity, 0.00 logMAR). (B) 25-year-old woman with maculopathy and peripheral areolar atrophies (WVA 0.5 logMAR). (C) 41-year-old woman with central maculopathy and central RPA changes (WVA 0.3 logMAR). (D) 52-year-old woman with maculopathy, pigmentary changes (WVA 1.2 logMAR), and advanced retinal degeneration with retinal atrophies.

2.2.2 Morphological changes in BD found with ocular computed tomography

A generalized early decrease of the central foveal thickness (Ø 1 mm) and the inner ring of the retina (Ø 3 mm) are shown with optical coherence tomography (Burstedt et al., 2010). In the outer ring (Ø 6 mm), the generalized thinning is seen predominately in the inferior regions of the OCT measurement and a trend of more preserved areas of the retinal thickness of the superior and nasal regions are observed. The total macular volumes in all ages of BD patients are low compared with those of controls. Comparisons of macular thickness in each region of the BD patients and age-matched controls are presented in Fig. 8.

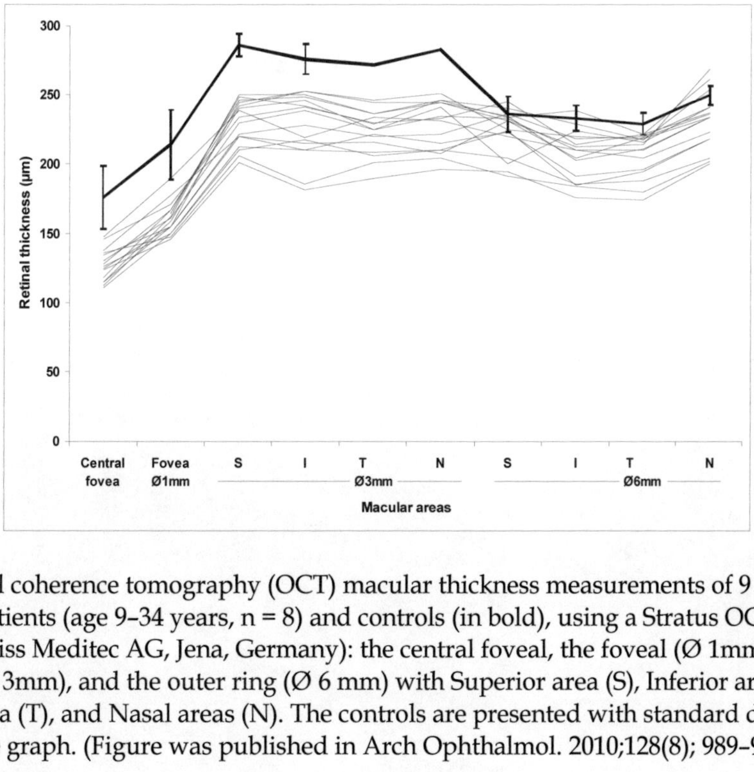

Fig. 8. Optical coherence tomography (OCT) macular thickness measurements of 9 areas in young BD patients (age 9–34 years, n = 8) and controls (in bold), using a Stratus OCT, model 3000 (Carl Zeiss Meditec AG, Jena, Germany): the central foveal, the foveal (Ø 1mm), the inner ring (Ø 3mm), and the outer ring (Ø 6 mm) with Superior area (S), Inferior area (I), Temporal area (T), and Nasal areas (N). The controls are presented with standard deviation shown on the graph. (Figure was published in Arch Ophthalmol. 2010;128(8); 989–995).

The cross-sectional morphology visualized by OCT presents a general thinning of cell layers and a reduced outer nuclear layer (ONL) in the youngest BD patients (9–34 years). Also, a third high-reflectance band, (3rd HRB), found in the younger cases, diminished in younger adults with BD, possibly representing the loss of the outer segment length of photoreceptors, predominately the cones in the fovea measured with OCT (Burstedt et al., 2010; Costa et al., 2004; Sandberg et al., 2005). This finding probably indicates an affection of the cone photoreceptors, and a possible degeneration of the outer segments of cones early in the course of the BD disease. The decreased retinal thickness and degenerative signs in the outer retinal layer were detected early in the course of the disease reported in a compound heterozygous patient with mutations in the *RLBP1* gene (R103W/R234W) (Nakamura et al., 2005). Similar to BD, prominent photoreceptor loss in the foveal and extrafoveal retina even in the youngest patients studied (6–17 years), with relative preservation localized in the superior-temporal and temporal pericentral retina and the ONL, were demonstrated in the patients with Leber congenital amaurosis, another retinal degenerative disease caused by mutations in *RPE65* gene encoding for a protein active in the visual cycle (Jacobson et al., 2008). How can an early foveal thinning, suggesting early degeneration of cone photoreceptors in BD patients possibly be explained? Studies show that not only the rods but the cones also incorporate 11-*cis* retinoids, derived from the rod and cone visual cycles, in their visual pigments, and when examining the visual cycle in the *RPE-65* and *LRAT* knock-out mice, diseases affecting the visual cycle, a key role for cell survival, was found to be 11-*cis*-retinal bound to cone opsins, important for retinal protein sorting, transport, and targeting (Collery et al., 2008; Zhang et al., 2008).

2.2.3 Morphological findings of retinitis punctata albescens (RPA)

The subretinal white lesions, retinitis punctata albescens, were initially observed in the teens with BD phenotype (Burstedt et al., 1999, 2001, 2010). The RPA spots often dominate in the macula area and adjacent to the arcades, varying from single to multiple generalized white lesions scattered over the posterior pole of the retina. Notably, these changes fade as the progressive retinal degeneration advances (Fig. 9).

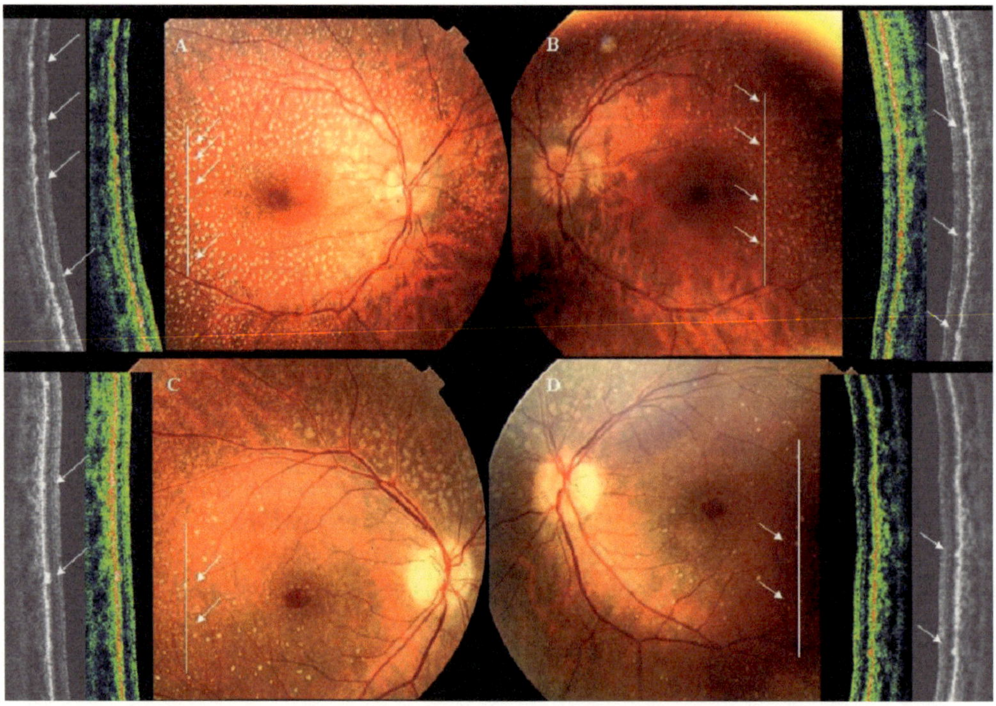

Fig. 9. Colour fundus photo and OCT. Top: 23-year-old man; below: 30-year-old woman. The vertical line of the binocular fundus photo with multiple generalized RPA traversing the retina at the temporal area of the macula between the arcades represents the scan lines of the corresponding OCT image presenting cross-sectional, visualized RPA (marked with arrows). (Figure published in Arch Ophthalmol. 2010;128(8);989-995).

RPA or subtle white lesions of the fundus have previously been described in several autosomal recessive RP cases with *RLBP1* mutations, and also in other progressive degenerative diseases, for example, the rhodopsin-related RP (Demirci et al., 2004; Eichers et al., 2002; Fishman et al., 2004; Katsanis et al., 2001; Nakamura et al., 2005; Souied et al., 1996). The localization of RPA lesions and their appearance may resemble more commonly known retinal lesions like drusen in age-related macular degeneration. However, the RPA lesions in BD do not present elevation, disruption, or detachment of RPE. Another finding in AMD is an accumulation of drusen between the retina and choriocapillaris that is shown to interfere with the exchange of nutrients and products close to the drusen, inducing RPE or neural retinal damage with overlaying photoreceptor cell layer thinning, predominately the photoreceptor outer segment affection (Holz et al., 2004; Pauleikhoff et al., 1990; Schumann et al., 2009). Since similar thinning or compression of the ONL overlaying the RPA lesions is observed in BD, a possible cause could be an accumulation of products in the RPE, possibly due to the higher affinity and impaired 11-*cis*-retinal release in the visual cycle in the BD phenotype shown in previous studies (Golovleva et al., 2003; He et al., 2009; Saari, 1990).

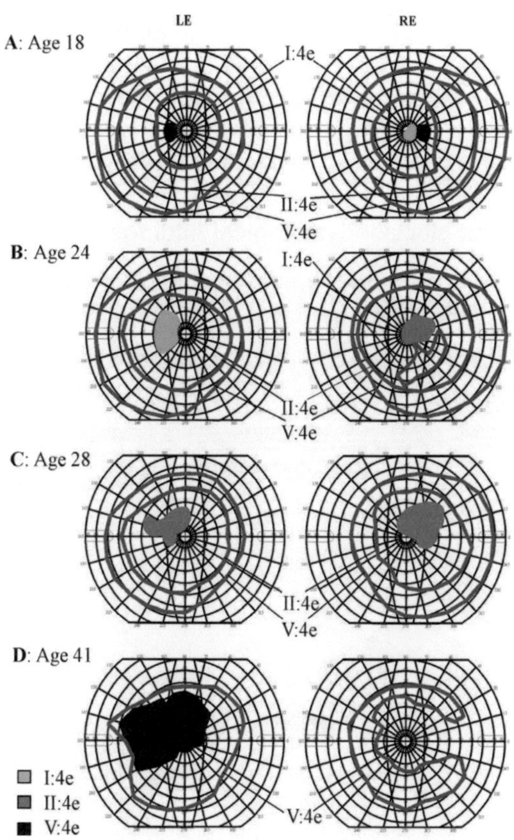

Fig. 10. Progression of visual field defects in a BD case. (A) Small central scotoma is noted in one eye at the age of 18. (B, C) Deeper and larger central-paracentral scotomas develop in young adulthood. (D) In middle age absolute central-paracentral scotomas are present and expanded, finally affecting the peripheral border. (Figure published in Arch Ophthalmol. 2001;119(2):260–267).

2.2.4 Psychophysical findings

Significant foveal depression was found early in BD by testing foveal threshold with Humphrey SITA standard 24-2. The mean deviations in all younger cases show significant loss, indicating an overall depression and/or loss of the central parts of the visual field in BD. Goldmann perimetries are unaffected in the BD cases under the age of 10, and relative parafoveal scotoma and/or ring scotoma is found in the teens, with additional large, deep to absolute central scotomas in both eyes, accompanied by a decrease in visual acuity in adulthood. The visual fields and the development of defects, registered over a time period of 23 years, are presented in Fig. 10.

In the fifth decade, extensive scotomas are present and only peripheral islets of the visual fields remain in middle age.

2.2.5 Angiographic findings

The fundus fluorescein angiograms in the early arteriovenous phase show a diffuse hyperfluorescence in the anatomic macular area, and locally, in the centre of the fovea, also presenting an early retinal thinning. As well as outside the arcades, corresponding to the atrophic areas in the colour fundus photograph, a general hyperfluorescence of granular type appears, indicating a gross atrophy of the pigment epithelium of the entire retina as a common clinical finding in this retinal degeneration (Burstedt et al., 2001).

2.3 Dark adaptometry and electrophysiological findings

2.3.1 Dark adaptometry and electrophysiological findings during standard dark-adapted conditions

Recovery of dark adaptation shows abnormalities of both rod and cone function (Fig. 11).

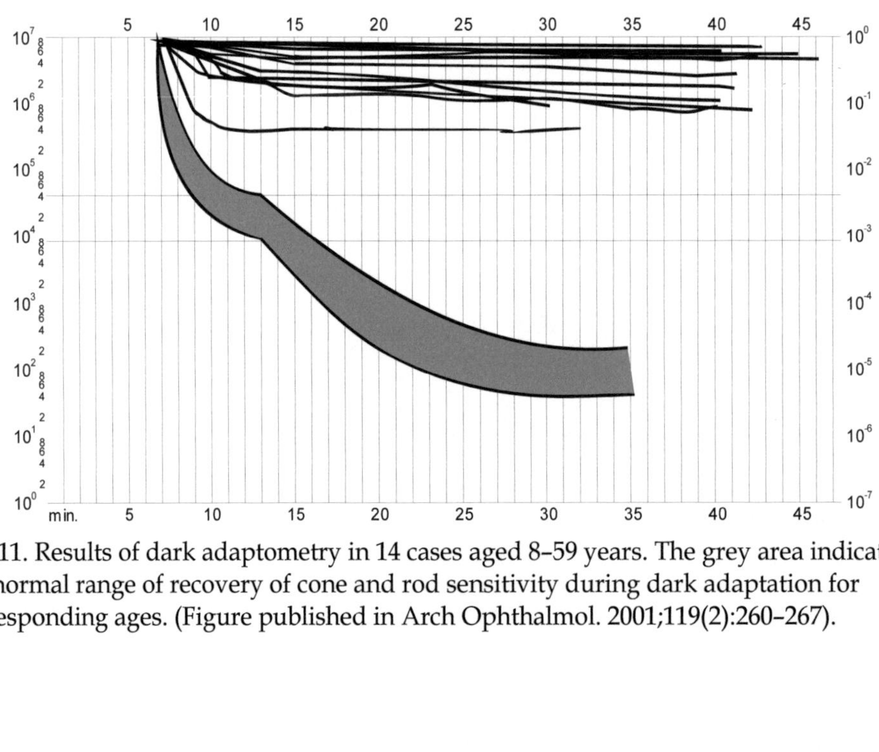

Fig. 11. Results of dark adaptometry in 14 cases aged 8–59 years. The grey area indicates the normal range of recovery of cone and rod sensitivity during dark adaptation for corresponding ages. (Figure published in Arch Ophthalmol. 2001;119(2):260–267).

In the younger patients the rod function is severely affected or absent and the cone adaptation often shows an extremely high, elevated final threshold, with the final dark-adapted sensitivity about four log units higher than a normal range. In elderly affected cases an even more pronounced cone dysfunction is found (Burstedt et al., 2001, 2003).

Full-field, single flash, and flicker electroretinograms (ERGs), including the oscillatory potentials (OPs) are recorded (UTAS-E 2000 LKC Technologies Inc., Gaithersburg, MD) using Burian-Allen bipolar electrodes during standard dark-adapted conditions, according to the recommendations of ISCEV (International Society for Clinical Electrophysiology of Vision). The outcome of the ERGs in all BD cases is subnormal or with non-recordable amplitudes of the rod-isolated b-waves with peak times either within the normal range or prolonged compared to controls (Burstedt et al., 2001, 2003, 2008). Representative full-field ERGs from five individuals from one family are presented in Fig. 12. The mixed rod-cone b-waves amplitudes are subnormal/non-recordable with comparatively short peak times in the younger cases. The amplitudes of the mixed rod-cone a-waves are found to be within the normal range in younger patients and subnormal to non-recordable with a prolonged peak time in adulthood. The amplitudes of the cone b-waves are better preserved and are within the normal range at the very young age, with peak times within the normal range, but prolonged in young adulthood and thereafter. Most of the younger patients had normal amplitudes and implicit times of the 30-Hz flicker ERGs that are within the normal limits, but already in early adulthood subnormal and delayed. The summed amplitudes of the individual oscillatory peaks, representing the Ops, show subnormal values at young age, decreasing with age and becoming non-recordable in BD cases older than 40 years of age.

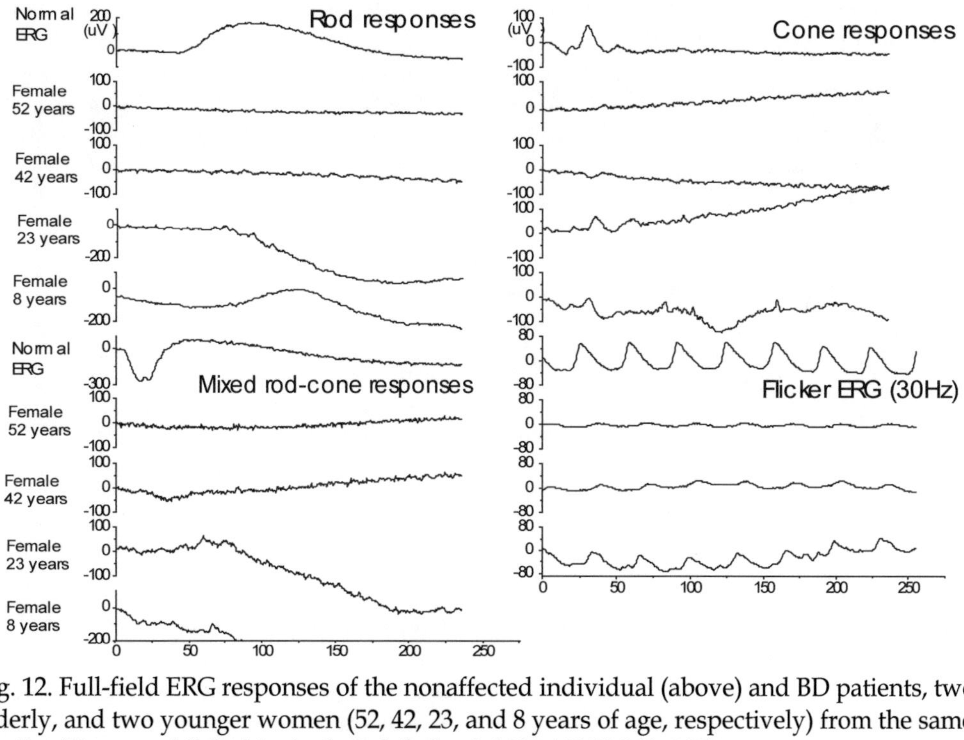

Fig. 12. Full-field ERG responses of the nonaffected individual (above) and BD patients, two elderly, and two younger women (52, 42, 23, and 8 years of age, respectively) from the same family. (Figure published in Arch Ophthalmol. 2001;119(2):260–267).

The ERGs recorded under standard conditions show that the rod and mixed rod-cone b-wave responses are relatively more affected than the mixed a-wave. The cone b-wave and the 30 Hz flicker amplitudes are significantly better preserved than the b-wave amplitudes of the rod and mixed rod-cone responses as well as the a-wave amplitude of the mixed rod-cone response, indicating later disturbance of the cones compared with the rods. At the same time the glial and inner retinal cell types seem to be affected at a relatively early stage in retinal degenerative disease (Burstedt et al., 2003).

2.3.2 Dark adaptometry and electrophysiology findings during 24 h prolonged dark-adaptation conditions

It has been shown that after illumination, the rhodopsin regeneration, 11-*cis*-retinal production, and dark adaptation are delayed by >10-fold in the visual cycle in *RLBP1* knockout mice (Saari et al., 2001). This could also be observed in humans, in six younger adults with BD, examined with a standardized Goldmann-Weekers adaptometer during an extremely prolonged dark adaptation of 24 hours (Burstedt et al., 2003). The extremely slow DA reaches steady state within 5 to 12 hours (Fig. 13); however, the final visual sensory thresholds do not return to normal levels after 24 hours of DA in most of the cases studied, probably affected by the disturbance in the normal function of CRALBP and lack of regeneration of 11-*cis* retinal in the RPE. An apparent plateau of recovery in the dark is observed, and duration for about 1 to 4 hours possibly represents a removal of bleached pigments, which has been suggested to occur in other retinal diseases affecting visual cycle function (Cideciyan et al., 1997). The 11-*cis*-retinal has been estimated to range from about 3.5% to 8% of that in normal subjects (Lamb & Pugh, 2004), with an average level of about 6% in the RPE in the BD phenotype.

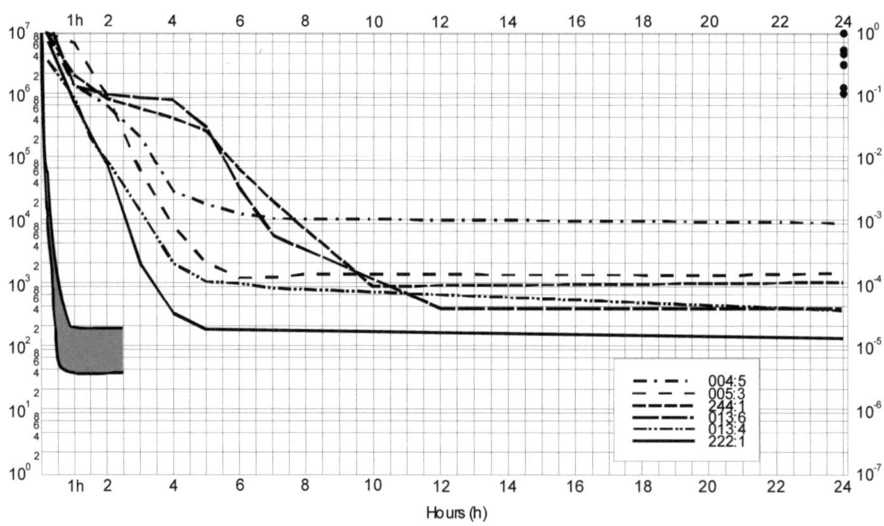

Fig. 13. Results of extremely prolonged (24 h) dark-adaptometry examinations in single eyes in BD patients, n = 6 (age 12–47 years). The final thresholds after 24 h were measured in both the patched single eye and in the unpatched contralateral eye. The values of the unpatched contralateral eye are indicated as filled symbols (•). The shaded area indicates normal range for corresponding age groups. (Figure published in Vision Research 2003:43(24):2559–2571).

Full-field ERGs after 24 hours of extremely prolonged DA were performed to evaluate the capacity of recovery of the whole retinal area and different cell types in BD disease. Six young cases (age 15–30 years) underwent full-field ERGs after 24 hours of DA in one eye and standard DA in the fellow eye. The results could be compared with the effect of the ERG after 10 hours' prolonged DA from a previous study (Burstedt et al., 2003, 2008). Enhanced rod-isolated b-wave after extremely prolonged DA (24 h) shows a sufficient number of rods able to function, generating responses of normal amplitudes even in young BD patients, although still with prolonged peak times (Fig. 14). Since the b-wave of the ERG is a glial response reflecting a depolarization of the Müller cells (Miller & Dowling, 1970), these findings may be correlated to an affected CRALBP function in the Müller cells of the retina or possibly a reversible effect on the second-order ON-bipolar cell function, as a consequence of a change in photoreceptor function.

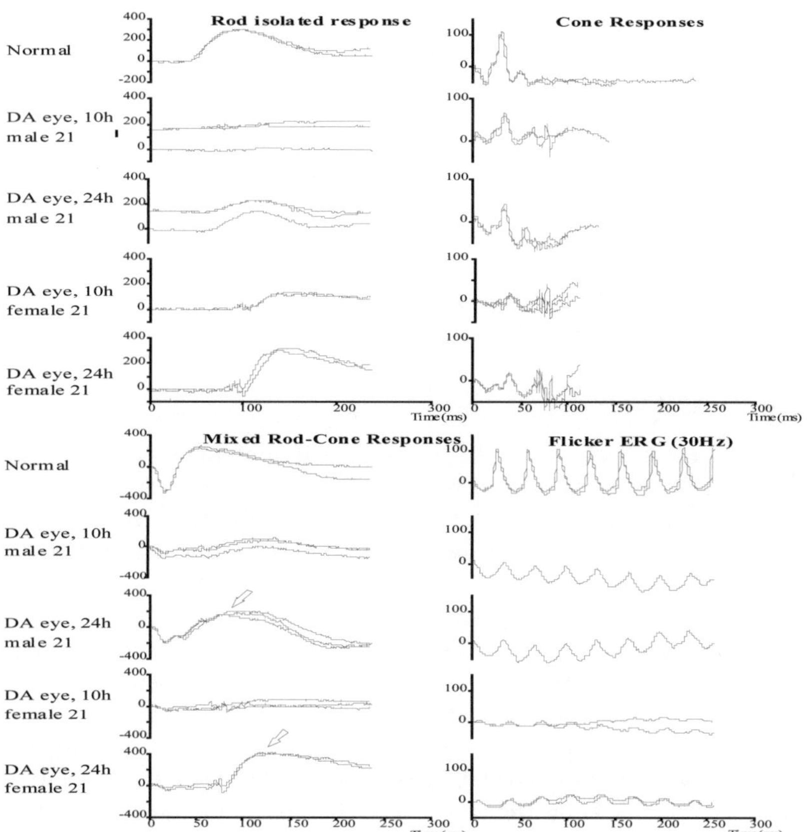

Fig. 14. Full-field electroretinograms of one eye, recorded after prolonged DA (10 h) and after extremely prolonged DA (24 h) in two BD patients (both 21 years old). A 'second', comparatively slowly rising positivity was observed in the mixed rod-cone response (arrows). For comparison, recordings of a normal subject are shown. (Figure published in Doc Ophthalmol. 2008;116(3):193–205).

The mixed rod-cone b-wave amplitude created by depolarization of the Müller and ON-bipolar cells in the inner retina is increased but still subnormal in the majority of patients.

After extended (24 h) DA, the mixed rod-cone a-wave response increases in amplitude to normal values in 4/5 cases with normal or somewhat delayed peak times. As the mixed a-wave shows normalized responses in the majority of the young BD cases examined, and the leading edge of the a-wave mainly represents a light-evoked hyperpolarization of the photoreceptors (Brown, 1968; Jamison et al., 2001; Robson et al., 2003; Tomita, 1965), these data suggest an additional, extremely slow regeneration of photopigments occurring even after 10 h DA. No obvious recovery of the cone b-wave is noted after the extremely prolonged DA (24 h); therefore, a relatively early damage to the cone system in BD patients cannot be excluded. Even though regeneration of opsin photopigments has been demonstrated in cone-dominant retinas, suggesting an interaction between Müller cells and cones in the recycling of visual chromophore (Mata et al., 2002), these electrophysiological results cannot confirm these findings.

In three younger BD patients a late evolvement in the mixed rod-cone response is observed (Fig. 14, arrows). The amplitudes are within the normal range of a mixed rod-cone b-wave, but the peak is extremely delayed (115 ms) compared to normal. This can be related to an enhanced scotopic activity associated with the slow and disturbed regeneration of photopigments. However, the exact origin of this late positive potential observed in BD patients is not known.

In summary, the continuous but slow regeneration of rod photopigments in *RLBP1* mutants presents an additional capacity for recovery of rod function and gain in activity in the inner retinal layers with extremely prolonged dark adaptation, possibly as a consequence of a change in photoreceptor function (Burstedt et al., 2003, 2008).

2.4 Outcome of visual function

Visual loss is an early sign of the BD disease, and individuals of working age may experience important socioeconomic consequences and interference with education as a result of their visual impairment. To provide insight into the perceived visual function of retinitis pigmentosa of Bothnia type, measurements of visual function were associated with the patients' self-assessment of their total self-reported visual function and health-related quality of life, measured with a questionnaire in 49 BD cases (Burstedt et al., 2010). Significant correlation was found between objective visual functions studied, and the subjective visual function. Almost 70% of the variability of the composite score could be explained by WVA and age alone. BD patients' responses to a majority of the questionnaire subscales significantly correlated with several of the clinical vision measures, especially those depending on central vision. Notably, the progressive declines in visual field area did not seem to affect significantly the self-perceived quality of life in patients with this phenotype. This finding might be an indication of ability to adapt to this type of gradual progressive visual field area loss, probably due to use of paracentral preserved areas. The expression of the disease has a significant impact on multiple domains of daily living, but there are no signs of worsening depression related to the increasing visual impairment.

2.5 Tinted contact lenses in BD

Could visual function be improved in BD? With the knowledge of an extremely prolonged dark adaptation (5–12 h) and even further gain of the ERG responses up to more than 12 h in this phenotype, outcome of wearing of tinted contact lenses during daylight was tested (Jonsson et al., 2007).

Twelve patients with BD were fitted with soft contact lenses tinted dark brown. Outcome of visual parameters, and visual-function questionnaire, were tested before the contact lens fitting and after one month. Visual function was improved by dark-tinted contact lenses, and it was observed that the BD cases with the lowest visual acuity described the most obvious improvement of their visual function and preferred the darker tinted contact lenses; the majority of BD cases from this study have also chosen to continue wearing the brown-tinted contact lenses for several years following the study, possibly indicating a continuous benefit in their daily life over time (authors' comments).

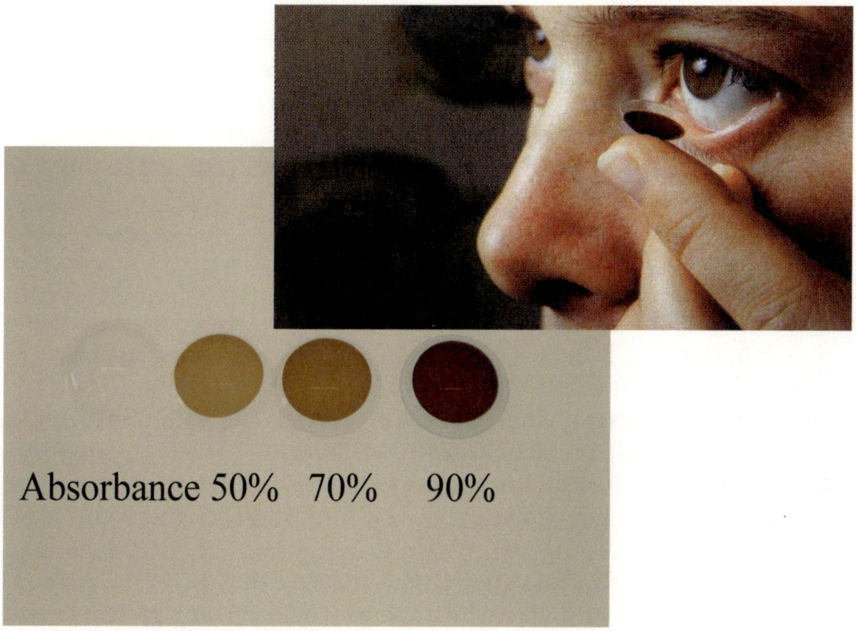

Fig. 15. Contact lenses with clear and different grades of tint were evaluated in retinitis pigmentosa of Bothnia type.

3. Conclusions

The RP population of northern Sweden has given us a unique opportunity to evaluate and compare the phenotypical expression of different *RLBP1* mutations over time. Despite genetic heterogeneity, the clinical expression of different *RLBP1* mutations in northern Sweden presents a unique phenotype of the retinal disease, clearly directing the molecular diagnosis and search for *RLBP1* mutations. It became possible to offer genetic testing among the families related to BD patients and also to the patients with a hereditary form of the recessive form of RP. In BD families we can offer risk assessment to future generations, providing genetic counselling based on molecular testing and clinical findings. There are several approaches to treatment of RP patients, although there are no established standards. Several drugs and nutritional supplements such as vitamin A palmitate, ascorbic acid, docosahexaenoic acid and others were evaluated with contradictory outcomes in different studies. Vitamin A palmitate, the most-used nutritional supplement, is shown to slow the rate of retinal degeneration, but this type therapy is not without controversy (Shintani et al., 2009). Gene therapy, which replaces or turns off the mutant disease-causing gene, represents another option for treatment. Several years of basic research of *RPE65*-Lebers congenital amaurosis, a retinal disease affecting the visual cycle, by several independent research groups, resulted in clinical trials of human gene therapies during recent years, demonstrating short-term evidence of visual gain (Jacobson & Cideciyan, 2010; Musarella & MacDonald, 2011). Therefore, we suggest that for treatment of BD patients, gene therapy is the most promising option among other concepts in the treatment of retinitis pigmentosa.

4. Acknowledgments

We acknowledge all BD patients and their families for their participation in all our studies. The authors express their thanks to all collaborators, and especially to Dr. Sandgren, for being a source of initiative and interest, and an engine in valuable discussions. This research was supported by funding from Crown Princess Margaretha's Foundation for Vision Research (KMA), the Swedish Medical Research Council, and grants from the County Council of Västerbotten.

5. References

Bridges, CDB., Foster, RG., Landers, RA., & Fong, S-L. (1987). Interstitial retinol-binding protein and cellular retinal-binding protein in the mammalian pineal. *Vis Res,* Vol. 27, No. 12, pp. 2049-2060, PMID: 3447356

Brown, KT. (1968). The electroretinogram: its components and their origins. *Vision Research,* Vol. 8, No. 6, (Jun), pp. 633–677, PMID: 4978009

Bunt-Milan, A., & Saari, J. (1983). Immunocytochemical localization of two retinoid-binding proteins in vertebrate retina. *J Cell Biol,* Vol. 97, Vol. 3, (Sep), pp. 703-712, PMID: 6350319

Burstedt, MSI., Sandgren, O., Holmgren, G., & Forsman-Semb, K. (1999). Bothnia dystrophy caused by mutations in the cellular retinaldehyde-binding protein gene (*RLBP1)* on chromosome 15q26. *Invest Ophthalmol Vis Sci,* Vol. 40, No. 5, (Apr), pp. 995-1000, PMID: 10102298

Burstedt, MSI., Forsman-Semb, K., Golovleva, I., Janunger, T., Wachtmeister, L., & Sandgren, O. (2001). Ocular phenotype of Bothnia Dystrophy, an autosomal recessive retinitis pigmentosa associated with an R234W mutation in the *RLBP1* gene. *Arch Ophthalmol,* Vol. 119, No. 2, (Feb), pp. 260-267, PMID: 11176989

Burstedt, MSI., Golovleva, I., Sandgren, O., & Wachtmeister, L. (2003). Retinal function in Bothnia Dystrophy. An electrophysiological study. *Vision Research,* Vol. 43, No. 24, (Apr), pp. 2559-2571, PMID: 12536144

Burstedt, MSI., Mönestam, E., & Sandgren, O. (2005). Association between specific measures of vision and Vision-Related Quality of Life in patients with Bothnia Dystrophy, a defined type of Retinitis Pigmentosa. *Retina,* Vol. 25, No. 3, (Apr-May), pp. 317-323, PMID: 15805909

Burstedt, MSI., Sandgren, O., & Wachtmeister, L. (2008). Effects on electrophysiological functions in the electroretinogram of extremely prolonged dark adaptation in patients with Retinitis Pigmentosa of Bothnia type. *Doc Ophthalmol*, Vol. 116, No. 3, (May), pp. 193-205. Epub 2007 Oct 6. PMID: 17922155

Burstedt, MSI., & Mönestam, E. (2010). Vision-related quality of life in patients with Bothnia Dystrophy, a defined type of Retinitis Pigmentosa. *Clin Ophthal*, Vol. 4, (Mar), pp. 147-154, PMID: 20390035

Burstedt, MSI., & Golovleva, I. Central retinal findings in retinitis pigmentosa of Bothnia type caused by *RLBP1* mutation. *Arch Ophthalmol*, Vol. 128, No. 8, pp. 989-995, (Aug), PMID: 20696998

Cideciyan, AV., Pugh, EN Jr., Lamb, TD., Huang, Y., Jacobson, SG. (1997). Rod plateaux during dark adaptation in Sorsby's fundus dystrophy and vitamin A deficiency. *Invest Ophthalmol Vis Sci*, Vol. 38, No. 9, (Aug), pp. 1786-1794. PMID: 9286267

Costa, RA., Calucci, D., Skaf, M., Cardillo, JA., Castro, JC., Melo, LA., Martins, MC., & Kaiser, PK. (2004). Optical coherence tomography 3: automatic delineation of the outer neural retinal boundary and its influence on retinal thickness measurements. *Invest Ophthalmol Vis Sci*, Vol. 45, No. 7, (Jul), pp. 2399–2406, PMID: 15223823

Collery, R., McLoughlin, S., Vendrell, V., Finnegan, J., Crabb, JW.,Saari, JC., & Kennedy, BN. (2008). Duplication and divergence of zebrafish CRALBP genes uncovers novel role for RPE- and Muller-CRALBP in cone vision. *Invest Ophthalmol Vis Sci*, Vol. 49, No. 9,(Sept), pp. 3812–3820, PMID: 18502992

Demirci, FY., Rigatti, BW., Mah, TS., Gorin, MB. (2004). A novel compound heterozygous mutation in the cellular retinaldehyde-binding protein gene (RLBP1) in a patient with retinitis punctata albescens. *Am J Ophthalmol*, Vol. 138, No. 1, (Jul), pp. 171–173, PMID: 15234312

Eichers, ER., Green, JS., Stockton, DW., Jackman, CS., Whelan. J., McNamara, JA., Johnson, GJ., Lupski, JR., & Katsanis, N. (2002). Newfoundland rod–cone dystrophy, an early-onset retinal dystrophy, is caused by splice-junction mutations in RLBP1. *Am J Hum Genet*, Vol. 70, No. 4, (Apr), pp. 955–964, PMID: 11868161

Eisenfeldt, AJ., Bunt-Milam, AH., & Saari, JC. (1985). Localization of retinoid-binding proteins in developing rat retina. *Exp Eye Res*, Vol. 41, No. 3, (Sep), pp. 299-304, PMID: 3905423

Fishman, GA., Roberts, MF., Derlacki, DJ., Grimsby, JL., Yamamoto, H., Sharon, D., Nishiguchi, KM., & Dryja, TP. (2004). Novel mutations in the cellular retinaldehyde-binding protein gene (RLBP1) associated with retinitis punctata albescens: evidence of interfamilial genetic heterogeneity and fundus changes in heterozygotes. *Arch Ophthalmol*, Vol. 122, No. 1, (Jan), pp. 70–75, PMID: 14718298

Futterman, S., & Saari JC. (1977). Occurrence of 11-cis-retinal-binding protein restricted to the retina. *Invest Ophthalmol Vis Sci, Vol.* 16, No. 8, (Aug), pp. 768-771, PMID: 560359

Golovleva, I., Battacharya, S., Wu, Z., Shaw, N., Yang, Y., Andrabi, K., West, KA., Burstedt, MSI., Forsman, K., Holmgren, G., Sandgren, O., Noy, N., Qin, J., &Crabb, JW. (2003). Disease causing mutations in the cellular retinaldehyde- binding protein tighter and abolish ligand interactions. *J Biol Chem*, Vol. 278, No, 14, (Apr), pp. 12397-12402. Epub 2003 Jan 20. PMID: 12536144

Haim, M. (2002). Epidemiology of retinitis pigmentosa in Denmark. *Acta Ophthalmol Scand Suppl.*, Vol. 80, pp. 1–34

He, X., Lobsiger, J., & Stocker, A. (2009). Bothnia dystrophy is caused by domino-like rearrangements in cellular retinaldehyde-binding protein mutant R234W. *PNAS,* Vol. 106, No. 44, (Nov), pp. 18545-18550. Epub 2009 Oct 21. PMID: 19846785

Humbert, G., Delettre, C., Senechal, A., Bazalgette, C., Barakat, A., Bazalgette, C., Arnaud, B., Lenaers, G., & Hamel, CP. (2006). Homozygous deletion related to Alu repeats in RLBP1 causes retinitis punctata albescens. *Invest Ophthalmol Vis Sci,* Vol. 47, No. 11, (Nov), pp. 4719–4724, PMID: 17065479

Jacobson, SG., Cideciyan, AV., Aleman, TS., Sumaroka, A., Windsor, EA., Schwarz, SB., Heon, E., & Stone, EM.(2008). Photoreceptor layer topography in children with Leber congenital amaurosis caused by RPE65 mutations. *Invest Ophthalmol Vis Sci,* Vol. 49, No. 10, (Oct), pp. 4573–4577. Epub 2008 Jun 6. PMID: 18539930

Jacobson SG.,& Cideciyan, AV. (2010). Treatment possibilities for retinitis pigmentosa. *N Engl J Med.,* Vol. 363, No. 17, (Oct), pp. 1669-1671, PMID: 20961252

Jamison, JA., Bush, RA., Lei, B., & Sieving, PA. (2001). Characterization of the rod photoresponse isolated from the dark-adapted primate ERG. *Vis Neurosci, Vol.* 18, (May-Jun), pp. 445–455, PMID: 11497421

Holz, FG., Pauleikhoff, D., Klein, R., & Bird, AC. (2004). Pathogenesis of lesions in late age-related macular disease. *Am J Ophthalmol,* Vol. 137, Vol. 3, (Mar), pp. 504-510, PMID: 15013875

Jonsson, Å., Sandgren, O., & Burstedt, MSI. (2007). Evaluation of dark tinted lenses i Bothnia Dystrophy, a defined type of retinitis pigmentosa. *Acta Ophthalmol Scand,* Vol. 85, No. 5, (Aug), pp. 534-539. Epub 2007 Mar 22. PMID: 17376191

Katsanis, N., Shroyer, NF., Lewis, RA., Cavender, JC., Al-Rajhi, AA., Jabak, M., & Lupski, JR. (2001). Fundus albipunctatus and retinitis punctata albescens in a pedigree with an R150Q mutation in RLBP1. *Clin Genet,* Vol. 59, No. 6, (Jun), pp. 424–429. PMID: 11453974

Köhn, L., Burstedt, M., Jonsson, F., Kadzhev, K., Haamere, E., Sandgren, O., & Golovleva, I. (2008). Carrier of R14W in carbonic anhydrase IV presents Bothnia Dystrophy phenotype caused by two allelic mutations in RLBP1. *Invest Ophthal Vis Sci,* Vol. 49, No. 7, (Jul), pp. 3172-3177, PMID: 11453974

Lamb, TD., & Pugh, EN, Jr. (2004). Dark adaptation and the retinoid cycle of vision. *Prog Retin Eye Res,* Vol. 23, No. 3, (May), pp. 307–380, PMID: 15177205

Mata, NL., Radu, RA., Clemmons, RC., & Travis, GH. (2002) Isomerization and oxidation of vitamin A in cone-dominant retinas: a novel pathway for visual-pigment regeneration in daylight. *Neuron,* Vol. 36, No. 1, (Sep), pp. 69–80, PMID: 12367507

Maw, MA., Kennedy, B., Knight, A., Bridges, R., Roth, KE., Mani, EJ., Mukkadan, JK., Nancarrow, D., Crabb, JW., & Denton, MJ. (1997). Mutation of the gene encoding cellular retinaldehyde-binding protein in autosomal recessive retinitis pigmentosa. *Nat Genet.* Vol. 17, No. 12, (Oct), pp. 198-200, PMID: 9326942

Miller, RF., & Dowling, JE. (1970) Intracellular responses of the Müller (glial) cells of mudpuppy retina: their relation to b-wave of the electroretinogram. *J Neurophysiol,* Vol. 33, No. 3, (May), pp. 323–341, PMID: 5439340

Morimura, H., Berson, EL., & Dryja, TP. (1999). Recessive mutations in the *RLBP1* gene encoding cellular retinaldehyde-binding protein in a form of retinitis punctata albescens. *Invest Ophthalmol Vis Sci,* Vol. 40, No. 5, (Apr), pp. 1000–1004, PMID: 10102299

Musarella, MA., & Macdonald, IM. (2011). Current concepts in the treatment of retinitis pigmentosa. *J Ophthalmol.* Epub 2010 Oct 11, doi: 10.1155/2011/753547, PMID: 21048997

Nakamura, M., Lin, J., Ito,Y., & Miyake, Y. (2005). Novel mutation in RLBP1 gene in a Japanese patient with retinitis punctata albescens. *Am J Ophthalmol*, Vol. 139, No. 6, (Jun), pp. 1133–1135, PMID: 15953459

Pauleikhoff, D., Harper, CA., Marchall, J., & Bird, AC. (1990). Aging changes in Bruch´s membrane: a histochemical and morphologic study. *Ophthalmology,* Vol. 97, No. 2, (Feb), pp. 171-178, PMID: 1691475

Phelan, JK., & Bok, D. (2000). A brief review of retinitis pigmentosa and the identified retinitis pigmentosa genes. *Mol Vis,* Vol. 6, (Jul), pp. 116–124, PMID: 10889272

Rebello, G., Ramesar, R., Vorster, A., Roberts, L., Ehrenreich, L., Oppon, E., Gama, D., Bardien, S., Greenberg, J., Bonapace, G., Waheed, A., Shah, GN., & Sly, WS. (2004) Apoptosis-inducing signal sequence mutation in carbonic anhydrase IV identified in patients with the RP17 form of retinitis pigmentosa. *Proc Natl Acad Sci U S A,* Vol. 101, No. 17, (Apr), pp. 6617-6622. Epub 2004 Apr 16. PMID: 15090652

Robson, JG., Saszik, SM., Ahmed, J., & Frishman, LJ. (2003). Rod and cone contributions to the a-wave of the electroretinogram of the macaque. *J Physiol,* Vol. 547, Pt. 2, (Mar), pp. 509–530, Epub 2003 Jan 24. PMID: 12562933

Rosenfeld, PJ., & Dryja, TP. (1995). Molecular genetics of retinitis pigmentosa and related retinal degenerations, In: *Molecular Genetics of Ocular Disease.* pp. 99-126, New York, Wiley-Liss

Saari, JC. (1990). Enzymes nd proteins of the mammilian visual cycle. In: *Progress in Retinal Research,* Osborn, N., & Chader, G., editors, pp. 363-381, Oxford, England: Pergamon Press

Saari, JC., Bredberg, L., & Noy, N. (1994). Control of substrate flow at a branch in the visual cycle. *Biochemistry,* Vol. 33, No. 10, (Mar), pp. 3106-3112, PMID: 8130225

Saari, JC,. Huang, J., Possin, DE., Fariss, RN., Leonard, J., Garwin, GG., Crabb, JW., & Milam, AH. (1997). Cellular retinaldehyde-binding protein is expressed by oligodendrocytes in optic nerve and brain. *Glia,* Vol. 21, No. 3, (Nov), pp. 259-268, PMID: 9383035

Saari, JC., Nawrot, M., Kennedy, BN., Garwin, GG., Hurley, JB., Huang, J., Possin, DE., & Crabb, JW. (2001). Visual impairment in cellular retinaldehyde binding protein (CRALBP) knockout mice results in delayed dark adaptation. *Neuron,* Vol. 29, No. 3, (Mar), pp. 739-748, PMID: 11301032

Sandberg, MA., Brockhurst, RJ., Gaudio, AR., & Berson, EL. (2005). The association between visual acuity and central retinal thickness in retinitis pigmentosa. *Invest Ophthalmol Vis Sci,* Vol. 46, No. 9, (Oct), pp. 3349–354, PMID: 16123439

Sarthy, V. (1996). Cellular retinaldehyde-binding protein localization in cornea. *Exp Eye Res,* Vol. 63, No. 6, (Dec), pp. 759-762, PMID: 9068383

Shintani, K., Shechtman, DL., & Gurwood, AS. (2009). Review and update: current treatment trends for patients with retinitis pigmentosa. *Optometry,* Vol. 80, No. 7, (Jul), pp.384-401, PMID: 19545852

Schuman, SG., Koreishi, AF., Farsiu, S., Jung, S., Izatt, JA., & Toth, CA. (2009). Photoreceptor layer thinning over drusen in eyes with age-related macular degeneration imaged in vivo with spectral-domain optical coherence tomography.*Ophthalmology,* Vol. 116, No. 3, (Mar), pp. 488-496. Epub 2009 Jan 22. PMID: 19167082

Souied, E., Soubrane, G., Benlian, P., Coscas, GJ., Gerber, S., Munnich, A., & Kaplan, J. (1996). Retinitis punctata albescens associated with the Arg135Trp mutation in the rhodopsin gene. *Am J Ophthalmol,* Vol. 121, No. 1, (Jan), pp. 19–25, PMID: 8554077

Tomita, T. (1965). Electrophysiological study of the mechanisms subserving color coding in the fish retina. *Cold Spring Harb Symp Quant Biol,* Vol. 30, pp. 559-566, PMID:5219504

Zhang, H., Fan, J., Li, S., Karan, S., Rohrer, B., Palczewski, K., Frederick, JM., Crouch, RK., & Baehr, W. (2008). Trafficking of membrane-associated proteins to cone photoreceptor outer segments requires the chromophore 11-cis-retinal. *J Neurosci,* Vol. 28, No. 15, (Apr), pp. 4008–4014, PMID: 18400900

Yang, Z., Alvarez, BV., Chakarova, C., Jiang, L., Karan, G., Frederick, JM., Zhao, Y., Sauve, Y., Li, X., Zrenner, E., Wissinger, B., Hollander, AI., Katz, B., Baehr, W., Cremers, FP., Casey, JR., Bhattacharya, SS., & Zhang K. (2005) Mutant carbonic anhydrase 4 impairs pH regulation and causes retinal photoreceptor degeneration. *Hum Mol Genet,* Vol. 14, No. 2, (Jan), pp. 255-265. Epub 2004 Nov 24. PMID: 15563508

26

Mechanisms of RDH12-Induced Leber Congenital Amaurosis and Therapeutic Approaches

Anne Kasus-Jacobi[1], Lea D. Marchette[1], Catherine Xu[1], Feng Li[1], Huaiwen Wang[1] and Mark Babizhayev[2]
[1]*Oklahoma University Health Sciences Center*
[2]*Innovative Vision Products, Inc.*
USA

To Finley: You made this work very special to us.

1. Introduction

Retinal dystrophies are characterized by the degeneration of vision-supporting photoreceptor cells of the retina, leading to irreversible blindness. It is a heterogeneous group of diseases that can be caused by mutations on more than 150 identified genes with diverse functions (http://www.sph.uth.tmc.edu/Retnet/home.htm). Retinal dystrophies can be classified based on whether the rod or the cone photoreceptor cells are affected first, and based on the onset and progression of vision loss [1]. Leber congenital amaurosis (LCA) is in clear contrast with other inherited retinal dystrophies in that both rod and cone photoreceptor cells are affected from the onset of the disease [1]. The second major characteristic of LCA is that the progression to complete blindness is fast, making it the most devastating form of inherited retinal dystrophies [1]. In most cases, visual handicap is diagnosed before one year of age and progresses to legal blindness in early adulthood [2]. Other signs of the disease are an extinguished or severely reduced scotopic and photopic electroretinogram, absent or diminished pupillary response to light, and nystagmus (roaming eye movements) [3]. It is a rare disease, affecting approximately 1:30,000 people worldwide but it is the first cause of inherited blindness in children [2].

During the past 15 years, our understanding of the genetic basis of LCA has greatly progressed [1]. Today, 14 different genes causing LCA have been identified [1]. Together they are responsible for approximately 75% of LCA cases, the remaining 25% of LCA cases being caused by mutations in unidentified genes. The identified LCA-causing genes are expressed in various cell types of the retina and are involved in a wide variety of developmental and physiological pathways [1]. Because the disease is induced by mutation on a single gene, LCA patients are potentially good candidates for gene replacement therapy. In recent years, exciting results have been obtained in clinical trials for LCA caused by mutations on the *RPE65* gene (LCA2), representing 3 to 16% of LCA cases [4]. Several other LCA-causing genes have received proof-of-concept validation for gene therapy in animal models [1]. We can anticipate that in the following years, patients with LCA induced by mutations on these genes will undergo clinical trials for gene replacement therapy.

In this chapter, we will concentrate on LCA13 caused by mutations in the *RDH12* gene. This gene encodes for an enzyme of the short-chain dehydrogenase/reductase superfamily. It was named retinol dehydrogenase 12 (RDH12) based on its similarity with the RDH11 enzyme (Figure 1) [5]. Gene replacement therapy is not currently available for LCA13 patients and may not be for several years. Thus, any alternative therapeutic approach would be beneficial. We will review our and other's findings regarding the function of RDH12, providing new insight into the mechanism of RDH12-induced LCA. We will discuss how understanding the role of RDH12 is allowing the development of alternative therapeutic strategies to gene replacement therapy for patients with LCA13. Finally, we will describe our encouraging preliminary results obtained in a mouse line with disrupted *Rdh12* gene, using an imidazole-containing peptide derivative, which could be rapidly developed into an effective therapeutic strategy to preserve retinal structure and function in LCA13 patients.

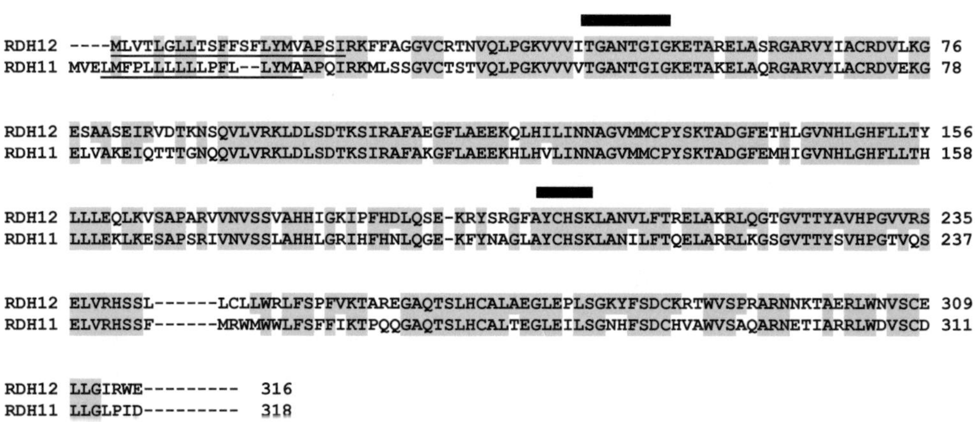

Fig. 1. **Alignment of human RDH12 and RDH11 sequences.** Residue numbers are shown on the *right.* Identical residues are *boxed. Overbars* denote the two signature sequences for the superfamily of short-chain dehydrogenase/reductases [6]. GenBank™ accession numbers for human RDH12 and RDH11 are NP_689656 and CAG33461, respectively. Stretches of NH2-terminal hydrophobic residues predicted to be inserted in the membrane are underlined.

2. RDH12 and Leber Congenital Amaurosis

In 2004, mutations in the *RDH12* gene were found in a subset of LCA patients [7, 8]. Since then, more than 30 *RDH12* mutations have been found in the homozygous or compound heterozygous state in LCA13 patients [7-11]. LCA13 is inherited in an autosomal recessive manner and represents about 4% of all LCA cases [2]. LCA13 appears to share a common clinical picture with other types of LCA characterized by a poor visual function in early life, followed by a progressive decline due to both rods and cones degeneration [9].

Interestingly, when compared with the RPE65-mutant retina that has a relatively well preserved structure with a disproportionate loss of photoreceptor function (as measured in 4 LCA2 patients; ages 17, 19, 19 and 23), the structure of RDH12-mutant retina appears disrupted at much younger ages (measured in 4 LCA13 patients; ages 8, 11, 13 and 21) [12].

A number of RDH12 mutations leading to LCA have been biochemically evaluated by expressing the mutants in cultured cells and by measuring the enzymatic activities of the recombinant enzymes [7-11]. These studies have shown that mutations in RDH12 result in decreased or abolished enzymatic activity due to a lower affinity for the substrate or a lower affinity for the coenzyme and/or to a decreased specific activity. In addition, most of RDH12 mutations resulted in low steady-state levels of the mutant proteins in cells [11, 13]. It was hypothesized that these mutants could be recognized as misfolded and targeted for accelerated degradation by the ubiquitin-proteasome system [13]. These studies strongly suggest that the loss of RDH12 function is the primary event causing the development of LCA13 phenotype (i.e. rapid loss of photoreceptor function and disruption of retinal structure). Thus, to determine the triggering event in LCA13 pathogenesis, and because RDH12 is an enzyme, the fundamental question is: what is the nature of the RDH12 substrate?

3. Enzymatic activity of RDH12

RDH12 is an oxidoreductase enzyme of the short-chain dehydrogenase/reductase superfamily [5]. Its substrate and coenzyme specificities have been elucidated *in vitro* [5, 14]. RDH12 was found to reduce all-*trans* retinal and other retinaldehydes (in *cis* configurations) to corresponding retinols, using the reduced form of nicotinamide adenine dinucleotide phosphate as cofactor [5, 14]. In addition, various aldehyde-containing molecules, including 4-hydroxynonenal (4-HNE), were found to be reduced by RDH12 to corresponding alcohols [14]. Thus, RDH12 has a double substrate specificity for all-*trans* retinal (and other retinaldehydes) and for 4-HNE (and other toxic aldehydes). In addition, the possibility that RDH12 could have other -yet unknown- substrates cannot be ruled out.

The existence of two groups of substrates for RDH12 suggests that this enzyme could have two distinct physiological functions *in vivo*. As mentioned, mutations of RDH12 associated with LCA resulted in a decreased enzymatic activity of RDH12, inhibiting the reduction of all-*trans* retinal and 4-HNE to the corresponding alcohols *in vitro* [7, 10, 11, 15].

4. Possible RDH12 function(s) in the retina

RDH12 is abundantly expressed in rod and possibly cone photoreceptor cells in the retina [16-19]. These cells are photosensitive; they detect the presence of photons through the 11-*cis* retinal chromophore bound to opsin protein (forming the photosensitive rhodopsin). When photobleaching of rhodopsin occurs, light isomerizes 11-*cis* retinal to all-*trans* retinal, which then dissociates from opsin. This photoisomerization is the initial event that triggers the visual transduction pathway, activation of second order neurons, and eventually transmission of the signal to the brain. Under constant illumination, 11-*cis* retinal has to be replaced (recycled) and all-*trans* retinal has to be removed from the surrounding of opsin so that photoreceptor cells continue to have an optimum sensitivity to light. The retinoid or visual cycle is the multi-step biochemical pathway that allows the recycling of 11-*cis*-retinal. The retinol dehydrogenases RDH8 (expressed in photoreceptor cells) and RDH5 (located in retinal pigment epithelium cells) were shown to directly participate in this essential pathway for maintenance of normal vision [20]. A possible function for RDH12 could thus be to reduce all-*trans* retinal, duplicating the RDH8 function, to keep photoreceptor cells in a state of high sensitivity to light.

We proposed another possible function for RDH12 in photoreceptor cells, in relation with its ability to reduce 4-HNE [15]. Reactive oxygen species formed within the mitochondria as byproducts of the electron transport chain can directly attack polyunsaturated fatty acids and initiate an auto-amplified chain reaction of lipid oxidation in cellular membranes. This causes the degradation of polyunsaturated fatty acids into a variety of oxidized products, including short- and medium-chain reactive aldehydes such as malondialdehyde, 4-hydroxyhexenal, and 4-HNE [21]. 4-HNE is the oxidation product of ω-6 arachidonic and linoleic fatty acids and is the most abundant and toxic end-product of lipid oxidation found in tissues [21-23]. It reacts readily with histidine, cysteine, and lysine to form Michael's adduct with these residues [24]. Oxidative modification of protein by 4-HNE leads to a variety of effects including inhibition of enzymatic activities; inhibition of protein functions; targeting of modified proteins for degradation; inhibition of protein, RNA, and DNA synthesis; cell cycle arrest; and apoptosis [21, 22, 25, 26]. When 4-HNE is reduced to the corresponding alcohol dihydroxynonene, its ability to form toxic adduct with proteins is abolished. Thus, we proposed that a possible function for RDH12 in the retina could be to detoxify 4-HNE by reducing it to dihydroxynonene [15].

When there is a loss of enzymatic function in cells, the substrate of the inactivated enzyme accumulates while the product of the reaction decreases. The next question is then whether it is the accumulation of substrate(s) or the disappearance of product(s), or both, that triggers the LCA13 phenotype. All-*trans* retinol, the product of all-*trans* retinal reduction, is not absolutely required for visual function because it is constantly supplied to the retinal pigment epithelium cells from the circulating blood. Therefore the most probable hypothesis is that accumulation of the substrate (all-*trans* retinal) rather than lack of product (all-*trans* retinol) might cause the retinal phenotype in LCA13 patients. Dihydroxynonene, the product of 4-HNE reduction, is not known to mediate any crucial biological function therefore in this scenario also, it seems that accumulation of the toxic substrate (4-HNE) rather than lack of product (dihydroxynonene) would cause the LCA13 phenotype.

5. Utilization of the *Rdh12* knockout mouse to determine the physiological substrate of RDH12

Identifying possible substrates for an enzyme *in vitro* is not enough to demonstrate that they are physiological substrates. *In vivo*, other considerations such as the localization and concentration of substrate relative to that of the enzyme are very important. Locations of the enzyme and substrate have to overlap and the substrate concentration has to be within a specific range for the enzymatic reaction to take place *in vivo*. The next step is thus to determine if there is accumulation of all-*trans* retinal and/or 4-HNE in the retina, in absence of RDH12. Mice with disrupted *Rdh12* gene have been generated [16, 19] and they have been useful to determine what substrate of RDH12 accumulates in the retina.

After bleaching of rhodopsin, a moderate delay in all-*trans* retinal clearance was found in the *Rdh12* knockout retina [19, 27, 28]. To explain the existing but surprisingly small delay in all-*trans* retinal clearance, it has been argued that RDH12 is located only in the inner segment of photoreceptor cells, while rhodopsin is located only in the outer segment. Thus, it was proposed that instead of participating directly (with RDH8) to the reduction of all-*trans* retinal released in the outer segment, RDH12 could reduce only a small portion of all-*trans* retinal overflowing to the inner segment after bleaching of rhodopsin [27, 28].

In our study, we found that retinas of both albino [15] and pigmented *Rdh12* knockout mice (Figure 2) accumulated more 4-HNE-modified proteins than the corresponding wild-type animals on the same genetic background. As shown in Figure 2, pigmented knockout mice have significantly more retinal 4-HNE-protein adduct than the wild-type when exposed to bright light, a condition that induces oxidative damage. Similarly, in the BALB/c albino mice, 4-HNE-protein adduct was 60% higher in *Rdh12* knockout than in wild-type retinas in 2-month old animals raised under dim cyclic light [15]. These results support the hypothesis that 4-HNE is a physiological substrate of RDH12 in rod inner segments.

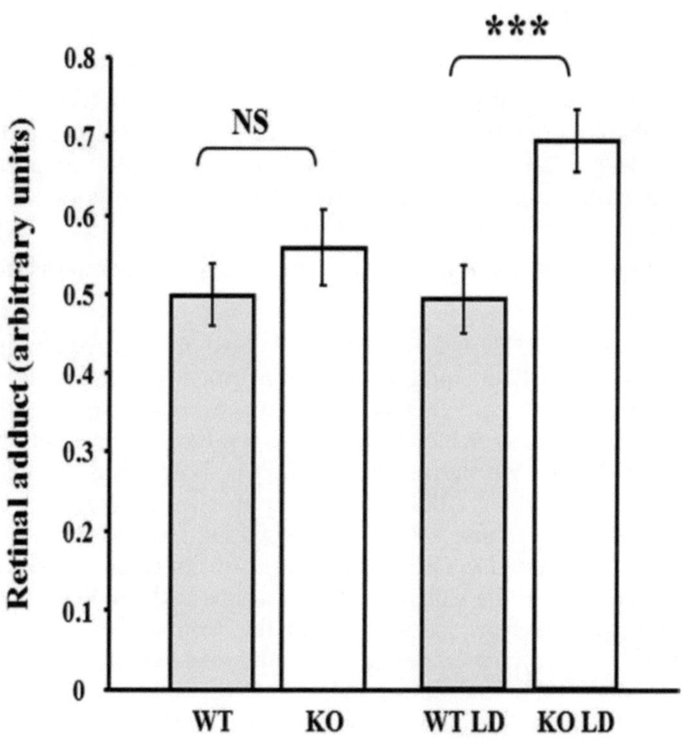

Fig. 2. **RDH12 protects against light-induced adduct formation in pigmented mouse retina.** Graph shows results for 6 mice per group. Littermates of wild-type and *Rdh12*

knockout mice were raised under dim (5-10 lux) cyclic light for 8 weeks. Control wild-type (WT) and knockout (KO) mice were killed 5 h after the (dim) light started. Light damaged (WT LD and KO LD) mice were killed after 48 h exposure to bright light (3,000 lux), without prior dilation of the pupils. Dissected retinas were homogenized in T-PER buffer (Pierce), according to the manufacturer's instructions. Protein concentrations were measured and dot blot analyses were carried out as described to quantify retinal adduct [15]. Equal aliquots (5 μg) of retinal protein were applied to a 96-well dot blot apparatus (Bio-Rad) and then transferred to a nitrocellulose membrane by vacuum filtration. Sample loading was monitored by staining the membrane with Ponceau red (Sigma). Membranes were blotted over night with a 1:1000 dilution of anti-HNE antibody coupled with horseradish peroxidase (abcam). Signals were quantified using SuperSignal West Femto Chemiluminescent Substrate (Pierce) and the digital Kodak Image Station 4000R.
Error bars denote SEM and Student's t test was used for significance.
NS, not significant ($p>0.05$); ***, $p<0.0001$.

The conclusion of these studies is that at least two physiological substrates of RDH12 coexist in photoreceptor cells; namely all-*trans* retinal and 4-HNE. The clearance of both of these substrates is delayed in the *Rdh12* knockout retina and it is now of crucial importance to determine which one, or if they can both, trigger the LCA13 phenotype.

6. Limitations of the *Rdh12* knockout mouse model to determine what substrate mediates photoreceptor damage

The main limitation to further determine whether accumulation of all-*trans* retinal or accumulation of 4-HNE is the triggering event in LCA13 is that, unlike LCA13 patients, the *Rdh12* knockout mouse does not develop a retinal phenotype [16, 19]. Thus the *Rdh12* knockout mouse is not an appropriate model for LCA13. We propose two possible explanations for the differences between mouse and human phenotypes.

6.1 Perhaps in mouse -but not in human- another enzyme is compensating for the loss of RDH12

In addition to RDH12, RDH11 and RDH13 are located in the inner segment of mouse photoreceptors. RDH11 and 12 are integral membrane proteins. Both enzymes are inserted in the membrane through a stretch of ~20 NH2-terminal hydrophobic residues (Figure 1) [5, 29]. RDH13 does not contain this stretch of hydrophobic residues and is a peripheral membrane protein. In previous studies, we showed that RDH11 is localized in the Golgi apparatus in spermatocytes [29] and in various cultured cells (unpublished observation). We performed a subcellular fractionation of mouse retinal tissues through ultracentrifugation on sucrose gradient [30]. RDH12 was found in Golgi- and endoplasmic reticulum-enriched fractions and RDH11 was detected only in the Golgi-enriched fractions [31]. Another study showed that RDH13 is a mitochondrial enzyme, localized within the intermembrane space, and associated with the inner mitochondrial membrane [32]. These different subcellular localizations suggest a specific role for RDH13 in the mitochondria, another specific role for RDH12 in the endoplasmic reticulum, but a possible redundant function for RDH11 and RDH12 in the Golgi. In the *Rdh12* knockout mouse photoreceptors, RDH11 may functionally compensate for RDH12 because these enzymes have overlapping localization and they have similar enzymatic activities and substrate specificities [17]. In humans on the other hand, RDH11 may not be expressed in photoreceptor cells [5] and thus may not compensate for the loss of RDH12 activity, possibly explaining the more dramatic phenotype in LCA13 patients.

6.2 Perhaps bright light is triggering the phenotype resulting from disruption of RDH12 enzymatic activity

Patients with LCA13 show an early disruption of their retinal structure [12]. The distorted laminar architecture of RDH12-mutant retinas seems to be a specific feature of some subtypes of LCA [12]. It has been suggested that such dysplastic retinal response could be triggered by some forms of photoreceptor damage induced by environmental conditions [12]. For example, light exacerbates the retinal dysplasia in a mouse model of LCA caused by *CRB1* mutations (LCA8) [33, 34]. Interestingly, the *Rdh12* knockout mice do not have a retinal phenotype when they are raised under a controlled dim (5-10 lux) cyclic light environment [15, 16, 19]. However, when they are challenged by exposure to bright light (3,000 lux for the *Rdh12* knockout mice under the BALB/c background), the *Rdh12*-null photoreceptors appear significantly more sensitive than the wild-type cells to light-induced apoptosis [15, 19]. Since *Rdh12* knockout photoreceptors degenerate only after exposure to bright light but do not have a spontaneous degeneration when raised under controlled dim cyclic light, it is possible that similarly, the LCA13 patients have retinal degeneration because they are regularly exposed to very bright light intensities (i.e. outdoor light during a sunny day). Anticipation of dysplastic retinal response and greater understanding of the pathway that triggers it could lead to specific therapy to prevent this process in LCA13 patients. Without such prevention, the amount of salvageable retina might quickly become so low that any gene replacement therapy would not be worth attempting.

It is likely that the compensation by other RDHs combined with the controlled lighting environment, and anatomical differences between mouse and human retinas explain the absence of retinal phenotype in the *Rdh12* knockout mouse, as opposed to the dramatic phenotype in LCA13 patients. In any case, it is difficult to use the *Rdh12* knockout mice to determine what substrate of RDH12 accumulating in absence of enzyme induces a retinal phenotype, because there is no phenotype. Retinal damage can be induced by exposure to bright light but this treatment exacerbates the production of both substrates of RDH12 simultaneously so it is impossible to distinguish which one triggers the hypersensitivity of *Rdh12*-null photoreceptor cells to light-induced damage. In addition, we cannot exclude the alternative possibility that the hypersensitivity to light of the *Rdh12*-null photoreceptors is not the specific result of accumulation of RDH12 substrate(s) but rather due to a non-specific effect of the gene inactivation.

7. Alternative strategy to determine what substrate mediates photoreceptor damage

An alternative strategy is to experimentally induce the production of all-*trans* retinal and 4-HNE simultaneously by exposure of the *Rdh12* knockout mice to bright light, while at the same time decreasing the level of 4-HNE using a molecule that can specifically scavenge 4-HNE and lower its concentration in the retina (Figure 3). This strategy allowed us to distinguish the relative participation of each substrate to the photoreceptor hypersensitivity to light.

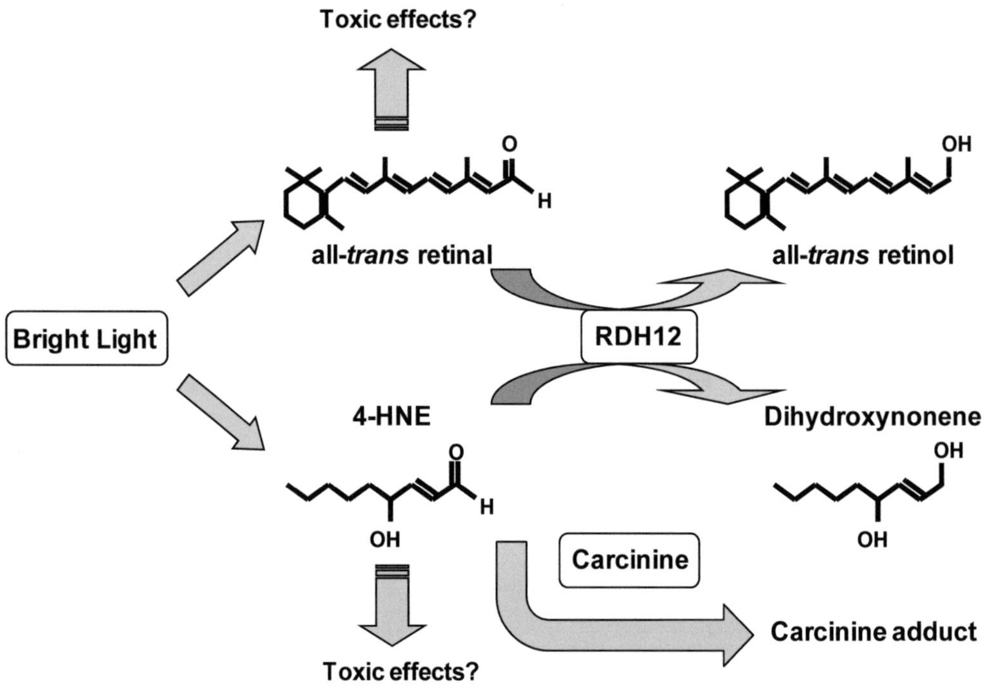

Fig. 3. **Experimental strategy to determine what substrate of RDH12 mediates photoreceptor hypersensitivity to light-induced damage.** Exposure to bright light exacerbates the production of both substrates (all-*trans* retinal and 4-HNE) simultaneously. In absence of RDH12, both substrates accumulate so it is impossible to distinguish which one triggers the hypersensitivity of photoreceptor cells to light-induced damage. Carcinine scavenges 4-HNE, forming 4-HNE-carcinine adduct, and thus can be used to lower 4-HNE independently of all-*trans* retinal. This allowed us to dissociate the effects of 4-HNE and all-*trans* retinal in the *Rdh12* knockout mouse retina.

Carcinine (β-alanyl-L-histamine) is a natural imidazole-containing peptide derivative that has antioxidant properties and can scavenge reactive aldehydes produced by lipid peroxidation [35, 36], thus preventing them from reacting with cellular proteins (manuscript submitted for publication). We have shown that intravitreal injection and systemic administration of carcinine protect wild-type photoreceptors from light-induced damage (manuscript submitted for publication). Photoreceptors are the first retinal cell type to show signs of damage after exposure to bright light. Light-induced apoptosis of photoreceptor cells is preceded by an increase of oxidative modification of retinal proteins [17, 37] and can be blocked by various types of antioxidants [38-40] including carcinine (manuscript submitted for publication).

We used carcinine to lower 4-HNE independently of all-*trans* retinal and dissociate the effects of these two molecules in mouse retina. Incubation of carcinine with all-*trans* retinal *in vitro* does not lead to any modification of the all-*trans* retinal molecule as determined by high-performance liquid chromatography analysis (unpublished observation) but incubation with 4-HNE leads to the formation of an adduct between carcinine and 4-HNE as determined by high-performance liquid chromatography and mass spectrometry (manuscript submitted for publication). Thus, carcinine is not expected to lower the retinal level of all-*trans* retinal or other retinoids under normal conditions or during exposure to bright light.

As shown in Figure 4A, without carcinine treatment (phospate buffered saline-injected eye), exposure of wild-type mice to bright light induces a decrease of rod-mediated visual function by approximately 50% for both a- and b-waves (black bars). As expected, the *Rdh12* knockout mice are more sensitive than the wild-type to light-induced damage, as shown by the 80 to 90% decrease of rod-mediated visual function for both a- and b-waves under the same conditions of light exposure (white bars). This result is consistent with previously published studies showing hypersensitivity of these knockout mice to light-induced damage [15].

Carcinine is expected to prevent light-induced damage mediated by oxidative stress and lipid peroxidation in photoreceptors. As shown in Figure 4A, with carcinine treatment (carcinine-injected eye), exposure of wild-type mice to bright light induce the decrease of rod-mediated visual function to about 25% loss instead of 50% loss without carcinine. In the *Rdh12* knockout mice, carcinine completely prevents the decrease of rod-mediated visual function. The remaining rod-mediated visual function after light damage goes from 10% without carcinine to 100% with carcinine, demonstrating a considerably beneficial effect of carcinine in these mice. The reason(s) why carcinine seems to protect more efficiently *Rdh12* knockout than wild-type photoreceptors is unknown. However, we can speculate that the disruption of *Rdh12* creates a "mild stress" in photoreceptors, inducing maybe some alternative protective mechanisms. The combination of enhanced compensatory protection and carcinine protection could be a possible explanation for this apparent higher efficiency of carcinine in the knockout than in the wild-type photoreceptors.

As shown in Figure 4B, cone-mediated visual function is more affected in the knockout than in the wild-type mouse by exposure to bright light (in phospate buffered saline -injected eye), and complete protection was provided by carcinine in both wild-type and knockout mice (carcinine-injected eye).

The fact that carcinine completely prevents light-induced damage in the *Rdh12* knockout mouse photoreceptors strongly suggests that the damage induced by light is mostly -if not only- mediated by oxidative stress and lipid peroxidation products accumulating in the *Rdh12* knockout photoreceptor cells. However, a mirror experiment in which all-*trans* retinal is specifically lowered independently of 4-HNE would further confirm our conclusion, if there was no protection. To specifically lower all-*trans* retinal independently of 4-HNE, a possible approach could be to overexpress the RDH8 enzyme in the *Rdh12* knockout photoreceptors because, as we have shown before, 4-HNE is not a substrate of RDH8 [29].

A- Rod response after light-induced damage

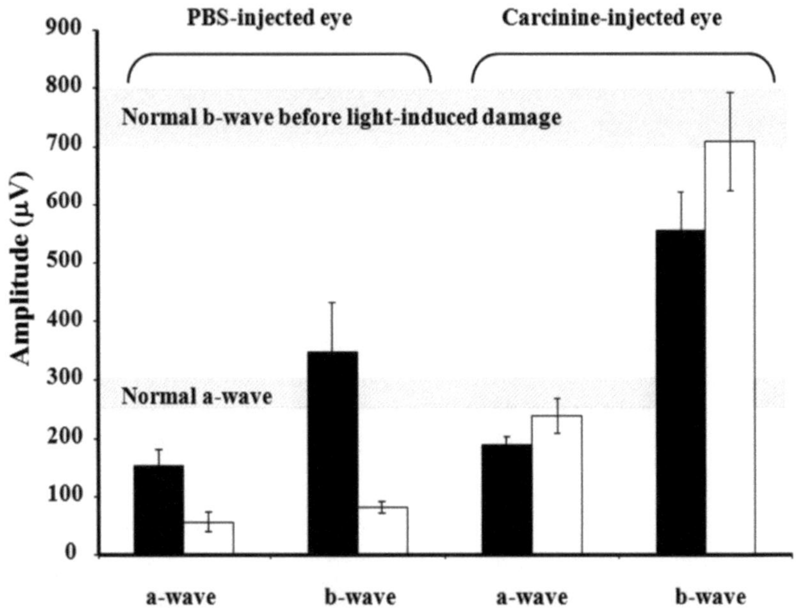

B- Cone response after light-induced damage

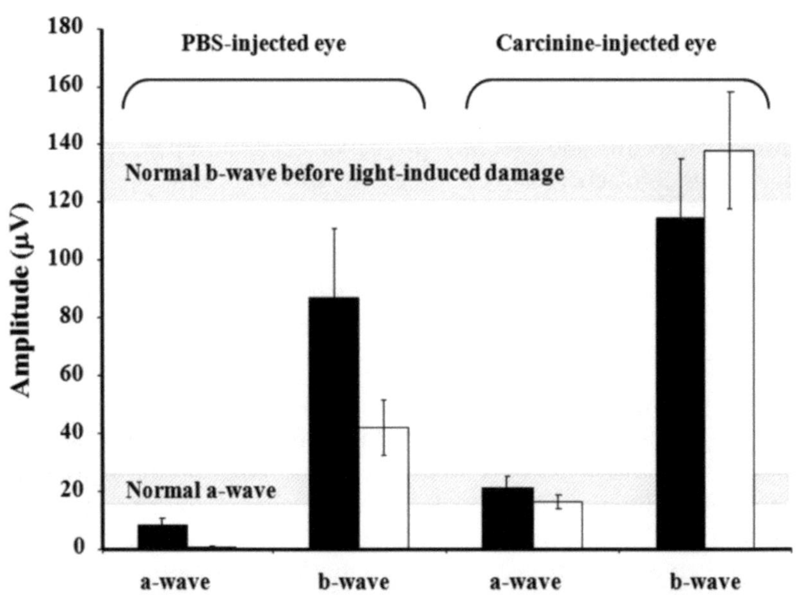

Fig. 4. **Carcinine protects visual function against light-induced damage in wild-type and *Rdh12* knockout mice.** BALB/c mice were raised in dim cyclic light for 8 weeks. Each

mouse was injected intravitreally in one eye with 1 µl phospate buffered saline (PBS) and in the other eye with 1 µl of 2 M carcinine diluted in PBS. Mice were returned in dim cyclic light for 48 h before light damage was initiated. Light damage was then induced in mice by 5 h exposure to 4,000 lux of white fluorescent light. After light exposure, mice are returned in dim cyclic light for 7 days to allow the retina to clear all dead cells. A. Scotopic electroretinographies were performed using saturating flash intensity. The a- and b-wave amplitudes of wild-type (black bars) and *Rdh12* knockout (white bars) are plotted to quantify rod-mediated visual function. B. Photopic ERGs were then performed to measure cone-mediated visual function. The a- and b-wave amplitudes are plotted to quantify cone-mediated visual function. Graphs show averaged results from 7 mice and error bars indicate SEM. Grey boxes show normal a- and b-waves recorded from PBS-injected eyes in mice that were not exposed to bright light.

8. Could decrease clearance of 4-HNE have toxic effects in photoreceptors?

Effects of 4-HNE in cells and its association with disease states have been increasingly well documented [23, 41]. Studies have shown that low, basal levels of the lipid aldehyde are present in cells (<5 µM), and at these concentrations, 4-HNE acts as a signaling molecule [42, 43]. It can activate cell growth and survival as well as stress response mechanisms, such as mitogen activated protein kinases, detoxification mechanisms, and inflammatory response, and by this way prepare the cells to overcome acute stress (protective effects) [41]. Under conditions of oxidative stress, 4-HNE concentrations increase above physiological levels; in membranes it accumulates at concentrations of 10 µM to 5 mM in response to oxidative insult [22, 23]. At such concentrations, the protective effect is lost; 4-HNE forms adduct with proteins inactivating their physiological functions, and activates intra cellular pathways promoting cell death [22, 23, 41].

The presence of 4-HNE-derived epitopes, including 4-HNE-protein adduct, has been reported in a growing number of diseases, including diabetes, cardiovascular, autoimmune, and neurodegenerative diseases, such as Alzheimer's disease, Parkinson's disease and amyotrophic lateral sclerosis [23]. The consistently growing evidence of increased 4-HNE tissue/blood levels in a great variety of human diseases certainly suggests a pathogenetic involvement of the aldehyde in their clinical expression and possible progression [41]. Recent studies have implicated 4-HNE in the pathogenesis of atherosclerosis and Alzheimer's disease [22, 41].

Oxidative stress, which induces lipid peroxidation and 4-HNE production, has been abundantly described to induce photoreceptor cell death [44-47]. Whether toxicity is mediated by 4-HNE and other lipid peroxidation products is unknown. We hypothesize that 4-HNE-mediated toxicity is inducing the rapid loss of vision in LCA13 patients. This hypothesis is based on the following evidences: (1) in cell culture, enzymatically active RDH12 protects against 4-HNE-induced cell death, while enzymatically inactive RDH12 does not [15, 37]. (2) Photoreceptor cells are particularly predisposed to oxidative stress because the retina has a high oxygen consumption, is chronically exposed to light, and contains several photosensitizers. This leads to an active production of reactive oxygen species. Furthermore, photoreceptors have a high content in polyunsaturated fatty acids, making their membranes particularly susceptible to lipid oxidation induced by reactive oxygen species. (3) In photoreceptor cells, 4-HNE production is induced by exposure to bright light, specifically in the inner segment, the compartment where RDH12 is located [15, 37]. (4) Disruption of RDH12 induces accumulation of 4-HNE-modified proteins in mouse retina, correlated with a hypersensitivity to acute light damage [15].

Taken together these results show a correlation between accumulation of 4-HNE in photoreceptor inner segments and loss of visual function, suggesting a possible cause-effect relationship. The cause-effect relationship has not been demonstrated but the mechanisms of 4-HNE toxicity have been abundantly documented in other cells types and disease states.

In LCA13 patients, it is likely that the loss of retinal structure and function is triggered by accumulation of RDH12 substrate(s). Two physiological substrates of RDH12 have been identified *in vitro* and *in vivo*. In absence of RDH12, accumulation of each of these substrates could theoretically mediate unwanted effects in photoreceptor cells.

9. Carcinine – A possible therapeutic agent for LCA13?

If 4-HNE is indeed involved in the LCA13 disease mechanism, then carcinine would clearly be beneficial based on its antioxidant and 4-HNE scavenging activities. Additionally, we recently found that carcinine has another effect that might be of significant interest for LCA13.

9.1 Carcinine protects RDH12 from degradation

In a previous study, we have shown that exposure to bright light induces a specific decrease of RDH12 protein level in the mouse retina while the closely related RDH11 protein remains stable [17]. This effect is not accompanied by a decrease of the *Rdh12* mRNA level so we hypothesized that the protein reduction was due to increased degradation rather than decreased production of RDH12 [17]. We further hypothesized that RDH12, like any other protein could be modified by 4-HNE (or maybe even more so because it has specific affinity for this molecule) and targeted for degradation [17]. Bright light would increase the endogenous production of 4-HNE and modification of RDH12, and the adduct would be quickly degraded. If not compensated by an increase in RDH12 synthesis, this would result in a net decrease of RDH12.

We used mouse retinal explants to test this hypothesis (Figure 5). Incubation of mouse retinas in a media containing 4-HNE leads to a 40% decrease of RDH12 in 4 h, while RDH12 level remains stable in retinas incubated in the same media without 4-HNE (Figure 5A). Total 4-HNE-modified proteins were then immunoprecipitated with anti-HNE antibody and immunoblotted using an RDH12 antibody. RDH12 was immunoprecipitated by the anti-HNE antibody (Figure 5B), demonstrating the modification of RDH12 by 4-HNE. The 4-HNE-RDH12 adduct accumulates first (at 1 and 2 h incubation with 4-HNE) and then decreases (at 4 and 6 h incubation with 4-HNE), supporting the hypothesis that the adduct is targeted for degradation. When compared with the total amount of 4-HNE-modified protein, the modification of RDH12 does not seem to happen significantly faster than the modification of the other proteins (Figure 5C). This result invalidates the idea that the specific affinity of RDH12 for 4-HNE would increase the rate of adduct formation. By contrast, the decrease of 4-HNE-RDH12 adduct is significantly faster than the decrease of the total amount of 4-HNE-modified protein (Figure 5C). This result suggests that RDH12 is particularly unstable (compared with other proteins) when subjected to oxidative modification.

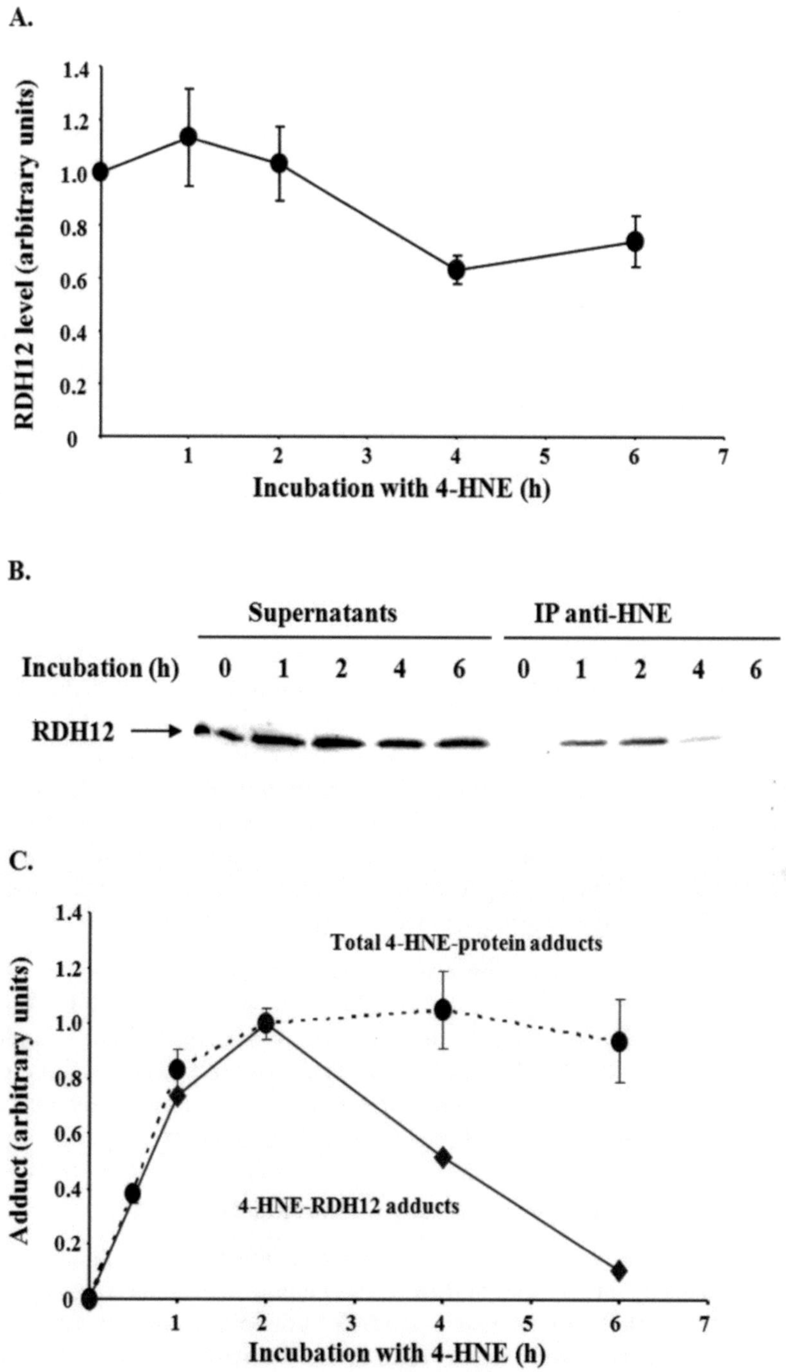

Fig. 5. **4-HNE modifies RDH12 and induces its degradation in retinal explants.** Retinas were dissected from 4- to 6-weeks-old pigmented wild-type mice. Retinas were incubated in Dulbecco's modified Eagle's medium, with or without 200 μM 4-HNE, at 37°C under 5% CO_2.

At indicated times, 6 retinas were removed from incubation, immediately washed in phosphate buffered saline, and frozen in liquid nitrogen for subsequent protein preparation. Frozen retinas were homogenized in T-PER buffer (Pierce), according to the manufacturer's instructions. A. Protein concentrations were measured and immunoblot analysis using anti-RDH12 antibody was performed using 30 μg of protein. The levels of RDH12 in retinal explants incubated with 4-HNE were expressed relative to those of RDH12 in retinal explants incubated without 4-HNE, arbitrarily defined as 1.0. B. Immunoprecipitation of 4-HNE-modified proteins was carried out as follow: equal amounts of protein were pooled from 6 retinas. 100 μg of pooled protein were incubated with 5 μl of anti-HNE antibody coupled with biotin (abcam) over night at 4°C, in a volume of 100 μl T-PER. 50 μl of streptavidin agarose resin (Pierce) was then added to each sample and incubated for 1 h at 4°C. After 3 washes with 1 ml T-PER, proteins were eluted in 50 μl Laemmli buffer and immunoblot analysis of supernatant and immunoprecipitated proteins were carried out with the anti-RDH12 antibody. C. Dot blot quantification of total 4-HNE-protein adduct was carried out as described in Fig. 2. with 2.5 μg of protein. The results from B were quantified and plotted on the same graph. At each time point the amounts of adducts are expressed relative to the highest level of adduct, arbitrarily defined as 1.0. Signals were detected using SuperSignal West Pico chemiluminescent or West Femto Maximum Signal Substrate (Pierce) and quantified using Kodak Molecular Imaging Software.

Interestingly, following intravitreal injection (Figure 6A) or systemic administration of carcinine (Figure 6B), the RDH12 protein level in mouse retina is stabilized and completely resistant to light-induced degradation. *In vivo*, the amount of 4-HNE-RDH12 adduct was undetectable (unpublished observation) so we could not determine whether carcinine was protecting RDH12 because it was opposing the 4-HNE-modification of RDH12 or through another mechanism. Absence of detectable 4-HNE-RDH12 adduct *in vivo* might be explained by the fact that endogenous production of 4-HNE as well as formation and degradation of adduct is an ongoing process, by contrast with the single dose of 4-HNE applied to the retinal explants creating a detectable "pulse" of 4-HNE-RDH12 adduct.

The stabilization of RDH12 protein by carcinine could enhance its therapeutic benefits for LCA13 patients. As discussed before, the RDH12 mutants associated with LCA are not only poorly active, but are also particularly unstable. The stabilizing effect of carcinine could keep the level of mutant RDH12 high enough to allow residual RDH12 enzymatic activity in photoreceptor cells. This, in addition with 4-HNE scavenging and antioxidant properties, could preserve the retinal structure and function in LCA13 patients.

9.2 Carcinine can be administered topically for chronic treatment

Treatment with carcinine would have to be started at the time of diagnosis and applied chronically to protect against 4-HNE and oxidative damage, which are ongoing processes in cells. We have investigated various modes of administration that could be compatible with a chronic treatment and measured the resulting level of carcinine in the retina (manuscript submitted for publication and unpublished results). Interestingly, topical administration through eye drop leads to detectable levels of carcinine in the retina (Figure 7). This result suggests that carcinine migrates from the cornea to the retina, following topical administration. The mechanisms of migration (simple diffusion versus transport) as well as the routes of migration (trans-corneal versus trans-conjonctival penetration, migration through the vitreous humor or by lateral diffusion through the sclera, etc) are currently under investigation. The possibility to administer carcinine through eye drops is promising because it is a non-invasive and particularly easy route of administration, compatible with chronic treatment.

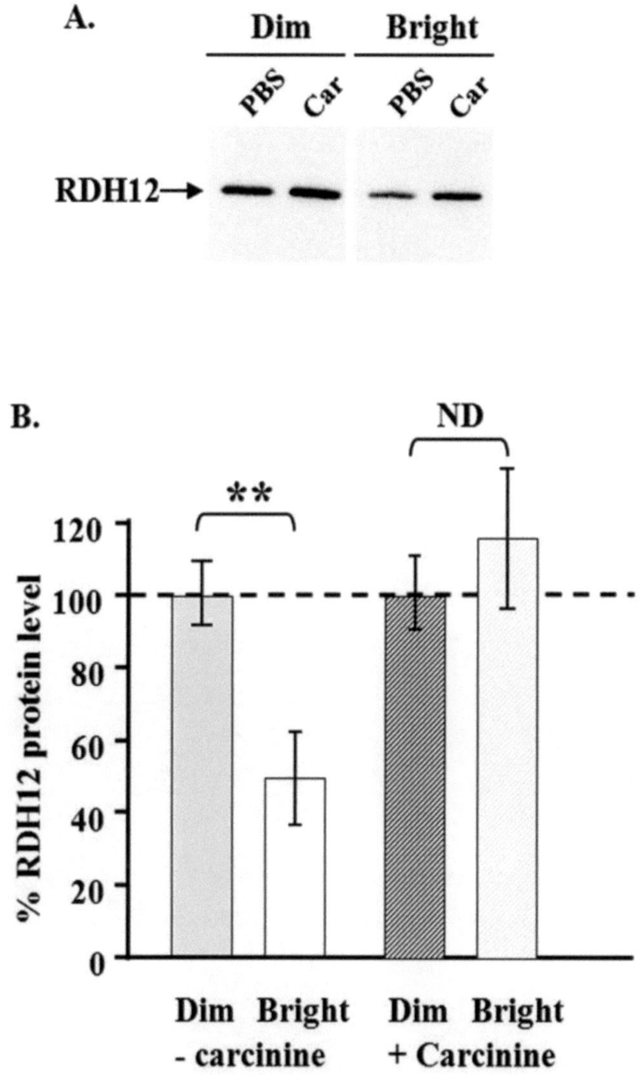

Fig. 6. **Carcinine protects RDH12 from light-induced degradation in mouse retina.** BALB/c mice were raised in dim cyclic light for 8 weeks before carcinine treatment. A. Mice were injected with carcinine or PBS and exposed to bright light as described in Fig. 4. For each group, 10 μg protein extract from 6 mice were pooled (60 μg final) and immunoblotted with anti-RDH12 antibody. B. Carcinine was administered through gavage (0 or 20 mg / mouse/ day) once a day for 5 days before light exposure. Mice were then exposed to bright white fluorescent light (3,000 lux) for 4h. Retinas were immediately frozen and proteins were extracted from one retina from each mouse (4 mice per group) using T-PER reagent. Protein

extracts from each mouse were individually quantified by immunoblot. RDH12 levels were normalized to β-actin first and expressed relative to the level of RDH12 in retinas of dim untreated mice, defined as 100%. Graph shows average and SEM values for 4 mice per group. Student's *t* test was used for significance; NS, not significant (>0.05); **=p<0.001.

A.

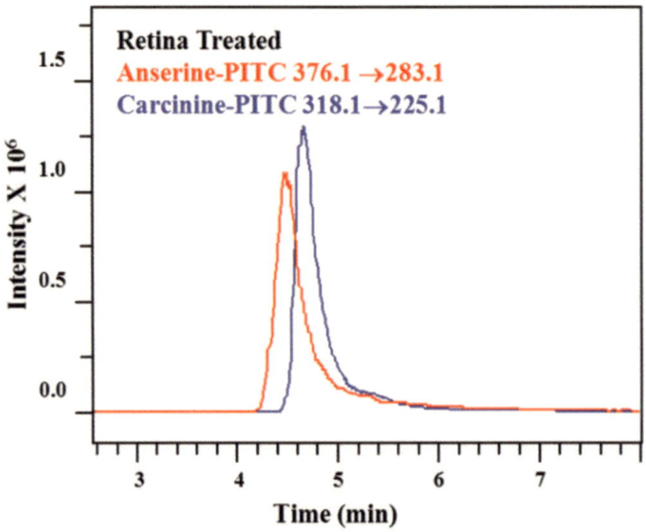

B.

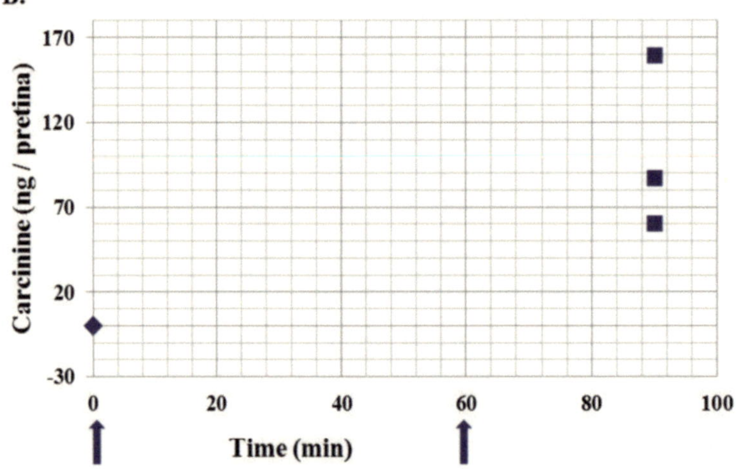

Fig. 7. **Topical administration of carcinine leads to detectable levels in the retina.** Mice received carcinine (0.2 M) dissolved in Can-C eye drop solution (Innovative Vision Products, Inc). To analyze and quantify retinal carcinine, 2 retinas were homogenized in 1ml of cold 0.01M HCl with polytron. One μg of internal standard anserine was added to the samples. Samples were extracted with acetonitrile and derivatized with phenylisothiocyanate (PITC). Samples were analyzed by high-performance liquid chromatography / mass spectrometry

(Michrom Bioresources Paradigm MSRB capillary HPLC, Bruker Daltonics HCT Ultra Ion trap MS). High-performance liquid chromatography was run on column Magic MS C18, 5m, 200 A, 0.5 x 150 mm with Solvent A (0.09% formic acid, 0.01% TFA, 2% acetonitrile, 97.9% water) and Solvent B (0.09% formic acid, 0.0085% TFA, 95% acetonitrile, 4.9% water). An isocratic program (15% B for 10 min) was used. The flow rate was 20 ml/min and detection wavelength was 215 nm. An ion trap mass spectrometer (HCT Ultra PTM discovery system, Bruker Daltonics) equipped with an electrospray ion source and operating under an Esquire data analysis system was used. The spray voltage was set at 4 kV in the positive mode. The heater temperature was maintained at 300 ° C. A, 0.2 M carcinine was administered in Can-C eye drop solution at 0 min and mice were killed 30 min later to collect retinas. B, Another set of mice received 0.2 M carcinine at 0 and 60 min (indicated by arrows) and were killed 30 min following the second administration (at 90 min) to collect retinas.

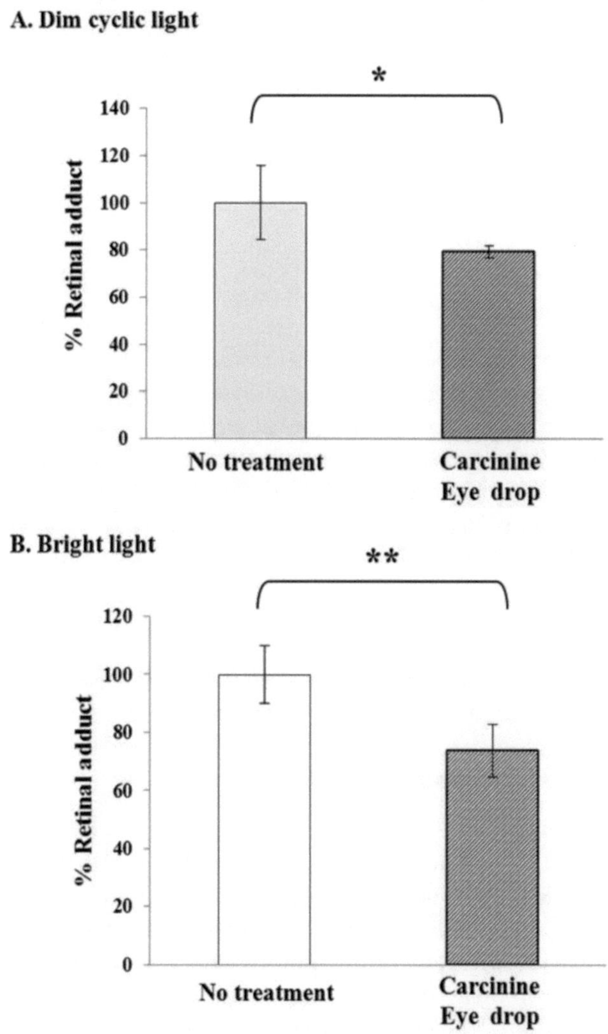

Fig. 8. **Carcinine decreases total 4-HNE-modified protein in mouse retina.** BALB/c mice were raised in dim cyclic light for 8 weeks before carcinine treatment. 0.2 M carcinine was

administered in Can-C eye drop solution (1 drop each 60 min, for 6 h) and mice were kept in dim light (A) or exposed to bright light (3,000 lux) for 4 h, starting right after administration of the second drop (B). Immediately after exposure to bright light, retinas were collected. Whole retinal homogenates were prepared and equal aliquots (10 μg) of retinal homogenates were analyzed by dot blot using anti-HNE coupled with HRP to quantify total 4-HNE-protein adduct. Five mice were used in each group, and the mean and SEM are plotted. Values were compared using Student's *t* test for significance; *=$p<0.05$; **=$p<0.001$.

9.3 Carcinine decreases the amount of 4-HNE-protein adduct in the retina

After administration of carcinine through eye drop, we found that the total amount of protein modified by 4-HNE in mouse retina is significantly decreased, both under dim and bright light (Figure 8). This result suggests that carcinine can scavenge 4-HNE *in vivo* after topical administration through eye drop. This implies that carcinine levels within the retina are adequate and that carcinine can enter the retinal cells to scavenge 4-HNE produced endogenously. Thus, carcinine could prevent the accumulation of toxic 4-HNE in RDH12-mutant retinas. We predict that carcinine, administered through eye drops, will prevent light-induced retinal damage in the wild-type and *Rdh12* knockout but these experiments have not been completed at this time.

10. Future directions

10.1 Developing therapeutic strategies

As shown by our preliminary experiments with carcinine, it is possible to start developing appropriate therapeutic strategies from the information already available on the function of RDH12. As discussed, exposure to bright light, as well as increased all-*trans* retinal levels, and increased oxidative damage particularly through 4-HNE modification are suspected to play a role in the disease mechanism. Accordingly, protection against these triggers can be developed with the goal to protect the retinal structure at least long enough to allow LCA13 patients to be eligible for gene replacement therapy.

10.1.1 Protection from light-induced damage

As discussed, the *Rdh12* knockout photoreceptors are more sensitive than the wild-type photoreceptors to light damage in mouse and exposure to bright light might be a trigger for the early dysplastic retinal response in LCA13 patients. Therefore, protection against light-induced retinal damage is an appropriate strategy.

Physical protection from bright light by wearing sun glasses should be encouraged for patients with LCA13. Compounds such as retinoid-like small molecules that provide chemical protection against light-induced retinal damage could also be beneficial [48, 49]. A number of studies have identified that photobleaching of rhodopsin is the essential trigger for retinal light damage [50, 51]. Genetically-modified mice that lack the opsin apoprotein or that have the opsin apoprotein but lack the ability to generate 11-*cis*-retinal are both protected against light damage [50-52]. A steady state rhodopsin level is achieved by the balance between its bleaching and regeneration. Therefore, the rate of rhodopsin regeneration is an important factor in light damage susceptibility. Fast regeneration of functional rhodopsin after bleaching increases retinal sensitivity to light damage, whereas slowing the flux of retinoids through the visual cycle increases the resistance of photoreceptors to light-induced insult. For example, slowing rhodopsin regeneration and inhibiting the visual cycle with 13-*cis*-retinoic acid prevents light damage in albino rats [53]. More recently, it has been shown that retinylamine provides efficient protection from light damage through a similar mechanism [48].

Most of the small molecules inhibiting the visual cycle are structurally similar to retinoids [49]. However, we recently identified α-phenyl-N-*tert*-butyl nitrone, a commonly used free radical spin trap, as another type of compound with no structural similarity with retinoids that interferes with rhodopsin regeneration during continuous illumination and protects against light-induced retinal degeneration [54]. The advantage that α-phenyl-N-*tert*-butyl nitrone may have over these retinol-related compounds is that it is not structurally similar nor a derivative of any of the visual cycle components and therefore may not have adverse effect by interacting with retinoid receptors and other components of the visual cycle.

10.1.2 Protection from oxidative damage

Because oxidative damage is likely to contribute to the LCA13 disease mechanism, compounds that inhibit oxidative damage or enhance endogenous protection against oxidative damage would be appropriate candidates for LCA13 treatment.

A wide variety of antioxidants are available as oral supplementations. Specific advantages of carcinine would be to combine antioxidant and 4-HNE scavenging activities. Thus, carcinine can offer an additional line of defense against oxidative damage by decreasing 4-HNE, a secondary product of oxidative stress that mediates and amplify the oxidative damage triggered by reactive oxygen species and that was shown to accumulate in mouse retina in absence of RDH12.

In addition, the main limitation for therapeutic utilization of antioxidants in retinal diseases is usually the poor targeting of the posterior segment of the eye (choroid, retinal pigmented epithelium, and retina) due to anatomical and physiological barriers that normally protect the eye. Most molecules cannot reach the posterior segment tissues upon topical administration in the form of eye drops. Periocular or intravitreal injections are more efficient routes of administration but they are invasive procedures, which are not compatible with a chronic preventive treatment. Oral supplementation of antioxidants is usually preferred but oral bioavailability and the necessity to cross the blood-retinal barrier limits the amount of compound reaching the target tissues, and therefore limits the prevention of oxidative damage in these tissues.

Carcinine is one of the very few compounds that can reach posterior segment tissues upon topical administration (less than 10 of such compounds have been reported to date) [55]. This method of administration represents the great advantages of being non-invasive, safer because it is used locally no systemic side effects are expected, and cheaper because it is used locally the amount needed is smaller than with systemic administration than any other methods. It is also compatible with a chronic treatment that could be administered by the patients themselves, or by their parents.

Drugs that upregulate the body's natural defense against oxidative stress would also be appropriate. Reactive oxygen species are constantly generated in cells as unwanted byproducts of aerobic metabolism. A wide variety of enzymatic as well as non-enzymatic cellular defense systems prevents and repair reactive oxygen species-induced damage to tolerable levels. Under ideal circumstances, the rate of production of oxidative damage should be comparable to that of its removal or repair. In LCA13, absence of the cellular defense mediated by RDH12 could perhaps be compensated by the enhancement of other cellular cytoprotective mechanisms through dietary or pharmaceutical manipulations. A wide variety of dietary polyphenols and other classes of phytochemicals have been reported to induce the expression of enzymes involved in cellular antioxidant defenses and detoxification mechanisms [56]. Such compounds would be appropriate candidates for LCA13 treatment as well.

11. Conclusion

Although generally described in the literature as an enzyme involved in all-*trans* retinal reduction, in this chapter we presented evidences for an additional detoxification role of RDH12 in photoreceptor inner segments, reducing the 4-HNE produced by lipid oxidation that takes place constantly in mouse retina. Loss of this function in patients with inherited retinal dystrophy due to mutations in *RDH12* might contribute to the dramatic and early onset loss of retinal structure and function in these individuals. Our preliminary experiments with carcinine show that this compound might be beneficial in LCA13 because it has antioxidant, 4-HNE scavenging, and RDH12 stabilizing effects in the retina. In addition, we showed that carcinine can be conveniently administered through eye drops to target the retina. Additional therapeutic strategies are developed for protection against bright light and all-*trans* retinal toxicity. Finally, the recent impressive clinical accomplishment of gene therapy for LCA2 patients laid the ground for using similar approaches to treat various types of LCA, including LCA13.

12. Acknowledgment

The authors thank Dr. Debra A. Thompson for her critical review of this manuscript. This work was supported by grants from the National Center for Research Resources (P20RR017703), the National Eye Institute (R21EY018907 and P30EY012190), the Oklahoma Center for the Advancement of Science and Technology, the University of Oklahoma College of Medicine Alumni Association, and by an unrestricted Grant from Research to Prevent Blindness, Inc. to the Ophthalmology Department of the University of Oklahoma Health Sciences Center.

13. References

[1] den Hollander, A.I., et al., *Lighting a candle in the dark: advances in genetics and gene therapy of recessive retinal dystrophies.* J Clin Invest, 2010. 120(9): p. 3042-53.

[2] Weleber, R.G., P.J. Francis, and K.M. Trzupek, *Leber Congenital Amaurosis.* GeneReviews, 2010.

[3] den Hollander, A.I., et al., *Leber congenital amaurosis: genes, proteins and disease mechanisms.* Prog Retin Eye Res, 2008. 27(4): p. 391-419.

[4] Stein, L., et al., *Clinical gene therapy for the treatment of RPE65-associated Leber congenital amaurosis.* Expert Opin Biol Ther, 2011. 11(3): p. 429-39.

[5] Haeseleer, F., et al., *Dual-substrate specificity short chain retinol dehydrogenases from the vertebrate retina.* J Biol Chem, 2002. 277(47): p. 45537-46.

[6] Kavanagh, K.L., et al., *Medium- and short-chain dehydrogenase/reductase gene and protein families : the SDR superfamily: functional and structural diversity within a family of metabolic and regulatory enzymes.* Cell Mol Life Sci, 2008. 65(24): p. 3895-906.

[7] Janecke, A.R., et al., *Mutations in RDH12 encoding a photoreceptor cell retinol dehydrogenase cause childhood-onset severe retinal dystrophy.* Nat Genet, 2004. 36(8): p. 850-4.

[8] Perrault, I., et al., *Retinal dehydrogenase 12 (RDH12) mutations in leber congenital amaurosis.* Am J Hum Genet, 2004. 75(4): p. 639-46.

[9] Schuster, A., et al., *The phenotype of early-onset retinal degeneration in persons with RDH12 mutations.* Investigative ophthalmology & visual science, 2007. 48(4): p. 1824-31.

[10] Sun, W., et al., *Novel RDH12 mutations associated with Leber congenital amaurosis and cone-rod dystrophy: biochemical and clinical evaluations.* Vision research, 2007. 47(15): p. 2055-66.

[11] Thompson, D.A., et al., *Retinal degeneration associated with RDH12 mutations results from decreased 11-cis retinal synthesis due to disruption of the visual cycle.* Hum Mol Genet., 2005. 14(24): p. 3865-75.

[12] Jacobson, S.G., et al., *RDH12 and RPE65, visual cycle genes causing leber congenital amaurosis, differ in disease expression.* Invest Ophthalmol Vis Sci, 2007. 48(1): p. 332-8.

[13] Lee, S.A., O.V. Belyaeva, and N.Y. Kedishvili, *Disease-associated variants of microsomal retinol dehydrogenase 12 (RDH12) are degraded at mutant-specific rates.* FEBS Lett. 584(3): p. 507-10.

[14] Belyaeva, O.V., et al., *Biochemical properties of purified human retinol dehydrogenase 12 (RDH12): catalytic efficiency toward retinoids and C9 aldehydes and effects of cellular retinol-binding protein type I (CRBPI) and cellular retinaldehyde-binding protein (CRALBP) on the oxidation and reduction of retinoids.* Biochemistry, 2005. 44(18): p. 7035-7047.

[15] Marchette, L.D., et al., *Retinol dehydrogenase 12 detoxifies 4-hydroxynonenal in photoreceptor cells.* Free Radic Biol Med, 2009.

[16] Kurth, I., et al., *Targeted disruption of the murine retinal dehydrogenase gene Rdh12 does not limit visual cycle function.* Molecular and cellular biology, 2007. 27(4): p. 1370-9.

[17] Kanan, Y., et al., *Retinol dehydrogenases RDH11 and RDH12 in the mouse retina: expression levels during development and regulation by oxidative stress.* Investigative ophthalmology & visual science, 2008. 49(3): p. 1071-8.

[18] Kanan, Y., et al., *Retinoid processing in cone and Muller cell lines.* Exp Eye Res, 2008. 86(2): p. 344-54.

[19] Maeda, A., et al., *Retinol dehydrogenase (RDH12) protects photoreceptors from light-induced degeneration in mice.* The Journal of biological chemistry, 2006. 281(49): p. 37697-704.

[20] Parker, R.O. and R.K. Crouch, *Retinol dehydrogenases (RDHs) in the visual cycle.* Exp Eye Res, 2010. 91(6): p. 788-92.

[21] Esterbauer, H., *Cytotoxicity and genotoxicity of lipid-oxidation products.* Am J Clin Nutr, 1993. 57(5): p. 779S-785S; discussion 785S-786S.

[22] Petersen, D.R. and J.A. Doorn, *Reactions of 4-hydroxynonenal with proteins and cellular targets.* Free Radic Biol Med, 2004. 37(7): p. 937-45.

[23] Uchida, K., *4-Hydroxy-2-nonenal: a product and mediator of oxidative stress.* Prog Lipid Res, 2003. 42(4): p. 318-43.

[24] Uchida, K. and E.R. Stadtman, *Modification of histidine residues in proteins by reaction with 4-hydroxynonenal.* Proceedings of the National Academy of Sciences of the United States of America, 1992. 89(10): p. 4544-8.

[25] Esterbauer, H., R.J. Schaur, and H. Zollner, *Chemistry and biochemistry of 4-hydroxynonenal, malonaldehyde and related aldehydes.* Free Radic Biol Med, 1991. 11(1): p. 81-128.

[26] Awasthi, Y.C., et al., *Role of 4-hydroxynonenal in stress-mediated apoptosis signaling.* Molecular aspects of medicine, 2003. 24(4-5): p. 219-30.

[27] Maeda, A., et al., *Limited Roles of Rdh8, Rdh12 and Abca4 on All-Trans-Retinal Clearance in Mouse Retina.* Invest Ophthalmol Vis Sci, 2009.

[28] Chrispell, J.D., et al., *Rdh12 activity and effects on retinoid processing in the murine retina.* J Biol Chem, 2009. 284(32): p. 21468-77.

[29] Kasus-Jacobi, A., et al., *Characterization of mouse short-chain aldehyde reductase (SCALD), an enzyme regulated by sterol regulatory element-binding proteins.* J Biol Chem, 2003. 278(34): p. 32380-9.

[30] Subramaniam, V.N., et al., *Biochemical fractionation and characterization of proteins from Golgi-enriched membranes.* The Journal of biological chemistry, 1992. 267(17): p. 12016-21.

[31] Saadi, A., et al., *Role of photoreceptor retinol dehydrogenases in detoxification of lipid oxidation products.* Studies on Retinal and Choroidal Disorders, To be published in 2012.

[32] Belyaeva, O.V., et al., *Human retinol dehydrogenase 13 (RDH13) is a mitochondrial short-chain dehydrogenase/reductase with a retinaldehyde reductase activity.* Febs J, 2007. 275(1): p. 138-47.

[33] Mehalow, A.K., et al., *CRB1 is essential for external limiting membrane integrity and photoreceptor morphogenesis in the mammalian retina.* Hum Mol Genet, 2003. 12(17): p. 2179-89.

[34] van de Pavert, S.A., et al., *Crumbs homologue 1 is required for maintenance of photoreceptor cell polarization and adhesion during light exposure.* J Cell Sci, 2004. 117(Pt 18): p. 4169-77.

[35] Babizhayev, M.A., *Biological activities of the natural imidazole-containing peptidomimetics n-acetylcarnosine, carcinine and L-carnosine in ophthalmic and skin care products.* Life Sci, 2006. 78(20): p. 2343-57.

[36] Babizhayev, M.A., et al., *L-carnosine (beta-alanyl-L-histidine) and carcinine (beta-alanylhistamine) act as natural antioxidants with hydroxyl-radical-scavenging and lipid-peroxidase activities.* Biochem J, 1994. 304 (Pt 2): p. 509-16.

[37] Tanito, M., et al., *Protein modifications by 4-hydroxynonenal and 4-hydroxyhexenal in light-exposed rat retina.* Investigative ophthalmology & visual science., 2005. 46(10): p. 3859-68.

[38] Organisciak, D.T., et al., *Protection by dimethylthiourea against retinal light damage in rats.* Investigative ophthalmology & visual science, 1992. 33(5): p. 1599-609.

[39] Tanito, M., et al., *Cytoprotective effect of thioredoxin against retinal photic injury in mice.* Investigative ophthalmology & visual science, 2002. 43(4): p. 1162-7.

[40] Tanito, M., et al., *Attenuation of retinal photooxidative damage in thioredoxin transgenic mice.* Neuroscience letters, 2002. 326(2): p. 142-6.

[41] Poli, G., et al., *4-hydroxynonenal: a membrane lipid oxidation product of medicinal interest.* Med Res Rev, 2008. 28(4): p. 569-631.

[42] Tanito, M., M.P. Agbaga, and R.E. Anderson, *Upregulation of thioredoxin system via Nrf2-antioxidant responsive element pathway in adaptive-retinal neuroprotection in vivo and in vitro.* Free Radic Biol Med, 2007. 42(12): p. 1838-50.

[43] Forman, H.J., *Reactive oxygen species and alpha,beta-unsaturated aldehydes as second messengers in signal transduction.* Ann N Y Acad Sci, 2010. 1203: p. 35-44.

[44] Cingolani, C., et al., *Retinal degeneration from oxidative damage.* Free Radic Biol Med, 2006. 40(4): p. 660-9.

[45] He, X., et al., *Iron homeostasis and toxicity in retinal degeneration.* Prog Retin Eye Res, 2007. 26(6): p. 649-73.

[46] Hollyfield, J.G., *Age-related macular degeneration: the molecular link between oxidative damage, tissue-specific inflammation and outer retinal disease: the Proctor lecture.* Invest Ophthalmol Vis Sci, 2010. 51(3): p. 1275-81.

[47] Kutty, R.K., et al., *Induction of heme oxygenase 1 in the retina by intense visible light: suppression by the antioxidant dimethylthiourea.* Proceedings of the National Academy of Sciences of the United States of America, 1995. 92(4): p. 1177-81.

[48] Maeda, A., et al., *Effects of potent inhibitors of the retinoid cycle on visual function and photoreceptor protection from light damage in mice.* Mol Pharmacol, 2006. 70(4): p. 1220-9.

[49] Travis, G.H., et al., *Diseases caused by defects in the visual cycle: retinoids as potential therapeutic agents.* Annual review of pharmacology and toxicology, 2007. 47: p. 469-512.

[50] Humphries, M.M., et al., *Retinopathy induced in mice by targeted disruption of the rhodopsin gene.* Nat Genet, 1997. 15(2): p. 216-9.

[51] Grimm, C., et al., *Protection of Rpe65-deficient mice identifies rhodopsin as a mediator of light-induced retinal degeneration.* Nat Genet, 2000. 25(1): p. 63-6.

[52] Redmond, T.M., et al., *Rpe65 is necessary for production of 11-cis-vitamin A in the retinal visual cycle.* Nat Genet, 1998. 20(4): p. 344-51.

[53] Sieving, P.A., et al., *Inhibition of the visual cycle in vivo by 13-cis retinoic acid protects from light damage and provides a mechanism for night blindness in isotretinoin therapy.* Proc Natl Acad Sci U S A, 2001. 98(4): p. 1835-40.

[54] Mandal, M.N., et al., *PBN ({alpha}-phenyl-N-tert-butyl nitrone) Prevents Light-induced Degeneration of the Retina by Inhibiting RPE65 Isomerohydrolase Activity.* J Biol Chem.

[55] Gaudana, R., et al., *Ocular drug delivery.* AAPS J, 2010. 12(3): p. 348-60.

[56] Surh, Y.J., J.K. Kundu, and H.K. Na, *Nrf2 as a master redox switch in turning on the cellular signaling involved in the induction of cytoprotective genes by some chemopreventive phytochemicals.* Planta Med, 2008. 74(13): p. 1526-39.

Part 6

Eye Plastics and Orbital Disorders

27

Eyelid and Orbital Infections

Ayub Hakim
Department of Ophthalmology, Western Galilee - Nahariya Medical Center, Nahariya, Israel

1. Introduction

The major infections of the ocular adnexal and orbital tissues are preseptal cellulitis and orbital cellulitis. They occur more frequently in children than in adults. In Schramm's series of 303 cases of orbital cellulitis, 68% of the patients were younger than 9 years old and only 17% were older than 15 years old.

Orbital cellulitis is less common, but more serious than preseptal. Both conditions happen more commonly in the winter months when the incidence of paranasal sinus infections is increased. There are specific causes for each of these types of cellulitis, and each may be associated with serious complications, including vision loss, intracranial infection and death. Studies of orbital cellulitis and its complication report mortality in 1- 2% and vision loss in 3-11%. In contrast, mortality and vision loss are extremely rare in preseptal cellulitis.

1.1 Definitions

Preseptal and orbital cellulites are the most common causes of acute orbital inflammation. Preseptal cellulitis is an infection of the soft tissue of the eyelids and periocular region that is localized anterior to the orbital septum outside the bony orbit. Orbital cellulitis (3.5 per 100,00) is an infection of the soft tissues of the orbit that is localized posterior to the orbital septum and involves the fat and muscles contained within the bony orbit. Both types are normally distinguished clinically by anatomic location.

1.2 Pathophysiology

The soft tissues of the eyelids, adnexa and orbit are sterile. Infection usually originates from adjacent non-sterile sites but may also expand hematogenously from distant infected sites when septicemia occurs. Preseptal cellulitis usually originates from skin infection with or without local trauma. It may also originate from structures inside the eyelid that are connected to the surface and become infected such as external and internal hordeolom. Chalazion is an example of internal hordeolom and these are all infected glands with surface connections. Glands with even partial preseptal location such as the lacrimal gland, in which the palpebral lobe is located preseptally, may also cause preseptal cellulitis.

Orbital cellulitis occurs in the following three situations:

- Spreading of an infection from the periorbital structures, usually from the paranasal sinuses, but also from the face, the globe and the lacrimal sac.

- Direct inoculation of the orbit from surgical trauma.
- Hematogenous spread from distant sites (bacteremia).

In case of local cutaneous infection, preseptal cellulitis can arise from the spread of a contiguous anterior eyelid infection such as a chalazion, local trauma resulting in infection such as insect bite, or a foreign body. The skin and, in some instances, the sinuses and lacremal mucosa, are colonized by various microorganisms. Orbital cellulitis following trauma is the consequence of a direct exposure of the orbital contents to these microorganisms. Open periorbital fractures, as well as closed fractures involving the sinuses or the nasal bone, may be a risk factor for orbital infections.

Orbital cellulitis, in contrast, usually arises from spread of infection from the paranasal sinuses. The ethmoid sinus is the most common source that extends to the orbit in children. In adults, pansinusitis is often accompanied by orbital cellulitis and its spread is believed to be caused through the ethmoid or frontal sinuses. The ethmoid sinus separeated from the orbit medially by the thinnest orbital bone - lamina papyracea. Often, the lamina contains congenital dehiscences through which sinus infections can easily spread into the orbit. This may support the frequency of orbital cellulitis secondary to ethmoiditis. The anterior and posterior ethmoidal foramina may also serve as potential passages for infection.

The orbital roof borders the frontal sinus. It is a diploeic bone and is thicker than the lamina papiracea. Infection may spread more easily through the valveless facial veins. Since the frontal sinus is adjacent to the anterior cranial fossa, it may serve as an intermediary for the spread of infection.

The orbital floor that borders the maxillary antrum also contain congenital dehiscences through which infection from the maxillary sinus can enter and facilitate infection spreading.

The posterior medial wall of the orbit borders the sphenoid sinus. Isolated sphenoiditis is rare. The sphenoid may be involved secondary to ethmoiditis. Sphenoethmoidal sinusitis has distinct clinical characteristics. Marked visual loss with or without ophthalmoplegia usually precedes the findings of proptosis and inflammatory orbital signs. This condition is rare due to the thick bony barrier and firm attachment of periorbita to the posterior orbital wall.

One dehiscence or more is often present in orbital walls, particularly in the thin-walled lamina papyracea and this facilitates the spread of infection to the orbit. Posteriorly, the optic nerve within the optic canal is adjacent to the lateral wall of the sphenoidal sinus. Dehiscence can also be found in the lateral wall of the sphenoidal sinus adjacent to the optic canal. The free valveless venous communication between the orbit and the sinus is another reason predisposing the orbit to the spread of adjacent sinus infection.

However, not all orbital cellulitis infections caused by sinus disease are secondary to acute sinusitis. Orbital fracture involving sinuses may allow spreading of an existing chronic sinus infection. Open fractures may also result in orbital cellulitis due to direct contact with the environment. Foreign bodies, such as a glass, wood or orbital floor implants, can cause orbital cellulitis. Infection can extend to the orbit from the eye, teeth, middle ear, or in neglected cases of preseptal cellulitis, from the eyelids and face.

Uncomplicated eyelid, strabismus, cataract surgery, glaucoma valve and retinal surgery may all expose the orbit to infection. Orbital implants that are imbedded and other foreign bodies, such as Molteno valve implant, may carry a risk for infection, especially if they are colonized or exposed. Orbital cellulitis secondary to keratitis may develop after radial keratotomy.

Advanced carries with secondary infection, poor dental work or an infected root or dental cyst can cause orbital cellulitis. Extraction of maxillary premolars, molars or canines exposes the patient to orbital infection. The most common pathway for odontico-orbital infections is through the paranasal sinuses. The apices of maxillary molars and premolars are in close proximity to the floor of the maxillary sinus and are, in fact, in direct contact with the maxillary mucosa. Direct fistula to the antrum may be caused by a floor fracture during dental extraction or maxillary mucosa disruption. Infection spreading from the sinus to the orbit can occur through congenital dehiscences in the medial orbital wall or through communication between the venous plexus of the maxillary mucosa and the ophthalmic veins, thereby causing thrombophlebitis.

Another pathway for the spread of infection is the thin buccal cortical plate of the alveolar processes.

Finally orbital cellulitis can occur secondarily from embolic spread in subacute bacterial endocarditis and from other distant organs.

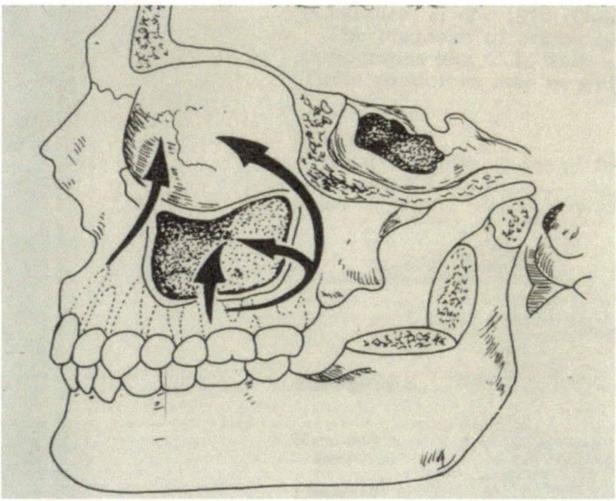

Pathway for odontico-orbital infections

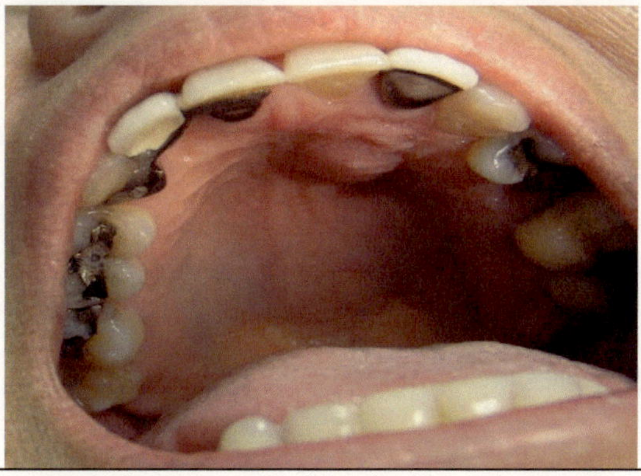

Dental abscess.Predisposing factors:poor dental care, advanced caries, root treatment, following dental extraction.

1.3 Classification

In 1970, chandler described a spectrum of progressive infectious changes in orbital cellulitis.

Chandler's Classification:

Stage I - Preseptal cellulitis

Ocasionally, edema may spread secondarily to preseptal cellulitis posterior to the septum without infection. In these cases chemosis may be present, but the extraocular movements and visual acuity remain intact.

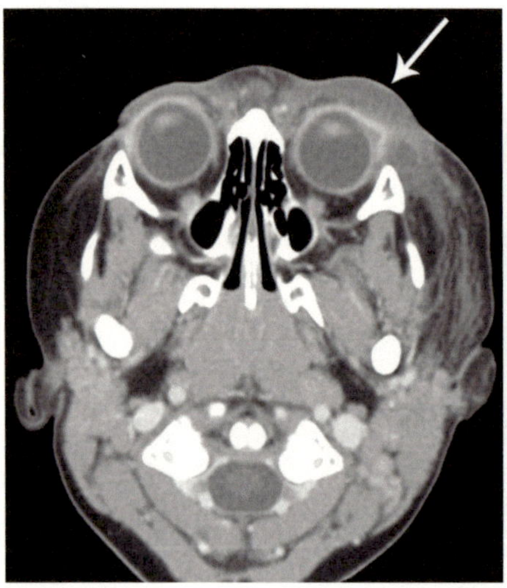

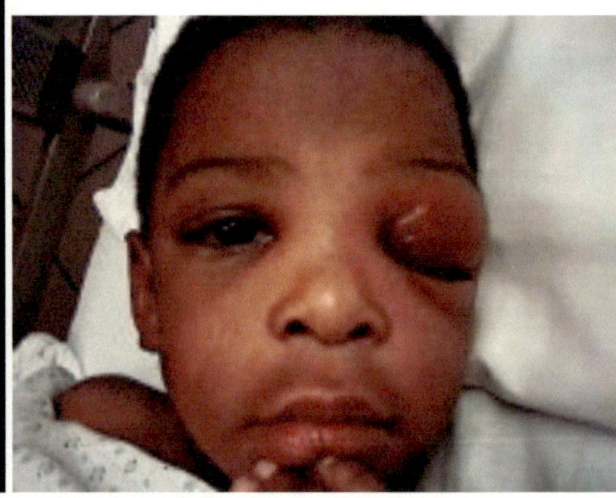

Stage II - Orbital cellulitis

Diffuse edema of orbital contents, with leukocytosis, fever, proptosis and impaired extraocular motility without discrete abscess formation.

Examples are shown in the images below:

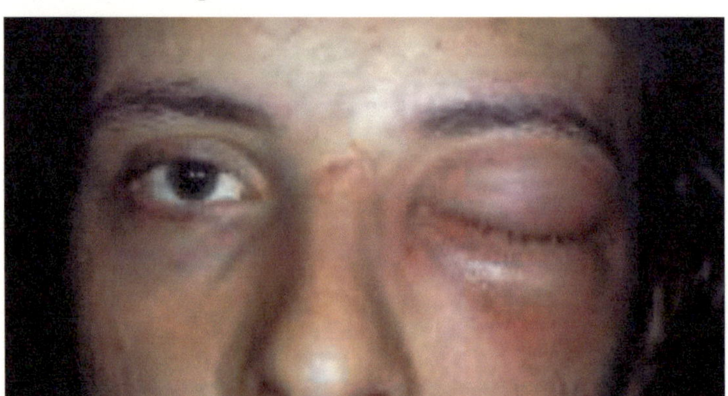

A male with left orbital cellulitis presented with proptosis, ophthalmoplegia, and edema and erythema of the eyelids. The patient also exhibited pain on eye movement, fever, headache, and malaise.

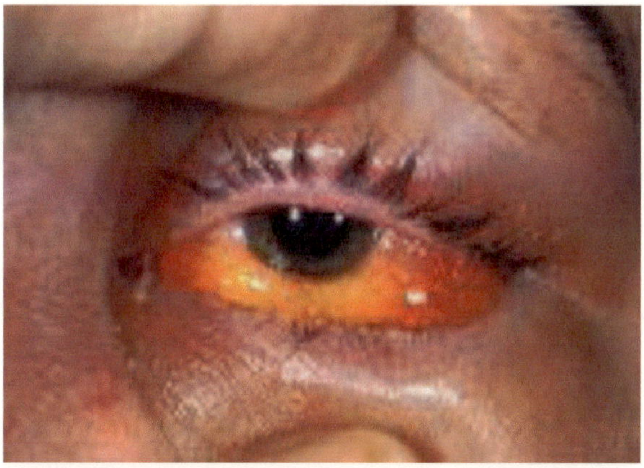

A male with left orbital cellulitis with proptosis, ophthalmoplegia, and edema and erythema of the eyelids. The patient also exhibited chemosis and resistance to retropulsion of the globe.

Stage III - Subperiosteal abscess

The globe is often displaced and limited in the field of gaze of the abscess.

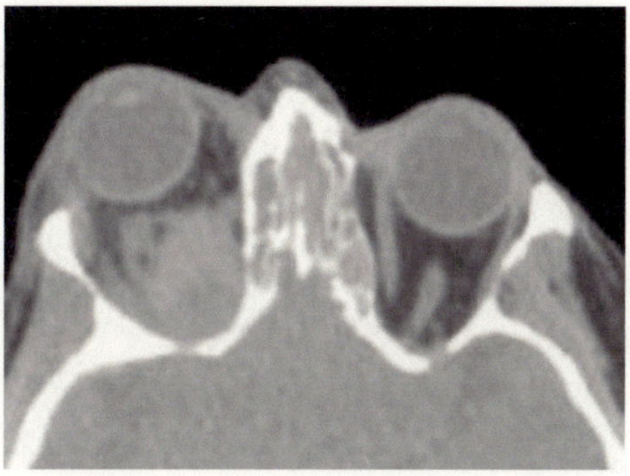

An axial computed tomography scan in a patient with a right orbital infection caused by streptococcus pneumoniae and a right superior orbital subperiosteal abscess that resulted in blindness.

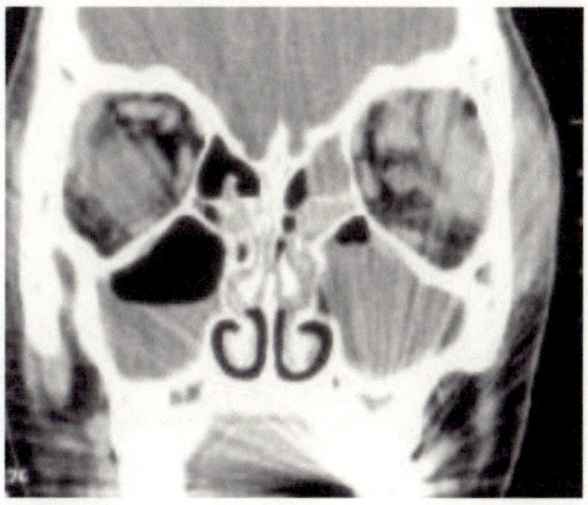

A coronal computed tomography scan of a child with pansinusitis as well as a left orbital and subperiosteal abscess.

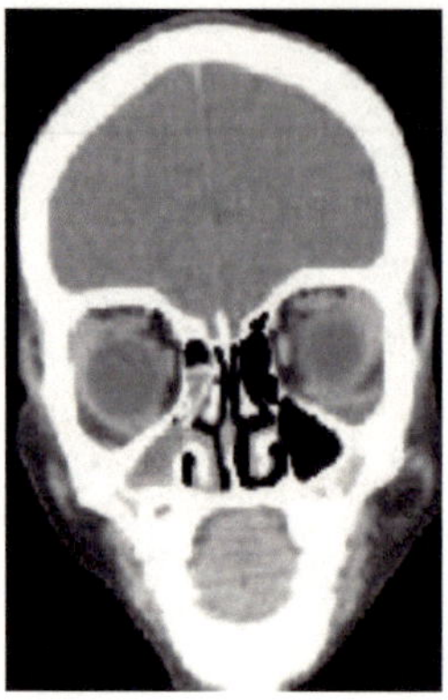

A coronal computed tomography scan in a patient with sickle cell disease. In this image, the patient has a left subperiosteal bleeding that mimiced the appearance of an infectious subperiosteal abscess.

Stage IV - Intraorbital abscess, purulent collection:

These patients have severe proptosis, chemosis, ophthalmoplegia and often visual loss.

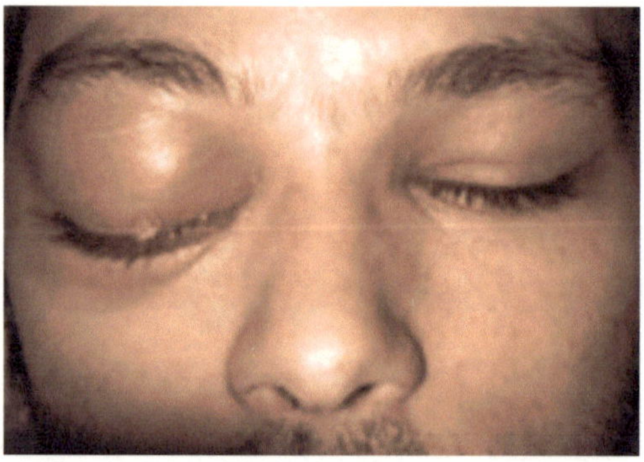

Frontal view of the patient with a right orbital abscess showing periorbital redness, swelling and proptosis.

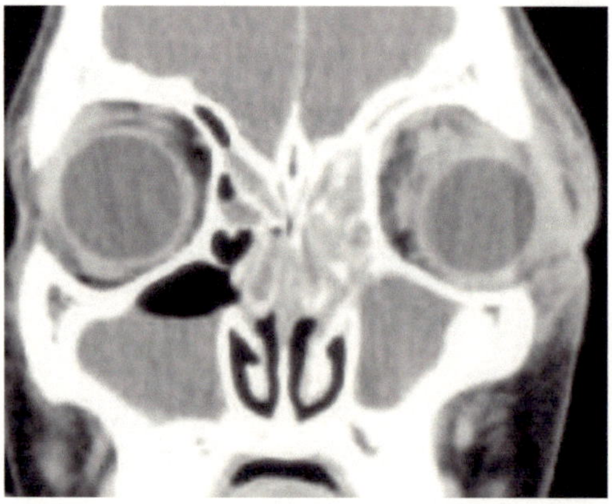

Coronal computed tomography scan in a pediatric patient with pansinusitis sinusitis and left orbital abscess.

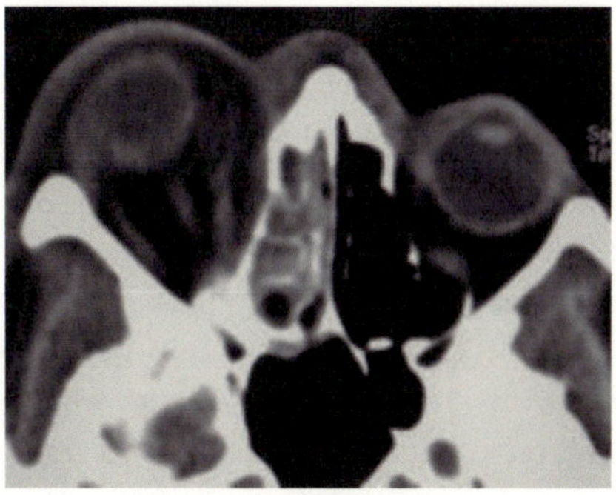

Axial computerized tomography scan shows a right classic proptosis associated with an abscess of the orbit, as well as displacement of the medial orbital tissues and tenting of the posterior.

Stage V - Cavernous sinus thrombosis (septic abscess)

In these instances, the orbital signs evolve in the fellow eye (bilateral) and other central nervous system signs supervene.

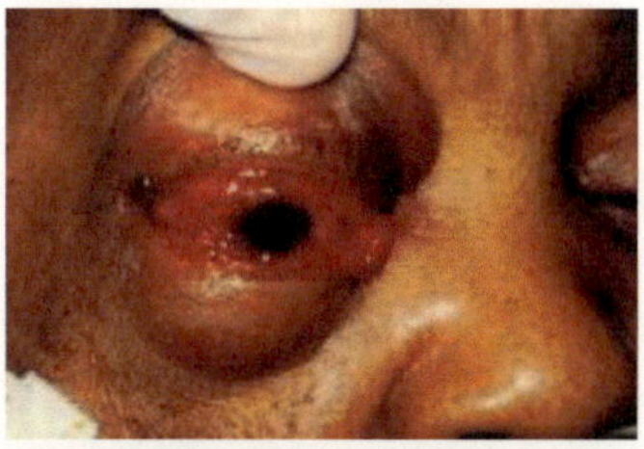

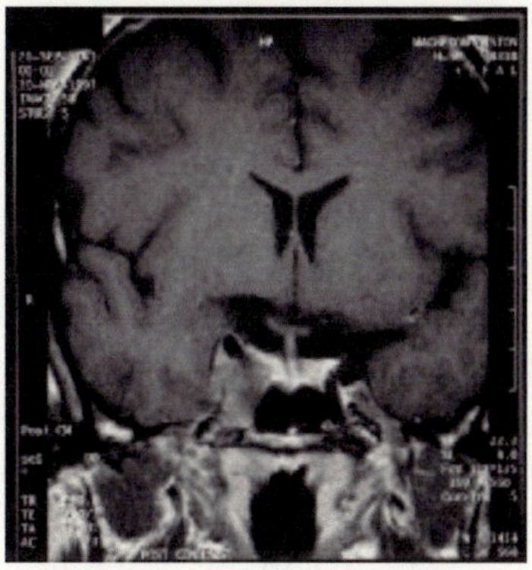

A T1 weighted coronal MRI demonstrating asymmetry between the caverenous sinuses with obliteration of the right cavernous sinus.

2. Preseptal cellulitis

Preseptal cellulitis is more common than orbital cellulitis. It can present with swelling and erythema of tissues surrounding the orbit, with or without fever. Preseptal cellulitis most commonly occurs from a contiguous infection of the soft tissues of the face and eyelids secondary to local trauma, foreign bodies or insect or animal bites. It is rare for untreated preseptal cellulitis to progress to orbital cellulitis by local extension. Defining the exact location of inflammation is essential for proper diagnosis and treatment.

2.1 Symptoms and signs

Patients with preseptal cellulitis often have a short history (days) of painless swelling of the eyelids. A history of early upper respiratory tract infection, trauma, insect or animal bite, conjunctivitis, or chalazion may be disclosed. Fever is an inconstant feature. The eyelid characteristically is erythematous, edematous, tender and warm. Vision and pupillary response are always unaffected and proptosis, globe displacement and limitation in ocular motility are never present. Concurrent preseptal cellulitis was discovered in the presence of many systemic diseases including, varicella, asthma, nasal polyposis and neutropenia. Preseptal cellulitis is more common among children than in adults.

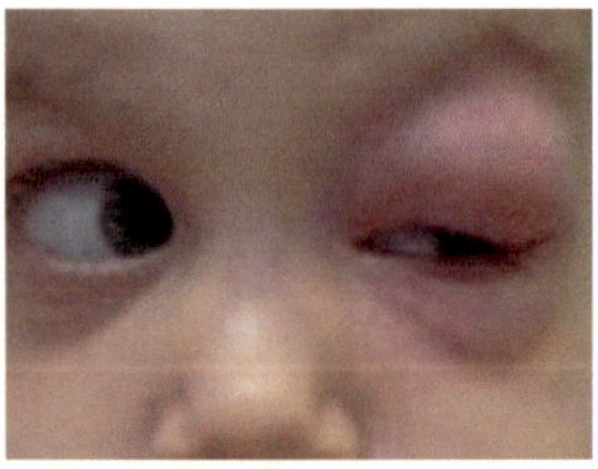

Preseptal cellulitis is more common in children than in adults.

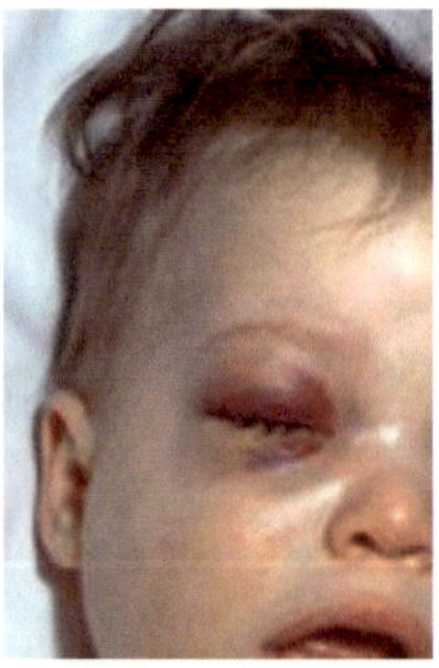

swelling and erythema of soft tissues surrounding the orbit.

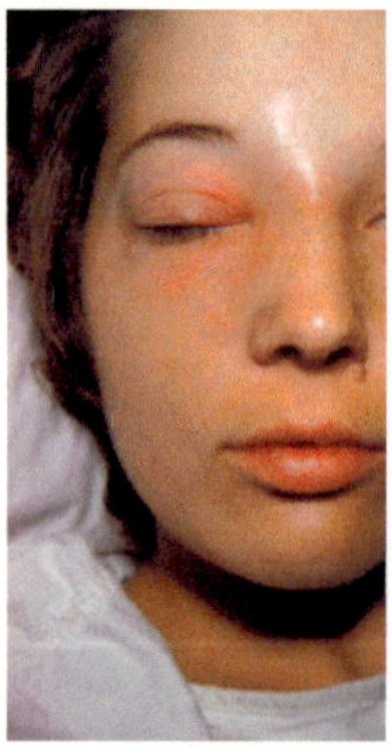

Eyelid swelling, erythema, local warmth, tenderness.no proptosis, limited ocular motility or optic nerve involvement.

2.2 Microbiology

The most common inciting microorganisms include *Streptococcus pneumoniae, Staphylococcus aureus*, other Streptococcus species and anaerobes. *Haemophilus infuenzae* type B was the most common cause in children under four years old. However, routine vaccination with conjugate *Haemophilus influenzae* vaccines since 1985 has dramatically decreased this infection in young children. Less commonly implicated microorganisms include Acinetobacter spp., *Nocardia brasiliensis, Bacillus anthracis, Pseudomonas aeruginosa, Neisseria gonorrhoea*, Proteus spp., *Pasteurella multocida, Mycobacterium tuberculosis* and Trichophyton spp.

2.3 Differential diagnosis

Conditions that might masquerade as preseptal cellulitis include allergic edema (anaphylactoid reaction) of the eyelids, severe blepharitis with scruffs (seborrheic), collarets(staphylococcal), sleeves(demodex) with or without erythema but no local warmth. The meibomianitis is characterised with eyelid swelling, pouting of meibomian gland orisices and discharge from orifices but no local warmth.

In addition dacryoadenitis, blunt trauma, thyroid eye disease, leukemic infiltrates, blepharochalasis syndrome and autoimmune inflammatory disorder such as lupus. Other disorders of less resemblance include orbital tumors/pseudotumours (, orbital vasculitis, necrotising fascitis and others.

2.4 Management

Treatment regimens cover the most likely organisms to cause infection in this setting and according to case series. Outpatient treatment should include broad-spectrum oral antibiotics and close observation. The author came to a conclusion that most cases of preseptal cellulitis can be safely managed as outpatients with oral antibiotics and follow-up until improvement is documented. If the condition does not improve or deteriorates 48 hours or more after oral antibiotic treatment, the patients should be admitted for intravenous antibiotic treatment and close observation. The average time of hospitalization is four days.

The appropriate antibiotics in adults include Amoxicillin–clavulinate (Augmentin) 875 mg every 12 h, and in children 90 mg/kg/day amoxicillin and 6.4 mg/Kg/day of clavulanate divided to two doses. Another option includes Cefpodoxime (Vantin) 200 mg every 12 h in adults, and 10 mg/kg/d divided every 12 h in children with maximum daily dose of 400 mg. Cefdinir (Omnicef) 600 mg daily in adults, and 14 mg/kg/d divided every 12 h in children with maximum daily dose 600 mg is another option.

Pediatric patients under 1 year of age and all more severe cases require the same approach as patients with orbital cellulitis, namely, intravenous broad-spectrum antibiotics and hospital observation .Blood cultures should be obtained if the systemic fever increases. The recommended duration of antimicrobial therapy is for 7-10 days. Occasionally, patients will continue to have local signs of cellulitis at end of treatment. Oral antibiotic therapy is recommended to be continued in these patients until resolution of the erythema. Children with preseptal cellulitis, no orbital involvement, and who do not appear toxic can be treated with intramuscular or oral antibiotics on a daily basis as outpatients. Preseptal cellulitis in adults can be managed on outpatient basis with oral antibiotics with frequent monitoring for progression.

3. Orbital cellulitis

Orbital cellulitis occurs in three settings:

i. Extension of infection from periorbital structures, such as the face, lacrimal sac and globe, but particularly from the paranasal sinuses. Acute sinusitis is complicated by orbital cellulitis in 1-3% of cases and the coexisting sinusitis is present in 73-94% of patients with orbital cellulitis. Ethmoid sinusitis and pansinusitis are most likely to progress to orbital cellulitis. The first ocular sign of sinusitis may be preseptal inflammation only. This can then quickly progress to the classic clinical picture of orbital cellulitis. Other causes include - orbital trauma, with fracture or a foreign body, dacryocystitis, and infection of teeth, middle ear or face.

ii. Direct inoculation from accidental trauma or from surgery. Orbital cellulitis is uncommon complication of ophthalmic surgery, being reported after strabismus surgery, blepharoplasty, radial keratotomy, retinal surgery and following peribulbar anesthesia. A special case is fungal orbital cellulitis, a relatively rare condition occurring in two principal forms - 1. Subacute infection due to genera of Zygomacetes (mucormycosis). 2. A more chronic orbital infection caused by species of Aspergillus. The distinction between these two may be difficult on clinical observation alone.
iii. Hematogenous spread (endogenous from bacteremia). The microorganisms responsible for most cases are aerobic non-spore forming bacteria.

3.1 Symptoms and signs

Orbital cellulitis as preseptal cellulitis can present with swelling and erythema. The cardinal signs and symptoms are proptosis, ophthalmoplegia and globe displacement. Pain on eye movement, vision loss (indicates orbital apex involvement), diplopia, conjunctival chemosis and elevated intraocular pressure are common but variable accompanying signs.

3.2 Microbiology

S. aureus and Streptococci are the most commonly identified organisms in culture-positive orbital cellulitis. Less common causes are *H. influenza* and non-spore forming anaerobes. However, many other common and rare bacterial pathogens include *Eikenella corrodens, Aeromonas hydrophilia, P. aeroginosa,* fungal and mycobacterial pathogens, including *Scedosporium apospermum, M. tuberculosis* and *Mycobacterium avium* complex. The prognosis of aspergillosis is poor. More than 80% of reported patients have died from this causative.

3.3 Differential diagnosis

Conditions that may mimic orbital cellulitis include:

- Anaphylactoid reaction can be characterised with eyelid swelling and erythema but no local warmthand no proptosis, limited ocular motility or optic nerve involvement.
- Cavernous sinus syndrome that is characterised by proptosis, complete ophthalmoplegia, optic nerve involvement, V2 involvement, evolve to bilateral condition and usually in debilitated patients (diabetics, drug abusers, HIV).
- The orbital apex syndrome is characterised with complete external ophthalmoplegia, optic nerve and V1 involvement with/without proptosis.
- Superior orbital fissure syndrome is a condition that is characterised with complete external ophlmoplegia, V1 involvement with or without proptosis.
- The orbital compartment syndrome and the orbital tumors can present with proptosis, limited ocular motility, optic nerve involvement and increased intraocular pressure but no local warmth.

3.4 Diagnosis

There have been no controlled trials examining the utility of radiologic studies (e.g. computed tomography scanning, orbital ultrasound, or magnetic resonance imaging) in the diagnosis of orbital cellulitis or in distinguishing preseptal from orbital cellulitis.

Computed Tomography scanning (CT)

CT can confirm extension of inflammation into the orbit, detect coexisting sinus disease, and identify an orbital or subperiosteal abscess. Whether every patient with suspected orbital cellulitis needs a CT scan is controversial. Some experts suggest that a CT scan be performed only in those patients who deteriorate or fail to respond to 48 hours of IV antibiotics, as the majority of patients with orbital cellulitis do well with conservative medical management. It is suggested that patients with suspected orbital cellulitis - those with proptosis, globe displacement, limitation of eye movements, double vision, vision loss, and those patients in whom the physician cannot accurately assess vision - usually patients less than one year of age, at presentation have a baseline CT scan.

Orbital Ultrasunography(US)

US provides higher-resolution details of orbital contents and is useful when sequential follow-up of an abscess or drained abscess is required. However, orbital sonography is not widely available and is dependent on the expertise of the sonographer.

Magnetic Resonance Imaging (MRI)

MRI is superior to CT in the resolution of soft tissue disease. However, it is not usually performed because of the need for sedation in pediatric patients and because MRI is rarely immediately available.

Microbiologic studies

The causative microorganism in orbital cellulitis may be difficult to identify due to normal flora contaminants, mixed infection, and prior antibiotic therapy. Cultures for aerobic and anaerobic organisms may be obtained from blood, sinus aspirates, and abscess. Because blood cultures are usually negative, some clinicians obtain cultures of eye secretions or pharyngeal culture. However, these cultures are likely to be contaminated with normal oropharyngeal flora and should not guide the choice of antibiotic therapy. Microbiologic data limited to microorganisms recovered by surgical drainage from orbital abscesses or involved sinuses and/or positive blood culture are the most reliable information. It is recommended that in patients with suspected orbital cellulitis, blood cultures should be obtained before the initiation of antibiotic treatment. If surgery is performed, culture of abscess material or sinus contents should be sent for aerobic, anaerobic and fungal cultures.

3.5 Complications

The complications of bacterial orbital cellulitis may be orbital or intracranial. Orbital complications of orbital cellulitis include subperiosteal or orbital abscess formation in 7-9%, permanent globe displacement, limited ocular motility that may cause diplopia, and vision loss in 1%. Orbital abscess may be clinically indistinguishable from orbital cellulitis. Proptosis and globe displacement tends to be more severe with orbital abscess than in orbital cellulitis, and patients are more likely to be systemically ill. The diagnosis of orbital abscess is confirmed by imaging or at surgery. The identification of an orbital abscess on the baseline CT scan is important since these patients almost always require surgery. Intracranial complications, which are encountered in 4% of orbital cellulitis secondary to sinusitis include meningitis in 2%, cavernous sinus thrombosis in 1%, intracranial abscess formation, epidural or subdural abscess or parenchymal brain abscess in 1%, and carotid artery occlusion. Intracranial involvement may be heralded by ophthalmoplegia, changes in mental status, contralateral cranial nerve palsy, or bilateral orbital cellulitis. Cavernous sinus thrombosis has become relatively rare in developed countries because of prompt and adequate treatment of most cases of acute sinusitis, but it still poses a major threat. The mortality rate of cavernous sinus thrombosis may exceed 50%.

Permanent vision loss may occur because of:

1. Corneal ulcer and perforation secondary to exposure or neurotrophic keratitis.
2. Destruction of intraocular tissues following neovascular or inflammatory glaucoma, endophthalmitis, septic uveitis or retinitis and exudative retinal detachment.
3. Various other mechanisms affecting the globe or posterior orbit, such as secondary glaucoma due to elevated orbital pressure, infectious optic neuritis or inflammatory optic neuritis , pressure effects the optic nerve, thrombophlebitis of ocular veins and central retinal artery occlusion.

Blindness can result from elevated intraorbital pressure causing optic neuropathy or extension of the infection to the optic nerve from the sphenoid sinus.

3.6 Management

Prompt administration of appropriate antibiotics is the key for successful treatment of orbital cellulitis. After appropriate workup, all periorbital and orbital infections should be treated with broad-spectrum antimicrobial agents. There have been no controlled trials examining the required duration of antimicrobial therapy in orbital cellulitis. Treatment regimens are based upon coverage of the most likely organisms to cause infection in this setting and treatment of case series. The initial empiric antibiotic treatment should consist of parenteral broad-spectrum therapy. Infection due to methicillin-resistant *S. aureus* is best treated with vancomycin, clindamycin and cefotaxime.

Fungal orbital cellulitis occurs and is primarily due to mucor and aspergillums species. It requires antifungals, such as amphotericin. Corticosteroids may be helpful in bacterial infections, but they should not be started before surgery and until the patient has been on appropriate antibiotics for 2-3 days to ascertain eradication of the microbial agents.

If secondary glaucoma develops, ocular anti-hypertensive agents should be initiated promptly. Prompt diagnosis and therapy are important since delayed intervention can result in sustained vision loss.

3.6.1 Antibiotic treatment

Due to increasing incidence of Methicillin-resistant *S. Aureus*, empiric therapy with Vancomycin (Vancocin) (15 mg/kg IV every 12 hours in adults, 10 to 15 mg/kg IV every 6 hours in children, maximum daily dose of 4gr) is recommended. If susceptibility testing reveals Methicillin-sensitive *S. aureus*, Vancomycin should be replaced with Nafcilin (Unipen), or Oxacillin (Bactocill) - (both agents are dosed at 2gr IV every 4 hours in adults, and 200 mg/kg per day IV in 4-6 divided doses in children, maximum daily dose of 12gr) since these agents have better CNS penetration than vancomycin.

One of the following should be added:

1. Ampicillin-sulbactam (Unasyn) 3gr IV every 6 hours in adults, 300 mg/kg per day in 4 divided doses in children, maximum daily dose of 12 gr.
2. Ticarcillin-clavulanate (Ticar), which covers most of the Gram-negative bacteria as well as Gram-positive organisms, including atypical *H. influenza,* and has also excellent anaerobic coverage. The dosage is 3.1gr IV every 4 hours in adults, 200-300 mg of ticarcillin component per kg per day in 4-6 divided doses in children of less than 60 kg. The maximum daily dose of ticarcillin component is 18 gr.
3. Piperacillin-Tazobactam 4.5gr IV every 6 hours in adults, 240 mg/kg per day in 3 divided doses in children, with a maximum daily dose of 16gr of piperacillin component.
4. Ceftriaxone (Rocephin) is effective agpenicillinase-producing *S. aureus,* most Gram-positive organisms, and most Gram-negative organisms except for Pseudomonas. Ceftriaxone also crosses the blood-brain barrier; therefore, it is an excellent choice if there is a suspicion of concurrent intracranial infection. 2gr IV every 12 hours in adults, 80-100 mg/kg per day in 2 divided doses in children, maximum dose of 4gr daily may be given.
5. Cefotaxime (Claforan), a third-generation cephalosporin that covers most of the common sinus pathogens with the exception of *Clostridium difficile,* may be given 2gr IV every 4 hours in adults, 150-200 mg/kg per day in 3-4 equally divided doses in children, with a maximum daily dose of 12gr.

Patients allergic to penicillin and/or cephalosporins may be treated with a combination of vancomycin and a flouroquinolon. For patients over 17 years of age, ciprofloxacin 500 mg twice a day or levofloxacin 500 mg daily may be prescribed. Flouroquinilones are not recommended for use in pediatric patients as first-line therapy for any infection because of the musculoskeletal side effects - The mildest side effects include muscle pain, called fibromyalgia. A more serious side effect, though also less common, is tendon damage. Fluoroquinolones can, in high doses, cause tendon damage, which can ultimately lead to rupture of the Achilles tendon (in addition gastrointestinal effects predominating (nausea, vomiting, diarrhea, or abdominal pain in 1.0%-5.0% of thepatients), followed byeffects onthecentral nervous system (dizziness, headache, and/or insomnia in 0.1%-0.3% of the patients) and skin (0.5%-2.2% of the patients). Elevation in levels of hepatic enzymes occurred in 1.8%-2.5% of thepatients, azotemia in 0.2%-1.3%, and eosinophilia in 0.2%-2.0%. Initial antibiotic therapy should be administered IV under hospitalization. Generally switching to oral therapy is done after the patient is afebrile and skin findings have begun to resolve, which usually take 3-5 days.

The duration of treatment depends on the response. Patients should be treated with parenteral antibiotics until they show clear evidence of clinical improvement as manifested by decrease in orbital congestive signs such as proptosis, gaze limitation, cellulitis and edema. Intravenous therapy should continue for a minimum of 3 days. Then oral antibiotic therapy may be instituted for a total course of 10 days to 3 weeks, depending on the severity of infection. Associated bacteremia, however, should be treated with 7-10 days of IV therapy.

As aforesaid, the oral regimen should be tailored based upon the results of the cultures. If the results are not available, reasonable empiric oral antibiotic choices include 1. amoxicillin

- clavulinate - 875 mg twice daily for adults or children over 40 kg, and 45 mg/kg/day divided every 12 hours for children over 3 moths and under 40 kg or 2. fluoroquinolone - (levofloxacin 750 mg once daily in adults). Linezolid (ZYVOX) - (600 mg twice daily in adults and children over 12 years of age, 10 mg/kg three times daily for children under 11 years) should be added if MRSA is suspected.

Careful follow-up is indicated in all patients who present with orbital cellulitis. This should include twice-daily examinations with attention to visual acuity, confrontation visual fields, exophthalmometry, motility and pupillary examination.

3.6.2 Antifungals

(Amphotericin B- Ambisome) 1 mg/kg IV q24h or Voriconazole (VFEND, Pfizer) 6 mg/kg IV q12h for 2 doses, then 4 mg/kg IV q12h or Voriconazole 200-300 mg PO q12h

Antifungal is the treatment of choice for fungal orbital cellulitis. It is administered IV and may be appropriately administered before laboratory confirmation of fungal infection in cases of severe infection and debilitated patients (diabetes mellitus, drug abusers, human immunodeficiency disease, metastatic cancer, prolonged administration of antibiotics and/ or corticosteroids).

3.6.3 Surgery

The timing for surgical intervention is critical. In cases of orbital cellulitis without abscess formation, in which visual acuity is 20/60 (Snellen notation), 6/15 (metric equivalent) or less, or declines with appropriate medical management, orbital exploration should be emergent. In cases in which the acuity is better than 20/60, the patient should be followed, expectantly, and frequently while more conservative management is initiated.

Orbital surgery is indicated if the patient:

1. Fails to respond
2. Deteriorates clinically despite treatment
3. Has worsening visual acuity or develops afferent pupillary defect
4. Develops an abscess, except selected pediatric cases with medial subperiosteal abscess, which may be successfully treated medically.

In patients older than 14 years of age, the author favours the latter approach because the risks of surgery are negligible compared with the visual and life-threatening risks of no intervention. In patients 9 years of age or younger, 25% of the subperiosteal abscesses are likely to resolve with antibiotic therapy alone. Several indications have been suggested for drainage of subperiosteal abscesses. These include age of 9 years or older, large abscess, frontal sinusitis, non-medial abscesschronic sinusitis, dental infection, optic nerve involvement, suspicion of anaerobic infection and recurrence after drainage. All other cases may be managed conservatively by intravenous antibiotics.

4. References

Abbott RL, Shekter WB: Necrotizing erysipelas of the eyelids. Ann Ophthalmol 11:381, 1979

Abou-Rayyah Y, Rose GE, Konrad H, et al. Clinical, radiological and pathological examination of periocular dermoid cyst:evidence of inflammation from an early age. Eye (Lond) 2002;16:507.

Adams WG, Deaver KA, Cochi SL, et al: Decline of childhood *Haemophilus influenzae* type b (Hib) disease in the Hib vaccine era. JAMA 269:221, 1993

Agarwal M, Biswas J, S K, Shanmugam MP. Retinoblastoma presenting as orbital cellulitis: report of four cases with a review of the literature. Orbit 2004;23:93.

Ailal F,Bousfiha A, Jouhad Z, et al. (Orbital cellulitis in children: a retrospective study of 33). Med trop (Mars) 2004; 64:359.

Allan BP,Egbert MA, Myall RW. Orbital abscess of odontologic origin. Case report and review of the literature. Int J Oral Maxillofac surg 1991;20:268.

Allen MV, Cohen KL, Grimson BS. Orbital cellulitis secondary to dacryocystitis following blepharoplasty. Ann Ophthalmol 1985; 17:498.

Ambati BK, Ambati J, Azar N, Stratton L, Schmidt EV: Periorbital and orbital cellulitis before and after the advent of haemophilus influenzae type B vaccination. Ophthalmology 107:1450, 2000

Antoine GA, Grundfast KM: Periorbital cellulitis. Int J Pediatr Otorhinolaryngol 13:273, 1987

Arjmand EM, Lusk RP, Muntz HR. Pediatric sinusitis and subperiosteal orbital abscess formation:diagnosis and treatment. Otolaryngol Head Neck Surg 1993;109:886.

Ataullah S, Sloan B. Acute dacryocystitis presenting as an orbital absvess. Clin Experiment ophthalmol 2002;30:44.

Bach MC, Knowland M, Schuyler WBJ: Acute orbital myositis mimicking orbital cellulitis. Ann Intern Med 109:243, 1988

Barkin RM, Todd JK: Periorbital cellulitis in children. Pediatrics 62:390, 1978

Barman Balfour JA, Lamb HM: Moxifloxacin, a review of its potential in the management of community-acquired respiratory tract infections. Drugs 59:115, 2000

Barone SR, Aiuto LT. Periorbital and orbital cellulitis in the Haemophilus influenzae vaccine era. J Pediatr Ophthalmol Strabismus 1997; 34:293.

Batson OV: Relationship of the eye to the paranasal sinuses. Arch Ophthalmol 16:322, 1936

Bergin DJ, Wright JE: Orbital cellulitis. Br J Ophthalmol 70:174, 1986

Botting AM, McIntosh D, Mahadevan M. Paediatric pre- and post-septal peri-orbital infections are different diseases. A retrospective review of 262 cases. Int J Pediatr Otorhinolaryngol 2008; 72:377.

Brannan PA, Kersten RC, Hudak DT, et al. Primary Nocardia brasiliensis of the eyelid. Am J Ophthalmol 2004; 138:498.

Brenner DJ, Elliston CD, Hall EJ, Berdon WE: Estimated risks of radiation-induced fatal cancer from pediatric CT. AJR 176:289, 2001

Brook I, Frazier EH. Microbiology of subperiosteal orbital abscess and associated maxillary sinusitis. Laryngoscope 1996; 106:1010.

Bullock JD, Fleishman JA: The spread of odontogentic infections to the orbit: diagnosis and management. J Oral Maxillofac Surg 43:749, 1985

Caça I, Cakmak SS, Unlü K, et al. Cutaneous anthrax on eyelids. Jpn J Ophthalmol 2004; 48:268.

Carter BL, Bankoff MS, Fisk JD: Computed tomographic detection of sinusitis responsible for intracranial and extracranial infections. Radiology 147:739, 1983

Casteel I, DeBleecker C, Demaerel P, et al: Orbital myositis following an upper respiratory tract infection: contribution of high resolution CT and MRI. J Belg Radiol 74:45, 991

Catalano RA, Smoot CN: Subperiosteal orbital masses in children with orbital cellulitis: time for a reevaluation? J Pediatr Ophthalmol Strabismus Surg 27:141, 1990

Chalumeau M, Tonnelier S, d'Athis P, et al: Fluoroquinolone safety in pediatric patients: a prospective, multicenter, comparative cohort study in France. Pediatrics 111:714, 2003

Chandler JR, Langenbrunner DJ, Stevens ER: The pathogenesis of orbital complications in acute sinusitis. Laryngoscope 80:1414, 1970

Chaudhry IA, Shamsi FA, Elzaridi E, et al. Inpatient preseptal cellulitis: experience from a tertiary eye care centre. Br J Ophthalmol 2008; 92:1337.

Chaudhry IA, Shamsi FA, Elzaridi E, et al. Outcome of treated orbital cellulitis in a tertiary eye care center in the middle East. Ophthalmology 2007; 114:345.

Chou SY, Tsai CC, Kau SC, et al. Aeromonas hydrophila orbital cellulitis in a patient with myelodysplastic syndrome. J Chin Med Assoc 2004; 67:51.

Claudia F E Kirsch, MD, Roger Turbin, MD, Devang Gor, MD, Barton F Branstetter IV, MD, Bernard D Coombs, MB, ChB, PhD, C Douglas Phillips, MD, Robert M Krasny, MD, James G Smirniotopoulos, MD (Orbital Infection Imaging) - Updated: May 27, 2011.

David G Hunter , MD, PhD, Michele Trucksis, Phd, MD, Stephen B Calderwood, MD, Morven S Edwards, MD, Jonathan Trobe, MD, Anna R Thorner, MD, Uptodate review version 19.2:2011 May.

Donahue Sp, Khoury JM, Kowalski RP: Common ocular infections. Drugs 52:526, 1996

Duane's Ophthalmology, William, M.D. Tasman, Edward A., M. Jaeger, Publisher: Lippincott Williams & Wilkins, ISBN: 0781725879 DDC: 617 Edition: Hardcover; 2000-09

Dudin A, Othman A. Acute periorbital swelling: evaluation of management protocol. Pediatr Emerg Care 1996; 12:16.

Eustis HS, Mafee MF, Walton C, Mondonca J: MR imaging and Ct of orbital infections and complications in acute rhinosinusitis. Radiol Clin North Am 36:1165, 1998

Filips RF, Liudahl JJ. Asymptomatic posterior orbital cellulitis resulting from ethmoid/maxillary sinusitis. J Am Optom Assoc 1997; 68:55.

Forstot SL, Ellis PP: Nontraumatic rupture of the globe secondary to orbital cellulitis. Am J Ophthalmol 88:262

Frederick J, Braude AI: Anaerobic infection of the paranasal sinuses. N Engl J Med 290:135, 1974

Galetta SL, Wulc AE, Goldberg HI, et al: Rhinocerebral mucormycosis: management and survival after carotid occlusion. Ann Neurol 28:103, 1990.

Gamble RE: Acute inflammations of the orbit in children. Arch Ophthalmol 10:483, 1933

Ganesh A, Venugopalan P. Preseptal orbital cellulitis following oral trauma. J Pediatr Ophthalmol Strabismus 2000; 37:315.

Gans H, Sekula J, Wlodyka J: Treatment of acute orbital complications. Arch Ophthalmol 100:329, 1974

Garcia GH, Harris GJ, Criteria for nonsurgical management of subperiosteal abscess of the orbit: analysis of outcomes 1988-1998. Ophthalmology 2000;107:1454-6.

Gellady AM, Shulman ST, Ayoub EM: Periorbital and orbital cellulitis in children. Pediatrics 61:272, 1978
Givner LB. Periorbital versus orbital cellulitis. Pediatr Infect Dis J 2002; 21:1157.
Gold SC, Arrigg PG, Hedges TR: Computerized tomography in the management of acute orbital cellulitis. Ophthalmic Surg 18:753, 1987
Goldberg F, Berne AS, Oski FA: Differentiation of orbital cellulitis from preseptal cellulitis by computed tomography. Pediatrics 62:1000, 1978
Goldfarb MS, Hoffman DS, Rosenberg S: Orbital cellulitis and orbital fractures. Ann Ophthalmol 19:97, 1987
Goodwin WJ, Weinshall M, Chandler JR: The role of high resolution computerized tomography and standardized ultrasound in the evaluation of orbital cellulitis. Laryngoscope 92:728, 1982
Greenberg MF, Pollard ZF. Medical treatment of pediatric subperiosteal orbital abscess secondary to sinusitis. J AAPOS 1998; 2:351.
Grossniklaus HE, Wojno TH: Leukemic infiltrate appearing as periorbital cellulitis. Arch Ophthalmol 108:484, 1990
Hajek M:Complications involving the orbit and visual organ. In Pathology and Treatment of Inflammatory Disease of the Nasal Accessory Sinuses. vol 2, 1926578–606
Handler LC, Davey IC, Hill JC, Lauryssen C: The acute orbit: differentiation of orbital cellulitis from periosteal abscess by computerized tomography. Neuroradiology 33:15, 1991
Harr DL, Quencer RM, Abrams GW: Computed tomography and ultrasound in the evaluation of orbital infection and pseudotumor. Radiology 142:395, 1982
Harris GJ. Age as a factor in the bacteriology and response to treatment of subperiosteal abscess of the orbit. Trans Am Ophthalmol Soc 1993; 91:441.
Harris GJ. Subperiosteal abscess of the orbit. Age as a factor in the bacteriology and response to treatment. Ophthalmology 1994; 101:585.
Harris GJ: Subperiosteal abscess of the orbit. Arch Ophthalmol 101:751, 1983
Hawkins DB, Clark RW: Orbital involvement in acute sinusitis. Clin Pediatr 16:464, 1977
Haynes R, Cramblett H: Acute ethmoiditis. Am J Dis Child 114:261, 1967
Hegde V, Smith G, Choi J, Pagliarini S. A case of gonococcal kerato-conjunctivitis mimicking orbital cellulitis. Acta Ophthalmol Scand 2005; 83:511.
Hemady R, Zimmerman A, Katzen BW, Karesh JW. Orbital cellulitis caused by Eikenella corrodens. Am J Ophthalmol 1992; 114:584.
Hirsch M, Lifschitz T: Computerized tomography in the diagnosis and treatment of orbital cellulitis. Pediatr Radiol 18:302, 1988
Hofbauer JD, Gordon LK, Palmer J. Acute orbital cellulitis after peribulbar injection. Am J Ophthalmol 1994; 118:391.
Hornblass A, Herschorn BJ, Stern K, Grimes C: Orbital abscess. Surv Ophthalmol 29:169, 1984
Howe L, Jones NS. Guidelines for the management of periorbital cellulitis/abscess. Clin Otolaryngol Allied Sci 2004; 29:725.
Hubert L: Orbital infection due to nasal sinusitis. NY State J Med 37:1559, 1937
Hutcheson KA, Magbalon M. Periocular abscess and cellulitis from Pasteurella multocida in a healthy child. Am J Ophthalmol 1999; 128:514.
Israele V, Nelson JD: Periorbital and orbital cellulitis. Pediatr Infect Dis J 6:404, 1987

Jacobs D, Galetta S. Diagnosis and management

Jain A, Rubin PAD: Orbital cellulitis in children. Int Ophthalmol Clin 41:71, 2001

Janakarajah N, Sukumaran K: Orbital cellulitis of dental origin: case report and review of the literature. Br J Oral Maxillofac Surg 23:140, 1985

Jarrett WH, Gutman FA: Ocular complications of infection in the paranasal sinuses. Arch Ophthalmol 81:683, 1969

Jarrett WH, Gutman FA: Ocular complications of infection in the paranasal sinuses. Arch Ophthalmol 81:683, 1969

John N Harrington, MD, FACS, Brian A Phillptts, MD, Franisco Talavera, PharmD, PhD, Mark T Duffy, MD, PhD, Lance L Brown, OD, MD. Chief Editor:Hampton Roy Sr, MD, Medscape review version (Preseptal and Orbital cellulitis), Oct 10 2011.

Jones J, Katz SE, Lubow M. Scedosporium apiospermum of the orbit. Arch Ophthalmol 1999; 117:272.

Karesh J, Lakhanpal V, Haney P, et al: Metastatic anaerobic orbital subperiosteal abscess: value of CT scanning. J Pediatr Ophthalmol Strabismus 19:52, 1982

Karkos PD, Karagama Y, Karkanevatos A, Srinivasan V. Recurrent periorbital cellulitis in a child. A random event or an underlying anatomical abnormality? Int J Pediatr Otorhinolaryngol 2004; 68:1529.

Kaufman SJ: Orbital mucopyoceles: two cases and a review. Surv Ophthalmol 25:253, 1981

Komolafe OO, Ashaye AO. Combined central retinal artery and vein occlusion complicating orbital cellulitis. Niger J Clin Pract 2008; 11:74.

Krohel GB, Kraus HR, Winnick J: Orbital abscesses: presentation, diagnosis, therapy, and sequelae. Ophthalmology 89:492, 1982

Krohel GB, Krauss HR, Christensen RE, Minckler D: Orbital abscess. Arch Ophthalmol 98:274, 1980

Kyprianou I, D'Souza A, Saravanappa N, et al. Referral patterns in paediatric orbital cellulitis. Eur J Emerg Med 2005; 12:6.

Langham-Brown JJ, Rhys-Williams S: Computed tomography of acute orbital infection: the importance of coronal sections. Clin Radiol 40:471, 1989

Lasko B, Lau CY, Saint-Pierre C, et al: Efficacy and safety of oral levofloxacin compared with clarithromycin in the treatment of acute sinusitis in adults: a multicentre, double blind, randomized study. J Int Med Res 26:281, 1998

Lemke BN, Gonnering RS, Harris J, Weinstein JM: Orbital cellulitis with periorbital elevation. Ophthalmic Plast Reconstruct Surg 3:1, 1987

Mair MH, Geley T, Judmaier W, Gassner I. Using orbital sonography to diagnose and monitor treatment of acute swelling of the eyelids in pediatric patients. AJR Am J Roentgenol 2002; 179:1529.

Malik NN, Goh D, McLean C, Huchzermeyer P. Orbital cellulitis caused by Peptostreptococcus. Eye (Lond) 2004; 18:643.

Maniglia AJ, Kronberg FG, Culbertson W: Visual loss associated with orbital and sinus disease. Laryngoscope 94:1050, 1984

Manning SC: Endoscopic management of medial subperiosteal orbital abscess. Arch Otolaryngol Head Neck Surg 119:789, 1993

Mathews D, Mathews JP, Kwartz J, Inkster C. Preseptal cellulitis caused by Acinetobacter lwoffi. Indian J Ophthalmol 2005; 53:213.

McKinley SH, Yen MT, Miller AM, Yen KG. Microbiology of pediatric orbital cellulitis. Am J Ophthalmol 2007; 144:497.

McLeod SD, Flowers CW, Lopez PF, et al. Endophthalmitis and orbital cellulitis after radial keratotomy. Ophthalmology 1995; 102:1902.

Miller J. Acinetobacter as a causative agent in preseptal cellulitis. Optometry 2005; 76:176.

Mills R. Orbital and periorbital sepsis. J Laryngol Otol 1987; 101:1242.

Mills RP, Kartush JM. Orbital wall thickness and the spread of infection from the paranasal sinuses. Clin Otolaryngol Allied Sci 1985; 10:209.

Milstone AM, Ruff AJ, Yeamans C, Higman MA. Pseudomonas aeruginosa pre-septal cellulitis and bacteremia in a pediatric oncology patient. Pediatr Blood Cancer 2005; 45:353; discussion 354.

Molarte AB, Isenberg SJ: Periorbital cellulits in infancy. J Pediatr Ophthalmol Strabismus 26:232, 1989

Morell A, Skvaril F, Hitzig WH, Barandum S: IgG subclasses: development of the serum concentrations in "normal" infants and children. J Pediatr 80:960, 1972

Morgan PR, Morrison WV: Complications of frontal and ethmoidal sinusitis. Laryngoscope 90:661, 1980

Nageswaran S, Woods CR, Benjamin DK Jr, et al. Orbital cellulitis in children. Pediatr Infect Dis J 2006; 25:695.

Newell FW, Leveille AS: Management and complications of bacterial periorbital and orbital cellulitis. Metab Pediatr Syst Ophthalmol 6:209, 1982

Noel LP, Clarke WN, Peacocke TA: Periorbital and orbital cellulitis in childhood. Can J Ophthalmol 16:178, 1981Jackson K, Baker SR: Clinical implications of orbital cellulitis. Laryngoscope 96:568, 1986

Okamoto Y, Hiraoka T, Okamoto F, Oshika T. A case of subperiosteal abscess of the orbit with central retinal artery occlusion. Eur J Ophthalmol 2009; 19:288.

Osguthorpe JD, Hochman M. Inflammatory sinus diseases affecting the orbit. Otolaryngol Clin North Am 1993; 26:657.

Partamian LG, Jay WM, Fritz KJ: Anaerobic orbital cellulitis. Ann Ophthalmol 15:123, 1983

Patil B, Agius-Fernandez A, Worstmann T. Hyaluronidase allergy after peribulbar anesthesia with orbital inflammation. J Cataract Refract Surg 2005; 31:1480.

Patt BS, Manning SC. Blindness resulting from orbital complications of sinusitis. Otolaryngol Head Neck Surg 1991; 104:789.

Patt BS, Manning SC: Blindness resulting from orbital complications of sinusitis. Otolaryngol Head Neck Surg 104:789, 1991

Pelton RW, Smith ME, Patel BC, Kelly SM. Cosmetic considerations in surgery for orbital subperiosteal abscess in children: experience with a combined transcaruncular and transnasal endoscopic approach. Arch Otolaryngol Head Neck Surg 2003; 129:652.

Powell KR: Orbital and periorbital cellulitis. Pediatr Rev 16:163, 1995

Quick CA, Payne E: Complicated acute sinusitis. Laryngoscope 82:1248, 1972

R Gentry Wilkerson, MD, Richard H Sinert, DO, Zach Kassutto, MD, FAAP, Elizabeth Fiedler, MD, Edmond A Hooker II, MD, DrPH, FAAEM, Francisco Talavera, PharmD, PhD, Douglas Lavenburg, MD, John D Halamka, MD, MS, Robert E O'Connor, MD, MPH (Chief Editor), eMedicine review (Periorbital infections),jul 10 2011.

Ragab A, Samaka RM. Department of ORL Head and Neck Surgery, Menoufyia University Hospital, (Is pyogenic ethmoidal osteitis the cause of complicated rhinosinusitis with subperiosteal orbital abscess?).PubMed, Eur Arch Otorhinolaryngol. 2010 Aug;267(8):1231-7. Epub 2010 Jan 13.

Rahbar R, Robson CD, Petersen RA, et al. Management of orbital subperiosteal abscess in children. Arch Otolaryngol Head Neck Surg 2001; 127:281.

Raina UK, Jain S, Monga S, et al. Tubercular preseptal cellulitis in children: a presenting feature of underlying systemic tuberculosis. Ophthalmology 2004; 111:291.

Raja NS, Singh NN. Bilateral orbital cellulitis due to Neisseria gonorrhoeae and Staphylococcus aureus: a previously unreported case. J Med Microbiol 2005; 54:609.

Rees TD, Craig SM, Fisher Y: Orbital abscess following blepharoplasty. Plast Reconstr Surg 73:126, 1983

Reynolds DJ, Kodsi SR, Rubin SE, Rodgers IR. Intracranial infection associated with preseptal and orbital cellulitis in the pediatric patient. J AAPOS 2003; 7:413.

Robbins JB, Schneerson R, Argaman M, Handzel ZT: *Haemophilus influenzae* type b: disease and immunity in humans. Ann Intern Med 78:259, 1973

Robie F, O'Neal R, Kelsey DS: Periobital cellulitis. J Pediatr Ophthalmol 14:354, 1977

Rubin SE, Rubin LG, Zito J, et al: Medical management of orbital subperiosteal abscess in children. J Pediatr Ophthalmol Strabismus Surg 26:21, 1989

Rubinstein A, Riddell CE. Posterior scleritis mimicking orbital cellulitis. Eye (Lond) 2005; 19:1232.

Rubinstein JB, Handler SD. Orbital and periorbital cellulitis in children. Head Neck Surg 1982; 5:15.

Rubinstein JB, Handler SD: Orbital and periorbital cellulitis in children. Head Neck Surg 5:15, 1982

Rudloe TF, Harper MB, Prabhu SP, et al. Acute periorbital infections: who needs emergent imaging? Pediatrics 2010; 125:e719.

Rumelt S, Rubin PAD. Potential sources of orbital cellulitis. Int Ophthalmol Clin 36:207, 1996

Russo G, Di Pietro M, La Spina M. Ocular involvement in neuroblastoma: not always metastasis. Lancet Oncol 2004; 5:324.

Ruttum MS, Ogawa G. Adenovirus conjunctivitis mimics preseptal and orbital cellulitis in young children. Pediatr Infect Dis J 1996; 15:266.

Ryan JT, Preciado DA, Bauman N, et al. Management of pediatric orbital cellulitis in patients with radiographic findings of subperiosteal abscess. Otolaryngol Head Neck Surg 2009; 140:907.

Saini JS, Mohan K, Khandalavala B: Wooden foreign bodies of the orbit. Orbit 8:139, 1989

Schmitt NJ, Beatty RL, Kennerdell JS. Superior ophthalmic vein thrombosis in a patient with dacryocystitis-induced orbital cellulitis. Ophthal Plast Reconstr Surg 2005; 21:387.

Schramm VL Jr, Curtin HD, Kennerdell JS. Evaluation of orbital cellulitis and results of treatment. Laryngoscope 1982; 92:732.

Schramm VL, Curtin HD, Kennerdell JS: Evaluation of orbital cellulitis and results of treatment. Laryngoscope 92:732, 1982

Schramm VL, Myers EN, Kennerdell JS: Orbital complications of acute sinusitis: Evaluation, management, and outcome. Trans Am Acad Otolaryngol 86:221, 1978

Schur PH, Rosen F, Norman ME: Immunoglobulin subclasses in normal children. Pediatr Res 13:181, 1979

Schwartz G. Department of Emergency Medicine, Vanderbilt University Medical Center, (Etiology, Diagnosis, and Treatment of Orbital Infections) - PubMed, Curr Infect Dis Rep. 2002 Jun;4(3):201-205

Scott PM, Bloome MA: Lid necrosis secondary to streptococcal periorbital cellulitis. Ann Ophthalmol 4:461, 1981

Sears JM, Gabriel HM, Veith J. Preseptal cellulitis secondary to Proteus species: a case report and review. J Am Optom Assoc 1999; 70:661.

Shapiro ED, Wald ER, Broznski BA: Periorbital cellulitis and paranasal sinusitis: A reappraisal. Pediatr Infect Dis J 1:91, 1982

Shields CL, Shields JA, Honavar SG, Demirci H. Primary ophthalmic rhabdomyosarcoma in 33 patients. Trans Am Ophthalmol Soc 2001; 99:133.

Shields JA, Shields CL, Suvarnamani C, et al: Retinoblastoma manifesting as orbital cellulitis. Am J Ophthalmol 112:442, 1991

Siber GR, Schur PH, Aisenberg AC, et al: Correlation between serum IgG-2 concentrations and the antibody response to bacterial polysaccharide antigens. N Engl J Med 303:178, 1980

Silver HS, Fucci MJ, Flanagan JC, Lowry LD: Severe orbital infection as a complication of orbital fracture. Arch Otolaryngol Head Neck Surg 118:845, 1992

Sirbaugh PE. A case of orbital pseudotumor masquerading as orbital cellulitis in a patient with proptosis and fever. Pediatr Emerg Care 1997; 13:337.

Slavin ML, Glaser JS: Acute severe irreversible visual loss with sphenoethmoiditis: 'posterior' orbital cellulitis. Arch Ophthalmol 105:345, 1987

Smith AT, Spencer JT: Orbital complications resulting from lesions of the sinuses. Ann Otol Rhinol Laryngol 57:5, 1948

Smith TF, O'Day D, Wright PF: Clinical implications of preseptal (periorbital) cellulitis in childhood. Pediatrics 62:1006, 1978

Sobol SE, Marchand J, Tewfik TL, et al. Orbital complications of sinusitis in children. J Otolaryngol 2002; 31:131.

Sorin A, April MM, Ward RF. Recurrent periorbital cellulitis: an unusual clinical entity. Otolaryngol Head Neck Surg 2006; 134:153.

Spires JR, Smith RJH: Bacterial infections of the orbital and perirobital soft tissues in children. Laryngoscope 96:763, 1986

Stammberger H: Endoscopic endonasal surgery: concepts in treatment of recurring rhinosinusitis. Otolaryngol Head Neck Surg 94:143, 1986

Stammberger H: Functional Endoscopic Sinus Surgery. p 68. Philadelphia: BC Decker, 1991

Starkey CR, Steele RW. Medical management of orbital cellulitis. Pediatr Infect Dis J 2001; 20:1002.

Swift AC, Charlton G. Sinusitis and the acute orbit in children. J Laryngol Otol 1990; 104:213.

Tannenbaum M, Tenzel J, Byrne SF, et al: Medical management of orbital abscess. Surv Ophthalmol 30:211, 1986

Thatcher DB: Necrotic choroidal melanoma presenting with severe inflammation. Surv Ophthalmol 12:247, 1967

Towbin R, Han BK, Kaufman RA, Burke M: Postseptal cellulitis: CT in diagnosis and management. Radiology 158:735, 1986

Uehara F, Ohba N: Diagnostic imaging in patients with orbital cellulitis and inflammatory pseudotumor. Int Ophthalmol Clin 42:133, 2002

Uzcátegui N, Warman R, Smith A, Howard CW. Clinical practice guidelines for the management of orbital cellulitis. J Pediatr Ophthalmol Strabismus 1998; 35:73.
Uzcategui N, Warman R, Smith A, Howard CW: Clinical practice guidelines for the management of orbital cellulitis. J Pediatr Ophthalmol Strabismus 35:73, 1998
Vail DT: Orbital complications in sinus disease: a review. Am J Ophthalmol 14:202, 1931
Varma D, Metcalfe TW. Orbital cellulitis after peribulbar anaesthesia for cataract surgery. Eye (Lond) 2003; 17:105.
Velazquez AJ, Goldstein MH, Driebe WT. Preseptal cellulitis caused by trichophyton (ringworm). Cornea 2002; 21:312.
von Noorden GK: Orbital cellulitis following extraocular muscle surgery. Am J Ophthalmol 74:627, 1972
Watters EC, Wallar H, Hiles DA, Michaels RH: Acute orbital cellulitis. Arch Ophthalmol 94:785, 1976
Weakley DR. Orbital cellulitis complicating strabismus surgery: a case report and review of the literature. Ann Ophthalmol 1991; 23:454.
Weber AL, Mikulis DK. Inflammatory disorders of the paraorbital sinuses and their complications. Radiol Clin North Am 1987; 25:615.
Weiss A, Friendly D, Eglin K, et al: Bacterial periorbital and orbital cellulitis in childhood. Ophthalmology 90:195, 1983
Welsh LW, Welsh JJ: Orbital complications of sinus disease. Laryngoscope 84:848, 1974
Westfall CT, Shore JW: Isolated fractures of the orbital floor: risk of infection and the role of the antibiotic prophylaxis. Ophthalmic Surg 22:409, 1991
Whitnall SE: The Anatomy of the Human Orbit and Accessory Organ of Vision. 2nd ed, pp 29–35.New York: Oxford University Press, 1932
Williamson-Nobel FA: Diseases of the orbit and its contents secondary to pathological conditions of the nose and paranasal sinuses. Ann R Coll Surg 15:46, 1954
Wilson ME, Paul TO: Orbital cellulitis following strabismus surgery. Ophthalmic Surg 18:92, 1987
Wulc AE, Adams JL, Dryden RM: Cerebrospinal fluid leakage complicating orbital exenteration. Arch Ophthalmol 107:827, 1989
Wulc, AC. Orbital infections. In: Duane's Ophthalmology 1999 CD ROM edition, Volume 2, Chapter 34.Williams BJ, Harrison HC: Subperiosteal abscesses of the orbit due to sinusitis in childhood. Aust NZ J Ophthalmol 19:29, 1991
Younis RT, Lazar RH, Bustillo A, Anand VK. Department of Otolaryngology, University of Miami School of Medicine, (Orbital infection as a complication of sinusitis: are diagnostic and treatment trends changing?) PubMed, Ear Nose Throat J. 2002 Nov;81(11):771-5.
Younis RT, Lazar RH, Bustillo A, Anand VK: Orbital infection as a complication of sinusitis: are diagnostic and treatment trends changing. Ear, Nose, Throat J 81:771, 2002
Youssef Z, Pennefather PM, Watts MT. Orbital cellulitis vs allergic reaction to hyaluronidase as the cause of periorbital oedema. Eye (Lond) 2005; 19:691.
Zhanel GG, Ennis K, Vercaine L, et al: A critical review of the fluoroquinolones. Drugs 62:13, 2002
Ziakas NG, Boboridis K, Gratsonidis A, et al. Wegener's granulomatosis of the orbit in a 5-year-old child. Eye (Lond) 2004; 18:658.
Zimmerman RA, Bilaniuk LT: CT of orbital infection and its cerebral complications. AJR 134:45, 198

28

Extended Applications of Endoscopic Sinus Surgery to the Orbit and Pituitary Fossa

Balwant Singh Gendeh
Department of Otorhinolaryngology – Head and Neck Surgery
UKM Medical Center, Jalan Yaacob Latif, Bandar Tun Razak, Kuala Lumpur
Malaysia

1. Introduction

There has been significant evolution over time from external headlight sinus surgery to endoscopic sinus surgery(ESS). ESS was pioneered by Messenklinger, who discovered that the sinuses had a predetermined mucociliary clearance pattern towards the natural ostium irrespective of additional openings into the sinuses. This philosophy of opening the natural ostium of the diseased sinus was then popularized by Stammberger and Kennedy. ESS is now accepted as the surgical management of choice for chronic sinusitis. Furthermore, as our knowledge of the anatomy of the sinuses has improved, other anciliary surgeries such as endoscopic lacrimal surgery, orbital decompression, applications to the pterygopalatine and infratemporal fossa, approaches from the sphenoid/sella extending to the cribriform, parasellar and clival region have evolved. Moreover, innovation in instrumentation has led to the acceptance of endoscopic management of benign endonasal tumors and more recently, on endoscopic management of malignant tumors of the nose and sinuses.

The current interest in ESS stems from several developments. The first is the advent of compact, multi-angled telescopes that allow excellent visualization of the nasal cavity for examination and of the sinuses during procedures, including such areas as the maxillary ostia and the frontal recess. Secondly, is the acceptance and appreciation of the great work of Messerklinger(1967) demonstrating that the anterior ethmoids are usually the key to persistent sinusitis. Thirdly, is the advent in radiological imaging. Endoscopic diagnostic examinations in conjunction with modern imaging methods, particularly CT scan, have proven to be an ideal combination and have been accepted as the "Standard of Care' for sinus disease. The CT scan can clearly identify anterior ethmoids disease which can easily be missed on a plain paranasal sinus X-ray. These developments make it possible to diagnose more accurately and treat sinusitis refractory to non-invasive therapy.

The technique of ESS was developed in Europe by Messerklinger and Wigand, who had two different goals designed for extremes of disease. The Messerklinger technique advocated in 1985 is an anterior to posterior approach which involves only the anterior ethmoids and the maxillary sinus ostium and can be extended into the posterior ethmoids, sphenoid and the frontal sinus anteriorly if necessary. Thus, the Messerklinger technique is ideal for patient with anterior ethmoid disease with or without maxillary or frontal sinus disease. On the contrary, the Wigand approach advocated in 1978 is posterior-to-anterior and routinely involves all the sinuses on the ipsilateral side and is ideal for patient with pan-sinusitis who has or is apt to fail the more limited Messerklinger approach. Both techniques are based on the assumption that the sinus mucosa is most likely reversibly diseased and will return to normal once ventilation has been established. No attempt is made to eradicate the sinus mucous membrane, as in the Caldwell-Luc procedure, but rather to reestablish drainage so the mucosa can return to normal and restore its proper function.

Although telescopes give the surgeon a clearer and magnified view of the nose and sinuses, the picture on the video monitor is not three-dimentional and depth perception and orientation can be difficult. Consequently there is a risk of getting lost and this may result in an injury to the orbit, its contents, the optic nerve and the intracranial cavity. To reduce this risk, surgeons should ensure that they are thoroughly familiar with the anatomy and the anatomical variations that can occur in the nose and sinuses. Therefore, radiological imaging is essential prior to surgical intervention.

A significant development for soft-tissue removal was the development of "through-cutting" instrumentation. Powered instrumentation using soft tissue shavers (Metronic, Xomed, USA) offer another significant advancement to the endoscopic sinus surgeon but with some risk to the orbit and cranium in inexperienced hands (Fig 1). Setliff and Parsons were the first to report the use of soft-tissue shavers in endoscopic sinus surgery (Setliff , 1994). ESS with its minimally invasive technique often reduces pain, bleeding and length of hospital stay and avoids external incision and thus reduces surgical cost compared to conventional techniques. Endoscopic surgery cannot replace every conventional external approach and we should never be embarrassed to employ or convert to these conventional approaches when necessary (Gendeh et al, 2007). However, not all cases are suitable for an endoscopic approach and the surgeon must be experienced in the full range of surgical options, the patho-physiology and natural history of disease processes, if optimum results are to be achieved. This is particularly true in the controversial area of sinonasal neoplasia.

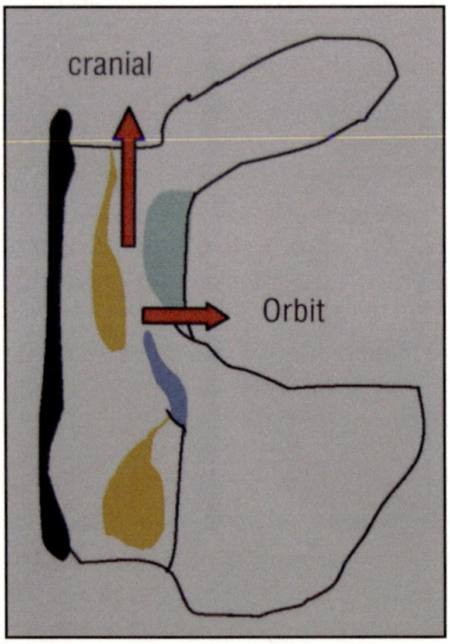

Fig. 1. Diagrammatic coronal section of paranasal sinuses showing the anatomical proximity of orbit and cranium to the nasal cavity in utilization of powered instrumentation and the risk involved.

This chapter will briefly outline the future trends in endoscopic skull base surgery. The Expanded Endonasal Approach(EEA) is a an extended endoscopic transnasal approach, providing access to the entire skull base from the epicenter, the sphenoid sinus.

It is important to define the word "endoneurosurgery" (Kassam et al, 2007). This is a new and emerging field and represents the use of the endoscope as the sole and only tool used to visualize the entire neural axis. In the case of EEA, only the endoscope is used to access the ventral skull via a completely transnasal route. As a joint team effort, this extended applications beyond the sphenoid sinus/sella needs a lot of surgical skills, planning and coordination for proper patient selection and optimal care. The EEA provides surgical access to the ventral skull base to resect a wide variety of intra-dural and extra-dural pathologies and allows the reconstruction of the resulting defect using a naso-septal flap. The evolution of these techniques has been enabled by technological advances including the design of specific endonasal instrumentation, surgical navigation technology and the development of new biomaterials for reconstruction. The incidence of tumor recurrence will be very much reduced with this minimally invasive ventral skull base technique. The use of powered instruments with navigational fusion imaging is most beneficial especially in revision cases.

2. Endoscopic dacryocystorhinostomy

Dacryocystorhinostomy(DCR) involves the formation of a bypass from the lacrimal sac into the nose. It is essential that with proper history and examination including syringing and probing, a correct diagnosis is made. Syringing and probing is performed only in congenital and acquired nasolacrimal duct obstruction (NLDO) and are indications for the procedure. They are not performed in acute and chronic dacryocystitis.

2.1 Indications (Table 1)

The main indication is when there is distal outflow obstruction to the nasolacrimal system which can clearly be demonstrated on a dacrocystogram. Endoscopic surgery is not indicated for obstruction of a punctum or a canaliculus for which there are other procedures. Often distal obstruction is mixed with varying degree of proximal obstruction and this need to be explained when counseling the patient. Syringing and probing is helpful in defining the site of obstruction. It is expected that in congenital and acquired NLDO, the epiphora would resolve and in acute and chronic dacryocysitis, the infection would be resolved without recurrences.

1. Primary acquired NLDO
2. Secondary acquired NLDO
    a. Infectious causes of secondary acquired lacrimal duct obstruction
    b. Inflammatory causes of secondary lacrimal obstruction
    c. Neoplastic causes of lacrimal obstruction
    d. Traumatic causes of lacrimal obstruction
    e. Mechanical causes of lacrimal obstruction

Table 1. Indications for Endonasal DCR(EDCR)

A dacrocystogram (Fig 2) is indicated if there is any mass within the sac and scintigraphy helps to define a functional problem. A functional problem is one issue for which a dacryocystogram is helpful. Lacrimal sac mass is another indication for dacryocystogram. A bloody discharge from the punctum is a symptom that needs investigating to exclude malignancy in the sac. The common symptoms are epiphora, recurrent dacryocystitis or swelling from a mucocele. It is unusual for intranasal pathology like Wegener granulomatosis and sarcoidosis to be the causative factor. Nasolacrimal duct obstruction can occur following a middle-third facial fracture. Distal nasolacrimal obstruction can be secondary to endoscopic sinus surgery if the Stammberger Rhinoforce Antrum Punch (Stortz, Germany) used to remove the uncinate process is placed too far forward.

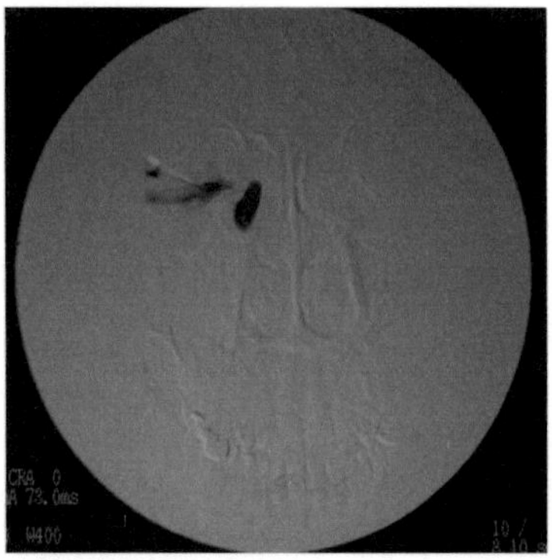

Fig. 2. A dacrocystogram showing distal obstruction of right nasolacrimal system on failure of penetration of dye into the inferior meatus in a patient with unilateral unresolving tearing.

2.2 Contraindications (Table 2)

A contraindication to DCR is the presence of a benign or malignant lesion in the lacrimal system or the surrounding tissues and active Wegener granulomatosis. Other causes are lacrimal sac diverticulum,, canalicular stenosis, lacrimal calculi and extensive midfacial trauma.

1. Known or suspected lacrimal system neoplasm
2. Large lateral lacrimal sac diverticulum
3. Common canalicular stenosis
4. Lacrimal system stones
5. Extensive midfacial trauma

Table 2. Contraindications for Endonasal DCR(EDCR)

2.3 Anatomy and pre-operative assessment

The lacrimal system comprises the lacrimal gland and its drainage system which commences with a punctum in each eyelid for 1mm at right angles to the lid margin. It continues as the upper and lower canaliculus which run parallel to the lid margin and then join to form a common canaliculus that drains into the lacrimal sac (Fig 3). Inferiorly the sac forms the nasolacrimal duct, which drains into the inferior meatus about 1cm posterior to the anterior end of the inferior turbinate (Fig 4). The lacrimal sac sits in the lacrimal fossa which is a very thin bone. Unlike its anterior margin, the anterior lacrimal crest, is made of very dense bone. In about 8% of patients, an anterior ethmoidal air cell lies medial to the lacrimal fossa which needs to be transverse before a rhinostomy can be created.

Topical anesthetic drops such as amethocaine are placed in the eye followed by dilatation of the upper and lower puncta performed with punctual dilator. The puncta are initially dilated with the instrument perpendicular to the lid margin, rotating it for the first 1 mm with the lid margin taut, before turning it medially parallel to the lid. Upon dilatation of the punctum, a "0" Bowman probe is passed through the dilated punctum and angled medially. As the probe enters the common canaliculus, a slight resistance may be felt as a "soft stop" and as it touches the medial wall of the sac, there is a "hard stop". The probe is then angled vertically down to feel whether there is any sac pathology or distal obstruction. This is a description for probing in children, which is preferably performed under general anaesthesia. It is avoided in adults because of the intolerable pain. Rigid 0.7 mm dacryocystoscopes can be used to inspect the fine obstructing membranes that can be found at the medial aspect of the upper and lower canaliculi (Wormald, 2002). These proximal membranes are the main cause of proximal obstruction, and a DCR is not indicated if this is the site of the obstruction. For surgeons becoming familiar with intranasal anatomy or a history of previous sinonasal surgery, it may be helpful to introduce a 20-gauge fiberoptic endoilluminator(Stortz, Germany) through the superior or inferior canaliculus after punctual dilator. The endoilluminator is then advanced gently until a hard stop signifying the lacrimal bone is identified (Woog, 2004). The location of the lacrimal sac may then be visualized endoscopically by transillumination (Fig 5 a, b).

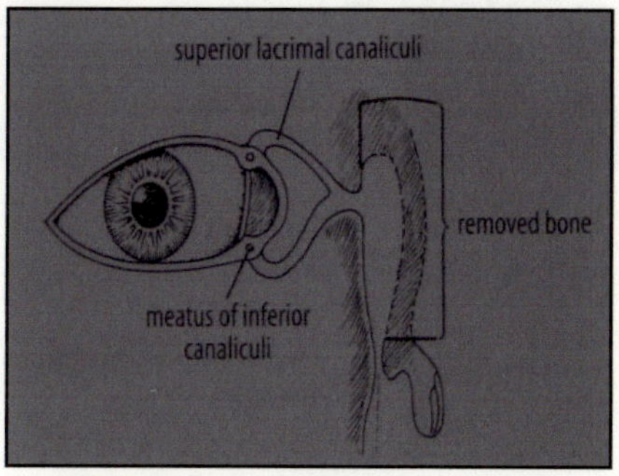

Fig. 3. Diagrammatic anatomical picture of nasolacrimal drainage system

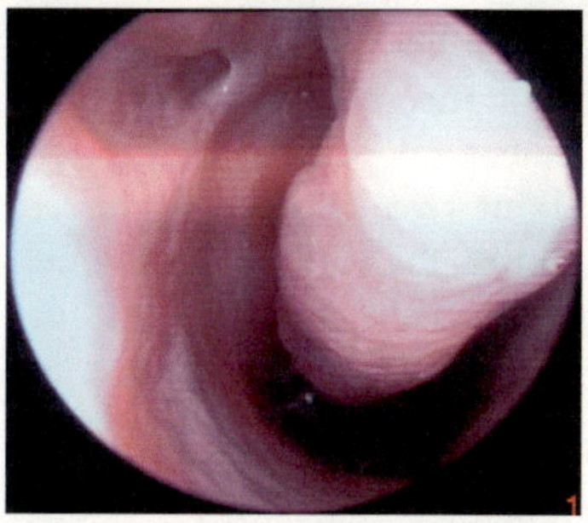

Fig. 4. Endoscopic view of a right nasolacrimal duct opening into an inferior meatus

Distal obstruction is diagnosed by probing and then syringing to see whether the fluid can initially pass through the canaliculi into the nose. If it refluxes through the other punctum, it indicates that there is distal obstruction. On the contrary, if there is reflux through the same punctum, then there is canalicular or common canalicular stenosis and this can be confirmed by gentle probing. There are many causes of dysfunction that requires a different treatment than DCR. The most common site of distal obstruction is where the sac becomes the duct. Some surgeons will offer a DCR to patients with a functional blockage where there is free flow on syringing but on scintigraphy the pump system does not work. Only 70-75% of the tears are drained through the inferior canaliculus. Lester-Jones Pyrex tube is required only in bi-canalicular extensive obstruction that cannot be managed by other procedures such as forced probing and silicone intubation.

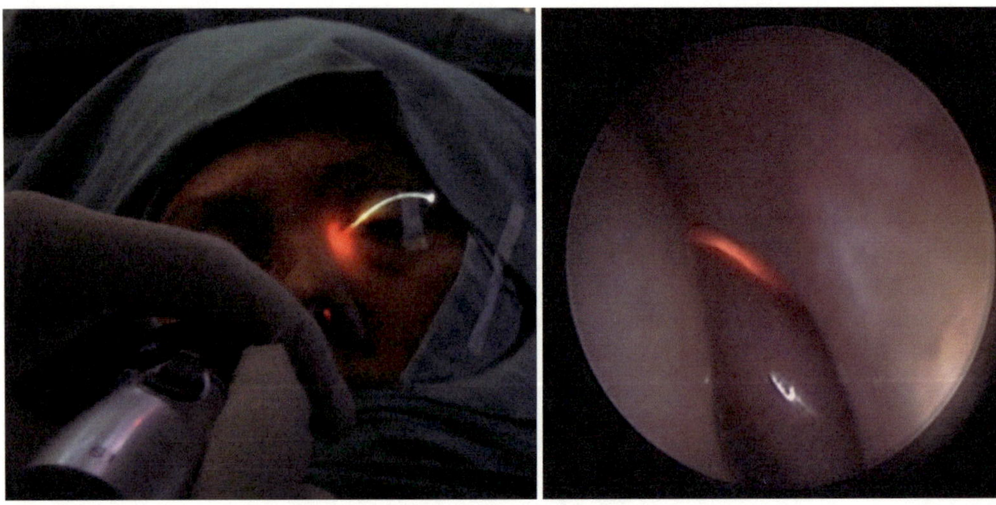

(a) (b)

Fig. 5. A picture showing a fiber-optic endoilluminator being introduced via the left inferior cannaliculus to illuminate the nasolacrimal sac(a) and a zero degree endoscopic view identifying the location of the illuminated lacrimal sac(b) in the same patient.

2.4 Surgical technique

Upon nasal decongestion with neuropatties and infilteration with lidocaine and adrenaline, a 15 scalpel blade is used for initial mucosal incisions. The first incision is made horizontally 1 cm above the axilla of the middle turbinate, commencing 3 mm posterior to the axilla and coming forward 1 cm onto the frontal process of the maxilla. The blade is then turned vertically and incision made about two thirds of the vertical height of middle turbinate, stopping just above the insertion of the inferior turbinate into the lateral nasal wall. The blade is then turned horizontally and the inferior insertion commenced at the insertion of the uncinate process and brought forward to meet the vertical incision.

A suction Freer's dissector (Stortz, Germany) is used to elevate the mucosal flap, ensuring that the tip of the sucker always maintains contact with the bone. Meanwhile the bone should be palpable so that the junction of the soft lacrimal bone and hard bone of the frontal process can be identified. The thin lacrimal bone is 2 to 5 mm wide before the insertion of the uncinate process is reached. The dissection stops at the uncinate. A round knife (Stortz, Germany) is used to flake the soft lacrimal bone away from the postero-inferior region of the sac.

A forward-bitting Hajek Koeffler punch (Stortz, Germany) is used to remove the lower portion of the frontal process of the maxilla (Fig 6). The tip of the punch is used to push the lacrimal sac away where the lacrimal bone has to be removed. The punch is engaged in the hard bone of the frontal process and this bone is removed. Care should be taken not to grasp the sac as the punch is closed during bone removal. Removal of the frontal process of the maxilla uncovers the antero-inferior portion of the lacrimal sac. Bony removal with punch is continued as far superiorly as possible until the bone becomes too thick for the punch to engage. At this juncture the 15 degree curved 2.9 mm rough diamond burr(Medtronic Xomed, Jacksonville, Florida, USA) is attached to the micro-debrider and used to remove the rest of the bone up to the superior mucosal incision (Jones,1998). Often, an agger nasi cell is present and the mucosa of this cell will be exposed as the sac is followed superiorly above the axilla of the middle turbinate thus exposing the frontal recess (Fig 7). The diamond burr can be brought into light contact with the lacrimal sac lining without damaging the sac. A cutting burr will remove the bone faster but may cause significant damage to the sac wall with development of hole in the sac wall.

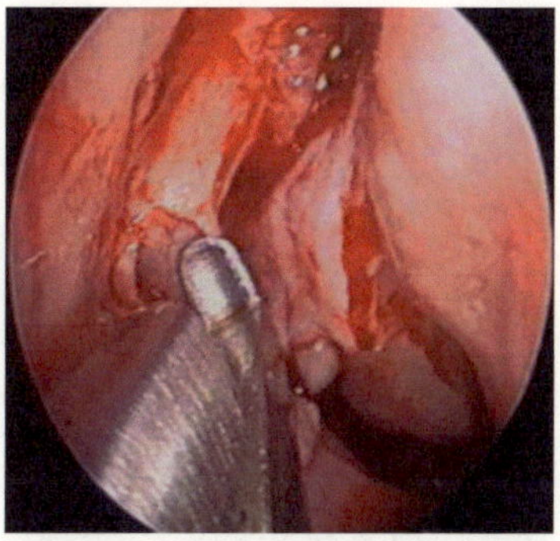

Fig. 6. Intraoperative endoscope view showing right dacrocystorhinostomy with initial removal of the thin lacrimal bone with Hajek Koffler sphenoid punch and subsequently the hard frontal process of maxilla with a microdrill

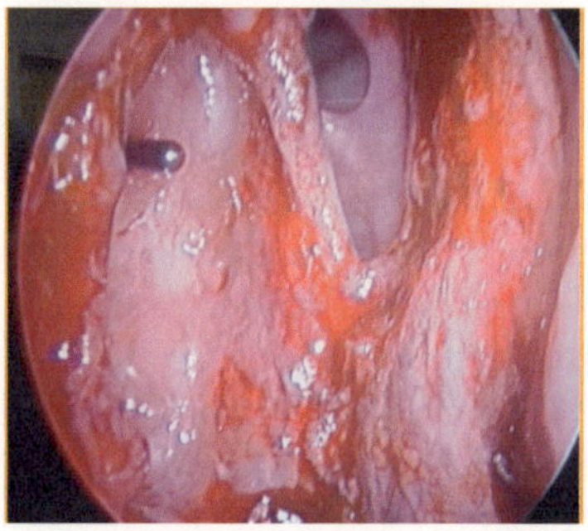

Fig. 7. Intraoperative endoscopic view showing a right dacrocystorhinostomy with wide exposure of the nasolacrimal sac with visible end of eye probe and removal of agger nasi cell exposing the frontal recess

Next, the inferior punctum is dilated with a punctum dilator and a Bowman's canalicular probe is passed into the sac. If the tip of the probe is not seen to move behind the thin sac wall, the probe is not in the lumen. The exposed sac is incised vertically with a DCR minisickle knife (Metronic Xomed, USA). Belucci scissors (Stortz, Germany) are used to make upper and lower releasing incisions in the posterior flap which is rolled out on the lateral nasal wall. The sac should now be completely marsupialized and lie flat on the lateral nasal wall. Approximating the lacrimal and nasal mucosa should result in a first intention healing rather than a secondary intention healing and should reduce the formation of granulation tissue and scarring. The puncta are dilated and Silastic lacrimal intubation tubes(O'Donoghue tubes) are placed through the upper and lower puncta and retrieved endonasally. Ligar clips are placed to secure the tubes in place (Fig 8). Before placing the clips ensure a loop of tubing is pulled in the medial canthus of the eye so that the tubes are not tight. If the loop is tight the tubes can cheese-wire through the punctum (Khairullah and Gendeh, 2011). A square of Gelfoam(Pharmacia NSW, Sydney, Australia) or Merogel (Metronic Xomed) is slid up the tubing and placed over the flaps to hold them in position.

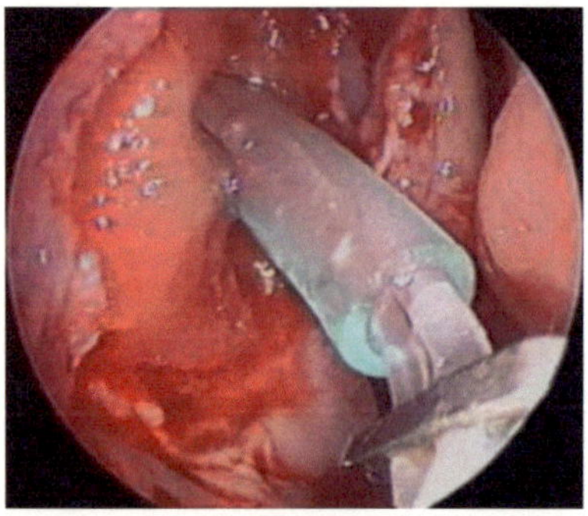

Fig. 8. Intraoperative endoscope view showing right dacrocystorhinostomy with stent in situ an adult patient presenting with unresolving right tearing.

Saline irrigation is started within 3 to 4 hours of surgery. The patient is commenced on broad spectrum antibiotics for 5 days and eye drops are used for 3 weeks. The O'Donoghue tubes are removed in the clinic after 4 weeks. It is rare to see any granulation tissue but if they are present they should be removed. The patient is reviewed for a further 18 months before discharge.

2.5 Laser assisted DCR

For osteotomy, laser was used exclusively in the early part of the series in 1992 and 1993. The preferred site for osteotomy was the thinnest bone located in the infero-posterior parts of the lacrimal fossa, which corresponds to the brightest area in the nasal cavity as demonstrated by the transilluminator. The authors concluded that the success rate of laser-assisted DCR was around 78%, which was much lower than that of conventional DCR. Beginning in 1999 and 2000, osteotomy was performed with either a drill, a punch, or both, which enabled removal of thicker bone. The site of the osteotomy was moved to the level of medial canthus, which was anterior and superior to that of previous surgeries. When the osteotomy was completed, the common internal punctum was visible on endoscopy. With this approach, the success rate improved to 92%(Lee et al, 2004).

In another interesting study in 65 patients with a mean follow-up of 74 months, the authors found the success rate of endoscopic laser assisted DCR has gradually declined over the years to 56%. The authors do not advocate the use of laser in endonasal DCR with epiphora (Umapathy et al, 2006).

3. Endoscopic applications in orbital surgery

3.1 Endoscopic blow out fracture repair

Fractures of the roof of the maxillary sinus with herniation of the orbital content (blow-out fracture), often produce strangulation of the inferior rectus or inferior oblique muscles and thereby impairing movement of eyeball (Fig 9). They can present with periorbital ecchymosis and subconjunctival hemorrhage. Those with fracture of medial wall of orbit without prior surgical intervention can present with enopthalmos.

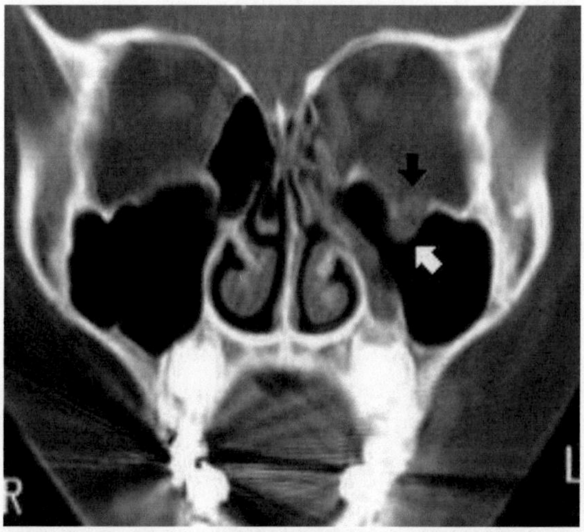

Fig. 9. Coronal CT scan of the paranasal sinuses showing a 'tear drop' sign resulting from a blunt trauma to the left eye in a patient presenting with diplopia

Passage of the endoscope through the intranasal maxillary antrostomy may provide superb visualization of the posterior orbital floor which is the most difficult area to view by transconjunctival or subciliary approach. Anatomically, this area of the orbital floor commonly lies behind the middle half of the globe on axial view. This posterior view may furthermore be obscured because the orbital floor angulates 15 degrees superiorly as one proceeds from the orbital rim toward the orbital apex. Therefore, the endoscope is an extremely useful means of safely and definitely identifying the posterior edge of the defect and ensuring that the posterior edge of the orbital implant do not compromise the optic nerve or other structures at the orbital apex (Hartstein et al, 2004). In many small fractures for which an implant is not required, endoscopic examination and reduction may be sufficient, thus avoiding an external incisional approach.

It is doubtful that endoscopy alone will replace standard CT scanning in the evaluation of orbital fractures. Thus, combining forced duction testing with endoscopic visualization of a fracture may prove to be useful diagnostic tool.

3.1.1 Indications

This include fractures with extension to the middle and posterior portions of the orbital floor, in delayed or secondary fracture repair.

3.1.2 Surgical technique

Orbital fracture repair is normally performed using general anaesthesia. Some author's have reported the use of purely endoscopic approach for the repair of orbital floor fracture (Ikeda et al, 1999). The procedure is commenced by enlarging the maxillary ostium and then introducing an angled endoscope. Bony fragmenst in the fracture site are removed endoscopically until an improvement in forced duction testing is noted. Subsequently, a uretheral balloon catheter is introduced through the ostium into the maxillary sinus. In some patients with trap-door-type fractures, successful fracture repair may be possible with endoscopic approach alone, with removal of the displaced bony fragment and relieve of the entrapment. Saline is used to inflate the balloon which elevates the contents out of the fracture site. The balloon is removed approximately two weeks after surgery.

Tips for successful surgery

Endoscopic visualization of fractures of the posterior aspect of the orbital floor and medial orbit may facilitate safe and secure implant placement and ensures that no residual orbital soft tissue is entrapped within the fracture site or beneath the implant. The endoscopic technique minimizers the uncertainty of implant placement posteriorly in both primary and secondary repairs. It may help to minimize the number of additional incisions required in the medial orbit, maxillary sinus and even the eyelid. The increased accuracy of implant placement may help to reduce the risks of residual exopthalmos postoperatively. This technique is useful in the more complex fractures involving the posterior orbital floor and medial wall.

3.2 Endoscopic orbital decompression of complications of thyroid-related orbitopathy

Graves' disease is an autoimmune disorder affecting the thyroid, orbit and skin. Approximately 50% of patients with this disorder develop orbital manifestation of dysthyroid orbitopathy. Fewer than 5% of such patients have disease that is severe enough to require surgical decompression of the orbit (Metson and Samaha, 2004). The extensive muscle enlargement limits globe movement in extremes of gaze which will cause diplopia. Visual loss in Grave's disease is uncommon, occurring in only 2 to 7% of patients (Kountantakis et al, 2000; Kuppersmith et al, 1997). Exopthalmos in Grave's disease is thought to result from the deposition of immune complexes in the intraocular mucles and fat which in turn leads to edema and fibrosis (Tandon et al, 1994). The resultant increase in intraorbital pressure pushes the globe forward causing proptosis. If this proptosis become severe enough, the eyelids cannot close properly and chemosis with or without exposure keratitis of the cornea may occur. Furthermore, the crowding of the orbital apex by the obviously enlarged extraocular muscles places pressure on the optic nerve. Stretching of the optic nerve by increasing proptosis may result in the development of optic neuropathy and visual loss. If medical treatment fails (high dose steroids with or without low-dose radiotherapy) , surgical decompression of eyelid is indicated(Cook et al, 1996).

Removing one or more of the bony walls can decompress the contents of the orbit. The least amount of decompression would be achieved with medial wall removal , but the most physiologic and least to cause complications like globe displacement and diplopia. Endoscopic orbital decompression affords maximal orbital decompression at the orbital apex, an area that is not fully accessible via the external or transantral routes (Metson et al, 1994). Many techniques have been described for decompressing the orbit but the order of the procedures is that orbital decompression first, then strabismus and lastly the eyelid.

3.2.1 Indications and contraindications

The primary indication for the surgery is exopthalmos, either for cosmetic reasons or when vision is deteriorating and steroids and radiotherapy treatment has failed. The most common indications for such surgery are exposure keratopathy and optic neuropathy that have been refractory to conservative measures. Patients with diplopia from dysthyroid orbitopathy may require decompression before strabismus surgery to reaccess the globe and improve the predictability of muscle adjustments. Some surgeons who consider aesthetically undesirable proptosis to be an indication for orbital decompression have performed such surgery for its cosmetic benefits.

Contraindications to endoscopic orbital decompression include acute sinusitis and anatomic abnormalities of the maxillary bone. Endoscopic decompression may be technically difficult in patients with very small maxillay sinuses or thick orbital walls. These features are easily identified on computed tomography(CT) scan of the orbit and sinuses, which should be obtained on all patients before surgery.

3.2.2 Useful instruments

- A long-shanked drill with a course diamond burr (Medtronic Xomed, Jacksonville, Florida, USA) and good irrigation system to keep the bone cool.
- Image guided surgery

3.2.3 Endoscopic technique

The patient is placed in a supine position with head slightly elevated. Packing that has been soaked in a 4% cocaine solution is placed in the nasal cavity to initiate mucosal vasoconstriction. Both eyes are exposed in the surgical field. If general anaesthesia is used, the corneas are covered with protective shells. Under endoscopic visualization, submucosal injections of 1% lidocaine with epinephrine are administered along the lateral nasal wall and middle turbinate. If a septal deviation precludes endoscopic access to the middle meatus region, a septoplasty is performed before orbital decompression.

The bones removed in endoscopic decompression include the medial wall of the orbit and the portion of the floor that is medial to the infraorbital canal. The procedure is initiated with an incision through the uncinate process. This incision is made just posterior to the maxillary line, a bony eminence that extends from the anterior attachment of the middle turbinate to the root of the inferior turbinate(Fig 10). The maxillary sinus ostium is then generously enlarged to provide optimal exposure of the orbital floor to prevent obstruction of the maxillary sinus by the decompressed globe. Bone is removed in the posterior direction to the level of the back wall of the sinus. Anterior removal is terminated at the thick bone of the frontal process of the maxilla, which protects the nasolacrimal duct. The ostium is enlarged superiorly to the level of the orbital floor and inferiorly to the root of the inferior turbinate. A 30-degree endoscope is used to identify the infraorbital nerve along the roof of the sinus (Fig 11).

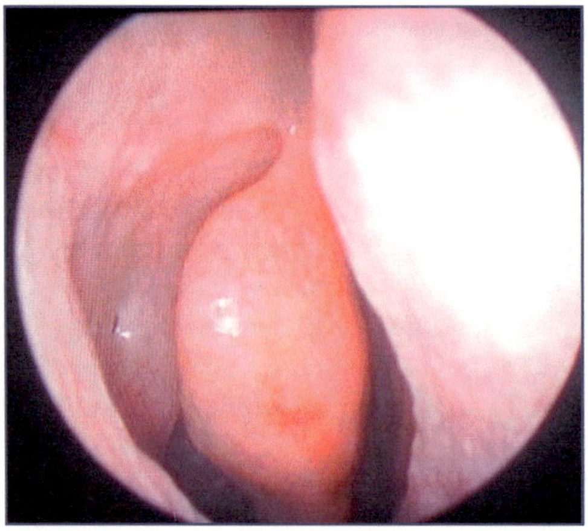

Fig. 10. A zero degree endoscopic view of left lateral nasal wall showing the maxillary line and uncinate process

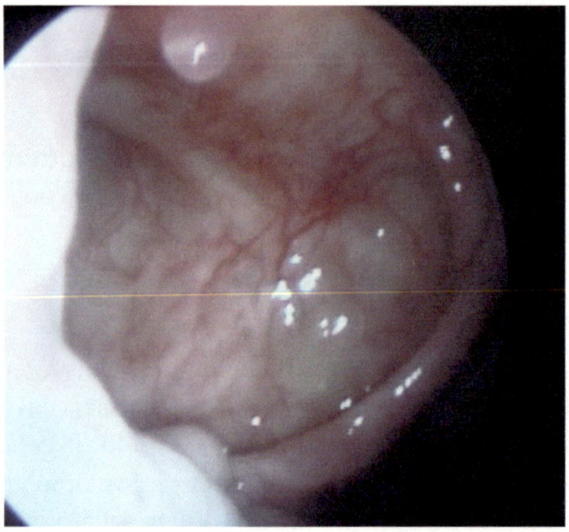

Fig. 11. A 30 degree endoscopic view showing evidence of wide right middle meatal antrostomy with infraorbital indentation in the roof of the maxillary sinus

An endoscopic sphenoethmoidectomy is then completed as described by Stammberger (1991) and Kennedy (1985). The degree of pneumatization of the sphenoid determines whether the optic nerve indents or even dehiscent in its lateral wall. Similarly, if the posterior ethmoid sinuses envelop the optic nerve before it reaches the sphenoid sinus, am Onodi cell may be present (Fig 12).The anterior and posterior ethmoid arteries are identified along the ethmoid roof. The middle turbinate that serves as a landmark during the sphenoethmoidectomy is removed before opening the lamina papyracea to optimize exposure to the medial orbital wall and facilitate postoperative cleaning. The skeletonized lamina papyracea is gently penetrated with a small spoon curette. Bony fragments of lamina papyracea is lifted in a medial direction to avoid perforation of the underlying periorbita. This elevation may also be performed with a periosteal elevator or delicate Blakesley forceps(Stortz, Germany). If surgery is performed using local anaesthesia, additional injections may be necessary to desensitize the medial orbital wall. Anaesthetic agent is injected just deep to the periorbita through the bony opening in the lamina.

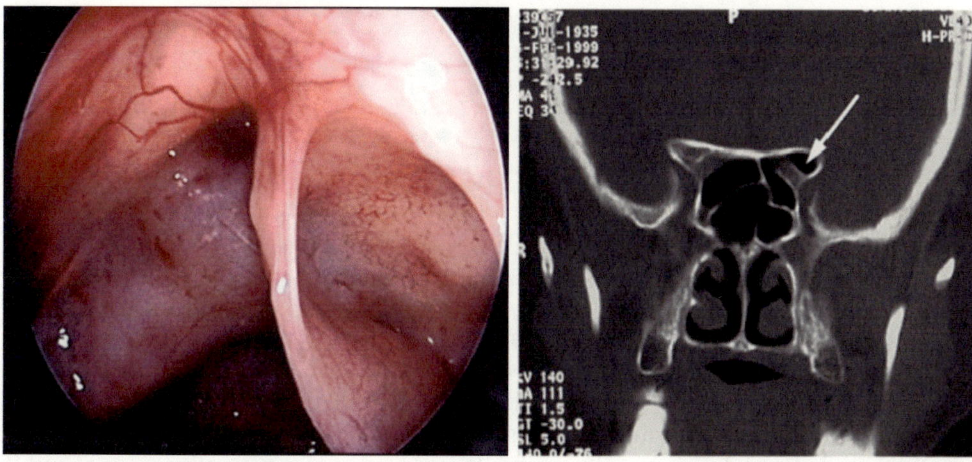

(a) (b)

Fig. 12. An intra-operative endoscopic view (a) and coronal CT scan view (b) showing an Onodi cell

Bone of the lamina papyracea is removed in a superior direction toward the level of the ethmoid roof. The frontal recess is the most anterior superior portion of the ethmoid sinus, which communicates with the frontal sinus. Removal of the lamina papyracea in this region can cause postoperative obstruction of the frontal sinus by herniated fat. As dissection continous in a posterior direction toward orbital apex, thicker bone and underlying periorbita are generally encounterd within 2 mm of the sphenoid face. This thickening represents the annulus of Zinn, from which the extra ocular muscles(EOMs) originate and through which the optic nerve passes (Fig 13). This landmark represents the posterior limit of dissection and does not need to be removed. In cases of neuropathy, bone removal proceeds more posteriorly and may extend to the lateral wall of the sphenoid sinus.

Fragments of bone are cleared from the anterior end of lamina papyracea where it joins the lacrimal bone. Dissection in this region may be facilitated by use of an angled spoon curette and 30-degree endoscope (Stortz, Germany). The thick white fascia of the lacrimal sac may be uncovered but should not be opened. Firm bone anterior to the maxillary line protects most of the sac, so it should not be removed. Removal of the bone along the medial orbital floor can be most technically challenging aspect of this surgery. A spoon curette is used to fracture the bone in a downward direction. This bone may break apart in several small fragments with a natural cleavage plane along the infraorbital canal. Use of a 30-degree endoscope may facilitate visualization within the maxillary sinus and aid in the identification of the infraorbital nerve which serves as the lateral limit of bone removal.

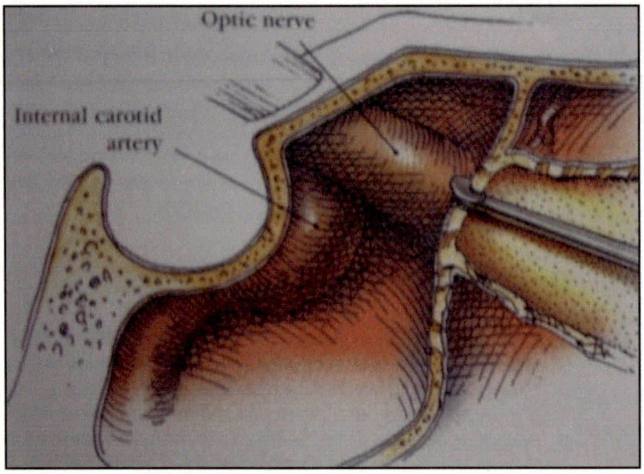

Fig. 13. A diagrammatic sagittal section of left sphenoid and posterior ethmoids showing the thick bone at the annulus of Zinn at the junction of the orbital apex and sphenoid sinus

After the periorbita has been fully exposed and cleared of bony fragments, it is opened with a sickle knife(Stortz, Germany). The incision is usually commenced in front of the sphenoid sinus. Care is taken to keep the tip of the blade superficial to avoid injury of the underlying orbital contents especially the medial rectus muscle, which may be enlarged secondary to dysthyroid orbitopathy. Incision of the periorbita is extended along the ethmoid roof and the orbital floor. A horizontal strip of periorbita overlying the medial rectus muscle is preserved (Fig 14). This fascial sling serves to decrease prolapsed of the muscle and is thought to reduce the incidence of postoperative diplopia (Metson and Samaha, 2002). However, in patients with optic neuropathy, maximal decompression is needed and the fascial sling is sacrificed to allow for wider excision of the periorbita which is removed eventually with angled Blakesley forceps. At the completion of the procedure, the generous prolapsed of the orbital fat into the opened ethmoid and maxillary sinuses should be observed(Fig 15)

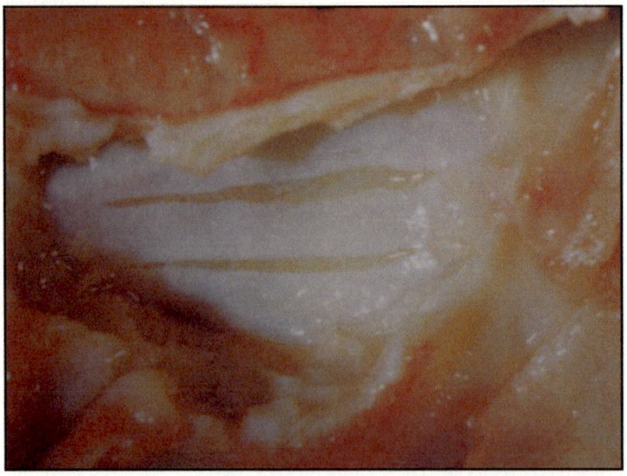

Fig. 14. A 70 degree endoscopic view showing an emergency horizontal orbital decompression incisions of the periorbita extending from the ethmoidal roof to the orbital floor for thyroid related orbitopathy

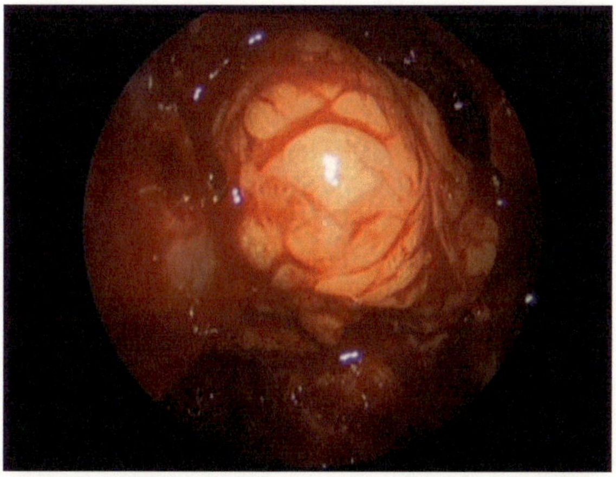

Fig. 15. A 30 degree endoscopic view showing prolapsed of orbital fat into the nasal cavity on balloting the right eye

A lateral orbital decompression may be performed at this time, depending on the extent of patient's disease and the degree of additional decompression desired. Due to the prior medial decompression, the orbital contents are easily retracted in a medial direction to provide excellent exposure of the lateral bony wall, which is removed or contoured. Concurrent excision of excess intraconal fat may also be performed if necessary. Bilateral orbital decompressions may be performed concurrently or as a staged procedure.

Nasal packing is avoided in order to prevent compression of the optic nerve, which is rendered increasingly vulnerable by the decompression. The patient is discharged the morning after surgery with a prescription for oral antibiotics and instructions to begin twice-daily nasal saline irrigations with a bulb syringe. During postoperative visit a week later, residual debri is cleared from the nasal cavity under endoscopic guidance.

In some cases, local anaesthesia may be preferred to general anaesthesia. These situations include patients who have an only-seeing eye, significant medical comorbidity, or a strong preference for local anesthesia.

The use of local anesthetic enables the surgeon to monitor the patient's vision on a continuous basis during the surgery and reduces the likelihood of occult injury to the optic nerve (Metson et al, 1994). Ideal sedation is achieved with intravenous bolus of propofol, 0.4 to 0.8mg/kg, administred before local injection, followed by maintenance infusion of 95 to 75 ug/kg during the procedure. Submucosal infilteration of 1% lidocaine with epinephrine 1:100,000 is performed exactly as described for the procedure utilizing general anaesthesia. Patients may report discomfort during removal of the lamina papyracea, and this may require a small additional infiltration of anaesthetic solution into the periorbita.

3.2.4 Complications

Diplopia is a relatively common sequela of endoscopic orbital decompression reported in 15 to 30 % of postoperative patients. This complication can be the result of change in the vector of pull of the EOMs. Diplopia that is present preoperatively is usually not improved by this surgery. Patients with preexisting or new-onset post-operative diplopia frequently require strabismus surgery. It is essential that all patients be informed of the possibility of postoperative double vision before undergoing orbital decompression.

Techniques to decrease the incidence of new-onset postoperative diplopia, including the preservation of the fascial sling of periorbita to prevent prolapsed of the medial rectus muscle, have been mentioned (Metson and Samaha, 2002). To decrease the incidence of postoperative diplopia, the use of balanced decompression technique is advocated. This technique involves performing external lateral wall decompression at the time of endoscopic medial wall decompression to reduce pressure on the medial rectus muscle while simultaneously increasing the degree of ocular recession.

Postoperative bleeding after endoscopic orbital decompression is managed by direct caurterization of the bleeding site. Nasal packing is avoided in these patients to avoid pressure in the region of the optic nerve. The incidence of sinonasal infection post-surgery is minimized with the routine use of postoperative antistaphylococcal antibiotics.

Postoperative epiphora may occur if the nasolacrimal duct is transected during the maxillary antrostomy. This complication is readily treated with an endoscopic DCR. Blindness and cerebrospinal fluid rhinorrhea are also potentially serious complications of orbital decompression but rare.

Endoscopic orbital decompression should be performed only by surgeons with extensive experience in endoscopic intranasal techniques. A team approach, which uses the skills of both an Otolaryngologist and an Opthalmologist during the performance of this procedure is highly recommended.

Tips for successful surgery

Orbital decompression for thyroid-related orbitopathy is an effective method for reduction of proptosis for cosmetic proptosis, eye complications from exposure of the cornea and visual loss. The amount of regression of proptosis is related to the number of walls removed during surgery. It is believed that three-walled decompression may give a more balanced decompression with less likelihood of postoperative diplopia.

3.3 Endoscopic orbital decompression for acute orbital hemorrhage

The procedure of choice is lateral canthotomy and inferior cantholysis with of course cold dry compresses as tolerable. This is performed for 'orbital compartment syndrome' due to orbital bleeding, emphysema or tumor. For orbital decompression, lateral canthotomy alone is not sufficient and the inferior eyelid should be completely free to allow anterior displacement of the globe. Drainage of any kind is only indicated if this is not helpful. The problem with drainage is that the bleeding is diffuse and not confined to one compartment. Endoscopic drainage is actually performed to remove adjacent orbital wall and open the periosteum to allow decompression of orbital soft tissues. It is important to note that the same can be achieved with the faster canthotomy and inferior cantholysis.

Invariably the anterior ethmoidal artery(AEA) can be located one cell behind the frontal recess(Fig 16 a, b). The size of the so called supra-orbital cell (Bolger & Mann, 2001) varies: it can be small or large. The AEA can often be seen on CT scan, (Fig 10) particularly as it enters the orbit where it produces a fluted defect in the lamina papyracea(LP). The more pneumatized the supra-orbital recess, the more vulnerable it is to damage. Often the ethmoidal bulla (EB) attaches to the skull base and the AEA lies within the roof and is 1-2 mm behind the attachment of the anterior wall of the EB to skull base. If the frontal recess (FR) does require opening, it is best approached anteriorly, away from AEA if the landmarks are poor owing to previous surgery or bleeding. As the AEA is sometimes dehiscent, it is advisable not to grasp polyps in this area if one is unable to identify the anatomy clearly. Often the FR can be found by following the intact anterior wall of the ethmoidal bulla superiorly.

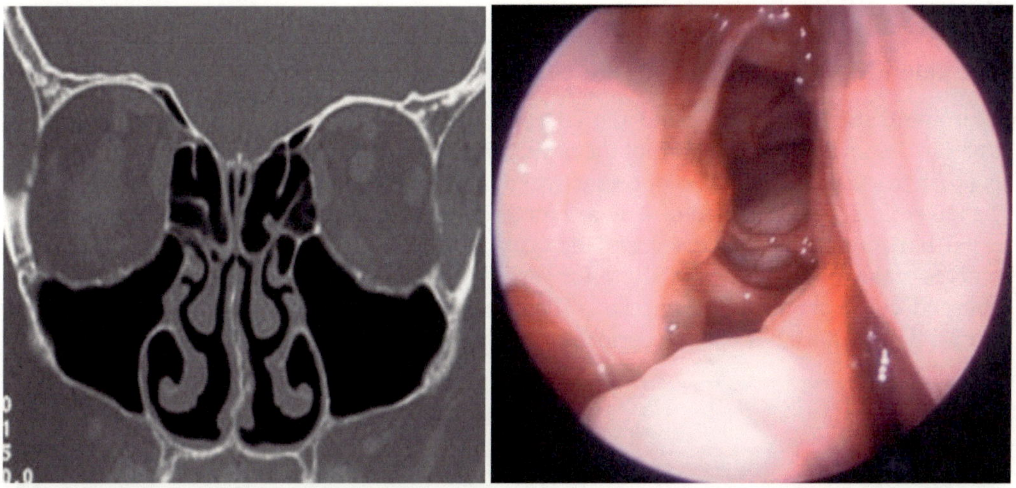

(a) (b)

Fig. 16. A coronal CT imaging showing an indentation of right anterior ethmoidal artery at the region of frontal recess (a) and a 70 degree endoscopic view showing indentation of the artery in the same patient(b).

The AEA is dehiscent at some point in the majority of patients (Lang, 1989). It is essential to avoid tearing it for it can cause marked bleeding. If it is transected and retracts into the orbit, a marked increase in pressure in the posterior compartment of the eye can occur and place the retinal artery and its supply to the retina at risk. If it is torn, gentle bipolar diathermy will arrest the bleeding but this should be performed with great care to avoid transecting the remaining segment of the artery.

3.3.1 Bleeding

If there is obvious bleeding into the posterior compartment of the eye, the eye will prop out, the orbit will become very firm and within a few minutes the swinging flash light test will reveal an afferent defect. An awake patient will complaint of discomfort and loss of vision. An orbital tourniquet should be tried on immediate recognition. This involves placing a cotton wool over the closed eyelid and applying an orbital tourniquet over the cotton wool and around the head and then inflating it to systolic pressure. This is performed for one minute and then it should be removed and the pupil reflexes and/or the vision checked. If the vision or pupil reflex has improved, the orbital tourniquet should be reapplied and the process repeated every minute for up to 5 minutes. If this is performed soon after injury, it may be sufficient to stop bleeding into the orbit and it can arrest the process.

It is advisable to monitor vision for 6 hours postsurgery to ensure that no further bleeding occurs into the posterior compartment. If this maneuver fails then the orbit must be decompressed. A lateral canthotomy and inferior cantholysis is quick and efficient technique for up to one hour and it is best to decompress the orbit as early as possible (Jones, 1997). Moreover, one should not wait for an opthalmological colleague to arrive unless they do so within an hour. Assessing the vascular supply of the retinal vessels with an opthalmoscope is inadequate.

3.3.2 Lateral canthotomy and inferior cantholysis

Local anesthetic is placed around the lateral canthus of eye and it is divided using small straight scissors down to the bone of the orbital rim and to the depth of the lateral sulcus of the conjunctiva. A corneal abrasion or conjuctival damage can be avoided by protecting the globe. The lower lid is then retracted downward for good expose. The scissors is angled at 45 degree to the horizontal axis and the lateral ligament and septum is divided and the globe and contents of the orbit will then prolapse forward (Fig 17). The pupil reflexes, the pressure of the orbit and vision should all be checked. The orbit will retract to its normal position over the next 2-3 days. Suturing is usually performed a week or so after the procedure.

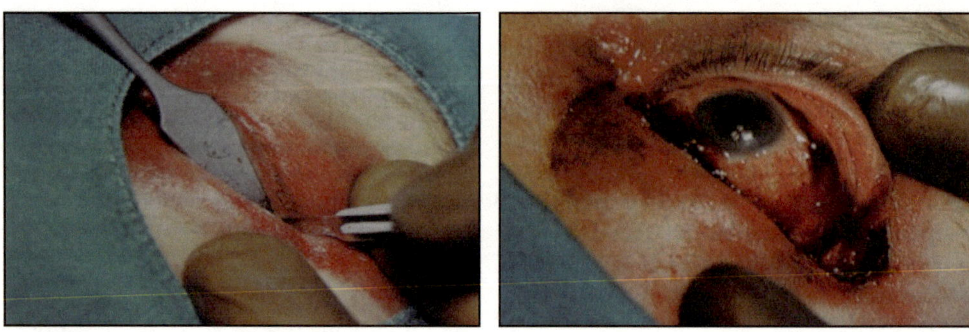

(a) (b)

Fig. 17. Picture showing an emergency left lateral canthotomy (a) and subsequent cantholysis (b) being performed in the same patient for iatrogenic orbital hemorrhage

This procedure is normally sufficient to decompress the posterior compartment of the eye. If inadequate a surgical decompression should be undertaken. It can be done either endoscopically by removing the LP widely and incising the orbital periosteum or externally via a Lynch-Howarth incision. Preserving vision takes priority over producing an external scar. If the orbit is decompressed by an external approach, the AEA will not be found as it will have retracted into substance of the orbit.

3.3.3 Medial rectus damage

Medial rectus damage occurs when there is disinsertion of the muscle, damage to the muscle nerve or intramuscular bleeding. In damage encountered during enscopic sinus surgery, a vigilant assistant should look out for movement of the globe which occurs unintentionally. As a precautionary measure, the assistant should repeatedly ballot the eye when the surgeon is operating on the lateral nasal wall. Anatomically the medial rectus muscle is located closer to LP posteriorly then anteriorly (Fig 18). The suction port of the powered shaver should preferably be directed medially away from the LP to minimize the risk of damaging the structures in the lateral nasal wall. Damage to medial rectus occurs through deeper penetration into the orbit. Unfortunately, it is very difficult to prevent the scarring and diplopia that are likely to occur if recognized then. Moreover, expert strabismus surgeons have difficulty in correcting the problems caused by damage to the medial rectus. It is a medical negligence and should preferably be settled out of court.

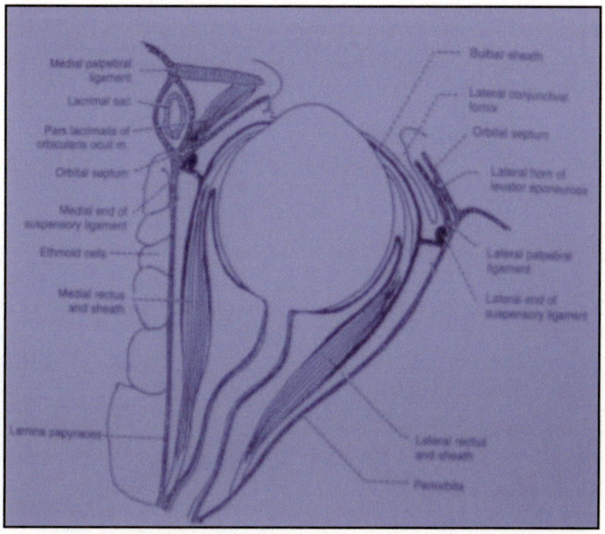

Fig. 18. Axial section of the relationship of right medial rectus and optic nerve to the lamina papyracea

3.3.4 Optic nerve damage

The optic nerve can be damaged by penetration of the orbit through the lamina papyracea. Therefore, it is important for the assistant to look for eye movements when the surgeon is operating on the lateral nasal wall. Moreover, the optic nerve can be damaged if it is exposed in a sphenoethmoid air cell(Onodi cell)(Fig 19). An Onodi cell should be identified on routine pre-operative imaging and care taken in removing polyps lateral to the sagittal plane of the medial wall of the maxillary sinus. It is advisable to identify the sphenoid sinus ostia medially and then work forward. The optic nerve indentation can be prominent in 20% of patients in the upper half of lateral wall of sphenoid sinus but is rarely dehiscent (Fig 20). The carotid artery lies in the lateral and inferior aspect of the sphenoid sinus. Therefore, it is advisable to avoid the lateral wall of sphenoid sinus by directing the suction port of the powered shaver medially away from the lateral wall of sphenoid sinus to minimize the risk of damaging the structures present there.

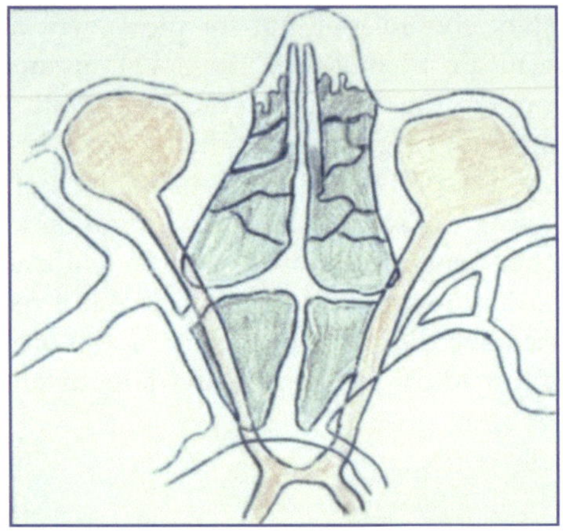

Fig. 19. A diagrammatic axial view of the paranasal sinuses showing a rare bilateral Onodi cell

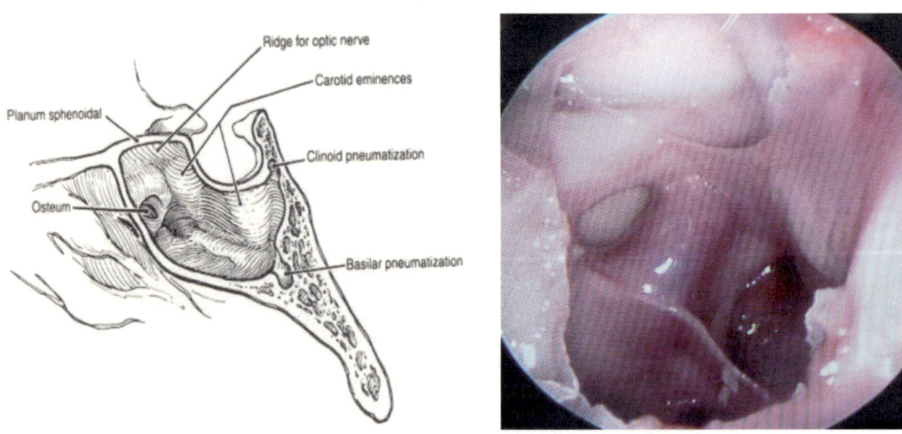

Fig. 20. Diagrammatic sagittal section and endoscopic view of the sphenoid sinus showing indentations of the lateral wall by internal carotid artery inferiorly and optic nerve superiorly

3.3.5 Post-operative complications

3.3.5.1 Bleeding

Sitting the patient 30% head up at end of procedure is often adequate for minor general ooze. Coughing during extubation will result in temporarily more bleeding due to increase in venous pressure. A nasal pack soaked in 1:10,000 epinephrine is helpful for more than minor ooze and removed in the recovery or left in position for 12 hours if oozing continues. Prophylactic antibiotics are advocated for nasal packs left in position for more than 24 hours. Rarely, torrential reactionary bleeding can occur in the first 12 hours due to these vessels initially going into spasm intra-operatively when the platelet plug and clotting factors block them but with due time either due to relaxation of artery or fibrinolysis reverses this process and bleeding commences. Usually it is impossible to locate the bleeding site. If a local nasal pack with vasoconstrictor and local anesthetic is not helpful to control the bleeding, then bipolar caurtery of the offending vessel may be helpful. If this too fails, then reinserting a nasal pack and/or balloon may be necessary to tamponade the bleeding until the spheno-palatine artery(SPA) can be ligated under general anesthesia. If a large sphenoidotomy has been performed, the bleeding could be due to the damaged septal branch as it crosses the anterior wall of the sphenoid (Fig 21).

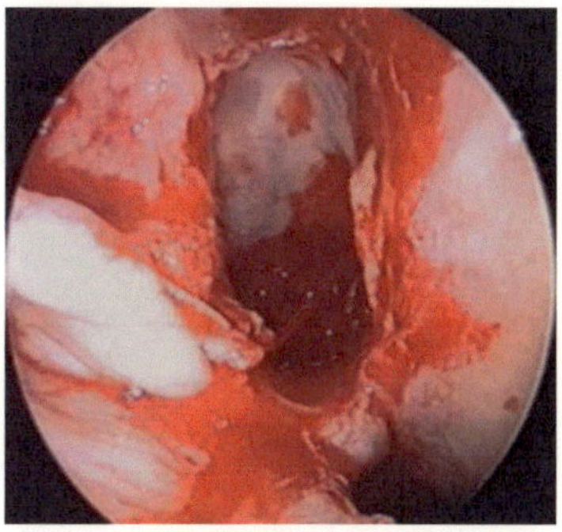

Fig. 21. Intraoperative Endoscopic view showing a right low sphenoidotomy with evidence of sphenopalatine bleed

3.3.5.2 Adhesions

Mucosal damage to adjacent surfaces can result in adhesions (Fig 22). Adhesions can be minimized by topical and local corticosteroids application. If adhesions are present pre-operatively, they need removal with a through-cutting punch followed by douching and debridement at one week.

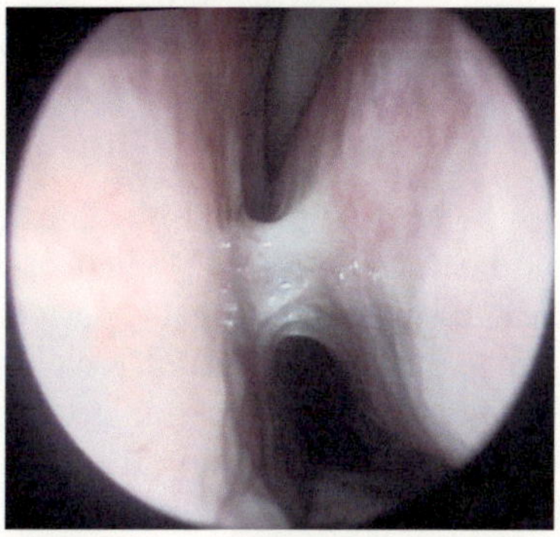

Fig. 22. Endoscopic view showing adhesions between left septum and inferior turbinate after nasal surgery

3.3.5.3 Epiphora

The lacrimal sac or naso-lacriminal duct can be damaged if the middle meatal antrostomy(MMA) is extended too far anteriorly. If middle meatus needs to be enlarged anteriorly to allow improved access or drainage, then the uncinate process (UP) is removed retrograde with Stammberger Rhinoforce antrum punch (Stortz, Germany). If patient complaints of watery eyes post surgery, it is best not to intervene as it will often resolve on its own. If the epiphora is persistent, an endo-nasal DCR will be helpful.

3.3.5.4 Periorbital emphysema

Peri-orbital emphysema or air in the soft tissues around the eye is due to intra-operative breach of the LP and the patient unknowingly blown their nose(Fig 23).The anesthetist should be advice to take care on extubating the patient and not to use too much force if patient needs to be ventilated with face mask. The emphysema will resolve in due time provided the patient does not blow any more air into the area. Prophylactic antibiotics are administered for active sinusitis or history of sinusitis.

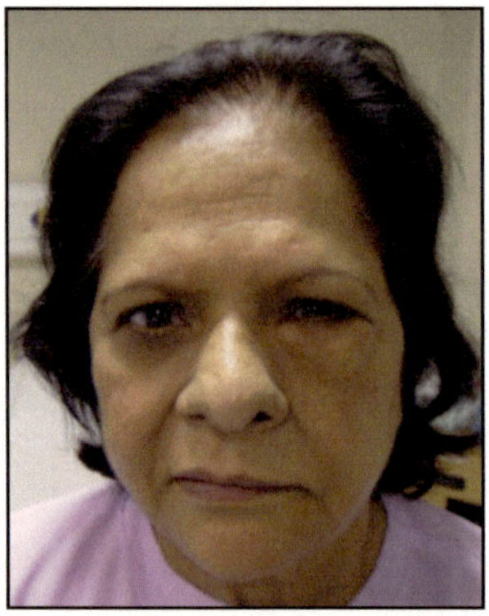

Fig. 23. Left periorbital emphysema post powered endoscopic sinus surgery which resolved spontaneously

3.3.5.5 Anosmia

Smell is a precious sense and every effort should be made to preserve or improve it. The olfactory mucosa extends from the cribriform plate to cover almost all the medial side of middle turbinate and the same area on the septum with a little inferior extension.

Pre-operative oral steroids are helpful in preventing damage to the mucosa, especially if polyps are medial to the middle turbinate (MT) when assessed as an outpatient. If the polyps remain medial to middle turbinate at surgery, perform an ethmoidectomy and then gently lateralize the MT to open the olfactory cleft which allows better access to topical steroid spray. If the patient has hyposmia or anosmia post-surgery and the MT is adherent to the septum, it is worth resecting and lateralizing the MT as an elective procedure when mucosal edema has settled down.

3.3.5.6 Frontal recess stenosis

The frontal sinus is often opaque on CT scan in nasal polyposis and it is normally due to retained secretions. It is rare to find polyps within the frontal sinus. Often opening the middle meatus and de-bulking polyps in region below the frontal recess with a shaver or through-cutting forceps (Stortz, Germany) followed by washing and topical nasal steroids may be adequate to allow the patients disease to be controlled.

It is essential not to denude the frontal recess of its mucosa since this may predispose to stenosis. If there is purulent disease within the frontal sinus causing symptoms, then it is advisable to open the recess, preserving as much mucosa as possible. This is ideally performed by dissecting the mucosa off the agger nasi cells with a ball probe and pulling it down on the shell of the cell and removing the fragments of bone and carefully preserving the mucosa. Any loose fragments of mucosa are best left alone. Large fragments of redundant mucosa around the frontal recess can be trimmed using a shaver or through-cutting forceps (Stortz, Germany). If there is a bony partition between the supra-orbital cell and frontal recess or a high frontal cell, the partition between them should be removed sub-mucosally.

3.3.5.7 Crusting

Crust results from mucosal damage. If there is full thickness mucosal damage, the mucus produced stagnates because there is no functioning cilia to clear it and it may take up to a year for the cilia to start to function synchronously again. Therefore, mucosal damage should be minimized and a full thickness defect should be avoided at all cost.

3.3.5.8 Infection

Superficial infection of stagnant mucus is common and usually resolves with douching. Sometimes, staphylococci multiply in a sump of mucus that collects in the maxillary sinus and may be slow to clear with douching alone. Topical nasal mupirocin ointment sniffed liberally after douching 6 times a day for 3 weeks can be very helpful.

3.3.5.9 Osteitis

Local osteitis due to exposure of bone is a rare complication resulting in severe pain. It produces a very dull, severe crippling nagging ache that causes tears to the patient. This condition is very distressing to the patient and worrying for the surgeon. Major analgesics are required and local treatment appears to provide little relief. Patients undergoing surgery for inverted papilloma where mucosal preservation is not practiced are at risk.

Tips for successful surgery

Intraobital hemorrhage should be managed with lateral canthotomy and cantholysis followed by orbital decompression with removal of the medial orbital wall. Orbital decompression can be performed without canthotomy and cantholysis if the complication is notice intraoperatively

3.4 Endoscopic orbital decompression for orbital sub-periosteal abscess

Rhinosinusitis in children is not a surgical disease, and therefore the treatment is medical with systemic antibiotics such as clavulinic acid and ampicillin(Augmentin). The priority should be safety in any treatment as the problem usually resolves with time without intervention. Growth and maturation of the immunological response to pathogens play a major role in resolution of the disease (Jones, 1999; Howe & Jones, 2004).

Patients presenting with orbital complications of sinusitis commonly have a degree of cellulitis and edema (chemosis) around the eye with associated proptosis (Fig 24). This may be associated with some restriction of eye movement. Patients typically present with history of nasal obstruction, purulent rhinorrhea and facial pressure or pain. Nasal endoscopy reveals an inflammed and oedematous nasal mucosa with usually presence of pus in the middle meatus.

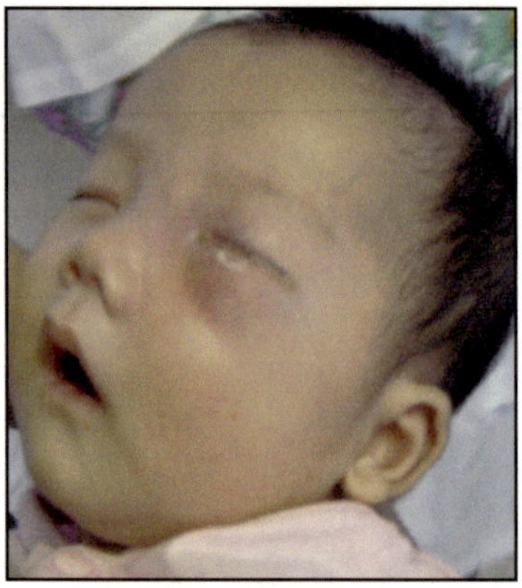

Fig. 24. Picture of a child with a left orbital cellulitis

If a subperiostal abcess is suspected, a CT scan of the parananasal sinuses with contrast will present a mass located on the lamina papyracea or in relation to the frontal sinus. The rim of the mass will enhance with the contrast. Moreover, the proptosis will be visible on the axial scans.

The external approach is quick and easy and the abscesss can usually be rapid and safely drained. If the surgeon is a skilled and experienced endoscopic sinus surgeon, endoscopic drainage of the subperiosteal abscess can be performed. The problem with this procedure is the significant vascularity that is associated with acute sinusitis. If the mucosal surface is touched with an instrument or endoscope, it will usually bleed and an inexperienced surgeon may lose orientation and complications may occur as a result of poor visibility during the surgery. Frequent packing with decongested soaked neuropatties throughout the procedure helps to minimize the bleeding but will not control it entirely. In a patient with acute sinusitis, the anaesthetist needs to optimize the patient's hemodynamics parameters to create an optimal surgical field.

The surgical approach is to perform an uncinectomy and enlarge the maxillary ostium to a moderate degree. Uncinectomy alone without antrostomy carries the risk of postoperative closure of the maxillary sinus because the inflammation and edema predisposes to scarring and adhesion formation. Clearance of the frontal sinus depends on whether the frontal sinus is thought to be the origin of the subperiosteal abscess. If the abscess is located adjacent to the ethmoidal sinuses, clearance of the bulla ethmoidalis and posterior ethmoids is performed with identification of the lamina papyracea. The lamina papyracea over the subperiosteal abscess is widely exposed and removed. If the abscess is related to the floor of the frontal sinus, it can still be drained endoscopically. A minitrephine is usually placed in the frontal sinus before dissection of the frontal recess. This aids in identification of the frontal outflow tract. The frontal recess is cleared and the frontal ostium identified. The lamina papyracea directly behind the the lacrimal sac is removed and using a curette, the orbital periostium is kept intact and gently pushed laterally while the curette advances into the subperiosteal abscess and the abscess drained (Wormald PJ, 2005).

A malleable suction (Medtronic Xomed, Jacksonville, Florida, USA) is introduced into the cavity and any fibrin within the cavity is removed. A corrugated Pendrose drain is slid into the abscess cavity and left in place, draining the abscess cavity into the ethmoid sinuses for 1 to 2 days before being endoscopically removed. Endoscopic removal of the subperiosteal abscess remains highly effective but it must be emphasized that the surgeon should be very experienced.

Although endoscopic drainage of subperiosteal and other orbital abcesses is becoming more common, the efficiency of narrow surgical drainage via an endoscopic approach has not been thoroughly been evaluated (Page and Wiatrak, 1996). Similarly, although endoscopic treatment of frontal sinus is less invasive than open frontal surgery, it also has a lower reported success rate (Metson and Gliklich, 1998).

Indications for CT scan

- Unable to accurately assess vision, gross proptosis, opthalmoplegia, deteriorating visual acuity or colour vision, bilateral edema, no improvement or deterioration at 24 hours or a swinging pyrexia that does not resolve within 36 hours

Tips for successful surgery

Endoscopic decompression of a subperiosteal abscess should only be performed by very experienced endoscopic sinus surgeons because the surgical field can be very bloody, which can significantly increase the degree of difficulty and the likelihood of complications. If the surgeon is not experienced, then the abscess should be drained via an external incision.

3.5 Endoscopic optic canal decompression

The most common indication for endoscopic optic canal decompression is traumatic optic nerve neuropathy(TON). Currently it is thought that 5% of severe head injuries will have concomitant injury to the optic nerve, optic tract or optic cortex (Tandon et al, 1994; Kountantakis et al, 2000; Kuppersmith et al, 1997). Since major brain injury takes precedence over traumatic optic neuropathy, it may result in the optic nerve injury being diagnosed somewhat later then the brain injury. Some authors feel that early diagnosis and treatment of traumatic optic neuropathy may be of greater benefit to the patient(Lubben et al, 2001, Sofferman, 1995) and advocate diagnosis of optic nerve deficit by the presence of an absolute or relative afferent pupillary defect supported by disc edema and congestion of the vessel walls. These findings in addition to CT scan and possibly MRI scan and visual evoked potentials are sufficient to undertake optic canal decompression. Currently there is no properly conducted randomized controlled trials comparing high-dose steroid therapy, surgical decompression and observation (Steinsapir et al, 2002).

Traumatic optic neuropathy is believed to result from two distinct injuries to the nerve. The primary injury is the result of either a direct contusive force on the optic canal and nerve or elastic deformation of the sphenoid, with transfer of the force on the intra-canalicular optic nerve disrupting the axons and blood vessels (Steinsapir & Goldberg, 1994). This primary injury may result in compression of the nerve by bony fragments or in hemorrhage into the nerve sheath. A secondary injury may occur if the primary injury is not treated in due time. Compression of the blood vessels occur if there is bleeding into the dura resulting in ischaemia and continued axon loss (Sofferman, 1995; Steinsapir & Goldberg, 1994).

We have adopted a conservative approach to traumatic neuropathy with all patients undergoing high-dose steroid treatment before being offered surgical intervention. The exception is when bony fragments are found to impinge on the optic nerve.

A randomized clinical trial demonstrated no benefit of either high-dose corticosteroids nor optic nerve decompression. Both are still employed because the alternative may be irreversible blindness. However, at the initial presentation, the visual performance of visual fields is correlated to the final outcome.

3.5.1 Medical therapy for traumatic optic neuropathy

Presently megadose intravenous methylprednisolone is helpful. Methylprednisolone 30mg/kg IV loading dose is given followed by 5.4 mg/kg/hr thereafter (Cook et al, 1996). The patient's visual acuity is monitored hourly and surgical intervention is considered if the patient shows or fails any of the criteria below:

- A dilated optic nerve on CT scan
- Fracture of optic canal on CT scan with vision less than 6/60
- Fracture of optic canal with vision more than 6/60 but the patient's vision deteriorates on steroids
- Vision is less than 6/60 after 48 hours of steroids with likely canal injury (indicated by the presence of fluid levels in the posterior ethmoids and sphenoids and/or the presence of fractures of the ethmoids, orbital apex and sphenoid).

3.5.2 Surgical therapy for traumatic optic neuropathy

Optic nerve decompression (OND) is an extension of orbital decompression when the optic nerve in the lateral wall of the sphenoid is decompressed.

3.5.3 Indications

Optic nerve injury is usually and should be recognized immediately by the existence of relative afferent papillary defect (RAPD) or inverse RAPD. It always appears in optic nerve injury even if visual acuity is relatively preserved initially. If it occurs in traumatic setting, the visual acuity will always deteriorate to no light perception. One should suspect this injury whether the ocular media are clear or opaque. It may be inappropriate for the patient to undergo surgery if they have a Glasgow coma scale of less than eight (Jones et al, 1997). Several studies suggest that with retro-orbital hemorrhage, decompression of the orbit needs to be done in less than one hour (Mason et al, 1998). However, where there is no hemorrhage, it is less understood under what circumstances it is beneficial to decompress the nerve pathway. If there is an anatomical constriction on CT scans affecting the course of the optic nerve and the patient is fit for anesthesia, then it seems reasonable to remove bone pressing on the nerve.

3.5.4 Useful instruments

- A long-shank drill with a course diamond burr and good irrigation system (Medtronic Xomed) to keep the bone cool.
- Image guided surgery

3.5.5 Surgical technique

The standard preparation of the nose is performed with decongestants and infilteration. An uncinectomy with exposure of the maxillary ostium is performed (Fig 25). An axillary flap is performed and the agger nasi cell removed for acess to skull base. The fovea ethmoidalis is exposed in the region above the bulla ethmoidalis. If there is disruption of the cells of the frontal recess, then this will be cleared. In some patients with severe sinus fracture, the entire skull base may be mobile.

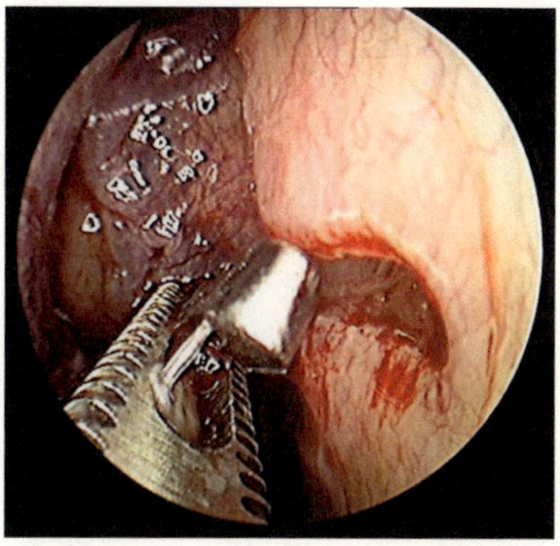

Fig. 25. A zero degree endoscopic view showing a left uncinectomy being performed

In majority of patients, the posterior ethmoid cells will be full of blood and when combined with mobility of lamina papyracea, the skull base surgeon can become disorientated. Thus, this surgery should be undertaken only by highly experienced endoscopic sinus surgeons. A posterior ethmoidectomy and sphenoidotomy should be performed. In the posterior ethmoids, the posterior lamina papyracea and fovea ethmoidalis should be identified. If significant disruption of the posterior ethmoids and lamina papyracea has occurred, then a large middle meatus antrostomy provides an extra reference point and lessens the likelihood of the surgeon becoming disorientated. The natural ostium of the sphenoid sinus should be identified and anterior face of the sphenoid widely opened.

The anterior face of the sphenoid needs to be taken as high as possible so that the roof of the sphenoid and the posterior ethmoids is continuous (Kuppersmith et al, 1997; Luxenberger et al, 1998; Chow and Stankiewicz, 1997). The sphenoid should be inspected and the optic nerve, carotid artery and pituitary fossa identified (Luxenberger et al, 1998; Chow and Stankiewicz, 1997). If there is significant disruption of the orbital apex or the lateral wall of the sphenoid, the identification of these basic structures can be difficult and image guidance may be helpful here.

The thick bone overlying the junction of the orbital apex and sphenoid sinus is known as the optic tubercle. This bone is normally too thick to flake off and an irrigated 15 degree angled diamond burr(Medtronic Xomed, Jacksonville, Florida, USA) is used to thin this bone down until it is almost transparent (Luxenberger et al, 1998; Chow and Stankiewicz, 1997). A blunt Free's elevator is pushed through the lamina papyracea 1.5 cm anterior to the junction of the posterior ethmoids air cell(s) and the sphenoid. While performing, care should be taken to keep the orbital periosteum intact, otherwise prolapsed of the orbital fat can severely obstruct the dissection of the optic nerve. The bone of the posterior orbital apex is flaxed off the underlying orbital periosteum (Luxenberger et al, 1998; Chow and Stankiewicz, 1997).

The bone over the optic canal is approached once the bone over the orbital apex is removed. This bone is usually quite thin and in majority of the cases can simply be flaked off the underlying nerve (Fig 26). Sometimes, the bone over the nerve can be too thick and will need to be thinned with diamond burr prior to removal. When the bone is thin enough to be flaked off the underlying nerve, suitable instruments like the Beale's elevator and the House curette, both from the ear tray should be used.

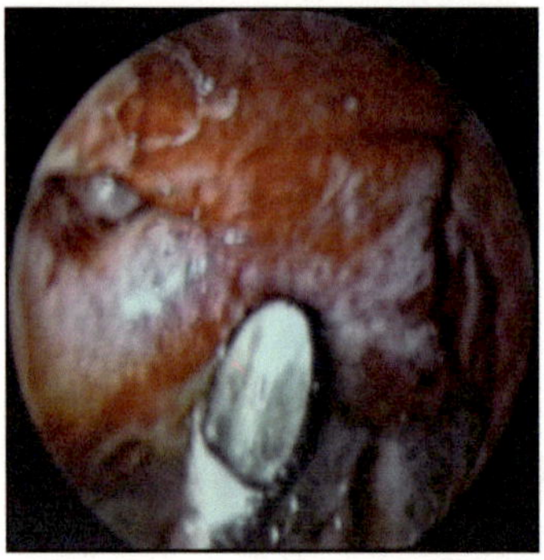

Fig. 26. A 45 degree endoscopic view showing bone being cleared off the optic canal with underlying optic nerve sheath clearly visible in a patient with traumatic optic neuropathy

When all the bone has been cleared off the optic canal and underlying optic nerve sheath is clearly visible, the sheath should be incised (Luxenberger et al, 1998; Chow and Stankiewicz, 1997). The location of the ophthalmic artery should be noted for it usually runs in the posteriorinferior quadrant of the nerve. Occassionally, this artery can migrate around the lower edge of the nerve and potentially into the surgical field (Steinsapir et al, 2002). However, if the nerve is incised in the upper medial quadrant, the risk to this artery should be minimal(Luxenberger et al, 1998; Chow et al, 1995). A sharp sickle knife is used to incise the sheath of the optic nerve. Usually the swollen nerve is under pressure and the sheath splits as it is incised and nerve will protrude through the incision.. The incision is continued onto the orbital periosteum of the posterior orbital apex with resultant protrusion of orbital fat. The orbital fat covering this area of the medial rectus muscle is thin and care should be taken to avoid injuring this muscle (Fig 27). No packs are placed on the nerve or in the sinuses.

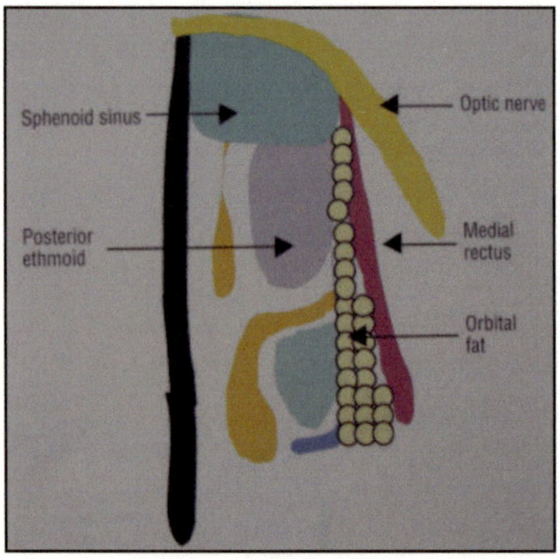

Fig. 27. A diagrammatic axial section of the paranasal sinuses and the orbit showing the anatomical relationship of the medial rectus muscle to fat and periorbita

It is vital to monitor the vision post-operatively quarter-hourly for one hour and then hourly for 4 hours. The immediate or early results of decompression are frequently extremely gratifying. The patient should be instructed not to blow their nose or sniffle sneezes for 4 days to avoid surgical emphysema.

Tips for successful surgery

Optic nerve decompression is a highly complex procedure and should be undertaken by endoscopic sinus surgeon with significant experience and skill. Potential injury to the skull base with a resultant CSF leak may occur and in addition an associated injury to the internal carotid artery may be present. Injudicious manipulation of bony fragments may have catastrophic consequences for the patient. A trial of medical therapy should be advocated before surgery is contemplated unless there is an obvious bony fragment impinging on the optic nerve. Literature review suggests that patients should be operated upon if medical therapy fails to improve the vision within 24 to 48 hours. Significant delays would seem to lessen the potential for success of the surgery. Great care should be considered in exposing the optic nerve especially when flaking the bone from the nerve. Injudicious use of inappropriate instruments has the potential to worsen the vision. In the hands of an experienced endoscopic sinus surgeon, this procedure is relatively safe with low morbidity and has the potential to improve and in some cases restore lost vision, especially after blunt trauma.

4. Endoscopic applications to the pterygopalatine and infratemporal fossa for resection of benign pathological lesions

The most common benign tumor involving the pterygo-palatine and infra-temporal fossa is the juvenile angiofibroma(Fig 28). These tumors originate in the region of spheno-palatine foramen and expand into pterygo-palatine fossa. Large tumors may extend into infra-temporal fossa and usually have a large intranasal component that may extend into nearby sinuses especially the sphenoid sinus. Other benign tumors in this region are inverting papilloma extending from the nasal cavity or rare tumors arising from the nerve sheath (schwannomas)(Fig 29), cartilage or muscle. Meningoceles extending into this area from the middle cranial fossa are rare.

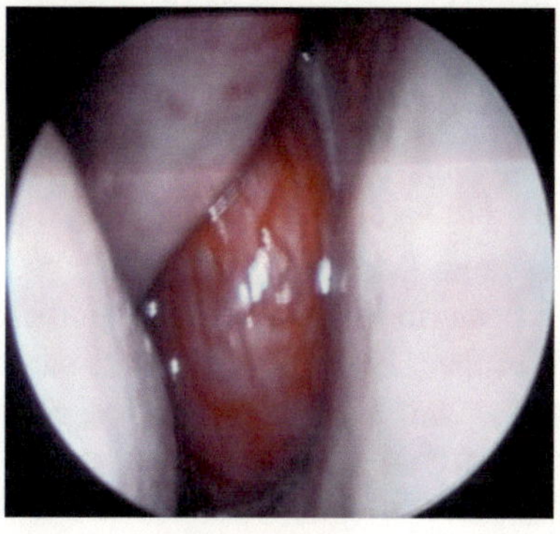

Fig. 28. Endoscopic view of a right juvenile angiofibroma in a teenage male presenting with recurrent epistaxis.

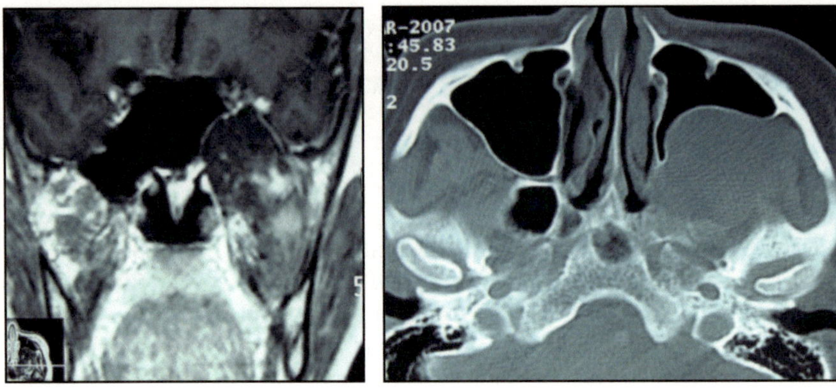

(a) (b)

Fig. 29. A coronal(a) and axial(b) MRI view of the paranasal sinuses showing a left maxillary nerve schwanomma

4.1 Surgical technique for endoscopic modified medial maxillectomy

The nasal cavity is prepared by placing cocaine and adrenaline-soaked neuropatties in the nasal cavity. The lateral nasal wall and septum are infiltrated with 2% lidocaine and 1:80,000 adrenaline. Using 2 ml of lidocaine and adrenaline, a pterygo-palatine fossa block is placed via the greater palatine canal which greatly helps to reduce vascularity during dissection of medial wall of the maxilla and pterygo-palatine fossa.

The initial step in endoscopic modified medial maxillectomy is to remove the uncinate process and perform a large middle meatal antrostomy. Moreover, the maxillary antrum is enlarged posteriorly up to posterior wall of maxillary sinus. This provides visualization of the medial orbital wall and aids in removal of residual medial maxilla without endangering the orbit. Majority of tumors of maxillary sinus and pterygo-palatine fossa will involve the posterior ethmoids and sphenoid. The bulla ethmoidalis is removed and a posterior ethmoidectomy and sphenoidotomy are performed. The inferior turbinate is medialized and its posterior two-thirds removed. A right angled phako-knife is used to make mucosal incisions from just below the orbit, through the anterior one third of the inferior turbinate onto the floor of the nasal cavity. The incision is continued along the floor of the nose to the posterior region of the inferior turbinate and on to the maxillary sinus. A sharp chisel is used to cut the bone under the mucosal incisions

If the bone forming the medial maxillary wall is mobilized, the naso-lacrimal duct will tether the bone anteriorly and the duct will be visualized which can be transected with a scalpel (Fig 30). Subsequently, a DCR spear knife (Metronic Xomed) is used to open the lower half of the sac, creating an anterior and posterior flaps and rolling these out (Wormald et al, 2003; Wormald & van Hasselt, 2003; Vrabac, 1994). This prevents stenosis of the sac postoperatively (Wormald et al, 2003; Wormald & van Hasselt, 2003). The edges of the resected maxilla are cleaned with micro-debrider (Metronic Xomed). Using a 70 degree endoscope the entire maxillary sinus can be visualized including the anterior wall and floor. The tumor can now be removed from the maxillary sinus under direct vision. A canine fossa puncture can be performed, if additional access is required which can be useful to access areas within the sinus that may otherwise be difficult to access. Malleable suction dissector's are useful because these instruments can be bent to the required angle for dissection in difficult areas like the anterior wall or antero-lateral region of the lateral wall of maxillary sinus.

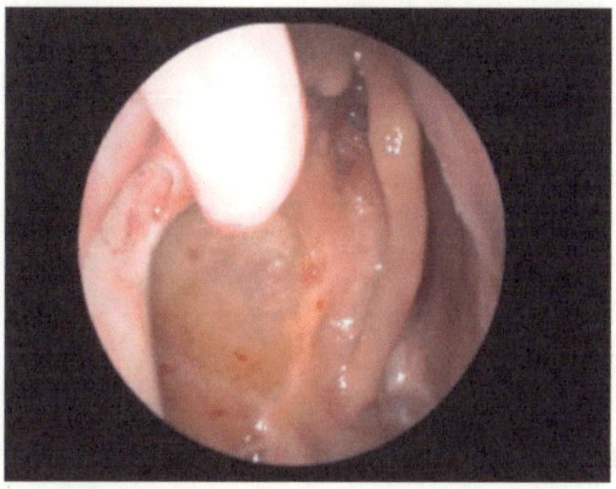

Fig. 30. A 30- degree endoscopic view showing evidence of right modified medial maxillectomy performed for an inverted papilloma.

4.2 Exposure of the pterygo-palatine fossa

Exposure of the pterygo-palatine fossa via a wide medial maxillary antrostomy is necessary for tumors the occupy the ptergo-palatine fossa and extending into the infra-temporal fossa. The mucosa from the posterior wall of the maxillary sinus is elevated and preserved and the exposed bone removed to access the pterygo-palatine fossa. A 45 degree through-bitting Blakesley forceps is used to remove the bone anterior to the spheno-palatine artery and continued to the posterior wall of the maxillary sinus exposing the contents of the pterygo-palatine fossa. Traction is vital for tumors that extend into the infra-temporal fossa because it allows the surgeon to identify the areas of attachment of the tumor to the surrounding tissues and to dissect these free with suction dissector. Thus the entire tumor can be mobilized and its pedicle identified.

Tumors that extend into the infra-temporal fossa will usually be closely associated with the maxillary nerve in the pterygo-palatine fossa. This nerve should be identified both distally and proximally early in the dissection and preserved. Suction dissection instruments are used to separate the nerve from the tumor. Fibrous tissue is easily divided with endoscopic soft tissue scissors.

Feeding blood vessels can either be caurterized with suction bipolar diathermy forceps or clipped and cut. Once the tumor is removed, the tumor bed can be closely inspected to ensure no tumor remnant remains. Once hemostasis is achieved with suction bipolar forceps, the preserved mucosa from the posterior wall of the maxillary sinus is replaced. Surgicel can be placed in the cavity if required. Finally, ensure that the lacrimal sac is adequately exposed to prevent postoperative stenosis and epiphora. The incidence of postoperative epiphora has been described as high as 30% (Bolger et al, 1992).

Endoscopic two-surgeon technique for tumors of the pterygo-palatine and infra-temporal fossa

The key to successful endoscopic removal of large tumors in this region is having two surgeons operating at the same time. This can be achieved by providing access to the tumor bed for the second surgeon through the septum from the opposite nasal cavity. A hemi-transfixation(Freer's) incision is made on the opposite site of tumor. Using standard septoplasty techniques, the mucosa is elevated off the cartilage of the septum which is preserved but most of posterior bony septum is resected. A horizontal incision is made in the opposite septal mucosa to allow instruments placed through the opposite nostril and into the Freer's incision to cross the septum and access the tumor on the contra-lateral side of the nose.

During tumor removal, the second surgeon can provide significant traction on the tumor and when the feeding vessel from the maxillary artery is cut, large volume suction in the field can allow the suction bipolar cautery to be used to identify and cauterize the large bleeding vessel.

4.3 Juvenile angiofibroma with pterygo-palatine and infra-temporal fossa extension

Angiofibromas that significantly extend into pterygopa-latine fossa can be removed after endonasal endoscopic medial maxillectomy (Kennedy et al, 1990) and embolization within the preceding 24 hours. This reduces the vascularity of the tumor and allows dissection around the tumor without major hemorrhage. The second surgeon can keep the surgical field clear using a large suction in the area of dissection while the other surgeon holds the telescope and suction dissection instrument.

4.4 Schwannoma involving the pterygo-palatine and infra-temporal fossa

Endoscoopic medial maxillectomy also provides access to other tumors that may involve the pterygo-palatine and infra-temporal fossa. Schwannoma of the maxillary nerve involves the entire ptrygo-palatine fossa and extends significantly into the infra-temporal fossa. Endoscopic medial maxillectomy allows access to the entire posterior wall of the maxillary sinus and after its removal, to the tumor.

4.5 Post-operative care

Douching of the nose with saline is started immediately postoperatively. Local and systemic antibiotics and corticosteroids are usually helpful. Crusting will usually continue for a few weeks until the cavity epithelializers but has not proved to be problematic in the long run. Benign tumors do not usually need any adjuvant treatment but malignant tumors may require postoperative radiotherapy.

5. Endoscopic resection of benign pathological lesions of paranasal sinuses

5.1 Mucoceles

Mucocele is a chronic, expansile, benign cystic lesion limited by the mucosa of the paranasal sinus, with thick, translucent mucous secretions (Fig 31). The most common are the frontoethmoidal mucoceles which presents with headaches and orbital symptoms. The expansile character of the mucocele promotes slow erosion of the adjacent bone via compression and consequent bone absorption. This disease is usually secondary to obstruction to sinus drainage, leading to stagnation of the secretion within the cavity. The predisposing factors can be fractures, mucosal edema, polyps, tumors, surgical trauma and chronic sinusitis. Mucoceles are classified according to the sinus of origin. The frontal sinus being the most common site, followed by the ethmoid, maxillary and sphenoid sinuses.

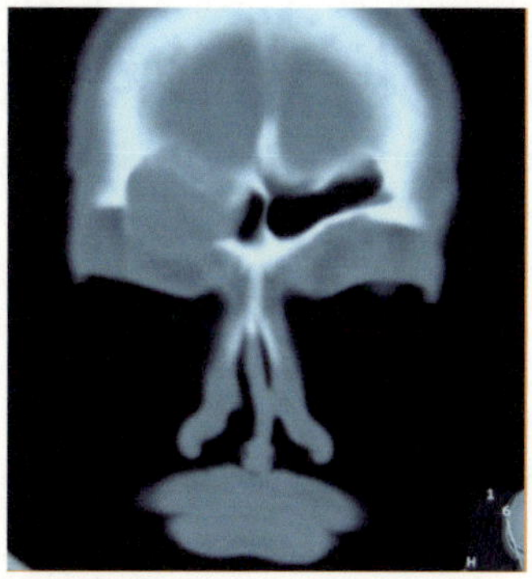

Fig. 31. Coronal CT imaging of the right frontal sinus with evidence of a right mucocele showing expansile erosion of right orbital floor with lateral extension

Fronto-ethmoidal sphenoidal and the rare maxillary sinus mucoceles are ideal cases for endoscopic approach provided wide marsupilization can be achieved (Hehar & Jones, 1997). Mucoceles accessible with the endoscope should be opened as widely as possible using through-cutting forceps in order to minimize the amount of scar tissue that forms around the edges and which might lead to recurrence. Coronal CT scan is helpful to show whether the lesion can be approached via the nasal cavity and whether it is unilocular or multilocular. In the frontal sinus, a small mucocele may be drained via the endoscopic approach (Fig 32) but mucoceles with lateral extension may be difficult to access via the nose. Therefore, an external and endoscopic approach can be usefully combined, preserving lateral support of the frontal recess and avoiding a stent.

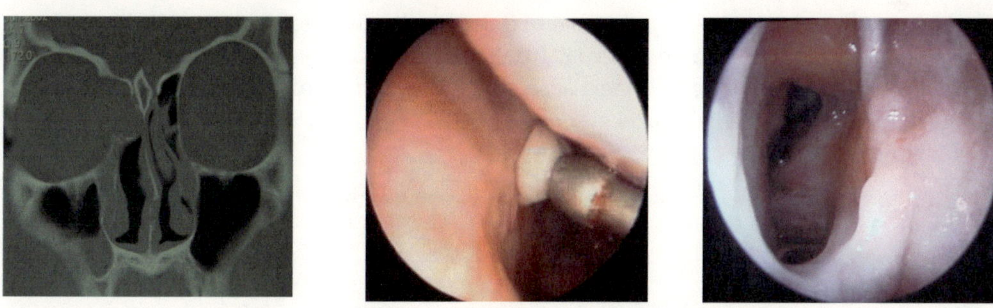

Fig. 32. Coronal CT imaging showing a right iatrogenic frontoethmoid mucocele and intraoperative endoscopic drainage and follow up a 3 months post surgery showing a patent frontal sinustomy in an adult presenting with frequent right headaches and heavy eyes

Preoperative evaluation of patients with frontal mucoceles should include careful evaluation of the lesion relative to the skull base. Endoscopic decompression is probably the best initial therapy for these lesions. It is particularly true of mucoceles that have eroded the posterior table of the frontal sinus and become adherent to the dura.An uncinectomy is performed with an axillary flap as advocated by Wormald PJ(2005). Often in surgery of these lesions, the skull base is identified within the posterior ethmoids and then followed anteriorly until the bone of the lesion is identified. The mucosal covered mass at the frontal recess area is opened with Blackesley's straight forceps (Stortz, Germany). As the lesion is approached or entered, mucoid or mucopurulent material is sucked out. The frontal sinustomy is enlarged upto about 2cm and the edges of exposed mucosa marsupilized. It is essential to remove all osteitic intersinus septa if recurrence of disease is to be avoided. If the bony margins are not flushed with the surrounding wall, narrowing of the opening, due to scarring and closure may occur (Kennedy et al, 1989). Once a frontal and/or ethmoid mucocele has been marsupilized, the expanded "shell" of bone that remains can be pushed manually to correct any bony swelling that may cause a cosmetic defect or displacement of the orbit intraoperatively. Sometimes a posteriorly placed mucocele may leave the orbit displaced even after marsupilization and then the orbit may need to be decompressed by removing its lateral wall (Conboy & Jones, 2003).

The majority of mucocels can be marsupilized endoscopically with minimal morbidity and long-term results as compared to other techniques. The wider the mococele is marsupilized, the better the result. Majority of mucoceles can be marsupilized well with the endoscope except those lying in the lateral aspect of the frontal sinus, those that are secondary to malignancy(require an en-bloc and a craniofacial resection) and those secondary to pathology like Paget disease of fibrous dysplasia (Kennedy et al, 1989; Beasley & Jones, 1995).

In the postoperative period, the mucosal lining the mucocele cavity may undergo significant hypertrophy and secretions may accumulate, necessitating suction from time to time. However, mucociliary clearance becomes reestablished, typically in a few weeks and the mucosal hypertrophy resolves over time (Kennedy et al, 1989). Hospitalization usually is less than 24 hours. As with other endoscopic sinus surgery, meticulous postoperative care is essential.

Relative contraindications for endoscopic marsupilization

- Abnormally thick bone (Paget's disease (Fig 33), fibrous dysplasia (Fig 34)).
- Revision surgery where an external fronto-ethmoidectomy was performed and if the recurrence is located lateral to area accessible via a median drainage procedure
- A laterally placed frontal mucocele
- Malignancy associated with a mucocele

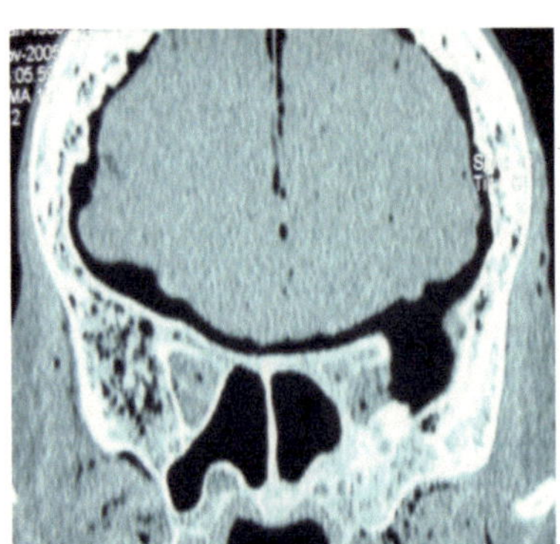

Fig. 33. A coronal CT scan view of paranasal sinuses and skull showing evidence of Pagets disease

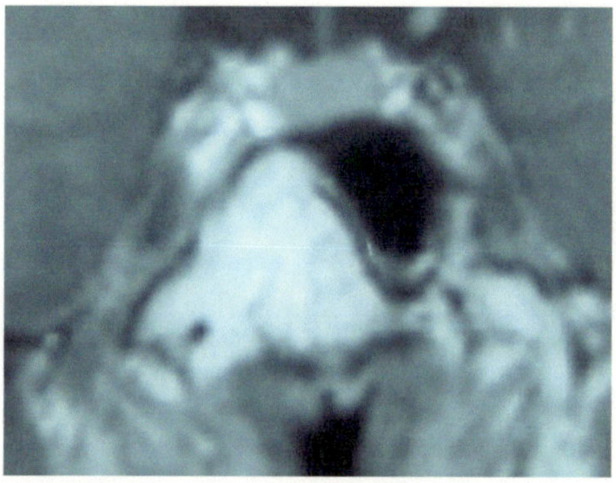

Fig. 34. A coronal CT scan of the paranasal sinuses showing evidence of fibrous dysplasia involving the sphenoid sinus

6. Endoscopic applications to the sellar, parasellar and clival for resection of benign pathological lesions

6.1 Endoscopic pituitary micro-adenoma and macro-adenoma surgery

6.1.1 The various approaches to the pituitary include

- Trans-septal, trans-sphenoidal
- Trans-nasal
- Transcolumellar approach(Fig 35)
- Via an external ethmoidectomy approach
- Through the upper buccal sulcus of the mouth and then trans-septal, trans-sphenoidal
- Via a craniotomy eg an anterolateral or a frontal approach

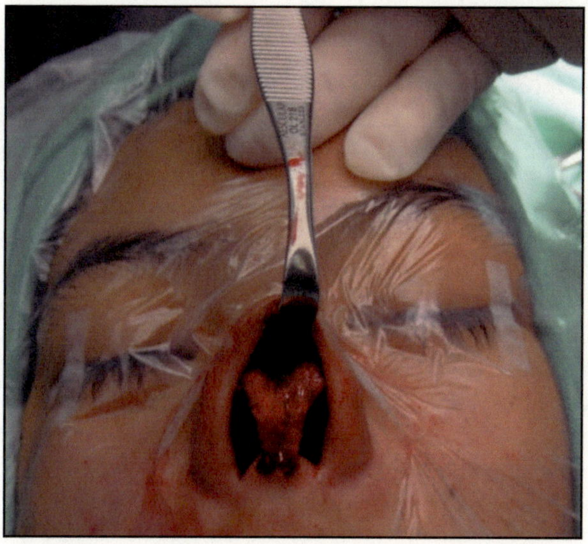

Fig. 35. A picture of transcolumella approach as an access route to the pituitary

6.1.2 Indications

Pituitary tumors occur in 9 in 10,000 pupulation and comprise 10% of intracranial tumors. The commonest pituitary tumors in patients under 35 years secrete prolactin and adrenocorticotropin whereas after 35 to 50 years they generally secrete growth hormone. In the latter, non-secreting tumors are more common. Symptoms can be caused by pressure on the anterior pituitary and hypo-pituitarism or by extra-sellar growth that can produce headaches, pressure on the optic chiasma or brain (Fig 36). Surgery is usually the treatment of choice. Surgery is the first-line treatment in acromegaly, where up to 90% of micro-adenomas are cured but the outcome is not as good as in large tumors.

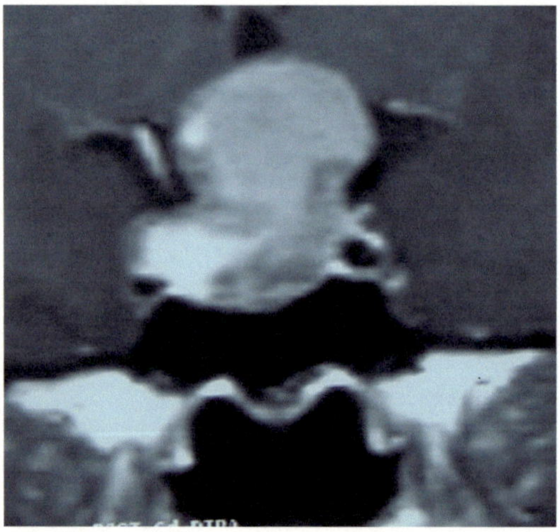

Fig. 36. A coronal MRI of the paranasal sinuses showing a suprasellar extension of a pituitary adenoma presenting with headaches and visual symptoms

Surgery for pituitary disease must be based on an assessment of the patient by a multidisciplinary team (Gendeh, 2006). The medical management of many pituitary tumors has reduced the frequency of the need for surgery in many patients. Medical management is rarely indicated in tumors that extend into the supra-sellar region and extending above the diaphragma sellae.

The endoscope gives excellent visibility within the sphenoid sinus and with a 45 degree endoscope it is possible to see more detail within the pituitary fossa than with the microscope. The advantages of the trans-nasal, trans-septal or lower buccal approach is that it avoids an external scar and by removing the posterior part of the septum, vomer and anterior wall of sphenoid, this approach allows wide access. In the endoscopic trans-nasal technique, mucosal preservation is an added advantage and allows the surgeon to work bimanually if necessary. The advantage of the two nostril technique is when there is moderate or severe bleeding, it can be controlled more readily. An external ethmoidectomy approach produces a scar and has the potential to cause stenosis of the frontal recess. Pituitary surgery has been routinely been performed with endoscopic endonasal approach at our referral center since 1990. (Gendeh, 2010)

6.1.3 Surgical anatomy

The vomer consistently joins the sphenoid in the mid-line and this is a very reliable landmark. The sphenoid inter-sinus septum is often asymmetric(more than 75%) and its essential to review the CT scans pre-operatively. The degree of pneumatization of the sphenoid sinus also varies greatly (Lang, 1989). A chonchal sinus is small and confined to the anterior aspect of the sphenoid in 5% of cases. A pre-sellar sinus extends to the coronal plane level with the anterior wall of the sphenoid in 28% of cases. In 67% of cases it is sellar type(Fig 37). Agenesis of the sphenoid sinus occurs in 0.7% of patients. The carotid artery bulges into its lateral wall and it can be dehiscent in up to 30% of patients. Axillary imaging cuts complement coronal sections and sagittal reconstruction helps. The natural sphenoid sinus is relatively high in the posterior wall of the sphenoid and is often placed at the level of the superior turbinate which may be readily visible after gentle lateralization of the middle turbinate. The bony anterior wall of the sphenoid sinus is often thin or deficient 1 to 1.5 cm above the posterior choana. The lateral wall of the sphenoid sinus has indentations from various structures (Fig 38):

- The optic nerve can indent its surface in the upper third
- The maxillary nerve can form an almost horizontal semicircular intrusion that may be mistaken for optic nerve in its medial third
- The degree of pneumatization of the sinus varies and influences how prominent structures are in its lateral wall. Pneumatization can extend to the clivus, the lesser wing and the root of the pterygoid process).
- The vidian nerve can bulge into its floor

1. Choncal (5%)
   - Common in children below 12 years
   - Area below sella is complete block of bone
2. Presellar (28%)
   - Posterior limit of air cavity is perpendicular to sella
3. Sellar (67%)
   - Commonest,
   - Air cavity extended into body of sphenoid below sella and may extend as posterior as clivus

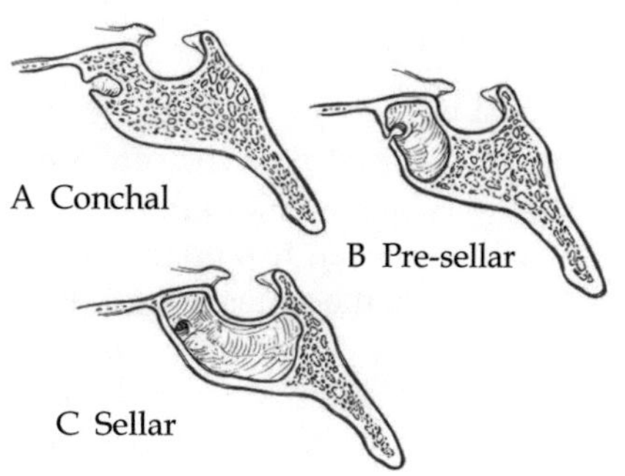

Fig. 37. Types of sphenoid sinus pneumatization

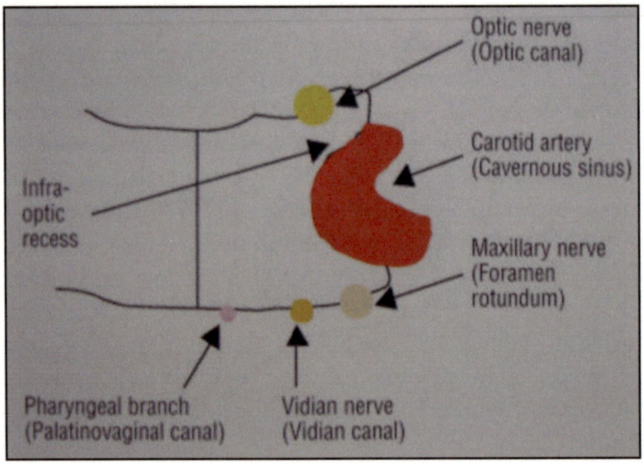

Fig. 38. A diagrammatic coronal section of the sphenoid sinus showing the anatomical indentaions of vital structures in its roof, lateral wall and floor.

6.1.4 Useful instruments

- Hajek-Koffler punch (Stortz, Germany) to remove thick bone. The rotating sleeve allows its jaws to be pointed in any direction and for the handle to be in a comfortable position for the operator
- A Kerrison punch (Stortz, Germany) allows fine controlled removal of small segments of bone and the slight reversed angle of its jaws help to remove the back of the vomer
- A long-shanked drill with a coarse diamond (Metronic Xomed) to remove any bone in the roof of the sphenoid bone in a controlled way
- A computer guided systems

6.1.5 Surgical technique

The trans-nasal endoscopic approach commences by making a sphenoidotomy on the side of the tumor or when it is in the midline opening, the side where the sinus is larger. The sphenoidotomy is opened up to the level of the skull base using a sphenoid punch. Suction diathermy will be needed to stop the bleeding from the posterior branch of spheno-palatine artery when opening the sphenoidotomy inferiorly. Any vomerine spur should be removed. After careful CT examination and endoscopically inspecting the sphenoid sinus to check on the proximity of the lateral structures, the lateral aspect of the anterior wall can be removed if necessary. A Kerrison antrum punch (Stortz, Germany) is useful for performing this as its small diameter means that the bone can be removed in small pieces with good visibility. If more space is required across the midline, the vomer can be fractured across or it can be incised 1cm in front of the sphenoid and removed. The vomer can be very thick where it joins the sphenoid but it rarely needs drilling (Fig 39). The pituitary often bulges into the roof of the sphenoid and the bone may be very thin (Fig 40). If the bone is thick, a course diamond burr (Metronic Xomed) should be used to thin it. A diathermy point is useful to open the dura by making a cross-shaped incision through it. A 45 degree endoscope gives excellent visibility and helps to avoid going through the diaphragm sellae. A Hajek punch (Stortz, Germany) helps to remove the bone over the pituitary. The tumor is often grey in colour, but occasional it can be vascular and ooze moderately. The pituitary fossa can be closed at the end of the procedure with raised naso-septal flap placed onto the bony defect. If there is a CSF leak, in addition an underlay duragen(collagen matrix graft) is placed before a naso-septal flap is placed as overlay flap and secured in position by Tisseel and gel-foam over it.

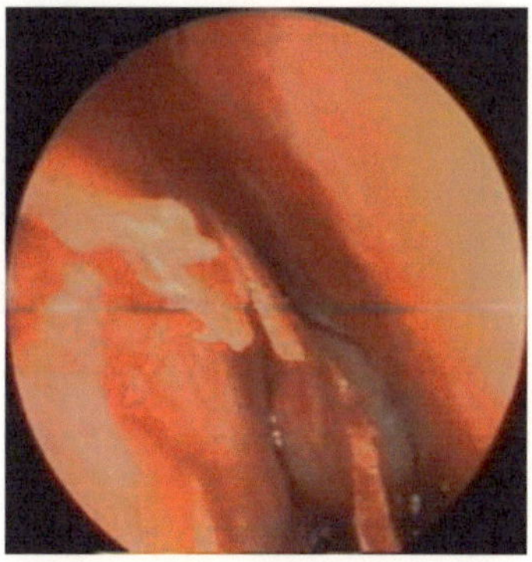

Fig. 39. Intraoperative endoscopic view showing a transseptal transsphenoidal approach to pituitary adenoma exposing the sphenoid rostrum

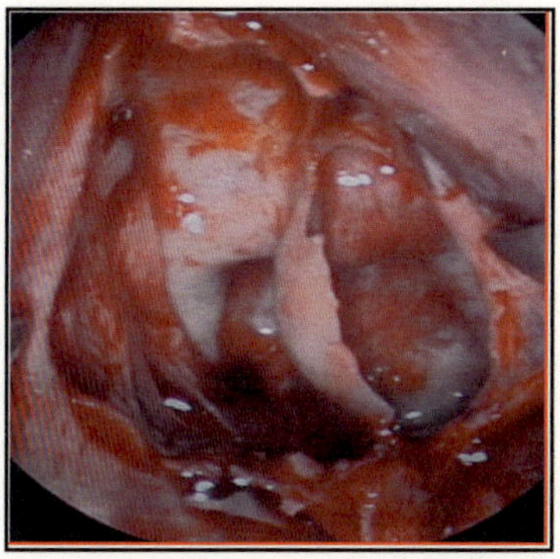

Fig. 40. A 45 degree endoscopic view of exposed sphenoid sinus showing a intersinus septum and an enlarged sella

It is possible to approach the pituitary via a limited sphenoidotomy, although it reduces access and visibility. It may be useful to trim the middle turbinate on one side for better access and visibility utilizing a four hand technique.

7. Endoscopic repair of skull base CSF fistula

CSF leak results from a breach in the dura, which may be spontaneous, secondary to a fracture, related to a surgical trauma or associated with pathology of the skull base and/or secondary to a high-pressure system (Fig 41).

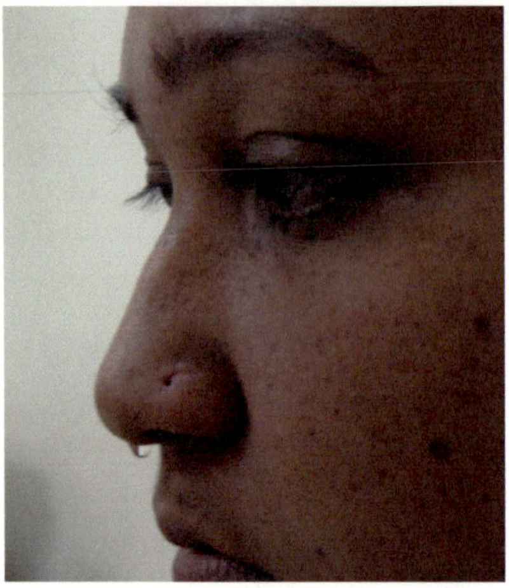

Fig. 41. Picture of an adult obese female presenting with unilateral clear watery spontaneous CSF rhinorrhoea on exertion

7.1 Indications

The main indications for repairing a CSF leak is its association with a 10% risk per year of developing meningitis (Gendeh et al, 1998). Those who have a leak from a fracture of the anterior skull base repaired still have a slightly increased risk of developing meningitis in the future but this is less than those whose leak stops spontaneously. Therefore, active leaks should probably be repaired at any stage.

7.2 Surgical anatomy

The skull base is made up anteriorly of the posterior wall of the frontal sinus, which is a thick frontal bone that extends posteriorly to form roof of ethmoid sinuses(fovea ethmoidalis) on either side of the cribriform plate. The cribriform plate joins the fovea through the lateral lamella and can be almost non-existent when the cribriform plate and fovea ethmoidalis are on the same plane or it can form the thin vertical bone connecting them, depending on how far the cribriform plate dips into the nose (Fig 42). Posteriorly, the sphenoid sinus and posterior ethmoidal air cells form the inferior relationship of the skull base.

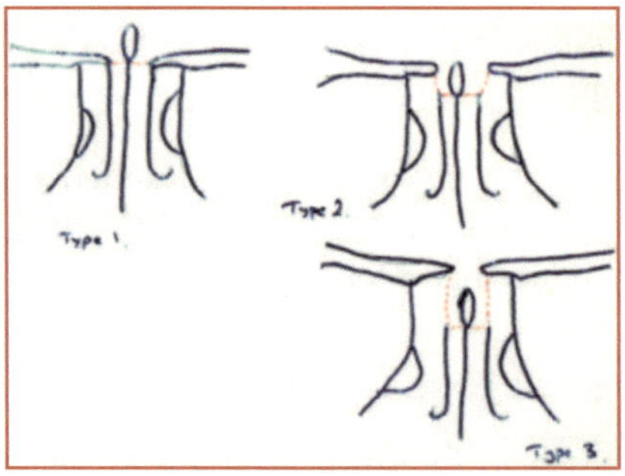

Fig. 42. Keros classification of the anatomy of the cribriform plate which may lie at different level in relation to the anterior skull base

The commonest site of a spontaneous CSF leak is the area of the cribriform plate where dura around the olfactory nerves appears to have extended through the cribriform plate and ruptured (Fig 43). The next most commonest leak is from a very well-pneumatized sphenoid sinus (Fig 44). A high-pressure system may be a contributing factor in these cases and a shunt or venrticulostomy may be required.

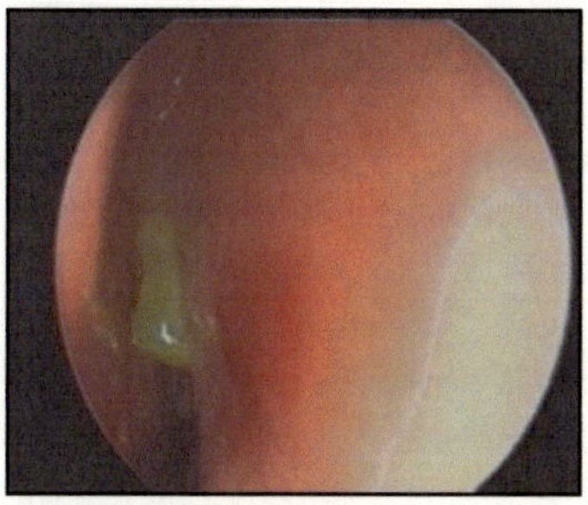

Fig. 43. Intraoperative endoscopic view showing arachnoid granulations arising from the left cribriform area in an obese female presenting with spontaneous cerebro-spina fluid rhinorrhea

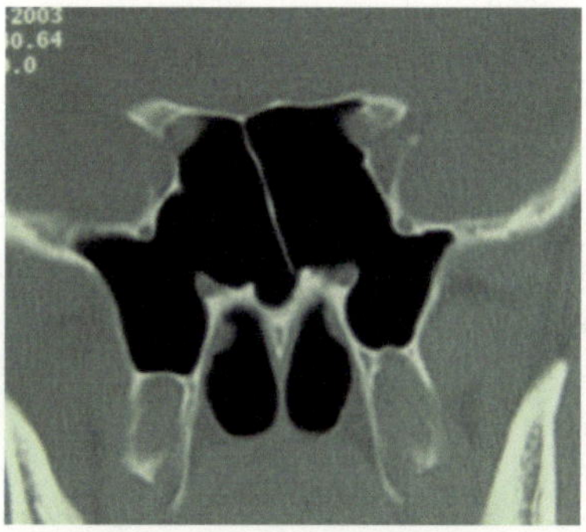

Fig. 44. A coronal CT scan showing a well pneumatized sphenoid sinus

Iatrogenic CSF leaks are often found around the lamina lateralis (the vertical thin bone joining the cribriform plate to the fovea ethmoidalis) near the anterior ethmoidal artery. Post neurosurgical procedure leaks most commonly follow pituitary surgery, come from the posterior wall of frontal sinus when it has not been cranialized and more likely if a peri-cranial flap has not been used to repair any dural defect.

7.3 Diagnosis

- It is vital to localize the site of a leak (Marshall et al, 2001)
- Fluid collected should be tested for immune-fixation of beta-2-transferrin
- Rule out any high- pressure system leak
- Successful closure depends on localizing the exact site of the fistula

It is essential to confirm the diagnosis with immune-fixation of beta-2-transferrin which is extremely specific and sensitive test (Eljamel, 1993). Unilateral autonomic rhinitis is unusual but can mimic CSF rhinorrhea.

Site of any defect should be defined using high-resolution coronal CT (Lloyd et al, 1994). If CT fails to define the site of the defect, T2-weighted MRI may help which has superseded CT cisternography (Stafford et al, 1996). In a few post-trauma patients the site of leak is uncertain or it could be that there is more than one leak. In dural defects less than 15mm, the 'bath plug' technique is encouraged which consists of introducing a fat plug with vicryl suture into the intra-dural space (Wormald & McDonough, 1997) It is believed that this technique would prevent high pressure from pushing the graft away from the defect (Gendeh et al, 2002). The fat pug can be harvested from the ear lobule. A 4 0 vicryl suture is knotted through one end of the fat plug and the suture is passed down the length of the fat plug. A free mucosal graft about 3 x 3 cm is harvested anterior to the middle turbinate from the contralateral lateral nasal wall. The fat plug is placed below the defect and the malleable frontal sinus probe (Metronic Xomed, Jacksonville, Florida, USA) is used gently to introduce the fat plug through the defect (Wormald and McDonough, 1997). Once the fat plug has been safely introduced through the defect, the plug is stabilized with the probe and the vicryl suture is gently pulled. The seal is tested by placing the patient head down and asking the anaesthetist to perform a forced-inspiration maneuver. No Fluorescein-stained CSF should be seen. The patient is placed head-up (15 degrees) and the free mucosal graft is slid up the vicryl suture until it covers the defect (Fig 45). Ensure that the graft is correctly orientated with the mucosal surface facing the nasal cavity. Fibrin glue is applied and the vicryl suture cut. Gelfoam is placed over the free mucosal graft and fibrin glue is reapplied. No other nasal packing is used.

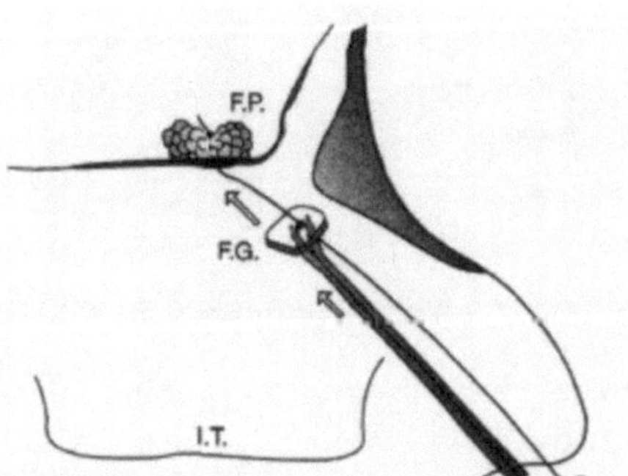

Fig. 45. A diagrammatic sagittal section of the nose showing the a free mucosal graft being slid up the vicry suture to cover the protruding fat plug and skull base defect. Adapted with permission from Wormald and McDonough. Americal J Rhinol 2003; 17:299-305

A diagnostic or pre-operative sodium fluorescein lumbar puncture will help define the source of leak(Fig 46 a). It is vital to ensure that there is a free flow of CSF before proceeding to inject any sodium fluorescein. The patient was skin tested with 2% sodium flourescein eye drops one day before surgery. A lumbar drain was inserted on the day of surgery and intrathecal sodium fluorescein 10%(0.1% of sodium flourescein is diluted with 10ml of withdrawn CSF) was given in a slow bolus over 10 minutes to identify site of fistula (Gendeh et al, 2005). The ideal time for the sodium fluorescein to be injected is one hour beforehand. It is a great help to place the patient in a 10 degree head-down position. The fluid will appear bright yellow, unless a blue filter is used when it appears fluorescent green (Fig 46 b). The systemic clearance of fluorescein is essentially complete by 48 to 72 hours from the patient's body.

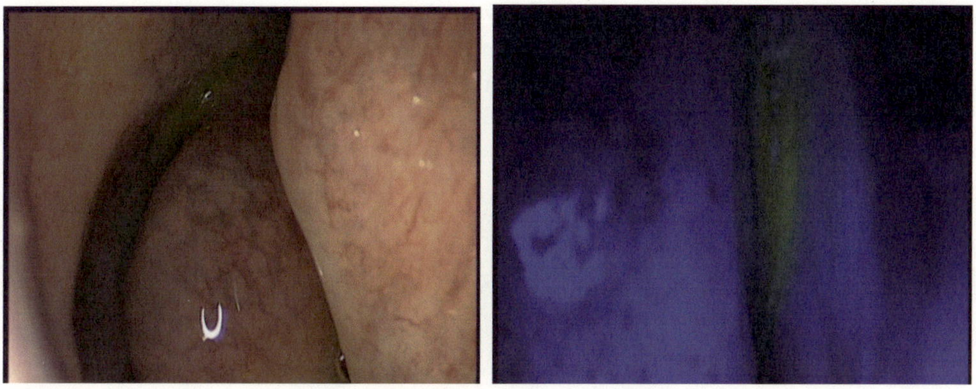

(a) (b)

Fig. 46. A 30 degrees endoscopic view showing a spontaneous CSF leak from the anterior cribriform plate using intrathecal sodium fluorescein(a) and highlighted using blue blue filter(b) in the same patient

The adverse reactions of intrathecal fluorescein administration are nausea, vomiting, gastrointestinal distress, headache, syncome and hypotention. Cardiac arrest, basilar artery ischaemia, severe shock, convultions, thrombophlebitis at the injection site and rare cases of death have been reported.

7.4 Surgical technique

Initially the repair of CSF fistula involved the use of multi-layered barrier comprised of free tissue grafts harvested from the nasal perichondrium or temporalis fascia. On top of the on lay graft, an abdominal fat graft was used as a bolster and a biological dressing. A fibrin sealant was applied to help fixate the fat graft. Sponge packing (Merocel tampons) were placed intra-nasally to support the fat graft and provide some compression.

We adopted the use of collagen matrix graft (duragen, Intra Life Sciences, USA), which was easy to maneuver, is soft and pliable, thus decreasing the risk of injuring any critical structures as we tuck the graft to overlap the surrounding dural edges of the defect. Duragen is an absorbable and sutureless collagen onlay indicated as dura substitute for the repair of dura mater. We eliminated the routine use of lumbar drains and reserved them for high-risk situations or secondary repairs.

The latest intervention to decrease CSF leaks employs vascularized mucosal flaps which hastens the healing process, especially in patients with prior radiation therapy and make patients more suitable for early postoperative radiation therapy. Hadad and Bassagasteguy from Argentina developed the nasoseptal flap, supplied by the posterior nasoseptal arteries which are branches of the posterior nasal artery. A mucoperichondrial/mucoperiosteal flap pedicle on the posterior nasal arteries provides a long flap that has a wide arc of rotation and a potential for area of coverage that is superior to any other flap previously described(Fig 47). The flap may be harvested to cover the entire anterior skull base from the frontal sinus to the sella or cover a clival defect from the sella to second cervical vertebra (C2). Use of this flap has to be anticipated in advance, since a posterior septectomy and a wide large slphenoidotomy removes the vascular pedicle. This flap is very reliable and is typically positioned over a fascial graft or fat graft and held in place with fibrin glue and a balloon catheter. We have not observed any significant donor site morbidity with the use of this flap and the septum becomes remucosalized within several months of surgery

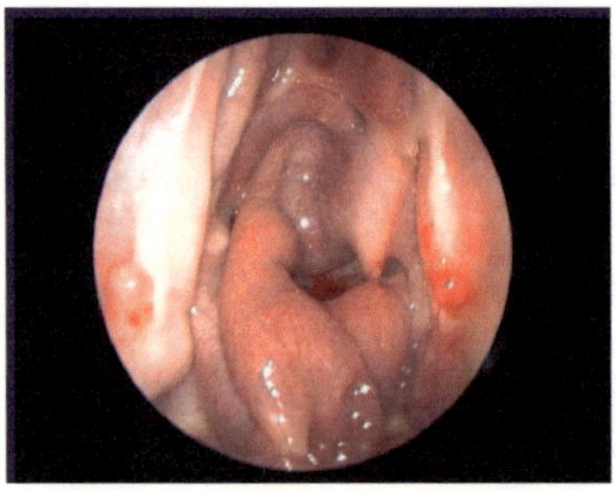

Fig. 47. Endoscopic view of a healed nasoseptal flap repair at 3 months post surgery for a pituitary macroadenoma with evidence of CSF fistula

8. Recent advances in technology and its application to anterior and ventral skull base lesions

There is an ongoing revolution in multiple surgical specialties with the introduction of minimally invasive techniques. A natural extension of ESS has been the application of endoscopic techniques for the surgical treatment of pathologic conditions of the cranial base. This has been driven by the ongoing development of endoscopic technology increasing consumer demand. Furthermore, as the limits of ESS is tested, the possibilities for cranial base surgery are expanded. Truly, it is a maximally invasive endoscopic surgery than minimally invasive surgery.

The Expanded Endo-nasal Approach(EEA) to the ventral skull base provides endoscopic access from the frontal sinus to C2 in the sagittal plane and from the midline to the jugular foramen, internal acoustic canal(IAC) and lateral mass of C2 in the coronal plane (Fig 48). Potential advantages of the EEA not only include improved cosmesis but more importantly, the potential for much less neurovascular manipulation in well selected cases. In pediatric patients, preservation of facial skeleton avoids disruption of growth centers and development of facial asymmetry with further growth. In contrast to an intracranial approach, an endo-nasal approach avoids the need for any brain retraction and may result in less damage to brain tissue. Improved visualization and better access to difficult sites may result in improved oncological outcomes.

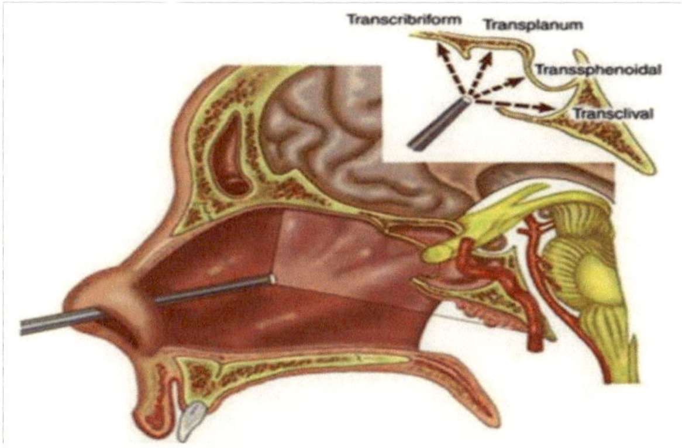

Slide Courtesy of the Pittsburgh Otolaryngologists & Neurosurgical team

Fig. 48. Expanded endonasal approaches to base of skull

Advances in cranial base surgery over the last two decades have only been possible with the collaboration of multiple surgical specialities (Kassam et al, 2007). This is more obvious with endoscopic skull base surgery. Rather than working sequentially as is often done with open approaches, surgeons from different speciality work together simultaneously as a team: one person maintaining a view with the endoscope and the other working bimanually to dissect the tissues. The benefits of the two team surgery include improved visualization, increased efficiency and the ability to deal with a crisis such as vascular injury. There is added value of having a 'co-pilot' for problem solving, avoiding complications and modulating enthusiasm.

The primary advantage of the endoscope compared to other methods is improved visualization which accounts for an increased access to difficult to reach areas and may facilitate complete tumor resection and avoidance of complications due to poor visualization. Other potential benefits of endoscopic surgery include improved cosmesis and decreased morbidity from tissue trauma and manipulation of vessels and nerves. The consequences of decreased morbidity are a faster recovery, shortened hospitalization and decreased cost of medical care (Gendeh, 2009).

Familiarity with endoscopic anatomy, proper instrumentation, an experienced surgical team and adherence to endoscopic surgical principles are essential ingrediants for avoiding severe complications. The basic principle of endoscopic cranial base surgery is internal debulking of tumor to allow extra-capsular dissection of tumor margin with early identification of neural and vascular structures. This principle is the same for open neurosurgical procedures and sharp dissection of tumor margins is performed without pulling on tumor. Adherence to these fundamental principles minimizes the risk of neural or vascular injury.

In the late 1970s and early 1980s, the combined effort between the Otolaryngologist and neurosurgeons worldwide, made significant strides in the surgical removal of tumors at the base of the skull and brain. These procedures were however disfiguring and painful for the patient. Furthermore, patients encountered long recovery periods and significant risk of complications because the procedures involved large incisions in the face and scalp and removal of parts of the skull to reach the abnormality at the cranial base.

In 1998, a group of Otolaryngologist and neurosurgeons at UPMC in Pittsburgh, USA initiated the first systemic approach to using the nose as a minimally invasive passageway to the brain. They began the extensive process of mapping anatomy and in collaboration with the medical device manufacturers, designed new instruments to make this idea a reality.

By 2000, the Pittsburgh team of doctors had developed the necessary tools and techniques to access tumors located inside the skull by the way of the nose known as EEA. In EEA, the surgeons use endoscopes with light source as well as other instruments especially designed, to treat various types of brain and spinal abnormality. Hence, today surgeons can take out baseball-sized growths without pulling on the brain or touching the normal tissue. This continued refinement of EEA now allows access to an expanded region of the brain, skull base and spine. The classification of endoscopic approaches to cranial base are listed in Table 3.

SAGGITAL PLANE

- Transfrontal
- Transcribriform
- Transplanum (Suprasellar/Subchiasmatic
- Transsphenoidal (Sellar/Medial transcavernous)
- Transclival
  - Posterior clinoid
  - Mid-clivus
  - Foramen magnum
- Transodontoid

CORONAL PLANE

- Transorbital
- Petrous apex (Medial transpetrous)
- Lateral transcavernous
- Transpterygoid
- Transpetrous
  - Superior
  - Inferior
- Transcondylar
- Parapharyngeal space

Snyderman CH.2007. Acquisation of surgical skills for endonasal skull base surgery: a training program. Laryngoscope 117(4): 699-705

Table 3. Classification of endoscopic approaches to cranial base

The collaborative effort has put the Otolaryngologist and the neurosurgeon to work closely via the nose using the two-nostril and four hand technique was first advocated by Prof. Dr Heinz Stammberger from Graz, Austria for endoscopic cranial base surgery.

Standardization of training and the adoption of modular, incremental training program are expected to facilitate the gradual training of endo-nasal surgeons in Otolaryngology and Neurosurgical disciplines. Stages of training are established for both surgical speciality based on level of technical difficulty, potential risk of vascular and neural injury and unfamiliar endoscopic anatomy. Mastery of each level is recommended before attempting procedures at higher level. Adherence to such a program during the growth phase of endoscopic skull base surgery may decrease the risk of complications as the surgeon's knowledge and surgical expertise develop (Snyderman et al, 2007).

Complications of EEA are the same as open approaches: neural and vascular injury, infection and CSF leak. Literature report of neural and vascular injury are fortunately rare accounting for 1% incidence. These can be avoided with attention to anatomical landmarks and proper dissection techniques. An experienced team can effectively control venous bleeding from the cavernous sinus or basilar plexus. Peri-operative antibiotic prophylaxis, multilayered repair of dural defects and aggressive management of postoperative CSF leaks are contributing factors. One of the biggest remaining challenges is repair of large dural defects and prevention of post-operative leaks. With the advent of the septal mucosal flap, the Pittsburgh group suggest an incidence of 6% of CSF leak. Developments that have decreased the incidence of postoperative CSF leaks include a multilayered closure, direct suturing of grafts to dural edges, use of biological glues, coverage with vascularized septal mucosal flap and supporting the reconstruction with an intranasal balloon catheter.

9. Acknowledgements

I wish to acknowledge with gratitude the co-operation of the Departments of Otorhinolaryngology - Head and Neck Surgery, Neurosurgery, Endocrinology and Ophthalmology of the National University Malaysia Medical Faculty (UKMMC).

10. References

Beasley N and Jones NS. 1995. The role of endoscopy in the management of mucoceles. *American Journal of Rhinology* 9(5): 251-256

Bolger WE, Parsons DS, Mair EA, Kuhn FA. 1992. Lacrimal drainage system injury in functional endoscopic sinus surgery: Incidence, analysis and preventions. *Archives of Otolaryngol Head Neck Surg* 118(11): 1179-1184

Bolger WE and Mann CB. 2001. Analysis of the suprabullar and retrobullar recesses for endoscopic sinus surgery. *Annals of Otology, Rhinology and Laryngology* Supplement 186 110(5 part 2): 3-14

Chow PI,Sadun A, Lee H. 1995. Vascular and morpheometry of the optic canal and intracanalicular optic nerve. *J Neuroopthalmol* 15: 186-190

Chow J and Stankiewicz. 1997. Powered instrumentation in orbital and optic nerve decompression. *Otolaryngol Clin North Am* 30: 467-478

Conboy PJ and Jones. 2003. The place of endoscopic sinus surgery in the treatment of paranasal sinus mucoceles. *Clin Otolaryngol* 28: 207-210

Cook M, Levin L, Joseph M, Pinczower E. 1996. Traumatic optic neuropathy: a meta-analysis. *Arch Otolaryngol Head Neck Surg* 122: 389-392

Eljamel MSM. 1993. The role of surgery and beta-2-transferrin in the management of cerebrospinal fluid fistula. *MD thesis*. University of Liverpool.

Gendeh, B.S, Selladurai B.M, Selvapragasam T, Khalid B.A.K, Said H. 1998. The transseptal approaches to pituitary tumours: Technique, rhinologic functions and complications *Asian J Surgery* 21(4): 259-265

Gendeh BS, Wormald PJ, Forer M, Goh BS, Misiran K. 2002. Endoscopic repair of spontaneous cerebro-spinal fluid rhinorrhoea: a report of 3 cases. *Med J Malaysia* 57(4): 503-508

Gendeh BS, Mazita A, Selladurai BM, Jegan T, Jeevanan J, Misiran K. 2005. Endoscopic repair of Anterior Skull Base Fistula: The Kuala Lumpur Experience. *J Laryngol Otol* 119: 866-874

Gendeh BS. 2006. Minimally invasive surgical approaches to the sphenoid sinus, sell, parasellar and clival region. Current and future perspectives. *Med J Malaysia* 61(3); 274-277

Gendeh BS, Salina H, Selladurai B, Jagan T. 2007. Endoscopic assisted craniofacial resection: A case series and post-operative outcome. *Med J Malaysia* 62(3); 234-237

Gendeh BS. 2010. Extended applications of endoscopic sinus surgery and its reference to cranial base and pituiatary fossa. *Indian J Otolaryngol Head Neck Surg* 62: S 68-S 80.

Gendeh BS, 2009. Advances in technology and its application to rhinology. In Gendeh BS Ed. Clinical atlas of nasal endoscopy. *UKM Publication*. Pg 114-117

Hartstein ME, Kokoska M. Woog JJ. 2004. Endoscopic techniques in orbital fracture repair. In Woog JJ, ed *Manual of endoscopic lacrimal and orbital surgery*. Butterworth Heinemann, pp 175-182.

Hehar SS and Jones NS. 1997. Fronto-ethmoidal osteoma: the place of surgery. *J Laryngol Otol* 111: 372-375

Howe L and JonesNS. 2004. Guidelines for the management of periorbital cellulitis/abcess. *Clin Otolaryngol* 29: 725-728

Ikeda K, Suzuki H, Oshima T, Tomonori T. 1999. Endoscopic endonasal repair of orbital floor fracture. *Arch Otolaryngology Head Neck Surg* 125; 59-63

Jones NS. 1997. Visual evoked potentials in endoscopic and anterior skull base surgery. *Journal of Laryngol and Otology* 111: 513-516(OMIT)

Jones NS, Bullock P, Hewitt s et al. 1997. Head injuries and the principles of craniofacial repair. In Jones NS, ed. *Craniofacial Trauma: An interdisciplinary approach.* Oxford: Oxford University Press, pp. 18-60

Jones NS. 1998. Microendoscopy in rhinology. *Minimally Invasive Therapy and Allied Technologies* 7: 149-154

Jones NS. 1999. Current concepts in the management of paediatric rhinosinusitis. *Journal of Laryngology and Otology* 113: 1-9

Kassam A, Snyderman, CH and Carrau RL et el. 2007.Introduction, Conclusion. In *The Expanded Endonasal Approach to the Ventral Skull Base: Sagittal Plane,* edited by Snyderman CH. Tuttlingen: Endo-Press

Kennedy DW. 1985. Functional endoscopic sinus surgery technique. *Arch Otolaryngol Head Neck Surgery* 111:643-649

Kennedy DW, Josephson JS, Zinreich SJ, Mattox DE, Goldsmith MM. 1989. Endoscopic sinus surgery for mucoceles: a variable alternative. *Laryngoscope* 99:885-889

Kennedy D.W, Goodstein M.L, Miller N.R, Zinreich. S.J. 1990. Endoscopic transnasal orbit decompression. *Archives of Otolaryngology Head and Neck Surgery.* 116: 275-282

Khairullah A, Gendeh BS. 2011. Tube extrusion and cheese wiring 5 years post dacryocytorhinostomy: case report. *Phillipine Intn J of Otolaryngol* 26(2): 34-36

Kountantakis S, Maillard A, El-Harazi S, Longhini L, Urso R. 2000. Endoscopic optic nerve decompression for traumatic blidness. *Otolaryngology Head Neck Surg* 123: 34-37

Kuppersmith R, Alford E, Patrinely J, Lee A, Parke R, Holds J. 1997. Combined transconjunctival/intranasal endoscopic approach to the optic canal in traumatic optic neuropathy. *Laryngoscope* 107: 311-315

Lang J. 1989. *Clinical anatomy of the nose, nasal cavity and paranasal sinuses.* Stuttgart: Georg Thieme Verlag

Lee TS, Shin JC, Woog JJ. 2004. Endoscopic dacryocystorhinostomy: An eastern perspective. In Woog JJ, ed *Manual of endoscopic lacrimal and orbital surgery.* Butterworth Heinemann, pp 123-133.

Lubben B, Stoll W, Grenzebach U. 2001. Optic nerve decompression in the comatose and conscious patients after trauma. *Laryngoscope* 111: 320-328

Luxenberger W, Stammberger H, Jebeles J, Walch C. 1998. Endoscopic optic nerve decompression: The graz experience. *Larygoscope* 108: 873-882

Marshall A, Jones NS, Robertson IJA. 2001. CSF rhinorrhoea: a multidisciplinary approach to minimise patient morbidity. *British Journal of Neurosurgery* 15(1): 8-13

Mason JDT, Haynes RJ, Jones NS. 1998. Interpretation of the dilated pupil during endoscopic sinus surgery *J of Laryngol and Otology* 112: 622-627

Metson R, Dallow R, Shore J. 1994. Endoscopic orbital decompression. *Laryngoscope* 104: 950-957.

Metson R, Gliklich RE. 1998. Clinical outcomes of endoscopic surgery for frontal sinusitis. *Otolaryngol Head Neck Surg* 124(10): 1090-1096

Metson R, Samaha M. 2002. Reduction of diplopia following endoscopic orbital decompression: The orbital sling technique. *Laryngoscope* 112: 1753-1757

Metson R, Samaha M. 2004. Endoscopic orbital decompression. In *Manual of endoscopic lacrimal and orbital surgery.* Editor Woog JJ. Butterworth Heinemann, Elsevier, pg 167-173

Page EL,Wiatrak BJ. 1996. Endoscopic versus external drainage of orbital subperiosteal abscess. *Arch Otolaryngol Head Neck Surg* 122(7): 737-740

Setliff R.C. 1994. The "Hummer": New instrumentation for functional endoscopic sinus surgery. *Am J Rhinol.* 8: 275-278.

Sofferman B. 1995. The recovery potential of the optic nerve. *Laryngoscope* 105: 1-38

Stafford JDB, Brenan P, Toland J, O'Dwyer AJ. 1996. Magnetic resonance imaging in the evaluation of cerebrospinal fluid fistula. *Clinical Radiology* 51:837-841

Stammberger H. 1991. *Functional endoscopic sinus surgery*: The Messerklinger Technique. Philadelphia: Brian C Decker

Steinsapir K, Goldberg R. 1994. Traumatic optic neuropathy. *Surv Opthalmol* 38: 487-518

Steinsapir K, Seiff S, Goldberg R. 2002. Traumatic optic neuropathy: where do we stand? *Ophthal Plast Reconstr Surg* 18: 232-234

Snyderman CH, Kassam A and Carrau RL et al. 2007. Acquisition of Surgical Skills for Endonasal Skull Base Surgery: A Training Program. *Laryngoscope* 117: 699-705

Tandon DA,Thakar A, Mahapatra AK, Ghosh P. 1994. Transethmoid optic nerve decompression. *Clin Otolaryngol* 19: 98-104

Umapathy N, Kalra S, Skinner DW, Dapling RB. 2006. Long-term results of endonasal laser dacrocystorhinostomy. *Otolaryngol Head Neck Surgery* 135(1): 81-84

Vrabac DP. 1994. The inverted Schneiderian papilloma: a 25 year study. *Laryngoscope* 104: 582-605

Woog JJ. 2004.Endoscopic dacryocystorhinostomy and conjunctivodacryostorhinostomy. In Woog JJ, ed *Manual of endoscopic lacrimal and orbital surgery.* Butterworth Heinemann, pg 105-121.

Wormald P, McDonough M. 1997. Bath plug technique for the endoscopic management of cerebrospinal fluid leaks. *J Laryngol Otol* 111: 1042-1046

Wormald P.J. 2002. Powered endoscopic dacryocystorhinostomy. *Laryngoscope.* 112(1): 69-72.

Wormald PJ and van Hasselt CA. 2003. Endoscopic removal of juvenile angiofibroma. *Otolaryngol Head Neck Surgery* 129: 684-691

Wormald PJ, Ooi E, van Hasselt CA, Nair S. 2003. Endoscopic removal of sinonasal inverted papilloma including endoscopic medial maxillectomy. *Laryngoscope* 113: 867-873

Wormald PJ. 2005. Endoscopic orbital decompression for exopthalmos, acute orbital hemorrhage and orbital subperiosteal abscess. In Wormald PJ, ed. *Endoscopic sinus surgery: Anatomy, three-dimentional reconstruction and surgical technique.* Thieme Medicl Publishes, Inc, New York. Stuttgart, pg135-140

Inhalt

Vorwort

Man kann annehmen, dass die Faszination des Menschen für den „Pflanzenrauch“ so alt ist wie die Nutzung des Feuers. Es gibt Hinweise, dass bereits vor über einer Million Jahren der *Homo erectus* den Umgang mit dem Feuer beherrschte und, dass vor etwa 32.000 Jahren der moderne *Homo sapiens* endgültig das Feuer gezähmt hatte. Er lernte die vielen Vorteile des Feuers zu nutzen. Untrennbar verbunden mit dem Feuer ist der Rauch. Bereits in den Zeiten, als sich der Mensch noch in Höhlen aufhielt, entstand das Interesse am Rauch des Feuers und die Menschen konnten beobachten, dass unterschiedliches Feuermaterial verschiedene Arten von Rauch hervorbrachte. Es war dann nur mehr ein kleiner Schritt zur Entdeckung des aromatisierten Rauchs von Pflanzen, die in die Glut geworfen einen unverkennbaren Duft entfalteten. Mit diesem Rauch konnten Schädlinge abgewehrt werden, er wirkte keimtötend und konnte zum Konservieren von Fleisch verwendet werden.

Mit dem Glauben an ein Jenseits und an Gottheiten, die über unserer Welt stehen, bekam der aromatische und in den Himmel aufsteigende Rauch neue Dimensionen. Es entwickelte sich der Begriff des Rauchopfers, bei dem der Rauch das Medium bildete, mit dem die Gebete der Gläubigen nach oben zu den Göttern getragen werden sollten. Diese Tradition des Rauches, um damit die Götter zu ehren und mit ihnen Kontakt aufzunehmen, ist ein transkulturelles Phänomen und entstand in allen Kulturen der Menschheit und fand den Weg über die griechische und römische Kultur auch zum Christentum, wo beim katholischen Gottesdienst das Räuchern mit dem Weihrauchfass bis heute eine bekannte Zeremonie darstellt. Hinweise auf das Rauchopfer finden sich im Alten Testament, z. B. im Psalm 141 der lautet: „Wie ein Rauchopfer steige mein Gebet vor dir auf; als Abendopfer gelte vor dir, wenn ich meine Hände erhebe“.

In den alpenländischen Heiltraditionen haben sich neben den Räucherritualen im Umfeld von religiösen Festen auch in der Volksmedizin magische Räucheranwendungen mit pflanzlichen und tierischen Produkten entwickelt, wobei aus heutiger Sicht teilweise skurrile Anwendungen entstanden sind. Aus dem 17. Jahrhundert ist überliefert, dass man Kleinkinder dem Rauch gewisser Heilpflanzen aussetzte, um das Nachtweinen zu bekämpfen. Räucherungen mit der Haut eines Igels wendete man zur Heilung von Rotlauf und Gesichtsrose an. Es kursierte die Vorstellung, dass gewisse „Würmer“ für die Entstehung von Krankheiten verantwortlich seien. So schreibt noch Hildegard von Bingen, dass man „Zahnwürmer“ mit dem Rauch von Aloe und Myrrhenharz bekämpfen kann. Das Räuchern mit Samen des Bilsenkrauts wurde bei Zahnschmerzen empfohlen, um den „Zahnwurm“ zu vertreiben.

Betrachtet man nun die derzeit sehr lebendige volksheilkundliche Tradition in Kärnten und in den anderen Gebieten der Alpenländer ist zu beobachten, dass die Durchführung von Räucherritualen wieder großes Interesse findet. Fast wären ja die überlieferten Anwendungen von Pflanzenmaterialien im Umfeld von Rauchanwendungen in Vergessenheit geraten. So entstand aber eine neue und interessante Szene im Grenzbereich zwischen Esoterik und wissenschaftlich fundierter Ethnobotanik. Der Rauch bildet jedenfalls eine sehr komplexe Welt zwischen Psychologie und Pharmakologie und er hat sich in den heilkräuterkundlichen Anwendungen von Pflanzen einen eigenen Bereich erobert. Es ist ein großes und dankeswürdiges Verdienst von Dr. Romana Seunig, dass sie mit ihrem Buch das altüberlieferte Wissen zur Anwendung von Pflanzen in Räucherritualen zusammengefasst hat und damit den an Heilpflanzen interessierten Menschen eine sehr gute und für eigene Anwendungen anregende Lektüre bietet. Romana Seunig hat über den theoretischen Zugang hinaus selbst eine große Erfahrung in der Durchführung von Räucherritualen. Dieses Wissen hat sie schon an viele Interessierte auf ihrem Bauernhof in Schwarz auf der Sattnitz weitergegeben.

Dr. Helmut Zwander
Botaniker und Vorstandsmitglied der FNL Kräuterakademie nach Ignaz Schlifni
Klagenfurt, 2024

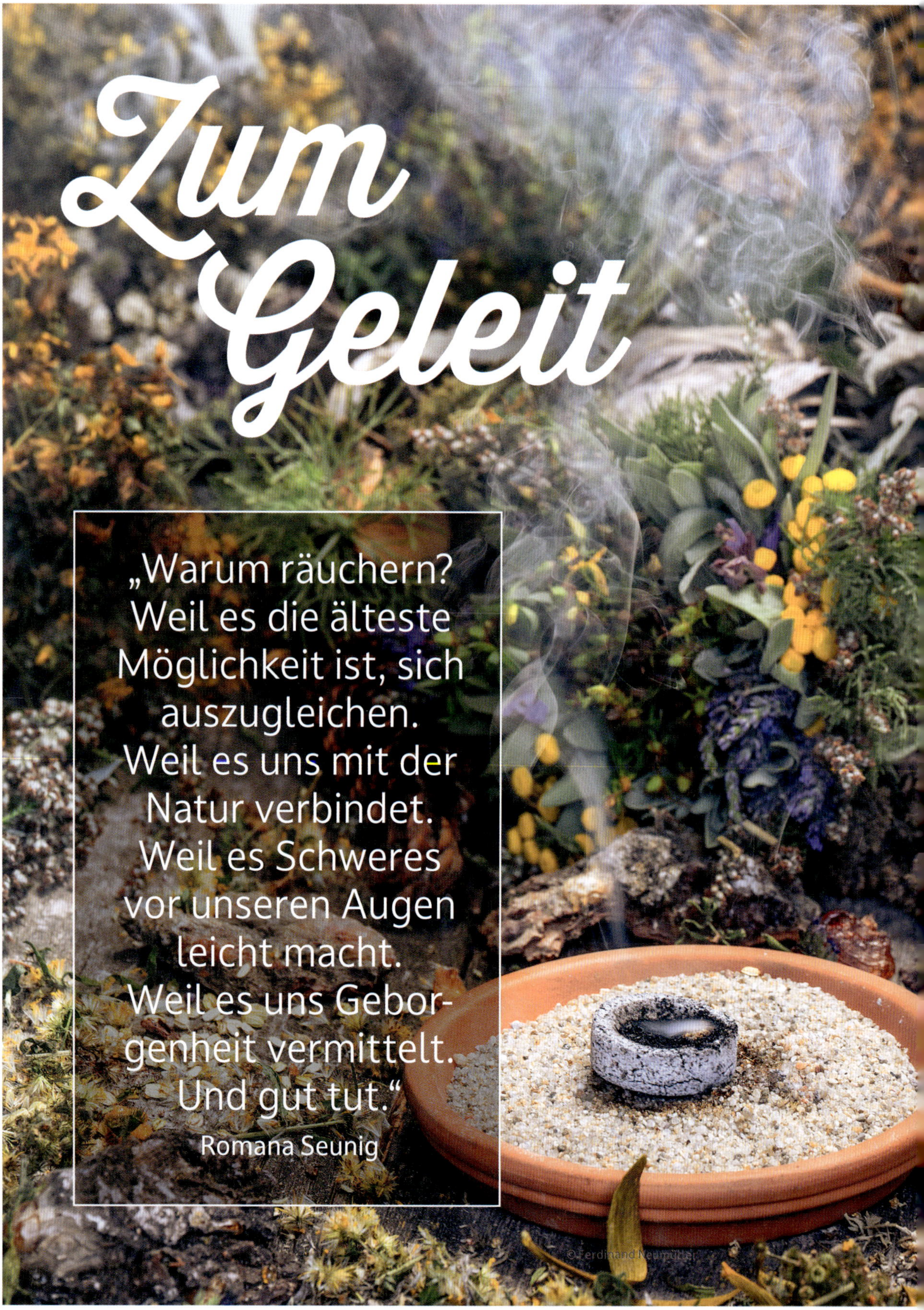

Zum Geleit

„Warum räuchern?
Weil es die älteste
Möglichkeit ist, sich
auszugleichen.
Weil es uns mit der
Natur verbindet.
Weil es Schweres
vor unseren Augen
leicht macht.
Weil es uns Geborgenheit vermittelt.
Und gut tut.“

Romana Seunig

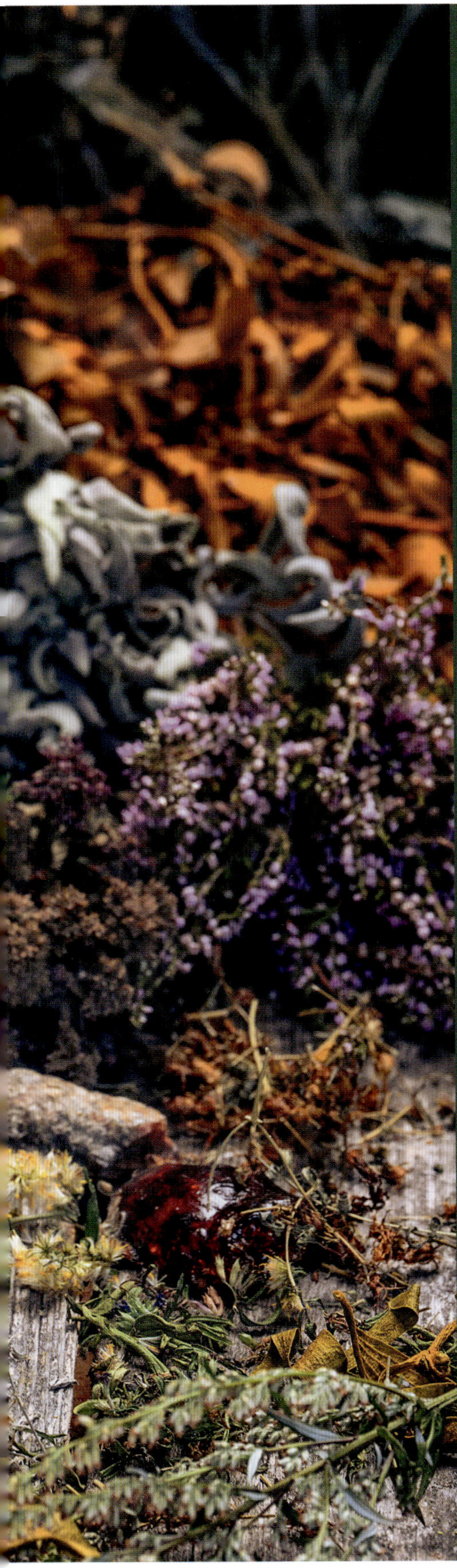

Die heimische Pflanzenwelt bietet eine wertvolle und schier unerschöpfliche Ressource an Räucherstoffen. Es hat viele Jahre gedauert, bis ich aus rund 200 verschiedenen Pflanzen aus den Wäldern und Wiesen meiner Umgebung sowie aus meinem Kräutergarten die vorliegende Auswahl zusammengefunden habe.

Es war ein langsamer, sich selbst immer wieder überlagernder und hinterfragender Prozess, bei dem es mir hauptsächlich darum ging, jene Pflanzen bzw. Pflanzenteile herauszufinden, die ihre Kraft und Informationen am deutlichsten im Rauch, also als Räucherstoff, weitergeben. Es war mir dabei besonders wichtig, die Resonanzfähigkeit der einzelnen Pflanzen eindeutig erspüren und lesen zu können, weil ich überzeugt bin, dass nur der Rauch von Pflanzen mit klaren Botschaften für Menschen zu einer helfenden Unterstützung in unterschiedlichen Lebensphasen werden kann.

Aus dieser Suche sind auch die zahlreichen Rezeptvorschläge hervorgegangen: Zu jeder Pflanze liegt mindestens ein Vorschlag für eine Räuchermischung vor, als Anregung und Impuls für weitere Ideen der Leserschaft.

In dieser Zeit der Suche haben mich immer mehr die Wurzeln der einzelnen Pflanzen als besonders wertvolle Räucherstoffe überrascht, was auch prompt zum umfangreichsten Kapitel geführt hat. Bis auf einige wenige Wurzel-Räucherungen ist der Räucherstoff „Wurzel" traditionell kaum präsent. Das sollte sich ändern und wir sind alle eingeladen, diese pflanzlichen Angebote anzunehmen. Denn gerade in schnelllebigen, oberflächlichen Zeiten setzt der Rauch von Wurzeln oft den ersehnten Kontrapunkt.

Mit großer Freude habe ich auch die jahrhundertealten Zuschreibungen und Erfahrungen mit den einzelnen Pflanzenpersönlichkeiten zusammengetragen. Die vielen Potenziale, heilsamen Kräfte und hoffnungsvollen Anwendungen unserer Vorfahren präzisieren den Charakter der einzelnen Pflanzen als Räucherstoff: Denn im Rauch fließen all diese Aspekte zusammen.

Dieses Buch soll eine Einladung sein, sich der heimischen Natur und ihren ausgleichenden Botschaften mittels Rauches anzunähern und ihre Begleitung zu genießen.

Romana Seunig, Herbst 2024

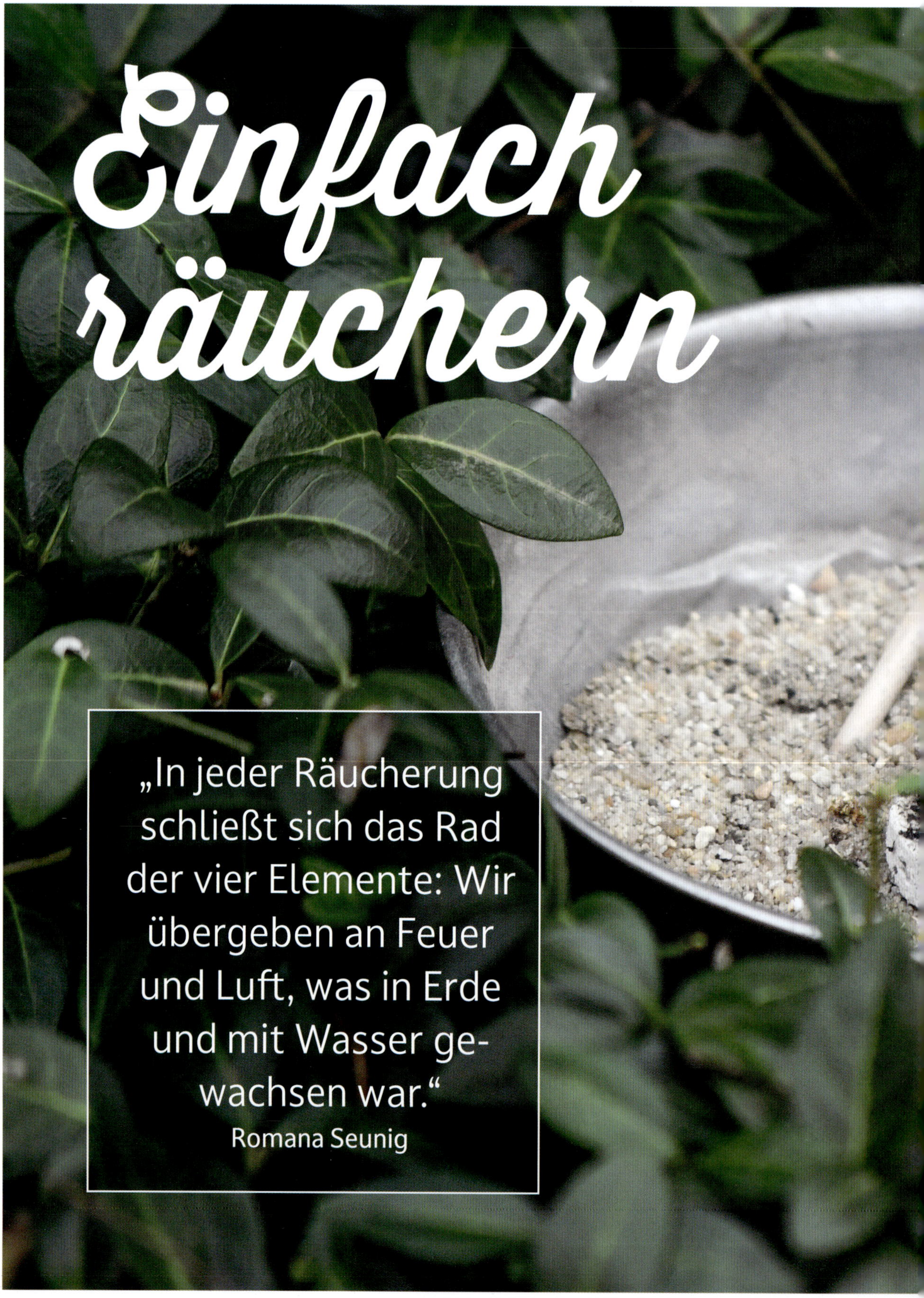

Einfach räuchern

„In jeder Räucherung schließt sich das Rad der vier Elemente: Wir übergeben an Feuer und Luft, was in Erde und mit Wasser gewachsen war.“

Romana Seunig

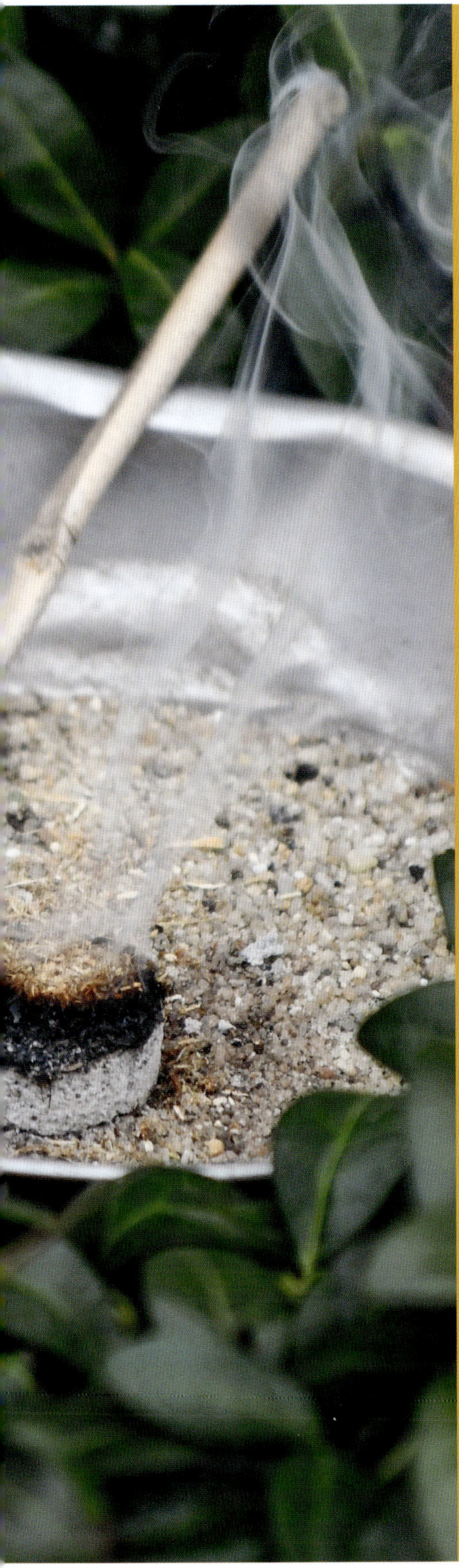

Rauch – Pflanzenatem zwischen Himmel und Erde

Rauch entzieht sich der Schwerkraft: Rauch steigt nach oben, direkt in den Himmel, wo immer schon die Götter saßen, von denen man sich Beistand erhoffte, in schwierigen Zeiten und für zahllose Anforderungen des täglichen Überlebens.

Räuchern ist verbunden mit lichtgebendem und wärmendem Feuer. Es geht darum, in der Dunkelheit Licht zu machen, um die Lebenden zu schützen. Doch der Schein des Feuers allein ist nicht genug – es braucht den Rauch von besonderen Hölzern und Pflanzen, die uns Menschen gegen die Dämonen der Finsternis helfen.

Der Rauch dient als Medizin der Seele, als Schutz und Abwehr dessen, was aus der Dunkelheit an Bedrohlichem auf uns zukommen könnte. Man dachte, so wie Tiere den Rauch meiden, würden auch grausame Wesen der Anderswelt oder erschreckende Phantasiegestalten den Rauch meiden und der Mensch wäre somit in Sicherheit.

Keep it simple – Gedanken zur Räucherpraxis

Es braucht nicht viel, um sich selbst mit passenden Räucherungen zu versorgen. An Ausstattung reichen ein oder zwei Blumentopfuntersetzer aus Ton, etwas Quarzsand, der die Wärme der Räucherkohle gut speichern kann, ein kleines Holzbrett und einen Putz-Stängel. Das Holzbrett fängt etwaige Hitze zuverlässig ab und der Putz-Stängel dient dazu, die Räucherkohle während der Räucherung von etwaigen Rückständen zu säubern. Ich nehme meistens Beifußstängel, weil sie sich leicht zurechtschneiden lassen und dem Rauch gleichzeitig die Information „Klärung und Schutz“ mitgeben.

Tipp *Die im Handel erhältliche Räucherkohle zieht Feuchtigkeit an, wodurch es sein kann, dass sie manchmal nur schwer oder gar nicht mehr zündet. Sollte dies einmal der Fall sein, dann bricht man die Kohle in der Mitte auseinander, wobei man sie ganz fest zusammendrückt, denn sonst zerbröselt sie. In der Mitte ist meist noch ausreichend Zünder vorhanden, so dass man die zwei Hälften verwenden kann. Im Übrigen ist für eine normale Räucherung in einer Wohnung meist bereits eine halbe Räucherkohle ausreichend.*

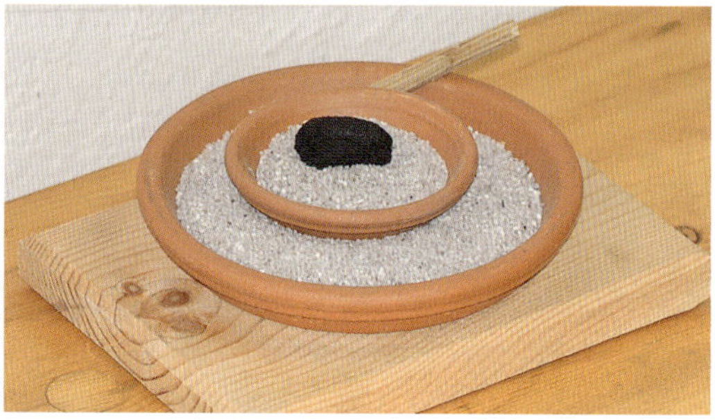

Grundausstattung zum Räuchern: Holzbrettchen, Tongefäße, Quarzsand und Putzstängel.

Räucherstoffe und Räuchermischungen

Da ich mit Räucherkohle und nicht mit Holzglut räuchere, bleibt das Räuchergefäß ruhig stehen und muss nicht für weitere Luftzufuhr bewegt werden, wie das bei der Holzglut-Räucherung der Fall ist. Gleichzeitig bedeutet das für diese Art des Räucherns aber auch, dass die Räucherstoffe feiner aufgearbeitet werden müssen. Wenn größere Räucherteile unbewegt auf der Kohle liegen, glühen sie nur kurz auf und brennen danach ab. Das heißt, das Dufterlebnis ist nur von sehr kurzer Dauer und danach kann es nicht nur für die Nase, sondern auch für das Wohlbefinden unangenehm werden.

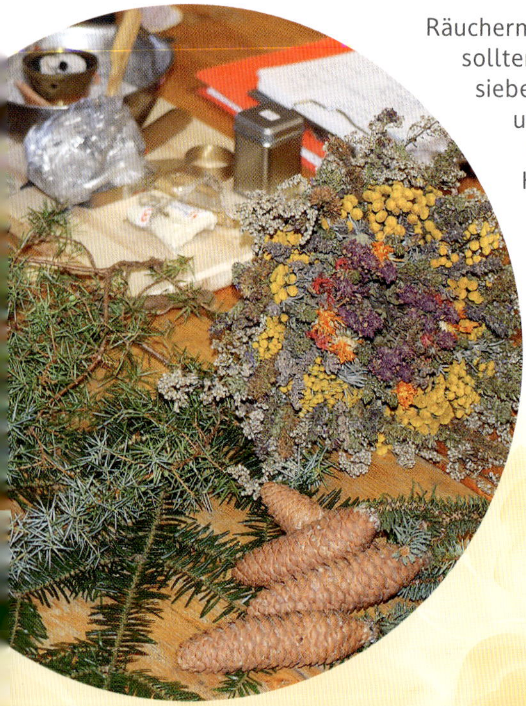

Räuchermischungen sollten aus bis zu sieben Pflanzen und mindestens einem Harz bestehen.

Das feine Aufarbeiten der pflanzlichen Räucherstoffe – bis auf das Harz – passiert entweder im Mörser oder in einer Kaffeemühle. Die Pflanzen- und besonders Wurzelteile sollten schon vor der Trocknung entsprechend zerkleinert werden, denn das erleichtert das Vermahlen.

Räuchermischungen bestehen aus einer Kombination von Harzen und bis zu sieben anderen Pflanzenbestandteilen. Es ist anzuraten, in jeder Räuchermischung zumindest ein Harz zu verwenden, weil die Bestandteile des Harzes die Pflanzenbestandteile gut ummanteln, damit diese im Verglühen noch ihren Duft freisetzen können. Diese Ummantelung geschieht im Mörser, wo man die fein gemahlenen Pflanzenteile mit den Harzbrocken so lange verarbeitet, bis sich ein feiner Räucherstoff ergibt.

Gewisse fette Samen und Früchte können in einer Räuchermischung die Rolle des Harzes übernehmen. So kann man beispielsweise durch Zugabe von Wacholderbeeren in einer Räucherung auf ein Harz verzichten. So gesehen bei Paracelsus (1493–1541) in einer Räucherung „wider die pestilentzische Lufft". Da aber die reinen Kräuter auf der Räucherkohle eher verbrennen als verglühen, wird sich in einer solchen Räucherung kein nachhaltig angenehmer Duft entwickeln.

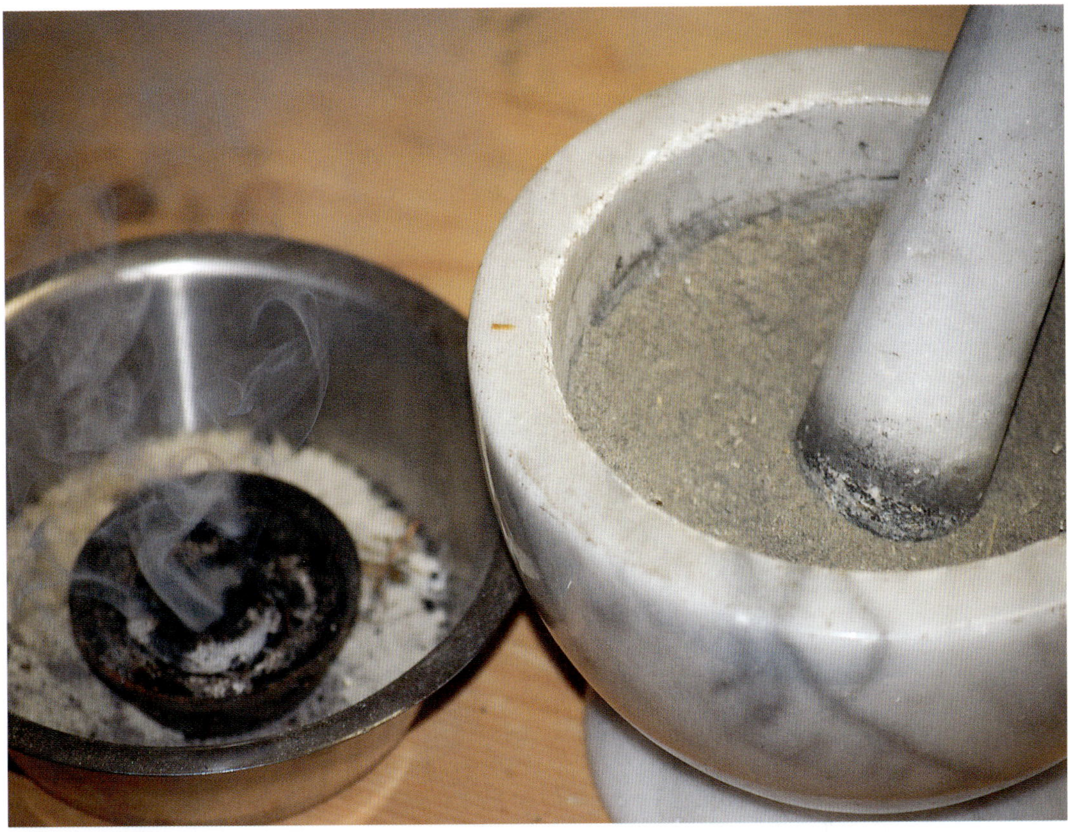

Im Mörser entsteht aus den fein gemahlenen Pflanzenbestandteilen und den Harzbrocken ein feiner Räucherstoff.

Selbstverständlich kann man auch mehrere Harze und mehr als sieben verschiedene Pflanzen mischen. Es geht immer darum, zu prüfen, ob die gewählte Ausrichtung noch sinnvoll ist.

Tipp *Die Vorschläge für Räuchermischungen, die ich bei den einzelnen Pflanzen angeführt habe, enthalten keine Bezeichnung des beizufügenden Harzes. Es ist mir besonders wichtig, hier die Möglichkeit für jeden offen zu lassen, für sich selbst das passende Harz dazuzugeben. Das Leitharz wäre hier Fichtenharz, aber manche greifen automatisch zu Weihrauch, für andere kommt nichts über Mastix, wieder andere bevorzugen ein leichtes Kopal. Alle diese Harz-Varianten sind möglich und geben den Räucherungen die persönliche Note.*

Alle können räuchern

Der Rauch macht frei und leitet einen sanft, wenn man sich auf die persönlichen Empfindungen während der Räucherung einlässt. Lassen Sie sich nicht vorschreiben, wie lange oder in welche Richtung geräuchert oder gelüftet werden sollte. Alle können räuchern – und sollte etwas als unangenehm empfunden werden: Aufhören zu räuchern, durchlüften, seine Räuchermischung überdenken und gegebenenfalls nachbessern.

Räuchermischungen herstellen

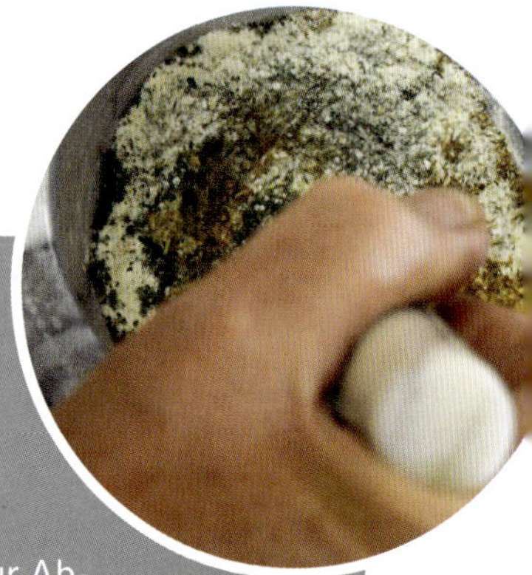

Ausgangsmaterial für eine feine Räuchermischung zur Sommersonnenwende

FEIN GEMAHLENE RÄUCHERMISCHUNG

Feine Räuchermischungen sind ideal für Räucherungen mit Räucherkohle.

Die Gerätschaften zur Herstellung einer feinen Räuchermischung:

- getrocknete Räucherstoffe nach Wahl und Anlass
- Gewürzmühle oder alte Kaffeemühle zum Zerkleinern aller pflanzlichen Bestandteile, außer dem Harz. Sollte keine Mühle vorhanden sein, wird alles nach und nach im Mörser verrieben
- Mörser zum Zerkleinern des Harzes sowie zum Verreiben mit den gemahlenen Kräutern
- Räucherschale mit etwas Quarzsand und Räucherkohle zum Ausprobieren der Mischung

Beispiel

Zu den Sonnenwenden finden neben Feuer-Ritualen häufig auch Räucherungen statt. Wir mischen hier eine Räucherung zu Sommer-Sonnenwende:

- Haselnussblätter – zur Abwehr gegen Blitzschlag, Feuer und Unwettergeschehen zur Erntezeit, sowie gegen krankmachende Praktiken
- Beifuß-Wurzeln und -blätter – die schützende Kraft der Übergänge in der Natur und im persönlichen Erleben
- Johanniskraut – das spannungsabbauende Wetterkraut, das dunkle Mächte fernhalten soll und zur Sonnenwende hilft im positiven Rhythmus zu bleiben
- Kleines Habichtskraut – die bodenbedeckende Pflanze vermittelt im Rauch einen besonderen Schutz vor negativen Übergriffen und Anhaftungen. Sie sorgt für Erdung und neue Energie.
- Fichtenharz unterstützt in dieser Mischung den Seelenfrieden, beruhigt die Nerven und macht frischen Mut, sodass die Wende gelingen kann.

Anfänglich empfiehlt es sich, mit annähernd gleichen Mengen der Zutaten zu starten und sich über die eigene Wahrnehmung dem persönlich passenden Rauch anzunähern. Jede so entstandene Räuchermischung lässt sich nachträglich noch verändern, indem man mehr von einem oder zwei Kräutern dazu vermörsert.

Wer schon erste Erfahrungen gesammelt hat, wählt die Mengen meist intuitiv aus. Es kann sich zu einem Kraut eine besondere Beziehung entwickeln, oder die Beschreibung im vorliegenden Buch entspricht dem momentanen persönlichen Bedarf.

Die gemahlenen Kräuter-Zutaten kommen zum Harz in den Mörser und werden verrieben. Es ist keine bloße Vermischung der Zutaten mit dem Harz, sondern es wird die gesamte Mischung kraftvoll gemörsert. Dadurch werden die Kräuter mit dem Harz ummantelt und können so in der Räucherung ihren Duft optimal entfalten.

Um den Duft zu testen, legen Sie eine Prise der Räuchermischung auf die Räucherkohle. Auch während der Räucherung sollten Sie stets nur kleine Mengen auf einmal verräuchern, damit sich der Rauch gut entwickeln kann. Zudem wächst die eigene Wahrnehmung, wenn Sie die Räucherkohle nicht überfrachten, sondern diese öfter bedienen müssen und so intensiv bei der Sache bleiben.

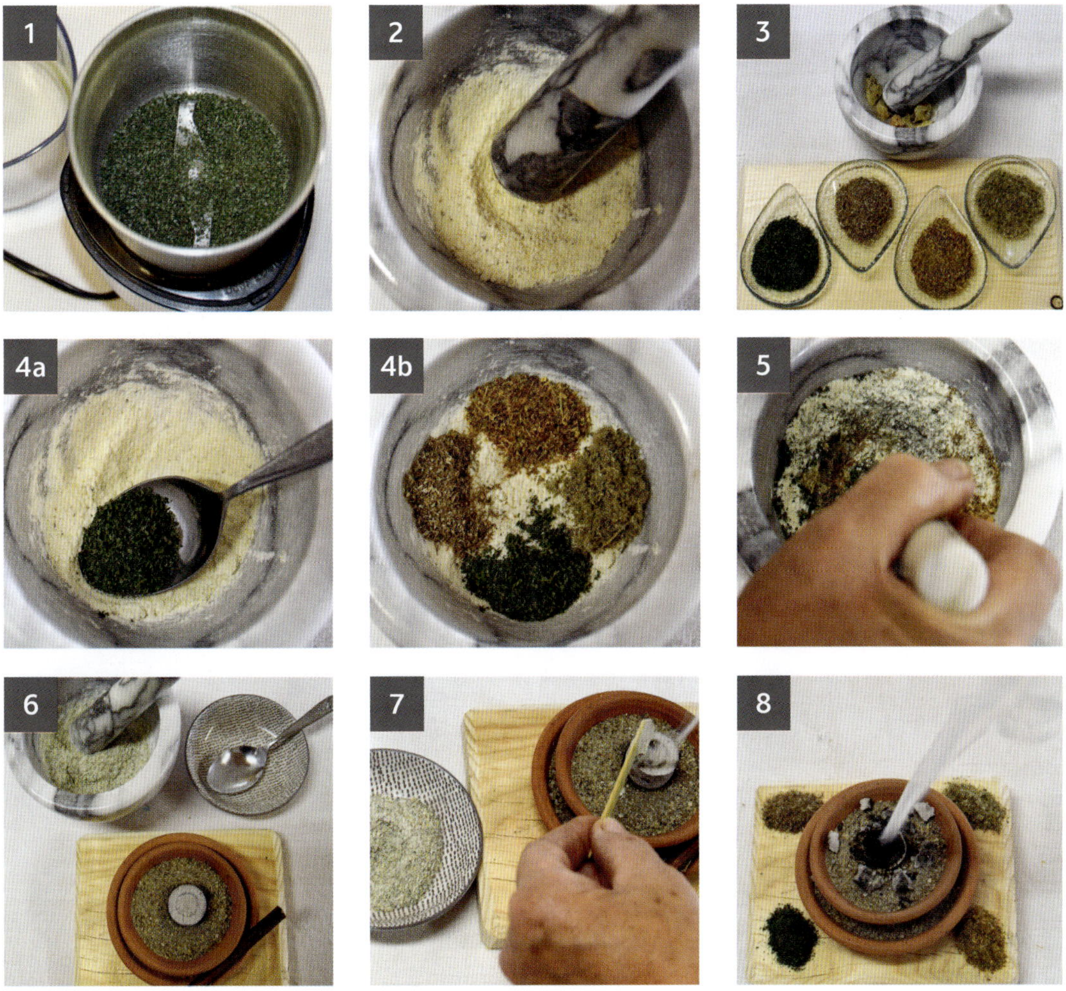

1 Die Räucherzutaten werden im ersten Schritt nacheinander in einer Gewürzmühle vermahlen.

2 Das Harz wird zunächst extra im Mörser zerkleinert, da die zähen Anteile des Harzes die Gewürzmühle, die sich ja mit großer Geschwindigkeit dreht, verkleben würden.

3 Nachdem die Grundzutaten zerkleinert wurden, folgt das Vermengen.

4 Anschließend kommen die Kräuter-Zutaten zum Harz in den Mörser.

5 Mörsern Sie danach die gesamte Mischung kraftvoll.

6 Jetzt ist die Räuchermischung fertig zum Probieren.

7 Um den Duft zu testen, legen Sie nur ganz wenig der Räuchermischung auf die Räucherkohle.

8 Nutzen Sie auch während der Räucherung stets nur kleine Mengen auf einmal, damit sich der Rauch gut entwickeln kann.

GROB GEREBELTE RÄUCHERMISCHUNG

Grobe Räuchermischungen eignen sich für Anwendungen im Räucher-Stövchen bzw. für Räucherungen mit Ofenglut. Viele bevorzugen den Kräuterduft vom Räucher-Stövchen, bei dem das Räuchergut nicht direkt mit dem Feuer in Berührung kommt. Die aufsteigende Wärme des Teelichtes sorgt dabei für eine angenehme Raumbeduftung. Für solche Anwendungen ist es wichtig, dass die Räucherstoffe grob gerebelt in einer losen Mischung zusammengefügt werden. Dazu werden die getrockneten Pflanzenstoffe mit einer Schere grob geschnitten und beispielsweise durch ein altes breites Nudelsieb gedrückt, um sie zu ähnlicher Größe zu bringen. Feine Räuchermischungen würden, aufgrund der Harz-Ummantelung rasch das Stahlsieb verkleben.

Auch bei Räucherungen in der Glutpfanne, wie sie früher mit Ofenglut gemacht wurden, bleibt das Räuchergut grob. Während des Räucher-Rundganges muss man die Glutpfanne immer wieder bewegen, damit der Sauerstoff die Glut erhält. So können auch größere Pflanzen- und Harz-Stücke verglühen und ergeben einen wunderbaren Duft.

Die Gerätschaften zur Herstellung einer groben Räuchermischung:

- getrocknete Räucherstoffe nach Wahl und Anlass
- Schere, ev. breites Nudelsieb
- Mörser zum Zerkleinern des Harzes
- Räucher-Stövchen mit Teelicht oder Räucherpfanne für ein Stück Ofenglut zum Ausprobieren

Beispiel

Der zweite große Wendepunkt im kosmischen Jahr, der seit Jahrtausenden von den Menschen mit Rauch-Ritualen begleitet wird, ist die Winter-Sonnenwende. Es sind die immergrünen Pflanzen, die den Überlebenswillen und die Hoffnung auf ein gedeihliches neues Licht im Rauch zum Ausdruck bringen. Hier ein Vorschlag für eine Räucherung in der dunklen Wende-Zeit:

- Tannennadeln – der große Schutzgeist für innere Balance und neuen Lebensmut
- Misteln – vermitteln die Lebenskraft der Sonne und helfen dunkle Phasen durchzustehen und wieder in den richtigen Rhythmus zu kommen.
- Johanniskraut – verscheucht Dämonen und bedrückende Phantasmata und ist ein erster goldener Hoffnungsschimmer hin zu neuem Licht
- Wacholder-Nadeln und -beeren – sorgen für neue Energie und wehren negative Übergriffe ab.
- Fichtenharz zur Klärung der Raumatmosphäre.

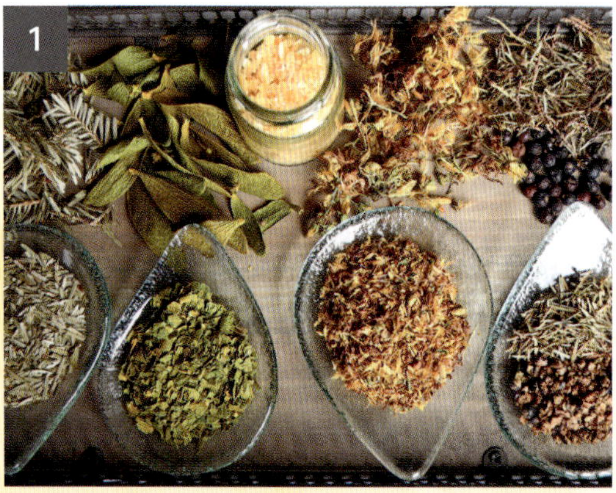

1 Ausgangsmaterialien für eine grobe Räuchermischung zur Winter-Sonnenwende

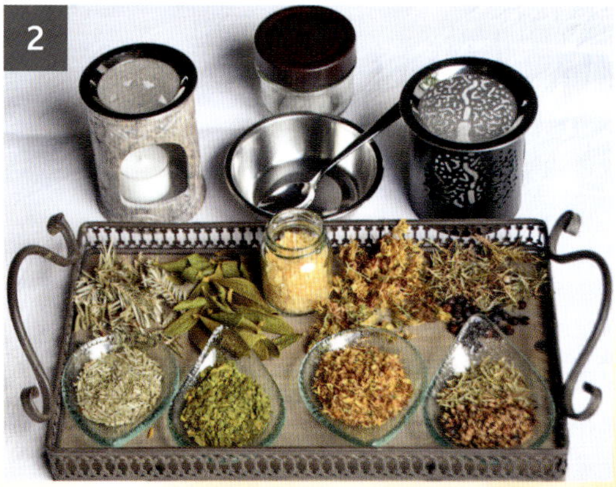

2 Materialien und Hilfsmittel zur Herstellung einer Räuchermischung fürs Stövchen

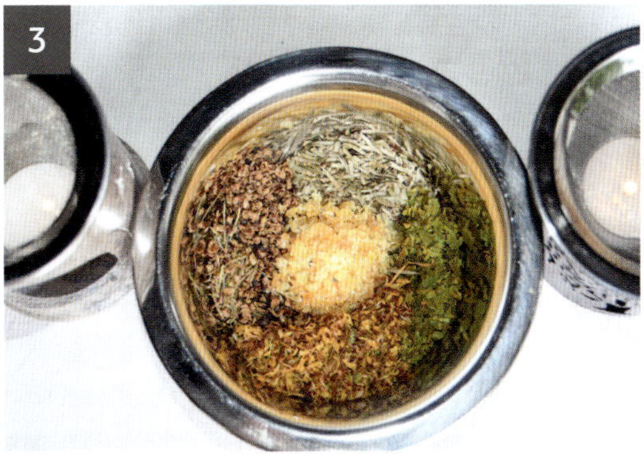

Vermischen Sie die grob verrebelten Kräuter mit dem Löffel.

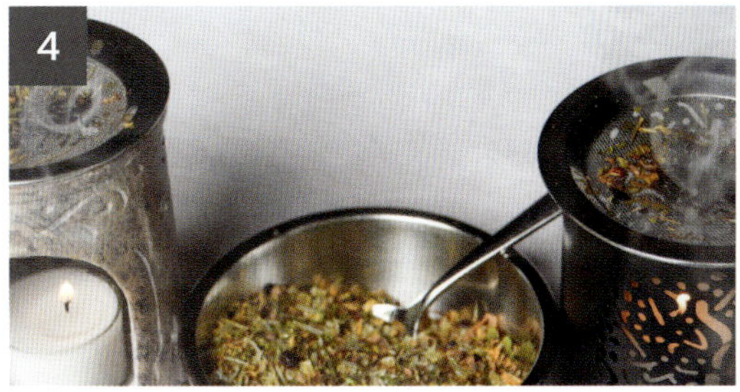

Bringen Sie die Kräutermischung kleinweise auf das Gitter des Räucher-Stövchens auf. Die ausgekühlten Sieb-Einsätze können anschließend mit einer kleinen Drahtbürste gereinigt werden.

Die salutogenetische Seite des Rauches

Möglicherweise waren es die Jahrtausende am offenen Feuer, die dazu geführt haben, dass Rauch uns augenblicklich körperlich, geistig und vor allem emotional anspricht. Das Tor zum Rauch tragen wir alle in uns, wie ein gemeinsames menschliches Erbe. Ob und wie weit man es öffnet, ist jedem freigestellt.

Der Rauch aus Natur und Garten zentriert uns, hält uns im Hier und Jetzt, er ist ein verlässlicher Schutzgeber und ein passender Begleiter in digitalen Zeiten. Die heimische Natur bietet uns ein unerschöpfliches Reservoir an hocheffizienten Räucherstoffen, die uns durch hektische und ruhige, durch fröhliche und ernste, durch glückliche und traurige Tage begleiten.

Rauch sorgt für genussvolle Momente, kleine Lichtfunken des Wohlbefindens, Augenblicke der Sorglosigkeit und des sich eingebunden Fühlens in ein großes Ganzes. Nicht mehr – aber auch nicht weniger.

Wie Räucherungen wirken

Bei einer Räucherung geht es einerseits um den vordergründigen Duft der Räuchermischung, andererseits jedoch um die eigentliche Auswirkung auf die persönliche Befindlichkeit sowie die Überlagerung der Raum- und Umgebungsatmosphäre.

Wie stark wir von Veränderungen der Raumatmosphäre sowie von Kraft- und Abtragungsfeldern beeinflusst werden bzw. wie klar wir solche wahrnehmen können, hängt davon ab, wie gut man sein persönliches feinstoffliches Sensorium zu öffnen bereit ist.

Mit jeder Räucherung wird unsere Befindlichkeit beeinflusst, aber auch die Atmosphäre des jeweiligen Ortes. Der Pflanzenrauch wirkt allgemein positiv unterstützend, lösend und heilsam für Menschen und Orte. Sowohl unser persönliches Kraftfeld als auch die Raumstimmung werden durch die Wellenlänge der Rauchschwaden, die von einer Räuchermischung aufsteigen, überlagert und verändert.

Wir alle leben an Orten und in Räumen mit unterschiedlichen energetischen Prägungen und vielleicht belastenden Geschichten, von denen wir möglicherweise nichts wissen. Dabei ist es wichtig zu beachten, dass das „Gedächtnis" von Orten weit zurückreichen kann und sich negative Energien nicht einfach von selbst auflösen können. Der Rauch hingegen kann immer wieder heilsame Überlagerungsarbeit leisten.

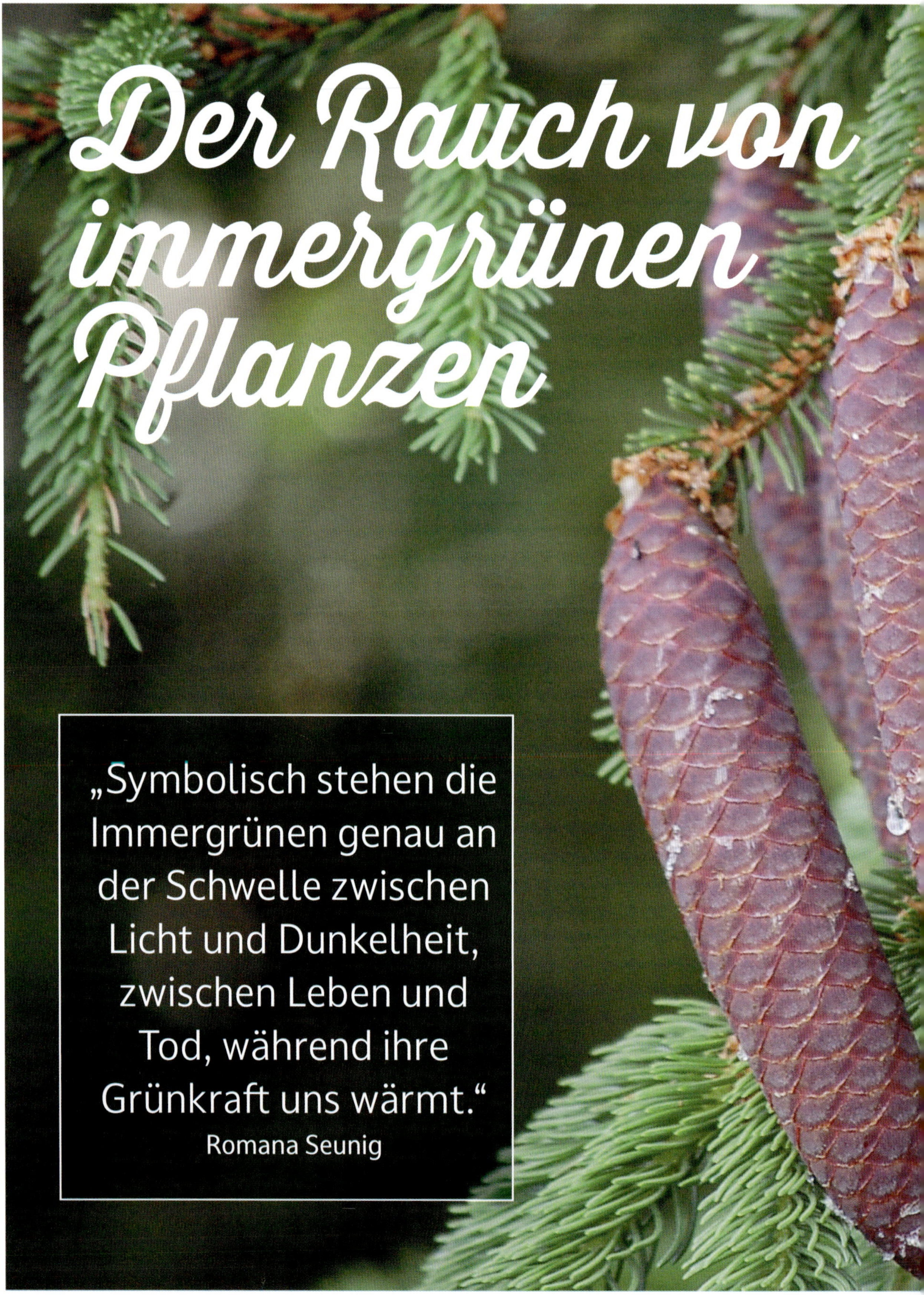

Der Rauch von immergrünen Pflanzen

„Symbolisch stehen die Immergrünen genau an der Schwelle zwischen Licht und Dunkelheit, zwischen Leben und Tod, während ihre Grünkraft uns wärmt.“

Romana Seunig

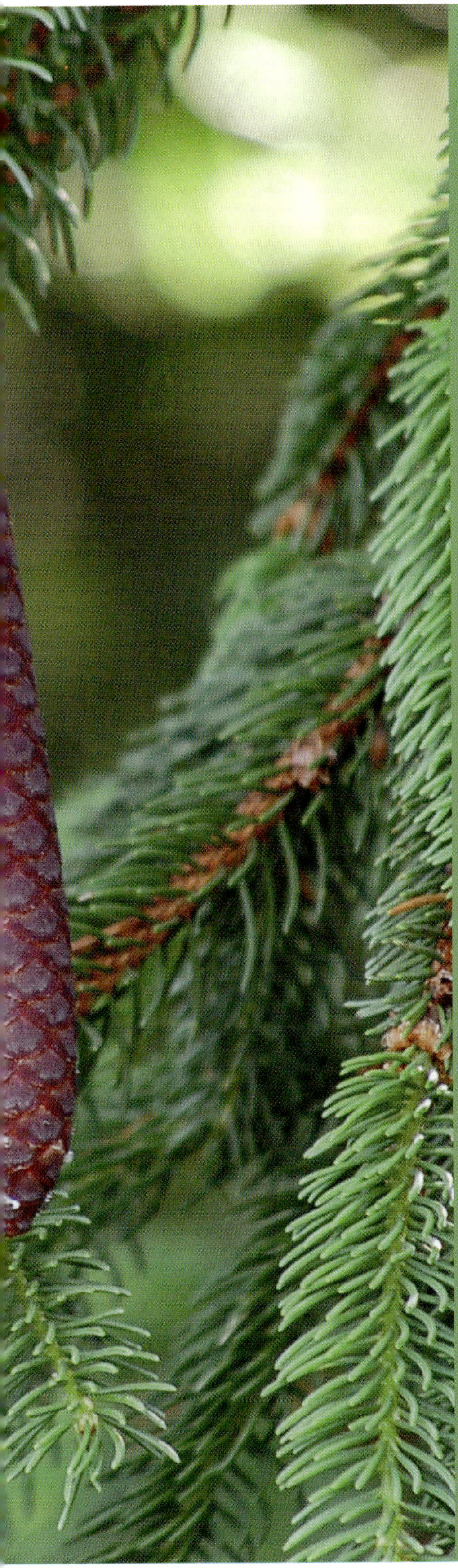

Botanisch gesehen stellen die immergrünen Pflanzen keine eigene Gruppe dar. Es sind unterschiedliche Pflanzen, mit ganz besonderen Lebens- und Erneuerungskräften: Anpassungsfähigkeit, Zähigkeit, Ausdauer sind nur ihre vordergründigen Eigenschaften, um im europäischen Alpenraum die Herausforderungen der wechselnden Jahreszeiten immergrün zu überstehen. Dahinter verbergen sich gezielte Überlebensstrategien, die jede immergrüne Pflanze für sich selbst entwickelt hat, und die das Wachstum und die Reife betreffen. Jedes Jahr pendeln diese Pflanzen so zwischen äußerstem Rückzug und vollem Wachstum, zwischen Stillstand und Aufwärtsstreben, zwischen unten und oben. So überwinden sie Jahr für Jahr extreme Polaritäten.

Immergrüne Pflanzen stehen symbolhaft für Treue und Unsterblichkeit. Ihnen werden saturnale Kräfte zugeschrieben: altes Wissen, Weisheit, die die Zeiten überdauert, Konzentration der Kräfte, sowie die Fähigkeit alles Unwesentliche los- bzw. ruhen zu lassen. Diese Bilder und Symbole brauchen wir gerade in der Winterzeit, um an ein Wiedererstarken der fruchtbaren Kräfte der Natur glauben zu können. Da stellen wir immergrüne Gestecke vor die Haustür und auf die Gräber unserer Angehörigen, winden einen immergrünen Adventkranz, holen uns den immergrünen Christbaum ins Haus. Im Winter steht in der Natur die Lebenskraft der immergrünen Pflanzen gegen die äußere Dunkelheit mit ihren Dämonen. Symbolisch stehen die Immergrünen genau auf der Schwelle zwischen Licht und Dunkelheit, zwischen Leben und Tod, während ihre Grünkraft uns wärmt.

Für jeden von uns gibt es auch Phasen von innerer Dunkelheit, die nichts mit den Jahreszeiten zu tun haben. Es sind dies Lebensabschnitte, in denen wir von Ängsten und Trauer, von Verwirrung und Niedergeschlagenheit dominiert und verunsichert werden.

Die Impulse, die diese Pflanzen im Rauch an uns weitergeben können, sind mit nichts zu vergleichen, weil sie so vielseitig und lebensbejahend sind. Sie richten uns auf, helfen uns in Zeiten der Schwäche, geben Mut und Selbstbewusstsein. Mit ihren Beispielen durchsetzungsstarker Lebensläufe sind sie oft Rettungsanker und Leuchtturm zugleich.

Buchsbaum

Lat. Name: *Buxus sempervirens*
Pflanzenfamilie: Buchsbaumgewächse

Die mächtige, jahrhundertealte Buchsbaumhecke, die das Stift St. Georgen am Längsee in Kärnten nach Westen hin umsäumt, ist nicht nur pflanzlich beeindruckend. In katholischer Lesart offenbart sie sich auch als mächtiger Schutzwall gegen jegliche Übergriffe böser Geister, die aus dem Westen kommen, jener Himmelsrichtung, in der die Sonne untergeht und aus der sich die tägliche Dunkelheit übers Land legt.

Das extrem harte Holz mit seiner eleganten, gelblichen Färbung, ist seit jeher begehrt für feinste Zier- und Gebrauchsgegenstände. Die Griechen nannten die aus diesem Holz hergestellten, seltenen Dosen „pyxos". Davon leiten sich Bezeichnungen wie Büchse oder Box ab. Auch Flöten und andere Holzblasinstrumente werden traditionell aus diesem Holz gedrechselt.

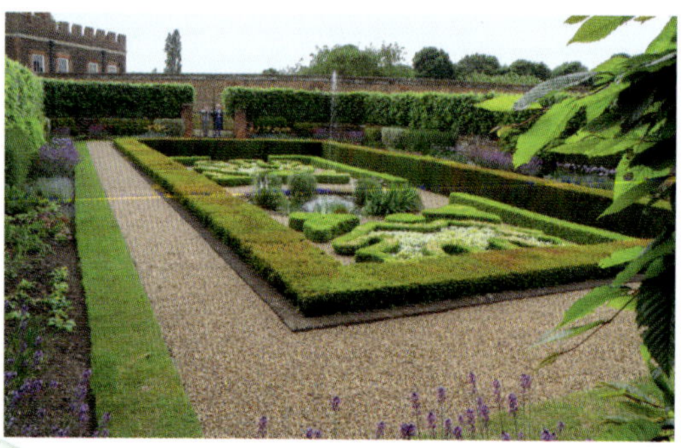

Buchsbaumhecken in Hampton Court Palace, London

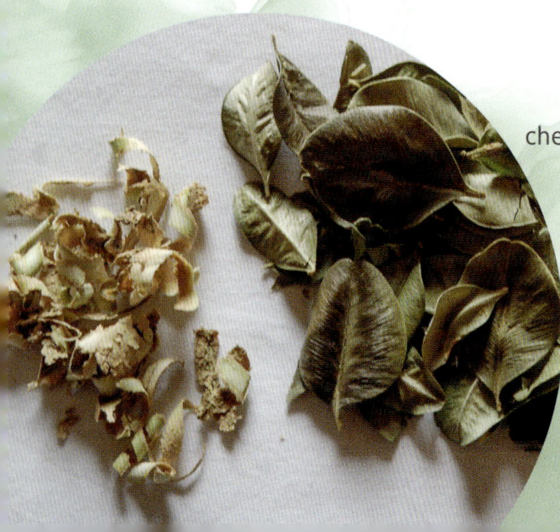

Zum Räuchern eignen sich die Blätter und die Rinde.

Der blickdichte Buchsbaum kann in Mitteleuropa im besten Fall bis zu fünf Meter hoch wachsen und mehrere hundert Jahre alt werden. Der Buchsbaum-Zünsler, ein gefürchteter Schädling, kann die Pflanze jedoch stark schädigen.

Rauch

Verwendete Pflanzenteile: Blätter, Rinde

Beste Sammel- und Erntezeit: Das ganze Jahr über.

Wirkung, Wahrnehmung: Sehr feines Aroma; nachhaltig wirkender Rauch; zum reinigenden Ausräuchern unruhiger Ecken im Wohnbereich. Abwehrrauch in geistig-seelischer Bedrängnis; eine gedankenklärende Wirkung kann meist erst Tage später auftreten, da der Rauch vordergründig als stark beruhigend und entspannend wahrgenommen wird; übergangslose, plötzliche Müdigkeit kann auftreten; die äußeren Grenzen halten Stand; Rückzug ins geschützte Innere wird möglich.

Hilfreich, um sich auf das Wesentliche zu beschränken; wenn man vor lauter Bäumen den Wald nicht mehr sieht.

Magisches zum Rauch: Als Symbol für die immer grünende Kraft des Lebens waren und sind die Buchsbaumblätter Bestandteil der Räucherungen um die Wintersonnenwende. Buchsbaumzweige, die traditionell in viele christliche Palmbuschen gebunden werden, werden mit diesen um die Weihnachtszeit verräuchert und stehen symbolisch für Standhaftigkeit, Ausdauer und Überlebenswillen.

Schwerpunkt, Anwendungen, Rezepte: Blätter und Rinde des Buchsbaumes sollten nur in geringer Menge in Räuchermischungen verwendet werden, denn sie können bei empfindlichen Menschen Kopfweh verursachen. Für Räucherungen in problembehafteten oder angstvollen Lebensphasen, wenn man nicht mehr abschalten kann, zusammen in Räuchermischungen mit anderen grenzziehenden Abwehrkräutern, wie Rainfarn, Beifuß oder Wermut, und einem Harz geeignet.

Mythologie und magische Praktiken

Für Homer ist es in seiner Ilias-Sage erwähnenswert, dass die Maultiere des König Priamos, des letzten Königs von Troja, ein Joch aus Buchsbaumholz trugen. Allein dieser, für uns wie nebensächlich klingende Hinweis, zeigt Homers perfekten Aufbau des trojanischen Dramas. Denn der Buchsbaum steht in der Antike aufgrund seines langsamen aber stetigen Wachstums für Unsterblichkeit. So wollte das trojanische Herrscherhaus gesehen werden. Unsterblich, in immergrüner Lebenskraft!

Der römische Liebesgott Amor soll nur Pfeile aus Buchsbaumholz verschossen haben, denn damit konnte er auch die Herzen jener durchbohren, die sich gegen die Liebe spreizten. Deshalb hielten die Römer den Buchsbaum für ein Symbol des Liebesschmerzes und der Liebe, die bis über den Tod hinausreicht.

Verwendung – gestern und heute

Ledrige Blätter, dicht belaubt und leicht formbar – diese Besonderheiten des Buchsbaumes inspirierten die antiken Völker rund ums Mittelmeer. Die Römer gestalteten wunderbare Beet-Einfassungen mit dem Buchsbaum. Plinius der Jüngere (61–115) schwärmt uns von seiner Villa Tusci und seinem Garten in der Toskana ausführlich vor. Dort habe er nicht nur alle möglichen Beet-Einfassungen, sondern auch Figuren aus Buchsbaum gestaltet sowie stufenartige Buchshecken als Übergang zur Landschaft außerhalb des Gartens.

Die mitteleuropäische Gartenkultur übernahm diese römischen Anregungen erst in der Renaissance (ca. 1400–1520). Ab da jedoch halten die Zierhecken aus Buchs Einzug in viele Kloster- und schließlich Bauerngärten.

Der Buchsbaum ist wegen seiner zahlreichen Alkaloide in allen Teilen giftig. In der Homöopathie werden Buchsbaum-Präparate gegen Rheuma und Altersleiden eingesetzt.

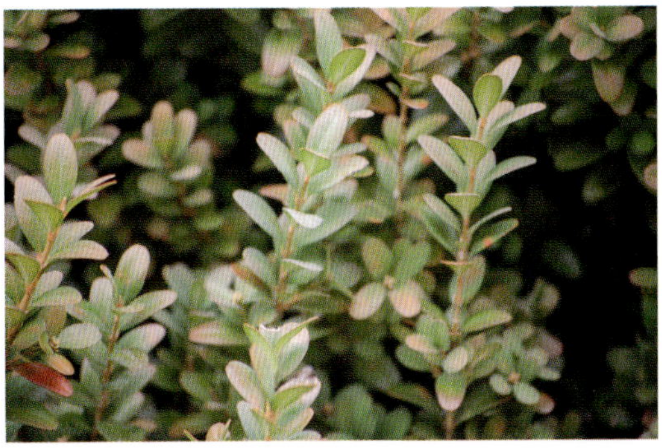

Blätter des Buchsbaums

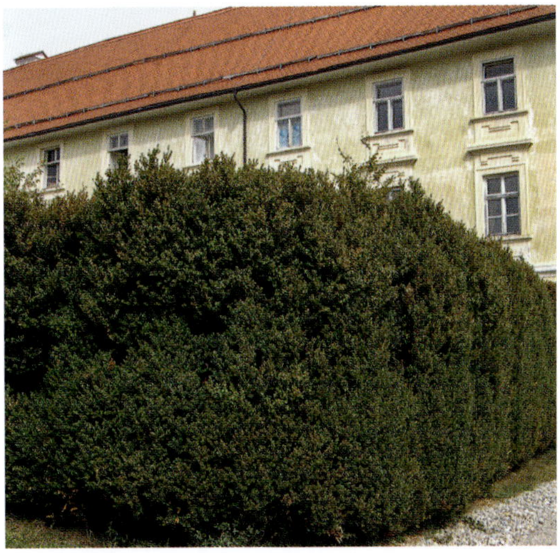

Buchsbaumhecke beim Stift St. Georgen am Längsee, Kärnten

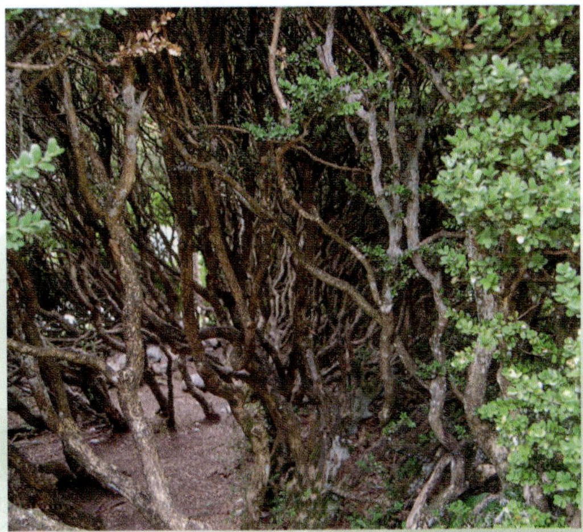

Beim Blick in die Buchsbaumhecke tritt das schöne Holz zutage.

Efeu

Lat. Name: *Hedera helix*
Botanischer Name: Gewöhnlicher Efeu
Pflanzenfamilie: Araliengewächse

Ziel dieser pflanzlichen Schlange scheint Licht und immer mehr Licht zu sein: Unaufhaltsam strebt sie aus der Tiefe nach oben. Der Efeu sucht sich ein Klettergerüst, das er zielstrebig hinaufkriecht. Es entsteht eine Nähe, die vom stützenden Baum wohl nicht gewollt ist. Obwohl der Efeu kein Schmarotzer ist, der die Rinde seiner Aufstiegshilfe mit Haftfüßchen verletzt, ist er in jedem Fall ein sehr naher Gegenspieler. Er zweigt im Wurzelbereich Wasser ab und ist im Stamm- und Kronenbereich ein lichtbeschränkender Konkurrent. Es gilt: Je schwächer der Wirtsbaum ist, desto schneller breitet sich der Efeu aus!

Die typische Suche der Efeuranken nach einem starken Partner, an den sie sich anlehnen und an dem sie emporwachsen können, wurde schon früh zum Symbol von Freundschaft, Treue und Liebe.

Als Araliengewächs vagabundiert der Efeu fernab von zu Hause. Diese Pflanzenfamilie besiedelt hauptsächlich die Südhalbkugel unserer Erde und dort eher die tropischen Gebiete. Der Efeu kann bis zu 20 Meter in die Höhe wachsen und erreicht oftmals ein Alter von mehreren hundert Jahren.

Rauch

Verwendete Pflanzenteile: Blätter.

Beste Sammel- und Erntezeit: Das ganze Jahr über.

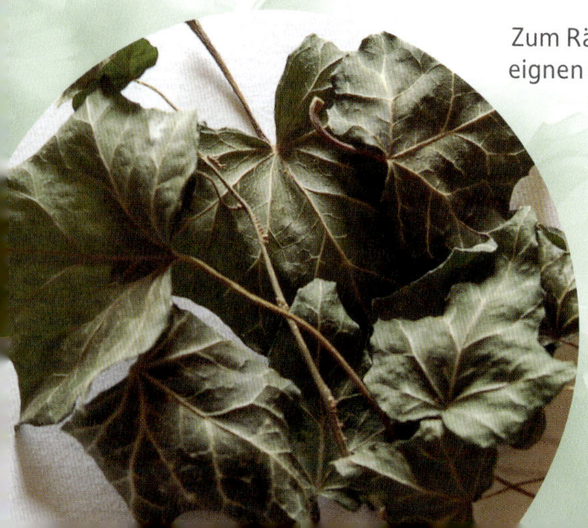

Zum Räuchern eignen sich die Blätter.

Wirkung, Wahrnehmung: Efeu kann räucherisch zu einer wichtigen Lehrerpflanze werden: Es geht um die Verbindung von Gegensätzen in uns, um leichter den eigenen Weg zu finden. Der Efeurauch vermittelt uns die Einsicht in das richtige Maß aller irdischen Beziehungen – das Festhalten und Nehmen und gleichzeitig das Loslassen und Geben.

Efeu wird im Rauch zum Schwellenhüter, der streng zwischen den Welten trennt. Efeurauch kann einen wie in Nebel einhüllen und die geistige Wahrnehmung während der Räucherung beeinflussen. Die Seelenreisen, auf die einen der Efeurauch mitnimmt, gehen immer sehr tief.

Schwerpunkt, Anwendungen, Rezepte: Efeu ist ein Symbol für ein langes Leben, für die Überwindung schlechter Zeiten durch die Kraft der lebensspendenden Sonne und gleichzeitig ein mahnendes Symbol für unsere eigene begrenzte Lebenszeit. Er wurde vielfach zu den Sonnenwenden verräuchert. Er passt gut in Räuchermischungen rund um eine Hochzeit, zusammen mit Harz und glücksbringenden Kräutern wie Fenchel, Thymian oder Vogelkirsche. Ebenso kann der Efeurauch in Abschiedszeremonien hilfreich sein, wenn es darum geht, eine Seele in aller Liebe gehen zu lassen. Hier mischt man zu den Efeublättern noch Eibe, Rosmarin und Beifußwurzel sowie Harz.

Mythologie und magische Praktiken

Im Volksglauben ist der Efeu gleichzeitig ein Glücks- wie auch ein Unglücksbringer: Efeu im Haus soll Unglück bringen und zwei Liebende würden sich trennen. Efeu im Garten oder am Haus steht für Bescheidenheit und Beständigkeit, aber auch lustvolle Geselligkeit.

Neben dem Buchsbaum ist auch der Efeu eine typische Friedhofspflanze, die von der Unsterblichkeit der Seele in Christus kündet, gleichzeitig aber auch symbolisch für die menschliche Liebe steht, die über den Tod hinausgeht. So ist wohl jene Szene aus der Geschichte von Tristan und Isolde zu deuten, in der König Marke von Cornwall die beiden Liebenden an verschiedenen Seiten der Kirche bestatten lässt, um sie auch noch im Tod zu trennen. Doch aus beiden Gräbern wachsen Efeuranken empor, die sich schließlich am Kirchendach vereinigen.

Die dreizackige saturnale Signatur hält uns unsere eigene Endlichkeit vor Augen und weist auf die zu erlangende Unsterblichkeit in Christus hin. So verwundert es nicht, dass frühe Christen auf Efeuranken aufgebahrt wurden, oder dass in den Katakomben Roms immer wieder Efeuranken in die Grababdeckungen gemeißelt wurden.

Verwendung – gestern und heute

Im europäischen Altertum war der Efeu heilig und galt sowohl bei den Griechen als auch bei den Römern als Symbolpflanze des Gottes des Weines, der Ekstase, des Wahnsinns, der Fruchtbarkeit: Dionysos und Bacchus. Man legte Efeublätter in Rotwein ein, um in den „dionysischen Wahn" zu verfallen. Dabei sorgten die giftigen Inhaltsstoffe der Efeuranken für wahnhafte Ausbrüche und ein ekstatisches Delirium, aus dem so mancher nicht mehr in die Realität zurückfand. Die solcherart Feiernden, Bacchanten genannt, bekränzten sich mit Efeuranken. Efeu ist für den Menschen in allen Teilen **giftig**. In der Homöopathie gibt es Anwendungen gegen akut entzündete Atemwege sowie gegen depressive Verstimmungen.

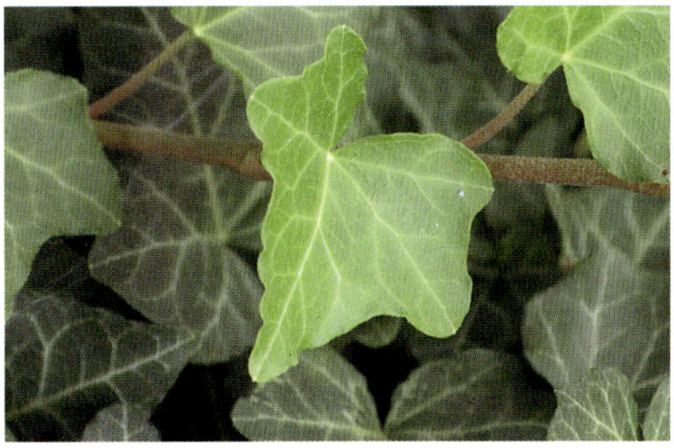

Blätter des Efeus

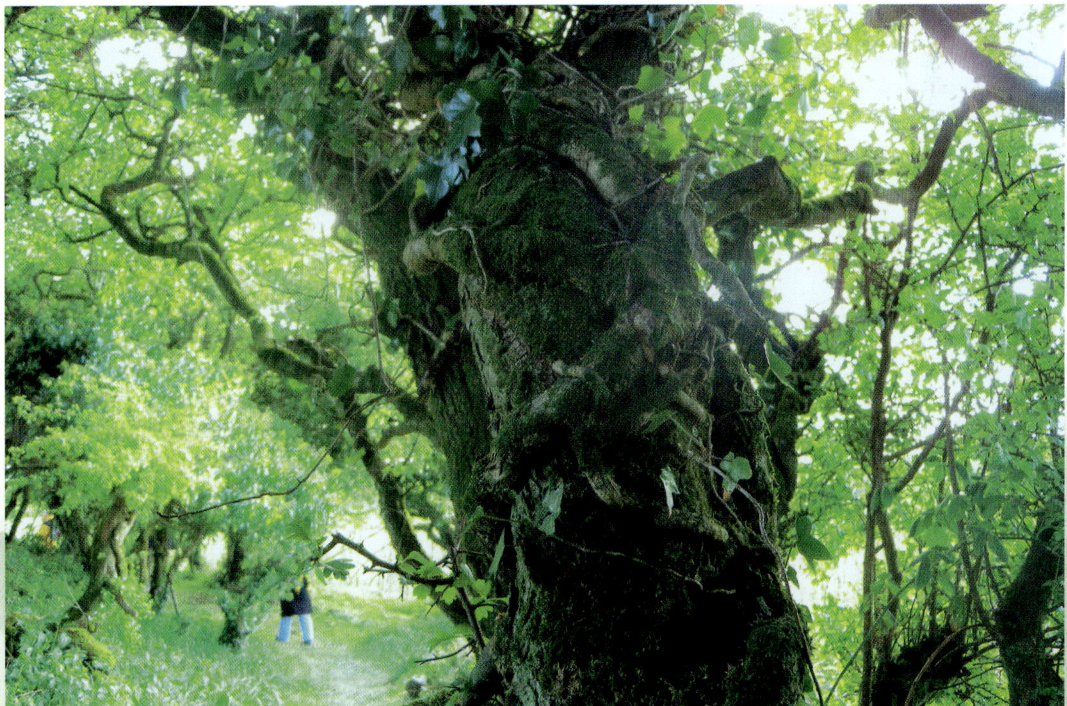

Efeuranken am Hill of Uisneach, Irland

Eibe

Lat. Name: *Taxus baccata*
Botanischer Name: Europäische Eibe
Pflanzenfamilie: Eibengewächse

Seit der Renaissance, etwa ab dem 16. Jahrhundert, wird die Eibe in herrschaftliche Gärten und Parkanlagen geholt, wo sie vor allem wegen der Formschnitte begehrt ist. Grenzenloses Staunen erfasste mich angesichts der „tanzenden" Eiben von Hampton Court in London (Foto Seite 24). Mit strenger Symmetrie in die Leichtigkeit eines üppigen Grüns eingebettet, gewaltig und leichtfüßig zugleich. Mühelos verbunden sind hier zwei Extreme.

Die Eibe ist im Unterschied zu anderen Nadelbäumen zweihäusig und harzlos, verfügt jedoch über ein sehr starkes **Gift**. Sie ist auch mit schlechten Standorten zufrieden. Weibliche Eiben tragen keine Zapfen sondern rote Früchte. Wegen ihres langsamen Wachstums kommt die Eibe heute kaum noch als mitteleuropäischer Waldbestand vor. So ist der Eibenwald von Paterzell, südlich von München in Bayern gelegen, eine echte Rarität.

Die Eibe passt sich erfolgreich an schwierige Umweltbedingungen an, hält Kälte, wochenlangen Wassermangel und wenig Sonnenlicht besser aus als alle anderen Nadelbäume. Ihr extrem langsames Wachstum lässt sie 10 bis 15 m hoch und weit über tausend Jahre alt werden.

Rauch

Verwendete Pflanzenteile: Nadeln.

Beste Sammel- und Erntezeit: Das ganze Jahr über.

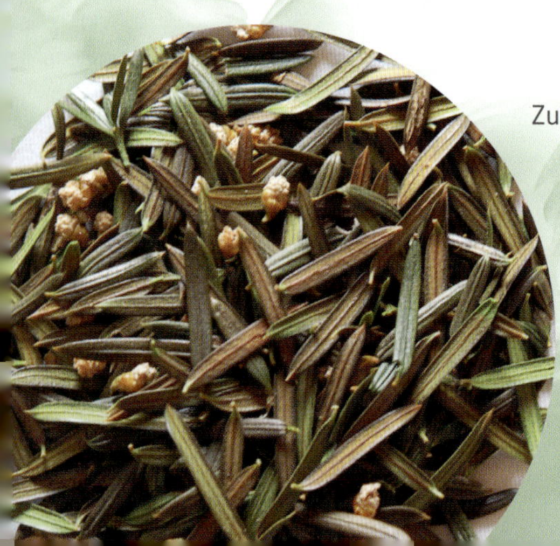

Zum Räuchern eignen sich die Nadeln.

Wirkung, Wahrnehmung: Symbol für Tod und Wiedergeburt; Ernsthaftigkeit und Vergänglichkeit; loslassen lernen; unterstützt das Sterben alter Dinge; hilft dabei Abschiede zu akzeptieren; mahnt zur Einkehr in einer lauten Zeit; schafft eine nachdenkliche Atmosphäre; konfrontiert uns mit Ohnmacht und unterdrückter Macht; Unwichtiges loslassen, sich auf das Kommende ausrichten; seine Begabungen und Talente erkennen; verhilft uns zu innerer Zufriedenheit; lehrt das Verlassen!

Wichtiger Räucherstoff für Transformationsrituale, Begleitung von Veränderungsprozessen, wenn das Alte noch zu stark anhaftet und man sich nicht im Guten lösen kann. Eibenrauch erleichtert eine Verbindung zu verstorbenen Seelen – man kann alles, was noch zu sagen bleibt, in diesen Rauch hinein loslassen.

Magisches zum Rauch: Eibenrauch soll vor Übergriffen böser Geister und anderer missgünstiger Wesen der Dunkelheit schützen.

Schwerpunkt, Anwendungen, Rezepte: Hildegard von Bingen (1098–1179) hielt den Rauch des Eibenholzes für heilsam bei Nasen- und Brustkrankheiten, „soweit sie von schlechten Säften herkommen".

Bei Abschiedsritualen werden zu den Eibennadeln noch Haselnussblütenkätzchen sowie Schlehenblüten und Harz in einer Räuchermischung vermörsert und entweder im Raum oder im Freien symbolisch in die vier Himmelsrichtungen verräuchert. Anschließend sollte man sich mit Fichtenharz freiräuchern.

Mythologie und magische Praktiken

In vielen Mythen gilt die Eibe als heiliger Baum der Toten und ist den jeweiligen Totengöttern geweiht. Sie hat eine düstere Ausstrahlung, gedeiht, auch wenn sie im Schatten steht und bringt mit ihrem Gift den sicheren Tod. Die schweigenden Eiben säumen den Weg zur Unterwelt.

Im vierten Buch von Ovids (43 v. Chr.–17 n. Chr.) „Metamorphosen" werden Menschen für die Missachtung des Bacchus-Festes bestraft: „... siehe den Weg, der sich senkt! Umdunkelt von tödlichen Eiben führt er hinab in die Tiefen der Erde durch düsteres Schweigen."

Die Warnungen vor dem Eibengift sind in der Antike allgegenwärtig: Gaius Julius Cäsar (100–44 v. Chr.) berichtet in seinem Werk „de bello gallico" (über den gallischen Krieg), dass sich der Kelten-Führer Cativulcus nach verlorenem Krieg mit Eibensaft selbst gerichtet habe. Weiters warnt der römische Dichter Vergil (70–19 v. Chr.) davor, Eiben in der Nähe von Bienenstöcken anzupflanzen. Auch solle der Wein, der aus einem Eibenbecher getrunken werde, tödlich sein.

Auch im Mittelalter waren die Menschen davon überzeugt, dass man bei einem längeren Aufenthalt unter Eiben sterben müsse. Heute weiß man, dass man danach besonders leicht einschlafen kann. Darauf bezieht sich auch William Shakespeare (1564–1616) in seinem Werk „Romeo und Julia", als er in der letzten Szene, in der Romeo stirbt, Balthasar sagen lässt: „... derweil ich unter dieser Eibe schlief, träumt ich mein Herr und noch ein anderer fechten..."

Die nordischen Mythen verehren vor allem die lebensbejahende Seite der Eibe: Sie gilt als heiliger Lebensbaum! In der Edda, der nordischen Göttersage, wird berichtet, dass der zentrale Marktplatz der Götterstadt Asgard mit Eiben umpflanzt sei. Dabei befinde sich Asgard in der Krone der Welten-Esche Yggdrasil und sei über die Regenbogenbrücke mit Midgard, der Erde, verbunden. Um diesen Bund zu stärken, fanden folgerichtig auf der Erde die entscheidenden Thingversammlungen (Volksversammlung nach germanischem Recht) unter Eiben statt.

Man fürchtete die Eibengegenden, weil dort Dämonen, Hexen und böse Geister ihre Tränke brauten und ihr Unwesen trieben. Gleichzeitig schrieb man dem Eibenholz bannende Kräfte gegen eben diese Unholde zu. Wenn man nur einen Eibenzweig auf den Weg legte, müssten alle bösen Geister umkehren.

Da dieser heilige Baum auf ganz besondere Weise mit der jenseitigen Welt in Verbindung steht, wurden aus seinem harten Holz verschiedene magische Gegenstände sowie besondere Zauberstäbe hergestellt. Denn vor Eiben kann kein böser Zauber bleiben!

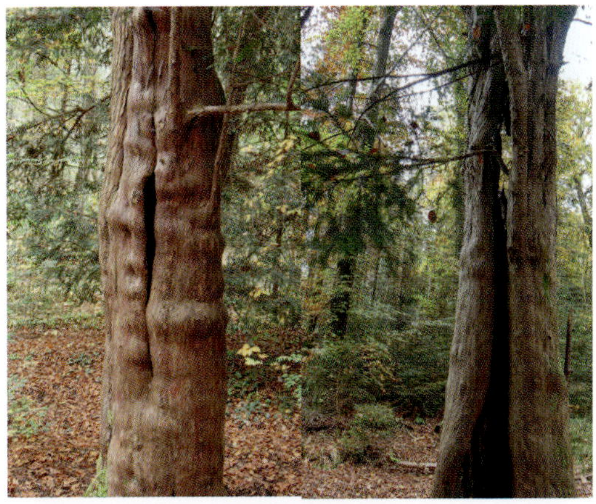

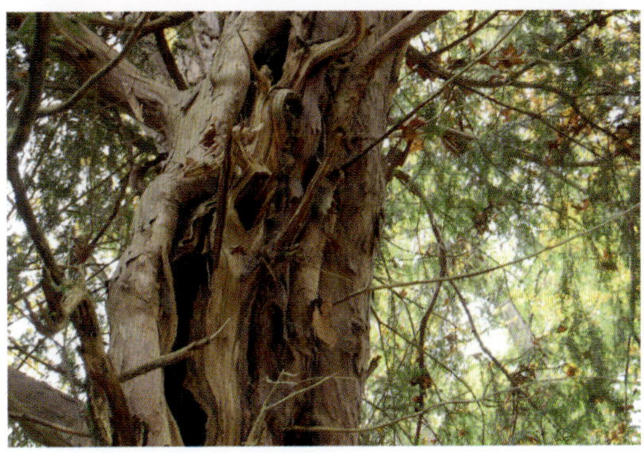

Im Eibenwald von Paterzell, Bayern

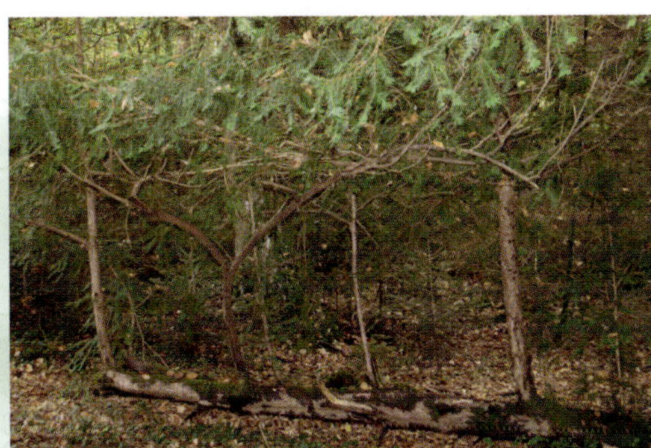

Die umgedrückte Eibe richtet ihre Zweige zu neuen Stämmen auf.

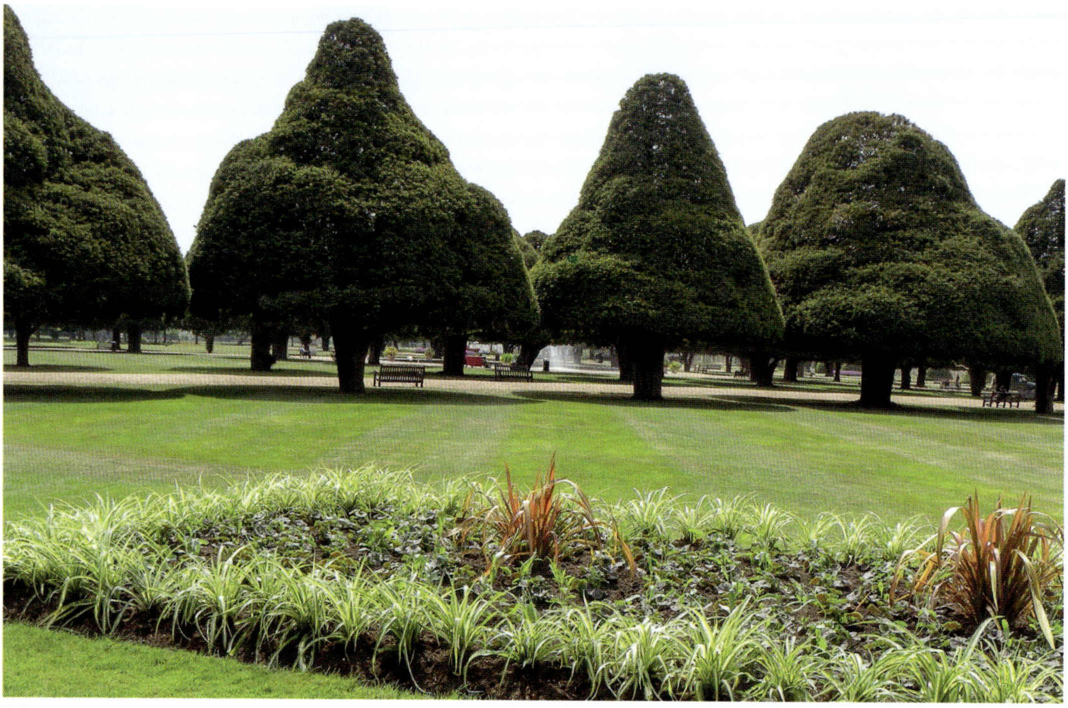

Die „tanzenden" Eiben im Park von Hampton Court Palace, London

Auf bretonischen Friedhöfen sind „les ifs", die Eiben, als stille Wesen präsent, die mit ihren Wurzeln das Reich der Toten vernetzen. Dem Volksglauben nach schützten die Friedhofseiben die Lebenden vor Wiedergängern, Untoten und vor jeder Unruhe, die aus dem Jenseits zurück in diese Welt zu dringen suchte. Das wollte man mit Eibenzweigen im Totentuch oder Eibenkränzen am Grab verhindern.

Verwendung – gestern und heute

Die Härte des Eibenholzes bei gleichzeitig großer Biegsamkeit ist ideal für die Herstellung von Pfeilen und Jagdbögen. Das erkannten und nutzten bereits die Menschen der Steinzeit, wie uns Ötzis Eibenbogen beweist. Immerhin hat der Mann aus dem Eis vor mehr als 5000 Jahren gelebt. Funde aus der jüngeren Steinzeit (um 3800 v. Chr.) an den Pfahlbauten am Mondsee in Oberösterreich belegen, dass schon sehr früh Gebrauchsgegenstände, wie Webschiffchen oder Kämme, aus Eibenholz hergestellt wurden. Die Kelten kochten aus den Eibennadeln ein starkes Nervengift, mit dem sie ihre Pfeilspitzen einrieben und tränkten. Im Mittelalter wurden Eibenwälder rund um Burgen angepflanzt, um das passende Holz für die besten Kriegsbögen nahe und unter Kontrolle zu haben.

Bis auf die roten Früchte sind alle Teile der Eibe tödlich **giftig**. Auch der schwarze Samen, der in jeder Frucht steckt ist giftig!

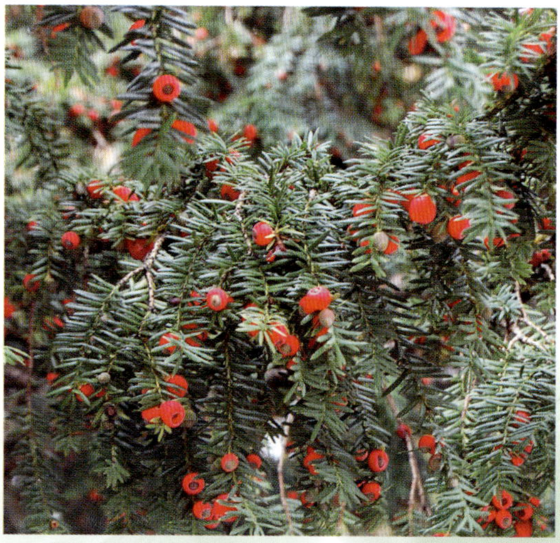

Die Eibe im Klosterhof von Wessobrunn in Bayern trägt besonders viele rote Früchte.

Fichte

Lat. Name: *Picea abies*
Botanischer Name: Gemeine Fichte
Pflanzenfamilie: Kieferngewächse

In Laastadt hinter Arriach, Kärnten, steht eine siebenwipfelige Kandelaber-Fichte, die um das Jahr 1518 (+/– 50 Jahre) gepflanzt wurde und derzeit wohl Österreichs älteste Fichte ist.

Die Kärntner „Feichtn“ prägt unser heimatliches Landschaftsbild und unser Wald-Verständnis bis heute. Doch die Folgen der menschlichen Massen-Baumhaltung treiben die heimischen Fichten zunehmend in die Krise. Aus dem Schutzbaum, der für viele Tiere nahrhaft ist und für Menschen ein breites heilsames Potenzial bietet, wurde in den letzten hundert Jahren ein reines Wirtschaftsholz. Aufgrund seiner Eigenschaften – geringes Gewicht und große Elastizität – eignet sich das Fichtenholz sowohl zur Papierherstellung, als Bauholz, für Spanplatten, als auch als Brennholz. Fichtenholz war für Waldbesitzer somit Garant für ein gutes Einkommen, was zur Aufforstung von Fichtenwald-Monokulturen führte. In Zeiten des Klimawandels schwächen längere Trockenphasen die feuchtigkeitsliebende Fichte immer mehr, sodass der Schädlingsbefall durch den Borkenkäfer mittlerweile in vielen Gebieten bestandsbedrohende Ausmaße angenommen hat. Orkanartige Winterstürme haben zudem im letzten Jahrzehnt in Kärnten und darüber hinaus enorme Fichtenbestände vernichtet. Dazu passt der Ausspruch eines deutschen Försters aus dem 19. Jahrhundert: „Willst du deinen Wald vernichten, pflanze Fichten, Fichten, Fichten!“ Damit wandte er sich damals gegen die Anlage von Fichten-Monokulturen im Tal, denn Fichten sind Kinder der Berge, die sich erst ab 900 m Seehöhe wohlfühlen.

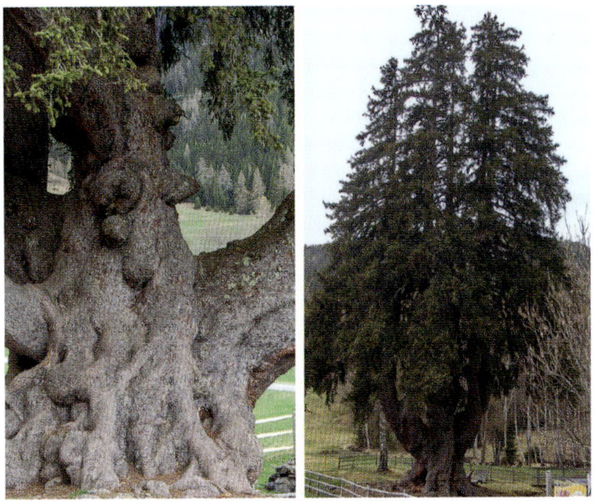

Siebenwipfelige Kandelaber-Fichte in Laastadt, Kärnten

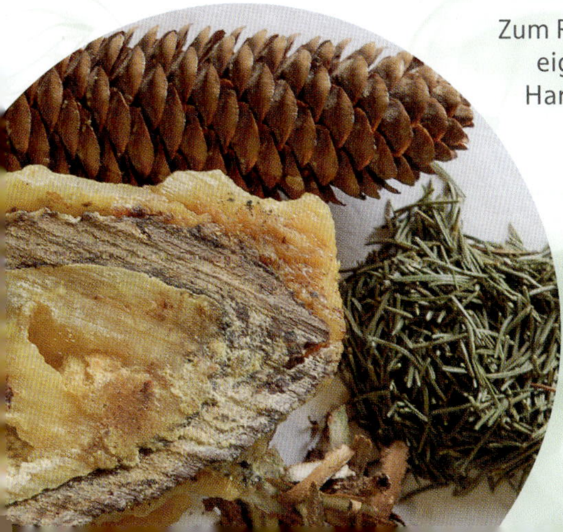

Zum Räuchern eignen sich Harz, Rinde, Nadeln, Zapfen und Samen.

Die Fichte ist ein sehr sensibles Wesen. Ihre Rinde kann sehr leicht verletzt werden und dann rinnen schier unaufhaltsam dicke Pechtränen den Stamm hinunter. Die Fichte ist buchstäblich „nahe am Wasser gebaut“. Sie trägt ihren Schmerz nach außen, hält nichts im Inneren zurück. Ihr Mut gründet in ihren frühen Jahren, denn sie keimt und wächst am liebsten auf dem Totholz ihrer Vorfahren. Dabei senken die Fichtenkinder ihre Wurzeln direkt durch das Holz der Vorgänger. Vom Wurzelcharakter her ist die Fichte flach verankert und hält sich in einem großen Kreis um den Stamm im Boden fest. In Hanglagen kann es schon einmal vorkommen, dass ihre kräftigen Wurzeln krampfaderartig am Waldboden zu Tage treten, um das Gleichgewicht besser ausbalancieren zu können.

Fichten werden bis zu 50 m, in manchen Lagen sogar bis zu 70 m hoch und erreichen ein Alter von mehreren hundert Jahren. Aufgrund der intensiven Fichtenholz-Nutzung erreichen die Bäume bei uns eine Höhe von etwa 35 m und ein Alter von kaum hundert Jahren.

Rauch

Verwendete Pflanzenteile: Harz, Rinde von Ästen, Fichtennadeln, Fichtenzapfen und -samen.

Beste Sammel- und Erntezeit: Das ganze Jahr über.

Wirkung, Wahrnehmung: Fichtenharz ist DAS heimische Räucherharz, universell einsetzbar, Waldweihrauch. Die Duftwahrnehmung reicht von angenehm süßlich bis beißend scharf, abhängig vom Trockengrad des Harzes. Die Fichte ist ein Baum des äußeren und inneren Winters, der für Durchhalten, Überleben und Rückzug auf das Wesentliche steht. Wirkt allgemein kräftigend, belebend, aufrichtend.

Wirkung im Außen: Reinigung und Klärung der Raumatmosphäre von alten Anhaftungen; überlagert zuverlässig negative Energien und Hinterlassenschaften in Räumen, unter Schreibtischen, in Schlafzimmern und hinterlässt ein ausgeglichenes Raumklima. Davon könnten auch Kindergärten, Schulklassen, Universitäten, Gerichtssäle usw. profitieren! Die Fichtenharz-Räucherung wirkt zusätzlich keimtötend und desinfizierend.

Wirkung im Inneren: Stärkt die Körper-Geist-Seele-Einheit; steigert die geistige Aufmerksamkeit und Konzentrationsfähigkeit; vertreibt dunkle, zornige Stimmungen; Seelenbalsam; erdet augenblicklich und richtet innerlich auf; hilft Ruhe zu finden; vermittelt Geborgenheit im Hier und Jetzt; hilft emotionale Wunden, die immer wieder aufbrechen, zu heilen.

Magisches zum Rauch: In der Ausgabe des Naturwissenschaftlichen Vereins für Kärnten „Carinthia II, Jahrgang 128“ aus dem Jahr 1938 wird ein Heilrauch aus einem „Pilfasknopf“ beschrieben. In der Gegend um Ebene Reichenau werde als Pilfas ein gebrochener, dann aber verknorpelt weitergewachsener Fichtenast bezeichnet. Ein „Pilfasknopf“ sei dabei die verdickte, weil verwachsene Stelle: „... der Pilfasknopf wird auch zerstoßen, das Pulver auf gesalzene Glut gestreut und damit die schmerzhaften Körperteile beräuchert. Eine Verbesserung dieses Räuchermittels besteht darin, dass man dem Pilfaspulver ein Gemenge von gedörrter, dann gemahlener Fichtenrinde, Almengras, Kardobenediktenkraut, Hanfsamen, Myrrhe, Harzkörnchen aus einem Ameisenhaufen*, Weizenmehl und Zucker beifügt.“

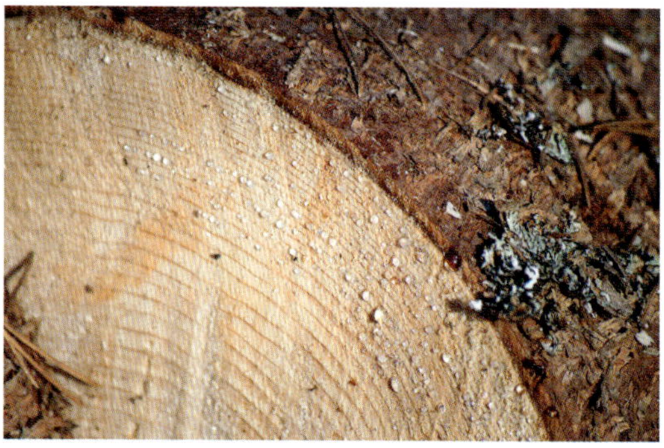
Fichtenholz

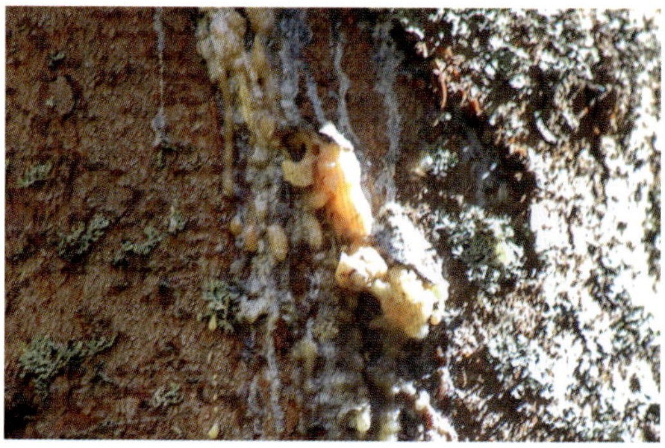
Fichtenharz

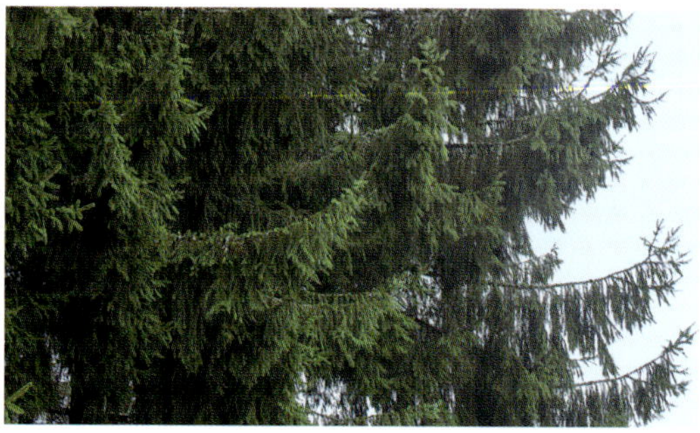
Fichtenzweige

** Wird Fichtenharz für ein paar Tage in die obere Schicht eines Ameisenhaufens gegeben, bewirkt die Ameisensäure einen Umwandlungsprozess, was zur Verfeinerung des Harzes führt. Die Räucherung mit einem solchermaßen behandelten Harz wird als balsamisch und weich empfunden.*

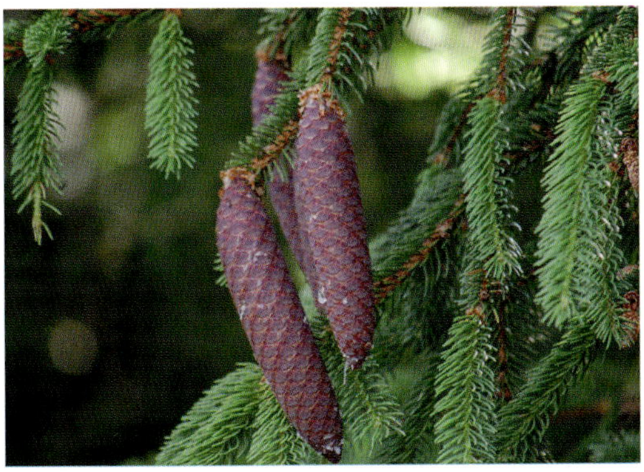

Frischer Fichtenzapfen

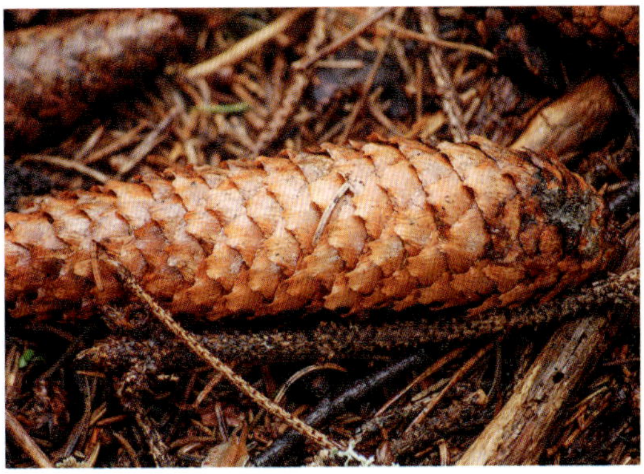

Fichtenzapfen getrocknet

Schwerpunkt, Anwendungen, Rezepte: Alle Bestandteile der Fichte wurden jahrhundertelang für körperlich heilsames Abräuchern bei Atemwegserkrankungen mit Ameisenharz, bei rheumatischen Beschwerden sowie bei verschiedenen Hautleiden verwendet.

Fichtenharz ist der heimische Weihrauch, der zu sämtlichen Räuchermischungen anstelle fremdländischer Harze genommen werden kann. Wichtig dabei ist, dass das Fichtenharz einigermaßen trocken ist. Das kann in unseren Wäldern sehr lange dauern. Durch und durch getrocknetes Fichtenharz hat eine hellgelbe Farbe und verglüht sehr rasch. Je feuchter das Harz ist, umso mehr Rauch entwickelt es auf der Räucherkohle. Das hat zwei Nachteile: Erstens kann es einen Hustenreiz auslösen. Dann sollte man sofort das Fenster öffnen und die Räucherschale ins Freie stellen. Zweitens beschlägt der Rauch von feuchtem Harz Fenster, Vorhänge und Wände mit einer mattierenden feinen Schicht. Es ist zu empfehlen, feuchtes Fichtenharz aus eigener Sammlung überwiegend im Freien zu verräuchern.

Mythologie und magische Praktiken

Wegen ihres kerzengeraden hohen Wuchses sahen unsere Vorfahren in der Fichte einen Mutter- und Schutzbaum, der die himmlische mit der irdischen Lebenskraft verbindet. So wurden im nordischen Brauchtum Fichtenfeste gefeiert, ähnlich den Birkenfesten, wobei geschlägerte Fichten zum Schutz in die Dörfer gebracht wurden. Auch heutzutage sind die allermeisten Maibäume Fichten!

Plinius der Jüngere (61 bis etwa 113) schreibt, dass nach dem Vesuvausbruch in Pompeij, 79 n. Chr., rund um die verwüsteten Gebiete Fichtenzweige als Zeichen der Trauer auf Türen gegeben wurden. Wilhelm Pelikan (1893–1981) meint, dass die Fichte im Unterschied zur Tanne eine besondere Erdenschwere besitze, die keine Misteln aufkommen lasse. In der Walpurgisnacht wurden in manchen Gegenden Fichtenzweige in den Misthaufen gesteckt, um Hexen und böse Geister vom Stall fernzuhalten.

Verwendung – gestern und heute

Hildegard von Bingen (1098–1179) war überzeugt, dass Fichten menschliche Krankheiten übernehmen könnten. Noch in der frühen Neuzeit versuchte man Gicht und andere körperliche Beschwerden mit entsprechenden Einritzungen und magischen Formeln oder Gebeten hinter die Fichtenrinde zu bannen!

Aus den Fichtensprossen wird traditionell eine Einreibung angesetzt, die gegen Gelenkschmerzen helfen soll. Der allseits bekannte Fichtenwipfel-Sirup kommt noch heute in vielen Familien bei Erkältungen und Husten zum Einsatz. Die jungen getrockneten Fichtennadeln ergeben einen nervenberuhigenden und schlaffördernden Duftpolster. Nicht zu vergessen die alte Pech-Salbe aus Fichtenharz, die im Alpenraum universell eingesetzt wird.

Heidekraut

Lat. Name: *Calluna vulgaris*
Pflanzenfamilie: Heidekrautgewächse

„Es ist kaum ein Gewächs in teütschen Landen, das die Biene lieber besucht als eben die blühende Heiden im Augustmonat ..." beginnt Hieronymus Bock (1498–1554) seine Beschreibung des Heidekrauts.

Der genügsame Zwergstrauch erfreut jeden Betrachter mit seiner zart-rosa Färbung vom Ende des Sommers bis weit in den Herbst hinein. Sein chaotischer Wuchs hilft ihm sich gegen Schnee und Kälte zu wappnen und sich an lichten Stellen des Waldes auszubreiten. Nach dem Motto „klein, aber oho" kann die Besenheide bis zu 30 cm hoch und 40 Jahre alt werden.

Rauch

Verwendete Pflanzenteile: Das blühende Kraut.

Beste Sammel- und Erntezeit: Ab August bis Oktober, in höheren Lagen oft bis Dezember.

Wirkung, Wahrnehmung: Stark reinigender und abwehrender Rauch nach außen und Seelentröster nach innen. Zur Abwehr von Unheil und Verwünschungen. Unterstützt das Durchhalten in schwierigen Phasen; fördert die gedankliche Beweglichkeit; positiv polend. Guter Weggefährte, wenn es um Veränderungen im Leben geht; hilfreich, um Dinge zu erkennen und bei der Auflösung von Täuschungen; hilft uns, zu biegen nicht zu brechen; Überlebenskräfte werden gestärkt, die geistige Abwehr wird mobilisiert. Hilft beim Loslassen.

Der Heidekrautrauch schützt vor seelisch-geistigen Vereinnahmungen. In diesem Rauch kann man kurz zur Ruhe kommen und Berufungen abwehren.

Magisches zum Rauch: Die besondere Kraft der Besenheide zeigt sich beim Ausräuchern von Vorratskellern und Viehställen: Die Vorräte bleiben länger frisch und die Kühe bleiben – im Gegensatz zu anderen Räucherstoffen – ruhig und geben mehr Milch. Als Wetterkraut wurde Heidekraut in das Herdfeuer gegeben oder die abgerebelten kleinen Blüten und Blätter auf die Herdplatte gestreut, um Blitz und Hagelschlag fernzuhalten.

Schwerpunkt, Anwendungen, Rezepte: Für glücksbringende Räucherungen wird die Besenheide mit Thymian, Fenchel und Tannennadeln sowie Harz gemischt.

Mythologie und magische Praktiken

Die Schutz- und Abwehrkraft, die diesem Strauch zugeschrieben wurde, zeigt sich in unterschiedlichen Formen: So verwehren Kränze aus Heidekraut an der Haustür allem Bösen den Eintritt; Heidekrautbüschel, die im Haus hinter Spiegel gesteckt wurden, schützten das Haus vor jedem Unwetter.

Aus der deutschen Heidelandschaft mit ihren großen Steinfindlingen und Wacholdersträuchern kommt die Sage, dass unter der Besenheide die Opfer großer Schlachten lägen, deren Blut die Heide rot gefärbt hätte.

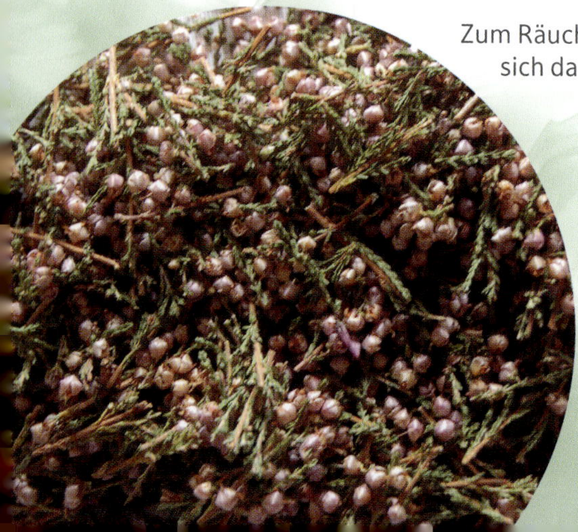

Zum Räuchern eignet sich das blühende Kraut.

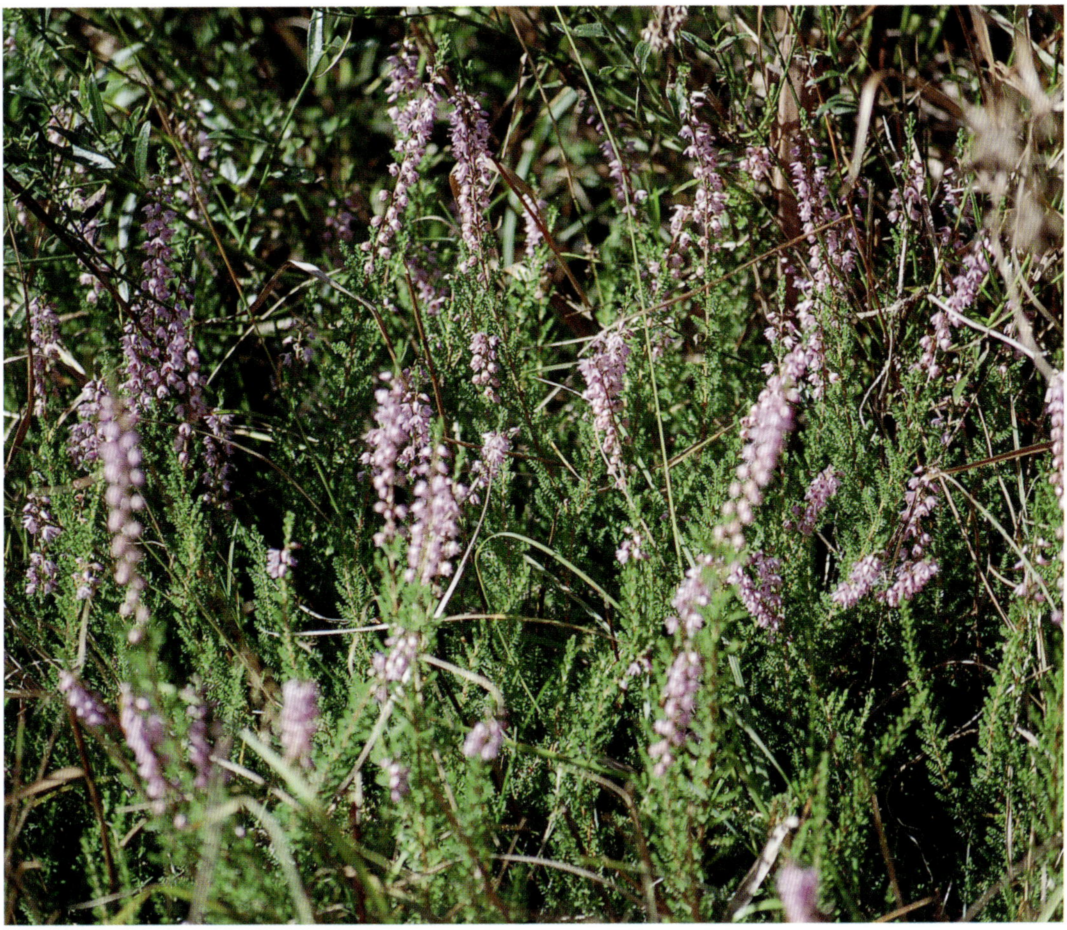

Heidekraut ist auch als Besenheide bekannt.

Verwendung – gestern und heute

Die Besenheide wurde wegen ihres störrisch sperrigen Wuchses zum namensgebenden Besen binden verwendet. Wer einmal versucht hat, eine Besenheide mit der Hand zu pflücken, weiß danach, was Zähigkeit bedeutet.

Die Bachblüte Nr. 14 „heather" – Heidekraut – hilft Menschen, die sich unentwegt mit sich selbst beschäftigen und immer im Mittelpunkt stehen wollen. Sie soll zu mehr Einfühlungsvermögen und Verständnis für andere führen.

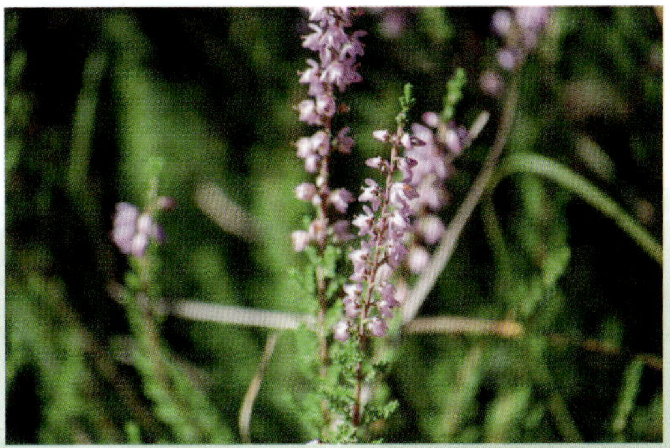

Blütenstand von Heidekraut

Kleines Immergrün

Lat. Name: *Vinca minor*
Pflanzenfamilie: Hundsgiftgewächse

Das wichtige antike Heilkraut mit den glänzenden Blättern und den stahlblauen, windradähnlichen Blüten ist heute als **giftig** eingestuft und führt so ein bescheidenes Dasein als immergrüner Bodendecker und als Friedhofspflanze. Es ist ein Kulturfolger alter Siedlungen und Burgen. So findet man es sporadisch auch in heutigen Waldbereichen, die in früheren Zeiten bewohnt gewesen sein mussten.

Die äußerst robuste langlebige Pflanze wird als kriechendes Wesen bis zu 15 cm hoch und kann Stängelausläufer von bis zu 75 cm ausbilden.

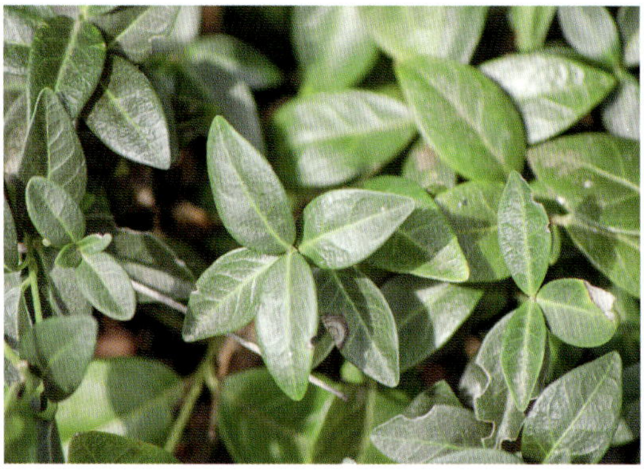

Blätter des Kleinen Immergrün

Rauch

Verwendete Pflanzenteile: Blätter, Stängel, Blüten.

Beste Sammel- und Erntezeit: Die Blätter ganzjährig, die Blüten ab März, oft bis in den Sommer hinein.

Wirkung, Wahrnehmung: Sinnbild des ewigen Kreislaufs von Vergehen und Werden, von Tod und Wiedergeburt; stärkt die Lebenskraft und vor allem den Überlebenswillen; trägt bei innerer Verunsicherung zur Beruhigung bei; stabilisiert die Körper-Geist-Seele-Einheit.

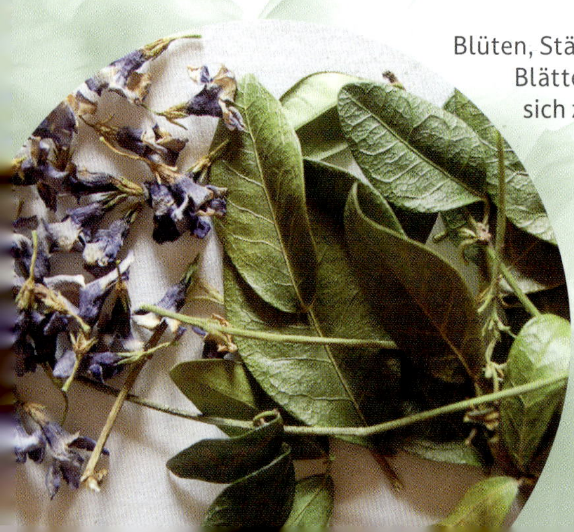

Blüten, Stängel und Blätter eignen sich zum Räuchern.

Magisches zum Rauch: Am Palmsonntag verräucherte Immergrün-Blätter sollen Kinder vor bösen Zaubern und Krankheitsgeistern schützen.

Schwerpunkt, Anwendungen, Rezepte: Wird in den Raunächten als Zeichen des grünenden Lebens in dunkler Zeit mit anderen immergrünen Räucherstoffen in Kombination mit Harz verräuchert.

Mythologie und magische Praktiken

Im Mittelalter traute man dem Immergrün zu, dass es vor Verhexungen und bösen Zaubern schützen könne. Kleine Kränze aus Immergrün wurden an Haus- und Stalltüren befestigt, um vor Blitzschlag und Unwetter zu schützen. Solche Kränze wurden auch Verstorbenen in den Sarg mitgegeben. Ein Kranz aus Immergrün zierte oft den Kopf der Braut, um die Kraft des Lebens zu symbolisieren und sie gleichsam unter den Schutz der wohlwollenden Kräfte der Natur zu stellen. Auch Wilderer vertrauten der Kraft des Immergrüns, wenn sie es in der Johannisnacht (24. Juni) ernteten, zusammen mit Eberraute in Essig auskochten und damit ihre Flinte säuberten, damit kein Schuss daneben gehe.

Verwendung – gestern und heute

Mit kleinen Kränzen aus Immergrün, die die Kraft der Wiedergeburt des Lebens symbolisieren sollten, schmückten die Römer ihre Toten. In Süd- und Mitteleuropa ist das Kleine Immergrün bis heute eine anspruchslose Friedhofspflanze.

Hieronymus Bock (1498–1554) empfiehlt trüben Wein damit zu klären: „So jemands trüben Wein hette, der neme des Krauts wenig oder vil, nach dem des Weins vil oder wenig ist, und leg das Kraut darein, schlag das Vaß zu, auff vierzehen Tag also gelegen, der Wein würt inn kurtzer Zeit schön lautter und hell."

Die Pflanze ist in allen Teilen **giftig**. Es gibt homöopathische Präparate aus dem Kleinen Immergrün.

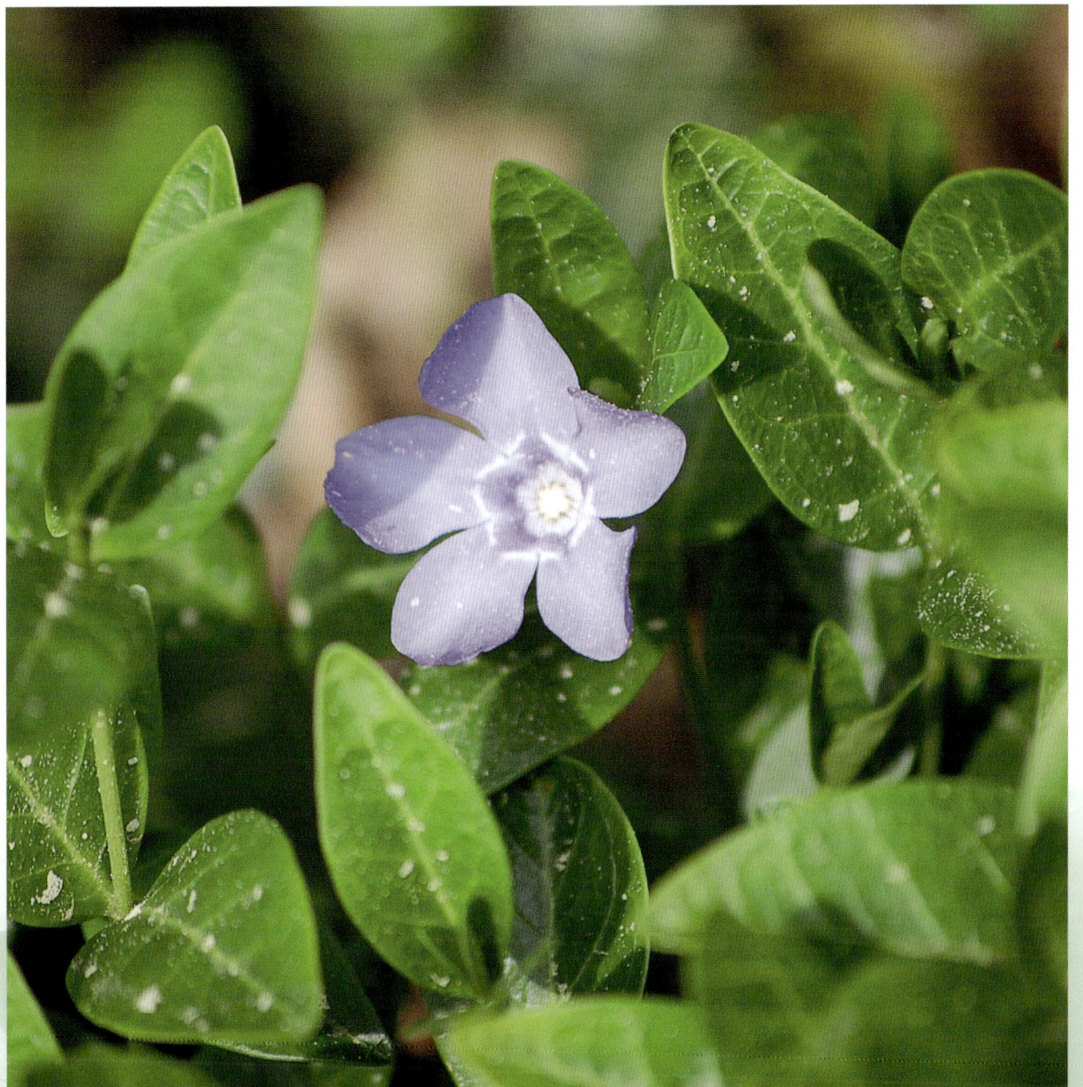

Blüte des Kleinen Immergrün

Kiefer

Lat. Name: *Pinus sylvestris*
Botanischer Name: Rot-Föhre
Pflanzenfamilie: Kieferngewächse

Meine lustige Kiefer steht zwischen Haselnuss, Weißdorn, Pfaffenhut und Birken am Rain. Sie ist der einzige Nadelbaum weit und breit, hat genügend Platz, Licht und Wasser und dennoch wächst sie nicht gerade, sondern macht alle möglichen Verrenkungen. In einem Jahr schießt sie voll Überschwang nach oben, doch ihre Krone, ihre Äste sind nicht stabil genug und verformen sich schon unter geringer Schneelast. Dann spaltet sie sich, macht plötzlich zwei Wipfel. Sie liebt es sich im Wachstum auszuprobieren und irgendwie scheint sie sich zu langweilen, so alleine am Rain. Ganz anders das Bild unter Kiefern im Wald – sie stützen und befeuern sich gegenseitig im Wachstum und ziehen meist so kerzengerade in die Höhe wie die Fichten.

Die Kiefer ist wohl die wichtigste Baumart der europäischen Forstwirtschaft. Zum einen liefert sie das meiste Bauholz, zum anderen gilt sie als Zukunftsbaum im Klimawandel. Sie ist anspruchslos, weitgehend schädlingsresistent und hat eine hohe Toleranz gegen Kälte, Trockenheit, Hitze und Umweltverschmutzung. Dabei kommt ihr ihre grobe, bei älteren Bäumen sich oft mehrfach überlagernde Borkenschicht zugute. Da kommt kein Tropfen Harz durch. Die Kiefer harzt nach innen, was das Holz in den vergangenen Jahrhunderten zum begehrten Feuerholz gemacht hat. Nicht zu vergessen die unverzichtbaren Kienspäne und Kiefernfackeln, die Burgen und Klöster schummrig erhellten. Kiefern besitzen eine vielfältige Heilkraft, aber auch die Kraft zur Umwandlung: Sie transformieren selbst karge Schotterböden in luftig heitere Kiefernwälder. Dabei werden sie bis 40 m hoch und können einige hundert Jahre alt werden.

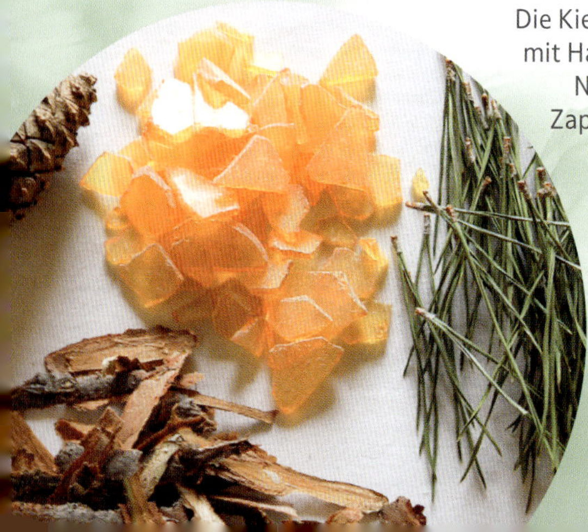

Die Kiefer liefert mit Harz, Rinde, Nadeln und Zapfen gleich mehrere Räucherausgangsstoffe.

Rauch

Verwendete Pflanzenteile: Harz, Rinde, Nadeln, Zapfen.

Beste Sammel- und Erntezeit: Nadeln, Rinde und Zapfen das ganze Jahr über; Kiefernharz selbst wird flüssig aus dem angebohrten Baumstamm gewonnen und für den Handel künstlich getrocknet.

Wirkung, Wahrnehmung: Starke Abwehrkraft, wichtigster heimischer Räucherstoff gegen Mobbing und alle geistigen Übergriffe. Mächtige Schutzkraft gegen Berufungen, Verwünschungen und krankmachende Praktiken durch andere. Bringt Ruhe für überstresste Rastlose; Geist und Seele können wieder Einklang finden; wirkt nachhaltig angstlösend und nervenberuhigend.

Vertreibt Trauer und Niedergeschlagenheit; besänftigt verletzte Seelen; eine Überwindung der belasteten Phase im Guten erscheint möglich.

Mit seiner wärmenden Wirkung stärkt eine Kiefernräucherung die Ausdauer bei extremen Belastungen. Macht Erholung und Stärkung möglich.

Magisches zum Rauch: Schwächliche Kinder wurden in einen Rauch aus Kiefernzapfen gestellt, um positive Energie auf sie zu übertragen. Kiefernnadeln wurden als wirkungsvoller Schutz gegen jede Art von Hexerei geräuchert und um negative Energien, Flüche und Dämonen zu bannen.

Schwerpunkt, Anwendungen, Rezepte: Lange Zeit wurde mit Kiefernharz bei Erkältungen und Husten geräuchert. Auch schmerzende Gelenke und gichtgeplagte Körperteile hielten unsere Vorfahren in den Rauch von Kiefernharz und -zapfen.

Mythologie und magische Praktiken

Die Kiefernzweige im winterlichen Gesteck vor der Haustür sind der eigentliche Schutz gegen alles Ungemach! Hier spürt man das schutzgebende Wesen, die machtvolle Verteidigerin. Das zeigt die Kiefer auch durch ihren Bezug zur Zahl fünf, der magischen Abwehrzahl, der Drudenfuß: Im Wachstum schiebt sich die Kiefer jährlich um ein Stockwerk mit fünf Trieben nach oben. Diese bilden sich weiter aus zu Ästen, von denen jeder jährlich wiederum fünf Zweige wachsen lässt.

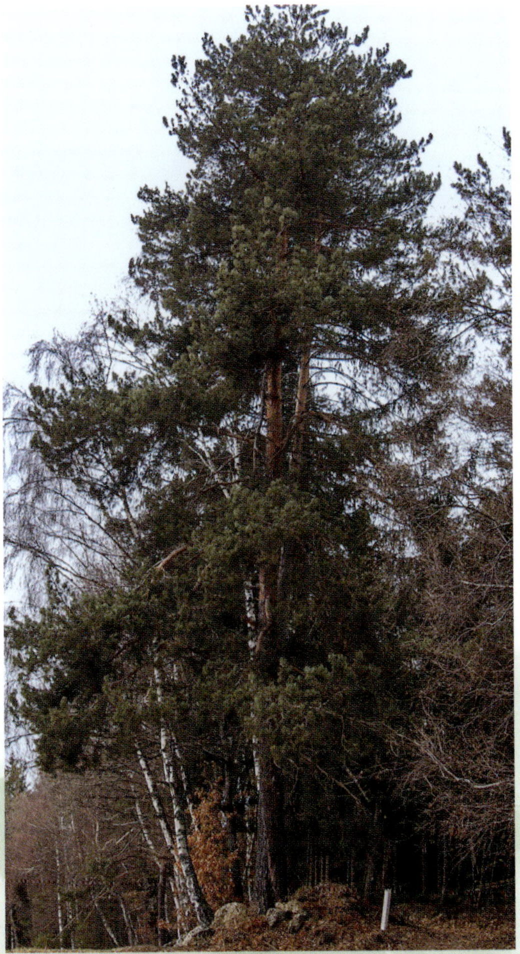

Kiefern erreichen eine stattliche Größe.

Verwendung – gestern und heute

Das alte Licht: Jahrhundertelang sorgten Kiefernfackeln für Licht in den menschlichen Behausungen.

Die Harzung, das Anbohren der Bäume, wird ab einem Baumalter von 90 bis 120 Jahren durchgeführt. Die Bäume können dann 30 bis 40 Jahre lang gepecht werden. Aus dem Kiefernharz werden die Rohstoffe Terpentinöl und Kolophonium mittels Wasserdampfdestillation gewonnen. Terpentinöl dient zur Herstellung und Verarbei-

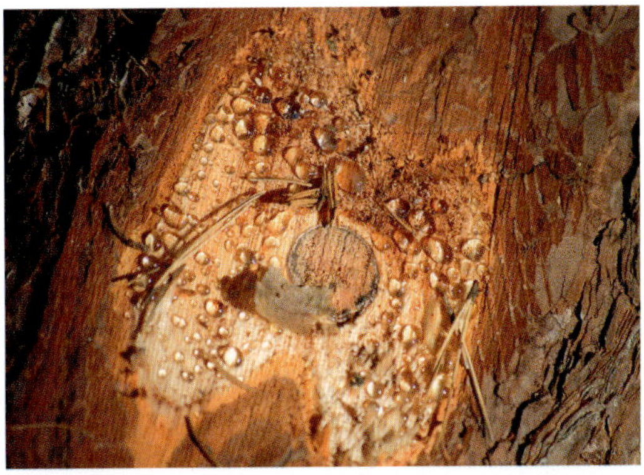

Das Harz der Kiefer ist unter der schuppigen Borke verborgen.

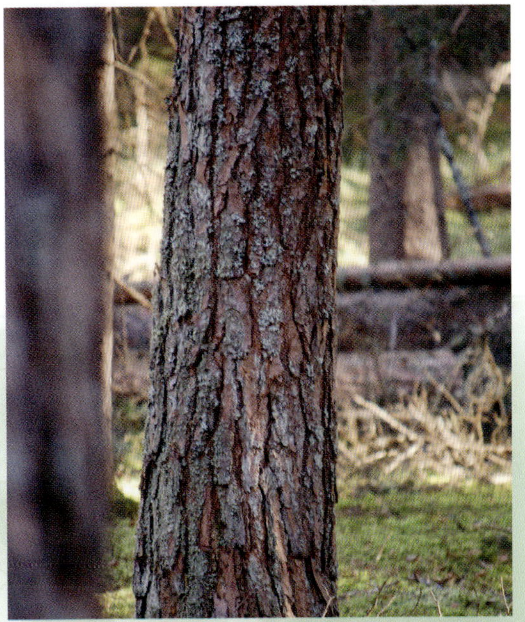

Die Rinde der Kiefer ist rötlich-braun.

tung von Farben und Lacken und wird auch in der Pharmaindustrie verwendet. Kolophonium nennt man die festen Bestandteile des Kiefernharzes, die glasartig und leicht brüchig im gepressten Zustand gehandelt werden. Kolophonium ist vor allem als Geigenharz bekannt. Mit siedendem Kiefernpech wurden Weinfässer ausgepicht. In Kärnten ist es als „Saupech" bekannt, das früher bei der Schlachtung von Schweinen zum äußeren Enthaaren eingesetzt wurde.

Bachblüte Nr. 24 „pine" – Gewöhnliche Kiefer – hilft gegen Schuldgefühle, Selbstvorwürfe und ein bedrückendes Lebensgefühl.

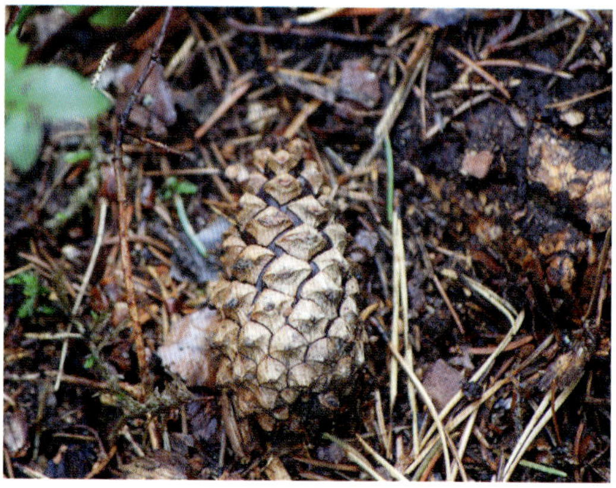
Kleine Zapfen sind kennzeichnend für die Kiefer.

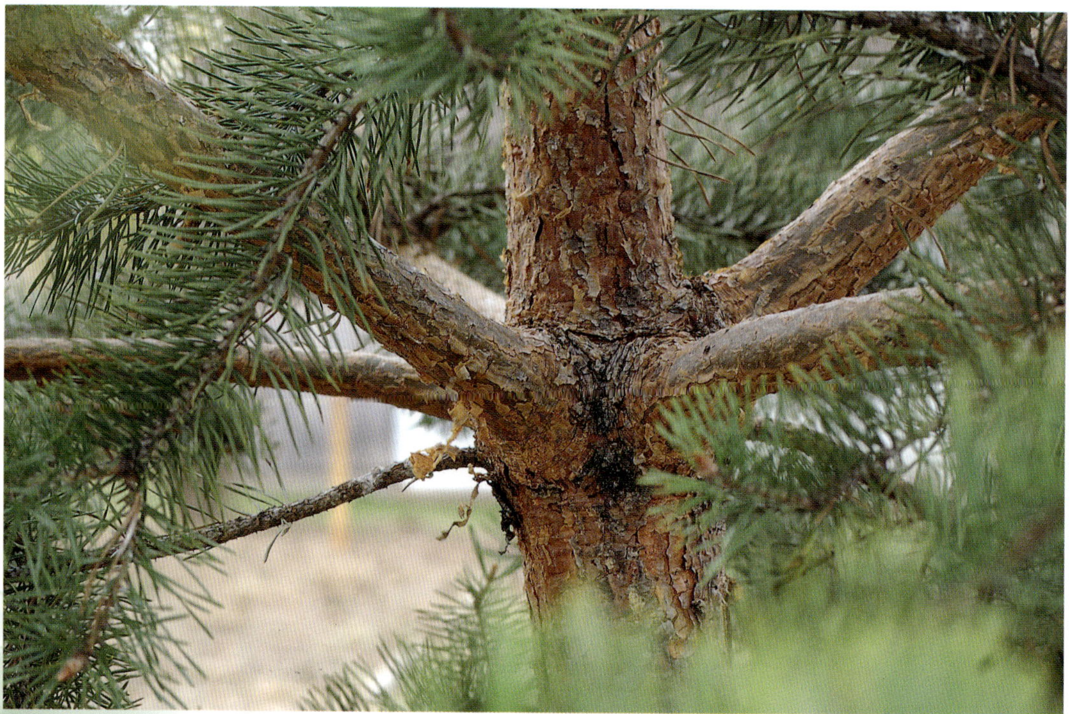
Kiefern haben einen starken Bezug zur Zahl fünf.

Latsche

Lat. Name: *Pinus mugo*
Botanischer Name: Bergkiefer
Pflanzengesellschaft: Kieferngewächse

Die Latsche ist ein Phänomen! Hier manifestiert sich die Anpassungsfähigkeit einer Art an einen extremen Standort, in der Bereitschaft zu ungewöhnlichen Lösungen: „Wenn das Wachstum in die Höhe zu beschwerlich wird, dann wachse ich in die Breite!" Schon die gewöhnliche Kiefer experimentiert gerne mit ihrem Wachstum, aber die Latsche schafft mit dieser Lösung für hohe Lagen zudem noch Schutzbereiche für viele Kleintiere und Pflanzen – und wer weiß, vielleicht auch für so manche Berggeister. Latschenkiefern werden bis zu vier Meter hoch und bis zu fünf Meter breit. Eine Latsche kann zehn Jahre alt werden. Sie wächst bis auf 2.700 m Seehöhe, fühlt sich aber unter Luxusbedingungen in Gärten und Parkanlagen auch sehr wohl.

Rauch

Verwendete Pflanzenteile: Nadeln, Zapfen.

Beste Sammel- und Erntezeit: Ganzjährig.

Wirkung, Wahrnehmung: Erdig und kraftvoll; raumfüllender Duft mit reinigender, klärender Kraft. Überlagert stark negative Raumenergien. Stärkt die eigene Widerstandskraft und die Hoffnung auf bessere Tage. Befreiende Wirkung – man kann die „Klammeraffen", die auf der Schulter zu hocken scheinen, abschütteln. Abwehr von Verwünschungen und Bannungen. Stärkt die positiven Energien, hebt die Lebenslust; lässt Phasen der Müdigkeit leichter überwinden; wirkt aufbauend und ausgleichend.

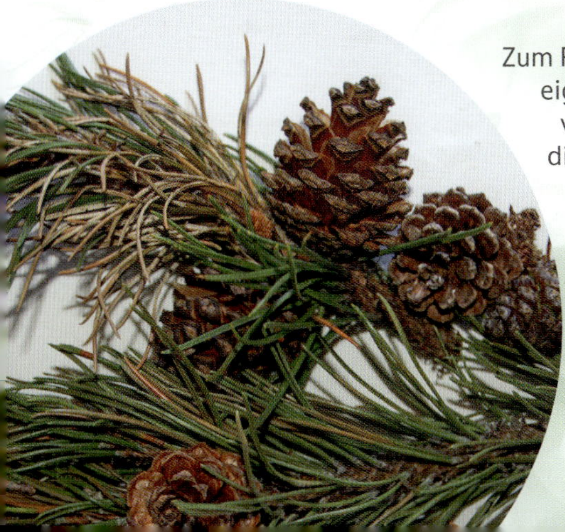

Zum Räuchern eignen sich vor allem die Zapfen und Nadeln.

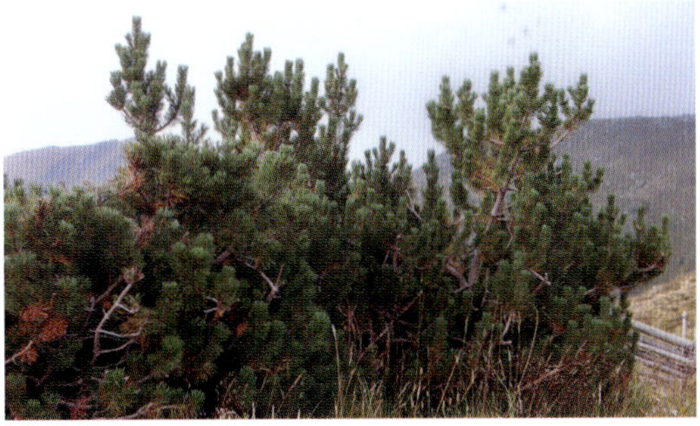

Latschen werden auch als Bergkiefern bezeichnet.

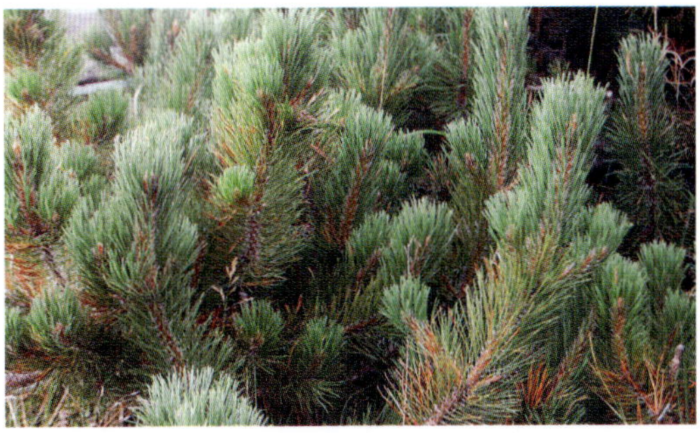

Die langen Nadeln der Latsche sind ein Erkennungsmerkmal dieses Baums.

Schwerpunkt, Anwendungen, Rezepte: Wird traditionell in den Raunächten geräuchert, als Schutz vor der wilden Jagd: Räuchermischung mit Latschen, Wacholder, Klettenwurzel und Fichte.

Mythologie und magische Praktiken

Auf den höheren Almen dienten die immergrünen Latschenäste zum Schutz vor ungewissen Bedrohungen durch eine oft gnadenlose Natur. Sie wurden an die Haus- und Stalltüren genagelt, um missgünstige Wesen davon abzuhalten, dort ihren vielfältigen Schadenszauber durchzuführen.

Verwendung – gestern und heute

Neben dem bekannten ätherischen Latschenkiefer-Öl kann aus den jungen Latschentrieben im Frühling auch ein wunderbarer Hustensaft gewonnen werden.

Mistel

Lat. Name: *Viscum album*
Botanischer Name: Laubholz-Mistel
Pflanzenfamilie: Sandelholzgewächse

Wenn im Herbst die Blätter fallen, taucht die Mistel wie aus dem Nichts plötzlich auf. Sie siedelt sich besonders gern auf Apfelbäumen, Pappeln, Birken und Linden an. Misteln auf Eichen sind sehr selten. Dagegen findet man Tannen- und Kiefermisteln meist erst, wenn der Baum gefällt ist. Sie ist ein Halbschmarotzer, lässt sich vom Wirtsbaum mit Wasser und Mineralstoffen versorgen und schert sich auch sonst wenig um pflanzliche Rahmenbedingungen. Sie wächst spektakulär nach unten, auch wenn alle anderen Pflanzen nach oben zum Licht wachsen. Sie fruchtet in der kalten Jahreszeit und sie „tanzt" ab Ende März: Jeden Tag orientieren sich ihre Blätter und Stängel in eine andere Richtung. Anfang Juli hat sie ihr Zentrum für diese Wachstumsperiode gefunden. Durch diese, in der Pflanzenwelt einzigartigen Bewegungen, bildet sich schließlich ihre kugelige Gestalt heraus.

Diese Eigenwilligkeiten und außergewöhnlichen Eigenschaften haben der Mistel einen zentralen Platz in der Mythologie, den Zauberkulten und magischen Traditionen vieler Völker beschert. Aus den Geschichten um Asterix und Obelix kennt man den Zaubertrank der Gallier, der unter Zugabe von Eichenmisteln gebraut wird und jedem Riesenkräfte verleihen soll.

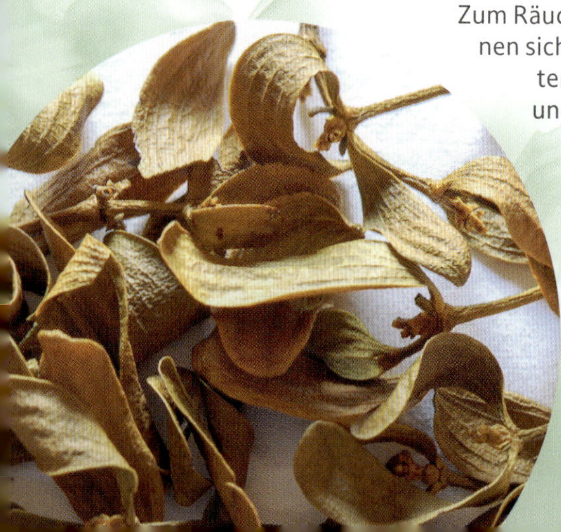

Zum Räuchern eignen sich die Blätter, Stängel und Beeren.

Die Mistel wächst sehr langsam, fruchtet im Alter von sieben Jahren das erste Mal und kann über 30 Jahre alt werden.

Rauch

Verwendete Pflanzenteile: Blätter, Stängel, Beeren.

Beste Sammel- und Erntezeit: Im Advent; nach altem Brauch durften Misteln nur an den beiden Sonnenwenden geerntet werden, ohne dabei ein Eisenwerkzeug zu verwenden. Nach dem Abbrechen durfte die Mistel nicht den Boden berühren, musste also in einem Tuch aufgefangen werden oder – noch besser – mit der linken Hand.

Wirkung, Wahrnehmung: Die Mistel strahlt wie ein Stern, eine kleine Sonne. Ihre kugelige Wuchsform ist ein Universum für sich, das gegen den irdischen Jahreslauf wächst und fruchtet. Die Mistel schwebt zwischen Himmel und Erde und hält die Verbindung von unten nach oben offen.

Der Mistelrauch unterstützt das zweite der sieben Gesetze des Lebens der Hermetik nach Hermes Trismegistos. Dieses Gesetz der Entsprechungen lautet zusammengefasst: „Wie oben so unten. Wie innen, so außen." Das bedeutet, dass man im Mistelrauch die Durchlässigkeit der verschiedenen Ebenen erkennen und vielleicht auch annehmen oder gar verstehen lernen kann. Das ist immer dann wichtig, wenn das Leben unerwünschte, nicht erwartete, plötzliche Wendungen nimmt und man damit nicht gut zurechtkommt.

Der Mistelrauch überlagert nachhaltig sämtliche negativen Anhaftungen, sowohl in Räumen als auch an Menschen und lässt wieder Ordnung und Ruhe einkehren. Er hat die Kraft Chaos, energetische Altlasten, Irrungen und Wirrungen, aber auch Ängste durch Überlagerung aufzulösen.

Als Pflanze des Übergangs vermittelt der Rauch der Mistel eine große Schutzkraft in dunklen Stunden; man empfindet diese lichtmehrende Kraft, die einen innerlich aufbauen kann, als sehr angenehm und lösend. Innere Klarheit und Zuversicht können wieder entstehen.

Magisches zum Rauch: Zahlreiche Abwehrzauber mit geheimen Handlungen unter Mistelrauch sind überliefert, durch welche Schadenszauber abgehalten oder aufgelöst werden sollen. So auch folgender Schutzzauber: „Thistil – Mistil – Kistil“ mit Rauch und Ritual gegen Schadenszauber durch böse Geister und Hexen. Mit Mistelrauch werden auch magische Abwehramulette aufgeladen. Das mit Silber eingefasste Mistelholz soll den Träger vor Albträumen und Dämonen schützen.

Schwerpunkt, Anwendungen, Rezepte: Die Mistel wird traditionell am Jahresende, in den Raunächten geräuchert, um den Übergang von der alten in eine neue Zeit schützend zu begleiten und diesen zwischen Himmel und Erde auszugleichen. Hier wird die Mistel mit Fichte, Wacholder, Stechpalme, Buchsbaum und den Kräutern des „Mariä-Himmelfahrt-Buschns“ geräuchert.

Als typischer Räucherstoff der beiden Sonnenwenden ist sie auch zur Sommersonnenwende am 21. Juni zu räuchern, um das Übermaß an

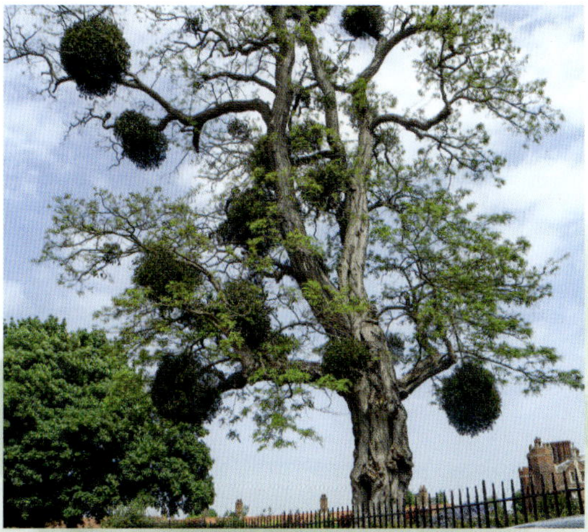

Die Misteln vor Hampton Court Palace, London

Licht einzufangen und einen geordneten Übergang zur Erntezeit zu ermöglichen. Die Räuchermischung umfasst hier neben Fichtenharz die Kräuter des „Johannis-Buschns“, wie Beifuß, Johanniskraut, Weinraute oder Baldrian.

Der Mistelrauch spielt auch im Ahnenkult eine zentrale Rolle. Wenn man die Verbundenheit mit seinen Vorfahren spüren oder sie als spirituelle Helfer um Beistand bitten möchte, könnte eine Räuchermischung mit Mistel, Eiben und Latschen hilfreich sein.

Mythologie und magische Praktiken

Da die Mistel offensichtlich keine Verbindung mit der Erde brauchte, hat man in ihr ein eigenständiges höheres Wesen gesehen. In der Mistel, der Gespensterrute, fühlen sich alle Geistwesen und Gespenster wohl. Sie hat in allen Kulturen einen starken Bezug zur Anderswelt.

Aeneas ist ein Held der griechischen, aber auch der römischen Mythologie. In seinem Epos Aeneas, im sechsten Buch „Aeneas in der Unterwelt“ beschreibt der römische Dichter Vergil (70–19 v. Chr.) die Mistel als magische Pflanze, mit der Kraft, das Tor zur Unterwelt zu öffnen. Dafür muss Aeneas erst den „goldenen Zweig“ finden um dann mit Sybille in die Unterwelt zu seinem Vater Anchises und wieder zurück auf die Erde zu gelangen. Bei der Suche nach dem goldenen Zweig helfen ihm zwei Tauben, die ihm seine Mutter Aphrodite geschickt hatte: „So wie die Mistel im Wald beim Froste des Winters mit neuem Grün sich belaubt, das nicht aus dem Stamme des Baumes entsprossen, und um den rundlichen Ast sich mit safranfarbenem Gezweig schlingt, so war der Schimmer des goldenen Laubs inmitten der dunkeln Eiche...“

In der skandinavischen Mythensammlung „Edda“ nimmt die Erzählung von Balders Tod eine zentrale Stellung ein: Balder, der Sonnengott aus dem Göttergeschlecht der Asen, zweiter Sohn von Odin und Frigga, ist der schönste, freundlichste und weiseste der Asen, was auch einige Neider auf den Plan ruft. Als er wiederholt von seinem nahen Tod träumt, nimmt Frigga allen Lebewesen der Erde das Versprechen ab, Baldur nicht zu töten. Beruhigt feiert man ein Fest zur Unverwundbarkeit Balders. Dabei überredet der tückische Loki den blinden Hödur, die Unverwundbarkeit Balders mit einer Mistel, von der kein Eid verlangt worden war, zu testen. Der gefrorene Mistelzweig durchbohrt den Sonnengott, er stirbt und fährt zu Hel in die Unterwelt. Der Vater stürmt über die Lande und versucht mit der wilden Jagd die Sonne wieder zurückzubringen. Deswegen muss zur Wintersonnenwende das Licht mit Räucheropfern unterstützt werden.

Die druidische Hochachtung der Mistel findet sich im englischen Spruch „no misteltoe, no luck" wieder. In der Weihnachtszeit werden Mistelzweige mit roten Bändern über Türen angebracht und darunter wird geküsst.

Verwendung – gestern und heute

Plinius der Ältere (23–79) berichtet in seiner „Naturalis historia" genau, mit welch strengen Ritualen die keltischen Druiden die Ernte von Eichen-Misteln vornahmen: „… denn nichts halten die Druiden –so nennen sie ihre Magier – für heiliger als die Mistel und den Baum auf dem sie wächst, sofern es nur eine Eiche ist…"

1500 Jahre später zitiert Hieronymus Bock (1498–1554), Botaniker, Arzt und lutherischer Prediger, Plinius wortgleich und resümiert: „Dann vil meinen noch, es haben die Eichen Misteln etwas krafft und gewalt für böse gespenst, henckens auch zum theil den jungen kinderen an die halß, der meinung, es soll den selben kindern kein zauberei oder gespenst schaden."

Um die Ausmerzung des heidnischen Mistelkultes durch die christliche Herrschaft geht es in dem Roman „Ekkehard", der von Josef Viktor von Scheffel (1826–1886) geschrieben wurde. Es handelt vom Leben und Wirken des Benediktinermönchs Ekkehard (verstorben im Jahr 990) aus St. Gallen und späteren Lehrer Otto II. (955–983). Untertanen der Herzogin von Schwaben hätten eine alte Waldfrau beim Verräuchern von Eichen-Misteln nach einem heidnischen Ritual beobachtet. Als Ekkehard davon erfährt und es seiner Herrin berichtet, lässt diese die Eiche fällen und die Waldfrau vertreiben.

Die Verwendung von Mistelpräparaten als Krebsbegleittherapie ist heute gängige Praxis. Entwickelt wurde sie in den Jahren 1916 bis 1927 vom Anthroposophen Rudolf Steiner (1861–1925) und der Ärztin Ita Wegmann (1876–1943).

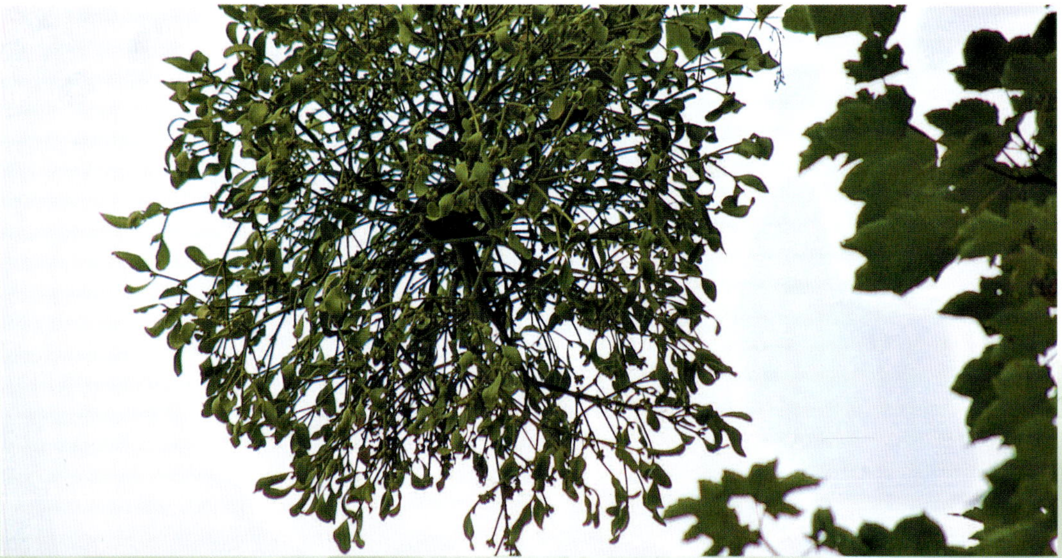

Misteln wachsen nach unten.

Preiselbeere

Lat. Name: *Vaccinium vitis-idaea*
Pflanzenfamilie: Heidekrautgewächse

Auf sauren Waldböden und rund um Moore gefällt es der immergrünen Preiselbeere besonders gut. Das leuchtende Rot der Beeren macht einen erst im Herbst auf die unauffälligen niedrigen Zwergsträucher aufmerksam. Die Preiselbeere besiedelt die ganze nördliche Halbkugel und wird meist nur 10–15 cm hoch.

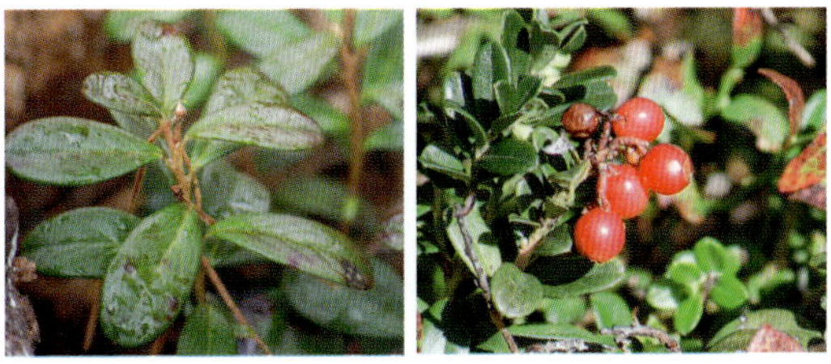

Blätter und Früchte der Preiselbeere

Rauch

Verwendete Pflanzenteile: Blätter und Stängel.

Beste Sammel- und Erntezeit: Ab dem Spätsommer bis in den Herbst hinein.

Wirkung, Wahrnehmung: Vielseitiger Schutzrauch, öffnet das Herz, macht einsichtig und nachgiebig; beruhigend bei innerer Unsicherheit, tiefsitzenden Zweifeln und unbestimmten Ängsten.

Im Rauch der Preiselbeerblätter wird man geneigt, ernsthaft über falsch gelaufene Dinge nachzudenken. Es wird die Wahrnehmung gestärkt, dass alles relativ ist und dass das Beharren auf bestimmten Positionen letztendlich ganz unwichtig sein wird. Hilft Vertrauen ins Leben zu stärken und einen positiven, liebevollen Zugang zu sich und zu anderen zu finden. Aufbauend bei Antriebs- und Kraftlosigkeit sowie für Menschen, die zu Resignation neigen.

Magisches zum Rauch: In Liebesräucherungen öffnet der Duft der Preiselbeere die Pforten zur Annäherung und Übereinstimmung.

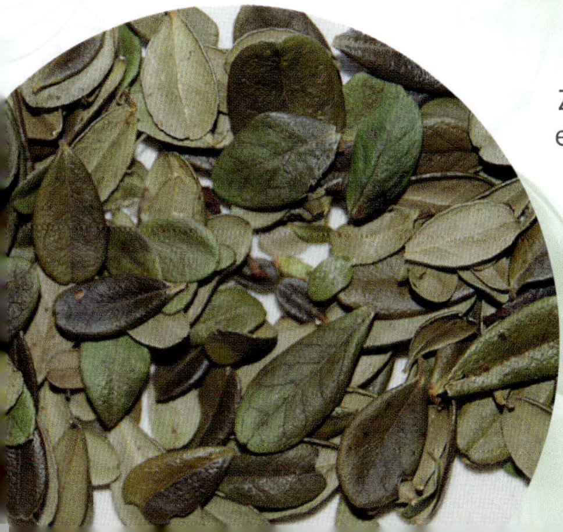

Zum Räuchern eignen sich die Blätter und Stängel.

Schwerpunkt, Anwendungen, Rezepte: Räucherung bei chronischer Überforderung: Bärenschote, Preiselbeerblätter und Salbei sowie Harz.

Räucherung zur Befreiung aus Perspektivenlosigkeit: Beifuß, Wirbeldost, Preiselbeerblätter und Ysop mit Harz.

Mythologie und magische Praktiken

In zwei nordischen Sagen wird die Preiselbeere mit Jungfrauen in Verbindung gebracht, die auf die Gottesmutter Maria hinweisen. In einer bretonischen Sage werden dem lieblichen Mädchen Kermaris beide Arme abgeschlagen. Doch durch ein Bad in einem Preiselbeer-Wasser wachsen die Arme wieder an und sie lebt seither glücklich für immer.

Im 50. Gesang des finnischen Epos „Kalevala“ aus dem 19. Jahrhundert wird die Jungfrau Marjatta durch das Essen einer Preiselbeere schwanger und bringt einen Sohn zur Welt, der von Geburt an weise und mächtig ist.

Verwendung – gestern und heute

Bereits in frühen Gesetzbüchern wird festgelegt, dass man auf fremdem Grund Preiselbeeren nur zum Verzehr von der Hand in den Mund sammeln, somit nicht mitnehmen, dürfe. Selbst in den bäuerlichen Pachtverträgen finden sich Regelungen hinsichtlich Nutzung oder gar Abgabeverpflichtung der Preiselbeeren an den Grundherren.

Zahlreiche Inhaltsstoffe, darunter Anthocyane, Beta-Carotin und viele Vitamine sorgen für eine zusammenziehende und entzündungshemmende Wirkung und machen die Preiselbeere zu einem wertvollen Begleiter bei verschiedenen Unpässlichkeiten.

Stechpalme

Lat. Name: *Ilex aquifolium*
Botanischer Name: Europäische Stechpalme
Pflanzenfamilie: Stechpalmengewächse

In der westlichen Kultur begleiten die Ilexzweige mit ihren knallroten Beeren seit Jahrtausenden die Geschehnisse rund um die Wintersonnenwende und sind auch noch heute nicht aus dem weihnachtlichen Pflanzenschmuck wegzudenken.

Der glänzende Auftritt der Ilex-Blätter erfreut das Herz das ganze Jahr. Dabei fällt auf, dass die unteren Blätter stacheliger sind als die Blätter, die weiter oben sitzen. Das hat sich die schlaue Hülse wohl so überlegt: Fraßschutz zum Selbstschutz. Im Winter wollen mehr kleine Tiere an ihre immergrünen Blätter als große.

Die Stechpalme, auch Hülse genannt, hat keine Probleme mit Hitze und längeren Trockenperioden, freut sich aber, wenn sie im Verband mit Buchen oder am Waldrand stehen kann. Sie gehört zur europäischen Urvegetation, ist jedoch heute kaum noch auf freien Waldflächen zu finden. Aber in so manchen Bauerngärten schützt sie meist die windige Nordseite.

Stechpalmen können strauchartig wachsen oder als Baum auftreten. Dabei werden von zwei bis zu zwanzig Meter hoch und mehrere hundert Jahre alt.

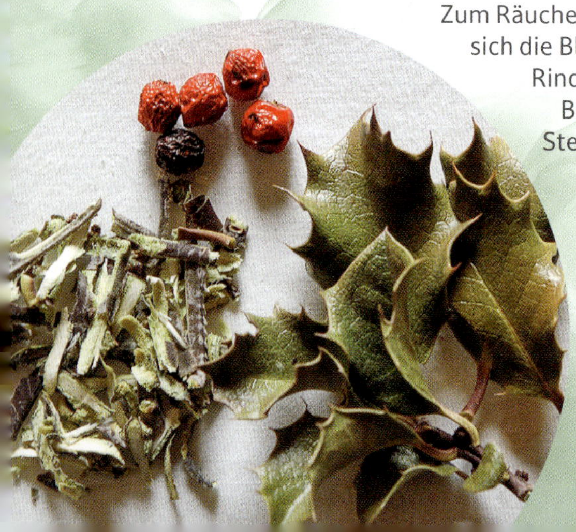

Zum Räuchern eignen sich die Blätter, die Rinde und die Beeren der Stechpalme.

Rauch

Verwendete Pflanzenteile: Blätter, Rinde, Beeren.

Beste Sammel- und Erntezeit: Die Blätter können ganzjährig genommen werden; die roten Beeren findet man meist schon vom Herbst weg bis ins Frühjahr hinein.

Wirkung, Wahrnehmung: Schutz- und Abwehrrauch; große Schutzkraft gegen alles Böse, diffuse Bedrohungen, die man zwar fühlt, aber nicht weiß, woher sie kommen oder was sie bedeuten. Schützt Lebensübergänge und Neuanfänge, vermittelt eine Atmosphäre des Gelingens. Gilt als Symbol von Glück, Freude und Gesundheit. Unterstützt die liebevolle Hinwendung zum Du; fördert Einsicht und Demut, Hoffnung und Liebe.

Magisches zum Rauch: Bei den Raunacht-Räucherumgängen wird sie getrocknet als Räucherstoff, wie auch grün als „Sprengzweigerl" fürs Weihwasser verwendet.

Schwerpunkt, Anwendungen, Rezepte: Die Stechpalme passt in Räuchermischungen, die einen unbelasteten Neubeginn unterstützen sollen, sowie, neben Wacholder und Mistel, in Räucherungen rund um Weihnachten – von Maria Empfängnis bis Mariä Lichtmess.

Mythologie und magische Praktiken

Die Stechpalme ist der Inbegriff des ewigen Lebens und spiegelt dies in vielen Ritualen rund um Geburt, Tod und Wiedergeburt wider. Keltische Stämme, Römer und Germanen verehrten die Hülse in diesem Sinne. Im nordischen Mythenkreis war sie der Unterweltsgöttin Hel geweiht. Die Römer widmeten sie Picus, dem Gott der Weissagung, der zwischen Stechpalmen auf dem Aventin wohnte.

Der römische Bacchuskult bezieht sich auf das Jenseits und folgt der Vorstellung, nach dem Tod von Gott Bacchus gerettet zu werden. Bei den Bacchanalien wurden die Türen mit Stechpalmenzweigen und Efeu geschmückt.

In europäischen Mythen trifft man auf einen Stechpalmenkönig und einen Eichenkönig, die Personifikationen von Winter und Sommer. Der Stechpalmenkönig ist der König des abnehmenden Jahres. Er wird zur Sommersonnenwende geboren, wird bei der Herbst-Tag- und Nacht-Gleiche immer stärker und regiert bis zur Wintersonnenwende. Dann wird er mit dem Verbrennen von Stechpalmenblättern verabschiedet und nimmt die Dunkelheit mit sich. Der Eichenkönig ist sein Zwillingsbruder und König des zunehmenden Jahres, des starken Lichtes. Er wird zur Wintersonnenwende geboren, wird bei der Frühlings-Tag- und Nacht-Gleiche immer stärker und regiert bis zur Sommersonnenwende. Dann verabschiedet man ihn mit dem Verbrennen von Eichenholz und gibt ihm so Kraft mit für seine Rückkehr.

Während der Wintersonnwend-Rituale kamen rote und weiße Beeren zusammen: Die roten Ilex-Beeren stehen für das weibliche Lebensblut und die weißen Mistelbeeren symbolisieren den männlichen Samen.

Die beerenbesetzten Zweige wurden an Häusergiebeln oder Türen befestigt, um Unheil und Unwetter abzuhalten. Aus ähnlichen Gründen werden zur Wintersonnenwende Zweige mit roten Beeren zu einem Kranz gewunden und im Haus aufgehängt, damit der Schutz der guten Geister ins Haus einzieht. Der Ilex-Schmuck sollte aber bis Ende Jänner aus dem Haus entfernt werden, da sich der Schutz der guten Geister, Elfen und Feen sonst in Unglück wandeln würde.

Durch das Auslegen von Ilex-Zweigen in Hühner- und Rinderställen wollte man dämonische Wesen der Nacht und Waldschraten fernhalten. Der berühmteste Spazierstock aus Stechpalmenholz gehörte wohl Johann Wolfgang von Goethe (1749–1832). Und der berühmteste Zauberstab aus Stechpalmenholz gehört Harry Potter. In Harry Potters Welt gehören die seltenen Ilex-Zauberstäbe zu den beschützenden, die

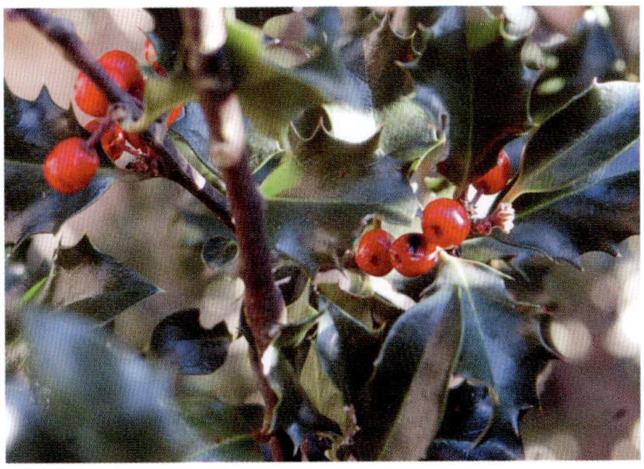

Früchte der Stechpalme

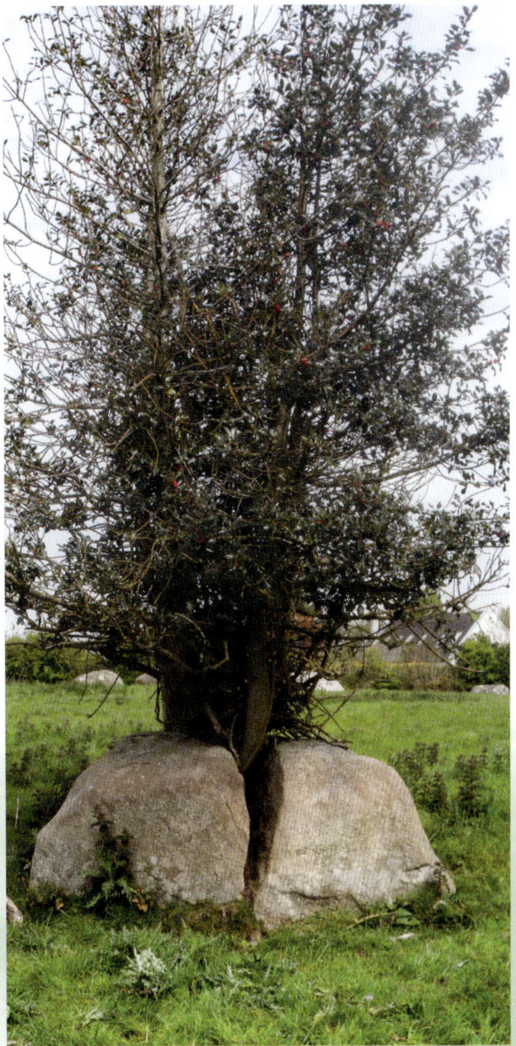

Ilex sprengt Steinkreis-Stein, Irland

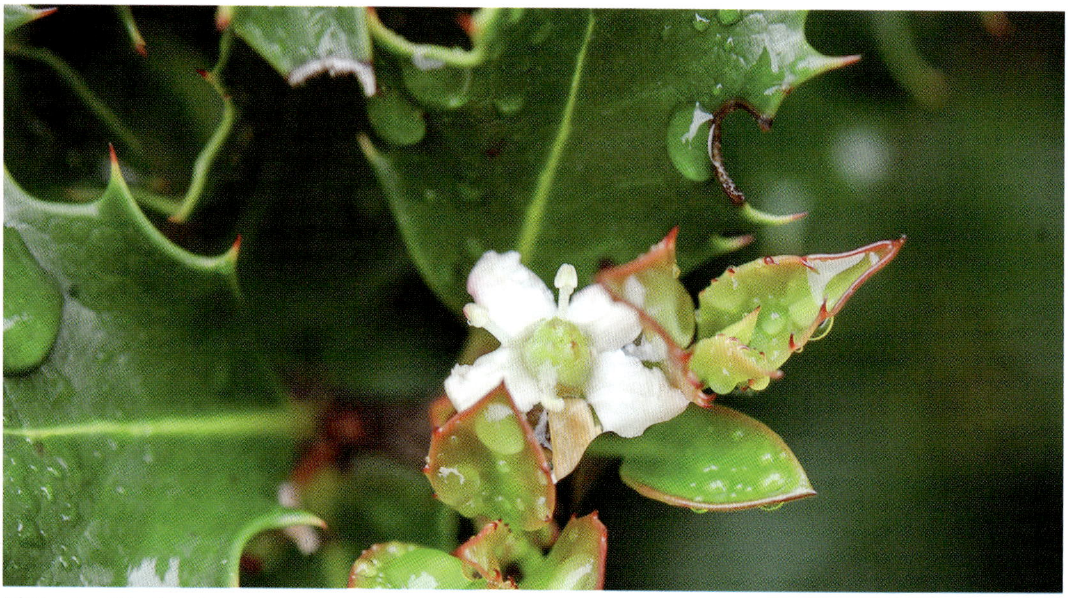

Blüte der Stechpalme

sich Besitzer aussuchen, die gefährliche spirituelle Aufgaben zu bewältigen haben. Und die berühmteste Filmstadt der Welt hat ihren Namen Holly-Wood (Stechpalmen-Wald) wohl von der dort wachsenden Hülse erhalten.

Verwendung – gestern und heute

Auch wenn die frühen Christen noch so gegen das gottlose Brauchtum rund um die Hülse wetterten, ganz verdrängen ließ es sich nicht. So wird die Pflanze schließlich in den christlichen Jahreslauf integriert und gehört in vielen Gegenden am Palmsonntag als immergrüner Kranz zum Brauchtum rund um den „Palmbuschn". Diesem Einsatz am Palmsonntag hat die Hülse auch ihren Namen Stechpalme zu verdanken: Denn, so die Umdeutung, nach der Verurteilung Jesu sei die Palme zur Stechpalme geworden. Jedenfalls soll der gesegnete Palm Mensch und Vieh vor bösen Geistern, Hexen und Blitzen schützen: „... alte Weiber glauben das gewiss, geweihte Zweige schützen vor Donnergschiss".

Bachblüte Nr. 15 „holly" – Stechpalme: Die Blüte der Herzöffnung; hilft stark negative Gefühle zu überwinden.

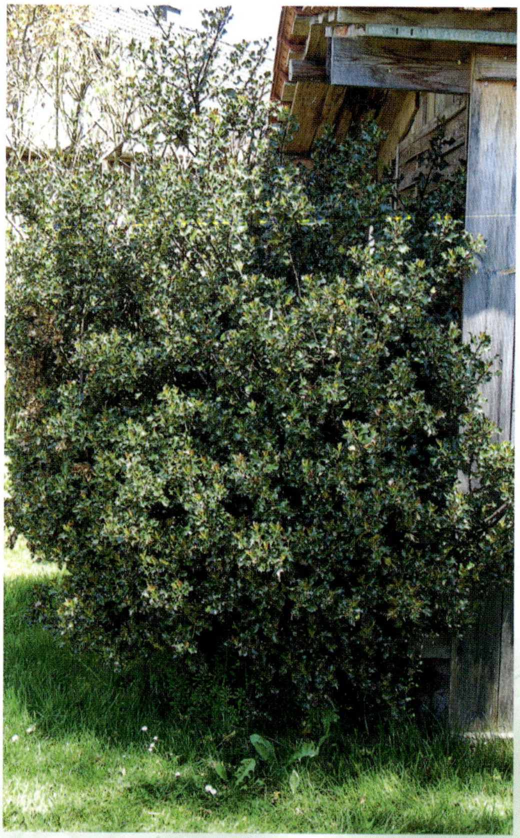

Ilex im Kräuterland, Kärnten

Wacholder

Lat. Name: *Juniperus communis*
Botanischer Name: Gewöhnlicher Wacholder
Pflanzenfamilie: Zypressengewächse

„Vor dem Holler zieht der Bauer seinen Hut, vor dem Wacholder kniet er nieder", lautet ein alter Merkspruch der Kräuterkundigen. Seit Jahrtausenden kommt dem Wacholder, dieser einsamen Gestalt unserer Wälder und Waldränder, eine besondere Stellung unter den heilkräftigen Gewächsen zu. Das zeigt sich allein schon darin, dass es mehr als 150 verschiedene volkstümliche Bezeichnungen für den Wacholder gibt – von Kranewitt bis feuer- oder Weihrauchbaum. Die Menschen glaubten, er sei von einer Muttergottheit beseelt, unter deren Schutz man vor allem Bösem gefeit wäre. Ein Schutz- und Lebensbaum also, der sehr langsam wächst und fruchtet und so für das Urprinzip des Überlebens steht. Neben den heilsamen, körperlich entgiftenden und aufbauenden Kräften wurde vor allem seine große spirituelle Schutzkraft verehrt, die abwehren, reinigen und mental stärken kann.

Gemeiner Wacholder ist auf der gesamten Nordhalbkugel verbreitet. Er blüht im Mai, seine Früchte reifen dann innerhalb von eineinhalb Jahren. Das führt dazu, dass der Wacholder immer Früchte unterschiedlichen Reifegrades trägt. Diese Früchte sind keine Beeren wie man, aufgrund ihrer fleischigen Hülle annehmen würde! Botanisch gesehen handelt es sich um Zapfen, was schon mehr zu den Nadelbäumen passt. Aus diesen Zapfen wird, im vergorenen Zustand, so manch bekömmlicher Wacholderschnaps destilliert.

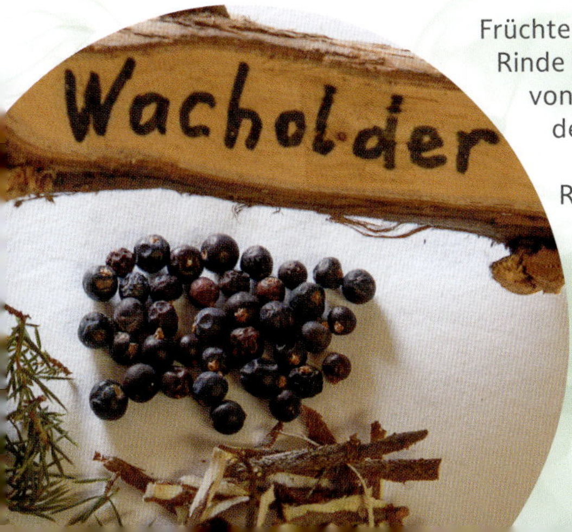

Früchte, Nadeln, Rinde und Holz von Wacholder eignen sich zum Räuchern.

Der Wacholder kann in unserer Region einige Meter hoch werden, in Gunstlagen über zehn Meter emporwachsen. Er hat keine Fressfeinde und kann aufgrund der Langsamkeit seines Wachstums zwischen 600 und 2000 Jahre alt werden.

Rauch

Verwendete Pflanzenteile: Früchte, Nadeln, Rinde, Holz.

Beste Sammel- und Erntezeit: Ganzjährig.

Wirkung, Wahrnehmung: Desinfizierender Reinigungsrauch; Räume und Gegenstände werden mit neuer Energie aufgeladen. Schutzrauch der Wintersonnenwende und in den Raunächten. Der Rauch aller Teile wirkt stark positiv polend. Die Nadeln wirken eher abwehrend, desinfizierend und entgiftend, während die Früchte uns eher erden und die Lebenskraft sowie die Ich-Kraft stärken. Bringt Licht ins Dunkel; alles Negative wird geschwächt und abgewehrt; schützt und begleitet alle wichtigen Übergänge im Leben; unterstützt das Erkennen und die Konzentration auf das Wesentliche.

Die große grüne Kraft, die negative Wesen und Gedanken fernhalten kann und die einen nachhaltig vitalisiert und stärkt. Der Rauch zieht Ruhe und Zuversicht sowie ein Gefühl des Gut-aufgehoben-Seins in dieser Welt nach sich.

Magisches zum Rauch: Wacholder wurde als teufelsscheuchendes Schutzmittel gegen böse Geister und Druden geräuchert. Ganzjährig, aber besonders zu Walpurgis und in den Raunächten: „... wo es nach Wacholder riecht, da hält sich der Teufel nit auf" überlieferten unsere Vorfahren. Oder auch: „Eichenlaub und Kranewitt, das mag der Teifel nit".

Während des gesamten Mittelalters galt der Wacholderrauch als ein unüberwindbares Mittel gegen Bannungen, Verwünschungen und

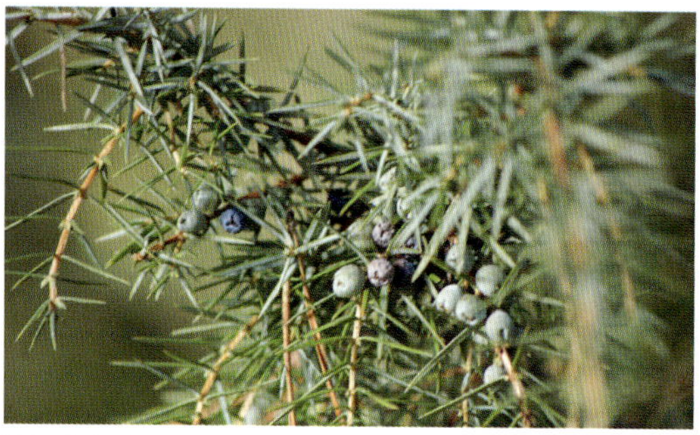
Die Früchte des Wacholderbaums

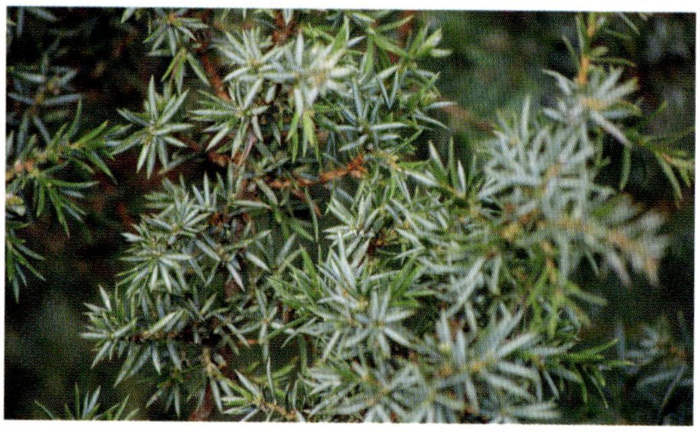
Wacholdernadeln

andere, laut ausgesprochene Schadenszauber. Dabei wurden meist ganze Wacholderzweige angezündet und die belasteten Orte und Menschen mit dem brennenden Holz freigeräuchert.

Schwerpunkt, Anwendungen, Rezepte: Der Allerseelen-Rauch: Bei allen Räucherungen in Erinnerung an Verstorbene und Vorfahren zentrales Räuchermittel in Form von Früchten, Nadeln und Holz.

In Europa seit jeher als Pest-Räucherung genutzt. 1548 berichtet der Schulmeister Schmeltzl aus dem pestverseuchten Wien: „... in den gassen und ringen, ettlich hundert feuer prinnen; von kranwitholz weihrauch dazu, damit die luft sich reinigen tu."

Wacholderrauch wirkt stark desinfizierend und kann als Schutzmittel in Ansteckungszeiten, aber auch im Krankenzimmer verräuchert werden: Für die Räucherung sollte der Kranke aus dem Zimmer gebracht werden. Dann wird die Räucherkohle mit Wacholdernadeln, die auch grün sein dürfen, bedeckt und circa eine Viertelstunde Rauch aufsteigen gelassen. Danach wird gut durchgelüftet.

Eine körperlich schmerzlindernde Anwendung des Wacholderrauches bei Gicht und Rheuma stammt aus dem späten 19. Jahrhundert: Hier sollen Lappen über den Rauch gehalten werden und dann sogleich um die schmerzenden Stellen gewickelt werden.

Bekannt ist auch das Abräuchern mit Wacholderbeeren bei verschiedenen Unpässlichkeiten, Wechselbeschwerden und Niedergeschlagenheit.

Mythologie und magische Praktiken

Die große Verehrung des Wacholders in der christlichen Welt beruht auf der Tatsache, dass jede Frucht ein Kreuzzeichen trägt. Man nahm an, dass der Strauch alle bösen Geister abwehren könne. Überdies wurde er im christlichen Umfeld als Gegenstück zum Paradiesbaum gesehen, als Symbol für die Lebenskraft Christi und dessen Überwindung des Todes.

Symbolisch ist der Wacholder, früher auch Frau Kranewitt genannt, in vielen Kulturen ein Mittler zwischen Leben und Tod. Bereits in sehr früher Zeit wurde sein Holz für Feueropfer, aber auch zur Totenverbrennung verwendet. Man meinte, dass er den Seelen der Verstorbenen als Aufenthaltsort diente und dass diese Seelen aus bestimmten Gründen auch wieder ins Leben zurückkehren wollten. Der Wacholder, der Wach-Halter, bezeichnet genau diese Schwelle des Übertritts. Er allein sei es, der eine Wiederkehr ermöglichen oder verhindern könnte. Aus diesem Grund glaubte man, er gelte zwar als Symbol des Todes, stehe aber gleichzeitig auch für Wiedergeburt und Neubeginn.

Aus heutiger Sicht sind das sehr tiefgreifende Bilder, die auch auf Lebensphasen, Beziehungen, Vorstellungen, Fixierungen übertragbar scheinen und die uns heutigen Menschen helfen können, die Angst und das Unbehagen vor Veränderungen zu überwinden. Denn der Wacholder führt uns nicht hinab in die endgültige Unterwelt, sondern begleitet uns in unserem inneren Wachstums- und Läuterungsprozess. Er führt uns zu unseren inneren Schatten, spiegelt unsere dunklen Seiten, damit dadurch eine Umkehr bewirkt werden kann. Er ist der einsame Pluto, der weiß, dass man solche Transformationsprozesse mit sich selbst ausmachen muss.

Die Menschen versuchten dem Wacholder mit verschiedenen magischen Reimen und Gebeten Krankheiten zu übertragen. So wie auch beim Holunder oder beim Weißdorn wird hier auf die heilende Kraft der archaischen Muttergottheit vertraut, die den Menschen stets wohlgesonnen und beschützend gegenübertritt.

Mit den Wacholderästen wurden verschiedene Abwehrzauber durchgeführt: Sie wurden als Knüppel gegen böse Geister verwendet und an den Eingangstüren festgemacht; mit ihnen wurde zur Abwehr eines Milchzaubers auf die Milchkannen geschlagen; mit ihnen konnte man unter Hersagen von magischen Formeln selbst Diebe dazu zwingen, das Diebesgut wieder zurückzugeben. Selbst als fruchtbarkeitsbringende Martinsgerte waren Wacholderäste in manchen Gegenden in Gebrauch. So zog man am 11. November in manchen Orten von Hof zu Hof und verteilte mit einem Wacholderast, der mit Eichenlaub geschmückt war, immergrüne Überlebenskraft und eicherne Zähigkeit.

Verwendung – gestern und heute

Im Papyrus Ebers, das ungefähr aus der Zeit von 1500 v. Chr. stammt, werden Wacholderbeeren als Heilmittel „für das Regeln des Harns" angeführt. Der Römer Cato der Ältere (234–149 v. Chr.) beschreibt in seinem Werk „de agri cultura", dass mit Wacholderbeeren ein Wein mit harntreibenden Eigenschaften angesetzt werden könne.

Die großen Heilkundigen von der Antike bis in die Neuzeit, von Hippokrates (460–370 v. Chr.) über Dioskurid (1. Jhd.), von Hildegard von Bingen (1098–1179) bis Paracelsus (1493–1541) und Sebastian Kneipp (1821–1897), widmeten sich ausführlich und voller Ehrfurcht der überdurchschnittlichen Heilkraft der Wacholderbeeren.

In den mehrfachen europäischen Pestzeiten schien der Wacholder das einzig potente Gegenmittel zu sein. „Esst Kranewitt und Bibernell, so sterbts ihr nit so schnell", lautete landauf, landab der Ratschlag für das einfache Volk. Hieronymus Bock (1498–1554) meint, dass die Wacholderbeeren ein besonderes Preservativ zur Zeit der Pestilentz seien und resümiert: „... im summa die würckung und tugent des Weckholterbaums seind zu beschreiben nit wol möglich".

Die Wacholderbeeren sind ein volksheilkundliches Allheilmittel, eine Art „Baum-Apotheke", die neben der körperlichen auch über eine besonders starke seelische Heilwirkung verfügen.

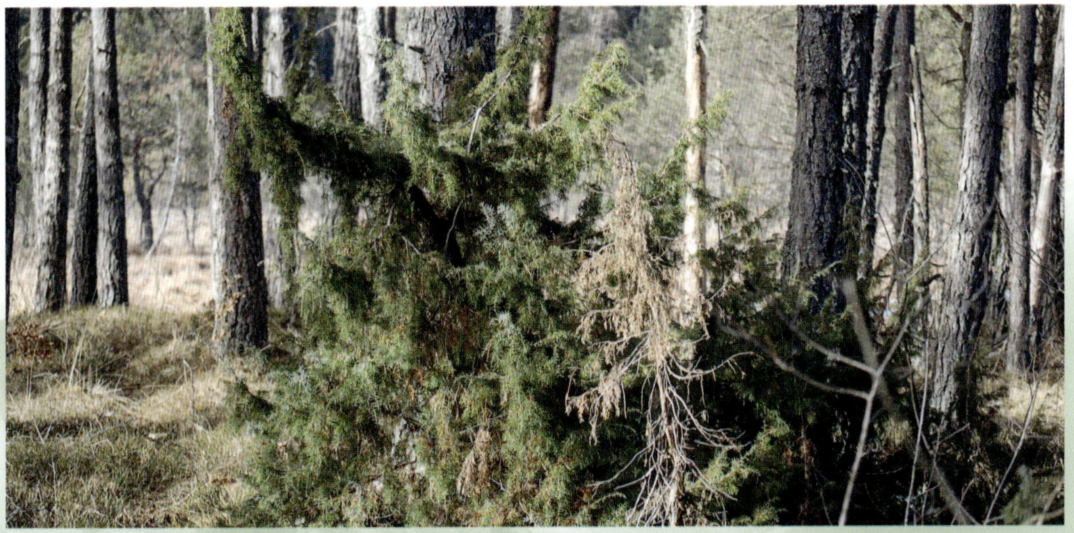

Tanzender Wacholder im Höflein Moor, Radsberg/Radiše, Kärnten

Weiß-Tanne

Lat. Name: *Abies alba*
Pflanzenfamilie: Kieferngewächse

Tannenbäume und Weihnachten – aus dieser Verbindung gibt es wohl kein Entrinnen. Die westliche Weihnachtskultur hat sich auf einen Tiefwurzler, einen Schattenbaum fixiert und ihn zum Symbol für Licht und neues Leben erhoben. Hildegard von Bingen (1098–1179) liefert eine Vorlage dazu: „… die Tanne ist mehr warm als kalt und enthält viele Kräfte. Sie ist ein Sinnbild der Stärke. Geister hassen Tannenholz und meiden Orte, an denen sich solches befindet!"

Wenn man an eine alte Tanne herantritt, spürt man eine besondere Kühle, die sich wie eine schützende Glocke über einen stülpt. Man verliert das Zeitgefühl, weil es sich so angenehm atmen lässt. Die perfekt geglättete, gräuliche Rinde, die weichen Nadeln, die aufrechtstehenden, harzenden Tannenzapfen erwecken den Anschein als stünde sie über den Dingen und nichts könne sie aus der Ruhe bringen. Ihre beruhigende Kühle unterstreicht ihr unaufdringliches, sanftes Wesen. An heißen Tagen sich an so einen Tannenstamm zu lehnen erfrischt Körper, Geist und Seele.

Tannen sind sehr empfindlich gegenüber Luftverschmutzung. Heimische Tannen werden bis zu 70 m hoch und bis zu 600 Jahre alt.

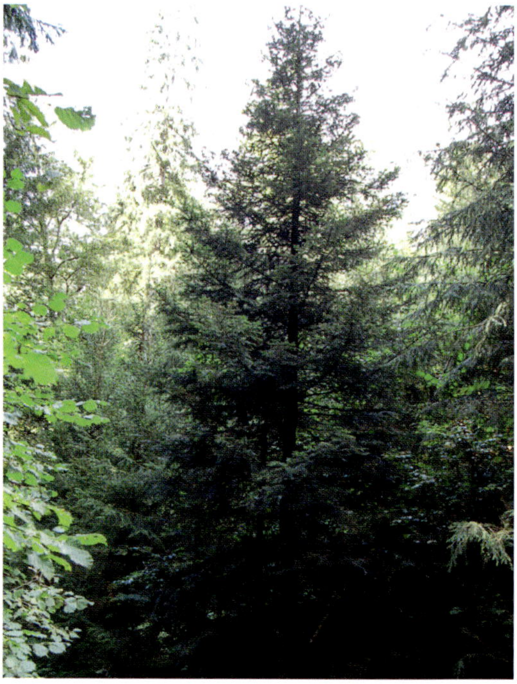

Tannen sind typische Weihnachtsbäume.

Rauch

Verwendete Pflanzenteile: Nadeln, Zapfen.

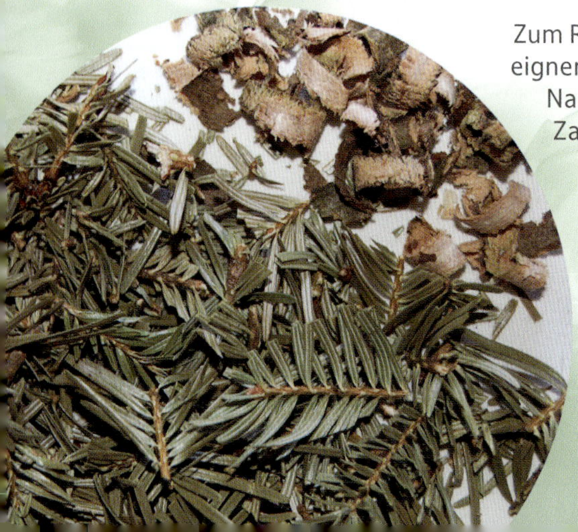

Zum Räuchern eignen sich die Nadeln und Zapfen der Tanne.

Beste Sammel- und Erntezeit: Die Nadeln das ganze Jahr über; die Zapfen ab August direkt vom Baum; die abgefallenen Nadeln des Adventkranzes bieten sich als Räucherwerk für die Raunächte an.

Wirkung, Wahrnehmung: Reinigungsrauch, überlagert und klärt jedes unangenehme, belastete Raumklima. Hellt dunkle Schatten auf; neue Lebenskräfte werden spürbar, Selbstheilungskräfte werden aktiviert; Schutz vor Krankheitsdämonen. Innere Balance finden; macht mutig und psychisch widerstandsfähiger; stärkt die Nerven und hinterlässt ein Gefühl von Sicherheit und Geborgenheit im Hier und Jetzt. Zuversicht und Angekommen sein sind die emotionalen Resonanzen, die der Tannennadel-Rauch hervorruft. Symbol für Entschlossenheit, Aufrichtigkeit, Standhaftigkeit und Ausdauer. Sie steht für Weisheit und Lösungskompetenz.

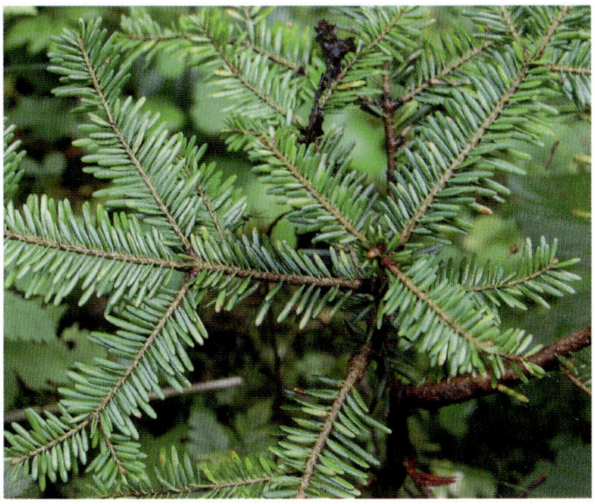

Tannenzweig

Magisches zum Rauch: Tannennadel-Rauch für Schutzrituale, wenn man vor Entscheidungen steht, diese aber wegen großer innerer Unsicherheit hinauszögert.

Schwerpunkt, Anwendungen, Rezepte: Gute Räucherung fürs Krankenzimmer, um den Überlebenswillen des Kranken zu stärken, zusammen mit Rosmarin, Thymian und Wacholderbeeren.

Tannenrauch wurde auch zur Linderung von rheumatischen Schmerzen und Gelenksproblemen verwendet. Dabei hielt man die schmerzenden Glieder über den Rauch oder setzte sich auf einen Stuhl und stellte das Räuchergefäß darunter. So saß man mitten im heilsamen Rauch.

Für eine Räuchermischung zum Stimmungsausgleich vermörsert man Tannennadeln, Fichte, Lärche und Eberesche in Kombination mit Harz.

Mythologie und magische Praktiken

Tannengirlanden sind ein Symbol des Todes und werden für Totenkränze gewunden. Hingegen begleiten Fichtengirlanden stets freudige Ereignisse.

Verwendung – gestern und heute

Bereits Kelten und Germanen holten sich zur Wintersonnenwende Tannenzweige in ihre Hütten, um den Lebenswillen zu stärken und als Symbol der Überwindung der Dunkelheit in der Natur.

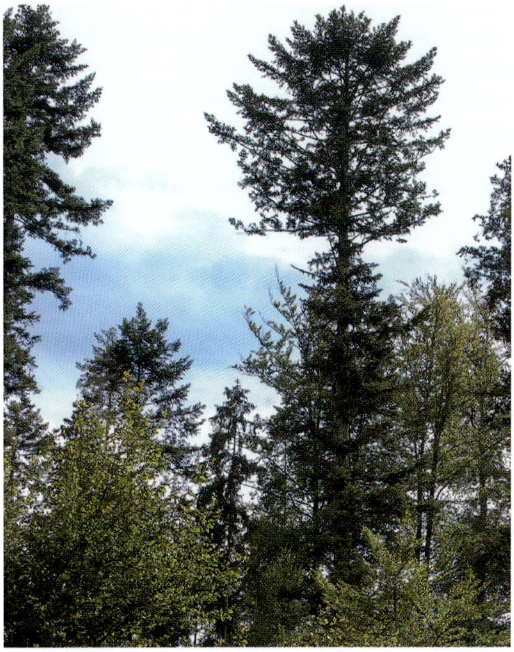

Tanne mit eigentümlichem Wuchs

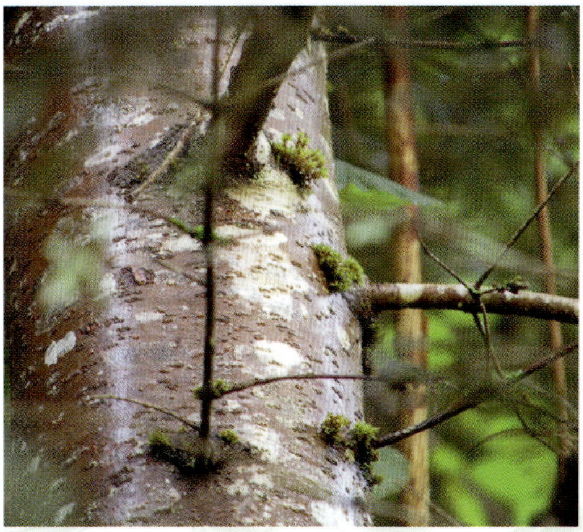

Tannenrinde

1539 soll im Straßburger Münster eine Tanne als erster, offizieller Christbaum gestanden sein. Nach anfänglicher Ablehnung von kirchlicher Seite, war der geschmückte Tannenbaum zur Weihnachtszeit nicht mehr zu stoppen.

Das ätherische Öl aus Tannennadeln wird in der Aromatherapie verwendet und hat eine desinfizierende Wirkung.

Der Rauch von Hölzern und Sträuchern

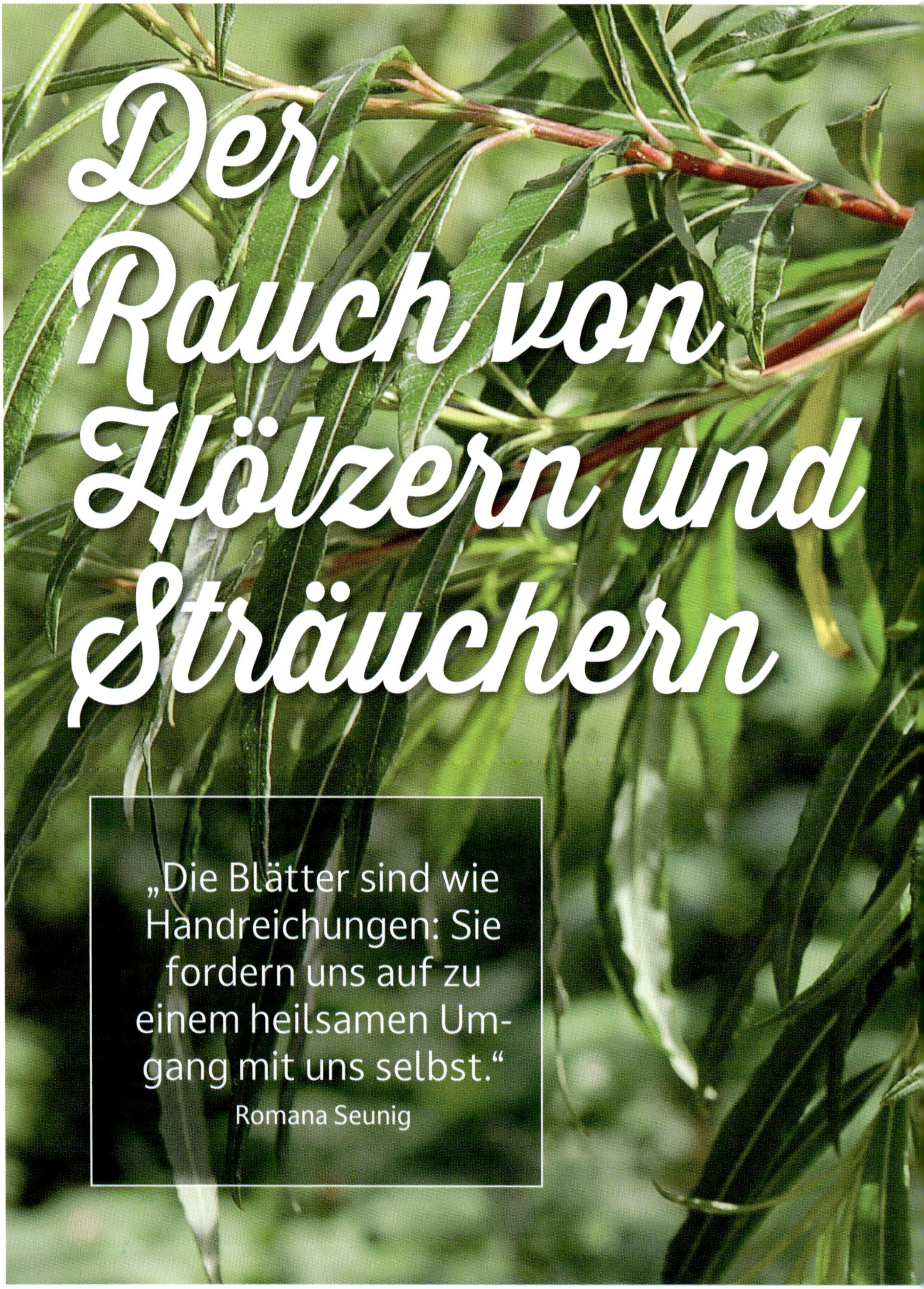

„Die Blätter sind wie Handreichungen: Sie fordern uns auf zu einem heilsamen Umgang mit uns selbst."

Romana Seunig

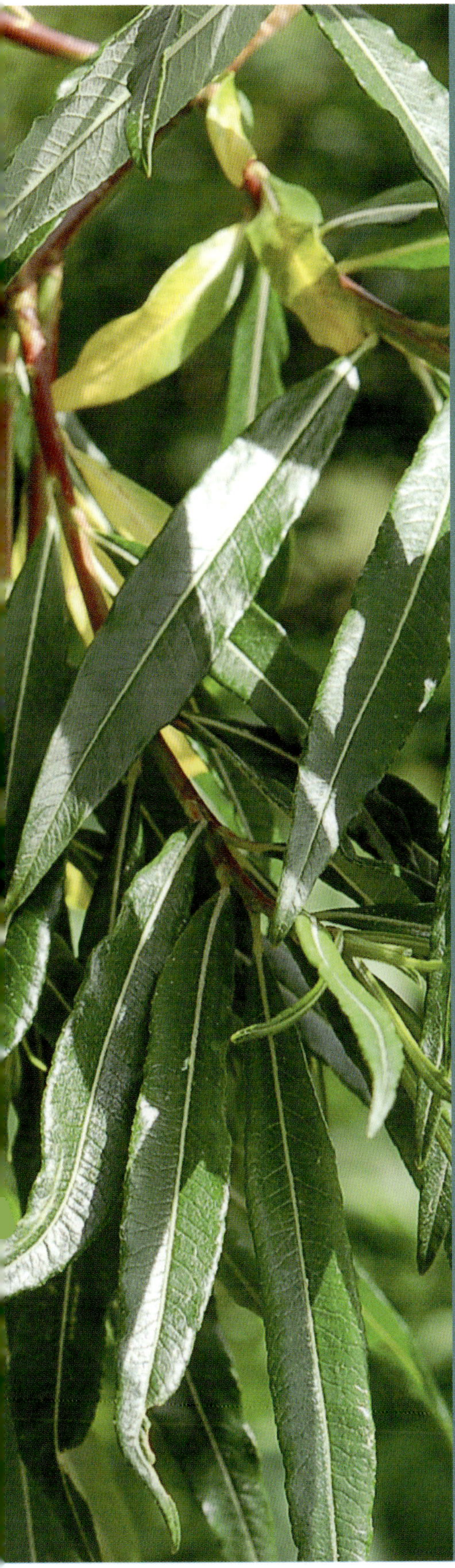

Die heimischen Gehölze und Sträucher sind eine zentrale Adresse für die Suche nach hilfreichen Räucherstoffen. Sie geben die Kraft aus ihren Lebensumwelten im Rauch an uns weiter. Dabei bringt jeder Pflanzenteil seine Prägung in die jeweilige Räuchermischungen mit ein:

Die Hölzer übernehmen klare Positionen. Sie fördern unsere Empathie und die soziale Ader, helfen die eigene Persönlichkeit besser zu erkennen und zu stärken. In den Räucherungen stehen sie für Schutz und Verantwortung.

Die Rinden können verschließen, aber auch erweiternd öffnen. Sie stehen für die schützenden Hüllen, die durch inneres Wachstum gefüllt werden wollen. Sie schwingen im Rhythmus des persönlichen Wachstums, führen uns oft zu den wichtigsten Gedanken.

Die Blätter sind wie Handreichungen: Sie fordern uns auf zu einem heilsamen Umgang mit uns selbst. Sie verhelfen uns zu einer positiven inneren Kommunikation. Sie machen uns die zahllosen Möglichkeiten des Seins deutlich und helfen die Rangfolge für unser Leben zu klären.

Die Blüten helfen einen guten Anfang zu setzen, sind Zeichen der Hoffnung in festgefahrenen Situationen, führen aus der Ausweglosigkeit, bösen Ahnungen, aus Existenzängsten und innerer Leere. Sie sichern uns den Weg bis zur Reife, helfen uns das Werden und Vergehen jeder Existenz anzunehmen.

Apfelbaum

Lat. Name: *Malus domestica*
Pflanzenfamilie: Rosengewächse

„Ein Apfelbaum unter Waldbäumen / ist mein Geliebter unter den Burschen. In seinem Schatten begehre ich zu sitzen. / Wie süß schmeckt seine Frucht meinem Gaumen!", heißt es im Hohelied Salomons. Die Erinnerung an das Paradies steht jedem Apfelbaum ins Geäst geschrieben, obwohl der biblische „Baum der Erkenntnis" nicht ausdrücklich als Apfelbaum benannt wird. Dennoch gilt der Apfelbaum in sämtlichen antiken Kulturen als magisches Symbol für Glück und Liebe.

Die Frucht, der Apfel selbst, spielt sowohl sprachlich als auch kulturhistorisch und mythologisch eine wichtige Rolle: vom paradiesischen Apfel bei Adam und Eva bis zum goldenen Apfel, der mit der Aufschrift „der Schönsten" unter den griechischen Göttinnen zum Zankapfel wurde und den Paris an die verheiratete Helena überreichte, um in ihr ewige Liebe für ihn zu entfachen. Der Apfel erscheint in Geschichten über Avalon, das nebelumhüllte keltische Apfelland im Jenseits, bis hin zum Reichsapfel und dem vergifteten Apfel im Märchen „Schneewittchen".

Die Römer sehen den Apfel eher zwiespältig: Einerseits betonen sie seine mythologisch durchaus dunkle Seite, indem sie den Apfel „malum" (schlecht) nennen und folgenden Sinnspruch prägen: „Malum ex malo" – alles Schlechte kommt vom Apfel. Andererseits sehen sie im Apfel ein Zeichen von Vollkommenheit. So ist für große Festmahle folgender Spruch überliefert: „ab ovo usque ad malo" (vom Ei bis zum Apfel). Die lukullischen Freuden reichten vom eingangs servierten Ei, dem Symbol der Schöpfung, bis zum abschließenden Apfel, dem Symbol der Vollkommenheit.

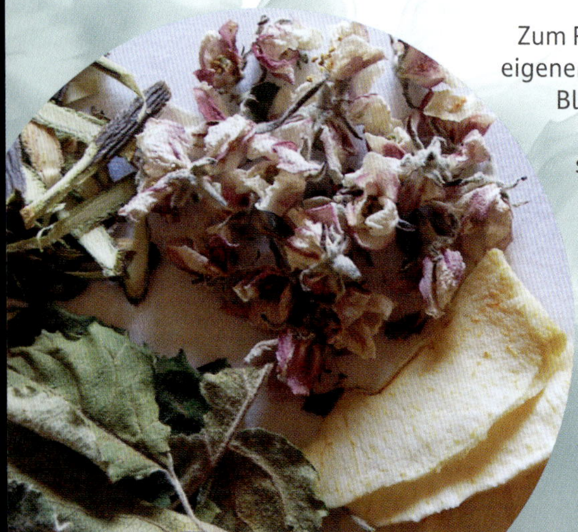

Zum Räuchern eigenen sich die Blüten und Blätter, sowie die Rinde und das Fruchtfleisch.

Dagegen gilt der Apfel in nördlicheren Breiten als Symbol der Erde, der nährenden Mutterbrust und somit des weiblichen Prinzips. Der Mythos Apfel reicht sogar bis zum „big apple" unserer Tage, dem Symbol für New York, für eine Stadt des Glücks und der ungeahnten Verheißungen. Im Apfel scheinen also, literarisch gesehen, alle schönen wie auch extrem unseligen Gefühle vereint zu sein, die man in Bezug auf Liebe und Glück nur haben kann.

Der flach wurzelnde Apfelbaum wird, je nach Sorte, bis zu 80 Jahre alt. Der bisher älteste Apfel wurde nahe Heilbronn gefunden und soll stolze 6000 Jahre alt sein. Im Vergleich dazu wirken die Apfelplantagen der Römer, die sie schon lange vor der Jahrtausendwende zur Versorgung Roms nutzten, fast schon modern. Fast 1000 Jahre später, um das Jahr 800, schreibt dann der Karolinger Kaiser Karl der Große (747–814) in seinem Werk „Capitulare de villis" mindestens vier Apfelsorten zum Anbau auf den königlichen Gütern vor. Neben der wichtigen Aufgabe der Winterversorgung wurde der Apfelgarten mittelalterlicher Klöster zum Paradiesgarten und als solcher zur Begräbnisstätte für die Mönche, die unter den weiß-rosa blühenden Apfelzweigen dem jüngsten Tag entgegen schlafen sollten.

Rauch

Verwendete Pflanzenteile: Blüten, Blätter, Rinde, Apfelspalten.

Beste Sammel- und Erntezeit: Die Blüten und Blätter sammelt man im Frühling und trocknet sie sorgsam. Die Rinde kann entweder unter Ausnutzung des Frühjahrsbaumschnitts geerntet werden oder das ganze Jahr über. Die getrockneten Apfelspalten oder Apfelscheiben werden gemörsert und unter Räuchermischungen gegeben.

Wirkung, Wahrnehmung: Bei Apfelräucherungen geht es immer um Zwischenmenschliches. Der Rauch der Apfelblüten wirkt lösend auf gedankliche Blockaden, fehlende Einsichten in Partnerschaftsthemen. Er lässt uns entspannen, sorgt für Harmonie und vielleicht wird eine andere Sichtweise möglich. Rinde und Holz haben eine stark reinigende, klärende, aufbauende Wirkung. Die Apfelscheiben geben einen sehr angenehmen, anregenden Duft und wirken besänftigend, ausgleichend und befördern liebevolle Gedanken.

Magisches zum Rauch: Der 30. November ist der Andreas-Tag, an dem früher unterschiedliche magische Praktiken hinsichtlich Partnerwahl durchgeführt wurden. In diesen Rahmen passt auch eine Räucherung mit Apfelblüten und Apfelspalten rund um das Thema „Partnerschaft“.

Schwerpunkt, Anwendungen, Rezepte: Zusammen mit Salbei, Mistel und Fichte eignen sich Apfelblätter und -rinde kombiniert mit Harz gut für eine Räuchermischung nach Streitigkeiten und anderem zwischenmenschlichen Verdruss.

Mythologie und magische Praktiken

Endlos scheint die Liste von Apfel-Bindezaubern und von Apfel-Liebeswahrsagerei, die je nach Region verändert werden. So sollen beispielsweise Apfelkerne unter der Fußmatte den Richtigen an die Bewohnerin des betreffenden Hauses binden. Apfelschalen, die über die Schulter geworfen werden, sollen den Anfangsbuchstaben des Zukünftigen verraten.

Verwendung – gestern und heute

Früher galt es für die Apfelernte Folgendes zu beachten: Die Äpfel durften, um die Haltbarkeit zu verlängern, lediglich im letzten Mondviertel geerntet werden und sollten bis zum 16. Oktober im Sack sein.

Reich an wertvollen Inhaltsstoffen lässt sich zum Apfel auch heute noch sagen: „an apple a day keeps the doctor away.“

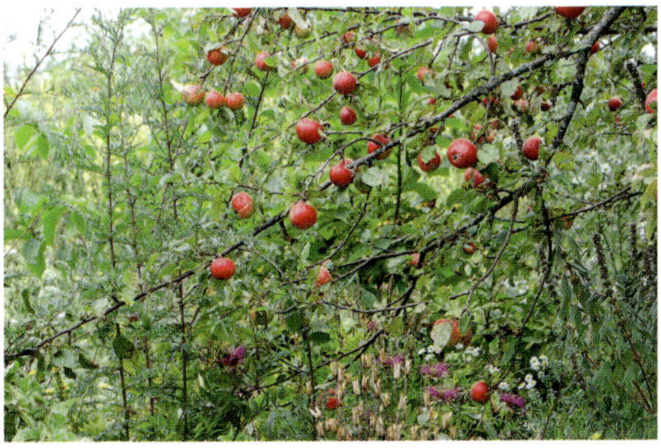

Die reifen Früchte

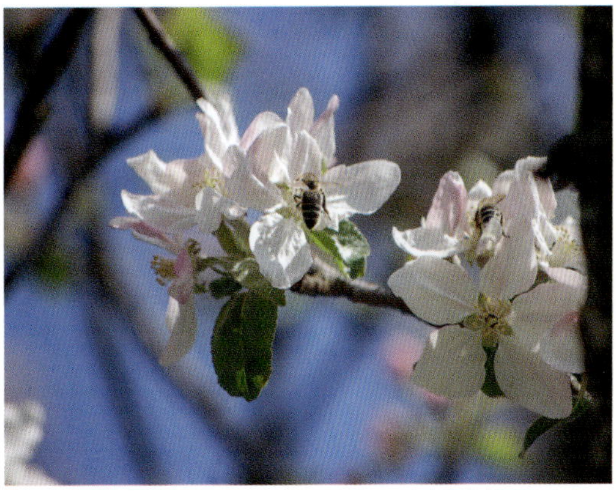

Apfelblüten

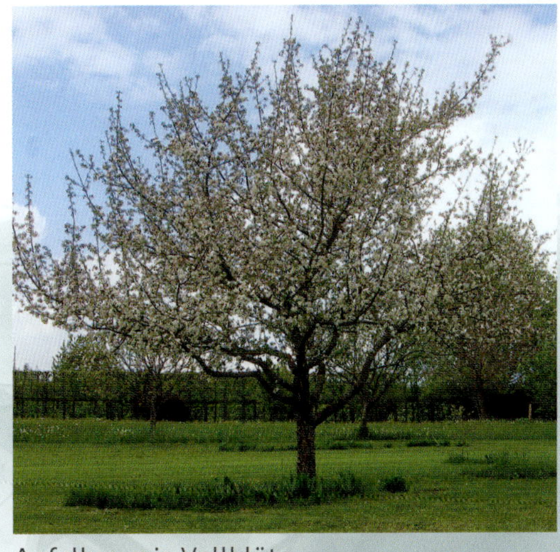

Apfelbaum in Vollblüte

Ahorn

Lat. Name: *Acer pseudoplatanus*
Botanischer Name: Berg-Ahorn
Pflanzenfamilie: Seifenbaumgewächse

Der Ahorn ist das große Glück! Mit seinem besonderen Grün wirkt er stets lichtdurchflutet, hell und voller Lebensfreude. Selbst als die massive Schneemenge meinem Ahorn die Baumkrone in mittiger Höhe abbrach, erschien sein Blätterkleid bereits im darauffolgenden Sommer wieder geordnet, seine ganze Gestalt symmetrisch und konkav nach oben geschlossen. Kein anderer Laubbaum steckt einen derart zentralen Verlust so leicht weg wie ein Ahorn! Ich schaue ihn nur an und schon überträgt er großzügig seine Leichtigkeit, seine liebevolle, aufmunternde Ausstrahlung. So viel angenehme Energie scheinen auch die Vögel zu spüren – drei Nester in einem Baum, bei genügend anderweitigem Angebot, sind bemerkenswert.

Der Ahorn ist in ganz Europa heimisch. Er wird bis zu 30 m hoch und bis zu 500 Jahre alt. Sein weißes Holz steht seit jeher für besondere Reinheit. Es vermittelt Harmonie und Gelassenheit.

Rauch

Verwendete Pflanzenteile: Blüten, Blätter und Früchte.

Beste Sammel- und Erntezeit: Der Ahorn blüht im Mai. Die Blätter werden über den Sommer gesammelt, die Früchte können bis spät in den Herbst auch noch trocken von den Ästen geholt werden.

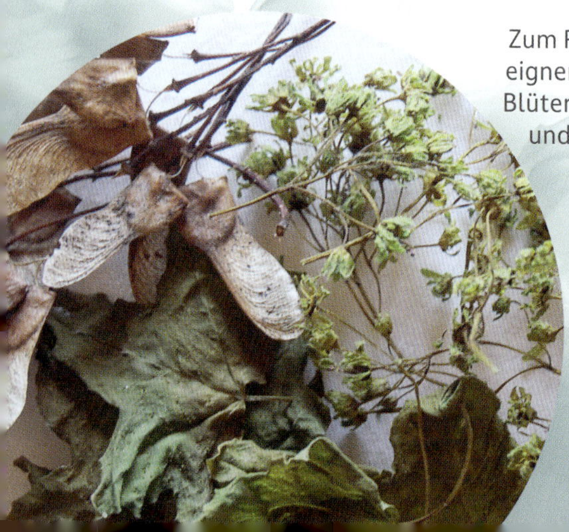

Zum Räuchern eignen sich die Blüten, Blätter und Früchte.

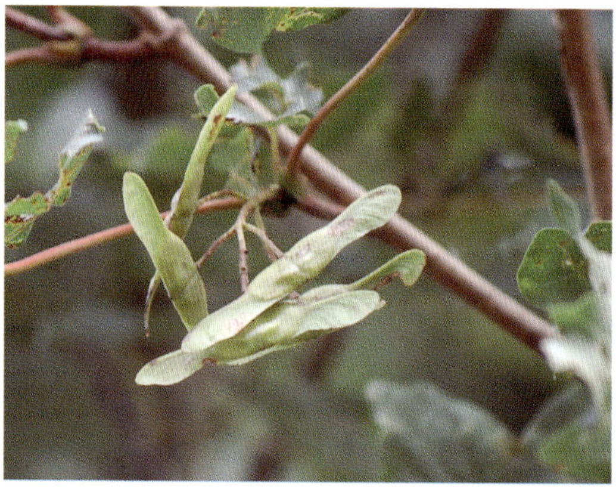

Ahornfrüchte

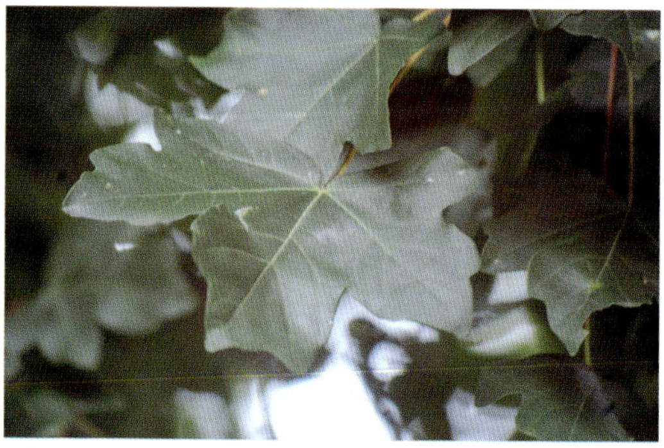

Ahornblatt

Wirkung, Wahrnehmung: Stimmungsaufhellend, entspannend bei emotionalem Durcheinander oder seelischen Verletzungen, vermittelt einen positiven Impuls für zurückhaltende Menschen, befreit von allzu bedrückenden Gedanken, vertreibt die schwarze Trud, die Angst und Beklemmungen verursacht, und hilft einem insgesamt in einen lebensbejahenden Rhythmus zurückzufinden. Hilfreich gegen das innere Leid in einer Arbeitswelt voller Misstrauen und Neid; gegen das täglich tropfende Gift unter Kollegen und Partnern.

Magisches zum Rauch: Wirksamer Schutzrauch gegen böse Geister und gefühlte Bedrohungen.

Schwerpunkt, Anwendungen, Rezepte: Unterstützt Räucherungen mit Lärche, Birke oder Eberesche kombiniert mit Harz in Richtung Ich-Stärkung und Erneuerung, Ausweg aus ungeschickten Lebensphasen.

Mythologie und magische Praktiken

Am Johannistag, den 24. Juni, werden Ahornzweige an die Haus- und Stalltür gesteckt, um für den Sommer Blitz, Feuer, Fledermäuse und andere Dämonen fernzuhalten. Zu ähnlichen Abwehrzwecken wurden kleine Stifte oder Zapfen aus Ahornholz angefertigt und in die Türschwelle, den Türrahmen oder das Türblatt verbohrt. Alles Negative, jeder böse Blick, soll daran abprallen.

Verwendung – gestern und heute

Der Ahorn wird bereits im Papyrus Ebers (etwa 1600 v. Chr.) als Heilsbaum genannt. Eine derart wertschätzende Bezeichnung gibt es in diesem Text nur noch für den Wacholder. Hildegard von Bingen empfiehlt fiebersenkende Bäder mit ausgekochten Ahornzweigen sowie bei Rheuma und Gicht das Auflegen von Ahornholz auf die erkrankten Stellen.

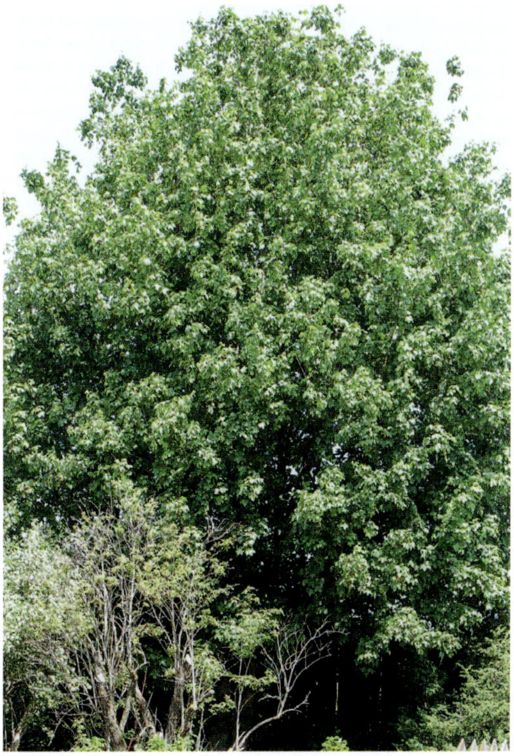

Stattlicher Ahorn im Kräuterland am Radsberg/Radiše

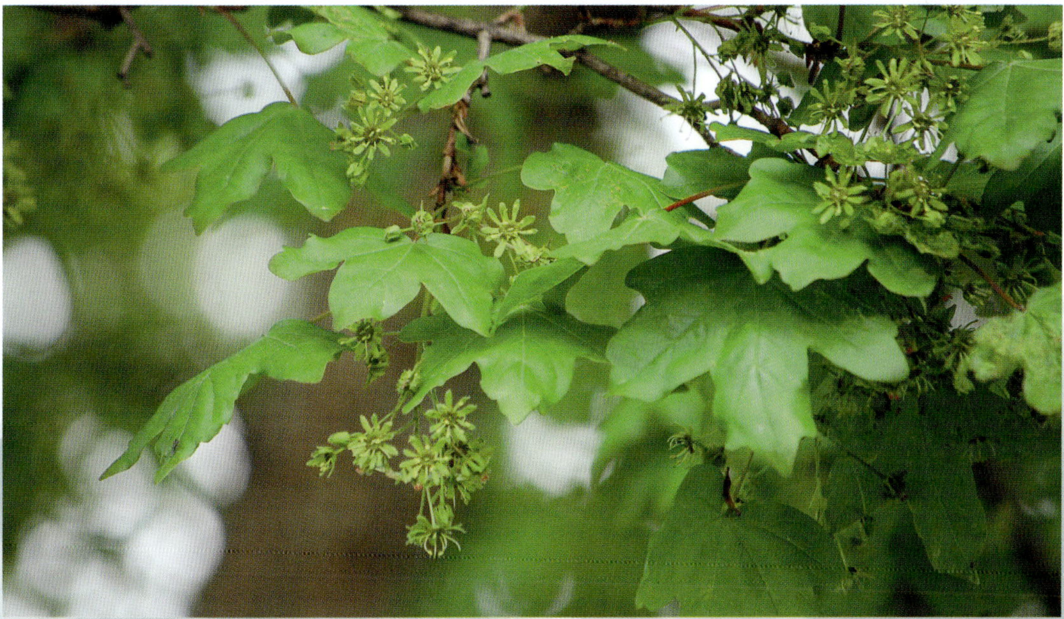

Ahornblüten

Birke

Lat. Name: *Betula pendula*
Botanischer Name: Hänge-Birke
Pflanzenfamilie: Birkengewächse

Die Birke beeindruckt durch ihr helles Leuchten im Frühjahr. Ohne Blätter, vielleicht mit noch etwas Schnee zu ihren Füßen, strahlt ihre weiße Borke hoheitlich und vollkommen rein. Genau das Richtige für einen neuen Anfang, für einen optimalen Start in einen neuen Lebenszyklus. Der Spruch „'Ich brauch' Tapetenwechsel', sprach die Birke…" aus Hildegard Knefs Lied zeigt diese Lust zur Veränderung gepaart mit der Kraft aufzubrechen, ja auszubrechen. Nicht umsonst gilt die Birke weltweit als heiliger Baum unter den Naturheilern. Für Tataren und Mongolen ist sie der Weltenbaum. Sie erscheint wie ein Wegweiser in eine andere Welt, bietet Treppen aus Birkenporlingen an, die den Suchenden hinauf, aber auch hinunter führen können, wo auch immer die Welt der Geister liegen mag. Die Birke vergesellschaftet sich gern mit bewusstseinsverändernden Fliegenpilzen und liebt unruhiges Gelände mit vielen Verwerfungen und Wasserstörzonen – kein Wunder, wenn sie pro Tag bis zu 70 Liter Wasser aus dem Boden pumpt. Neben Pilzen und Flechten sind Birkenzeisig und Birkhuhn ihre tierischen Begleiter. Es ist immer viel los rund um die Birke.

Der Baum wird bis zu 30 m hoch und kann bis zu 120 Jahre alt werden. Dabei wird ihre Rinde mit zunehmendem Alter rissig und immer weißer.

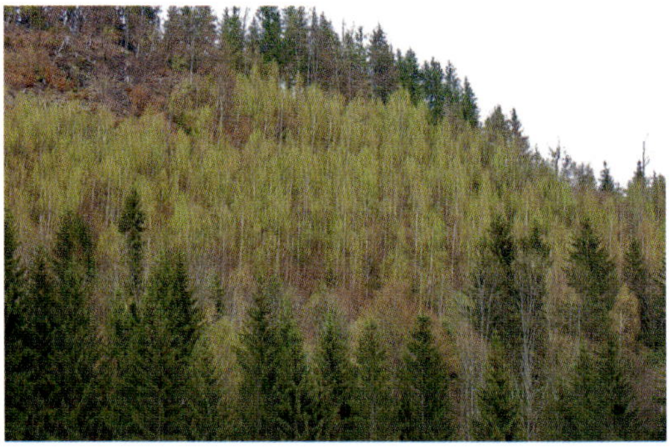

Birken sind Pionierpflanzen.

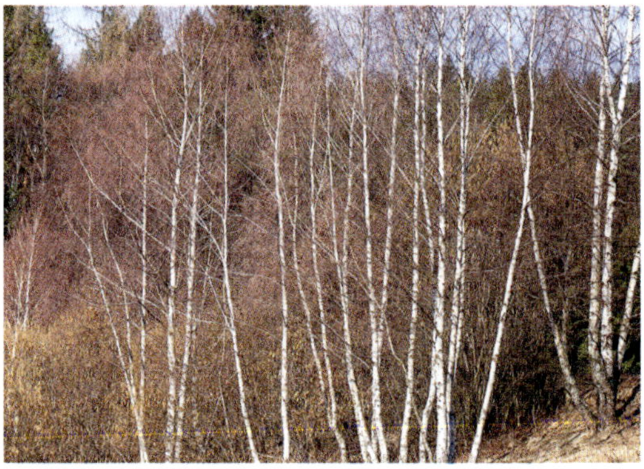

Ihre weiße Rinde ist unverkennbar.

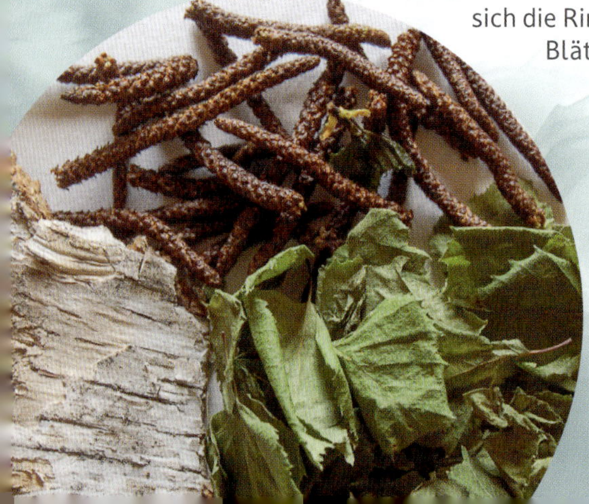

Zum Räuchern eignen sich die Rinde, die Blätter und Blüten.

Rauch

Verwendete Pflanzenteile: Blätter, Blütenkätzchen, Rinde.

Beste Sammel- und Erntezeit: Die Blätter können das ganze Jahr über gesammelt werden, wobei die Frühlingsblätter im Rauch am intensivsten duften; die Blütenkätzchen werden bis Ende Mai gesammelt; die rissigen weißen Rindenstückchen können das ganze Jahr über vom Stamm älterer Birken gelöst werden.

Wirkung, Wahrnehmung: Der Rauch reinigt das Raumklima, wirkt allgemein entlastend. Er klärt die Gedanken, sodass leichter Ideen und Pläne fließen können und Platz für Neues entsteht. Es ist ein aufbauender Rauch, der Licht und Hoffnung in dunkle Stunden bringen kann.

Der Birkenrauch unterstützt jeden Neuanfang, bringt Dinge in Bewegung und bläst einem erstaunlich frische Gedanken in den Kopf!

Der Blüten- und Rindenrauch der Birke beruhigt schmerzende Glieder und wird körperlich als sehr angenehm empfunden. Die Rinde allein kann zu kleinen Kegeln gedreht, auf dem Räucherstövchen angezündet und ausgeblasen werden. Die schmerzende Stelle, Fuß oder Handgelenk, wird ein paar Minuten lang über den aufsteigenden, schmalen Rauchfaden gehalten.

Magisches zum Rauch: Wenn es zu viel blitzt und donnert, wurden früher Birkenzweige verbrannt und getrocknete Birkenblüten auf die Herdplatte geworfen.

Schwerpunkt, Anwendungen, Rezepte: Für eine klassische Frühjahrsreinigungsräucherung mischt man zu den Birkenblättern noch Giersch-Wurzeln und Weide sowie Harz.

Mythologie und magische Praktiken

Die Birke gilt als Lebensbaum, als Sinnbild der erwachenden Natur, die alles Böse abwehren und vertreiben kann: So soll das erste Bett eines neuen Erdenbürgers aus Birkenholz sein. In alten Kulturen wurde Anfang Mai ein Birkenfest als Fest der Urmutter gefeiert, zur Erweckung der Fruchtbarkeit in der gesamten Natur. Das heutige Maibaum aufstellen ist ein ferner Abglanz dieser Festlichkeit, auch wenn unsere heutigen Maibäume keine Birken mehr sind.

Die Weiße prägt die Mythologie sämtlicher nordischer Völker: Bei den Kelten galt sie als Muse der Weisheitssuchenden und Heiler. Slawische Völker sahen in ihr weißgefiederte Schwanenjungfrauen, die sich hin und wieder mit den Heilern vermählten. Bei den Germanen ist die Birke der Göttin Freya zugeordnet, der schönsten und begehrtesten aller Göttinnen und Gefährtin Odins, die für Fruchtbarkeit, Frühling, Glück und Liebe steht.

Heilige Orte wurden mit einem Kultbesen aus Birkenzweigen saubergefegt, um alle bösen Geister zu vertreiben. Später wird dieser Kultbesen zum Hexenbesen, mit dem Hexen allgegenwärtig sein können und mit welchem sie zu ihren Versammlungen fliegen. Angst zu machen vor den unheimlichen Kräften der Natur war ein Merkmal der Umbruchsjahrhunderte von heidnischem Denken zum christlichen Glauben. Die zentrale mythologische Stellung der Birke ließ sich jedoch nicht zur Gänze auslöschen. Heute

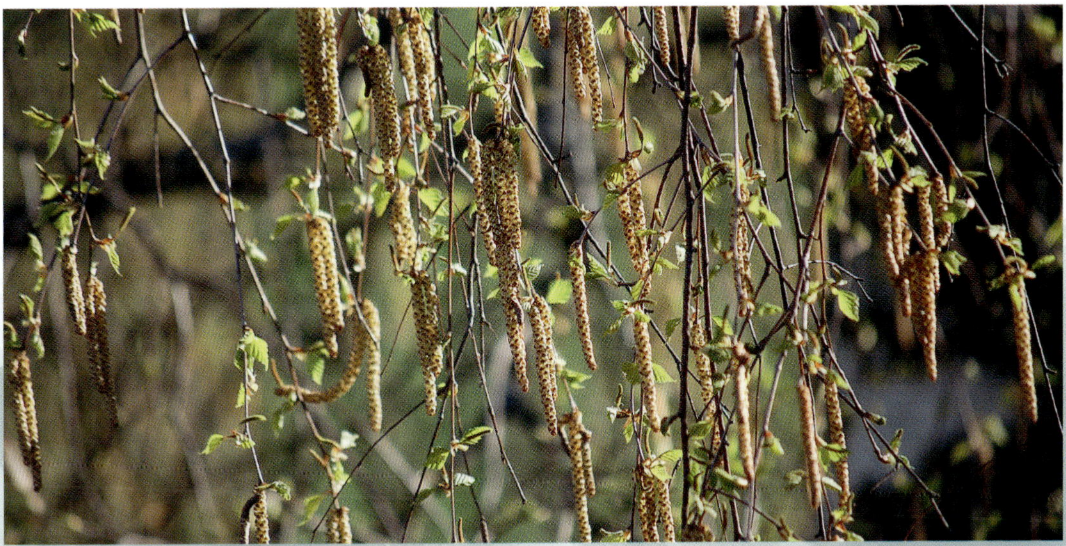

Blütenstand der Birke

ist Birkenschmuck zumindest bei zwei Anlässen im christlichen Kirchenjahr selbstverständlicher Begleiter: bei den Fronleichnamsprozessionen an jedem Stationsaltar im Freien und zu Pfingsten an jedem Haus, um den Heiligen Geist in die Stuben hineinzuwehen und gleichzeitig alles Böse draußen zu halten. Mit dem Laub solcherart „geweihter" Birkenzweige wurden mancherorts die Ställe gegen Schadenszauber ausgeräuchert. Das Laub verfütterte man auch an kranke Tiere, um diese zu stärken.

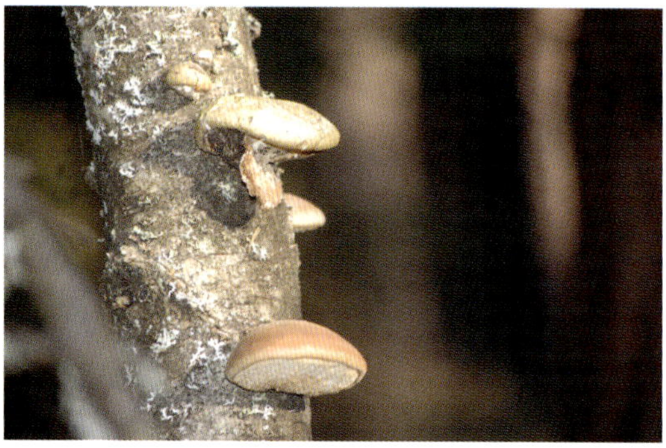

Der Birkenporling ist ein Pilz, der diese Baumart als Lebensraum erkoren hat.

Verwendung – gestern und heute

Im Norden steht die Birke für Weiblichkeit, Freiheit, Heilung. Die Römer jedoch bemächtigten sich der Symbolik der Birke mit der ihnen eigenen Geradlinigkeit: Bei der Amtseinführung von höheren Beamten trugen dessen Liktoren, sprich Leibwächter, ein rot geschnürtes Birkenreisigbündel voran, in dessen Mitte ein Beil steckte. Es sollte wohl die säubernde Kraft des neu bestellten Magistratus öffentlich hergezeigt werden. Nach dem Motto: Neue Besen kehren gut.

Hildegard von Bingen (1098–1179) nutzt die Birkenrinde als Räucherkegel, der auf die Haut aufgesetzt wird, um Rücken- und Eingeweideschmerzen zu lindern. Lonicerus (1528–1586) schreibt in seinem „Kreuterbuch" von dem Birkenbaum: „... sein Gebrauch ist gering in der Artzney...", er weiß hingegen: „bei den Römern vor Zeiten in großen Ehren gewesen, welche sie der Obrigkeit vorhergetragen. Ist auch noch heutzutag in großer Ehr, dieweil sie die böse und ungehorsame Kinder und Jugend strafet. Daher man in deutschen Reimen sagt: „Oh du gute Birken Ruth, du machst die ungehorsam´ Kinder gut."

Die Birke ist eine der zentralen Pflanzen der Volksheilkunde. Sie war über viele Jahrhunderte das Universalheilmittel aller nordischen Völker. Heute wird in den USA der hohe Betulingehalt der Birkenrinde im Kampf gegen Hautkrebs erforscht.

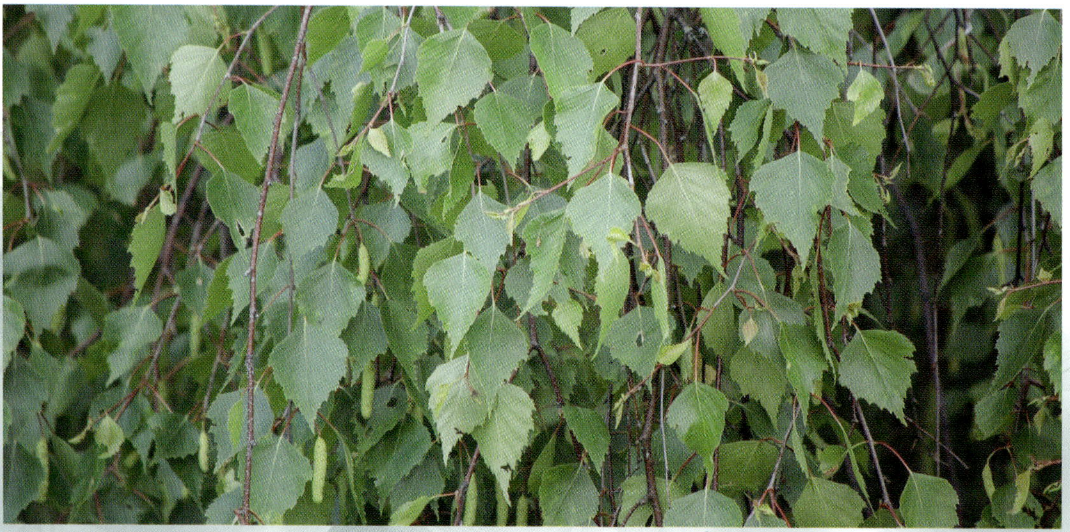

Birkenblätter

Buche

Lat. Name: *Fagus sylvatica*
Botanischer Name: Rot-Buche
Pflanzenfamilie: Buchengewächse

Die Buche ist die graue Eminenz des Waldes. Bei ihr läuft alles zusammen und von ihr geht alles aus – sie ist die Dirigentin, die alle anderen Bäume tanzen lässt. Nichts keimt unter ihr und noch weit über den Bereich ihrer Arme hinaus. Sie ist die unumstrittene Herrscherin.

Hätten wir nicht in unsere europäischen Wälder forsttechnisch eingegriffen, wären wir heute wohl überwiegend von Buchenwäldern umgeben. Buchenholz ist wegen seiner besonderen Härte nicht nur als Brennholz oder als geschmacklich angenehmes, eher neutrales Holz zum Räuchern von Fleischwaren begehrt, sondern vor allem als Bau- und Möbelholz.

Über Jahrhunderte waren die Früchte der Buchen, die Bucheckern, als Tierfutter in der Schweinemast unverzichtbar. Erst im Alter zwischen 40 und 80 Jahren bringt die Buche erstmals ihre Früchte hervor. Das ist angemessen früh, wenn man bedenkt, dass eine Buche bis zu 300 Jahre alt und zwischen 30 und 40 m hoch werden kann.

Rauch

Verwendete Pflanzenteile: Blätter, Rinde von Ästen und vom Stamm, Bucheckern.

Beste Sammel- und Erntezeit: Blätter und Rinde in der ersten Jahreshälfte, die Früchte im Herbst bis in den Winter hinein.

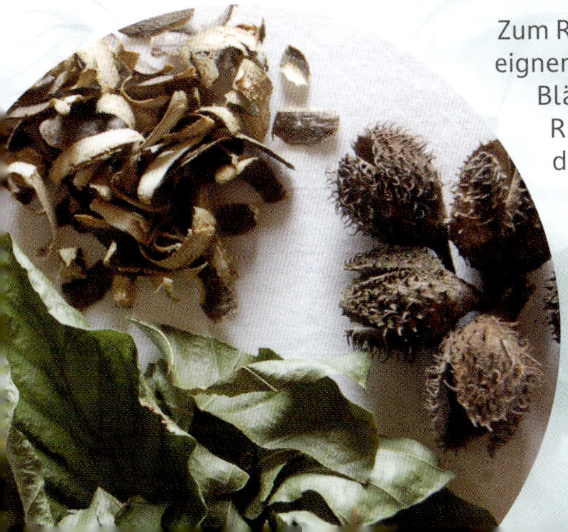

Zum Räuchern eignen sich die Blätter, die Rinde und die Früch-

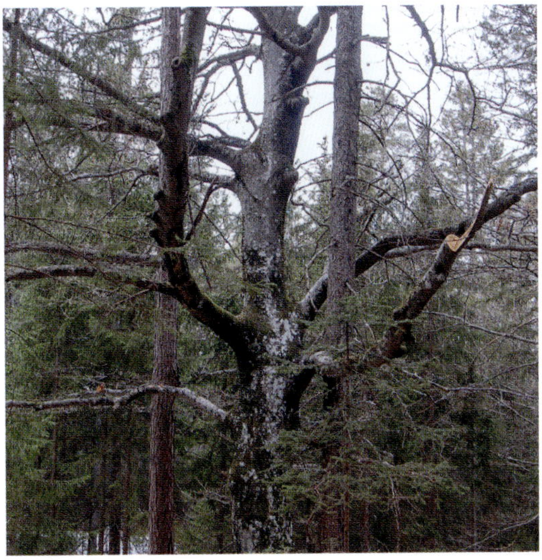

Buche im Winter

Wirkung, Wahrnehmung: Die Buche schweigt, hat mir nichts zu sagen. Gibt mir nichts Mütterliches, wie es in den Büchern steht; gibt mir kein Wissen, von dem die Schriftlosen träumten. Wendet sich ab von mir, schließt ihren Kreis. So sehr beschäftigt mit ihren Familiengeschichten: Als Leitfigur des Waldes trägt man schwer, muss seine Nachkommen richtig platzieren, muss mit ihnen Verbindung halten, muss sie lehren, muss geben, immer geben. Keine Zeit für lästige Menschen. Welche Anmaßung ihr etwas in die Rinde zu schnitzen und sie muss dafür geradestehen!

Buchenräucherungen gehen sehr tief; berühren Lebensthemen; helfen vielleicht auch diese zu tragen; vermitteln eine oft beängstigende Stille. Es erscheint mir, als würde im Inneren für einen Moment alles stillstehen und jede Äußerlichkeit bedeutungslos werden. In solchen Momenten kann man sich gefahrlos selbst in Frage stellen. Ernste Botschaften also.

Sie regt uns zum Nachdenken darüber an, dass wir in dieser Existenz ins Morgen nie ohne unser Gestern werden gehen können; offenbart uns aber auch die Verbindungen in der Zeit, in unserem Schicksal, wenn etwas, das wir hinter uns zu haben glaubten, tief drinnen noch pulsiert.

Magisches zum Rauch: Auch bei körperlichen Schmerzen hat man sich früher in den Buchenrauch gestellt oder die erkrankten Stellen über den Rauch gehalten – so bei Fieber, Husten, Hauterkrankungen, Wunden und Geschwüren, Rheuma und Gicht.

Schwerpunkt, Anwendungen, Rezepte: Mit Buche sollten überwiegend Harze (Fichte, Lärche) verräuchert werden, um ihre Wirkkraft klar zu transportieren. Buchenräucherungen helfen in Phasen, in denen Entscheidungen gut überlegt und vorbereitet werden müssen.

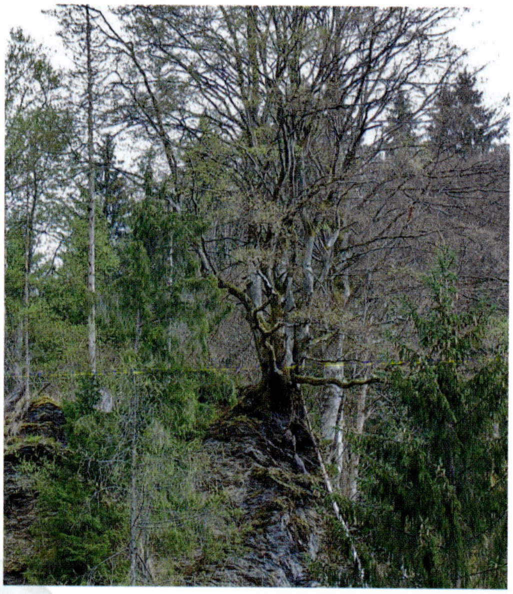

Rot-Buche am Felsgrat vor Arriach, Kärnten

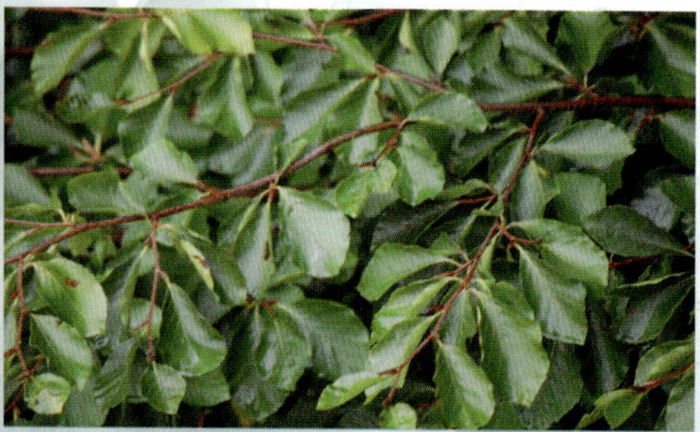

Blätter

Mythologie und magische Praktiken

Unter Buchen hörten keltische Druiden das Raunen des Großen Geistes und schnitzten es mit verschiedenen Zeichen, den Runen, in Buchenstäbe. Der römische Geschichtsschreiber Tacitus (58–120) berichtet über das Orakeln mit Buchenstäben bei den Germanen: „Von einem Zweig werden mehrere Stäbe abgebrochen, darauf werden Zeichen geritzt und dann wird alles auf ein weißes Tuch geworfen. Das Ergebnis war das „raedelse“, das Rätsel: Es werden drei Stäbe herausgenommen und gedeutet.“

Verwendung – gestern und heute

Die Überzeugung, dass die Buche eine unübertroffene spirituelle Kraft habe, spielt in der Vorstellung aller heidnischen Völker eine große Rolle. So wurde beispielsweise die christliche Bibel das „BUCH“ genannt, also von „Buche“ kommend.

Bachblüte Nr. 3 „beech“ – Rot-Buche – fördert Toleranz und Nachsicht und gilt als Heilmittel für überkritische Menschen.

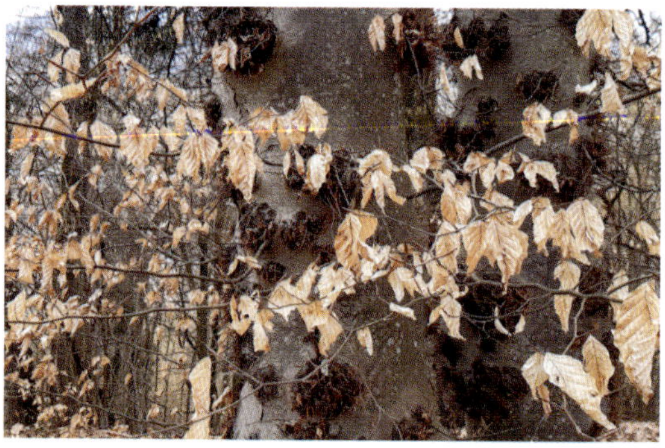

Buchenrinde

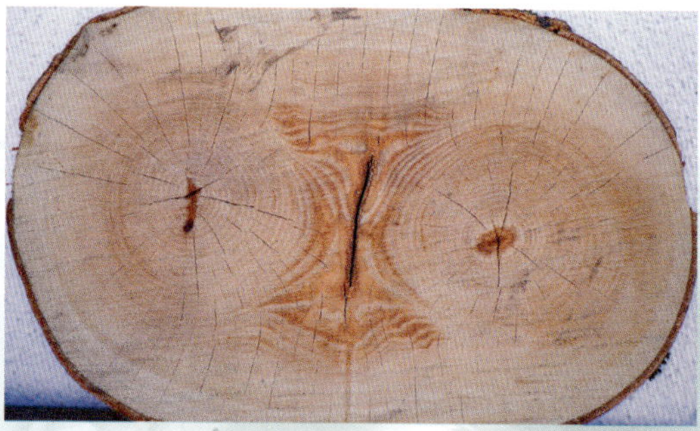

Frisches Buchenholz

Eberesche

Lat. Name: *Sorbus aucuparia*
Pflanzenfamilie: Rosengewächse

Man sollte sie nicht unterschätzen – so filigran und verspielt die Eberesche oder Vogelbeere nach außen hin auch wirken mag, die ihr zugeschriebenen Schutz- und Abwehrkräfte sind gewaltig! Sie war, neben der Eiche, dem germanischen Gott Thor geweiht, der die Urgewalt der Natur symbolisiert. Immerhin hatte sie ihn ja vor langer Zeit aus einem reißenden Fluss gerettet, indem sie ihm ihre Zweige entgegenstreckte, an denen er sich festhalten konnte.

Die Eberesche lebt bevorzugt am Waldrand, bildet den ersten Schutzwall vor der dunklen Ernsthaftigkeit des Waldes, winkt im Herbst mit fröhlichem Orange und verspricht vielen Vögeln ein opulentes Mahl. Tatsächlich besagt ihr lateinischer Name „aucuparia" = *aves capere* (Vögel fangen), dass ihre unwiderstehlichen Beeren früher zum Vogelfang verwendet wurden. Die Eberesche wird bis zu 15 m hoch und kann schon 120 Jahre alt werden.

Wer sich ihr nähert, spürt sofort ihre Leichtigkeit, die nichts Flatterhaftes hat, sondern auf tiefster Ausgeglichenheit zu beruhen scheint. Man nimmt ihr menschenzugewandtes und kommunikatives Wesen wahr und kann sich über so viel positive Energie nur freuen. „Und gib ihr eine Wasserfläche, sie sieht sich so gerne selbst!" rät mir die irische Eberesche vor langer Zeit, als ich zu ihren Füßen saß und ihr von der Eberesche in meinem Garten erzählte.

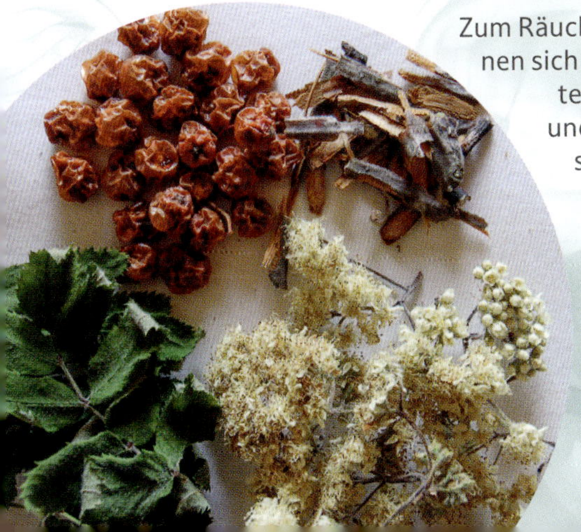

Zum Räuchern eignen sich die Blätter, Blüten und Beeren sowie die Rinde.

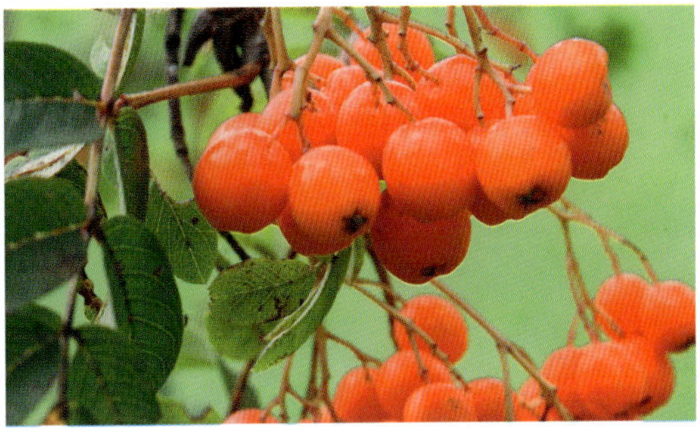

Die Früchte der Eberesche werden auch als Vogelbeeren bezeichnet.

Rauch

Verwendete Pflanzenteile: Blüten, Blätter, Rinde und vor allem die getrockneten Beeren.

Beste Sammel- und Erntezeit: Blätter und Blüten im Frühling, Rinde das ganze Jahr über und die Beeren werden im Herbst gesammelt und getrocknet.

Wirkung, Wahrnehmung: Große Schutzkraft vor Unheil und negativen Energien von außen sowie gegenüber negativen Gedanken. Unterstützt das geordnete Denken, die geistige Fruchtbarkeit und die Anpassungsfähigkeit in Übergangsphasen oder bei Lebensumbrüchen. Sie hilft einem, das Innere vom Äußeren zu trennen und dabei das Eine verborgen und das Andere stark zu halten.

Der wunderbar honigartige Geruch der getrockneten und verräucherten Blüten umhüllt einen wie ein Schutzmantel. Man ist sofort bereit, sich ganz diesem Duft hinzugeben. So wird so mancher vergeistigte Zeitgenosse wieder geerdet und so manch erkaltetes Herz wird erwärmt.

Der Rauch der Beeren wirkt Verwünschungen und Flüchen entgegen. Was der Blütenrauch schon andeutete, wird im Beerenrauch noch verstärkt: Er hilft dem „verschlossenen Herz" von der Kälte in die Einsichtsfähigkeit zurück. Der Rauch von Blättern und Rinde ist aufbauend und kann neue Energie übertragen. Er stärkt die

Aura und macht sie undurchdringlich für jeden negativen Angriff von außen – somit zu empfehlen zur seelischen Stärkung bei Mobbing, sozialer Ausgrenzung und sonstigen Dämonen und bösem Zauber unserer Tage.

Magisches zum Rauch: Im Dachstuhl wurden früher oft Kränze aus Ebereschenlaub aufgehängt, um das Haus gegen Blitzschlag zu schützen. Bei heftigen Gewittern holte man davon einige Zweiglein und warf sie auf den Herd, um die Atmosphäre zu entladen. Um die Wesenheiten der Natur gnädig zu stimmen, wurden im Freien Räucherungen mit Eberesche, Wald-Geißbart und Vogelkirsche durchgeführt.

Schwerpunkt, Anwendungen, Rezepte: Für neuen Schwung sorgt eine Räuchermischung aus Lärche, Eberesche, Löwenzahnwurzeln und Birkenrinde mit Harz.

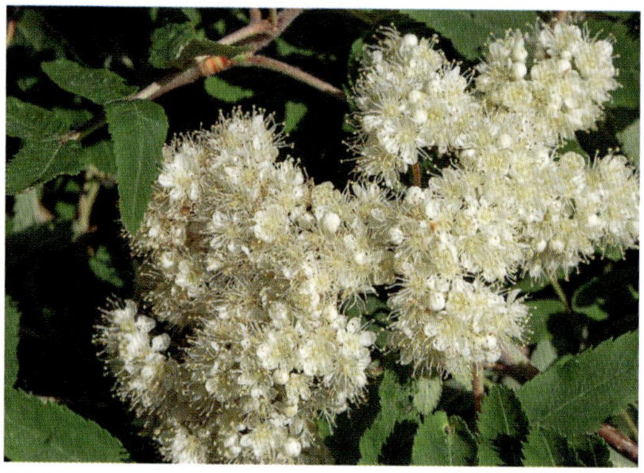

Blüten

Mythologie und magische Praktiken

Die Kelten glaubten, dass die erste Frau aus einer Eberesche entsprungen sei, der erste Mann einer Erle. Wie die Birke galt sie als Baum des Lebens und des Wiederwachens der Natur. Die Ritualstäbe der Druiden waren aus Ebereschenholz oder

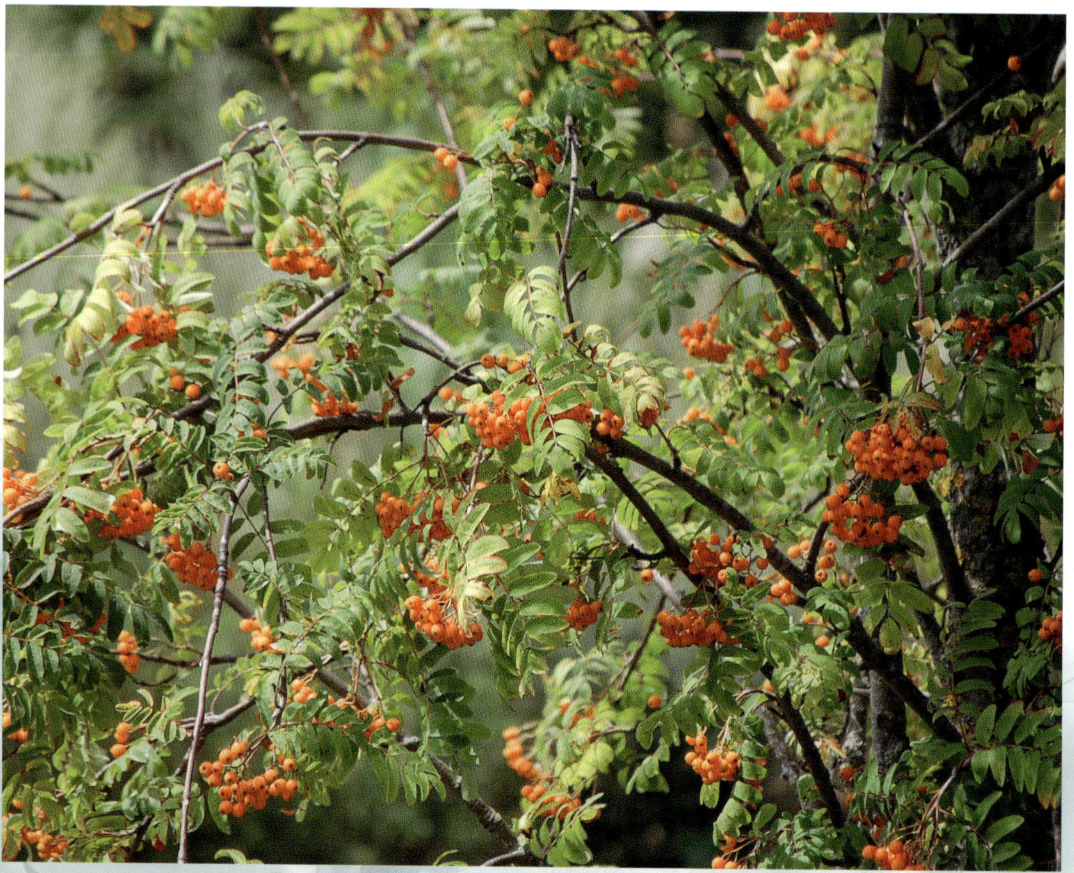

Fruchtstände

Eschenholz gefertigt. Aber viel wichtiger noch war für die Druiden die alles Unheil abwehrende Kraft dieser Bäume. So setzten sie Ebereschen als Außenbegrenzung um ihre Kultplätze, damit sie den heiligen Raum dicht machten: hart nach außen, beruhigt und harmonisch nach innen.

Die Eberesche steht für Gesundheit und Fruchtbarkeit. Dies versuchte man durch „quicken und quecken“ mit gleichzeitigem Hersagen von Beschwörungsformeln auf Menschen und Tiere zu übertragen. Die fruchtenden Zweige oder auch nur ein Stück Holz über die Wiege gelegt, an Haus- oder Stalltür befestigt, schützen alle Bewohner vor jedem Ungemach – vor Krankheit, Blitz und Verwünschungen. Solche magischen Praktiken werden nach dem Übergang von heidnischer zu christlicher Weltsicht verboten: Das Holz wird zu Hexenholz erklärt und darf nicht mehr ins Haus gebracht werden, da es dort Unglück brächte.

Verwendung – gestern und heute

Zu den Beeren schreibt Hieronymus Bock (1498–1554) in seinem Kreutterbuch: „... sie sind eines seltsamen, unlustigen Geschmacks, so man deren zu viel isst, machen sie Unwillen...“

Volksmedizinisch wurden Blätter und Blüten gegen Husten und Magenverstimmung verwendet, die getrockneten Beeren bei Durchfall. Die Iren vermeinten, wenn man einige Beeren verzehrte, würde man sein Leben um ein weiteres Jahr verlängern.

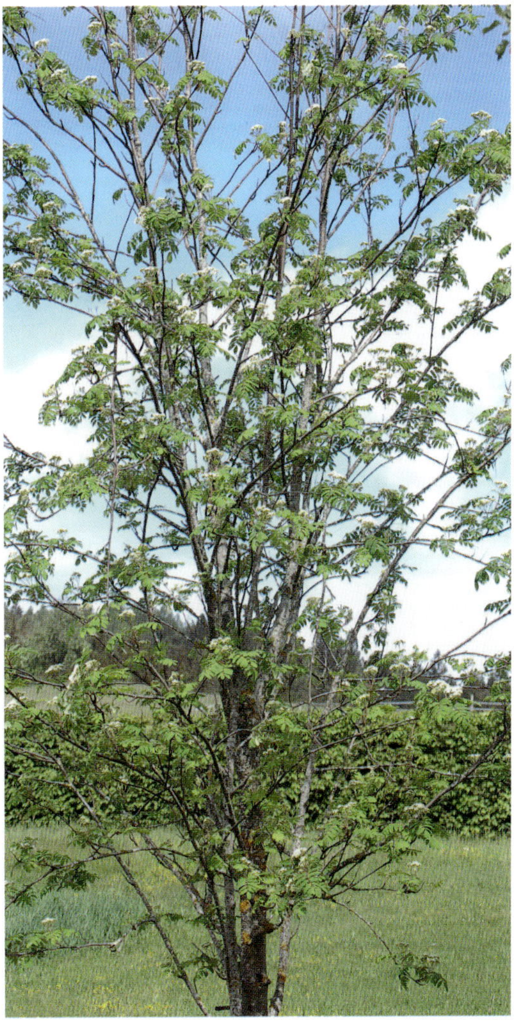

Eberesche

Eiche

Lat. Name: *Quercus robur*
Botanischer Name: Stiel-Eiche
Pflanzenfamilie: Buchengewächse

Eine Eiche entfaltet sich erst richtig, wenn sie alleine steht. Dann erst fahren ihre eigenwilligen Äste breit in den Himmel, dann erst zeigt sich ihre Mächtigkeit, ihre Unbezwingbarkeit. Es wird wohl dieses Bild gewesen sein, das unsere Vorfahren vor Jahrtausenden schon beeindruckte und dazu führte, dass sie in ihren Mythologien die Eiche stets der obersten Gottheit zuordneten. Die Eiche steht für Kraft und Willensstärke, Belastbarkeit, Ausdauer, Gerechtigkeit, Durchsetzungsfähigkeit und Mut.

Diese Zuschreibungen korrespondieren mit der Tatsache, dass Eichenholz zu den widerstandsfähigsten und härtesten Hölzern Europas zählt. Die Eiche sucht ihren Standort bevorzugt dort, wo es Störzonen gibt, wie auf kleinen Abhängen, an Waldrändern und manchmal auch auf freiem Feld. Von diesen Störzonen leitet sie große Erdkräfte nach oben und gibt diese auch gerne ab: Eichen-Coaching sozusagen. Bei ihr kann man sich Kraft holen, wenn man einmal nicht weiter weiß. Die Eiche lässt einen spüren: Auf, auf! Kopf hoch!

Und nicht von ungefähr ist auch die Zauberflöte in Wolfgang Amadeus Mozarts (1756–1791) Oper „Zauberflöte" aus dem Holz einer 1000-jährigen Eiche geschnitzt. Ihr Klang bietet Schutz gegen Dunkelheit und Verdammnis und mächtige Führung in größter Gefahr.

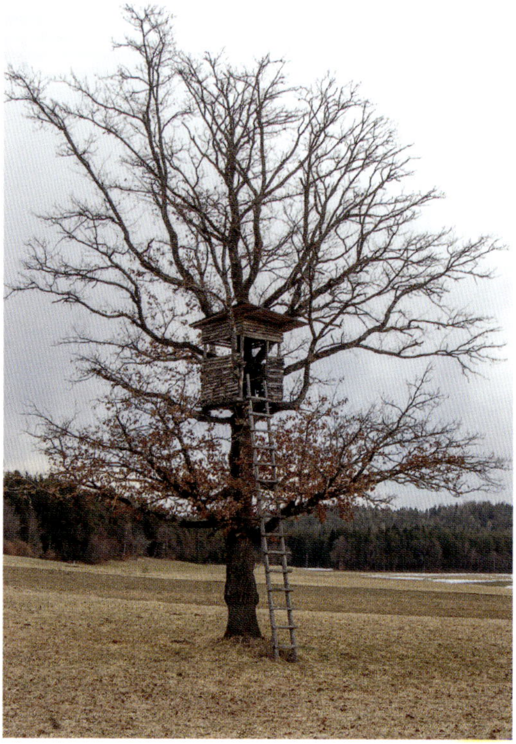

Hochsitz in der Eiche am Radsberg/Radiše

Als Baum der Wildnis ist sie Heimat für zahlreiche Tierarten: vom Eichelhäher über das Eichhörnchen und die Gallwespe bis zum Käfer namens Eichenbock. Lange vor Aufkommen der Eichelmast von Schweinen zählte ein Eichelbrei zu den menschlichen Grundnahrungsmitteln. Eine Eiche kann 30 bis 40 m hoch werden und bis zu unvorstellbare 1000 Jahre alt: Davon verbringt sie 300 Jahre in der Jugend, 300 Jahre in der Reife und die letzten Jahre im Alter.

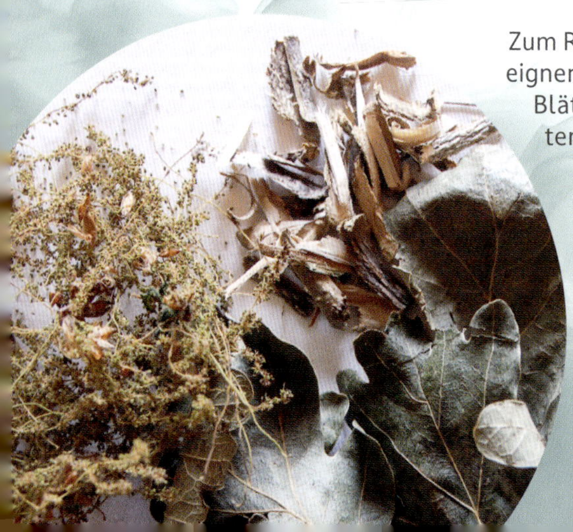

Zum Räuchern eignen sich die Blätter, Blüten und die Rinde.

Rauch

Verwendete Pflanzenteile: Blätter, Blüten, Rinde.

Beste Sammel- und Erntezeit: Die Blüten im Frühling, Blätter und Rinde können das ganze Jahr über beerntet werden, am besten aber in der zweiten Augusthälfte.

Wirkung, Wahrnehmung: Die Eiche spricht zu mir: „Was kommst du mit gesenktem Kopf zu mir? Kopf hoch und schau mich an! Ich will keine Unterwürfigkeit, ich brauche keine Zurückhaltung und keine Scheinheiligkeit. Was ich dir geben kann, bekommst du immer von mir, bedingungslos. Und spürst du ein Ziehen in dir, das dich an mich erinnert, dann komm einfach her und hol dir was du brauchst. Ich bin an deiner Seite."

Energetisch stark reinigend, lösend für jede negative Raumatmosphäre, klärt die Gedanken, hilft beim Konzentrieren, verbessert die geistige Ausdauer, unterstützt das Durchhalten und Umsetzen der eigenen Pläne. Das Vertrauen in die eigenen Fähigkeiten steigt. Das getrocknete Eichenlaub wirkt auch dämonenbannend und geistig aufbauend.

Der Rauch der Eichenrinde stärkt Willenskraft, sorgt für Erfolg und ein langes Leben. Hier sollte Salbei und Blutwurz mitverräuchert werden.

Magisches zum Rauch: „duir" ist das keltische Wort für Eiche. Die Druiden waren also Eichengeweihte. Somit galt: keine kultische Handlung ohne vorhergehende Eichenlaubräucherung! Wie bei den Kelten so ist es auch noch heute angebracht, den Raum mit einer Eichenräucherung zu klären, ehe man ein bestimmtes Räucherritual abhält.

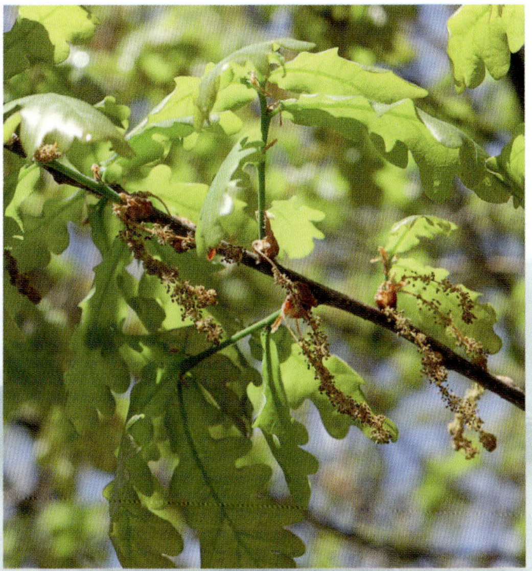

Eichenblüten

Schwerpunkt, Anwendungen, Rezepte: Die überwiegende Zahl meiner Räucherkurs-Teilnehmer hat während der Corona-Zeit intuitiv zum vermahlenen Eichenlaub gegriffen, als es darum ging, für sich selbst drei Räucherstoffe auszuwählen. Eine Eichenlaub-Räucherung mit Harz ist wie ein fester Anker in unsicheren Zeiten, der hilft, stark und positiv gestimmt zu bleiben.

Wenn es um weitgehende Entscheidungen geht, passen Salbei, Haselnussblätter und -rinde und/oder Holunderbeeren zum Eichenrauch.

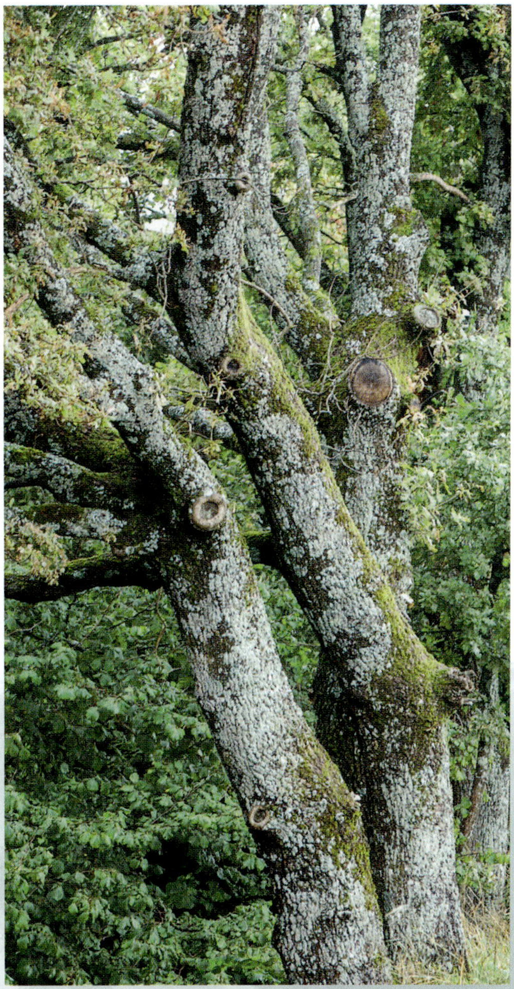

Eichenrinde

Mythologie und magische Praktiken

Bei den Griechen und Römern galt die Eiche als der ursprünglichste aller Bäume. Man glaubte, dass Eichen die Mütter der ersten Menschen waren. Zeus verkündete seinen Willen durch das Rauschen des Eichenlaubes und weiß gekleidete Priesterinnen hatten daraus dann einen Orakelspruch abzuleiten. Sokrates pflegte „bei der Eiche" zu schwören und griechische Verträge jener Zeit wurden unter der Eiche unterzeichnet, dem Symbol für Sicherheit und Gerechtigkeit.

Als Bonifatius (673–754) im Jahr 723, im Rahmen der zweiten Christianisierung des Abendlandes, die heilige Donar-Eiche in Fritzlar fällte, um mit ihrem Holz an Ort und Stelle eine Kapelle zu errichten, musste er um sein Leben fürchten, denn erstens durften sich ihr ausschließlich die heidnischen Priester nähern. Und zweitens wurden Menschen, die heilige Bäume fällten, seit Jahrhunderten mit dem Tod bestraft. So sang es auch der britische Barde Taliesin (534 bis ca. 599): „Drei Wesen ohne Atem sind nur mit atmenden Wesen zu bezahlen: Apfelbaum, Haselstrauch, Eichenhain". Und noch im 11. Jahrhundert schreibt ein Mönch des Regenburger Klosters St. Emmeram: „Es gibt Bauern, die es für einen Frevel halten, in einem Wald Bäume zu fällen, unter denen einst Heidenpriester geweissagt haben!"

Die ganze gnadenlose Macht der Obrigkeit bekamen die Menschen zu sehen, wenn in späterer Zeit Delinquenten an den Gerichtseichen aufgehängt wurden und dort zur Abschreckung hängen blieben.

Verwendung – gestern und heute

Die Bachblüte Nr. 22 „oak" – Eiche – hilft Kämpfernaturen und Workaholics Schwächen zuzulassen und sich einmal auch Erholungsphasen zu gönnen.

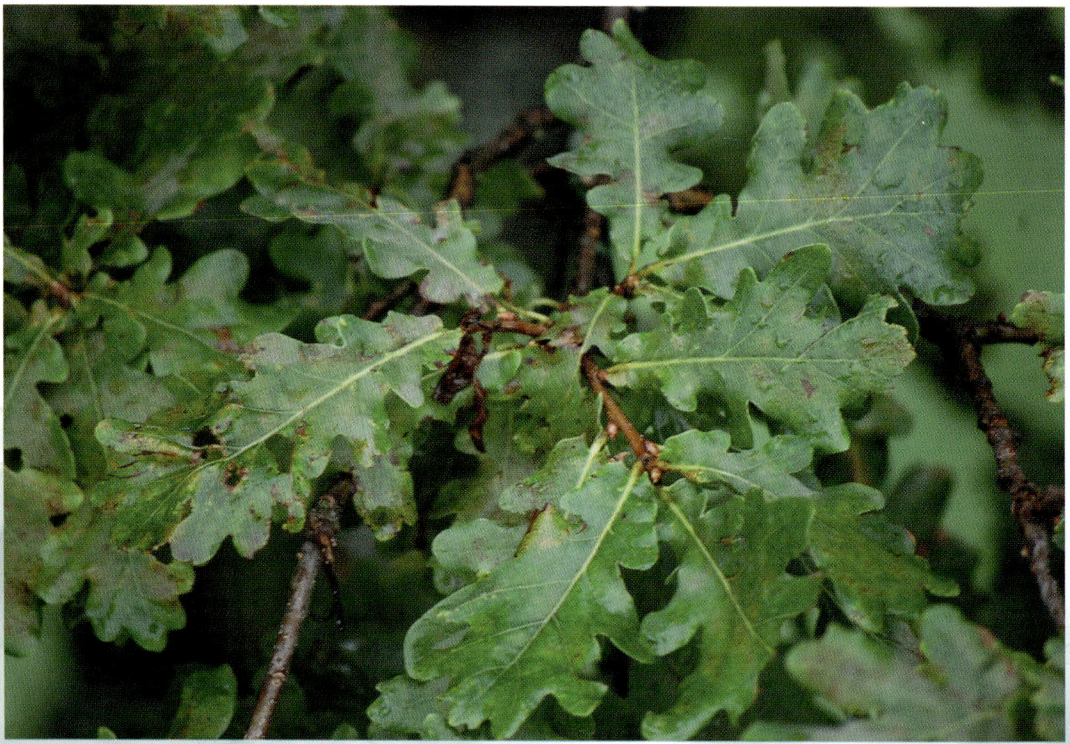

Eichenblätter

Erle

Lat. Name: *Alnus glutinosa*
Botanischer Name: Schwarz-Erle
Pflanzenfamilie: Birkengewächse

Die dunkle Schwester der Birke zieht es in dauerfeuchte Gegenden, in morastige Sumpf- und Überschwemmungsgebiete. In Kärnten, nahe Klagenfurt, hat die Gurk zwischen Sillebrücke und Rain neben ihrem normalen Flussbett einen solchen Fleck geschaffen, der „Haz“ genannt wird und an dem nur Erlen aufkommen. Dicht an dicht, aber dabei mitten aus dem Wasser, ragten ihre Triebe wie Kinderärmchen, bogen sich aufgeregt hin und her bei jeder kleinen Welle und beim geringsten Windhauch. Als Kind durchstreifte ich das nahe Dickicht besonders leise mit dem mulmigen Gefühl es könnte jederzeit etwas Beängstigendes passieren. Damals kannte ich die zahlreichen Geschichten nicht, die davon berichteten, dass in Erlenlandschaften Wassergeister, Nebelfeen, Moorgeister oder gar Irrlichter lebten. Auch wusste ich nichts von der Erlenfrau, Else genannt, die Wanderer auf falsche Spuren führt, damit sie sich verirrten. Oder vom Erlenkönig, der in verzweifelter Hetzjagd um das Leben seines Kindes kämpft.

Im Gegensatz dazu begleiten beeindruckend große Schwarz-Erlen die Gurk vor Grafenstein. Dunkel und gewaltig steigen sie empor und es ist, als wollten sie einen mitziehen, auf ihrem Weg in den Himmel. Und wieder ganz anders der Eindruck jener mächtigen Erlenbäume, die sich wie eine schwarze Perlenkette um das Südufer des Wörthersees legen und mit ihren Wurzeln genussvoll im Seewasser schwelgen.

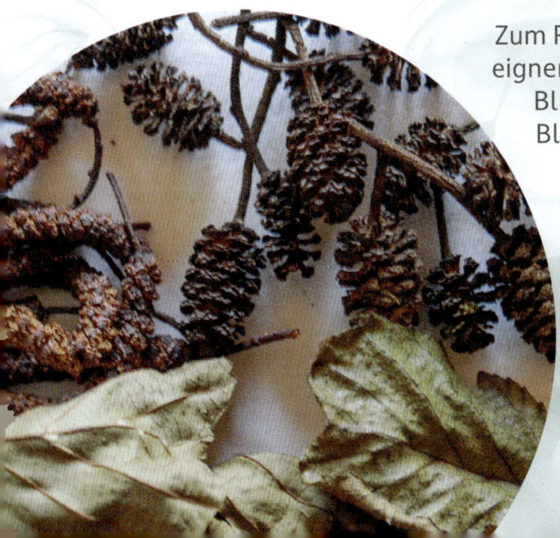

Zum Räuchern eignen sich die Blätter, die Blüten und Früchte.

Als Tiefwurzler macht es Erlen nichts aus, dass ihre Wurzeln dabei in durchnässtem, dauerfeuchtem Erdreich stehen. Die Schwarz-Erle kann schon 30 m hoch werden und ein Alter von bis zu 100 Jahren erreichen. Neben der Esche ist die Erle der einzige Laubbaum, der seine Blätter bereits im grünen Zustand abwirft.

Rauch

Verwendete Pflanzenteile: Blütenkätzchen, Blätter, Früchte.

Beste Sammel- und Erntezeit: Vom Frühjahr beginnend die Blüten, die Blätter bis Ende August und die kleinen, abgerundeten zapfenartigen Früchte im Herbst und Winter.

Wirkung, Wahrnehmung: Die Schwarz-Erle spricht zu mir: „Weil ich meine Wurzeln ein Leben lang in morastigen Grund stecke, kenne ich mich mit allem Dunklen aus; ich weiß um die Kraft der Erde und des Wassers; ich sehe, wo andere nicht sehen; ich höre jedes leise Plätschern in ständiger Erwartung der Urgewalt des Wassers. Ich weiß von der Finsternis und der Kälte, von der Ausweglosigkeit und der ungewollten Begrenzung. Ich habe mein Reich gewählt und liebe es von Grund auf bis zur höchsten Astspitze. Von dort oben hole ich mir das Wenige, das ich vom Himmel brauche.“

Im Rauch erfährt man eine stark lösende Kraft; bringt stockende Energien wieder in Fluss – auch in Räumlichkeiten, Büros oder Küchen; macht Schweres ertragbar, steigert die geistige Beweglichkeit, wirkt oft spontan befreiend, befördert das Loslassen und die innere Erneuerung. Erlenrauch fördert unser Verständnis für Übergänge in verschiedenen Lebensphasen; hilft zu einer ausgeglichenen Sichtweise zu kommen; lässt Belastendes davonziehen.

Einige Stunden nach einer Erlen-Räucherung fällt es leichter komplizierte Arbeiten fortzusetzen oder zu lernen.

Magisches zum Rauch: Mit Erlenrauch versuchte man früher das Wetter zu beeinflussen. Erlenzweige schützen gerade am Ende des Winters Haus und Hof vor Krankheit und anderen Dämonen: Am Karfreitag werden Schwarz-Erlenzweige gesammelt, zu kleinen Kreuzen verarbeitet und im Haus aufbewahrt. Sie sollen die Häuser vor der Feuersbrunst und Blitzschlag beschützen und wurden auch bei jeder anderen Gefahr im Herdfeuer verbrannt.

Schwerpunkt, Anwendungen, Rezepte: Die gemörserten Früchte in Kombination mit Harz wirken geistöffnend, mit der Chance, dass das Brett vor dem Kopf weggeht.

Mythologie und magische Praktiken

Die Erle symbolisiert die alte Göttin, die zwei Seiten hat: die helle, fruchtbarkeitsverheißende, dem Leben zugewandte Seite und die dunkle, todbringende, der Unterwelt, der Dunkelheit zugewandte Seite. So erklärt sich auch, dass Erlengründe oft Toten- und Opferstätten waren.

In der griechischen Mythologie liegen Orakelstätten oft am Wasser oder auf einer Insel und werden von Erlengebüsch umschlossen. Odysseus braucht sieben Jahre, um sich von der Nymphe Kalypso zu trennen, die in einer geheimnisvollen, erlenumstandenen Höhle haust. Die Lex Salica (um 510), das älteste fränkische Gesetzbuch, berichtet über ein Verbannungs-Ritual, das mit Erlenzweigen durchzuführen war: Über dem Haupt eines aus seiner Sippe ausgestoßenen Menschen wurden vier Erlenzweige zerbrochen. Diese warf man dann in die vier Himmelsrichtungen. Damit war der Verstoßene endgültig von der Sippe gelöst und sein Haus zur Wüstung freigegeben. Davon leitet sich der heutige Ausdruck „über jemanden den Stab brechen" ab.

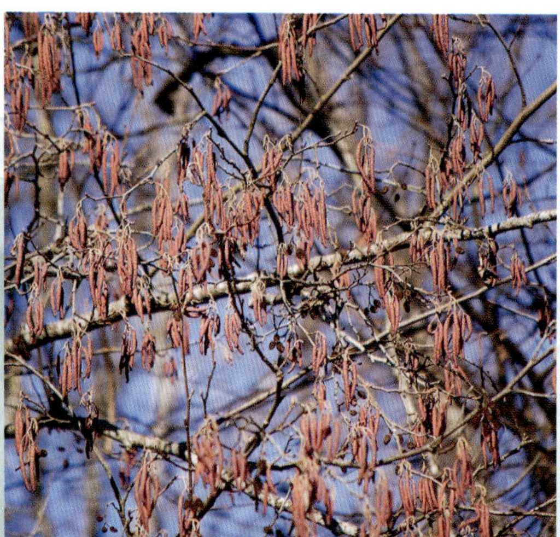

Blüten

Verwendung – gestern und heute

Lonicerus (1528–1586) schreibt in seinem Kreutterbuch: „...das grüne Laub ist äußerlich gut zu hitzigen Schäden. Also grün in die Schuh gelegt und darauf gegangen, zeucht es die Schmerzen, Hitz und Müdigkeit der Füße heraus..."

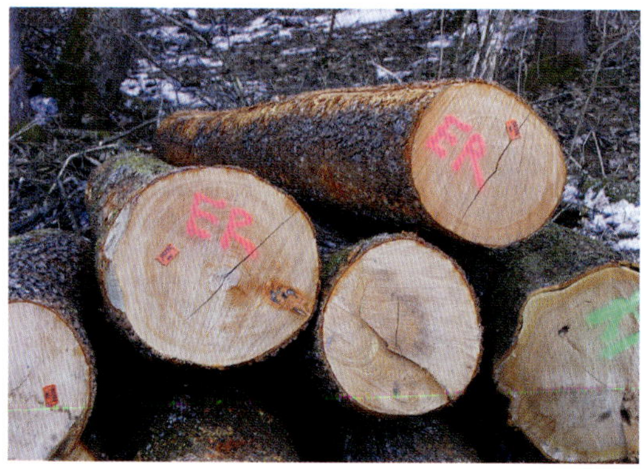

Erlenholz

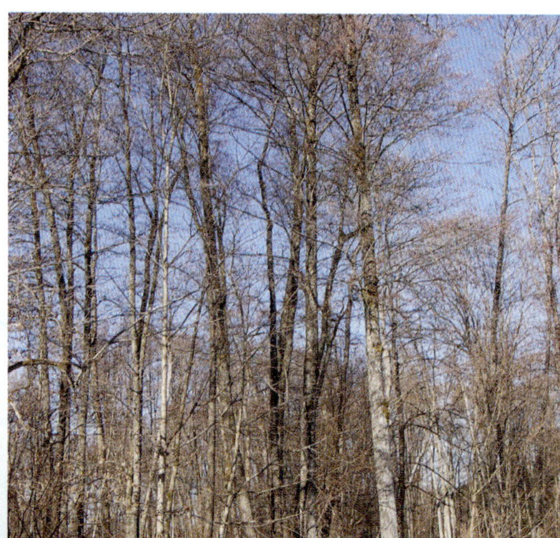

Erlen im Winter

Esche

Lat. Name: *Fraxinus excelsior*
Botanischer Name: Gemeine Esche
Pflanzenfamilie: Ölbaumgewächse

Es ist so, als verabschiede sich ein großer Schutzbaum, der Baum des Wissens und des Geistes, langsam aus unseren Wäldern! Verschiedene eingeschleppte Baumpilzarten haben in den letzten zwanzig Jahren den europäischen Eschenbestand so massiv vernichtet, dass sein Überleben gefährdet scheint – und es ist keine Hilfe in Sicht. Das Sterben vollzieht sich lautlos und blitzschnell: heute noch eine blühende Hoffnung und morgen schon fallen verwelkende Blätter vom Baum. Wo sind ihre großen Tage, die in altisländischer Sprache in den Edda-Mythen beschrieben werden? Yggdrasil, die Weltenesche, die die drei Welten, Ober-, Unter- und Zwischenwelt, verbindet – wo ist sie geblieben? Und die drei Nornen, die Schicksalsgöttinnen, die unter ihrer Wurzel wohnen?

„... eine Esche, weiß ich, heißt Yggdrasil. Den hohen Baum netzt weißer Nebel; davon kommt der Tau, der in die Täler fällt. Immergrün steht er über Urds Brunnen. Davon kommen Frauen, vielwissende. Drei aus dem See dort unterm Wipfel. Urd heißt die eine, die andre Verdandi. Sie schnitten Stäbe. Skuld hieß die dritte. Sie legten Lose. Das Leben bestimmten sie. Den Geschlechtern der Menschen das Schicksal verkündend..."

Einige Jahre nach dem Orkantief 2017, das einen Großteil unserer Waldflächen am Radsberg/Radiše, Kärnten, niedergemäht hat, kommen dort, wo bisher Fichten standen, zahllose Eschentriebe aus dem Boden, so eng an eng, dass man durch diese Flecken nicht durchgehen kann. Ihre überlangen, peitschenartigen Triebe tragen nur an der Spitze wenige Blätter. Kann das eine Lösung fürs Überleben sein? Immerhin sollte daraus ein Baum von bis zu 40 m Höhe werden, der früher einmal 250 Jahre alt werden konnte.

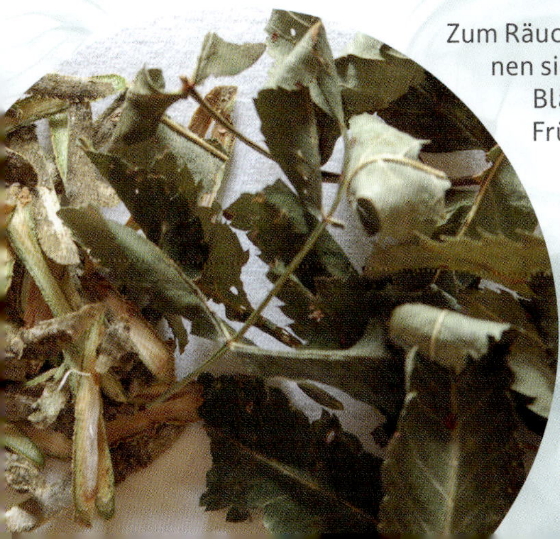

Zum Räuchern eignen sich Rinde, Blätter und Früchte der Esche.

Rauch

Verwendete Pflanzenteile: Blätter, Rinde, Früchte.

Beste Sammel- und Erntezeit: Blätter und Rinde das ganze Jahr über, die kleinen Nuss-Früchtchen verbleiben ab Oktober den ganzen Winter auf der Esche, manchmal auch noch darüber hinaus.

Wirkung, Wahrnehmung: Man fühlt sich sofort beschützt, lichtdurchflutet; vermittelt Standfestigkeit und große gedankliche Klarheit.

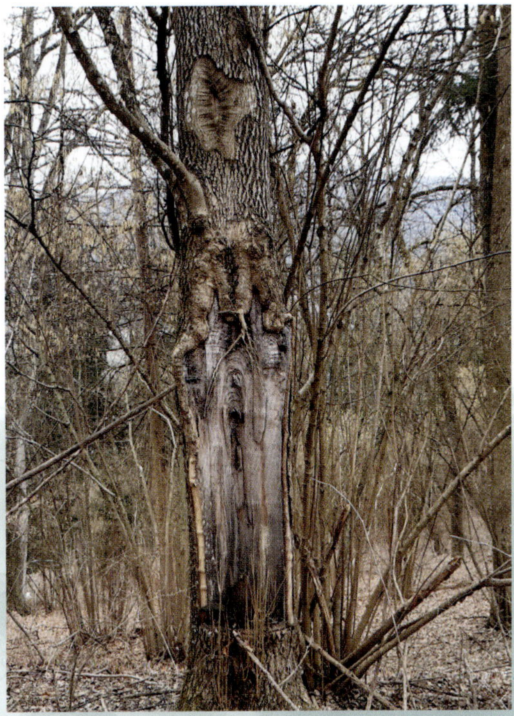

Eschenstamm

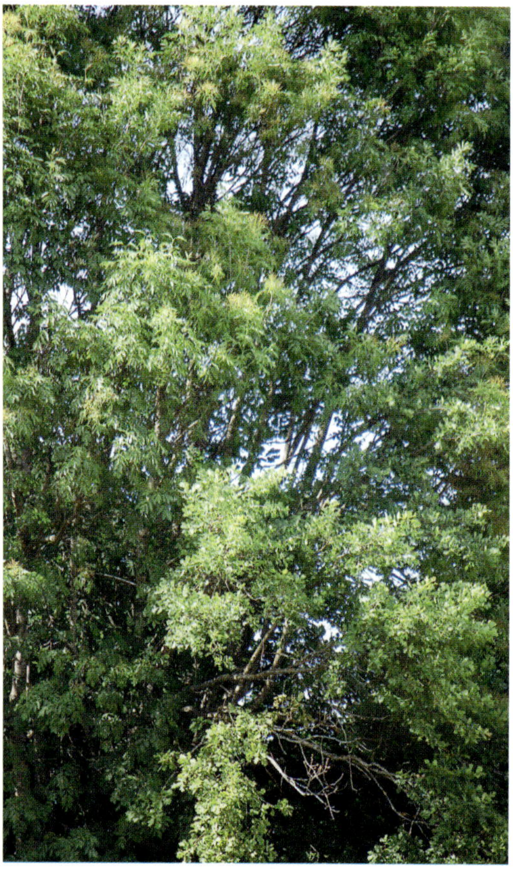

Eschenkrone

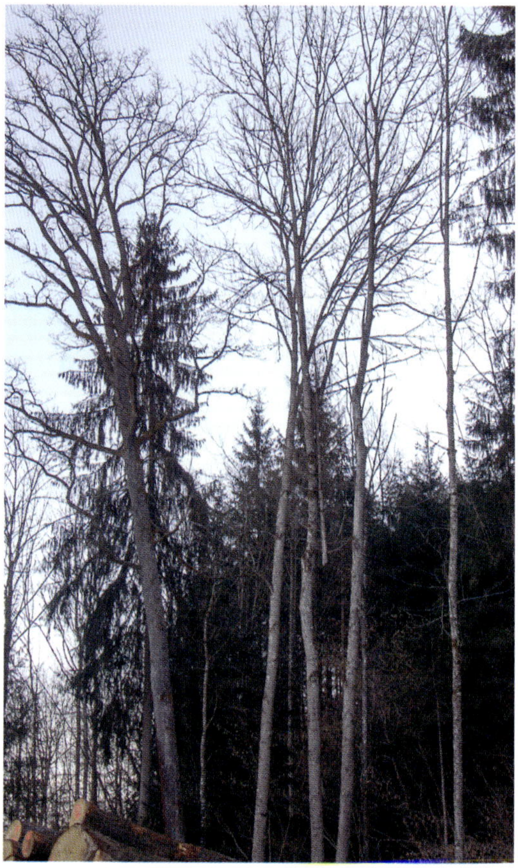

Esche im Winter

Unterstützt das Selbstwertgefühl in negativen Lebensphasen; stärkend bei seelischen Belastungen wie Mobbing; dämonenbannend und erhellend, wenn man das Gefühl hat, manipuliert zu werden. Hilft beim Durchschauen von unklaren Zuständen.

Magisches zum Rauch: Die Esche symbolisiert die Macht des Wassers. Für ihren Regenzauber verräucherten keltische Druiden Eschenlaub und Eschenholz unter Hersagen von Beschwörungsformeln und unter Verwendung eines Ritualstabes aus Eschenholz!

Schwerpunkt, Anwendungen, Rezepte: Eine abwehrende, weißmagische Eschenräucherung sollte aus nicht mehr als vier verschiedenen Räucherstoffen bestehen: Esche, Salbei, Fichten (Harz), Erlenfrüchte.

Mythologie und magische Praktiken

Besondere Wander- und Hüte-Stäbe werden ausschließlich am Tag der Wintersonnenwende aus dem Geäst der Esche geschnitten. Auf schwierigen Wegen geben sie stets Zuversicht und Kraft in die Hand des Wanderers. Sie halten einen auf sicheren Pfaden, schützen vor hinterlistigen Nebelgeistern und falschen Trittspuren, die einen in die Irre führen können.

Eschenblätter würden auch hervorragend in einen Liebesstrauß passen, als Zeichen für Großzügigkeit, Verbundenheit, Leichtigkeit und Treue.

Verwendung – gestern und heute

Die meisten Speer-Waffen der Antike wurden aus Eschenholz hergestellt. So fand die Esche auch Eingang in die Ilias, Homers weltbekanntes Werk über den trojanischen Krieg: Der berühmteste Eschenspeer wurde vom Kentauren Cheiron angefertigt, der dazu die heilige Esche am Berg Pelion gefällt hatte. Cheiron war der Ziehvater des beinahe unverwundbaren griechischen Helden Achilles. Im trojanischen Krieg tötete Achilles mit diesem Eschenspeer Hektor, den Heerführer und Thronfolger Trojas.

Dem britischen Barden Taliesin (534 bis ca. 599) wird das Gedicht „vom Krieg der Bäume" zugeschrieben, in welchem er das Kampfverhalten der Esche wie folgt skizziert: „...grausam gar der Eschenbaum, weicht doch keinen Fuß beiseite und zielt direkt aufs Herz..."

Nach so viel historischem Schlachtenlärm doch noch etwas Versöhnliches: Auch Amor´s Pfeile sollen seinerzeit aus Eschenholz gewesen sein... Hippokrates (460–370 v. Chr.) empfiehlt, eine Packung von überkochten Eschenblättern bei Rheuma und Gicht auf die schmerzenden Glieder aufzulegen.

Volksheilkundlich sind verschiedene Entwässerungstees mit Eschenblättern überliefert. Um 1750 galten Eschenblätter-Anwendungen sogar als Allheilmittel. Heute kennt man in Frankreich noch die Frenette als Lebenselixier.

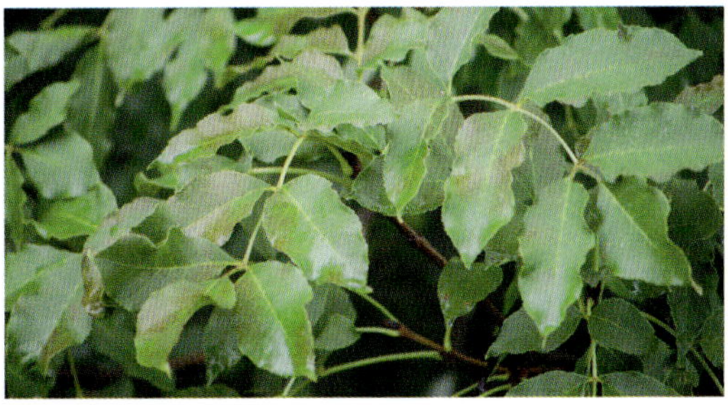

Eschenblätter

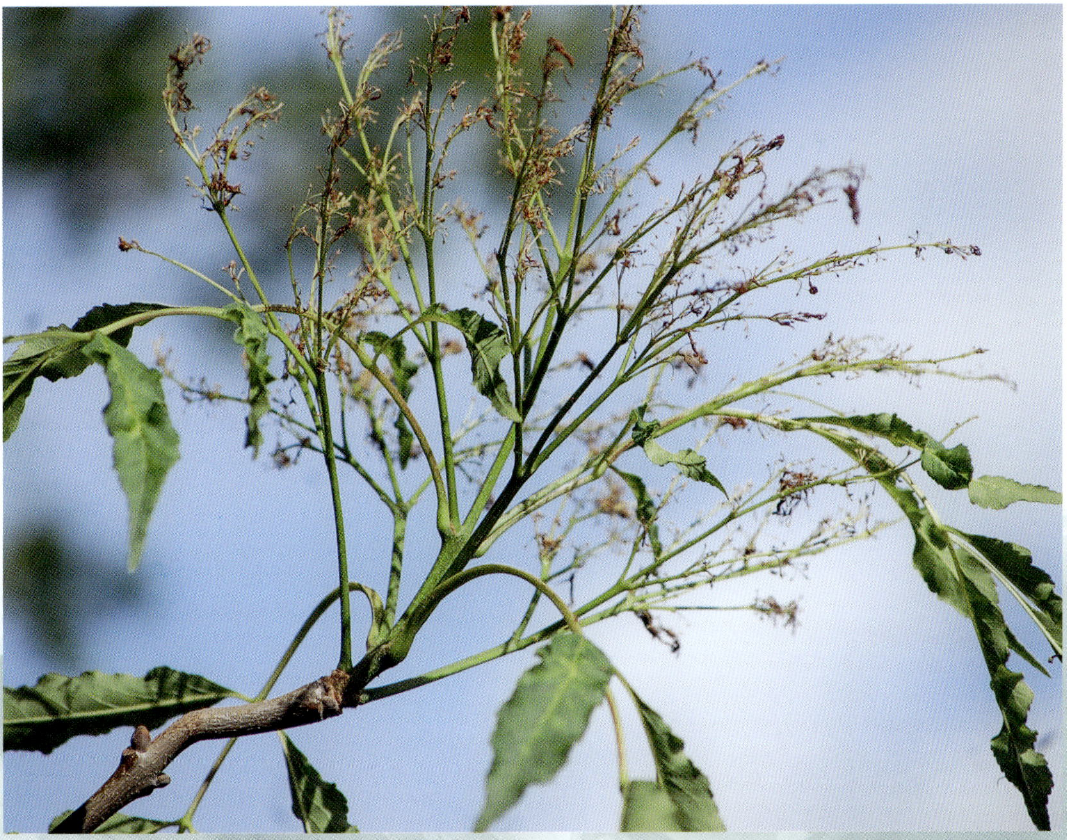

Eschenblüte

Faulbaum

Lat. Name: *Rhamnus frangula*
Pflanzenfamilie: Kreuzdorngewächse

Wie ein unscheinbares Mauerblümchen fügt sich der Stinkbaum in die wasserliebende, wilde heimische Sträuchervielfalt ein. Schon der Name allein macht ihn nicht unbedingt sympathisch. Dieser ist darauf zurückzuführen, dass die frische Rinde faulig riecht. Dennoch hat er so seine Besonderheiten, die ihn, zumindest für Insekten, unwiderstehlich machen. Da wären einmal seine zahlreichen, perfekt konstruierten Miniaturblüten, die ganze Scharen von Bienen anlocken und ernähren. Dann sind da seine Blätter: Neben den nahe verwandten Kreuzdornblättern, sind die Blätter des Faulbaumes die einzigen Blätter, auf die sich die Zitronenfalterraupe spezialisiert hat.

Der in ganz Europa beheimatete Faulbaum wird kaum höher als vier Meter und kann ein Alter von 60 bis 80 Jahren erreichen.

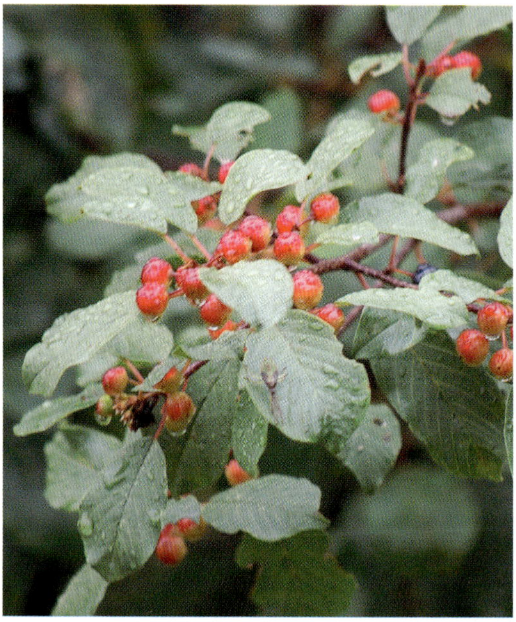

Früchte

Rauch

Verwendete Pflanzenteile: Blätter, Rinde.

Beste Sammel- und Erntezeit: Das ganze Jahr über können Blätter und die Rinde der Faulbaum-Äste geerntet werden.

Wirkung, Wahrnehmung: Sehr angenehmer Rauch, mit dem man gut Veränderungsprozesse begleiten kann. Entspanntes Loslassen; sich aus dem Gewohnten herausdenken, in Bewegung kommen, Ausgleich finden, aus jedem Zuviel wieder in einen harmonischen Verlauf kommen.

Schwerpunkt, Anwendungen, Rezepte: Unaufdringlicher Duft, der einen träumen und entspannen lässt. Geeignet für eine seelenschmeichelnde Räucherung aus Faulbaumblättern, Rosenblüten, Wacholderbeeren und Engelwurz-Samen.

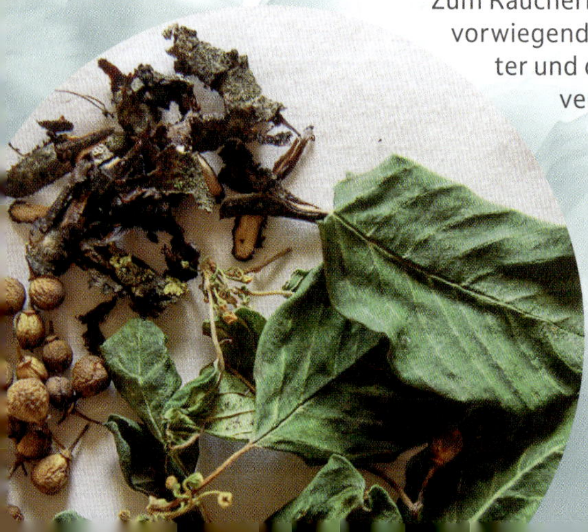

Zum Räuchern werden vorwiegend die Blätter und die Rinde verwendet.

Mythologie und magische Praktiken

Aus dem Holz des Faulbaumes wurde hochwertige Holzkohle hergestellt. Aber nicht nur das: Der Legende nach soll der Franziskanermönch Berthold der „Schwarze“ – so genannt wegen seines Hanges zu alchemistischen Experimenten – durch Zufall gegen Ende des 14. Jahrhunderts das „Schwarz“-Pulver erfunden haben. Er mischte die Holzkohle vom Faulbaum, Salpeter und Schwefel, verschloss den Mörser und stellte ihn warm, was nach einer gewissen Zeit zu einer heftigen Explosion führte.

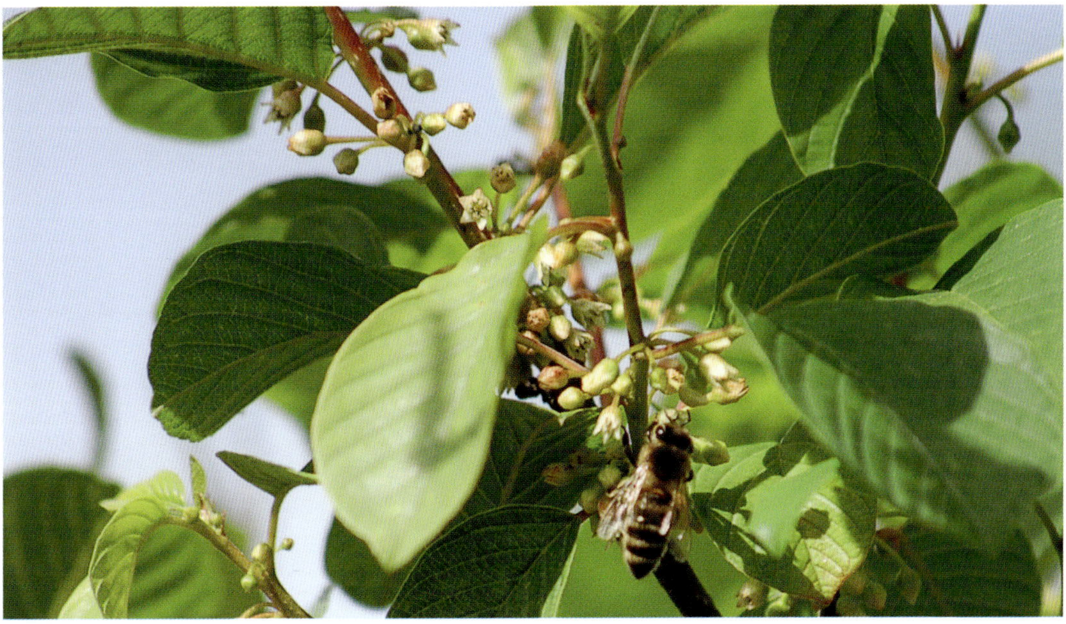

Blüten

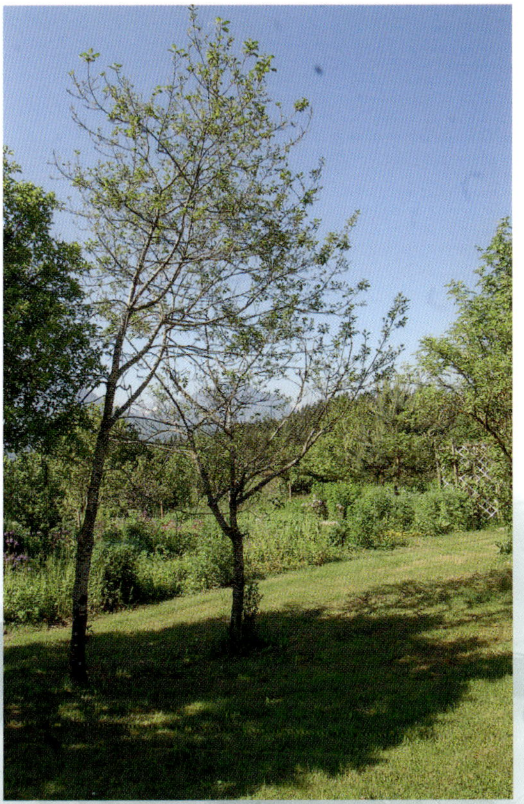

Faulbaum

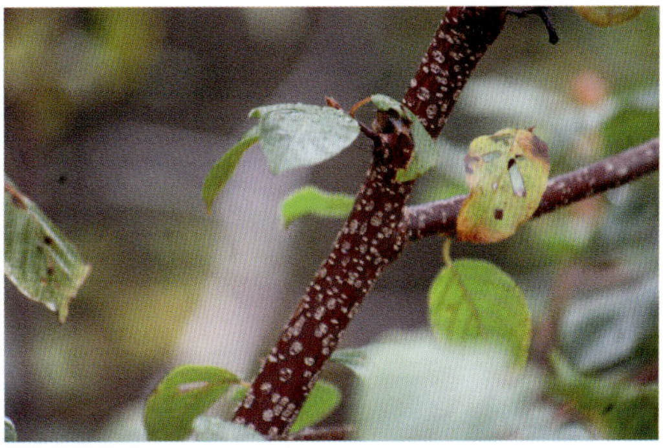

Rinde

Verwendung – gestern und heute

Die mittelalterliche Bezeichnung „Purgier- und Scheißbeere" ist der Einnahme von frischen Beeren geschuldet, was zu heftigen Ausscheidungsreaktionen führte. Heute sind die Blätter, die Beeren sowie die frische Rinde als **giftig** eingestuft.

Felsenbirne

Lat. Name: *Amelanchier ovalis*
Pflanzenfamilie: Rosengewächse

Im Süden meines Kräutergartens verläuft eine Hecke aus Rosengewächsen, die ein reiches Vogelleben angezogen hat: Schlehen und Weißdorne wechseln sich ab und dazwischen, zurückhaltend und unspektakulär die Felsenbirnen. Oft denke ich, sie halten sich so schmal und wachsen so dünn, weil sie mitten unter dornigen Gesellen stehen. Doch weit gefehlt! Sie verfügen über geringe Mengen an Blausäure in Blatt, Rinde und Samen – eine unsichtbare und somit auch raffiniertere Abwehrkraft. Als uns der Winter mehr als einen halben Meter Schnee auf einmal bescherte, traf es diese Hecke besonders stark: Alle Bedornten wurden niedergerissen – gespaltene Stämme der Weißdorne sowie niedergebogene und abgerissene Zweige der Schlehe verschwanden unter Schneemassen. Die bis zu 3,5 m hohen schlanken Felsenbirnen dazwischen waren schneefrei und aufrecht, als wäre nichts geschehen! Sie ragten leicht und elegant in die Höhe und erschienen mir wie Rufzeichen in der ausgezahnten Hecke: Es lebe die Leichtigkeit!

Der anspruchslose Strauch ist extrem winterhart und wird zwischen 70 und 80 Jahre alt. Die Felsenbirne wächst bis auf 2000 m Seehöhe und liebt felsige, kalkhaltige und sonnige Standorte.

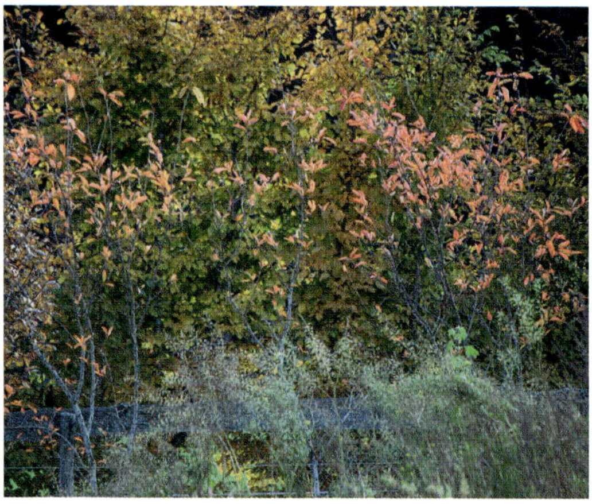

Felsenbirne im Herbst

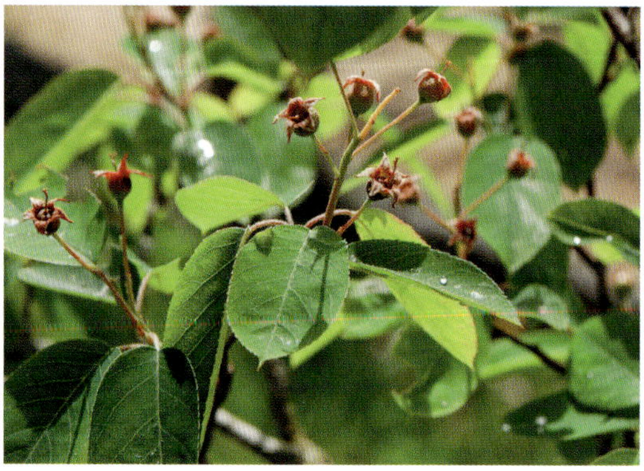

Fruchtstand

Rauch

Verwendete Pflanzenteile: Früchte, Blüten, Blätter.

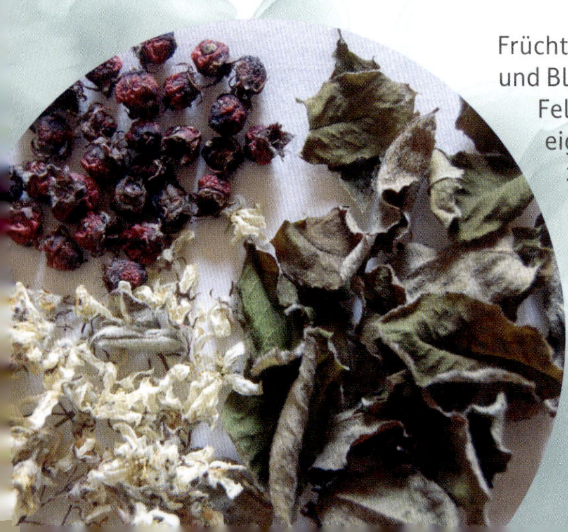

Früchte, Blüten und Blätter der Felsenbirne eignen sich zum Räuchern.

Beste Sammel- und Erntezeit: Die voll aufgeblühte Blüte im Mai, die Blätter ganzjährig.

Wirkung, Wahrnehmung: Schutz- und Segensrauch. Erinnert an die schönen Seiten des Lebens; hilft uns wieder durchlässig zu werden, verkrampfte Haltungen zu überdenken, in den positiven Fluss des Lebens zurückzukehren. Jeder Teil dieser Pflanze vermittelt im Rauch Geborgenheit, Zutrauen zu sich selbst und stärkt das Ich-Bewusstsein. Unterstützt die Überwindung seelischer Verletzungen; wärmt und beschützt von innen heraus. Der Rauch stimmt uns auf Meditationen ein; lässt uns von angenehmen Dingen träumen.

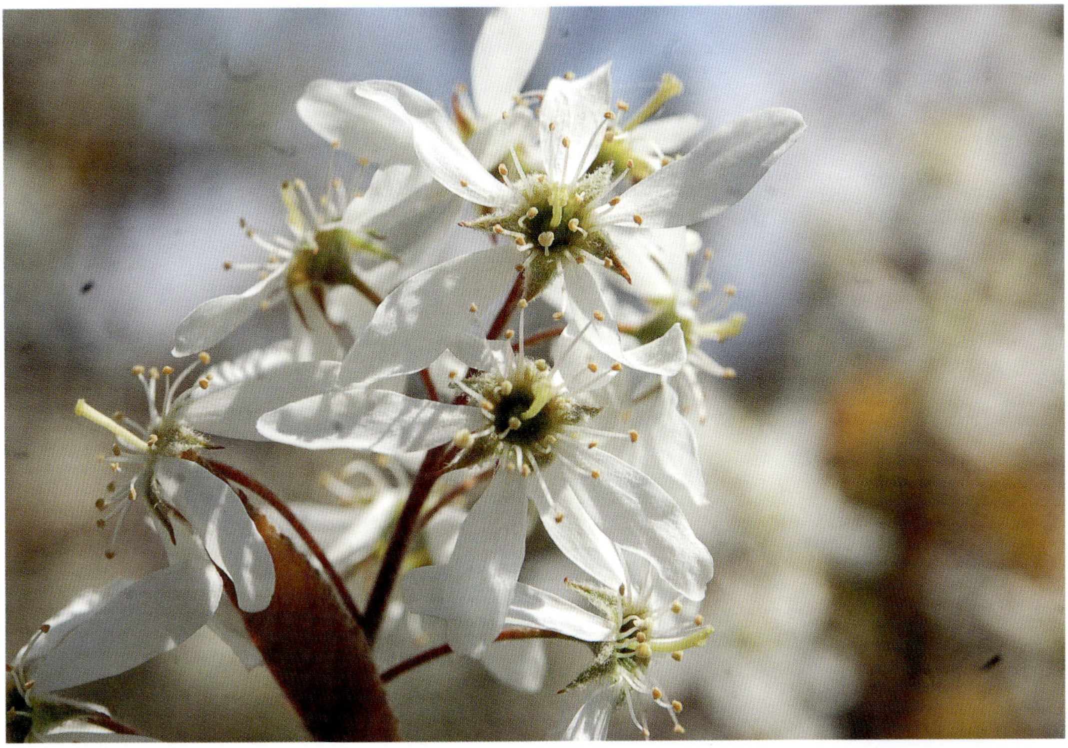

Blüten

Schwerpunkt, Anwendungen, Rezepte: Für eine wunderbare Entlastungsräucherung zur Abendzeit mischt man Felsenbirnenblüten und -früchte, Ahornblätter sowie Ebereschenblüten und -früchte, oder auch Vogelkirschenblüten mit Harz.

Gut geeignet für Räucherungen, in denen man etwas im Guten zu Ende bringen möchte: vielleicht kombiniert mit Harz in einer Mischung mit Lavendel und Mädesüß.

Verwendung – gestern und heute

Die Mehrzahl der Felsenbirnen-Arten ist in Nordamerika heimisch, wo ihre Früchte von den Indianern gegen Magenprobleme genommen sowie getrocknet als Kraftnahrung verwendet wurden.

Bei uns war die Nutzung als Rosinen-Ersatz bekannt: Dazu wurden ihre süßen Früchtchen getrocknet und dann entweder ganz oder ver-

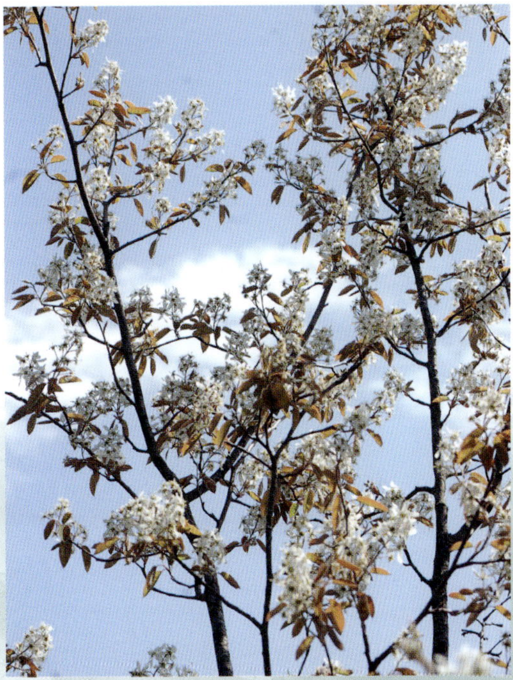

Blühende Felsenbirne

Drei besonders verbundene Pflanzen

In den menschlichen Vorstellungen gab es von Anfang an mehrere Welten. Es sind sichtbare und unsichtbare Bereiche, die miteinander verbunden sein mussten, damit das Leben gelingen konnte. Unsere Vorfahren waren überzeugt, dass sich die Wesen der unsichtbaren Welt in der sichtbaren Natur spiegelten und dort auch wahrgenommen werden konnten.

Weit verbreitet war die Annahme, dass sich die Wesenszüge von Gottheiten oder deren Helfern in Bäumen und Sträuchern manifestierten. So erklärt sich auch die alte Zuordnung der drei Räucherstoffe Hainbuche – Haselnuss – Schwarzer Holunder. Jahrtausendelang gab es in allen vorchristlichen Kulturen Europas die Vorstellung von drei Schicksalsgöttinnen bzw. einer Schicksalsgöttin in drei Gestalten, die das menschliche Dasein lenken.

Zuschreibungen der Schicksalsgöttinnen in verschiedenen Kulturen, die mit Hainbuche, Haselnuss und Schwarzem Holunder assoziiert sind

Kultur:	Die drei...			
griechisch	**Moiren**	Klotho	Lachesis	Atropos
römisch	**Parzen**	Nona	Decima	Morta
nordisch	**Nornen**	Skuld	Verdandi	Urd
keltisch	**Bethen**	Wilbeth	Ambeth	Borbeth
christlich	**Madln**	Hl. Katharina mit dem Radl	Hl. Margareta mit dem Wurm	Hl. Barbara mit dem Turm
Zuordnungen:				
Alter		**Die Junge**	**Die Mittlere**	**Die Alte**
Tätigkeit		spinnt den Faden	bemisst die Fadenlänge	schneidet den Faden ab
Farbe		weiß	rot	schwarz
Zeitqualität		Zukunft	Gegenwart	Vergangenheit
europäische Wildpflanze		**Hainbuche**	**Haselnuss**	**Schwarzer Holunder**

Hainbuche, Haselnuss und Schwarzer Holunder helfen im Rauch sehr unmittelbar und beeinflussen positiv und wohltuend unsere angeschlagene seelische Befindlichkeit. Sie sind die heilsamen Begleiter zerstörter Seelenlandschaften und gleichzeitig die wirkungsvollen Coaches hin zum inneren Überleben, hin zu neuer Lebensfreude.

Hainbuche

Lat. Name: *Carpinus betulus*
Botanischer Name: Gewöhnliche Hainbuche
Pflanzenfamilie: Birkengewächse

Der Eisenbaum ist seit einigen Jahrtausenden in Mitteleuropa nachweisbar. Sein extrem schweres Holz fand vielfältige Anwendung: als Waffenholz, als Bauholz, für Webstühle oder Spinnräder, was auch wieder auf das Attribut der Hl. Katharina (mit dem Radl) verweist. Die aus der Hainbuche gewonnene Holzkohle brennt so heiß, dass man mit ihrer Hitze sogar Eisen zu schmelzen vermag.

Wegen ihrer unerreichten Ausschlagkraft und Unbezwingbarkeit ist die Hainbuche jahrtausendelang die gebräuchlichste Feld- und Landbegrenzung. Sie überlebt die größten Verstümmelungen mit einer bewundernswerten Überlebenskraft. So erstaunt es nicht, dass die „Hage-Buche" mythologisch zum Sitz der „Hagezussen" wird, der früher hochangesehenen Baumreiterinnen und später verteufelten Hexen. In der Vorstellungswelt unserer Urahnen waren die Hagezussen das Bindeglied zwischen der wilden, furchteinflößenden Natur außerhalb der Hecke und der menschlichen Geborgenheit innerhalb derselben. Sie wurden gleichermaßen bewundert und gefürchtet, da man ihnen das Wissen um die unbändigen Kräfte der Natur zuschrieb. So konnten sie den Menschen gegenüber sowohl positiv (heilend) als auch negativ (krankmachend und verfluchend) auftreten.

Als Baum wird die Hainbuche bis zu 25 m hoch und kann ein Alter von 150 Jahren erreichen. Meist wird die Hainbuche jedoch als dicht belaubte Hecke gesetzt. Sie ist sehr gut in der Lage auch Trockenzeiten zu überstehen, da sie entlang ihrer tiefreichenden Herzwurzeln Wasser anlagern kann.

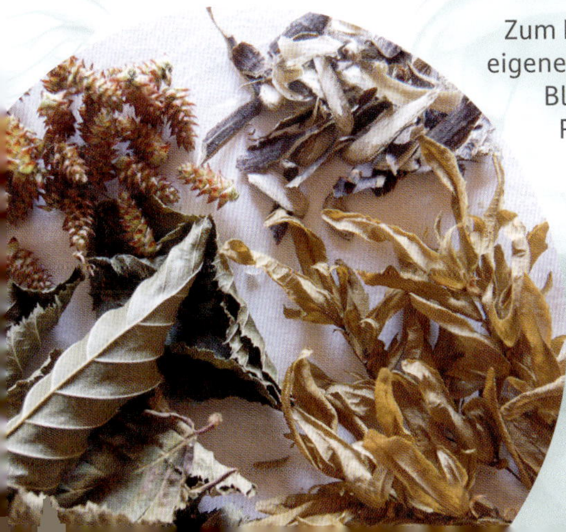

Zum Räuchern eigenen sich die Blätter, die Rinde, die Fruchtstände und Blüten.

Rauch

Verwendete Pflanzenteile: Blüten, Blätter, Fruchtstände, Rinde.

Beste Sammel- und Erntezeit: Blüten im Frühling, die Fruchtstände ab Mitte Mai, Blätter und Rinde vom Frühling bis in den Herbst.

Wirkung, Wahrnehmung: Es geht um Umbruchs- und Erneuerungsprozesse; unterstützt uns in Momenten, wo man sagt: „Jetzt ist es genug, es muss etwas anders werden", in Momenten, in denen man aufbricht in die Veränderung. Hilft morsche Dienstverhältnisse zu verändern und überwinden. Es geht um Grenzen, die man nicht klar genug gesetzt hat: Abgrenzung finden, Belastungen leichter zurückweisen, Übergreifern Grenzen setzen, um in Ruhe wachsen zu können. Führt zur Ich-Stärkung, stärkt und weckt die seelischen Überlebens- und Lebensgeister, baut einen nach bitteren Erkenntnissen und Niederlagen wieder auf. Stärkend, aufbauend, ausgleichend bei innerer Unruhe, harmonisierend bei innerer Zerrissenheit und Stress, lichtgebend bei lähmender Traurigkeit.

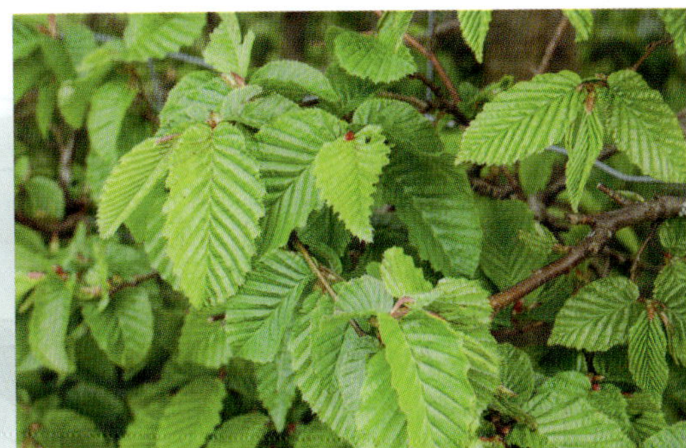

Blätter der Hainbuche

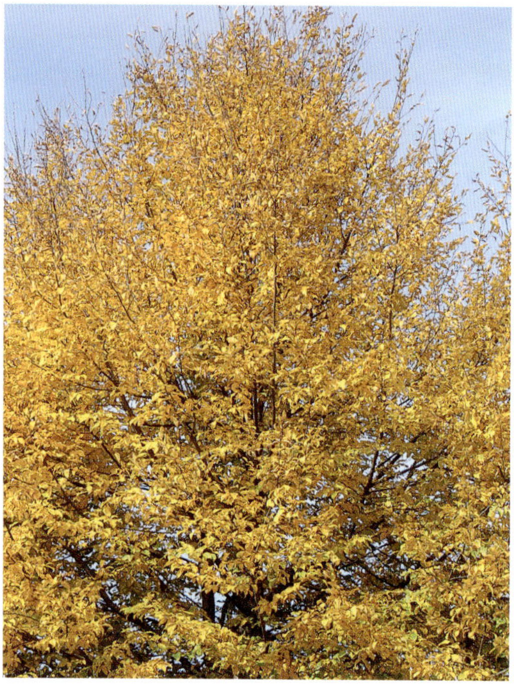

Hainbuche im Herbst

Magisches zum Rauch: Magisches Räuchermittel für unterschiedliche Abwehrrituale. Mein „Grenzbaum"-Ritual findet unter meinen Kursteilnehmern seit Jahren einen sehr hohen Identifikationsgrad: Die Räucherung besteht aus Hainbuchenblättern, Holunderbeeren, Blutwurz-Wurzel mit Fichtenharz. Im Freien sucht man sich einen passenden Platz, zieht mit einer Haselnussrute einen Kreis um sich selbst und stellt die Räucherschale vor sich auf den Boden. Nach einer als angenehm empfundenen Zeitspanne öffnet man den Kreis wieder, indem man mit der Haselnussrute den Kreis an einer Stelle symbolisch „ausradiert" und beendet die Räucherung.

Schwerpunkt, Anwendungen, Rezepte: Eine Räuchermischung von Hainbuche und Traubenkirsche kombiniert mit Harz verdeutlicht einem die Halbherzigkeit, mit der man oft wichtige Bereiche zur Seite schiebt. Hier kann man lernen, für sich selbst einzustehen. Bei schmerzenden Gliedern wird der Rauch der Hainbuchenblätter als sehr angenehm wahrgenommen. Wenn es mental wieder aufwärts gehen soll, unterstützt eine Räuchermischung aus Hainbuche, Odermennig, Heidekraut und Braunwurz mit Harz.

Mythologie und magische Praktiken

In den Schriften der Heiligen Hildegard von Bingen (1098–1179), Benediktinernonne, spätere Äbtissin ihrer Klostergründung am Rupertsberg (an der Nahe-Mündung, Deutschland), finden sich auch Ratschläge für Alltagsmagie, die dem christlichen Weltbild ihrer Zeit nicht zu widersprechen scheinen. So schreibt sie vom Hainbuchen-Holz: „... auch ist es dem Menschen gut und nützlich, immer (ein Stück) Holz von diesem Baum bei sich zu haben. Wenn die Hainbuche und andere Hölzer, an denen die Zeichen von Wohlergehen bemerkt werden, in einem Hause im Feuer verbrennen, dann weichen von dort die Luftdämonen und teuflische Vorspiegelungen und diese fliehen entsetzt, weil sie dort etwas Glücksbringendes verspüren."

Verwendung – gestern und heute

Von keltischen und germanischen Stämmen bis in den dreißigjährigen Krieg (1618–1648) wurden in ganz Europa Wehrhecken aus Hainbuchen als natürliche Verteidigungs- und Grenzlinien angelegt. Zu diesem Zweck wurden Hainbuchen-Hecken gesetzt und in einer gewissen Höhe umgehackt. Die Bruchstellen der Hainbuche bleiben über Jahre wie eiserne Lanzenspitzen zurück und die Hainbuche selbst schlägt wieder aus. Manchmal verstärkte man diese kaum überwindbaren Anlagen noch, indem man Weißdornsträucher dazwischen setzte. Bereits Caesar und Tacitus beschreiben diese Landwehren als gefürchtetes, weil unüberwindliches Hindernis für die römischen Legionen.

Hildegard von Bingen (1098–1179) empfiehlt zur Beseitigung von weißen Hautflecken angewärmte Hainbuchenspäne auf diese zu drücken. Bachblüte Nr. 17 „hornbeam" – Hainbuche – wird gegen Übermüdung und mentale Erschöpfung eingesetzt; wenn man vermeint den Alltag nicht mehr bewältigen zu können.

Haselnuss

Lat. Name: *Corylus avellana*
Botanischer Name: Gewöhnliche Haselnuss
Pflanzenfamilie: Birkengewächse

In der Hasel pulsiert das Leben in all seinen fruchtbaren Facetten! In ihrem Schatten gibt es kein Ausruhen oder gar Schlafen. Ihre starke Beziehung zum Wasser zeigt sich in ihrer blitzableitenden Kraft, aber auch ihrer Eignung als Wünschelrute. Unaufhörlich leitet die Hasel Energieströme nach oben. Kinder spüren das – bei all meinen „Wohnungsspielen" im Freien mit meinen Enkelinnen verorteten sie Badezimmer und Küche ausnahmslos unter der Hasel, niemals ein Wohn- oder gar Schlafzimmer.
Wie die Archäobotanik nachweisen konnte, gab es bereits vor 8.000 Jahren, also in der Steinzeit, eine „Haselzeit" in Mitteleuropa: Die Hasel hatte offensichtlich einen sehr hohen Stellenwert als Nahrungsmittel und war zu dieser Zeit in waldmäßiger Dichte über weite Landesteile verbreitet.
Die Hasel hat ein dem Menschen zugewandtes Wesen und stellt sich mit ihren vielfältigen Kräften und Gaben gern in unseren Dienst. Der mehrstämmige Strauch wird fünf bis zehn Meter hoch und schafft mit 60 bis 80 Lebensjahren ein Menschenalter.

Rauch

Verwendete Pflanzenteile: Haselkätzchen, Blätter, Rinde, Holz.

Beste Sammel- und Erntezeit: Blütenkätzchen ab Februar, Blätter bis Juni, Rinde und Holz das ganze Jahr über.

Zum Räuchern eignen sich die Blüten, die Blätter, die Rinde und das Holz.

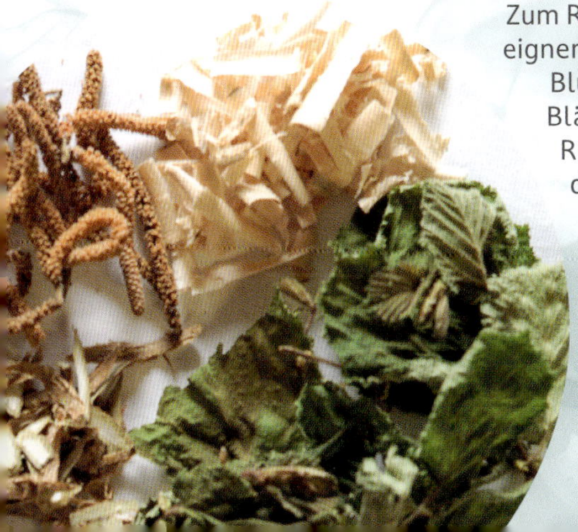

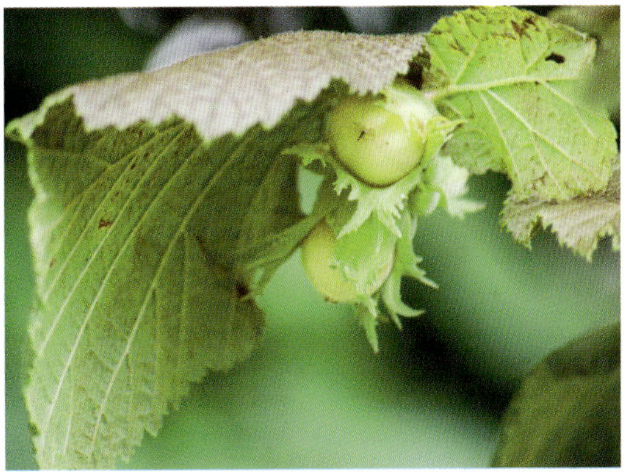

Blätter und Fruchtbildung

Wirkung, Wahrnehmung: Rauch der Sommersonnenwende; im Rauch sind viele unterschiedliche Impulse möglich, die sich zum Teil auch nach den übrigen verwendeten Räucherstoffen ausrichten können. Schutz und Förderung der geistigen Fruchtbarkeit; verhilft zu neuer Umsetzungsenergie; Energie für Vorhaben, die ins Stocken geraten sind; hilft einem „die Ernte einzufahren"; hilft Entscheidungen zu treffen; man kehrt leichter um, wenn man sich verrannt hat. Schutzrauch gegen chaotische Kräfte; große klärende Kraft, die den Ungeist vertreibt, man kann wieder geradeaus denken; befreiende Kraft, die die mentale Befindlichkeit stärkt; Flexibilität und geistige Beweglichkeit werden unterstützt. Fördert die Lust aufs Leben und Lieben; Leichtigkeit und Fröhlichkeit werden vermittelt.

Magisches zum Rauch: Der Rauch der Sommersonnenwende enthält verschiedene Wetterpflanzen, in jedem Fall aber Haselnussblätter und wird in alle vier Himmelsrichtungen im Garten verräuchert.

Schwerpunkt, Anwendungen, Rezepte: Um sich mit guter Energie aufzuladen, stellt man sich in einen Rauch aus Haselnuss, Salbei, Wacholder und Tannennadeln.

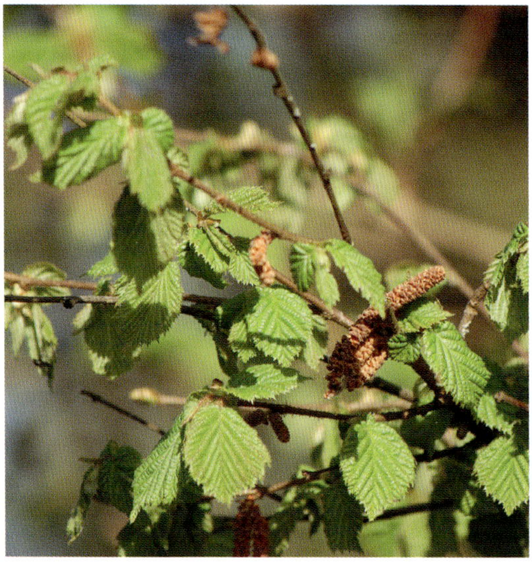
Haselkätzchen

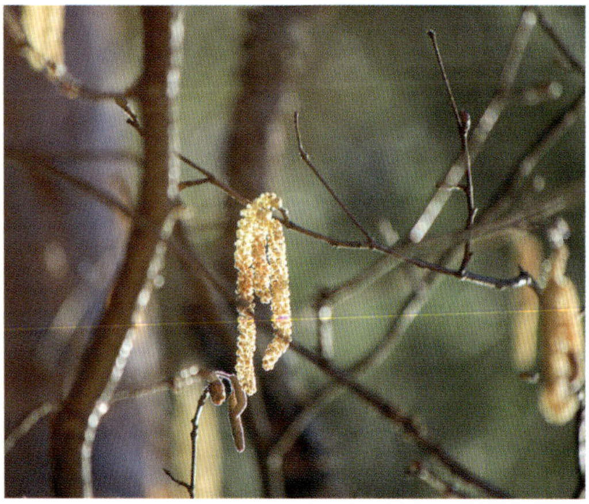
Blütenstand der Haselnuss

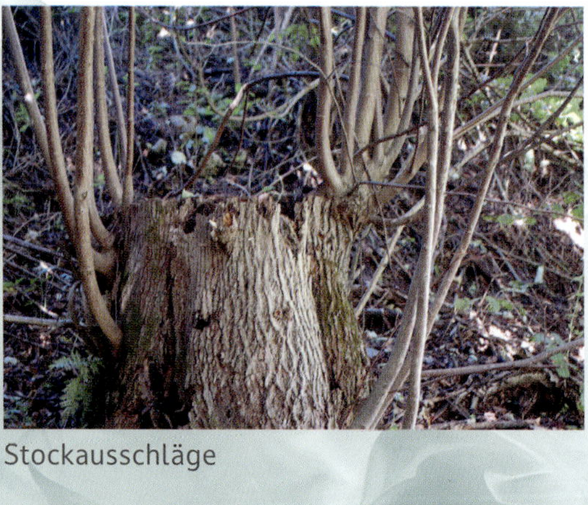
Stockausschläge

Eine Räuchermischung für positive Gedanken und zündende Ideen besteht aus Haselnuss, Beifußwurzel, Eberraute, Rosmarin und Eisenkraut.

Mythologie und magische Praktiken

Aus vorchristlicher, naturreligiöser Sicht wohnt unter der Hasel der Haselwurm, eine Art Schlangenkönig, der die Verbindung zur Anderswelt aufrechterhalten und der einem Macht über Geister und Schätze verleihen kann.

Hier erklärt sich auch die Zuordnung der Hasel zur Hl. Margareta (gestorben ca. 305) mit dem Wurm (siehe Kapitel „Drei besonders verbundene Pflanzen"): Hinter der volkstümlichen Bezeichnung „Wurm" verbirgt sich das lateinische Wort „draco", was mit Schlange oder Drache übersetzt wird. Im spätantiken und frühmittelalterlichen christlichen Glauben symbolisiert der Drache das Heidentum, welches es zu überwinden gilt. So ist es auch im Benediktinerkreuz als Leitspruch festgeschrieben: „crux sacra sit mihi lux, non draco sit mihi dux". Übersetzt: „Das Heilige Kreuz sei mein Licht, nicht der Drache sei mein Führer". Da die Hl. Margareta dem „draco" widerstanden hat, ist dieser „Wurm" zu ihrem Attribut geworden.

Eine erstaunliche Übereinstimmung gibt es auch noch zur mythologischen Frühzeit: Der Lebensstab mit dem Lachesis, die mittlere griechische Schicksalsgöttin, den gesponnenen Lebensfaden abmisst, war stets aus Haselholz. Dem Schlange-Hasel-Mythos wird in vielen Erzählungen entsprochen. Der Stab, den Moses vor den Pharao hinwirft und der zur Schlange wird, war ebenfalls aus Haselholz.

In der keltischen Gerichtsbarkeit saß der Druide wohl unter der Hasel. Denn sie hatte die magische Kraft, eine Verbindung mit der jenseitigen Welt und ihren weisen Führern herzustellen. So vermeinte man ein möglichst gerechtes Urteil zu gewährleisten oder eine zutreffende Weissagung zu ermöglichen. Im Märchen „Aschenputtel" macht der auf das Grab der Mutter gepflanzte Haselnussstrauch dem Aschenputtel die Verbindung zur verstorbenen Mutter möglich. Die Römer hielten die Hasel für eine Friedensbringerin mit vermittelnden Fähigkeiten. In den Volksrechten germanischer Stämme spielte die Hasel, hier auch Frau Hasel genannt, ebenfalls eine zentrale Rolle. „Die Hasel hat den Frieden" meinten sie und dementsprechend mussten sich friedenssuchende Unterhändler mit einem geschälten Haselzweig ausweisen. Dieses leuchtende Weiß sollte später zur berühmten weißen Fahne werden, die noch heute im Falle einer Kapitulation dem Kampfes- oder Kriegsgegner, wenn auch nur mehr symbolisch, überreicht wird.

Der Rechtsbegriff der „Haselung" stammt ebenfalls aus dieser frühen Zeit heimischer Stammesrechte und bedeutete, dass Thingstätten durch einen Zaun aus geschälten, also weiß leuchtenden sowie gekreuzten Haselruten eingegrenzt werden mussten.

Die „Frau Haselin" durfte sowohl diesseits als auch jenseits des Ärmelkanals nicht gefällt werden. Es musste wohl ein Tieropfer als Sühne für die Freveltat durchgeführt werden. Der britische Barde Taliesin (534 bis etwa 599) berichtet: „... drei nicht atmende Dinge werden ausschließlich mit atmenden Dingen bezahlt – ein Apfelbaum, eine Hasel, eine heilige Eiche..."

Um eine wirksame Wünschelrute zu erhalten, sollte man einige Rituale beachten: „sine ferre" (ohne Eisen) müsse der Ast gebrochen werden, am Hin- und Rückweg müsse man vollkommen stumm sein, man dürfe den Ast nur an besonderen Tagen im Jahr holen und zwar am Karfreitag oder am Johannistag (24. Juni) und diese Tage müssten noch dazu auf einen bestimmten Wochentag fallen donnerstags oder freitags. Nicht zu vergessen wären auch die – allerdings geheimen – Beschwörungsformeln mit denen man den Ast der Hasel erst abbitten und dann für sich quasi in Betrieb setzen musste.
Mit einem Haselnussstab kann man sich gegen Schlangen, Blitze, Verwünschungen und böse Geister schützen und mit Haselzweigen am Hut soll man vor Blitzeinschlägen gefeit sein, wenn man im Freien von einem Unwetter überrascht wird.

Eine Haselstange gehört vielerorts zum unverzichtbaren Bestandteil der österlichen Palmbuschen: Als Schutzzeichen und Fruchtbarkeitssymbol wird der „Haselstecken" (Stab) mitgeweiht und schützt so das Haus und seine Bewohner vor bösen Mächten, Blitzschlag und Feuersbrunst.

Verwendung – gestern und heute

Als um das Jahr 800 durch Kaiser Karl den Großen (747–814) eine Verordnung in 69 Kapiteln zur wirtschaftlichen Führung seiner Königshöfe erlassen wurde, umfasste das 70. Kapitel eine Liste von 73 Gartenpflanzen sowie 16 fruchttragenden Bäumen und Sträuchern: Darunter findet sich an der neunten Stelle „avellanarios", die Haselnuss. Haselnussblätter zählen zu den sogenannten Maiblättern und ergeben einen angenehmen Kräutertee.

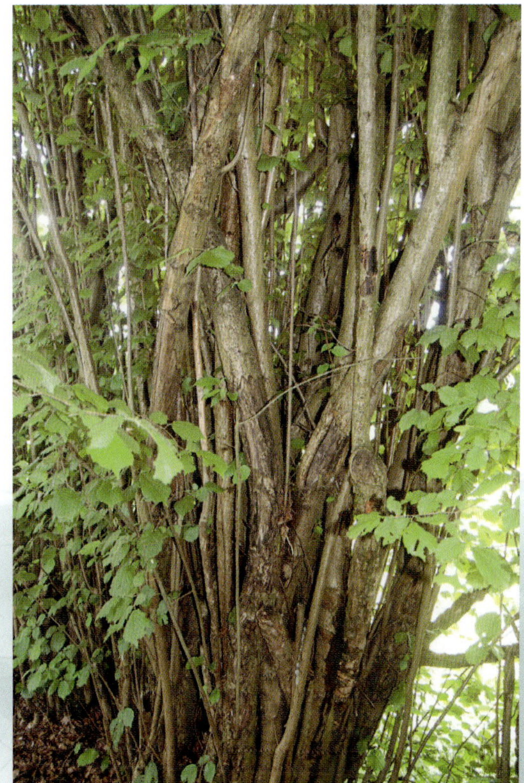

Haselnussstrauch

Schwarzer Holunder

Lat. Name: *Sambucus nigra*
Pflanzenfamilie: Moschuskrautgewächse

Mensch und Holunder sind ein gutes Gespann! Das konnte man bereits in steinzeitlichen Siedlungen nachweisen. Für viele mitteleuropäische Kulturen galt der Holunder über Jahrtausende als Lebens- und Sippenbaum, in welchem die schützenden Hausgeister wohnen. Als solcher ist er ein treuer Haus- und Hofbegleiter geworden. Man glaubte, dass er negative Energien und Krankheiten in die Erde, in die Unterwelt ableiten und sie so unschädlich machen konnte. Aus diesem Grund war er stets mit Lappen und anderen Zeichen überwundener Krankheiten behängt. Diese Übertragungszauber sind aus vielen Teilen Europas bekannt. Sie setzen ein großes Vertrauen der Menschen in das Vorhandensein einer heilsamen, unbändigen Verwandlungskraft des jeweiligen Baumes voraus. Neben dem Holunder wurde diese Transformationskraft nur noch dem Weißdorn zugetraut.

In Menschennähe sucht er sich seine Standorte gerne selbst, scheint aber nicht überall glücklich zu werden. Man denke nur an die, von Strauch zu Strauch ganz unterschiedlich großen Holunderblütendolden. Seine heilsamen und nährenden Gaben werden seit Jahrtausenden von den Menschen genutzt. Der Holunderstrauch ist eine Hausapotheke und füllt die Vorratskammer.

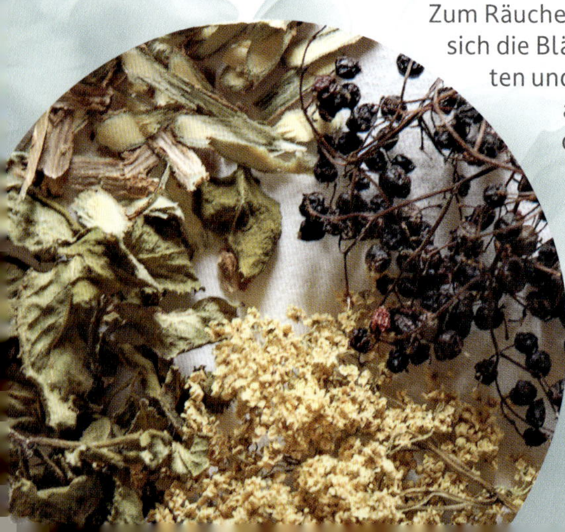

Zum Räuchern eignen sich die Blätter, Blüten und Früchte, aber auch die Rinde, das Holz und das Mark.

Er ist ein Ausbund an lebensbejahender Heilkraft und ein Meister in der Überwindung von Gegensätzen: Er vereint in sich Prinzipien einer schützenden Muttergottheit, aber auch die einer Todesgöttin. Dementsprechend erscheint sie einmal als strahlende, weiße Göttin und ein anderes Mal als gebücktes, schwarz gekleidetes, stummes Wesen.

Jenseits der mythologischen Gegensätze ist auch der Strauch selbst bipolar: leichtes Holz – schwere Düfte. Der erschreckend dumpfe, extrem erdige Rauch der Holunderblüten steht in eklatantem Gegensatz zu ihrer lieblichen Erscheinung.

Der Holunderstrauch wird bis zu sieben Meter hoch und erreicht ein Lebensalter von maximal 30 Jahren.

Rauch

Verwendete Pflanzenteile: Blüten, Blätter, Beeren, Rinde, Mark, Holz.

Beste Sammel- und Erntezeit: Nur ganz aufgeblühte Blüten im Frühjahr sammeln; Blätter, Rinde, Mark und Holz ganzjährig; die Beeren, die eigentliche Steinfrüchte sind, werden im Herbst geerntet, getrocknet und vor der Räucherung vermahlen.

Wirkung, Wahrnehmung: Räucherisch geht es hier immer um ernste Themen – wie Abschied nehmen, Veränderungen durchstehen. Erdung in schwierigen Zeiten; die Kraft des Mondes führt uns symbolisch durch die Nacht in einen neuen Tag, in eine neue Welt; Abwehr von negativen Energien.

Besonders wichtiger Räucherstoff bei allen Übergängen im Leben; der Coach der Veränderung lehrt uns das richtige Tun zur richtigen Zeit; heilsamer Begleiter in Umbruchsphasen und Lebensübergängen, unterstützt das Anneh-

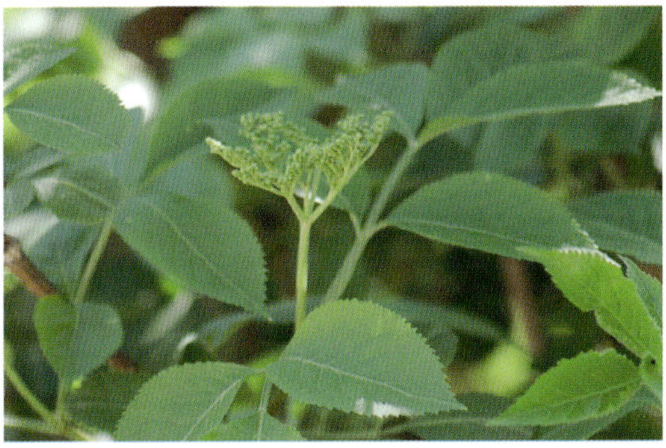

Holunderblätter

men von Werden und Vergehen! Erleichtert die Auseinandersetzung mit veränderten Lebensumständen; das eigene Zutrauen wird gekräftigt, sodass Entscheidungen getroffen werden können. Schutz und Stärkung wird vermittelt; der Beeren-Rauch wirkt aufbauend, stimmungserhellend; die Lebensgeister werden gestärkt. Es fällt einem wieder leichter innere Balance zu halten. Der Rauch der schwarzen Beeren, der Zuordnung zur Hl. Barbara, hilft einem den Lauf der Dinge anzunehmen. Vermittelt Schutz in der eigenen inneren Dunkelheit.

Der Holler ist keine Alltagsräucherung, man sollte sehr bewusst damit umgehen und sich jedenfalls einen passenden Ablauf zur Holunderräucherung überlegen.

Eine Holunder-Blütenräucherung zeigt uns die begrenzte Zeit an, die wir auf Erden haben. Ihr dumpfer Anfangsduft hinterlässt nach ein bis zwei Stunden eine beruhigende Grundstimmung, besonders bei großer seelischer Unruhe.

Magisches zum Rauch: Schutzamulette gegen Krankheiten und ständig negative Gedanken werden mit der Rinde und dem Mark des Holunders beräuchert.

Schwerpunkt, Anwendungen, Rezepte: In einer Holunderbeeren-Räucherung mit Harz und Beifuß können blockierte Emotionen gelöst werden. Bei Umzug in neue Räumlichkeiten kann ein Rauch mit Holunderblüten und -mark alte, negative Hinterlassenschaften in der Raumstruktur bannen und den Weg ins Neue freimachen. Zu einer derartigen Räucherung gehören noch Koriandersamen und Mistel sowie Harz.

Eine Räuchermischung in Zeiten des Wandels besteht aus Holunder, Eschenblättern, Lavendel, Mistel und Weinraute.

Mythologie und magische Praktiken

In der mitteleuropäischen Vorstellungswelt ist der Holunder der Baum der Erdgöttin Hulda oder Holda, die auch Frau Hel oder Frau Ellhorn oder Frau Holle genannt wird. Sie ist die ursprünglich germanische Göttin der Unterwelt, die das Leben schützen und Krankheiten heilen konnte. Bei ihr ruhen die Seelen der Verstorbenen und warten auf ihre Wiedergeburt. Frau Holle ist eine Schwellengottheit: Sie begleitet die Toten in die Anderswelt hinüber und sie hilft den Babys in diese Welt herüber! Sie ist eine zweifache Gestalt, sie ist weiß und schwarz. Das Märchen der Frau Holle symbolisiert also die Verbindung von oben und unten, von Leben und Tod, von weiß und schwarz. Es steht für das zyklische Denken unserer Vorfahren, als verschiedene Naturwesenheiten untrennbar mit menschlichen Schicksalen verbunden schienen. Die „hohe Frau" zieht zur Zeit der Wintersonnenwende über die Erde, um die lebensfeindlichen Kräfte niederzuringen und wieder neues Leben zu ermöglichen. Die weißen Schneeflocken waren ein Zeichen ihrer Anwesenheit.

In Südkärnten wird die Frau Holle zur „Pehtra Baba" und steht symbolisch für den dunklen Aspekt der großen Muttergottheit. In den Raunächten zieht sie übers Land und sammelt an den Wegkreuzungen die armen Seelen ein, die den Weg in die Unterwelt noch nicht gefunden haben. Sie wird als stumme, schwarz gekleidete Gestalt dargestellt. Im Rosental betritt sie am Vorabend des Heiligen Dreikönigstages, am 5. Jänner, sogar die Häuser – und zwar auf allen Vieren kriechend oder humpelnd. Ihr Gesicht ist mit einem schwarzen Tuch verhüllt. Sie trägt eine zweizinkige Gabel mit sich, auf die die Hausleute Würste hängen, damit sie von Krankheit und Unheil im neuen Jahr verschont blieben. Als Gabe schüttet die Pehtra Nüsse, Äpfel, gedörrte Zwetschken, Rüben und Erdäpfel aus ihrer Schürze auf den Stubenboden und verlässt schweigend, wie sie gekommen ist, wieder das Haus.

Neben dieser europaweit verbreiteten Geschichte der Frau Holle gibt es aber noch mehr Sagenhaftes rund um den Holler-Busch. Unsere Vorfahren vermeinten, dass das Unterwelt-Tor, das zwischen den Wurzeln des Holunders liege, nicht nur von der Frau Holle genützt, sondern auch noch von anderen Wesenheiten frequentiert werde. Es herrsche stets reges Treiben unter dem Holunder, verschiedene Erdwesen würden auf- und absteigen, die den Menschen zwar wohlgesonnen wären, aber dennoch eine gewisse Unruhe verbreiten würden. Man denke an folgendes Kinderlied: „Ringel, Ringel, Reihe, sind der Kinder dreie, sitzen unterm Hollerbusch, rufen alle husch, husch, husch." Man war zwar froh einen Holunder am Hof oder in der Nähe zu haben, nutzte seinen Schatten aber nie als Ess- und Rastplatz oder schob gar die Kleinsten zum Schlafen in seinen Schatten. Denn hätte man dies getan, wäre unter den Erwachsenen sehr bald Streit ausgebrochen und die Kinder hätten geschrien, weil sie, ob des lauten Getrappels nicht hätten schlafen können.

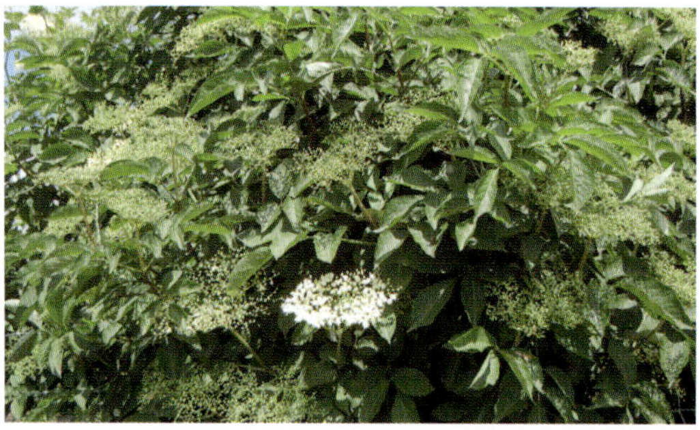

Schwarzer Holunder in Blüte

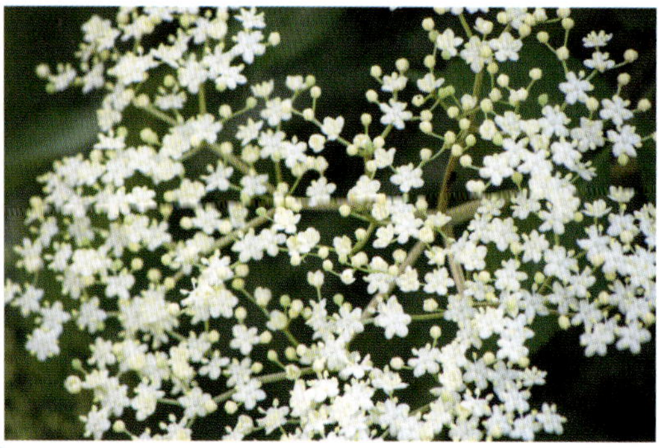

Holunderblüten

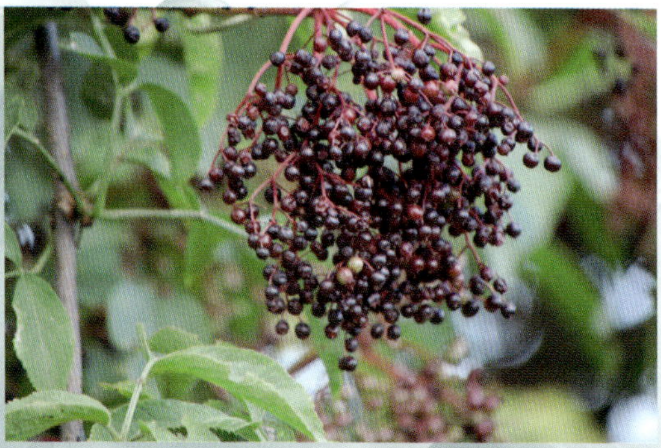

Holunderbeeren

Noch heute sagt man in manchen Gegenden, dass Holunderblütensträuße nicht mit ins Haus genommen werden sollten. Sie würden Unglück über die Bewohner bringen.

Hingegen ist seine Kraft als Schatzhüter legendär: Musste man einmal flüchten und sein Hab und Gut zurücklassen, vergrub man dieses schnell unter dem Holunderbusch und hackte ihn danach bodennah kahl. Man konnte getrost hoffen, dass er wieder austreiben und man seine Wertsachen nach der Rückkehr unter dem neuen/alten Holunder finden würde.

Verwendung – gestern und heute

Leonhart Fuchs (1501–1566) verweist in seinem „Neuen Kräuterbuch" von 1543 auf die wassertreibende, aber für den Magen schädliche Wirkung des „Holder". Nebenbei bemerkt er: „Der Saft von den Beeren angestrichen, macht das Haar schwarz".

Lonicerus (1528–1586) listet in seinem „Kräuterbuch" zahlreiche äußere Anwendungen mit Holunderblättern auf. Unter anderem: „Wenn man einem Roß im Reiten ein Holderzweiglin auf den Kopf steckt, so schadet ihm kein Trinken in der Hitz".

Später zählt der Holunder zu den Universalheilmitteln: „Rinde, Beeren, Blatt und Blüte, jeder Teil ist Kraft und Güte, jeder davon segensvoll!" Heute werden seine Blüten und gekochten Beeren zur Stärkung des Immunsystems und Vorbeugung von Erkältungskrankheiten genutzt.

Lärche

Lat. Name: *Larix decidua*
Botanischer Name: Europäische Lärche
Pflanzenfamile: Kieferngewächse

Eine Lärche kann augenblicklich unsere Stimmung aufhellen. Sie lebt ausschließlich im Hier und Jetzt. Sie strahlt beschwingte Leichtigkeit und tänzelnde Lebensfreude aus. Mit ihren feingliedrigen Ästen, die kleine schwebende Zapfen zu balancieren scheinen, ist sie Ausdruck großer feinstofflicher Energie. Nicht überraschend, dass sie als Lichtgestalt des Waldes seit jeher auch als beseelt von Saligen Frauen (weiße, durchscheinende Frauengestalten in der Mythen- und Sagenwelt der Alpenregion) und guten Waldgeistern gesehen wurde. Ihre, beinahe an Leichtsinnigkeit grenzende Unbekümmertheit zeigt sich auch darin, dass sie als einziger Nadelbaum unserer Breiten jährlich im Winter ihre Nadeln abwirft. Sie zeigt ihr riesiges Vertrauen in das Zukünftige, in Abläufe und permanente Erneuerungsvorgänge, die für sie nur gut ausgehen können. Unbeschwert in den Winter, heiter in den Frühling und unbeschadet von Blitzen durch den Sommer, denn es gibt kaum Lärchen, in die der Blitz eingeschlagen hätte. Ihr heilsames Harz zirkuliert wohlverborgen im Inneren. Wilhelm Pelikan (1893–1981) meint in seiner Heilpflanzenkunde, dass sie ihren Lebensrhythmus ganz dem Sonnenrhythmus angeglichen habe.

Die Lärche ist ein Tiefwurzler und extrem kälteresistent. Sie wird auch als Sturmanker des Waldes bezeichnet und wächst bis in 2.000 m Seehöhe. Die Lärche ist die große Überlebenskünstlerin, die auf geniale Weise Leichtes und Schweres verbindet! Sie wird 40 bis 50 m hoch und kann ein Alter von bis zu 500 Jahren erreichen.

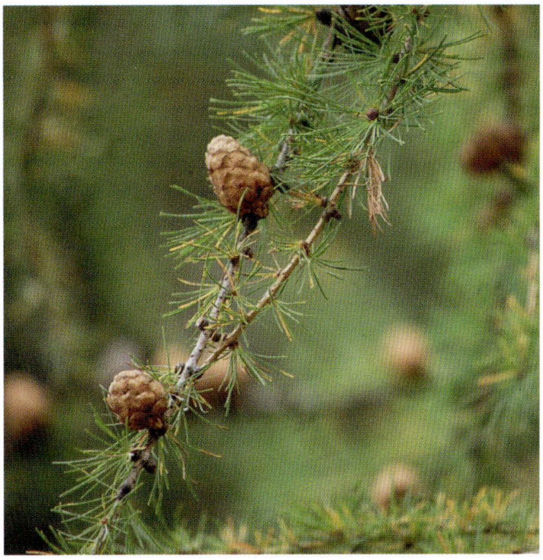
Lärchenzapfen

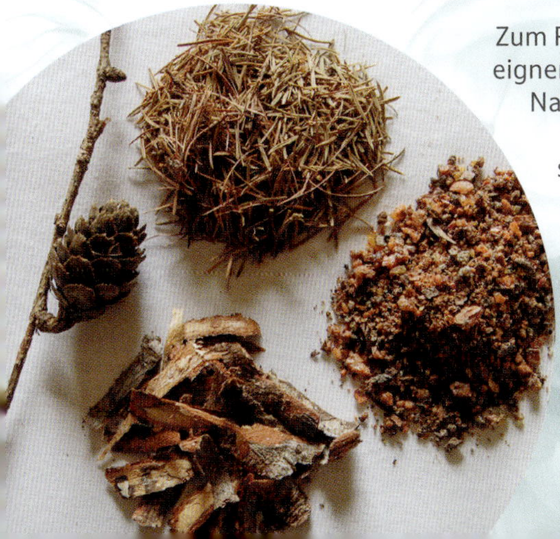
Zum Räuchern eignen sich die Nadeln und Zapfen sowie die Rinde und das Harz.

Rauch

Verwendete Pflanzenteile: Nadeln, Zapfen, Rinde, Harz.

Beste Sammel- und Erntezeit: Die Nadeln sollte man bis Ende Juni abgestreift haben; die übrigen Räucherstoffe der Lärche können das ganze Jahr über gesammelt werden.

Wirkung, Wahrnehmung: Egal welchen Pflanzenteil der Lärche man verräuchert, es überwältigt einen sofort ein stark aufbauender und extrem erdender Duft, so als bräuchte es zur Leichtigkeit, die nach außen zur Schau gestellt wird, einen Gegenpol, eine Tiefe, die nur im Inneren zu spüren ist. Nach dieser doch überraschenden Duftwahrnehmung stellen sich sogleich Gefühle von Altvertrautem, von Geborgenheit, Wohlbefinden, ja Demut und Dankbarkeit ein. Diese Umkehr von Erscheinen

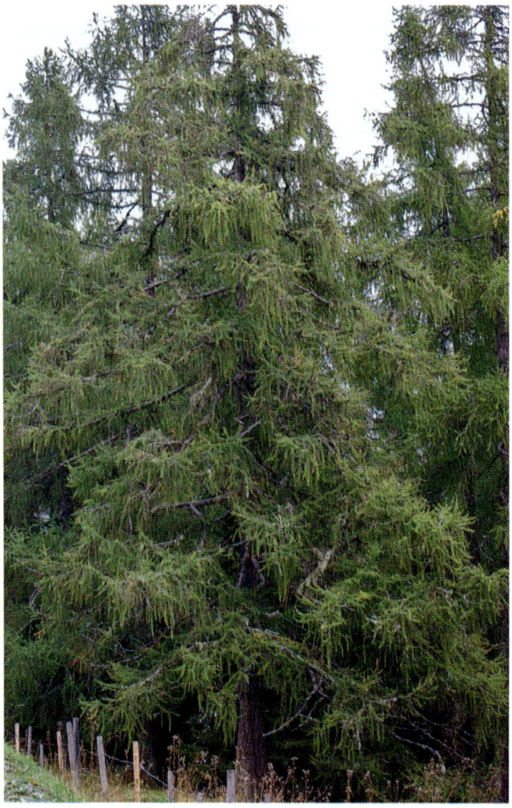
Lärche am Hochrindl, Kärnten

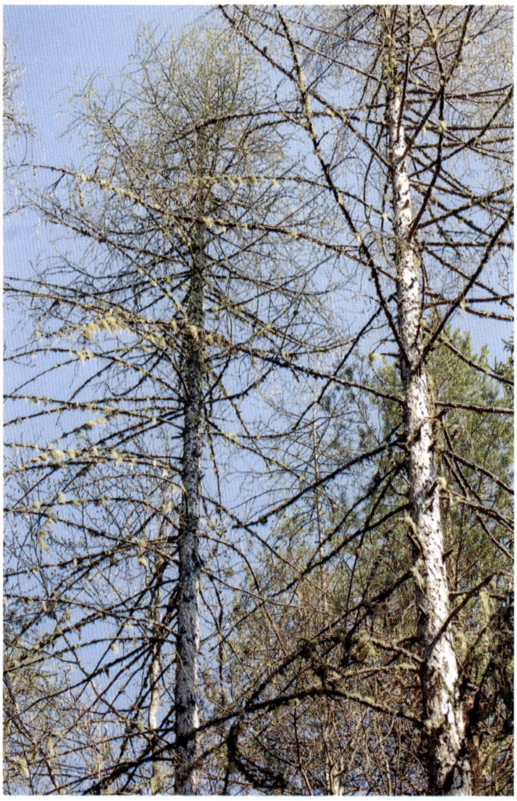
Lärche im Winter

und Dufterlebnis stelle ich auch bei anderen großen Schutzpflanzen fest, wie beispielsweise beim Schwarzen Holunder.

Alles geht leichter; sich angenommen fühlen; das Akzeptieren von schweren Dingen fällt leichter; an der eigenen Uneinsichtigkeit kann gearbeitet werden. Zur Reinigung nach Streitigkeiten. Hilft aus tiefer Verzweiflung und Lebensunlust; wirkt entkrampfend, erwärmend, lösend; hilft die eigene Individualität anzunehmen. Kräfte der Erneuerung werden angeregt; Aufgestautes wird zum Fließen gebracht; Blockaden werden gelöst; der Frühling in uns! Große Schutzkraft für Haus und Hof!

Magisches zum Rauch: Werden Räume und Häuser mit Lärche ausgeräuchert, entsteht eine positive Atmosphäre des Gelingens, des Zutrauens, des Friedens.

Schwerpunkt, Anwendungen, Rezepte: Eine Räucherung mit Lärchenpech (Harz) kann lindernd und lösend bei Erkältungen wirken und die Atmungsorgane stärken. Dazu wird das zähe Lärchenpech mit vermahlener Rinde oder vermahlenen Zapfen vermengt und als kleine Kugel auf die Räucherkohle gegeben.

Mythologie und magische Praktiken

Um die Lärche ranken sich zahlreiche heimische Sagen und Erzählungen, die das Naturverständnis unserer Vorfahren widerspiegeln. So wurde angenommen, dass die „Saligen Frauen" und andere Waldgeister in den Lärchen wohnten. Um sie herum würden sich die Tanzplätze der Wald- und Bergfeen befinden: Wenn der Mensch ihren Lebensraum respektiere und die Gesetze der Natur nicht verletze, würden sie es ihm reichlich lohnen.

Die Saligen und die Waldfrauen sind als Wesen beschrieben, die den Menschen stets wohlgesonnen gegenüber auftreten und ihnen in jeder Not zu Hilfe kommen. Besonders Frauen und Kinder stehen unter ihrem Schutz. Die Saligen verhelfen den Frauen zu einer guten Schwangerschaft. Wenn sie gerufen werden, stehen sie den Frauen bei schweren Geburten bei.

Eine am Radsberg/Radiše überlieferte Erzählung zeigt, dass die Saligen auch von sich aus Kontakt zu den Menschen suchen: Es wurden Lärchen gefällt und der Mensch ist in ihren Lebensraum eingedrungen. Da zeigt sich eine Salige in höchster Not dem Bauern, der mit seiner Hacke im Wald steht: „Bauer, mach Kreuz, mach Kreuz", ruft sie mehrmals und ist wieder verschwunden. Seit damals ist es angeraten, in den verbleibenden Lärchenholzstor (der nach dem Schlägern verbliebene Baumstrunk) mit der Hacke ein Kreuzzeichen hinein zu hacken, damit sich die Saligen und die Waldfrauen auf diese Store retten können, wenn sie von bösen Geistern und Dämonen gejagt und verfolgt werden.

Verwendung – gestern und heute

Kaiser Tiberius (32 v. Chr. bis 37 n. Chr.) ließ Unmengen von Lärchenstämmen als Bauholz nach Rom transportieren. Sicherlich waren die Römer angetan von der wunderbaren rötlichen Färbung des Lärchenholzes und seiner besonderen Stabilität.

Aus dem Lärchenpech, auch Lörgat oder Luagat genannt, wird im gesamten Alpenraum seit alters her eine besonders hilfreiche Wund- und Heilsalbe hergestellt. Heute weiß man, dass das Lärchenharz antibakteriell und entzündungshemmend wirkt.

Die Bachblüte Nr. 19 „larch" – Lärche – stärkt das Selbstvertrauen und die Selbstakzeptanz, tröstet bei Mutlosigkeit oder Verzweiflung.

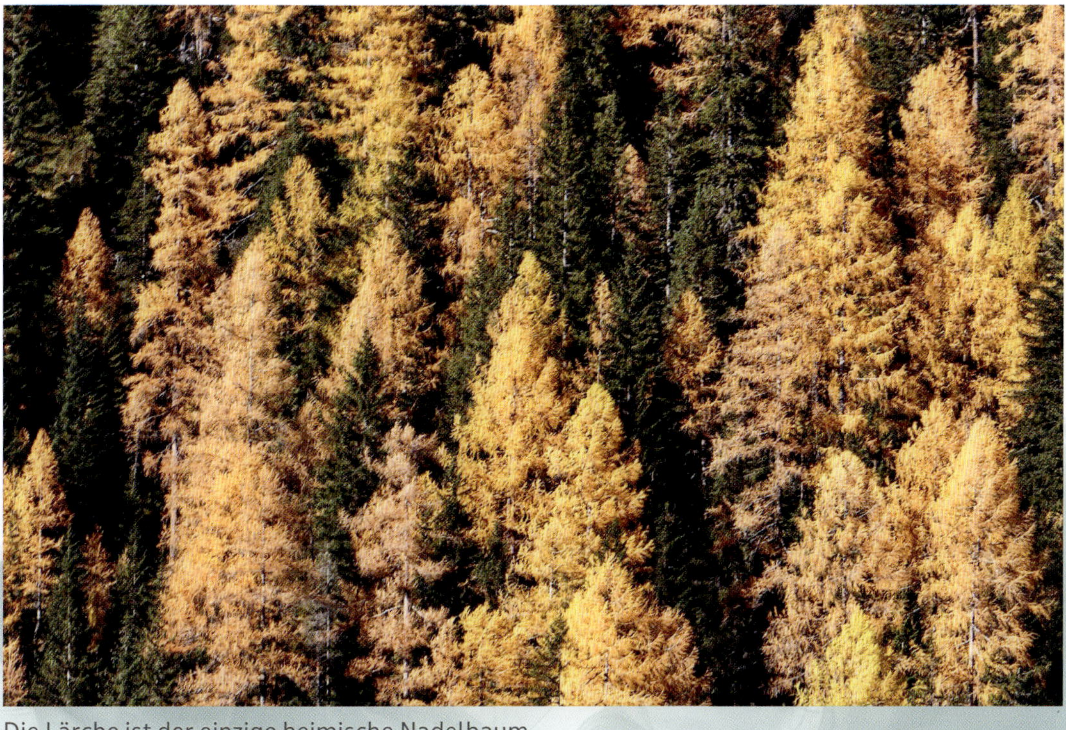

Die Lärche ist der einzige heimische Nadelbaum, der sich im Herbst verfärbt und dann seine Nadeln verliert.

Edelkastanie

Lat. Name: *Castanea sativa*
Pflanzenfamilie: Buchengewächse

Die Edelkastanie ist eine wahre Kämpferin. Als meine Edelkastanie nach ihrem zweiten Winter auf 800 m Seehöhe einen tiefen Riss in der jungen Rinde aufweist, verstreiche ich zwar provisorisch die Wunde, denke aber, das wird nichts mehr. Heute ist der Baum zehn Jahre alt und übertrifft sich jährlich an Lebenslust und Fruchtbarkeit!

Die Edelkastanie wird je nach Standort von 10 bis zu 20 m hoch, ihre Früchte werden erst in einem Alter von 25 Jahren nutzbar. In Westeuropa können diese Bäume bis zu 1000 Jahre alt werden; im Alpenraum maximal 200 Jahre.

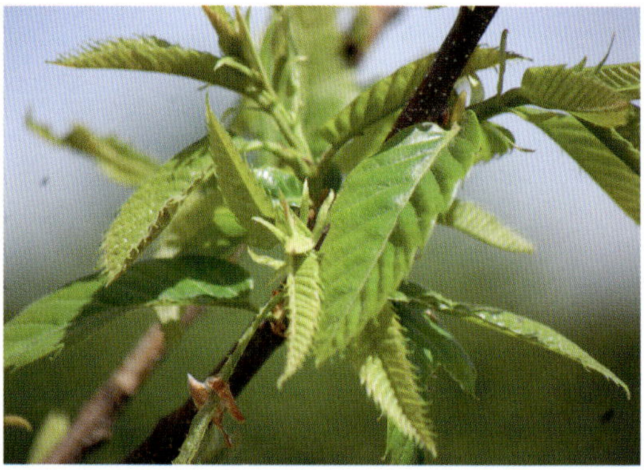

Blätter der Edelkastanie

Rauch

Verwendete Pflanzenteile: Blüten, Blätter.

Beste Sammel- und Erntezeit: Die Blüten im Frühjahr; die Blätter können das ganze Jahr über gesammelt werden.

Wirkung, Wahrnehmung: Angenehm entkrampfende Wirkung auf Geist und Körper, wirkt regulierend bei Unruhe und extremer Nervosität. Pulsiert mit starker Lebenskraft; hilfreich in Zeiten von allgemeiner Schwäche, bei Zwangsgedanken, Konzentrationsschwäche.

Magisches zum Rauch: Mit dem Blütenrauch aus Kastanien-, Waldgeißbart- und Mädesüßblüten können Schutzamulette für Kinder verstärkt und positiv aufgeladen werden.

Schwerpunkt, Anwendungen, Rezepte: Eine meiner Lern- und Prüfungsräucherungen besteht aus Edelkastanienblättern, Baldrianwurzel, Rosmarin und Tannennadeln in Kombination mit Harz.

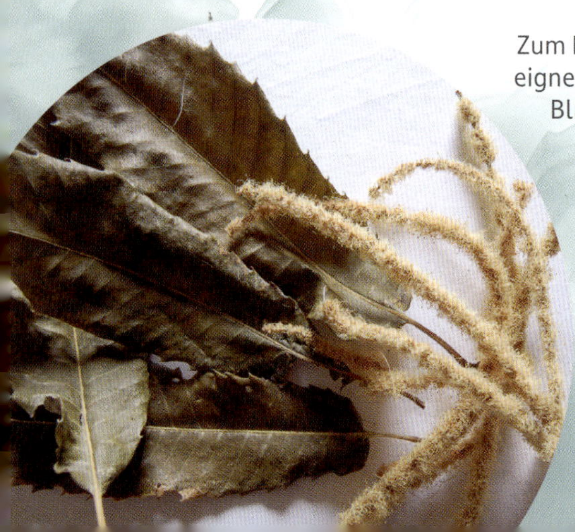

Zum Räuchern eignen sich die Blätter und Blüten.

Mythologie und magische Praktiken

Hildegard von Bingen (1098–1179) ist hellauf begeistert von den besonderen Kräften dieses Baumes, was sich in zahlreichen Rezepten niederschlägt. Die Maronen werden zu einem zentralen Lebensmittel in ihrer Ernährungslehre. Bemerkenswert auch nachfolgendes Rezept: „Ein Mensch, dem das Gehirn durch Trockenheit leer ist und der davon im Kopf schwach wird, dem koche die inneren Fruchtkerne dieses Baumes in Wasser und gebe sonst nichts dazu. Und wenn das Wasser ausgegossen ist, soll er sie oft nüchtern und nach dem Essen nehmen, und sein Hirn wächst und wird gefüllt und seine Nerven werden stark und so wird der Schmerz im Kopf weichen."

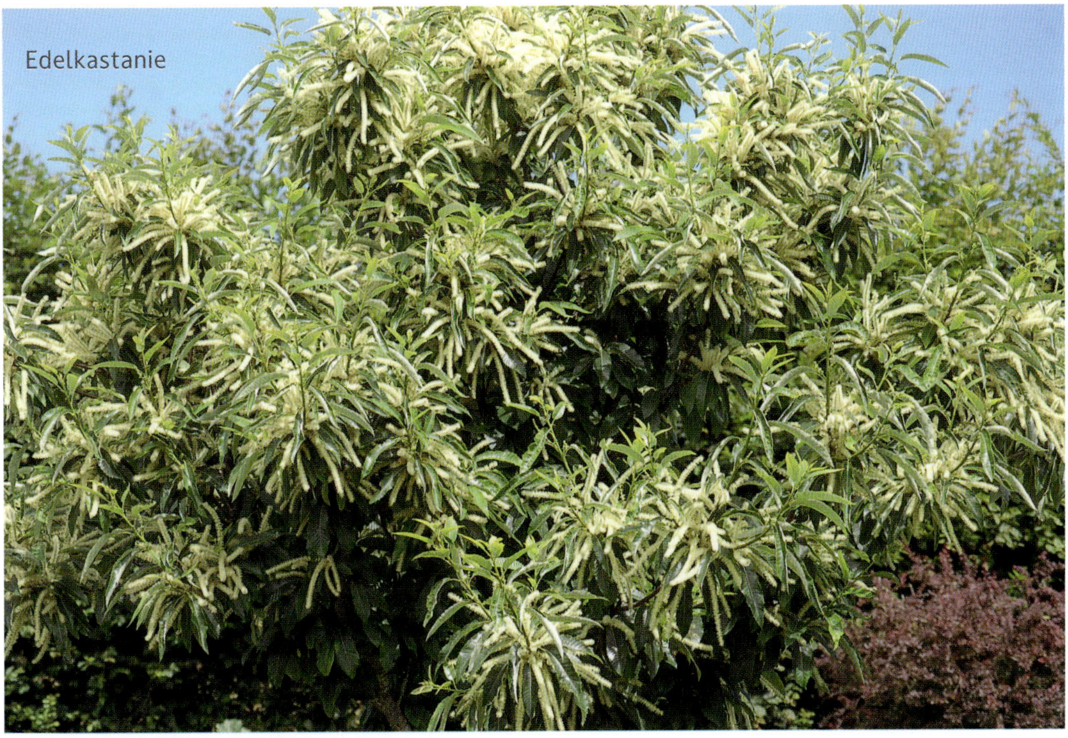

Edelkastanie

Verwendung – gestern und heute

Die Edelkastanie kommt mit den Römern zu uns und mit im Gepäck ist auch gleich das Kochbuch des Apicius (25 v. bis 42 n. Chr.) mit einem wunderbaren Maronen-Gericht. Es besteht aus Maronen mit Linsen und zahlreichen Gewürzen. Die Anbauverfügung Karls des Großen (747–814), erlassen um ca. 800 und bekannt unter dem Namen „Capitulare de villis vel curtis imperii", umfasst das wirtschaftliche Regelwerk für die Königshöfe des karolingischen Reiches. Nach 69 Kapiteln mit detaillierten Vorschriften folgt als Schlusskapitel – Nummer 70 – eine Pflanzenliste: Darin sind 73 Gartenpflanzen sowie 16 fruchttragende Bäume und Sträucher zum pfalznahen Anbau aufgelistet. An der sechsten Stelle werden „castanarios", Edelkastanien, zum Anbau vorgeschrieben.

Die Bachblüte Nr. 30 „sweet chestnut" – Edelkastanie – auch als Erlösungsblüte bekannt, kann aus innerer Ausweglosigkeit helfen, um wieder Tritt zu fassen und bereit zu werden für eine seelische Wandlung.

Nachgewiesen ist, dass die vielen ungesättigten Fettsäuren der Maroni Entzündungsherde im Körper günstig beeinflussen können.

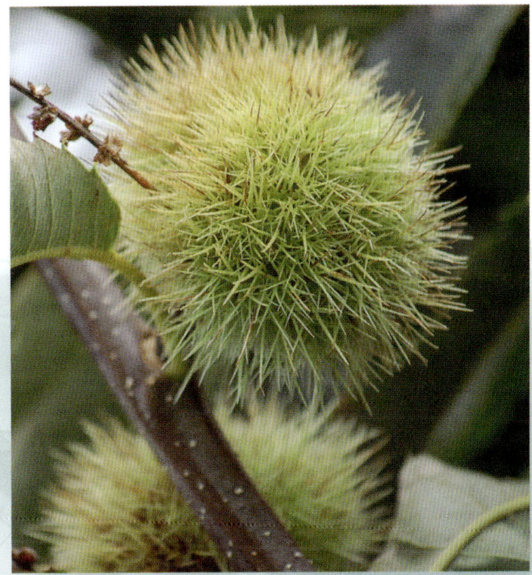

Früchte der Edelkastanie

Ross-kastanie

Lat. Name: *Aesculus hippocastanum*
Pflanzenfamilie: Seifenbaumgewächse

Pracht und Prunk des Hofes sollten sie vermitteln, jene Rosskastanien-Alleen die Ludwig XIV. (1638– 1715) pflanzen ließ. Knappe 100 Jahre zuvor war der Baum erst durch die Türkenkriege vom Osten nach Mitteleuropa gelangt. Mit diesen exklusiven Alleen verband Ludwig XIV. offensichtlich sein Renommee als moderner, absolutistischer Herrscher.

Die Rosskastanie ist nicht nur wegen ihres extrem dichten Laubes zum klassischen Gastgartenbaum aufgestiegen. Es hat auch etwas mit ihrer gemütlichen, leicht behäbigen Ausstrahlung zu tun, die einen bequem sitzen lässt und förderlich für jede Art von Genuss und Geselligkeit zu sein scheint.

Selbst wenn sie über und über von zart-rosa Blütenständen geschmückt ist, wirkt meine Rosskastanie immer etwas behäbig und schwer, mit der sprichwörtlichen „Rossnatur" behaftet. Das hat schon Karl Heinrich Waggerl (1897–1973) beflügelt: „Rosskastanie. Wie trägt sie bloß ihr hartes Los. In Straßenhitze und Gestank. Und niemals Urlaub, keinen Dank! Bedenke, Gott prüft sie nicht nur, er gab ihr auch die Rossnatur."

Die Rosskastanie wird bis zu 25 m hoch und kann, falls sie nicht von der Rosskastanienminiermotte befallen wird, bis zu 200 Jahre alt werden.

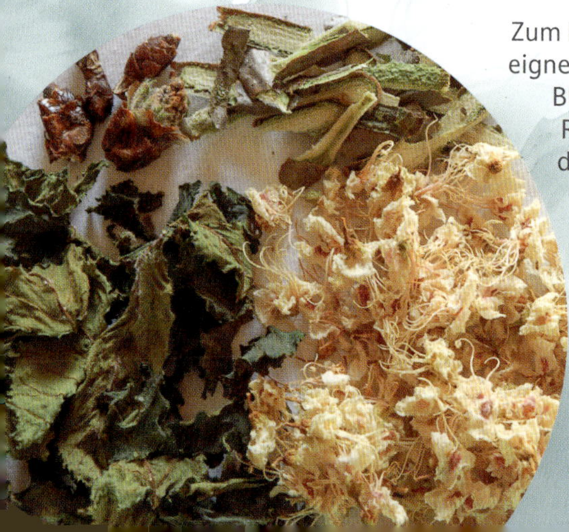

Zum Räuchern eignen sich die Blüten, die Rinde und die jungen Blätter.

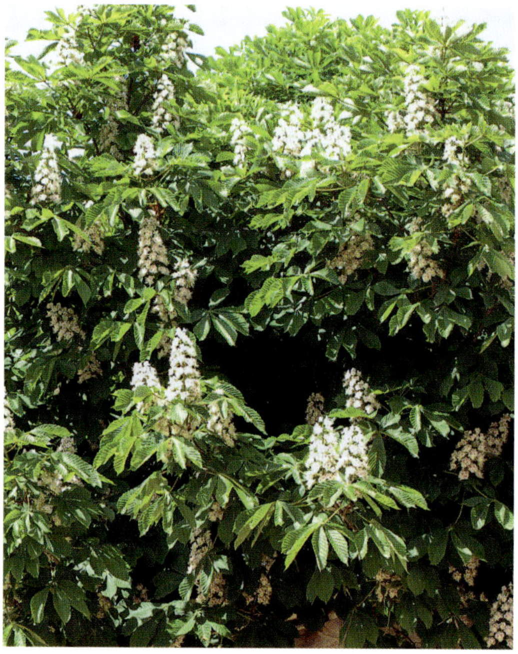

Blühende Rosskastanie

Rauch

Verwendete Pflanzenteile: Blüten,Blätter, Rinde.

Beste Sammel- und Erntezeit: Blüten und die noch kleinen Blätter im Frühling.

Wirkung, Wahrnehmung: ihr Rauch umfasst einen wie eine heilsame Umarmung durch einen lieben Menschen; stark erdend und tröstend; Arbeitsmäßig überstresste Menschen erleben den Rauch rhythmusverlangsamend und ausgleichend; das DU wird wieder möglich.

Schwerpunkt, Anwendungen, Rezepte: Für stimulierende Partnerschaftsräucherungen mit Harz und weiteren Blüten mischen, wie sinnlichen Rosenblüten und herzöffnenden Lindenblüten.

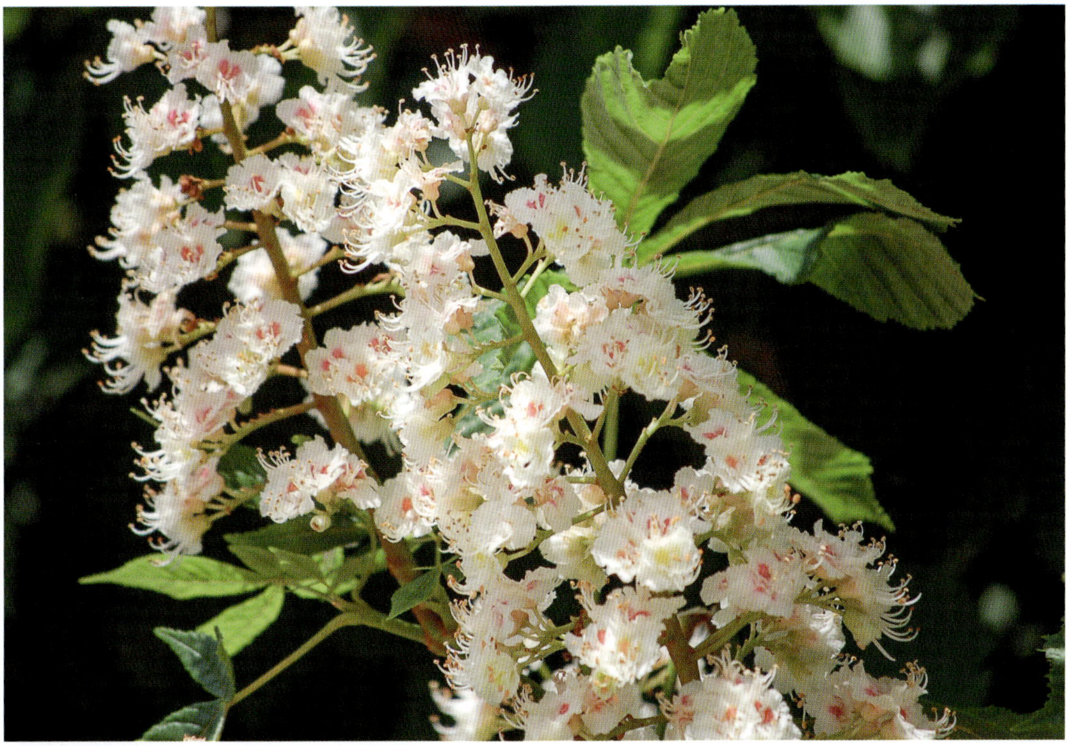

Blüten der Rosskastanie

Mythologie und magische Praktiken

Um für einen guten Schlaf zu sorgen, sollte man einige Kastanien unters Bett legen. Oder vielleicht in der Hosentasche mit sich tragen, um Rheumaschmerzen vorzubeugen.

Verwendung – gestern und heute

Es ist bemerkenswert, dass aus der gewöhnlichen Rosskastanie gleich zwei Bachblütenauszüge mit unterschiedlichen Energien hergestellt werden: Bachblüte Nr. 7 „chestnut bud" – Kastanienknospe – hilft Menschen, denen das Lernen schwerfällt – vor allem das Lernen aus den eigenen Fehlern. Die Bachblüte Nr. 35 „white chestnut" – Rosskastanie – hingegen verhilft wieder zu geistiger Ruhe und Klarheit.
Werden geviertelte Kastanien in Schnaps drei Wochen lang ausgezogen, erhält man eine Einreibung gegen müde Beine.

Kornel-kirsche

Lat. Name: *Cornus mas*
Pflanzenfamilie: Hartriegelgewächse

Das in Slowenien gebräuchliche Sprichwort „zdrava kot dren“ (gesund wie eine Kornelkirsche) bedeutet kerngesund zu sein, eine stählerne Abwehrkraft zu haben. Einer der vielen Sträucher dessen heutiges Ansehen in keinem Verhältnis zu seiner früheren Wertschätzung steht. Belege ihrer intensiven Nutzung als besonderes Lebensmittel finden sich von der Steinzeit bis in die Spätantike. Die Kornelkirsche liefert wertvolle Früchte, die einen wichtigen Beitrag für das körperliche Wohlbefinden unserer aufgeregten, überstressten und überzuckerten Gesellschaft leisten könnten. Intensive biologische Forschung an Kornelkirschen-Kulturen findet heute in der Ukraine statt.

Das hoffnungsfrohe Gelb ihrer frühen Blüten strahlt bereits ab Mitte März im sonst noch kargen Garten. Sie versorgt unsere Bienen mit ausreichend Nektar zu einer Zeit, zu der sie sonst kaum Nahrung finden. Oft summt die ganze Kornelkirsche wie ein übergroßer Bienenstock. Sie beschert mir jedes Jahr zuverlässig eine reiche Ernte.

Die Kornelkirsche, auch Dirndl genannt, wird bei uns etwa drei Meter, an guten Standorten und in Südeuropa bis zu acht Meter hoch und kann, dank ihres besonders harten Holzes, bis zu 100 Jahre alt werden.

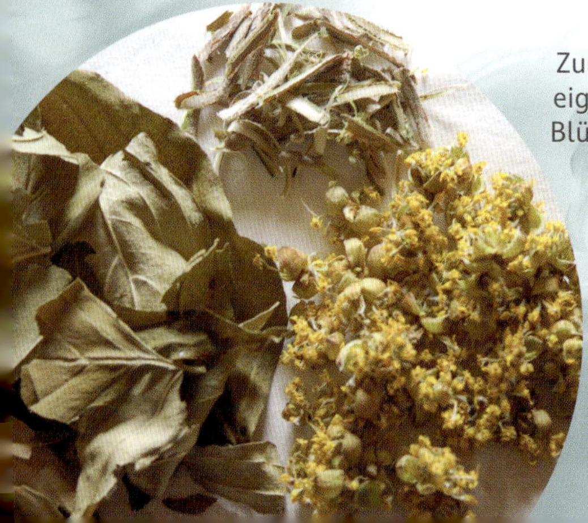

Zum Räuchern eignen sich die Blüten, Blätter und die Rinde.

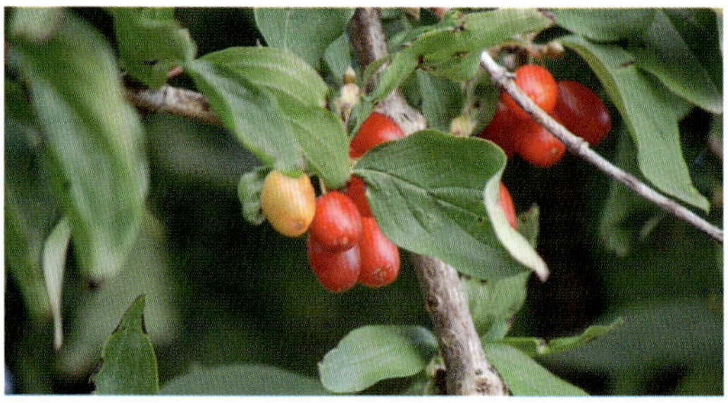

Früchte der Kornelkirsche

Rauch

Verwendete Pflanzenteile: Blüten, Blätter, Rinde.

Beste Sammel- und Erntezeit: Die Blüten im Frühling; Blätter und Rinde der Äste das ganze Jahr über.

Wirkung, Wahrnehmung: Hilfreich bei Unsicherheit und unbestimmten Angstgefühlen; bei seelischen Belastungen; der Rauch macht hellwach und hebt die Konzentrationskraft. Erdet nachhaltig und holt einen aus Hirngespinsten in die Realität zurück. Reinigend und schutzgebend für große Räume mit vielen Menschen – wie Kindergärten, Schulklassen, Seminarräume: Es bleibt eine angenehme Leichtigkeit und Frische zurück.

Magisches zum Rauch: Für Rituale bei besonderen Anliegen, zur Klärung und Unterstützung der eigenen Pläne.

Schwerpunkt, Anwendungen, Rezepte: Bei Abwehrräucherungen Blüten und Holz verwenden. Bei persönlichen Anliegen mit Rainfarn und Odermennig verräuchern; bei familiären Anliegen mit Salbei, Eberraute und Traubenkirsche gemeinsam räuchern; bei stark negativen Eintragungen in Räumen mit Beifuß, Speik und Wurzeln (siehe dort) mischen. Auf das Harz nicht vergessen!

Mythologie und magische Praktiken

Am Balkan und im vorderasiatischen Raum wurde das Holz der Kornelkirsche seit Jahrtausenden für Abwehrzauber verwendet: Das Holz sollte geburtsbeschleunigend wirken, wenn man damit über den Bauch der Gebärenden streicht. Aus Kornelkirschenholz geschnitzte Figuren sollen Krankheitsgeister und böse Dämonen vertreiben.

In Südeuropa gilt sie auch als Glücksbringer: Mit einem Kornelkirschenzweig ausgestattet wünschen dort die Kinder zwischen Weihnachten und Neujahr den Erwachsenen Glück und Gesundheit fürs neue Jahr.

Der gordische Knoten, mit dem der phrygische König Gordios Pferd und Streitwagen unauflöslich verbunden hatte, soll aus dem Bast der Kornelkirsche geknotet gewesen sein. Alexander der Große (356–323 v. Chr.) hat diesen gordischen Knoten einst mit einem Schwerthieb durchtrennt und für eine, noch heute gebräuchliche Redewendung gesorgt.

Bei den Römern ist die Kornelkirsche direkt mit dem Gründungsmythos Roms verbunden: 753 v. Chr. soll Romulus am Palatin seine Lanze aus Kornelkirschenholz als Grenzzeichen für die neue Stadt Rom in den Boden gestoßen haben. Aus dieser Lanze sei ein Strauch gewachsen.

Verwendung – gestern und heute

In Italien wurden Kerne der Kornelkirsche in den Überresten steinzeitlicher Pfahlbauten gefunden. Die Kornelkirsche als Genussmittel und als extrem hartes Lanzenholz war so alltäglich und gleichzeitig unverzichtbar, dass sie praktisch in allen großen Erzählungen der Antike vorkommt.

In Homers zehntem Gesang der „Odyssee" verwandelt die Zauberin Kirke die Gefährten des Odysseus in Schweine: „Weinend ließen sie sich einsperren, da schüttete Kirke ihnen Eicheln und Bucheneckern und Kornellen vor, das gewöhnliche Futter für Schweine".

Das extrem harte Holz eignete sich nicht nur zur Herstellung von langlebigen Werkzeugen, Stielen oder Speichen, es war auch ein hervorragendes Holz für militärische Zwecke. Durch starke und bruchsichere Lanzen aus Kornelkirschenholz erzielten damalige Einzelkämpfer und Heere eine größere Angriffs-, aber auch Abwehrkraft. Es war schließlich Philipp II. von Makedonien (382–336 v. Chr.), der mit Hilfe dieser Lanzen eine neue Militärstrategie initiierte: die Phalanx. Die Kornelkirschen-Lanzen und die neue Heeresformation leisteten sicherlich einen großen Beitrag zu den grandiosen Erfolgen seines Sohnes, Alexander des Großen (356–323), bei dessen Eroberungsfeldzügen im Osten.

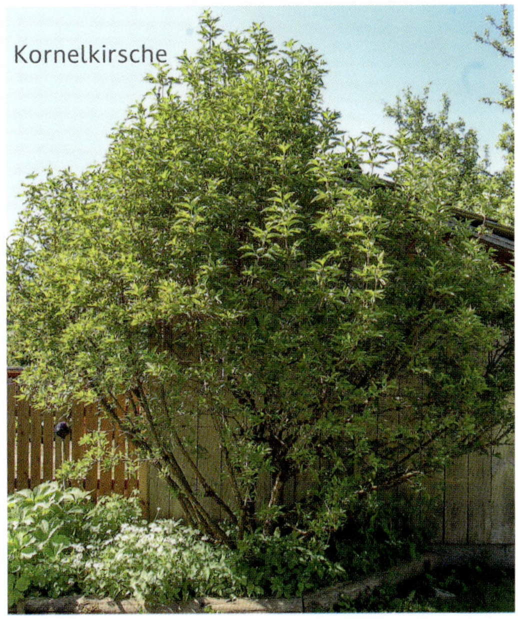
Kornelkirsche

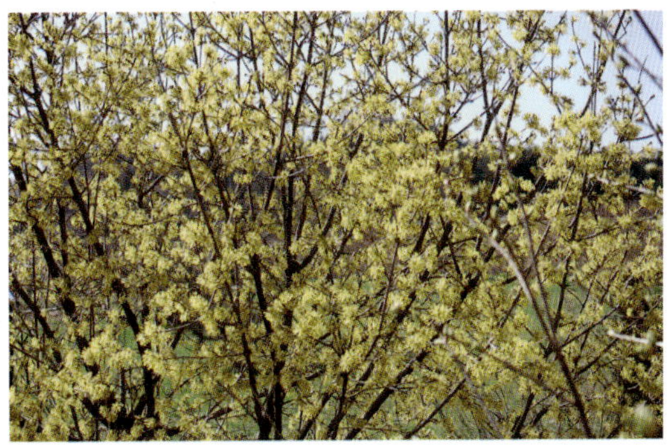
Kornelkirsche in Blüte

Hildegard von Bingen (1098–1179) schreibt: „Die Frucht dieses Baumes schadet dem Menschen nicht, wenn man sie isst, aber sie reinigt und stärkt den kranken und auch den gesunden Magen, sie nützt dem Menschen für die Gesundheit."

Kreuzdorn

Lat. Name: *Rhamnus cathartica*
Pflanzenfamilie: Kreuzdorngewächse

Irgendwie ungemütlich fühlt sich der Kreuzdorn in meinem Garten. Er steht direkt hinter seiner Verwandtschaft, dem Faulbaum, will sich aber am liebsten wegdrehen. Er bevorzugt Auenwälder und Moore, also feuchte Standorte. Das kann ich ihm leider nicht bieten. Aber von Schmetterlingen und Vögeln wird er umschwärmt und bis spätestens Dezember sind alle, wirklich alle seiner schwarzen Beeren von ihnen verzehrt.

Seit Jahrtausenden wird ihm eine große Abwehrkraft gegen Ungemach und böse Geister nachgesagt, was wohl mit den oft unheimlichen Standorten zu tun hat.

Seine Rinde und seine Beeren sind **leicht giftig.** Der Kreuzdorn wächst als Strauch bis drei Meter hoch, als Baum bis zu fünf Meter hoch und kann ein Alter von 100 Jahren erreichen.

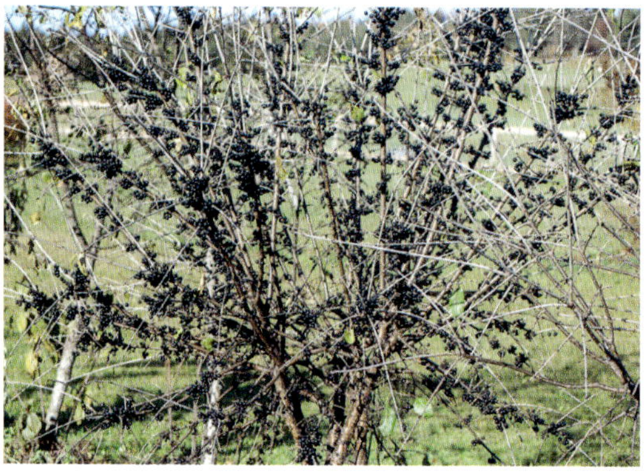

Früchte des Kreuzdorns im November

Rauch

Verwendete Pflanzenteile: Blätter, Beeren, Rinde.

Beste Sammel- und Erntezeit: Blätter das ganze Jahr; die Beeren werden im Herbst abgenommen und getrocknet. In die Räucherung kommen sie fein vermahlen.

Wirkung, Wahrnehmung: Sehr dumpfe, erdige Note; die Glut tut sich schwer mit diesem Räucherstoff; personenbezogen eher lähmend; man kommt kaum bis gar nicht in Resonanz mit dem Räucherstoff.

Sollte hauptsächlich in Räucherungen verwendet werden, die raumbezogen sind oder die im Freien, um die Gebäude herum, stattfinden. Für Abwehrräucherungen in Haus und Hof in Krankheits- oder Pandemiezeiten.

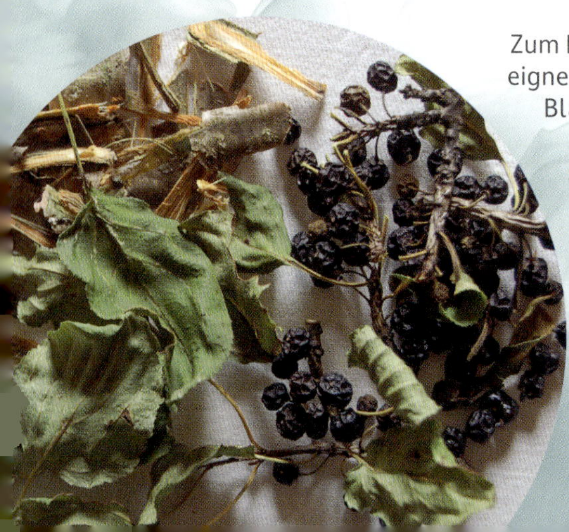

Zum Räuchern eignen sich die Blätter und Beeren sowie die Rinde.

Magisches zum Rauch: Der römische Philosoph Theodosius (385–430) überliefert, dass die Etrusker, die ab ca. 800 v. Chr. kulturell in Erscheinung getreten waren, durch das Abbrennen und Verräuchern von Kreuzdornbeeren sowie anderer schwarzer Beeren drohendes Unheil abzuwenden versuchten.

Schwerpunkt, Anwendungen, Rezepte: Bei Abwehrräucherungen mit Ergänzungen anderer Hölzer in der ersten Jahreshälfte und Wurzeln in der zweiten Jahreshälfte. Harz nicht vergessen!

Eine Räuchermischung zum neutralisieren des Hauseingangs und der Türschwelle ist die Mischung aus Kreuzdorn, Königskerze, Rainfarn und Blutwurz in Kombination mit Harz.

Mythologie und magische Praktiken

Dioskurides, ein angesehener römischer Arzt des 1. Jahrhunderts n. Chr., erwähnt, dass Kreuzdornzweige, die an der Haustüre angebracht werden, zauberabwehrende Kraft besäßen. In das gleiche Horn stößt 1.500 Jahre später Lonicerus (1528–1586): Zweige über der Tür vertreiben „allerlei Gift und Zauberei“.

War in den zahlreichen antiken Zuschreibungen von antidämonischer und zauberabwehrender Kraft die Rede, so wurde im christlichen Mittelalter nur mehr von hexenwidrigen Kräften gesprochen. Besonders wirksam sei es demnach, bei angehexten Viehkrankheiten, in der Johannisnacht (24. Juni) Zweige vom Hexendorn zu holen und damit, unter Hersagen eines Bannspruches, jedem Vieh drei Mal auf den linken Hinterfuß zu schlagen. Diese und ähnliche Anweisungen gab es viele, um dem Treiben der bösen Hexen Einhalt zu gebieten.

So konnte man sich beispielsweise zu Walpurgis (30. April/1. Mai) mit Kreuzdornzweigen Hexen vom Leib halten. Gelang das nicht oder sah man sich einer ganzen Schar von Teufeln und Hexen gegenüber, war es von Vorteil einen Stock aus Kreuzdornholz bei sich zu haben. Mit diesem zog man schnell am Boden einen Bannkreis um sich, verblieb ruhig darinnen stehen und schon war die Hexengefahr vorbei.

Verwendung – gestern und heute

Der Kreuzdorn wird auch Christusdorn genannt, weil man glaubte, er sei – neben Weißdorn und Schwarzdorn – die dritte Pflanze der Dornenkrone. Auch kam der Glaube auf, dass das Kreuz Christi selbst aus dem Holz des Christusdornes gewesen sei.

Begehrt waren Rinde und Beeren auch zum Färben von Wolle. Ein Baum – viele Farben, das ist in unseren Breiten nicht noch einmal zu finden. Vom Gelb der frischen Rinde bis zum Braun der getrockneten Rinde, vom Rot der halbreifen Beeren bis zum Braunrot der überreifen Beeren reicht die erstaunliche Farbpalette.

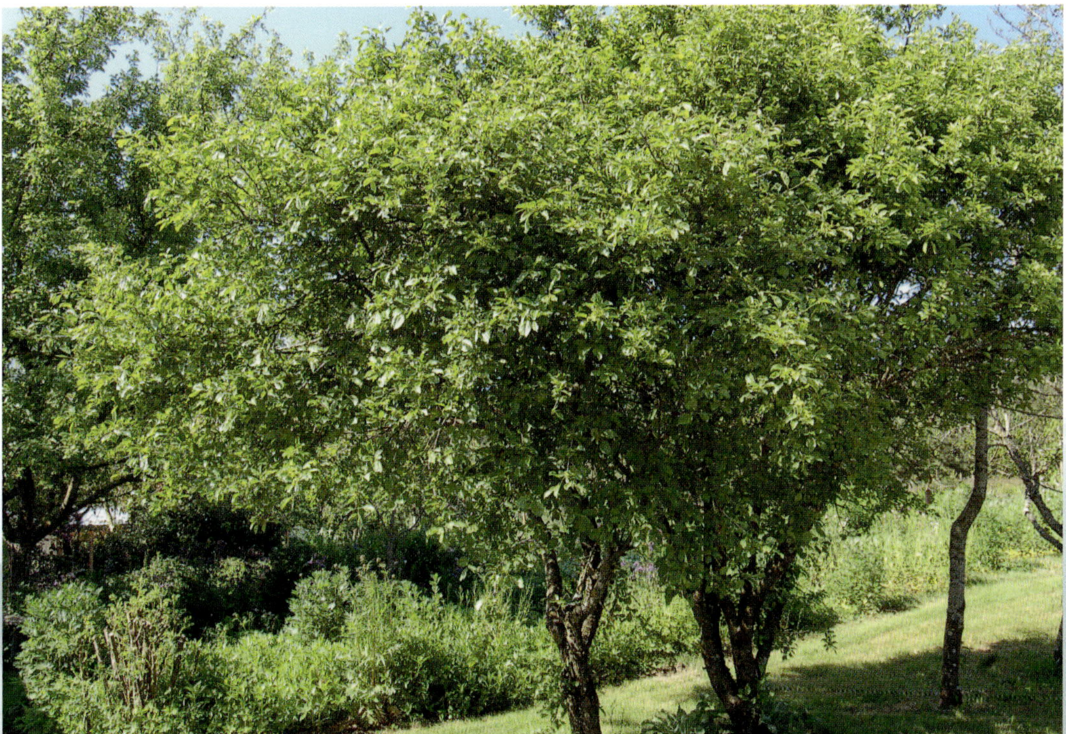

Kreuzdorn

Linde

Lat. Name: *Tilia* sp.
Botanischer Name: Winterlinde *(T. cordata)*, Sommerlinde *(T. platyphyllos)*
Pflanzenfamilie: Malvengewächse

Der große Schutzbaum der Liebenden, der Geselligkeit, der menschlichen Gemeinschaft. Viele Lieder und Gedichte wurden über die Linde geschrieben und stets wird ihr freundliches, beschützendes, ausgleichendes Wesen hervorgehoben. Zwei Texte sind zu einem echten Kulturgut geworden: das mittelalterliche Liebesgedicht von Walter von der Vogelweide (1170–1230), das mit folgenden Worten beginnt: „under der linden, an der heide, da unser zweier bette was …"; und das 1822 von Wilhelm Müller geschriebene und 1827 von Franz Schubert (1797–1828) vertonte Gedicht „am Brunnen vor dem Tore, da steht ein Lindenbaum…".

Es herrscht eine innige Beziehung zwischen Mensch und Lindenbaum. Noch bis ins frühe 20. Jahrhundert ist die Linde vielerorts Treffpunkt des Dorflebens. Unter ihr wird gespielt, gefeiert und getanzt. Zahlreiche Gasthäuser tragen die Linde in ihrem Namen.

Winter- und Sommerlinden können bis zu 40 m hoch werden. Eine Linde kann sehr alt werden, in Ausnahmefällen wird sie 1.000 Jahre alt. So alt wird man nur, wenn man sich zu helfen weiß: Im hohen Alter kann die Linde neue Innenwurzeln bilden, die vom Stamm aus in die Tiefe wachsen. Sie kann auch ihre Baumkrone erneuern, wenn die alte vergeht. Wie bei der Eiche gibt es auch bei der Linde einen 300-er Spruch: Die Linde kommt 300 Jahre, steht 300 Jahre, vergeht 300 Jahre.

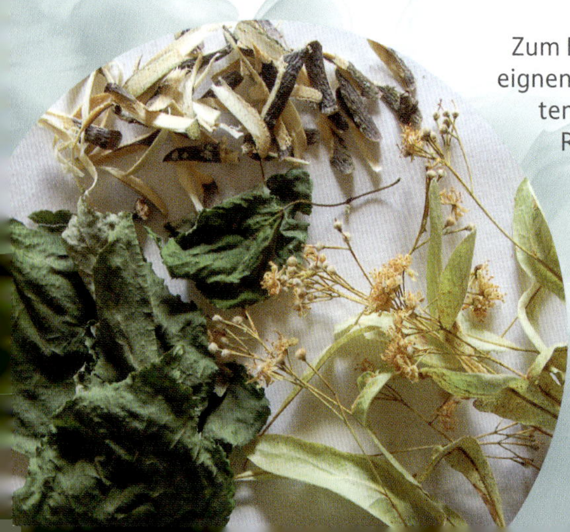

Zum Räuchern eignen sich Blüten, Blätter, Rinde und Holz.

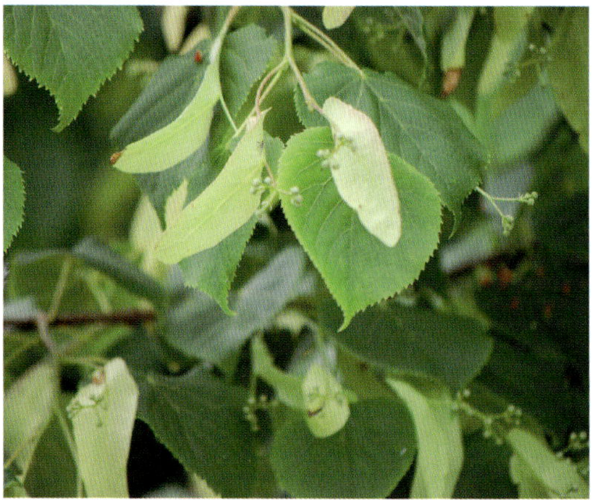

Blätter und Früchte der Linde

Rauch

Verwendete Pflanzenteile: Blüten, Blätter, Rinde, Holz.

Beste Sammel- und Erntezeit: Die aufgeblühten Blüten im Frühsommer; Blätter und Zweige für die Rinde und das Räucherholz können das ganze Jahr über gesammelt werden.

Wirkung, Wahrnehmung: Lindenrauch erwärmt das erstarrte Herz; steigert das Wohlbefinden; fördert Offenheit; Entspannung wird möglich; eine große Beruhigung tritt ein. Lindenblüten können Kindern alle Arten von Ängsten nehmen; der Rauch schenkt Urvertrauen, Gottvertrauen. Auch Beziehungsängste werden ruhiger. Der Rauch von Lindenblättern vermittelt Geborgenheit und Wärme für verletzte Seelen. Lindenholz stärkt das innere Kind, hilft frühe Verletzungen und Traumata zu ertragen. Manchmal überträgt sich die liebevolle und beständige Kraft des Lindenholzes auch dadurch, dass man ein Stück Lindenholz in der Tasche mit sich trägt.

Magisches zum Rauch: Aus dem „lignum sacrum" werden nicht nur gerne Heiligenfiguren geschnitzt, es ist zusammen mit Weihrauch und Myrrhe am Karfreitag auch eine alte Räucherung für den Herrgottswinkel.

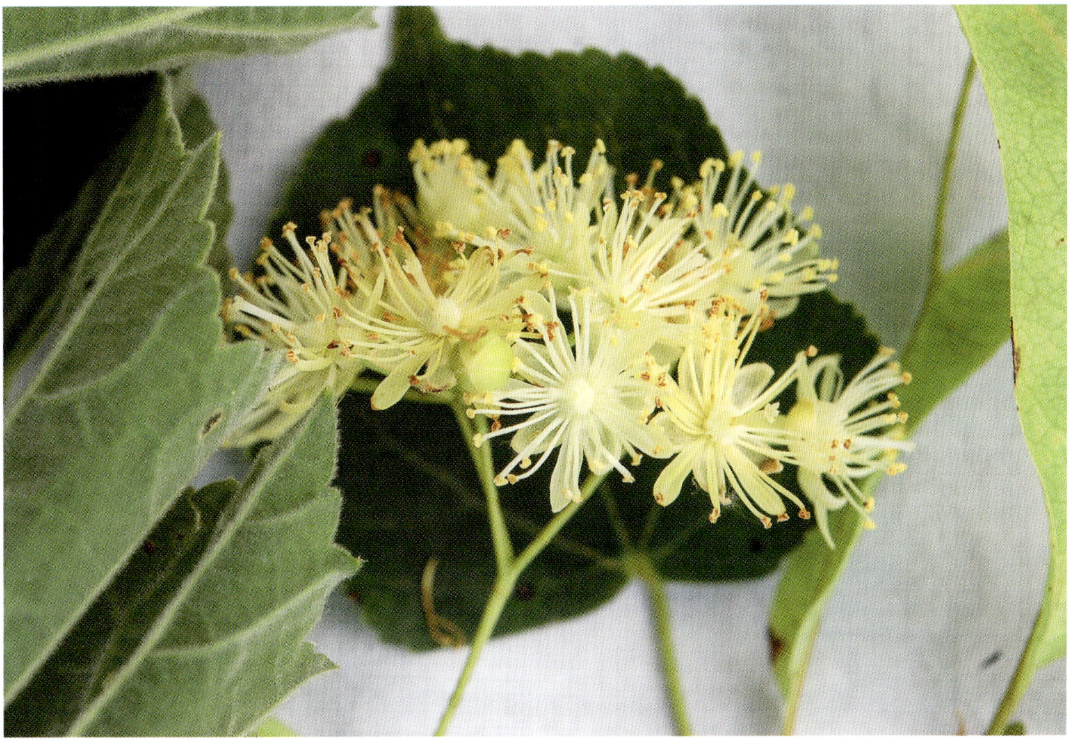

Lindenblüte

Schwerpunkt, Anwendungen, Rezepte: Eine schlaffördernde Räucherung ergibt sich mit Lindenblüten, Lavendel, Rosenblüten und Hagebutten. Bei Kopfschmerzen und Unruhezuständen kann folgende Räuchermischung Abhilfe bringen: Lindenblüten, Sanddornblätter, Heilziest und Lavendel. Stets mit Harz kombinieren.

Mythologie und magische Praktiken

Linden sind ein fester Bestandteil der mitteleuropäischen Mythologie und Kulturgeschichte: Unter den Linden hat der verliebte Zwergenkönig Laurin, Similde, die Tochter des Königs an der Etsch, entführt. Doch die Recken ihres Vaters, allen voran Dietrich von Bern, befreiten sie und nahmen Laurin gefangen.

Im Nibelungenlied beginnt Siegfrieds Glück und Ende unter einer Linde: Als er im Blut des erlegten Drachen badet, um unverwundbar zu werden, fällt ein Lindenblatt auf seine Schulter und verhindert so seine Unsterblichkeit.

Der römische Dichter Ovid (43 v. Chr. bis 17 n. Chr.) überliefert in seinen „Metamorphosen" die Geschichte von Philemon und Baucis, die aus der griechischen Mythologie stammt: Nachdem Zeus und Hermes, hier Jupiter und Merkur, bei einem armen, alten Paar zu Abend gegessen hatten, fragten sie die beiden, ob sie einen Wunsch hätten. Die Alten waren eigentlich mit allem zufrieden, äußerten dann aber doch einen Wunsch: Sie wollten gemeinsam sterben. Und das erfüllte ihnen der Göttervater. Als ihre Zeit gekommen war, verwandelte er Philemon in eine Eiche und die sanfte Baucis in eine Linde.
Bei den Germanen und Slawen war die Linde ein heiliger Baum. Ihr Holz wurde auch zur Einäscherung von Toten verwendet, denen man auf ihrem letzten Weg noch Liebe mitgeben wollte. Im Kartenspiel steht das symbolische Lindenblatt für den freien Bauernstand.

Verwendung – gestern und heute

In den vorgeschichtlichen Pfahlbauten wurde Lindenbast für Matten und Seile verwendet. Unter der Linde sollte nur die Wahrheit gesprochen werden! Vermutlich auch deswegen fand die mittelalterliche Rechtssprechung oft unter den Linden statt: „iudicium sub tilia". Wegen des ausgleichenden Wesens der Linde mag dies wohl mancherorts auch für „gelinde" Urteile gesorgt haben. Wer immer unter der Linde Schutz suchte, durfte nicht mehr verfolgt werden. Hingegen wurde ein unter der Feme-Linde Verurteilter sofort an ihr aufgehängt oder galt als „Verfemter" vogelfrei.

Linden wurden traditionell auch auf Kirchplätzen angepflanzt. Dort versammelten sich die Menschen vor und nach der Messe und dort fanden auch die Verkündungen der weltlichen Obrigkeit statt.

Wallensteins spektakuläres Tausend-Linden-Projekt erregte Aufsehen: Auf seinem Schloss Gitschin in Böhmen ließ Wallenstein (1583–1634), General des deutschen Kaisers und der katholischen Liga im dreißigjährigen Krieg, eine vierreihige Allee ansetzen. Dazu befehligte er tausend Soldaten an Ort und Stelle und gab mit einem Kanonenschuss das Kommando für das gleichzeitige Einsetzen der tausend Linden! Zufall war das sicher keiner, dass gerade ein kriegstüchtiger General tausend Bäume des Friedens pflanzen ließ.

Die Verwendung der Lindenblüten als Absud bei Erkältungen beginnt erst recht spät, im 17. Jahrhundert. Sie aktiviert die körpereigenen Abwehrkräfte. Davor sprechen die Kräuterkundigen von gebranntem „Lindenwasser" gegen Bauchschmerzen.

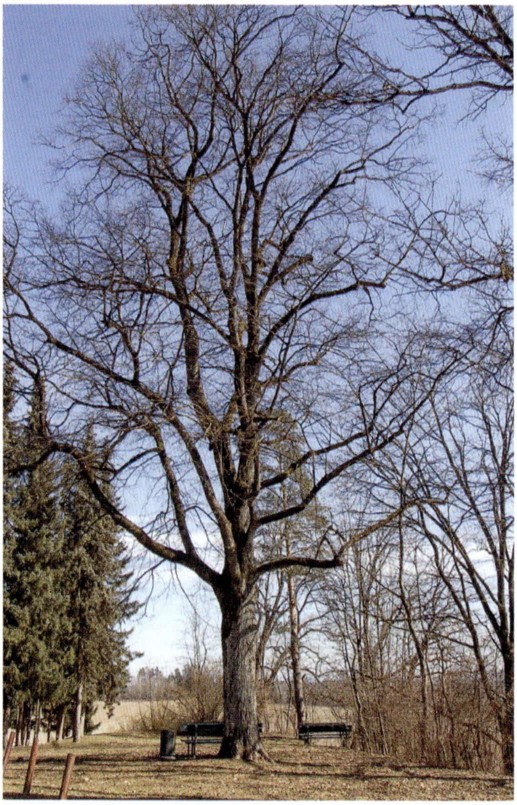

Friedhofslinde in Hörtendorf, Kärnten

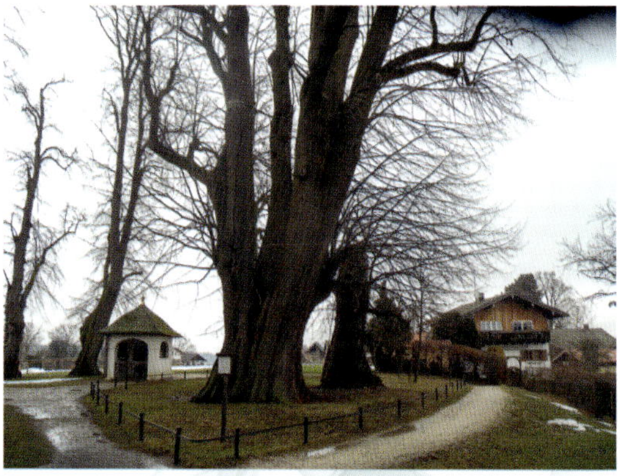

Tassilo-Linde auf der Fraueninsel im Chiemsee, Bayern

Schneeball

Lat. Name: *Virburnum opulus*
Botanischer Name: Gewöhnlicher Schneeball
Pflanzenfamilie: Moschuskrautgewächse

Nach den weißen Blütenkränzen des Frühjahrs leuchten im Herbst die saftig gefüllten knallroten Beeren vom Schneeball verführerisch. Aber irgendwie will sie keiner so gern haben. Für die Menschen sind sie roh giftig und auch die Vögel scheinen zu zögern und so hängen die Beeren oft bis ins Frühjahr am Strauch. Wenn man die Beeren zwischen den Fingern zerdrückt, kommt ein heller, leicht herzförmiger Kern zum Vorschein, der dem Schneeball auch seinen volkstümlichen Namen „Herzbeere" gegeben hat. Ich erinnere mich noch gut an den unangenehmen Geruch, den die Beeren im ganzen Haus verbreiteten, wenn meine Großmutter sie stundenlang einkochte. Heraus kamen ein bis zwei kleine Gläser Marmelade, die sie stets versteckt hielt und von der sie einen halben Teelöffel nahm, wenn sie an Kurzatmigkeit litt oder ihr die „Trutta mora" wieder auf der Brust saß.

Die Herzbeere liebt eher feuchte Böden und siedelt sich gerne in Auwäldern an. Das hat ihr ihren zweiten volkstümlichen Namen „Wasserholder" gegeben. Der genügsame Strauch wird zwischen zwei bis vier Meter hoch und kann bis zu 70 Jahre alt werden.

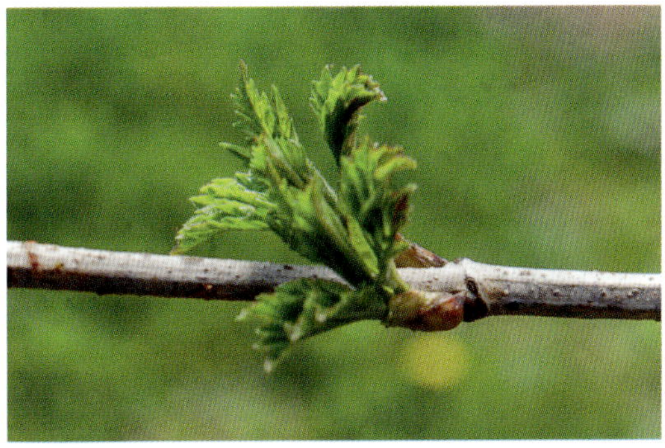
Schneeball beim Austreiben der Blätter

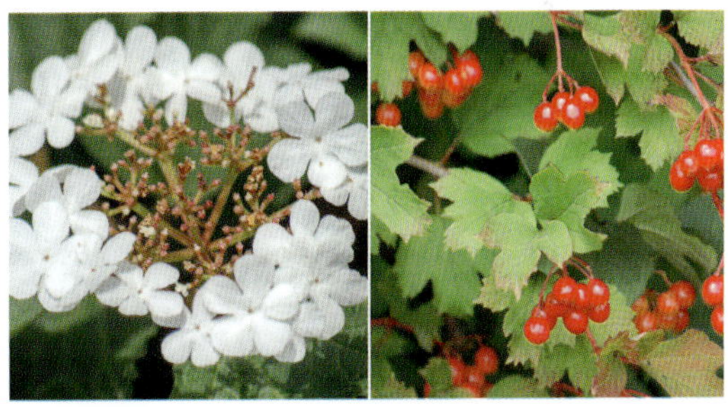
Links Blüten, rechts Früchte des Schneeballs

Rauch

Verwendete Pflanzenteile: Blüten, Blätter, Rinde.

Beste Sammel- und Erntezeit: Die weißen Blüten im Frühling; die Blätter können das ganze Jahr über gesammelt werden. Die Rinde wird von den Zweigen des Frühjahrs- oder Herbstschnittes genommen.

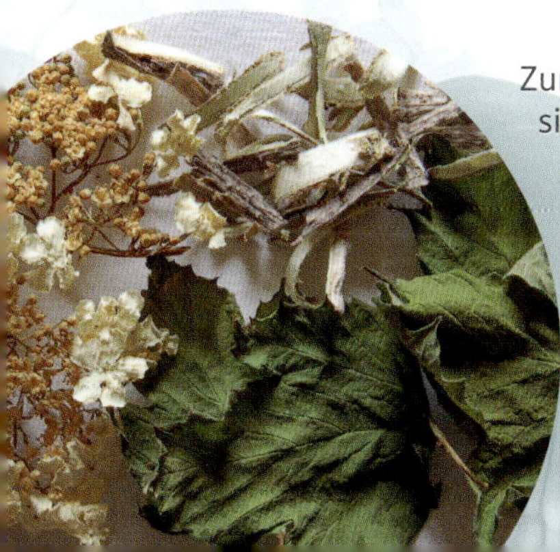
Zum Räuchern eignen sich die Blüten, Blätter und die Rinde.

Wirkung, Wahrnehmung: Der Rauch bringt schnell einen leicht unangenehmen Geruch mit sich; man spürt rasch die sedierende Wirkung. Beruhigend selbst für die größten Zappelgeister; man kommt in einen angenehm empfundenen Schwebezustand.

Schwerpunkt, Anwendungen, Rezepte: Für eine Abendräucherung zum besseren Einschlafen mischt man Schneeballblätter und Wald-Geißbart mit Harz.

Verwendung – gestern und heute

Das bruchfeste und gleichzeitig biegsame Holz der Zweige wurde als Holz für Pfeile verwendet. Der 5.300 Jahre alte Mann aus dem Eis, Ötzi, hatte vierzehn Pfeile aus Schneeballholz in seinem Köcher.

Achtung: Aufgrund des Glykosids Viburnin gelten alle Pflanzenteile als **giftig.**

Rose

Lat. Name: *Rosa canina*
Botanischer Name: Hundsrose, Heckenrose
Pflanzenfamilie: Rosengewächse

Fünf Blütenblätter, kreisrund angeordnet, jedes einzelne davon in einer angedeuteten Herzform, ein dezenter Duft: Das ist sie, die wohl berühmteste aller Blüten! Seit Jahrtausenden beflügelt sie die menschliche Phantasie: Ihre runde Form ist Symbol des Kreises, des Rades und nährt die Vorstellung von zyklisch wiederkehrenden Phasen in der Natur wie auch im Menschenleben. Die Zahl fünf vollendet das Pentagramm, ist dem Mars zugeordnet und gilt als Zahl der Alchemisten. Die fünf ist aber auch die Zahl der Magie! Und aus den herzförmigen Blütenblättern springt uns die Liebe entgegen. Und letztlich dreht sich bei der Rosensymbolik alles um Liebe: Irdische Liebe und Leidenschaft verbinden sich in ihr mit himmlischer Liebe und Vollkommenheit.

Sappho (ca. 630–570 v. Chr.), die berühmte Dichterin der griechischen Antike, betitelt die Rose als „Königin der Blumen" und schreibt in ihrer Ode an die Liebesgöttin Aphrodite unter anderem: „... Allmächtige komm vom Äther herab ...zu deinem Tempel, einst von Kretern erbaut. Unter den Apfelbäumen des heiligen Hains, als sie dir Opfer brachten auf den Altären, schwelten damals der kühlenden Quelle entlang, Wolken von Weihrauch. Immer noch rinnt das Wasser, von Zweigen beschattet, zum Garten hinab und tränkt mir die Rosen der Laube, wo ich voll Seligkeit, während sie lautlos entblättern, Kypris erwarte..."

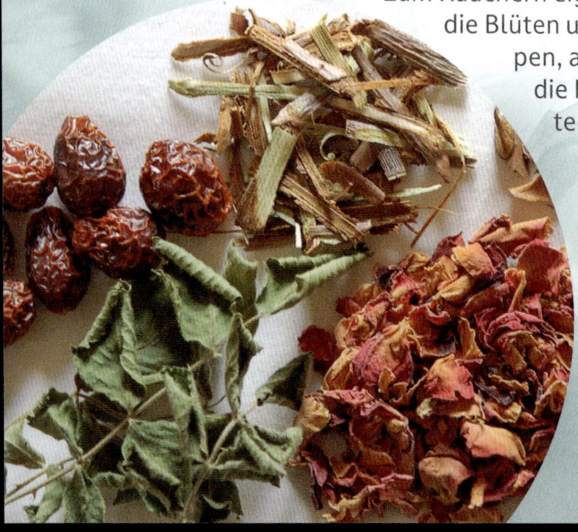

Zum Räuchern eignen sich die Blüten und Knospen, aber auch die Hagebutten und die Blätter, die Dornen und die Rinde.

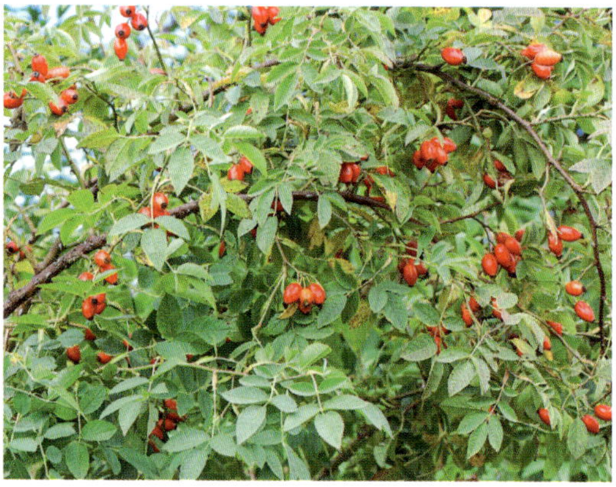

Blätter und Früchte der Rose

Im Gegensatz dazu reimt ein Kinderlied: „Ein Männlein steht im Walde, ganz still und stumm. Es hat vor lauter Purpur ein Mäntlein um. Sag wer mag das Männlein sein, das das steht im Wald allein, mit dem purpurrotem Mäntelein." Mit der Heckenrose betreten wir eine unerschöpfliche Vorstellungswelt, in der immer wieder die Extreme von Zeit und Ewigkeit, Leben und Tod in Liebe vereint werden können. Sie ist auf der ganzen Nordhalbkugel heimisch und wird heute noch als Grundlage für Veredelungen genommen. In den USA, in Oregon hat man eine 40 Millionen Jahre alte fossile Rose gefunden! Sie wächst bis in 1.600 m Seehöhe und wird teils über drei Meter hoch. Als Tiefwurzler kommt sie gut über Trockenphasen hinweg und kann ein Alter von 300 Jahren erreichen.

Rauch

Verwendete Pflanzenteile: Rosenblüten und -knospen, Hagebutten, ergänzend Blätter, für magische Rituale auch Dornen und Rinde.

Beste Sammel- und Erntezeit: Die Rosenblüten im Juni mit etwa 2 cm Stiel und die Hagebutten, ohne Stiel, im Herbst. Die Blätter, sowie Rinde und Dornen ganzjährig.

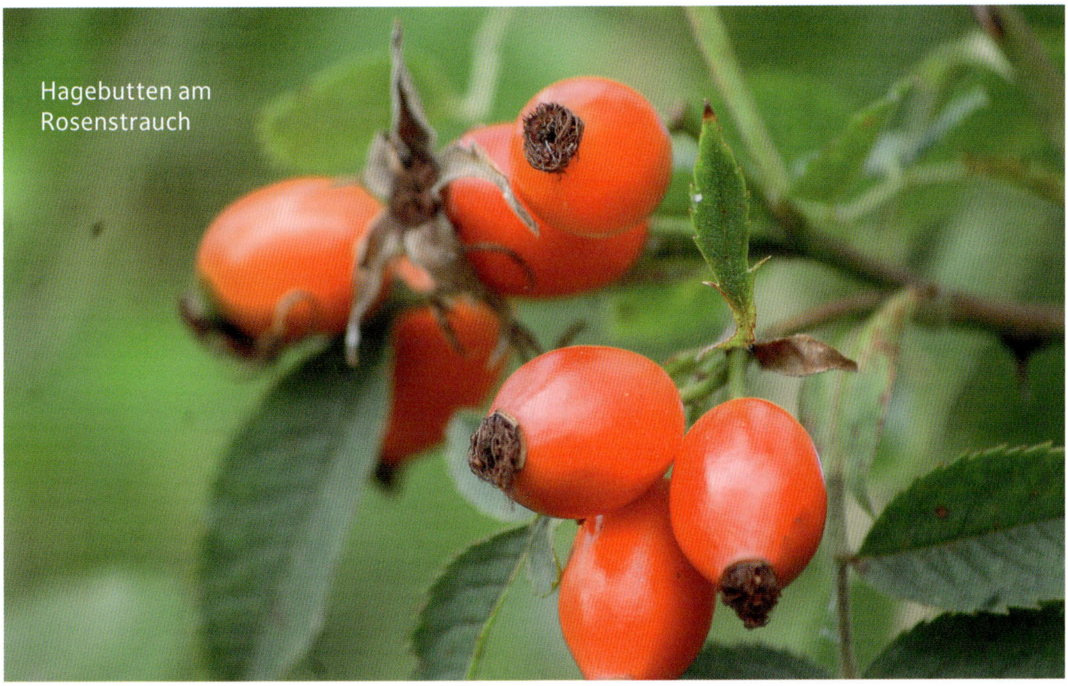
Hagebutten am Rosenstrauch

Wirkung, Wahrnehmung: Stärkung der Körper-Geist-Seele-Einheit und der inneren Zufriedenheit. Generell zur geistig/seelischen Entgiftung und Energetisierung.

Rosenblüten: Der Duft von Rosenblüten findet sich kaum im Rauch. Was bleibt, ist die Wahrnehmung, dass durch das Verräuchern von Rosenblüten der innere Frieden gestärkt und das Loslassen negativer Gefühle wie Neid, Missgunst, Eifersucht möglich wird. Wirkt stimmungsaufhellend, aufrichtend und ausgleichend; verhilft zu neuer Lebenslust, steigert den Lebenshunger und verbreitet eine lebensbejahende Fröhlichkeit. Neues kann in Liebe aufblühen! Öffnet das Herz für Annäherung und Verzeihung; auch für Versöhnung mit sich selbst! Man wird geneigter mit belastendem Alten in Frieden abzuschließen.

Hagebutten: Der Rauch der gemahlenen Hagebutten ist sanft reinigend und verbreitet eine versöhnliche und entspannte Atmosphäre; zieht Glück ins Haus; positive Kräfte und Gedanken können sich durchsetzen. Unterstützt die Liebe und das gegenseitige Verstehen; aber auch das Abschiednehmen in Güte. Nimmt das Brennen von der Seele, das den Prozess des Nicht-Loslassen-Wollens oder -Könnens so schmerzhaft macht. Am Ende von Beziehungen, am Ende des Lebens steht das fünffache Loslassen in Liebe. Und dabei ist der Hagebuttenrauch ein wichtiger Taktgeber!

Magisches zum Rauch: Die Heckenrose soll mit ihren Dornen vor Verzauberung schützen, aber im Rauch zusammen mit anderen Räucherstoffen zauberlösende Kräfte freisetzen: Dazu werden Dornen, Holz und Rinde zerkleinert und mit Traubenkirschenholz, Wermut und Eberraute sowie einem Harz vermischt und rituell verräuchert. Die Vorstellung von der Undurchdringlichkeit der Heckenrose macht hier den Abwehrzauber aus.

Schwerpunkt, Anwendungen, Rezepte: Für einen ausgleichenden und beruhigenden Rosenrauch mischt man Hagebutten, Rosenblüten, Felsenbirne und Fenchelblüten. Wie ein sanfter Engelsflügel berührt uns eine Räuchermischung aus Rosenblüten, Lavendel, Mädesüß und Wald-Geißbart. Harz hinzufügen.

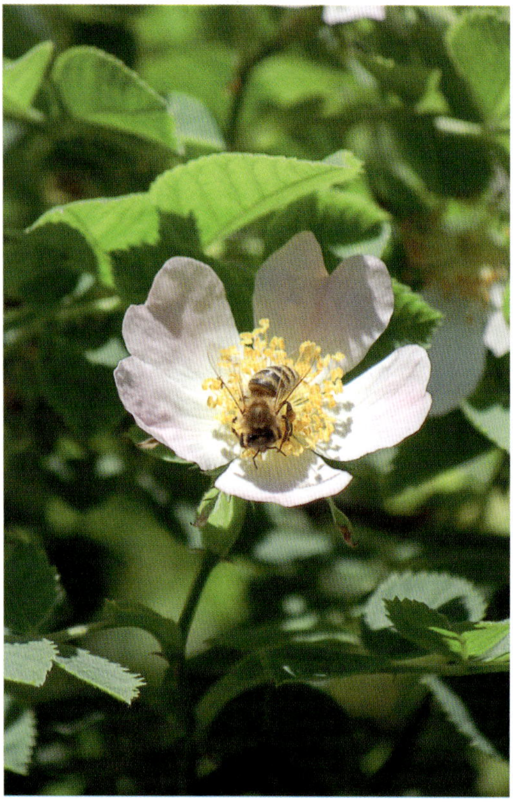

Rosenblüte

Mythologie und magische Praktiken

Seit nachgewiesenen 6.000 Jahren beschäftigt sich die Menschheit mit Rosenmagie: in Form von Bindezaubern, um einen geliebten Menschen an sich zu binden; in Form von Rosenorakeln, um die Zukunft in der Liebe vorherzusagen; in Form von Abwehrritualen, um nicht verzaubert oder in der Walpurgisnacht verführt zu werden; in Form von Märchen wie dem Dornröschen, wo die Rosenhecke zu blühen beginnt, als endlich der richtige Prinz kommt. Für derartige magische Zwecke soll die Blume des Liebeszaubers immer freitags, am Tag der Venus, mit einem Kupferwerkzeug geschnitten werden. Wie Weißdornzweige wurden auch Rosenzweige für den Milch- und Stallzauber verwendet.

Die ersten Abbildungen von Rosen finden sich 2800 v. Chr. auf sumerischen Tontafeln sowie ab etwa 2000 v. Chr. in der minoischen Kultur auf Kreta. Griechen und Römer weihten die Rose ihrer jeweiligen Liebesgöttin Aphrodite und Venus. Bei den Römern waren die Rosen einerseits Sinnbild für Laster, Trinkgelage und sexuelle Ausschweifungen, spielten aber auch im Totenkult eine zentrale Rolle: Zwischen 11. Mai und 15. Juli begingen die Römer ein Totenfest, die „dies rosae" (Rosentage). Dabei wurden Rosenblüten verschwenderisch auf die Gräber der Verstorbenen gestreut und auch den Hausgöttern, den Manen, geopfert.

Dieser Bezug zum Tod findet sich auch in den keltischen und germanischen Rosengärten. Gemeint sind damit Todesfelder, Orte, an denen blutige Kämpfe stattgefunden haben. Im Mittelalter bezeichnete man Schlachtfelder als Rosengärten, wo viele ihr Leben lassen mussten und die Erde vom Blut der Sterbenden durchtränkt ist. Diese Pflanze spielt auch eine zentrale Rolle in einem mittelhochdeutschen Gedicht rund um die Rosengärten des Zwergenkönigs Laurin, die unter den Trümmern der Burg Hauenstein bei Meran liegen sollen.

In vorchristlicher Zeit ist die Rose der großen Göttin geweiht, die den ewigen Kreislauf alles Lebendigen repräsentiert und die Menschen bei wichtigen Übergängen im Leben begleitet und schützt: Geburt, Hochzeit und Tod.

Nach anfänglicher Zurückhaltung, wohl wegen des römischen Rosen-Hypes hat sich die christliche Mystik später mit voller Wucht der Rosensymbolik bemächtigt. Ab dem Hochmittelalter wird sie Maria zugeordnet und gilt als Symbol für die irdische Vergänglichkeit und die Unsterblichkeit der Seele. In einem alten Marienlied heißt es: „... Maria du zarte, du bist ein Rosengarte, den Gott selber gezieret hat, mit dem der von dir geboren ward ..."

In mehreren Heiligenlegenden wird von Rosenwundern berichtet: so bei der Hl. Dorothea, der Hl. Elisabeth von Thüringen und dem Hl. Dominikus. Der einzige englische Papst Hadrian IV. (1100–1159) ließ in Anlehnung an eine römische Sitte, als Zeichen der absoluten Verschwiegenheit weiße Rosenmotive an den Beichtstühlen anbringen. Was „sub rosas" (unter den Rosen) gesagt wurde, durfte nicht nach draußen dringen.

Luzifer wollte einst über den Rosenstrauch wieder zurück in den Himmel schleichen, doch Gott-Vater verhinderte das, indem er der Rose Dornen verlieh!

Die riesigen Rosettenfenster der gotischen Dome bezeugen ab der Mitte des 12. Jahrhunderts die phänomenale europäische Baukunst jener Zeit. Da sie jeweils im Westwerk eingelassen sind, erfüllen sie aber auch eine wichtige Abwehrfunktion gegen Dämonen und böse Geister: Man war überzeugt, dass die Verderbnis, alles Unheil und die ewige Finsternis aus dem Westen kommen, von dort, wo die Sonne untergeht und wo auf ewig die bedrohliche Nacht herrscht.

Im späten 15. Jahrhundert brachte der Dominikaner Alain de la Roche (1428–1475), der sich als Verlobter Mariens bezeichnete, die Gebetsform des Rosenkranzes in die christliche Welt. Und schließlich wurde die Rose, mit folgendem Spruch auch zu Martin Luthers (1483–1546) Wappenblume: „Ein Christenherz auf Rosen geht, wenn´s mitten unterm Kreuze steht." Die Lutherrose war im 17. Jahrhundert auch symbolgebend für den Rosenkreuzer Orden.

Verwendung – gestern und heute

Um das Jahr 800 erließ Kaiser Karl der Große (747–814) einen Bewirtschaftungskodex für alle Höfe und Königshöfe seines Reiches, das sogenannte „Capitulare de villis vel curtis imperii". Im letzten Kapitel findet sich eine Pflanzenliste von 73 Kräutern und Gemüsesorten sowie 16 fruchttragenden Bäumen und Sträuchern. An der zweiten Stelle der Pflanzenliste sind Rosen zum Anbau im königlichen Pfalzgarten vorgesehen, als Symbolpflanze seiner königlichen Macht und Wehrhaftigkeit. Durch ihre Platzierung am Beginn der Liste verbindet die Rose, die

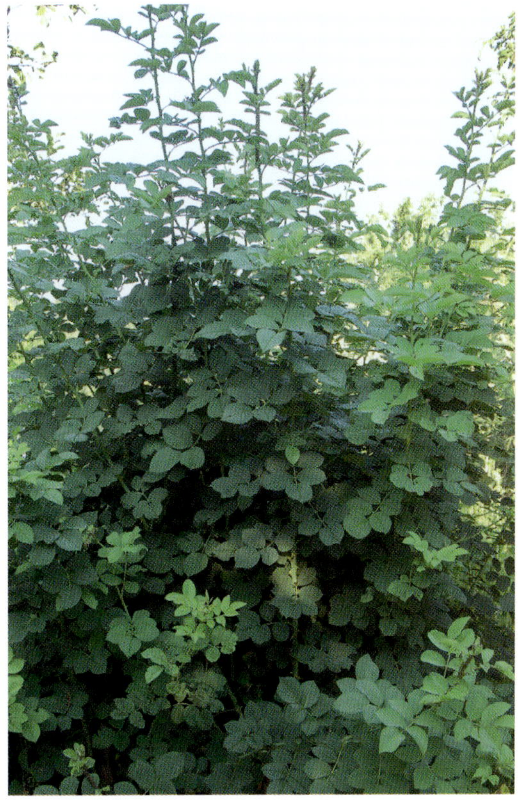

Rosenstrauch

auch als alte römische Kaiserpflanze gegolten hatte, den Glanz der Vergangenheit mit dem gegenwärtigen Ruhm des Kaisers. So huldigt der geschichtlich kundige Schreiber-Mönch seinem weltlichen Herrn.

Die Bachblüte Nr. 37 „wild rose" – Hundsrose – steht für das Überwinden innerer Teilnahmslosigkeit und führt hin zu neuer Lebenslust.

Rosenblüten waren in der Antike allgemein gebräuchliches Heilmittel gegen Kopfschmerzen und Epilepsie. Die Hagebutten dienen mit ihrem hohen Gehalt an Vitamin C zur Vorbeugung in Grippezeiten. Eine dänische Forschergruppe hat im Jahr 2003 den thermolabilen, fettlöslichen Inhaltsstoff Galaktolipid im Hagebuttenpulver entdeckt, der hilfreich bei Gelenksproblemen sein soll und weiter beforscht wird.

Roter Holunder

Lat. Name: *Sambucus racemosa*
Pflanzenfamilie: Moschuskrautgewächse

Als ich vor Jahren voller Freude einen roten Holunder im Kräutergarten ansetzte, war er wenige Wochen später komplett niedergefegt, d. h. das Wild rieb sich daran. In unmittelbarer Nähe standen andere, ebenso frisch angesetzte Sträucher. Sie alle waren unversehrt. Nur der rote Holunder schien es dem Rotwild wert zu sein, sich vom doch einigermaßen weit entfernten Wald aus auf den Weg zu machen, um in den Genuss des Rindenduftes zu kommen. Aus den zu Boden gedrückten dünnen Ästen trieb der kleine Strauch tapfer wieder aus. Mit dem zwischenzeitig errichteten Zaun, gelang es uns, ihn einige Jahre zu schützen. Doch er kam nicht recht voran, war bald brüchig und schien getrieben von einem starken Erneuerungs- und Veränderungswillen. So ging es etwa 15 Jahre, in denen er unterschiedlich präsent war, bis er nach einem schneereichen Winter komplett verschwand. Dann ein zarter Neubeginn, augenblicklich gefolgt von einer neuerlichen Verfegung – trotz Zaunes und obwohl er nur eine eher kümmerliche Rute in die Höhe gestreckt hatte. Der rote Holunder ist ein zurückhaltendes, sehr filigranes und eher scheues Gewächs. Seine roten Beeren sind bereits mitten im Sommer reif. Der Strauch wird bis zu drei Meter hoch und ist nach etwa zehn Jahren so brüchig, dass er selbst geringe Schneelasten im Winter nicht mehr halten kann. Ab einem Alter von fünf bis sechs Jahren ist jährlich eine steigende Erneuerung durch neue Wurzelaustriebe zu beobachten.

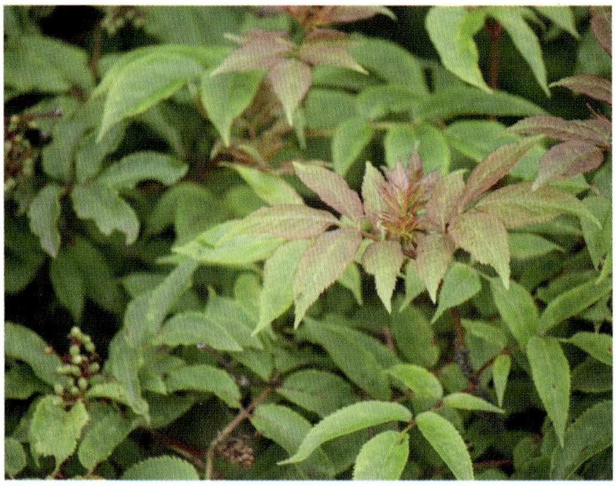

Blätter des Roten Holunders

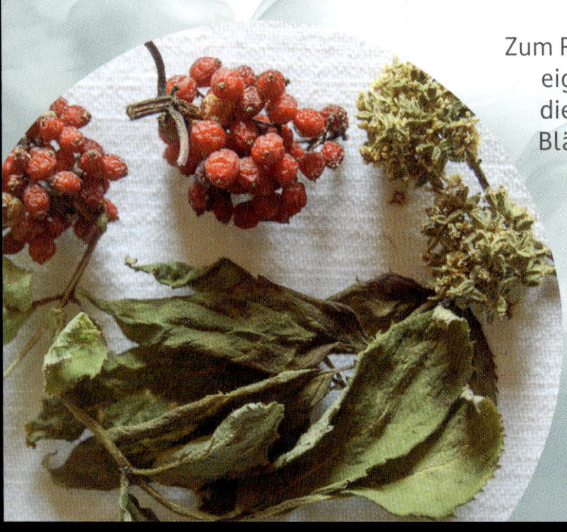

Zum Räuchern eignen sich die Beeren, Blätter und Blüten.

Rauch

Verwendete Pflanzenteile: Blüten, Blätter, Beeren.

Beste Sammel- und Erntezeit: Die Blüten im Frühling; zur gleichen Zeit können die frühen, eher rötlich gefärbten Blätter gesammelt werden; später ändern die Blätter ihre Farbe in grün. Auch in diesem Stadium können sie zum Räuchern genommen werden. Die Beeren im Sommer.

Wirkung, Wahrnehmung: Sehr angenehmer, ausgleichender Duft; nach einem hektischen Tag kann man in diesem Rauch gut abschalten. Die Hektik des Tages fällt ab, Ängste beruhigen sich, unruhige Gedanken können sich auflösen, eine wohlige Schwere zieht ein.

Schwerpunkt, Anwendungen, Rezepte: Macht leicht müde, also eher für Abendräucherun-

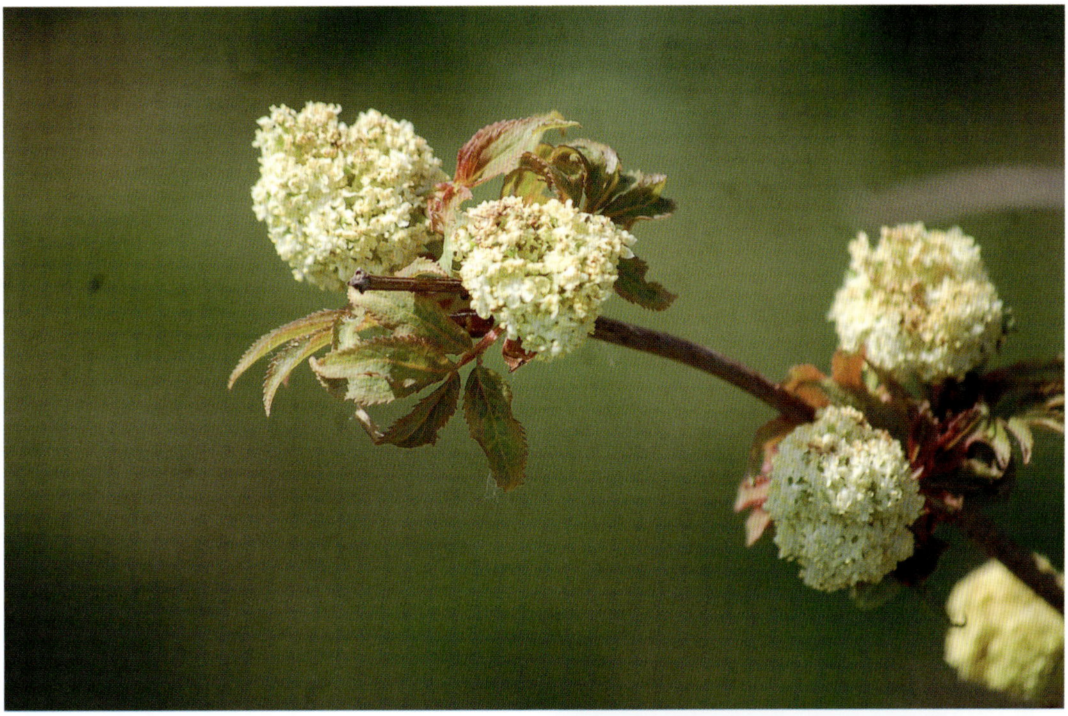
Blüten des Roten Holunders

gen zu verwenden. Passt zu Gelbem Salbei und Waldgeißbart in einer wunderbar ausgleichenden Räucherung kombiniert mit Harz.

Verwendung – gestern und heute

Als Erster der „Kreuttermeister" des frühen 16. Jahrhunderts beschreibt Hieronymus Bock (1498–1554) den Berg-Holder in seinem „Kreuterbuch". Er hat beobachtet, dass das Rot-Wild die Blätter des roten Holler bevorzugt frisst und dass die Blätter auch Medizin in der Schweinezucht sein können. Er berichtet, dass zwei von drei Kindern, die vielleicht aus Hunger zu viel Beeren roh gegessen hätten, verstorben seien. In bester wissenschaftlicher Tradition schließt er höchst ehrenhaft: „... die Kraft und roten Beeren des Wald-Holders habe ich noch nicht versucht noch wahrgenommen."

In der heimischen Volksheilkunde wurde früher aus den Beeren des roten Berg-Holunders stundenlang ein roter Fiebersaft ausgekocht.

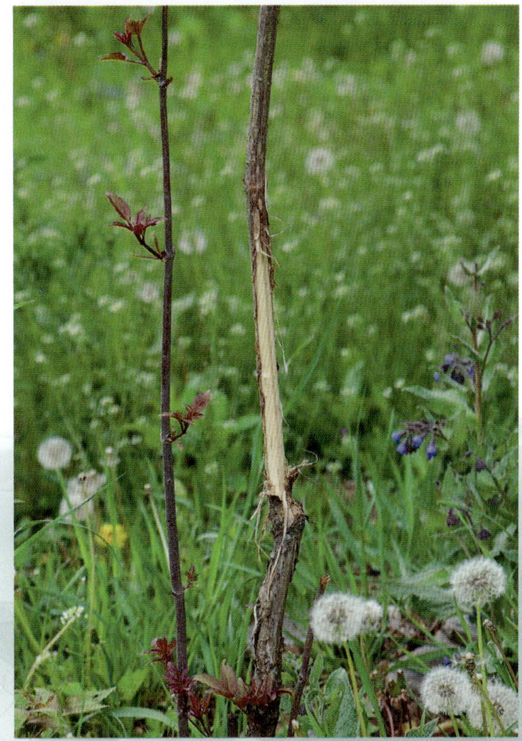
Wildschaden durch Fegen

Sanddorn

Lat. Name: *Hippophae rhamnoides*
Pflanzenfamilie: Ölweidengewächse

Der Sanddorn ist zweihäusig, das heißt es gibt männliche Sträucher, die die weiblichen befruchten und weibliche Sträucher, die die Beeren tragen. Dabei liegt Distanz zu halten wohl in seiner Natur: vor einigen Jahren hat ein fürchterlicher Wintersturm meinen männlichen Sanddorn beinahe umgeweht. Zumindest wurde er so weit entwurzelt, dass der obere Wurzelstrang aus dem Boden ragte, was den Strauch in eine starke Schieflage, hin zum weiblichen Strauch, brachte. Die beiden waren sich so nahe gerückt, dass sich ihre Äste fast berührten. Im ersten Jahr änderte sich nicht viel, der weibliche Strauch trug zwar insgesamt weniger Frucht, was aber im natürlichen Rhythmus der Pflanze vorkommen kann. Im zweiten Jahr allerdings grünte jener Bereich des weiblichen Strauches nicht mehr, der die männlichen Zweige fast berührte. Die Äste blieben, ohne offensichtliche Verletzung, braun und abgestorben. Sie zog sich zurück, während er an dieser Stelle zwar weiter grünte, aber erstaunlicherweise nicht weiter an Längenwachstum zulegte.

Der Sanddorn, auch rote Schlehe oder Zitrone des Nordens genannt, wächst in unseren Breiten problemlos und fruchtet jedes Jahr zuverlässig. Dadurch, dass man ihn nach bzw. mit der Ernte stark zurückschneidet, breitet er sich über die Jahre auch nicht wesentlich aus, was in kleineren Gärten von Vorteil sein kann. Ein männlicher Sanddorn kann fünf weibliche Sträucher befruchten.

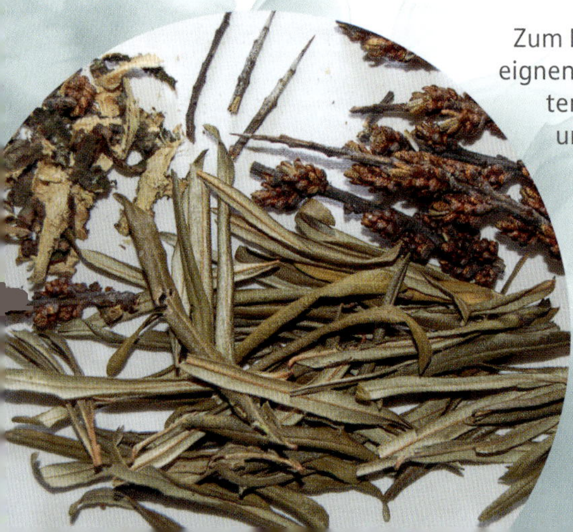

Zum Räuchern eignen sich Blüten, Blätter und Rinde.

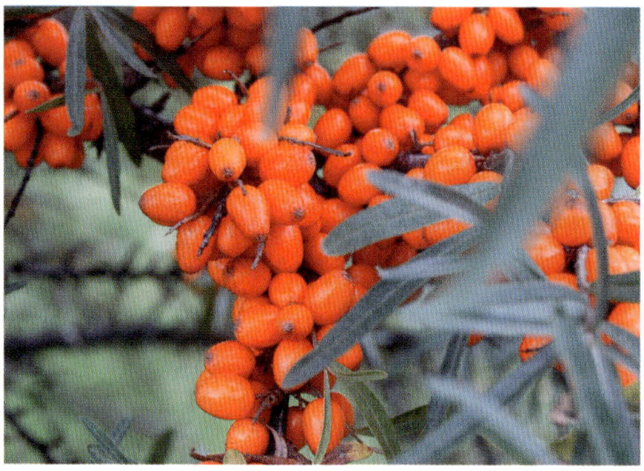

Früchte des Sanddorns

Seine ursprüngliche Heimat liegt in Nepal, von wo er durch eiszeitliche Verschiebungen westwärts gedrängt wurde. Er kann eine Höhe von bis zu drei Metern erreichen und wohl 40 Jahre alt werden.

Rauch

Verwendete Pflanzenteile: Blüten, Blätter, Rinde.

Beste Sammel- und Erntezeit: Die Blütenansätze im Frühling; die Blätter beider Geschlechter können das ganze Jahr über gesammelt werden. Am besten ist ein Gemisch von beiden Sträuchern. Rinde vom Rückschnitt nach der Ernte im Herbst.

Wirkung, Wahrnehmung: Angenehmer Rauch, bringt einen dazu, sich hinzusetzen und sich seinen Gedanken hinzugeben; sonnenhafte Wärme durchströmt einen. Es geht darum zu lernen, Abstand in vereinnahmende Beziehungen zu bringen; Konsequenzen für sich alleine ziehen und auch umsetzen; unterstützt den Versuch, sich starker Beeinflussung durch andere zu entziehen. Hebt die Selbstachtung; stärkt die persönliche, geistig-seelische Abwehrkraft; schützt vor negativen geistigen Bildern und Visionen.

Schwerpunkt, Anwendungen, Rezepte: Eignet sich besonders für Räucherungen, nach hektischen Tagen oder wenn man sich unter Druck gesetzt fühlt – zusammen mit Dost, Johanniskraut, Ebereschenfrüchten und vielleicht Rotem Holler (Harz nicht vergessen.)

Mythologie und magische Praktiken

Wegen der stark bedornten Zweige hielt man den Sanddorn bereits in der Antike für eine wichtige Pflanze zur Abwehr von negativen magischen Kräften. Man befestigte seine Zweige über Türen und Fenstern, um damit böse Geister und Dämonen aufzuhalten. Dort, wo es im europäischen Raum im Mittelalter Sanddornsträucher gab, wurden diese als rote Schlehe bezeichnet und ebenso wie diese zur Hexenabwehr über Türen genagelt.

Verwendung – gestern und heute

In frühen tibetischen Medizinwerken aus dem 8. Jahrhundert werden bereits über 300 Sanddorn-Anwendungen beschrieben. Im 13. Jahrhundert kam dann dieses Volksheilmittel des Ostens mit den mongolischen Reiterheeren nach Europa. Der Legende nach soll Dschingis Khan (1155–1227) seinen Pferden und Reitern Sanddorn verordnet haben – den einen zur Steigerung der Ausdauer und für ein schönes Fell, den anderen zum Durchhalten der wochenlangen Ritte.

Seine griechische Bezeichnung „hippophae rhamnoides“ bedeutet übersetzt „leuchtender Pferdedorn“, was wohl darauf zurückzuführen ist, dass man in der antiken Tiermedizin den Pferden Sanddornblätter ins Futter mischte, um ihr Fell glänzender zu machen und Parasiten abzuwehren.

In weiten Teilen Europas führte der Sanddorn lange Zeit ein Schattendasein. Nicht so im italienischen Friaul. Entlang des Flusses Tagliamento findet man wild wachsende Sanddornsträucher. Nach dem Zweiten Weltkrieg ernteten die Frauen mit Gabeln die orangen Früchte und verkauften die Säfte. Mit dem eingenommenen Geld bezahlten sie dann die Aussteuer ihrer Töchter. So wurde der Sanddorn als „Aussteuer-Beere“ bezeichnet.

Weiter nördlich wurde Mitte des 20. Jahrhunderts in der seinerzeitigen DDR der Anbau von Sanddorn zur Hebung der Volksgesundheit gefördert. Das erklärt auch den traditionellen Anbau und die Vermarktung von Sanddornprodukten auf der Insel Rügen. Heute betreibt China mit über einer Million Hektar weltweit die größten Anbauflächen.

Die Sanddornfrüchte enthalten unter anderem einen extrem hohen Vitamin C-Anteil, antioxidative Carotinoide sowie das in Pflanzen seltene Vitamin B12, das die gesunde Zellteilung fördert.

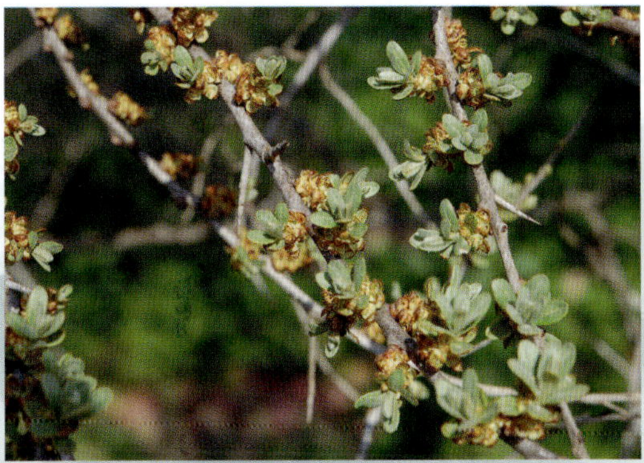

Sanddorn in Blüte

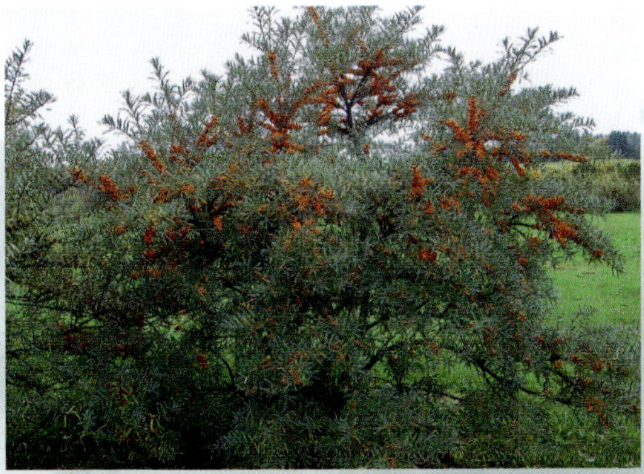

Fruchttragender Sanddorn

Schlehe

Lat. Name: *Prunus spinosa*
Pflanzenfamilie: Rosengewächse

Die Schlehe, auch Schwarzdorn genannt, ist seit Urzeiten ein menschlicher Kulturbegleiter. Funden von Schlehenkernen nach zu schließen, war sie bei den Menschen der Jungsteinzeit vor ca. 5.500 Jahren ein begehrtes Lebens- und Heilmittel. Gleichzeitig beschützte ihr undurchdringliches Gestrüpp die Siedlungen als pflanzliches Abwehrschild. Jedes Mal, wenn ich einen Schlehenkern in der Hand halte, frage ich mich, wie es die steinzeitlichen Menschen in ihren Pfahlbauten am Bodensee vor 3.300 Jahren geschafft haben können, diese kleinen harten Kerne zu durchbohren, um sie wohl als magisches Schutzamulett oder vielleicht nur als schmucke Halskette bei sich zu tragen.

Die Schlehenhecke in meinem Garten bietet zahlreichen Vögeln sicheren Schutz, darunter mittlerweile auch drei Paaren Neuntöter. Während der Brutzeit ist das Neuntöter-Männchen ein angriffslustiger Bewacher, der manchmal laut schimpfend direkt auf meinen Kopf zufliegt und mich zu vertreiben versucht, wenn ich dem Nest zu nahekomme. Die unerbittlichen Dornen der Schlehe helfen ihm bei der Vorratshaltung von zu viel gefangenen Insekten, die er dort aufspießt.

Die Schlehen verbreiten sich sehr gerne und wachsen, wenn man ihnen nicht Einhalt gebietet, gewaltig in die Breite. So können richtige Schlehenkolonien mit großer Erneuerungskraft entstehen, die weit über das Einzelalter von 40 Jahren hinaus für einen intakten, bis zu drei Meter hohen Bestand führen können.

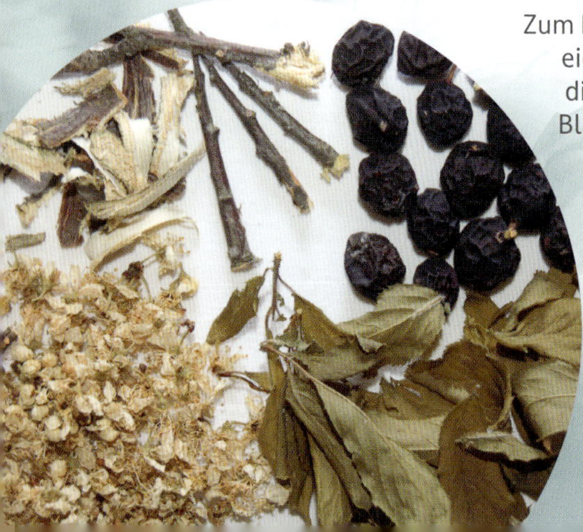

Zum Räuchern eignen sich die Blüten, Blätter und Früchte.

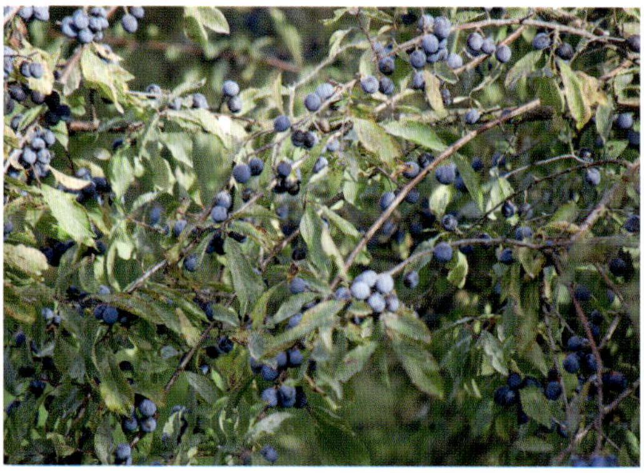

Früchte der Schlehe

Rauch

Verwendete Pflanzenteile: Blüten, Blätter, Früchte.

Beste Sammel- und Erntezeit: Die weißen Blüten im April, die schwarzen Früchte zu ihrer Zeit im November; die Blätter können das ganze Jahr über gesammelt werden.

Wirkung, Wahrnehmung: Vermittelt die Magie von Schwarz und Weiß und deren Überwindung; es geht um Auseinandersetzung und Wachstum und darum, Grenzen anzuerkennen. Hilfreich, wenn man in Bedrängnis geraten ist; abwehrstärkend und aufbauend für Phasen des Getrieben-Seins. Befähigt sich gedanklich zu formieren und für Übelwollende unberechenbarer zu werden. Stärkend in Angstphasen; treuer Begleiter in angstvollen Stunden; reicht dir eine schützende Hand. Die Pflanze der Percht wehrt böse Zauber ab und senkt unsere Angst vor Verlusten.

Magisches zum Rauch: Der Schlehenrauch schützt gegen Hexen, Unheil und alles Böse. In der Walpurgisnacht wurde mit Schlehe geräuchert, es wurden Schlehenkreuze angefertigt und diese in den Mist gesteckt.

Schwerpunkt, Anwendungen, Rezepte: Verwendung für Abwehr-Räucherungen wird durch

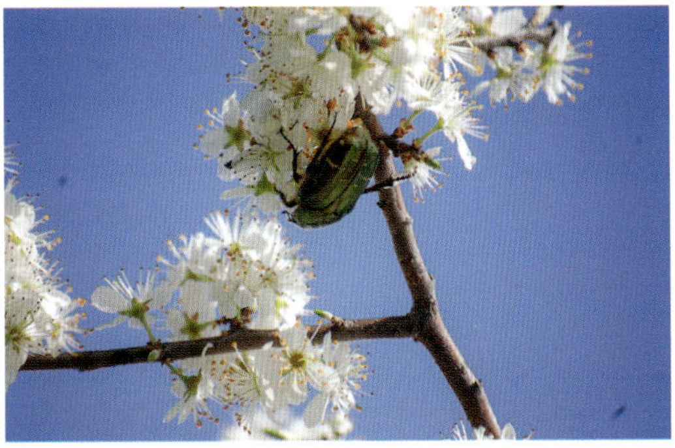
Blüten der Schlehe

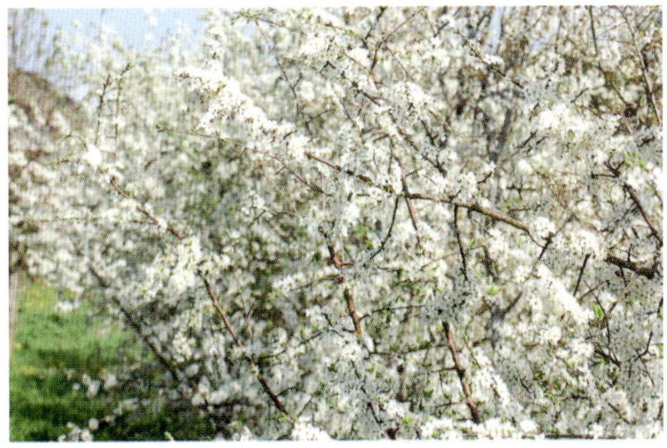
Blühende Schlehe

die Signatur nahegelegt: Räuchermischung mit Schlehenfrüchten, Wacholder, Beifuß und Weinraute. Diese Räucherung kann auch kritische Stunden in Projekten und anderen Unternehmungen überwinden helfen. Auch für Anrufungsräucherungen, wenn man von anderen Wesenheiten, den Saligen, Heiligen oder Engeln, Schutz und Hilfe erbittet.

Mythologie und magische Praktiken

Als magisches Sympathiemittel soll man die ersten drei Schlehenblüten im Frühling essen, um dadurch das ganze Jahr über vor Krankheiten, Fieber und Sodbrennen geschützt zu sein. Es gibt zahlreiche bäuerliche Wetterorakel mit der Schlehe: „So viel Tage die Schlehe vor Georgi (24. April) blüht, so viel Tage vor Jakobi (25. Juli) geht man zur Ernte" (Getreideernte). Oder: „Ist die Schlehe weiß wie Schnee, ist es Zeit, dass man die Gerste säe". Weiters vermeinte man, dass in einem Jahr mit besonders vielen Schlehenfrüchten ein strenger Winter drohe. Am 5. Februar, dem Tag der Hl. Agatha, holte man ein fingerlanges Zweigstück von der Schlehe, das sogenannte Agathen-Hölzl: Es sollte die Kraft haben, Wunden und Geschwülste zum Verschwinden zu bringen, wenn man mit ihm darüberstrich.

Kelten verehrten den Schwarzdorn wie den Weißdorn. Für sie war der Schwarzdorn die schwarze Göttin, die den Tod symbolisierte, der Weißdorn stand für die erneuernde Kraft der weißen Göttin.

Im christlichen Mittelalter trat immer mehr der dunkle Aspekt des Schwarzdorns in den Vordergrund. Schon die Dornen galten als giftig, da sie zu eiternden Wunden führen könnten. Man war überzeugt, dass mit Schwarzdornblüten böser Zauber bewirkt werden könne; mit Weißdornblüten hingegen könne dieser Zauber abgewehrt und gebrochen werden. Selbst das Essen von Schlehenfrüchten wurde Christen verboten und galt als sündhaft: Drei Schlehenfrüchte an einem Freitag gegessen hätten empfängnisverhütende oder gar abtreibende Wirkung.

Um gegen Hexen und Vampire und sonstige schreckliche Wesen der Nacht geschützt zu sein, nähte man sich dornenbewehrte Zweige der Schlehe in die Gewandsäume ein. Im 17. Jahrhundert wurden die Gräber von Wiedergängern (Untoten) geöffnet und man stieß ihnen mit einem Schwarzdornstecken ins Herz, um sie endgültig ins Jenseits zu verbannen.

Verwendung – gestern und heute

Hieronymus Bock (1498–1554) empfiehlt folgende Anwendung der Beeren: „Schlehen in Honig eingebeizt, sollen nit allein zum Schlaftrunk aufgetragen werden, sondern vielmehr denen helfen, die an der Ruhr oder Durchfall erkrankt sind. Zu diesen Gebrechen soll man auch einen wohlbereiteten Schlehenwein wohl bis in den August aufbewahren, wann die rote Ruhr am allermeisten regieret."

Heute werden die antioxidativen und immunsystemstimulierenden Inhaltsstoffe der Schlehenbeeren in Säften, Marmeladen und alkoholischen Auszügen genutzt.

Trauben-kirsche

Lat. Name: *Prunus padus*
Botanischer Name: Gewöhnliche Traubenkirsche
Pflanzenfamilie: Rosengewächse

Die Traubenkirsche sucht Störzonen an Hangabbrüchen, an Waldrändern und wuchert in Auwäldern. Im Verhältnis zu anderen typischen Wildsträuchern wächst sie sehr schnell und sehr hoch, bricht allerdings ziemlich leicht bei Wind- und Schneelasten, die für ihre pflanzlichen Nachbarn kein Problem darstellen. Der Haupttrieb der Traubenkirsche auf unserem Rain war so umgebrochen, dass seine Krone gerade den Boden streifte. Aus dieser Position heraus gelang es ihr im gleichen Jahr wieder auszutreiben und die Kronenäste, die nach dem Bruch ja nach unten gezeigt hatten, in so ein Wachstum zu versetzen, dass sie am Ende des Sommers wieder nach oben zeigten. Die improvisierte Rettung ihres erhobenen Hauptes hielt drei Jahre, bis der nächste schneereiche Winter sein Werk vollendete und sie endgültig zerbrach.

Mit voller Kraft startet die Traubenkirsche in den Frühling! Von weitem schon sieht man sie an den Waldrändern herausleuchten, wenn sie sich überschwänglich ihr weißes Blütenkleid anlegt. Beim Näherkommen lässt einen dann ihr wunderbarer Duft staunen. Nicht von ungefähr glaubten unsere Vorfahren, dass in ihrer frühen Blütenpracht schützende Wesenheiten wohnen.

Die Traubenkirsche wird schnell 15 m hoch und kann unter günstigen Bedingungen auch 50 Jahre alt werden.

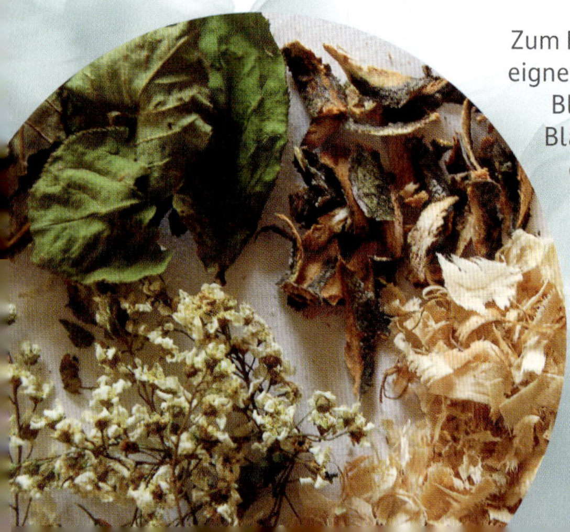

Zum Räuchern eignen sich die Blüten, die Blätter und das Holz.

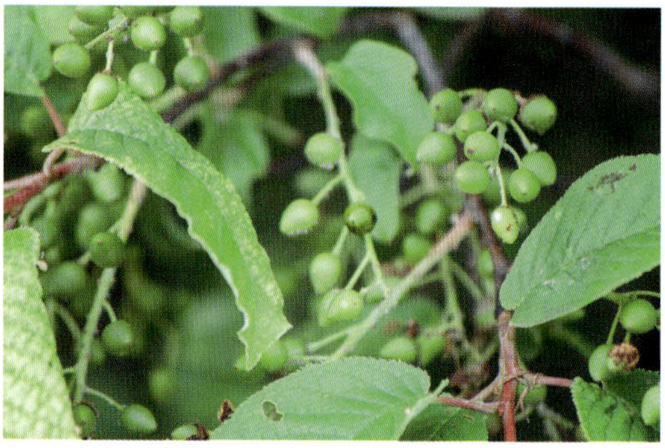

Früchte der Traubenkirsche

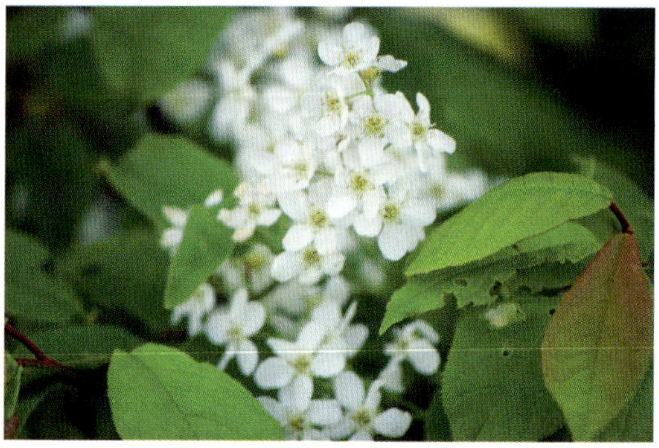

Blüten der Traubenkirsche

Rauch

Verwendete Pflanzenteile: Blüten, Blätter, Holz.

Beste Sammel- und Erntezeit: Die Blüten ab Ende März bis in den Mai; Blätter und Holz können das ganze Jahr über gesammelt werden.

Wirkung, Wahrnehmung: Sehr angenehmer Duft, der versöhnlich stimmt; man ist wunschlos glücklich und möchte nur immer weiter in diesem feinen Rauch bleiben. Große Schutzkraft; motiviert zu guten Lösungen; wer sich neuen Herausforderungen stellen muss, den unterstützt der Rauch von Blüten und Holz. Hilfreich, um aus Täuschungen und verzerrten Vorstel-

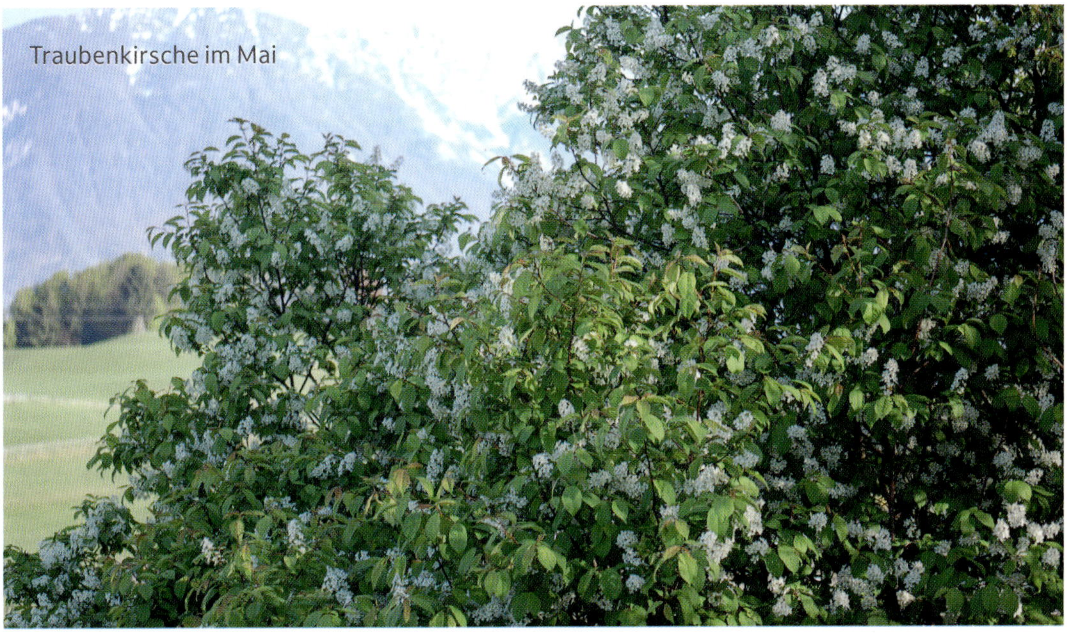
Traubenkirsche im Mai

lungen herauszufinden; man gewinnt langsam eine andere Perspektive und kann wieder neuen Mut fassen.

Magisches zum Rauch: Man glaubte, mit einer Traubenkirschen-Räucherung könne man Unholde und böse Menschen erkennen, da diese den Blütenrauch nicht aushalten würden.

Schwerpunkt, Anwendungen, Rezepte: Zur Unterstützung einer entspannten und friedvollen Atmosphäre räuchert man Traubenkirsche, Fenchel, Thymian und Rosenblüten mit Harz.

Mythologie und magische Praktiken

Mit der Traubenkirsche gibt es unterschiedliche magische Praktiken, die mit der Abwehr von Hexen und Dämonen in der Walpurgisnacht oder mit dem Erkennen von Hexen in der Karfreitagsmesse zu tun haben.

Männern wurde geraten, zur Hochzeit ein Zweigerl der Traubenkirsche in die Tasche zu stecken, um ja noch rechtzeitig zu erkennen, ob er wohl die richtige Frau vor den Altar führte. Würde es sich nämlich um eine Hexe handeln, dann würde das eingesteckte Taubenkirschenholz ihm ihr richtiges Wesen vor dem Altar enthüllen.

Man glaubte, ein Stück Traubenkirschenholz an die Stalltür genagelt oder gar ein Stallriegel aus diesem Holz, schütze vor jeder Verzauberung. So könne auch der viel gefürchtete Milchzauber bei Kühen nicht mehr wirken.

Man hielt das Holz auch für Verpflockungen geeignet, damit es quasi als magischer Türriegel, das Böse am Eintritt in das Haus hinderte: Dabei bohrte man ein Loch in den Türrahmen oder in die Türschwelle selbst und verschloss dieses, unter Hersagen verschiedener Zaubersprüche und Gebete, mit einem kleinen Holzkeil aus Traubenkirschenholz. In alten Kärntner Bauernhäusern wurden, nach dem gleichen Prinzip, auch Krankheiten verpflockt, wobei meist auch ein Symbol der Krankheit in das Loch gegeben wurde. Man findet noch heute die entsprechenden, mit einem anderen Holz verfüllten, runden Bohrlöcher in Türpfosten. Außerdem war man überzeugt, dass ein Kreuz, das aus diesem Holz gefertigt sei, die Macht habe, vor Verzauberung zu bewahren.

Verwendung – gestern und heute

Aus ihren angenehm duftenden Blüten lassen sich erfrischende Sirupe oder angenehm fruchtig schmeckende Blütenessige herstellen.

Vogel-kirsche

Lat. Name: *Prunus avium subsp. avium*
Pflanzenfamilie: Rosengewächse

Die Vogelkirsche oder Waldkirsche ist in Mitteleuropa heimisch und trägt ihre Bestimmung schon im Namen: Sie ernährt von der Biene bis zum Dachs viele Tiere und kommt mit ihrer Zähigkeit selbst neben Buchen und Eichen gut zurecht.

Vor zwei Jahrzehnten hat sich der Keimling einer Vogelkirsche an eine ungemütliche Wegecke vor meinem Fenster gesetzt. Nicht nur das abschüssige Terrain ist als Standort unbequem, direkt dahinter befindet sich auch noch eine Pferdeweide. Jahrelang haben die Pferde den aufkommenden Schössling benagt. Aber die Vogelkirsche hat mit unvorstellbarer Zähigkeit dagegen gehalten und ist einfach immer weiter gewachsen. Im Bereich der ärgsten Verbissstellen macht ihr Stamm heute eine leichte Ausweichbewegung. Ansonsten ist sie meine ganze Freude: Sie blüht leidenschaftlich im April, trägt reiche Frucht im Juli, erfreut mich den ganzen Herbst über mit ihrem sensationellen Farbspiel und liefert im November noch weiche Einstreu für viele Tiere am Hof.

Die Vogelkirsche wird 15 bis 20 m hoch und kann durch ihre Zähigkeit ein Alter von bis zu 120 Jahren erreichen.

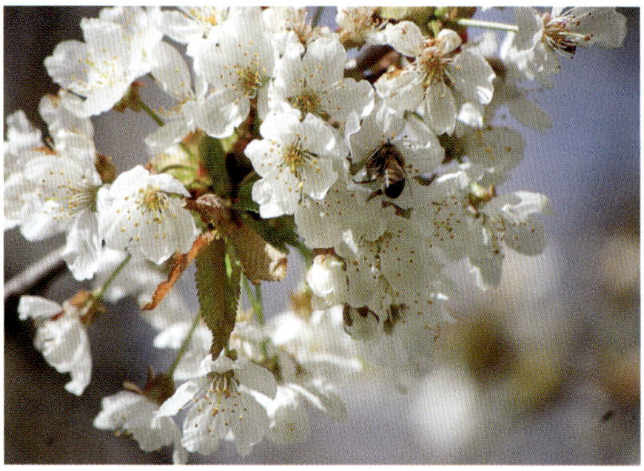

Blüte der Vogelkirsche

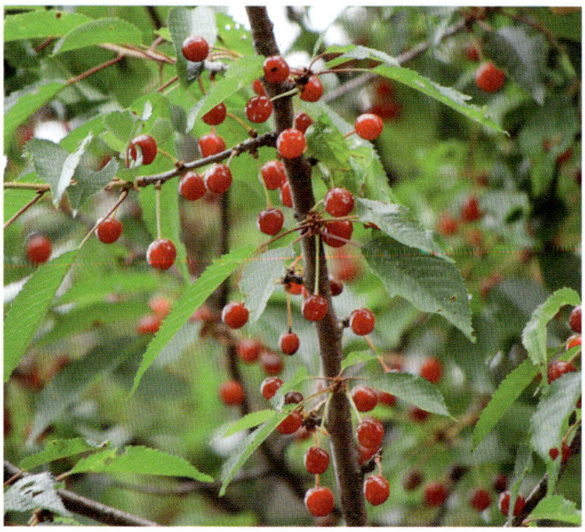

Früchte der Vogelkirsche

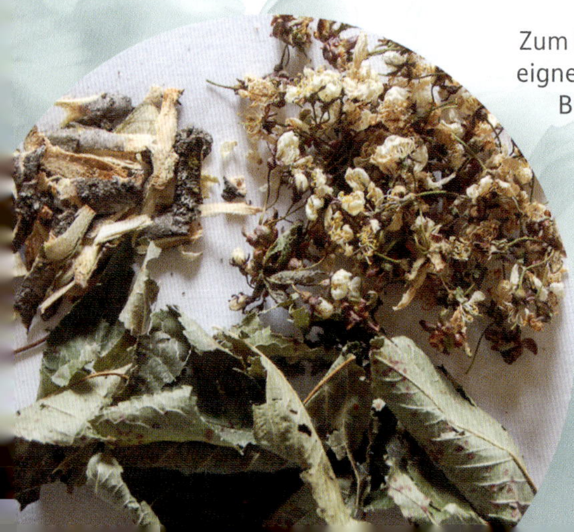

Zum Räuchern eignen sich die Blüten und Blätter sowie die Rinde.

Rauch

Verwendete Pflanzenteile: Blüten, Blätter, Rinde.

Beste Sammel- und Erntezeit: Die Blüten im April; Blätter und Rinde kann übers Jahr gesammelt werden.

Wirkung, Wahrnehmung: Für innere Ruhe und Stärke; wenn man im Leben aus der Bahn gewor-

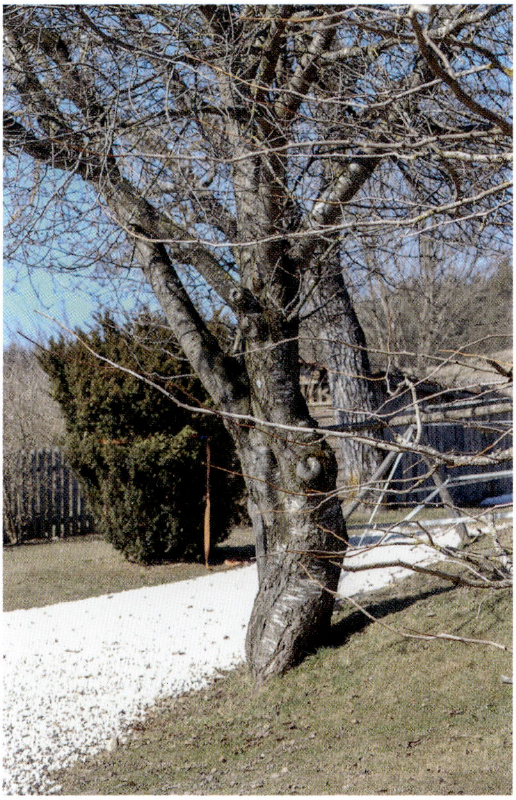
Stamm einer Vogelkirsche

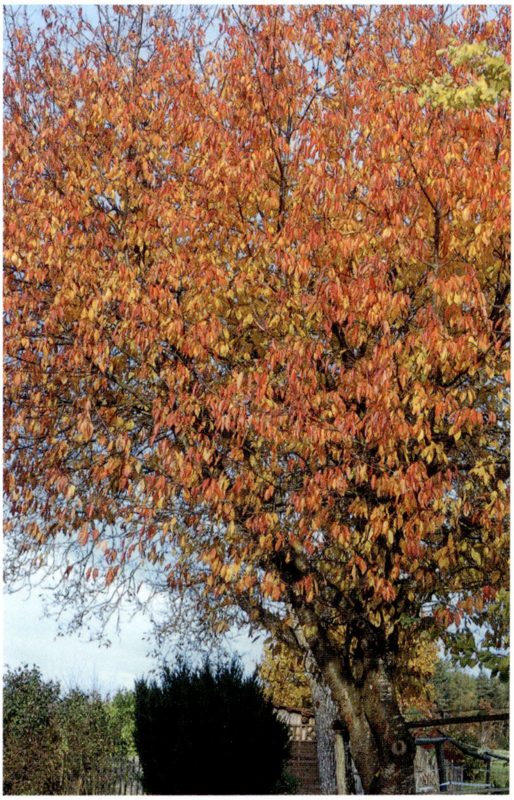
Vogelkirsche im Herbst

fen wird, kann dieser Rauch erden und beruhigen. Sorgt für seelischen Ausgleich; man fühlt sich getröstet, angenommen und umarmt. Ruhe und Gelassenheit werden vermittelt. Liebevolle Begegnungen werden unterstützt; wirkt positiv polend auch in Räumen, in denen viel Unruhe und auch negative Raumeinträge vorhanden sind.

Schwerpunkt, Anwendungen, Rezepte: Eine beruhigende Räuchermischung erhält man mit Vogelkirschenblüten, Apfelblüten und Kleinem Habichtskraut kombiniert mit Harz.

Mythologie und magische Praktiken

Die weißblühenden Bäume galten bei allen vorchristlichen Kulturen als Sitz von Frühlings- oder Fruchtbarkeitsgöttinnen. Die Vogelkirsche hat außerdem noch ein besonderes Blühverhalten: Innerhalb einer Woche hüllen tausende Blüten die meist noch kahlen Äste in strahlendes Weiß! So glaubten die Kelten, dass während dieser Zeit, Feen unter ihr tanzten.

Verwendung – gestern und heute

Die kleinen säuerlichen Kirschen wirken verdauungsfördernd und allgemein stärkend.

Walnuss

Lat. Name: *Juglans regia*
Pflanzenfamilie: Walnussgewächse

Der mächtige Vertreter Jupiters auf Erden ist gerne ein Einzelgänger und sorgt auch dafür, dass ihm kein anderer Baum zu nahe kommt. Plinius der Ältere (23–79) hielt fest, dass der Nussbaum andere Pflanzen zerstöre. Erst Matthiolus (1501–577) und dann auch Lonicerus (1528–1586) führen wortgleich aus: „Man sagt, dass eine solche Uneinigkeit unter dem Nussbaum und dem Eichbaum sei, dass er, neben einem Nussbaum gepflanzt, ganz verderbe". Aus solchen Beobachtungen ergeben sich über Jahrtausende hinweg symbolische Zuordnungen von Überlegenheit, Standhaftigkeit und Durchhaltevermögen.

Das Wesen des Walnussbaumes ist aber vielschichtiger. Er gehört zu den empfindsamsten und extrem vorsichtigen Hölzern, die im Gegensatz zum männlichen Äußeren schon einmal weibliche Botschaften in ihrem Inneren verborgen halten können, wie auf dem Foto vom Walnussholz zu sehen.

Im Frühjahr ist der Nussbaum der letzte, der es wagt seine Blätter sprießen zu lassen. Meistens umgeht er so noch die eine oder andere verspätete Frostnacht. Sollte ihn aber nach dem Austreiben doch noch ein Frost erwischen, gibt es in diesem Jahr keine Nussernte. Ständige Erschütterungen durch weidende Pferde bringen den sensiblen Baum so stark aus dem Rhythmus, dass er binnen weniger Jahre aufgibt.

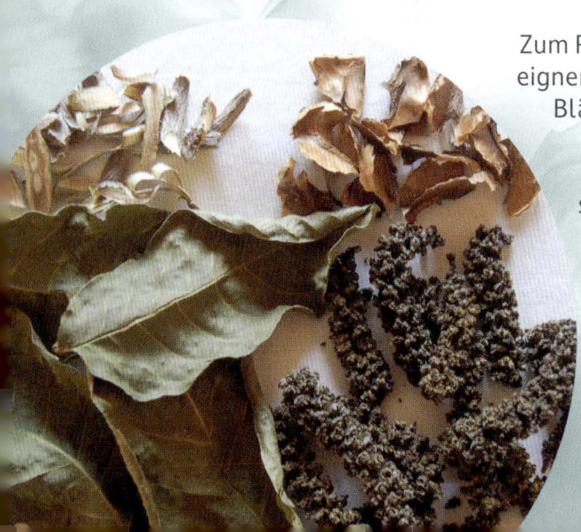

Zum Räuchern eignen sich die Blätter und Blütenkätzchen sowie die Rinde und Nusskämben.

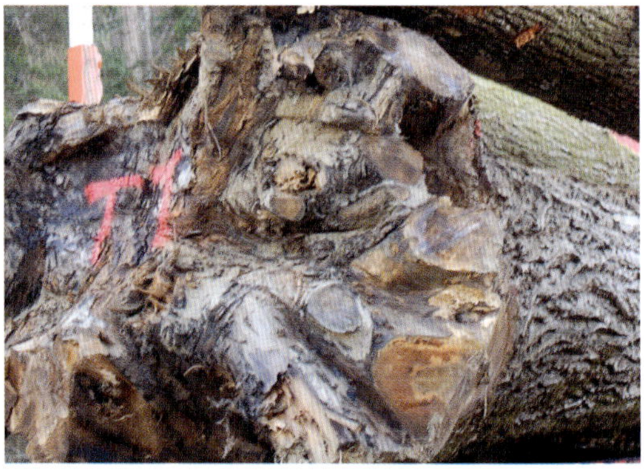

Geschlägerter Walnussbaum

Der Walnussbaum stammt ursprünglich aus dem Gebiet um das Schwarze Meer. Er wird bis zu 30 m hoch und kann, unter der Voraussetzung ungestörter Alleinherrscher an seinem Standort zu sein, ein Alter von bis zu 160 Jahren erreichen.

Rauch

Verwendete Pflanzenteile: Blätter, Blütenkätzchen, Rinde, Nusskämben.

Beste Sammel- und Erntezeit: Die Blüten im Frühling; einen Ast für die Rinde kann man das ganze Jahr über abschneiden; die Blätter sollen in der zweiten Jahreshälfte gesammelt werden; die Nusskämben (holzige Leisten zwischen den Nusshälften) holt man im Herbst aus den aufgeschlagenen Walnüssen, zerkleinert und trocknet sie.

Wirkung, Wahrnehmung: Der Rauch geht rasch in Resonanz zu unserer Feinfühligkeit; hilfreich für alle, die aus der Bahn zu fallen fürchten; bei Selbstzweifeln ebenso wie bei übertriebenem Perfektionsstreben. Konzentrationsfördernd, rhythmusgebend; spiegelt uns die richtigen Zeitpunkte im Leben. Der Rauch verbreitet ein großes Kraftfeld und schützt vor Energielosigkeit; hebt das Selbstvertrauen.

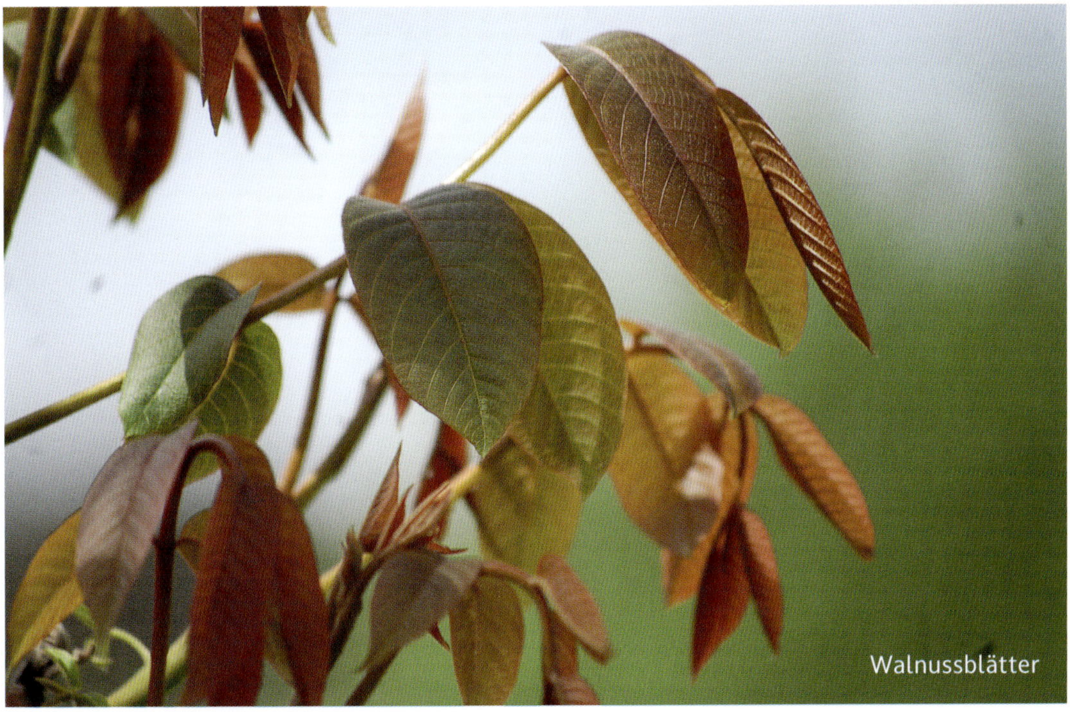
Walnussblätter

Magisches zum Rauch: Die feine Schwingung der Nussbaumblätter zieht Überspannungen an und erdet sie. Der Rauch soll Blitzeinschlag und Unwetter abwehren. Die getrockneten Nussbaumblätter wurden immer wieder gegen ansteckende Krankheiten verräuchert. So soll auch folgende Mischung vor der „pestilentzische Lufft" schützen: Verräuchern von Nusskernen oder Walnuss-Kammerwänden (Nusskämben) mit Wacholderbeeren und Weinraute.

Schwerpunkt, Anwendungen, Rezepte: Wichtiger Räucherstoff für schwierige Übergänge im Leben; neben Salbei, Eiche, Engelwurz, Eisenkraut. Zur Insektenabwehr hat sich eine Räuchermischung aus Nussbaumblättern mit Rainfarn und Harz als sehr wirkungsvoll herausgestellt.

Mythologie und magische Praktiken

Der Walnussbaum steht in Verbindung zum heidnischen Sonnwendkult, was sich schon früh im christlichen Johannisbrauchtum fortsetzt. So sind die jungen Nussblätter die äußeren Hüllblätter des „Sieben-Kräuter-Johannisbuschn", mit welchem man versuchte neidvolle Geister abzuwehren und gleichzeitig um Schutz in der Erntezeit zu bitten. Auszug aus meinem Buch „Kräuterbuschn" (2016): „Es galt sich vor Unwettern, Hagelschlag, Schädlingsplagen zu schützen und zu signalisieren, dass dieser Schutz im Einklang mit der Natur, ja, im Bewusstsein ihrer Übermacht, erbeten wurde." Zu Johanni (24. Juni) gepflückte Nüsse galten als heilkräftig!

Verwendung – gestern und heute

In zahlreichen mitteleuropäischen Pfahlbauten der Jungsteinzeit (ab ca. 11500 v. Chr.) wurden kleine Nüsse gefunden und belegen die Nutzung als frühes menschliches Nahrungsmittel. Auf dem Magdalensberg in Kärnten wurden schon etwas größere Nüsse gefunden, die aus der Latène-Zeit (um ca. 450 v. Chr.) stammen.

In der Antike wird der Walnussbaum überwiegend als Symbol der Fruchtbarkeit gesehen. Um 500 v. Chr. wurden bei Hochzeiten in Griechenland Walnüsse unter die Hochzeitsgäste gestreut.

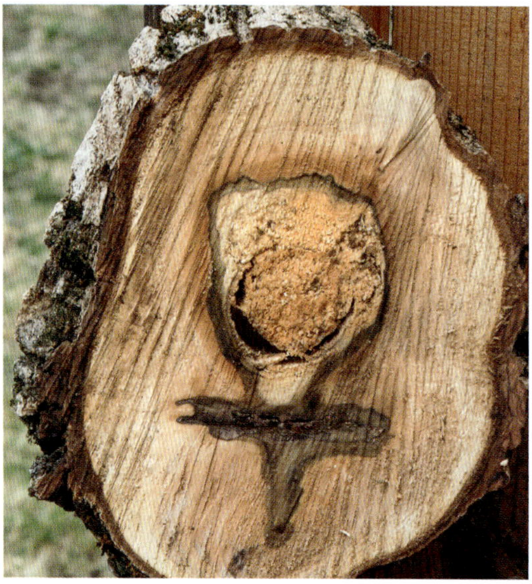

Verborgen im Walnussholz das Zeichen der Venus, der Weiblichkeit

Einen durchaus lustbetonten Zugang zum Walnussbaum zeigen uns auch die sinnenfrohen Römer. Sie nannten den Baum „jovi glans", Eichel des Jupiters! Von dem bedeutenden römischen Dichter Vergil (70–19 v. Chr.) ist der Spruch überliefert, der für einen Kinderwunsch steht: „sparge marite nuces"! (streue die Nüsse, Gatte). Übrigens wissen wir heute, dass Walnüsse für Männer fruchtbarkeitssteigernd wirken können, indem sie die Anzahl der Spermien erhöhen.

Karl der Große (747–814) schrieb in seinem „Capitulare de villis vel curtibus" (um ca. 800) unter den 16 genannten Bäumen an 15. Stelle „nucarios", also Walnussbäume zum Anbau auf seinen königlichen Gütern vor. Hingegen fiel auf der Piazza del Populo in Rom ein alter Walnussbaum in päpstliche Ungnade: Da sich hartnäckig der Glaube hielt, dass in seinen Ästen Geister hausten, sprach Papst Paschalis II. (Papst von 1099–1118) den Bann über den Baum, ließ ihn daraufhin fällen und an dieser Stelle eine Kirche erbauen.

In den darauffolgenden Jahrhunderten galt der Nussbaum immer öfter als unheilvoller Versammlungsort von Hexen und anderer Dämonen.

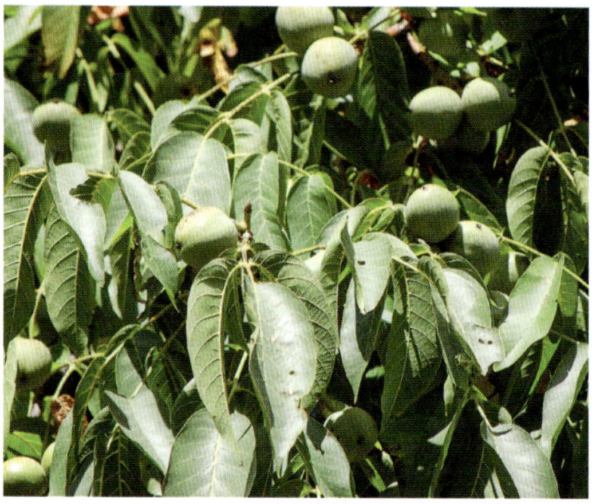

Reifende Walnüsse

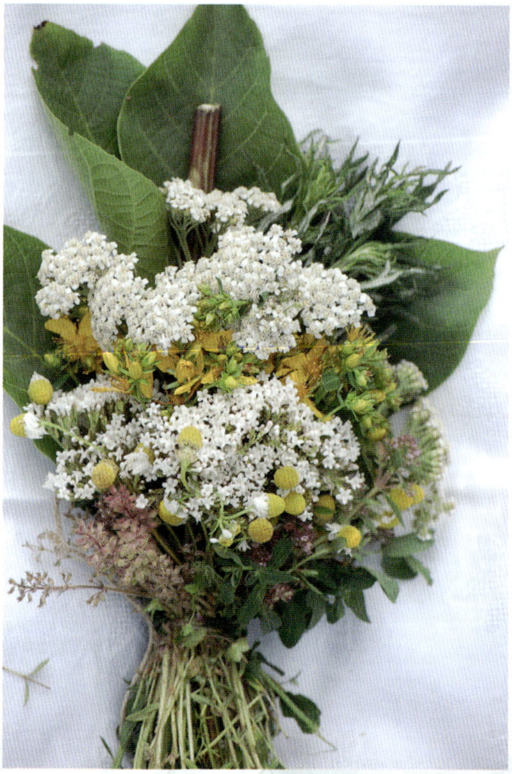

Der Sieben-Kräuter-Johannisbuschn besteht aus Walnussblättern, Beifuß, Schafgarbe, Johanniskraut, Baldrian, Kamille und Quendel.

Bachblüte Nr. 33 „walnut" – Walnuss – hilft die Entscheidungskraft bei Neuanfängen zu stärken und Beeinflussungen von außen hintan zu halten.

Weide

Lat. Name: *Salix sp.*
Pflanzenfamilie: Weidengewächse

In alten Kulturen wird die Weide als Symbol der Fruchtbarkeit und der Wiedergeburt in der Natur verehrt. Doch die Weide hat zwei Gesichter: ein helles, dem Leben zugewandtes und ein dunkles, dem irdischen Vergehen entsprechendes. Wie die Erle hat auch die Weide einen starken Bezug zum Wasser, ist aber insgesamt mehr dem Menschen zugewandt.

Von prähistorischer Zeit bis in unsere Tage sprechen Millionen von Weidenkörben für ihren kulturbildenden Beitrag. Bei den Weidenzweigen kommt aber auch gleich wieder eine dunkle Seite zum Vorschein: Die Züchtigung mit Weidenruten hat in der Menschheitsgeschichte schon für viel Schmerz und Ungemach gesorgt! Mit der Wachstumsgeschwindigkeit der Weide können andere Bäume kaum mithalten. Sie fügt sich nicht in waldähnliche Strukturen ein, sondern beansprucht Einzelplätze, die ihr viel Sonne und sehr viel Wasser bieten. Sie wird bis zu zehn Meter hoch, aber, als Tribut an ihr schnelles und intensives Leben, nur bis zu 40 Jahre alt.

Rauch

Verwendete Pflanzenteile: Weidenkätzchen, Blätter, Rinde.

Beste Sammel- und Erntezeit: Die Weidenkätzchen im Frühjahr. Es können sowohl die samtigen, weißen „Palmkatzerl“ als auch die schon aufgeblühten Kätzchen genommen werden;

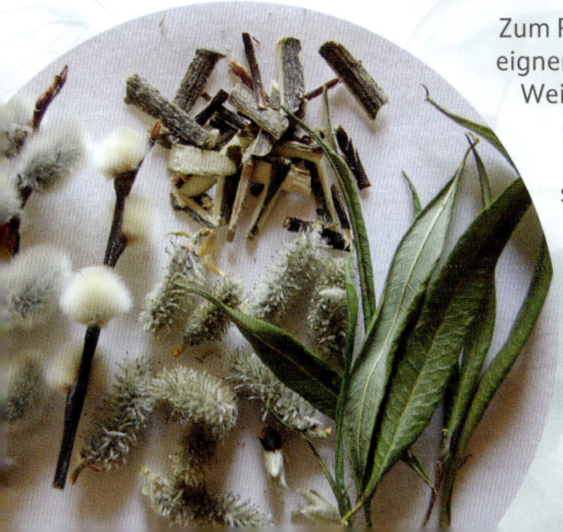

Zum Räuchern eignen sich die Weidenkätzchen und Blätter sowie die Rinde.

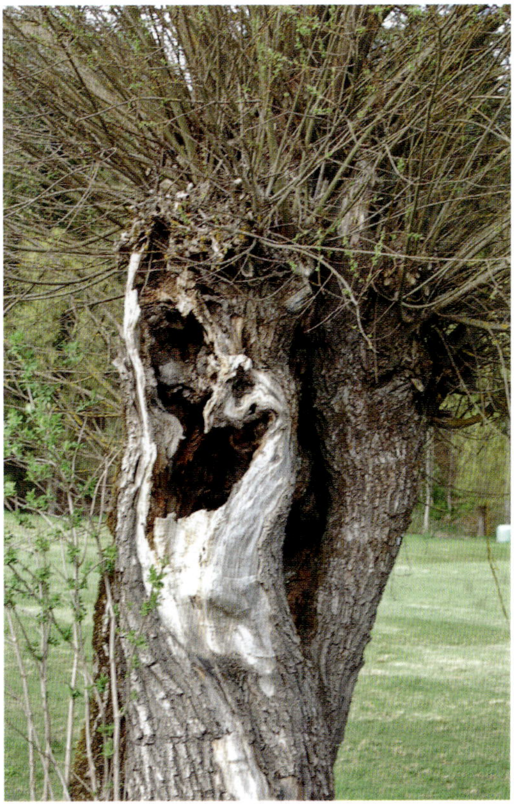

Weidenholz

Blätter und Rinde können das ganze Jahr über gesammelt werden.

Wirkung, Wahrnehmung: Die Weide spricht zu mir: „Im Wasser erkenne ich mich, der Mond beleuchtet die verwirrende Flut in meinem Inneren. Vergänglichkeit ist kein Maß für mich und meine Kinder. Wilde Lebenslust treibt mich heute an, lockt mich zur Sonne, aber morgen schon, morgen zieht mich der Nebel sanft ins vertraute Dunkel!“

Reinigende und gedanklich klärende Wirkung. Ihr Rauch steht symbolisch für Wandlungsfähigkeit und geht in Resonanz mit unserer Bereitschaft aufzubrechen, einen neuen Anfang unter widrigen Umständen zu wagen. Große

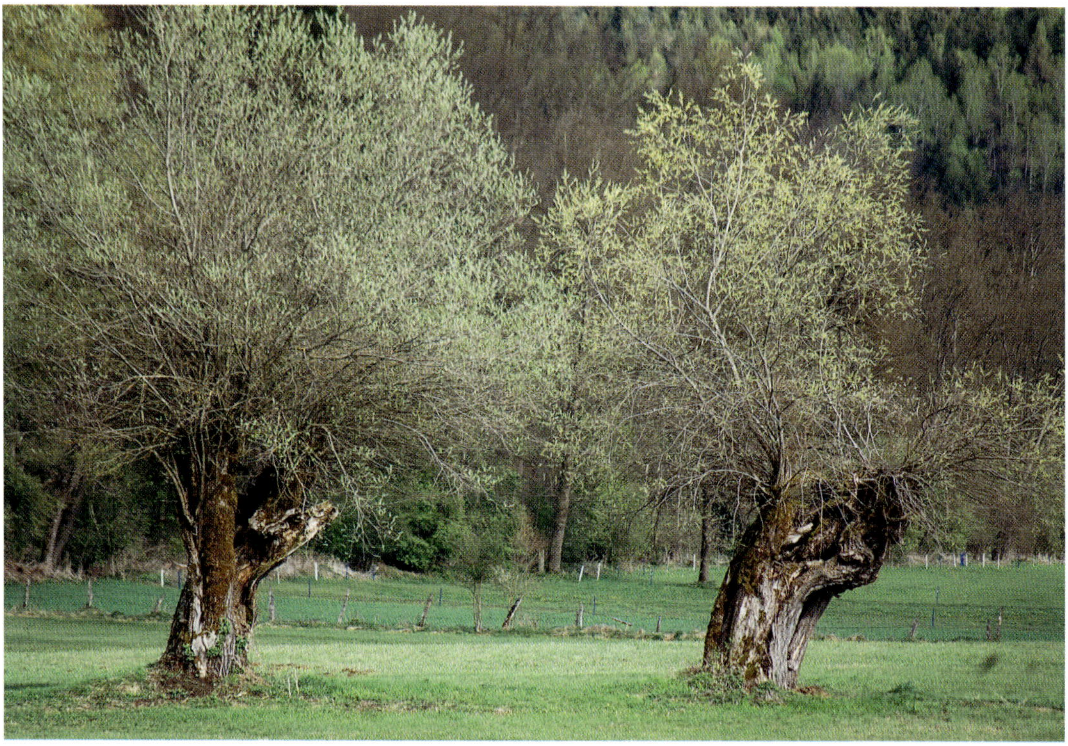

Kopfweiden bei Glanegg, Kärnten

Transformationskraft; es geht um Erneuerung und Lebenskraft; lehrt einen, sich zu biegen, um nicht zu brechen; mit Rückschlägen umgehen lernen. Fordert uns auf zur Beweglichkeit, um die eigenen starren Positionen zu überdenken! Verhindert mit ihrer Kraft ein zu frühes Aufgeben; Quelle neuer Kraft; Durchhalten, wenn nötig auch gegen den Strom.

Mit Weidenrauch kann man darüber nachdenken, dass sich in unserem Leben jederzeit alles ändern kann: Lädt uns ein, die uranischen, plötzlichen und schicksalhaften Veränderungen in unserem Leben anzunehmen und damit zurechtzukommen. Stark erdend und ausgleichend; aktiviert Selbstheilungskräfte; man hat das Gefühl, der Kopf sei wieder frei, man sei wieder Herr der eigenen Sinne.

Magisches zum Rauch: Ein Rauch mit Weide, Traubenkirsche, Baldrian und Wacholder solle einem, an bestimmten Tagen um Mitternacht geräuchert, Antworten eingeben, wer die Hexe mit ihren bösen Absichten sei.

Schwerpunkt, Anwendungen, Rezepte: Hilfreicher Rauch bei verschiedenen Lebensübergängen mit Holunder, Beifuß, Schlehe, Weißdorn, Efeu, Fichte als mögliche weitere Räucherzutaten.

Mythologie und magische Praktiken

In der antiken Mythologie wird das zwiespältige Wesen der Weide immer wieder thematisiert. Ganz prominent darf sie, als Symbol des ewigen Lebensstromes, über die Geburt der griechischen Göttereltern Zeus und Hera wachen.

Die Weide ist der heilige Baum der Demeter, der griechischen Göttin des Ackerbaus, der Fruchtbarkeit und des Wachstums. Manchmal erscheint aber auch deren Tochter Persephone in der Weide, die Göttin des Todes und der Wiedergeburt. Nach der Entführung ihrer Tochter durch Hades, den Gott der Unterwelt, hatte sich Demeter auf die Suche nach ihr begeben. Endlich verriet ihr Helios, der Sonnengott, ihren Aufenthalt und bestimmte, dass Persephone

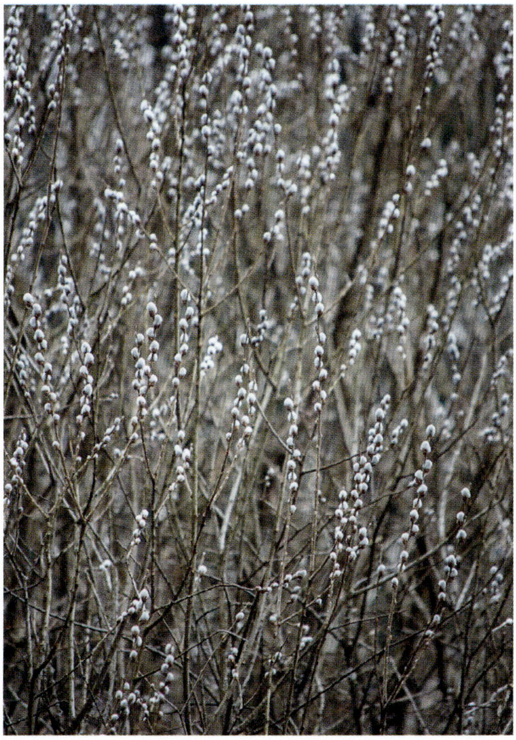

Blüten der Weide

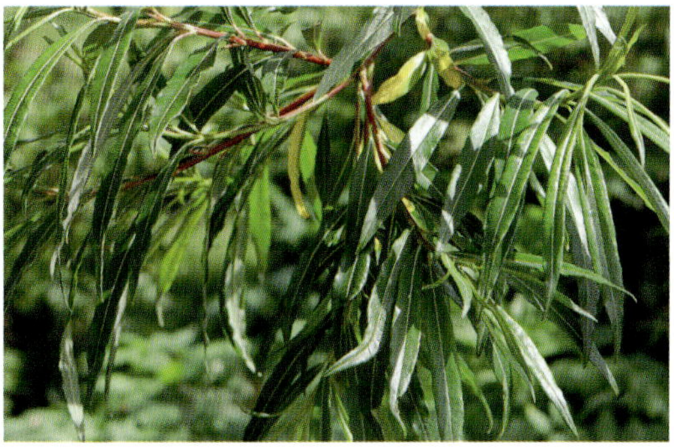

Weidenblätter

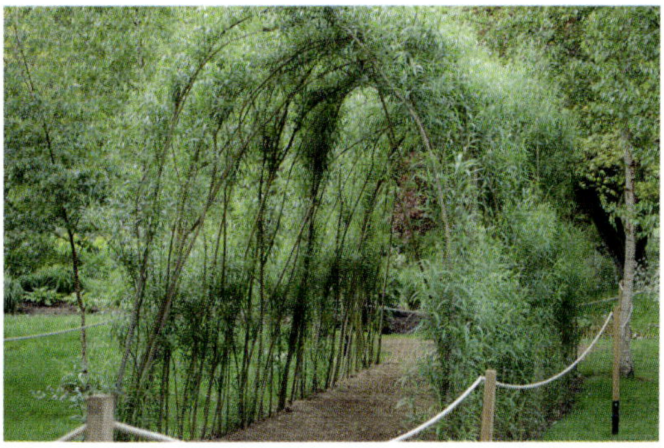

Weidendurchgang in Mozirje, Slowenien

selbst ihren zukünftigen Lebensraum wählen sollte. Da sich Persephone aber in der Zwischenzeit in Hades verliebt hatte, entschied sie sich dafür, die Hälfte des Jahres in der Unterwelt, bei ihrem Gatten zu leben und die andere Hälfte des Jahres bei ihrer Mutter Demeter.

Die keltische Kultur sah in der Weide ausschließlich einen heilenden Baum, der Krankheiten und Unheil in sich aufnehmen könne und so die Menschen beschütze. An den Weiden konnten Krankheiten abgestreift werden. Noch heute werden aus den Weidenzweigen des Palmbuschens kleine Kreuze gemacht und in die Felder und Fluren gesteckt, um für Fruchtbarkeit zu sorgen und Unheil, wie Hagelschlag, von ihnen abzuwenden.

Im christlichen Narrativ wurde die Weide zum Todesbaum für Selbstmörder, weil sich Judas in einer Weide erhängt haben soll.

Die Hexenangst Mitteleuropas führte auch zu folgender Vorstellung: Hexen und böse Geister würden als schöne Frauen in der hohlen Weidenstämmen verschwinden und als fauchende schwarze Katzen wieder hervorkommen. So wurden in der Zeit der Hexenverfolgung Hexen und ihre Verbündeten stets unter alten Weiden vermutet.

Verwendung – gestern und heute

Auf den germanischen Gerichtspulten der Freigrafen lag neben dem Schwert auch die Weidenrute, als Symbol der strafenden Gerechtigkeit. Und wenn es hieß „das sollst du an der Weide büßen“, erwartete einen die entwürdigende Strafe des öffentlichen Tragens von Weidenzweigen.

Bachblüte Nr. 38 „willow“ – Weide: die Schicksalsblüte. Hilft Menschen sich nicht als Opfer ihres Schicksals zu sehen.

Weidenrinde, geschabt und getrocknet, enthält Salicylsäure, die Urform aller schmerzstillenden Medikamente, und galt jahrhundertelang als das Fiebermittel der Volksheilkunde.

Weißdorn

Lat. Name: *Crataegus monogyna*
Pflanzenfamilie: Rosengewächse

Es ist immer der 17. Mai – jedes Jahr aufs Neue bin ich fasziniert von der Genauigkeit, mit der mein Weißdorn zu blühen beginnt. Egal ob es bis spät ins Frühjahr Schnee und Kälte gegeben hatte, oder ob es schon von Februar an warm gewesen war. Der große Auftritt der weißen Göttin findet in meinem Garten seit Jahrzehnten an diesem Tag statt.

Die Weiß- und Schwarzdornsträucher bilden den Schutzwall um jungsteinzeitliche Siedlungen: Nahrung, Heilmittel und undurchdringliches Dornengeäst in einem. In jene Zeiten ist ihre besondere mythologische Hochachtung zu verorten. Erst wenn der Frühling richtig Fuß gefasst hat, zeigt sich die weiße Göttin in ihrem Blütenkleid und lädt ein zu Fruchtbarkeit und sicherem Überleben.

Der Weißdorn kann sowohl als Strauch als auch als richtiger Baum wachsen. Dementsprechend variiert seine Höhe zwischen 2 und 13 m. Er kann ein Alter von mindestens 100 Jahren erreichen.

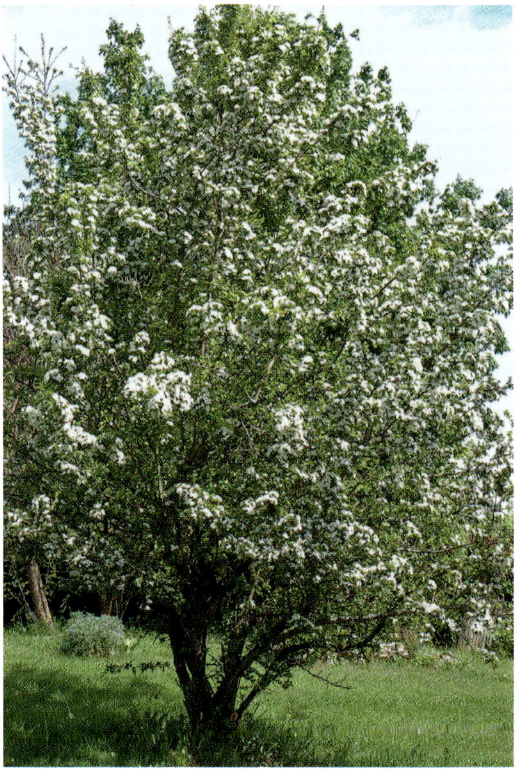
Weißdornstrauch

Rauch

Verwendete Pflanzenteile: Blüten, Blätter, Früchte, Rinde, Holz.

Beste Sammel- und Erntezeit: Blüten im Mai, Früchte im Herbst; Blätter, Rinde und Holz können das ganze Jahr über gesammelt werden.

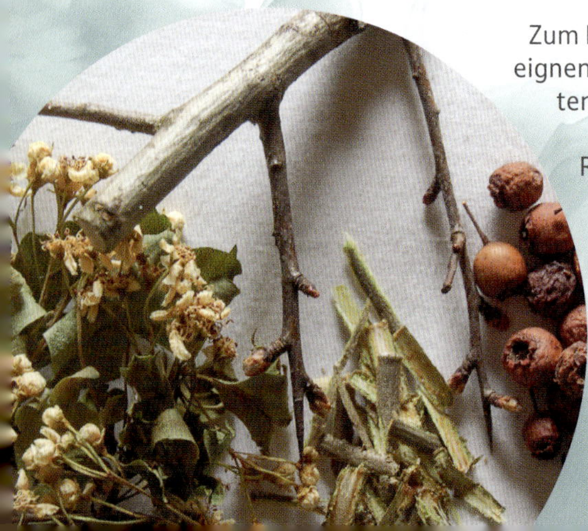
Zum Räuchern eignen sich Blüten, Blätter, Früchte, Rinde und Holz.

Wirkung, Wahrnehmung: Inbegriff von Schutz und Sicherheit im Rauch: hilfreich bei jeder Erschütterung im Lebenslauf; bei der Bewältigung von Schicksalsschlägen; bei gebrochenem Herzen und bei psychischen Traumata. Festigt den sprichwörtlichen „Boden unter den Füßen", um sich nicht ganz zu verlieren. Entspannt und löst emotionale Stauungen; zentriert und aktiviert neue Lebenskräfte (v. a. die Früchte). Er wird körperlich sehr wohltuend und entkrampfend erlebt.

Weißdornrauch ist die Brücke über den Abgrund, quasi eine ganzheitliche Erstversorgung im Krisenfall, ohne Zeit zu geben, in die Tiefe zu blicken. Der Blütenrauch fördert einen guten Beginn von Arbeiten, von bewusst gesetzten Veränderungen und neuen Lebensphasen.

Magisches zum Rauch: Das Holz des Weißdorns scheint für rituelle Abläufe und magische Handlungen besonders geeignet.

Schwerpunkt, Anwendungen, Rezepte: Weißdorn gehört – neben Tannennadeln, Thymian und Mistelkraut – in eine klassische Krankenräucherung. Für eine rhythmusgebende Räucherung werden die Kräfte der vier Elemente vereint: Weißdorn, Diptam, Esche und Birke. Harz nicht vergessen.

Mythologie und magische Praktiken

Das Holz galt auch als Amulett-Holz gegen den bösen Blick! Der Weißdorn war das Brautkleid der großen Muttergottheit. Sein einzigartiger intensiver Duft brachte die Sinne in Wallung und überzog die keltischen Frühlingsfeste mit lustvoller Sexualität und orgiastischen Paarungen.

Bei Griechen und Römern war die Braut mit Weißdornblüten geschmückt und das Weißdornholz war die Hochzeitsfackel. Bei den Römern musste der Bräutigam erst der Göttin Cardea opfern, bevor er seine Gattin über die Türschwelle heben durfte. Cardea war die Hüterin der Türschwellen und Türgriffe. Sie hatte aber auch die Aufgabe, über die Geburt zu wachen: Mit dem Weißdornholz konnte sie die Geburtswege öffnen und Neugeborene gegen blutsaugende Dämonen schützen.

Im Mittelalter gibt es einen Gebärzauber mit dem Holz des Weißdorns: Dabei werden Dornen des Weißdornes drei Mal auf den Bauch der Gebärenden fallen gelassen oder sie trägt ein Säckchen mit Dornen des Weißdornes an ihrer linken Seite bei sich.

Weißdornzweige gelten als mächtiger Schutz gegen jede Art von Übergriffen durch Hexen: ob als Türschmuck und als Büschel an der Stalltür angebracht zu Walpurgis oder als Schlagwerkzeug gegen den Milchzauber dämonischer Wesen.

Im Westen Europas verbindet der Weißdorn ab dem 5. Jahrhundert die keltische Spiritualität mit den christlichen Glaubensvorstellungen. Der Weißdorn ist das erzählerische Bindeglied und hat in Großbritannien und Irland seine außergewöhnliche Stellung bis heute behalten. Viviane, die Herrin vom See und magische Gestalt der Artussage, bannt den greisen Merlin unter einem Weißdornstrauch, nachdem er ihr alle Zaubergeheimnisse verraten hatte. Dort soll er schlafen, bis seine Zeit wiederkommt und ihn Vivianes Zauber nicht mehr bindet.

Der Weißdorn ist der britisch-irische Feenbaum. An Orten, an denen drei Weißdornsträucher zu-

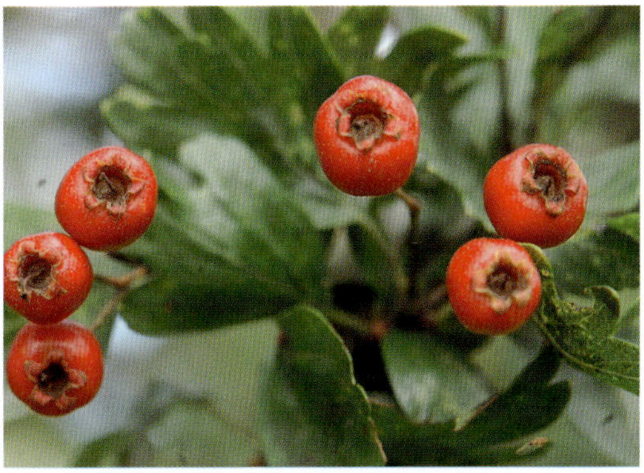

Früchte des Weißdorns

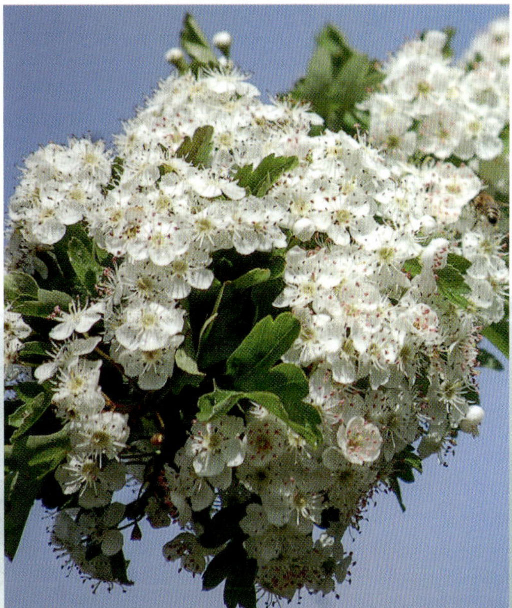

Blüten des Weißdorns

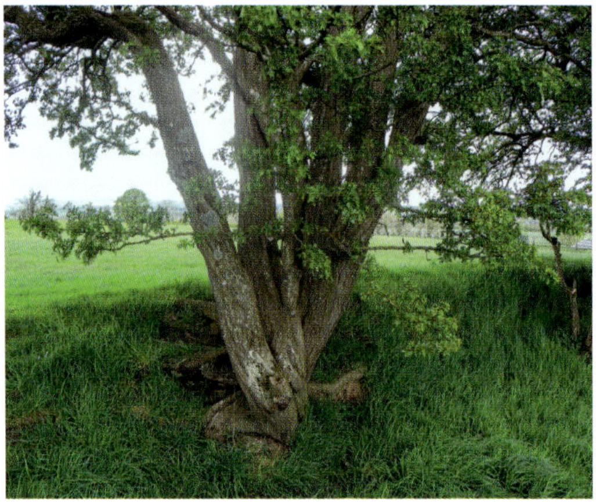
Weißdorn am Hill of Tara, Irland

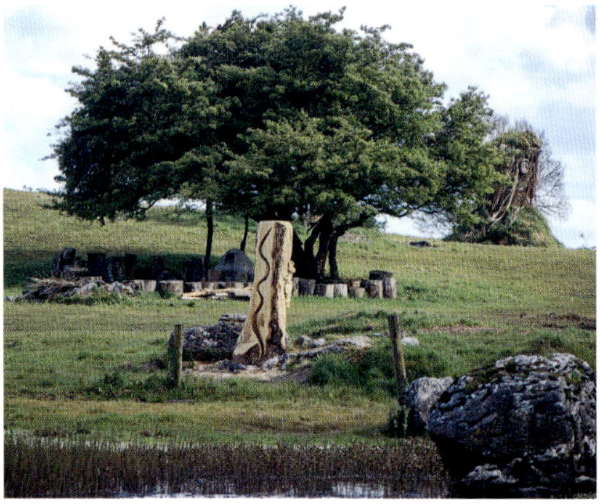
Weißdorn in Uisneach, Irland

sammenstehen, würde man Feen zu Gesicht bekommen, meinten die einen. Die Iren hingegen fürchteten in das Feenreich gezogen zu werden, wenn sie sich Anfang Mai unter einem Weißdorn aufhielten. Weiters bringe es Unglück einen Weißdorn zu fällen: Dann könnten Tiere verenden oder gar kleine Kinder sterben! Deswegen legt man in diesen Gegenden Wert darauf, Wege und Straßen tunlichst um einen Weißdorn herum zu führen und ihn nicht zu schlägern.
In Irland sind manche Weißdorne mit rosaroten und blauen Bändern und anderen Baby-Utensilien behängt – wohl um der weißen Göttin für eine glückliche Geburt und ein gesundes Kind zu danken.

Die gelungenste Transformation von heidnisch zu christlich fand in Glastonbury, England, statt: Glastonbury, inselartig inmitten einer gefährlichen, meist umnebelten Sumpflandschaft gelegen, ist ein zentrales keltisches Quellheiligtum. Aus seiner Quelle fließt rötliches, wohl eisenhältiges Wasser, das als Menstrualblut der großen Göttin gedeutet wird. Hier am ultimativen Übergang vom Diesseits ins Jenseits ist ihre pulsierende Lebenskraft zu spüren, übermittelt sie ihre Botschaften und fordert sie ihre Opfergaben ein. Und dann landet, der Legende nach, Joseph von Arimathäa vom Heiligen Land kommend auf britischem Boden in Glastonbury. Als geheimer Jünger Jesu habe er dessen Blut, das am Kreuz aus der Seite Jesu geflossen war, im Abendmahlkelch aufgefangen. Nachdem der Leichnam Jesu nach dessen Auferstehung verschwunden war, wurde Joseph beschuldigt und verhaftet und musste 40 Jahre im Gefängnis verbringen. Als nunmehr alter Mann habe er seiner Heimat den Rücken gekehrt und sei mit dem Abendmahlkelch, in dem sich das Blut Christi befunden hätte, nach Britannien gekommen, habe in Glastonbury eine Kapelle errichtet und den Kelch darin verwahrt. Joseph von Arimathäa ist somit der Begründer der Gralslegende, die zahllose mittelalterliche Recken in späteren Jahrhunderten auf die Suche nach dem wundertätigen Heiligen Gral schicken sollte, denn die Kapelle in Glastonbury sei 1184 abgebrannt und der Gralskelch verschwunden.

Jedenfalls soll Joseph von Arimathäa beim Betreten britischen Bodens seinen Wanderstab aus Weißdornholz in den Boden gesteckt haben. Aus diesem sei ein riesiger Weißdornstrauch erwachsen, der zwei Mal pro Jahr blühte: im Mai und zu Weihnachten. Von da an, bis zum heutigen Tag, wird dem britischen Königshaus zu Weihnachten ein blühender Weißdornzweig von Glastonbury überbracht! Die Botschaften: Erstens die christliche Kraft im Umgang mit der Natur ist doppelt so groß wie die heidnische

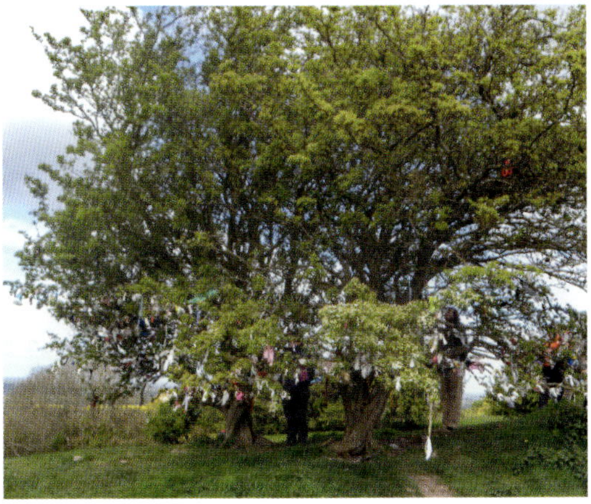

Dankes-Weißdorn am Hill of Tara, Irland

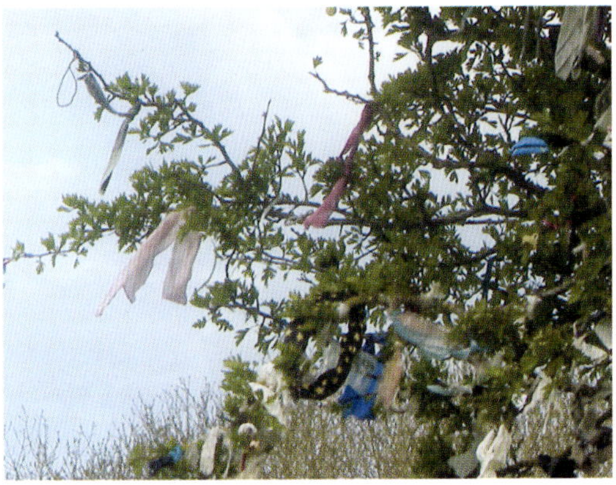

Die Stoffe am Weißdorn sind Dankesgeschenke für die weiße Göttin.

Kraft. Und zweitens werden die weiße weibliche Göttin und ihre fordernde Lebenskraft von einem alten, gebrechlichen männlichen Abgesandten des neuen Gottes dominiert und gezähmt! Drittens ist die christliche Lehre zum frühesten Zeitpunkt (um ca.70 n. Chr.) und exklusiv nach Britannien gekommen, womit auch das spätere Sendungsbewusstsein irischer, schottischer sowie englischer Mönche in der zweiten Christianisierungswelle einen legitimen Hintergrund bekommt.

Im Frühmittelaltermuseum Carantana in Molzbichl, Kärnten ist ein Sensationsfund aus dem 10. Jahrhundert zu sehen: das Skelett einer Frau, die nach ihrem Tod im Herzbereich gepfählt wurde. Aus Angst vor untoten Wiedergängern und blutsaugenden Vampiren wurden verschiedene, vermutlich schon zu Lebzeiten eher eigenartige Personen, mit dem doppelten oder dreifachen Tod endgültig zur Ruhe gebracht und für die Lebenden ungefährlich gemacht. Für die Toten-Pfählungen wurden Weißdornpflöcke im Brust- bzw. Herzbereich durch den Leichnam geschlagen.

So hat die weiße Göttin auch eine dunkle Seite, die eher Morrigan, der keltischen Geistergöttin entspricht, der Göttin für Krieg und Kampf. Das Hagedornholz wurde zum Einäschern der Toten verwendet und auch die Hackstöcke, auf denen die zum Tode Verurteilten hingerichtet wurden, waren Hagedornstrünke.

Im christlichen Kontext wird die große Macht der weißen Muttergöttin gebrochen, gleichzeitig aber in eine positive Symbolik umgewandelt und integriert: Der Weißdorn steht jetzt für unantastbare Keuschheit und Jungfräulichkeit, der die Treue in allen Bereichen zu schützen vermag und so auch das Zölibat unterstütze.

Verwendung – gestern und heute

Quercetanus (1544–1609), Arzt und Verfechter der paracelsischen neuen Medizin, lag schon richtig, als er für den französischen König Heinrich IV. (1553–1610) einen „Syrupus senelorum", einen „Senioren-Sirup" mischte und als Hauptzutat Weißdorn dazu verwendete.

In zahlreichen Studien konnte die herzstärkende Wirkung des Weißdorns belegt werden. Und so gilt auch noch heute: „Der Weißdorn, das weiß jedes Kind, stärkt Herz und Nerven ganz geschwind" oder auch: „Der Weißdorn mit seinen Blüten und Beeren, kann deinem Herzen viel Kraft bescheren".

Der Rauch von Halbsträuchern und krautigen Pflanzen

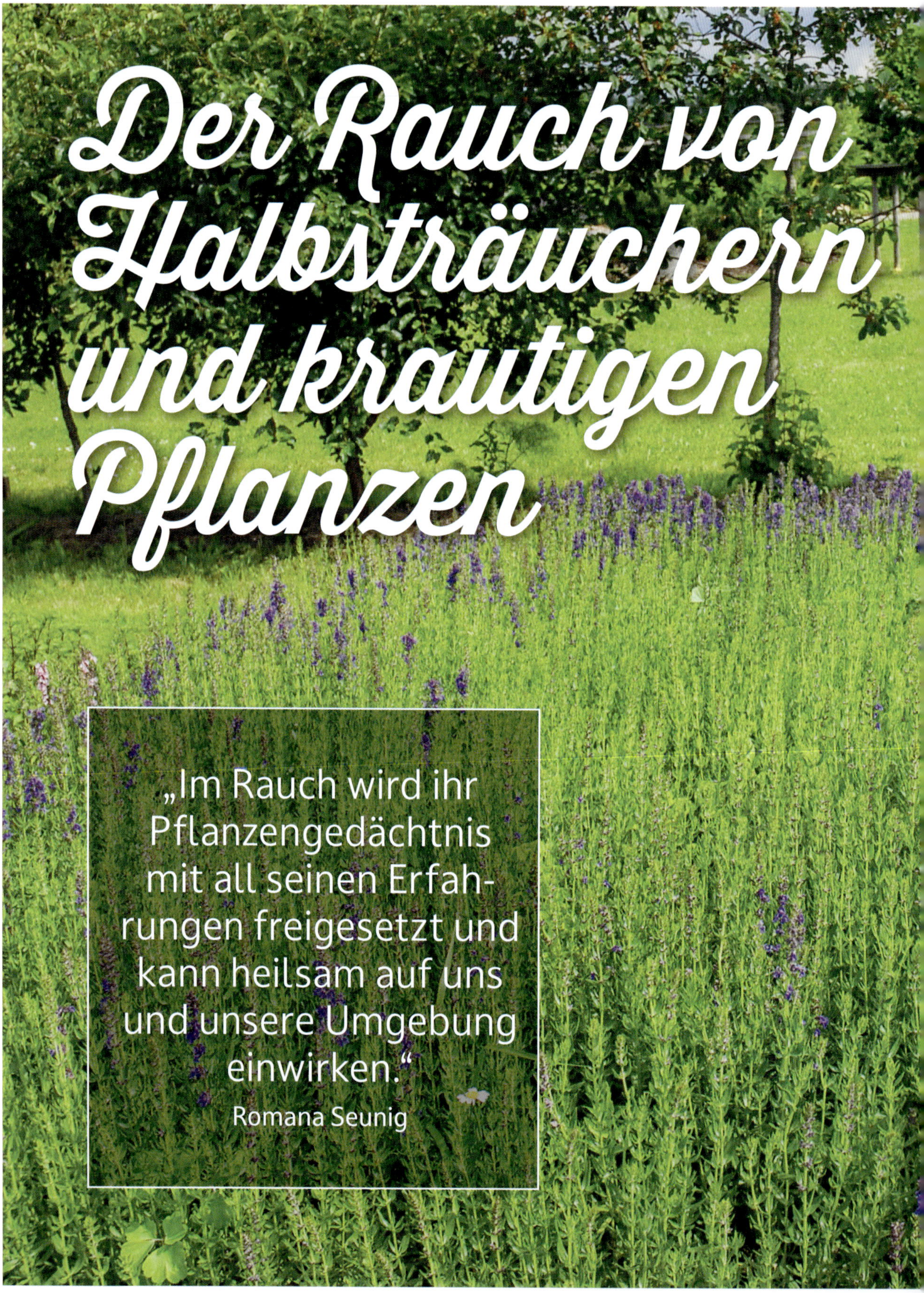

„Im Rauch wird ihr Pflanzengedächtnis mit all seinen Erfahrungen freigesetzt und kann heilsam auf uns und unsere Umgebung einwirken.“

Romana Seunig

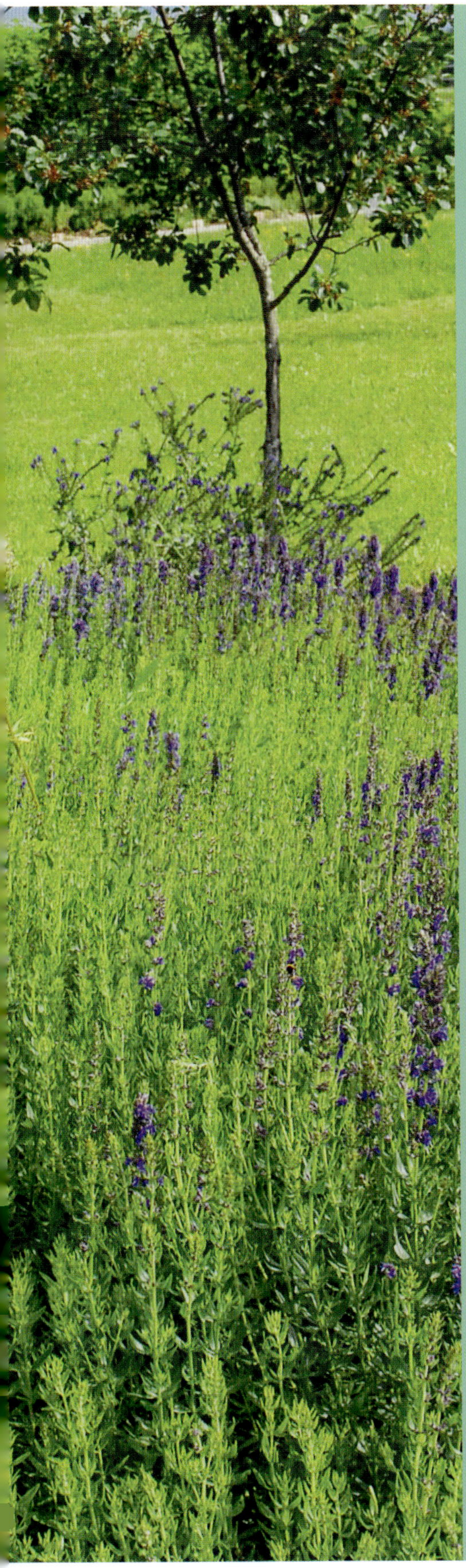

Halbsträucher und krautige Pflanzen sind über mehrere Jahre hinweg den Einwirkungen der Elemente ausgesetzt. Sie verarbeiten diese Einflüsse unterschiedlich: Die einen bündeln ihre Kräfte durch beginnende Verholzung, die anderen durchlaufen wiederholt den Prozess von „Stirb und Werde“ und erlangen so ihre spezielle Wesenstiefe.

Im Rauch wird ihr Pflanzengedächtnis mit all seinen Erfahrungen freigesetzt und kann heilsam auf uns und unsere Umgebung einwirken. Das macht diese Pflanzen zu besonders wertvollen Räucherstoffen!

Berg-Bohnenkraut

Lat. Name: *Satureja montana*
Pflanzenfamilie: Lippenblütler

Das Bergbohnenkraut ist ein drahtiger, widerstandsfähiger Halbstrauch, der etliche Winter mit Schnee und Eis mühelos überdauern kann. Gleich im Frühjahr treibt es wieder aus und hat bis Mitte Juli wieder seine leicht kugelförmige Gestalt ausgebildet. Mit der anschließenden Blüte ist es erntefertig und dient als intensives Küchengewürz, das so manche Speise bekömmlicher machen kann. Im Unterschied zum einjährigen Bohnenkraut (*Satureja hortensis*), das eine verzweigte Gestalt annimmt und sich im Garten meist von selbst weiter ausssät, ist das Bergbohnenkraut (*Satureja montana*) deutlich intensiver im Geschmack. So harmlos es aussieht, so wird doch schon in den ältesten Kräuteraufzeichnungen von seiner aphrodisierenden Kraft berichtet. Neben verdauungsförderlichen, wohltuenden und beruhigenden Eigenschaften gilt hier ganz besonders, dass Liebe wohl durch den Magen geht. Das Bergbohnenkraut ist mehrjährig und wird bis zu 30 cm hoch.

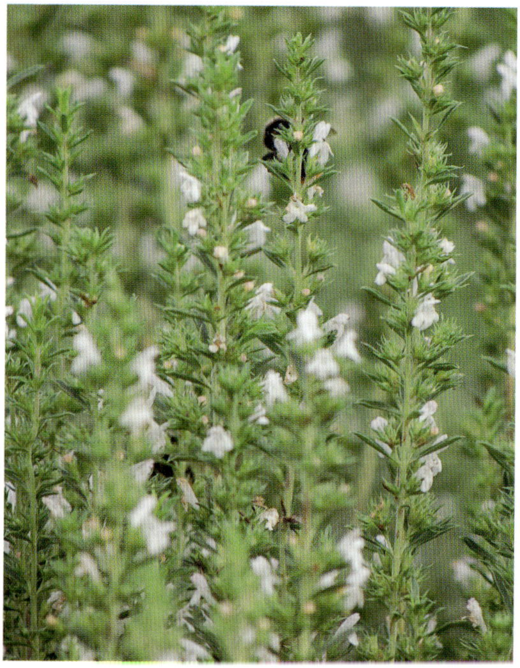

Blüten des Bergbohnenkrauts

Rauch

Verwendete Pflanzenteile: Das ganze Kraut.

Beste Sammel- und Erntezeit: Kann das ganze Jahr über geschnitten werden.

Wirkung, Wahrnehmung: Im Rauch entfaltet das Bergbohnenkraut einen großen energetischen Impuls! Es hat eine reinigende, klärende Wirkung, die einen wachrüttelt und so manches besser verstehen lässt. Der Rauch wirkt stärkend auf die Lebenslust, hält uns auf der positiven Seite, wenn die Zeiten wieder einmal rauer werden. Negative Gedanken werden verscheucht und verschreckte oder traurige Seelen wieder aufgebaut.

Magisches zum Rauch: Durch seine positiv stimmende Wirkung kann eine Räucherung mit Bohnenkraut gut zur Vorbereitung auf verschiedene Rituale geräuchert werden.

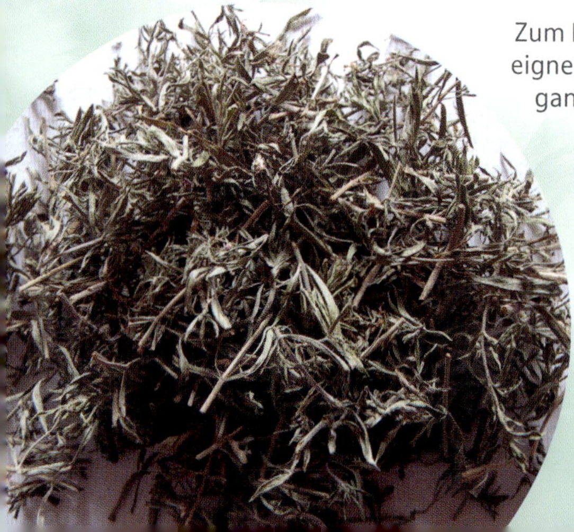

Zum Räuchern eignet sich das ganze Kraut.

Schwerpunkt, Anwendungen, Rezepte: Ideal für Herzenstrost-Räucherungen, die neben der geistigen, eine stark seelisch-sinnliche Seite in uns ansprechen wollen: Bohnenkraut zusammen mit Rose, Lavendel und Eisenkraut kombiniert mit Harz.

Verwendung – gestern und heute

Während der Hl. Isidor (560–636), Erzbischof von Sevilla schreibt: „Man glaube, dass es geneigt zur Liebe mache", klingt es bei Bartholomäus, Arzt und Medizinlehrer im 12. Jahrhundert schon eindeutiger. Seine Medizinhandschrift wurde das ganze Mittelalter hindurch in den Klöstern abgeschrieben und fand so europaweite Verbreitung. Nachzulesen im „Admonter Bartholomäus", einer Abschrift aus dem 15. Jahrhundert: „Wer Unkeuschheit pflegen und schimpflich mit den Frauen leben will, der trinke Bohnenkraut-Wurzel mit Wein, das macht den Mann begierig."

Der Arzt und Kräuterkundige Matthiolus (1501–1578) meinte in seinem Kräuterbuch von 1568 zum Bohnenkraut: „... benimpt den ungelust und das wüllen, bringt die unkeusche begirde auff die ban, darumb ettliche meinen, sie haben den namen von den geylen Satyris."

Nach Matthiolus verweise die lateinische Bezeichnung „*Satureia*" auf die Satyrn, die in der griechischen Mythologie als Mischwesen (Mensch und Ziegenbock) Dionysos, den Gott des Weines, der Freude und der Extase begleiten.

Bis heute gilt also für das Bohnenkraut: Magen erwärmen, Verdauung fördern und eheliche Werke befördern.

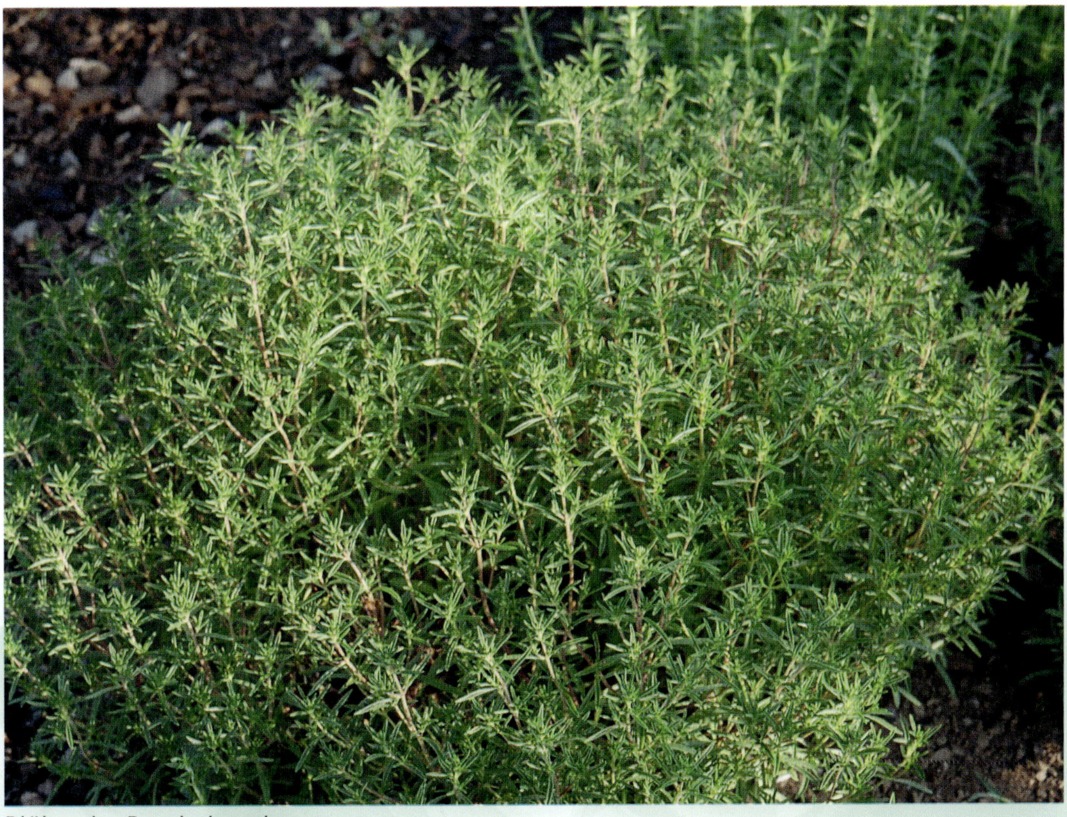

Blühendes Bergbohnenkraut

Dost

Lat. Name: *Origanum vulgare*
Pflanzenfamilie: Lippenblütler

Ein ganz besonderes Kraut wächst gern büschelweise zusammen auf extensiven Rainen und Wiesen, blüht ab Mitte Juli bis in den September und ziert verlässlich die Kräuterbuschn zu Mariä Himmelfahrt. Der als „Krampfkraut" oder „Kräutlein Wohlgemuth" bezeichnete Dost ist ein hoch angesehenes Schutzkraut. Der Dost ist mit vielen ätherischen Ölen ausgestattet, was ihn sowohl zu einem Gewürz- wie auch zu einem wunderbaren Heilkraut macht.

Rauch

Verwendete Pflanzenteile: Blatt, Stängel, Blüten.

Beste Sammel- und Erntezeit: Blätter und Stängel können das ganze Jahr über gesammelt werden; zur Blütezeit (Mitte Juli bis September) ist seine Kraft am größten.

Wirkung, Wahrnehmung: Abwehrrauch und Reinigungsrauch; große weißmagische Kraft! Der Rauch vertreibt nachhaltig negative Fremdenergien und zwar sowohl in Räumen und an Orten, als auch bei persönlichen Anhaftungen. Schutzrauch für die Seele bei Belastungen, Verunsicherungen; hält einen bei Lebensübergängen im hellen, warmen Licht und wehrt negative Einflüsse ab. Hoffnungsbringender Rauch, der dunkle Mächte von suchenden Seelen fernhält. Legt einen Schutzmantel um den Räuchernden.

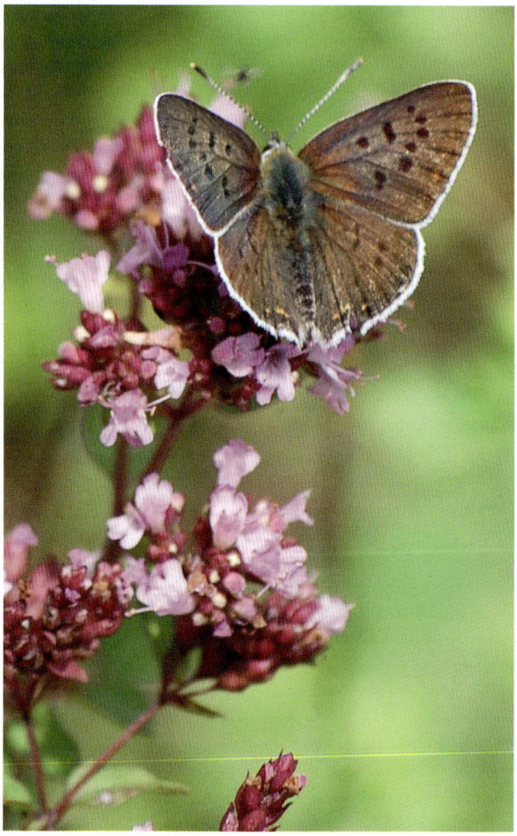

Blühender Dost

Stärkt die eigene Persönlichkeit, gibt Kraft für neue Entwicklungen und sorgt für sanfte Übergänge. Hilft Kummer zu überwinden und gibt neuen Lebensmut!

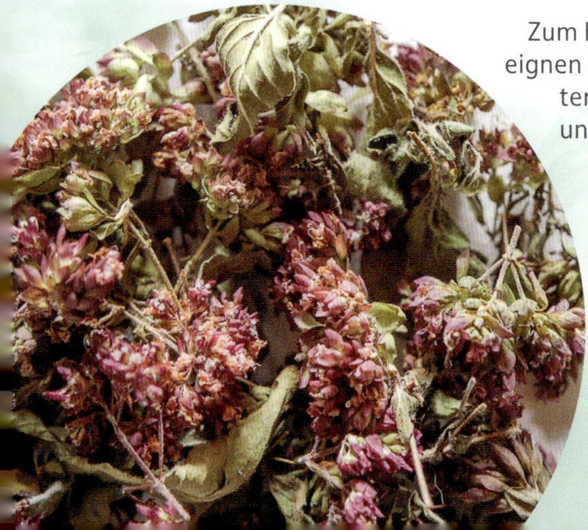

Zum Räuchern eignen sich Blätter, Stängel und Blüten.

Magisches zum Rauch: In einer Mischung mit Johanniskraut und Wermut wird gegen befürchteten Schadenszauber und schwarze Magie geräuchert. Seit der Antike als dämonenabwehrender Rauch beschrieben!

Schwerpunkt, Anwendungen, Rezepte: Zum Auflösen von Verwünschungen und anderem Schadenszauber mischt man Harz mit Dost sowie Odermennig, Klettenwurzel, Weinraute und Heilziest.

Mythologie und magische Praktiken

Im gesamten Mittelalter galt der Dost als hexenabwehrendes und teufelsscheuchendes Kraut. Diese zentrale Bedeutung zeigt sich noch heute in der Vielzahl von überlieferten Sinnsprüchen: „Hätt´st nit Dorant (Andorn) und Dosten, tät´s dich dein Leben kosten!“ oder: „Nimm Dost und Johannesblut, das ist für alle Kranken gut!“

In einer Sage aus Oberkärnten klagt der durch ein Dost-Büschel am Kleid der begehrten Jungfrau abgewehrte Teufel: „Roter Dost! Hätt ich das gewosst, hätt ich dich vernomme, wär ich nit dahergekomme!“

Dost, Dill und Johanniskraut wurden gemeinsam im Garten angesetzt, um Haus und Hof, um Mensch und Vieh vor Schaden zu bewahren. Sie mussten stets bereit sein für Räucherungen oder wurden frisch als Sprengwedel im Weihwassergefäß verwendet.

Verwendung – gestern und heute

Dioskurid berichtet bereits im 1. Jahrhundert n. Chr. vom Dost als einem erwärmenden Heilmittel. Auch Leonhart Fuchs (1501–1566) hält etliche Dost-Arzneien fest und rät unter anderem: „mit essig/öl und gersten meel vermengt und übergestrichen verzert die kröpff.“ Seine ausgleichende Wirkung macht den Dost auch heute zum beliebten Tee- und Gewürzkraut.

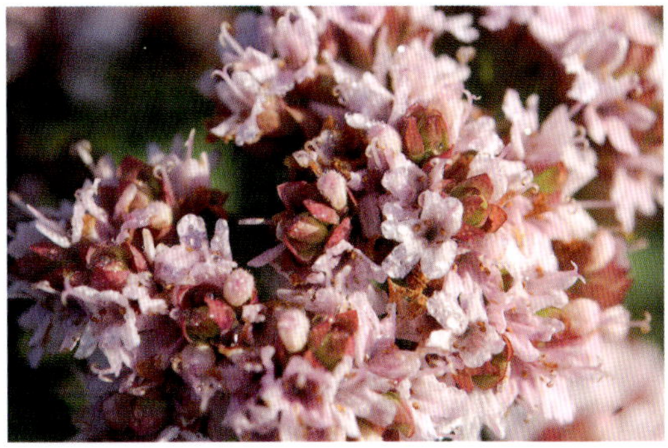

Blüten des Dosts

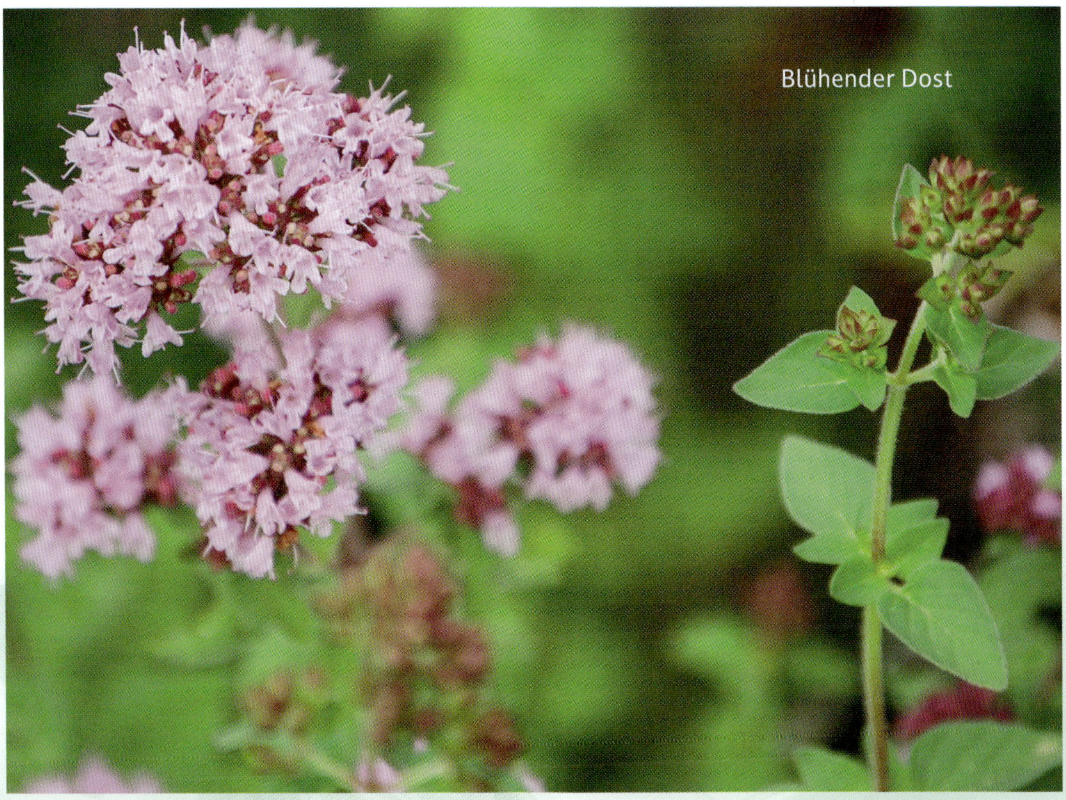

Blühender Dost

Eberraute

Lat. Name: *Artemisia abrotanum*
Pflanzenfamilie: Korbblütler

Wie ein getreuer Wächter stand die Eberraute in alten Bauerngärten gleich neben dem Eingang. Ihre Aufgabe war es, den Garten, seine Gewächse und die Menschen, die darin arbeiteten, vor Übergriffen des Teufels und vor jedem Schadens- und Neidzauber von Fremden oder Nachbarn, die über den Zaun schauten, zu schützen. In einigen Kärntner Sagen hat die „Obrot" ihre teufelsscheuchende Kraft unter Beweis gestellt und so manche unschuldige junge Frau vor den Nachstellungen des Gehörnten bewahrt.

Die Eberraute, früher auch Stabwurz genannt, ist ein Halbstrauch und kann leicht durch Stecklinge vermehrt werden. Da sie zum Verholzen neigt und nach jedem Jahr der holzige Astanteil länger und der grün beblätterte Nachwuchs kürzer wird, sollte sie einmal pro Jahr geschnitten werden. Meist passiert das im Rahmen der Sommerernte. Die Eberraute stammt aus dem Mittelmeerraum und wird bis zu einem halben Meter hoch. Gewisse Arten können jedoch auch bis zu einem Meter hoch werden.

Rauch

Verwendete Pflanzenteile: Das ganze Kraut.

Beste Sammel- und Erntezeit: Die Ernte kann bis Ende August erfolgen; dann sollte die Pflanze nicht mehr geschnitten werden, um gut über den Winter zu kommen.

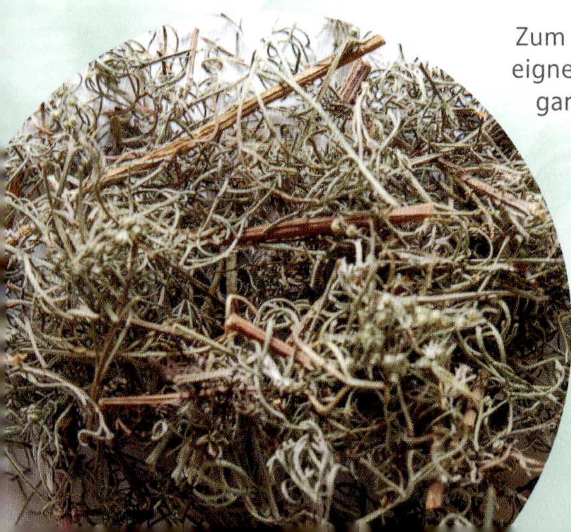

Zum Räuchern eignet sich das ganze Kraut.

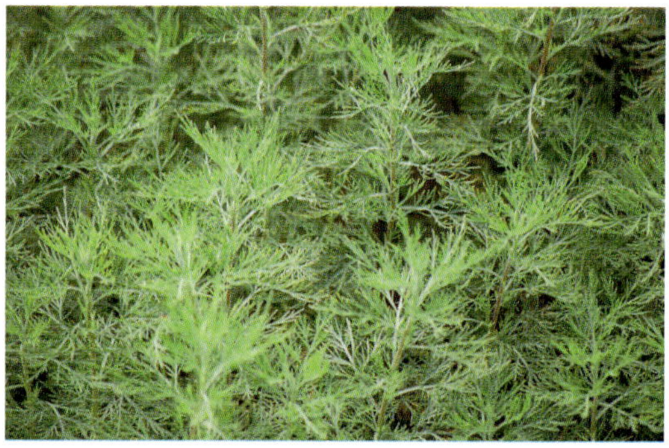

Blattwerk der Eberraute

Wirkung, Wahrnehmung: Eberraute wirkt konzentrationsfördernd, klärend und insgesamt aufbauend und vitalisierend. Der Rauch vermittelt Wachheit und Aufmerksamkeit, hilft Dinge in Angriff zu nehmen. Hervorragendes Räuchermittel bei Kraftlosigkeit und Überforderung; wie alle Artemisia-Arten trägt auch der Rauch der Eberraute dazu bei, die Dinge in einem verträglichen Rhythmus zu halten. „Immer weiter" lautet die Devise.

Magisches zum Rauch: Dort, wo man Schlangen und Ungeziefer vermutete oder fand, machte man mit Eberraute einen intensiven Rauch, um sie zu vertreiben.

Schwerpunkt, Anwendungen, Rezepte: Tabernaemontanus (1522–1590) rät bei Erkältung und verstopfter Nase Eberrauten-Rauch durch die Nase aufzuziehen, um diese wieder frei zu bekommen.

Mythologie und magische Praktiken

Die Eberraute war ein wichtiges Kraut des „Würtzwischen", des Kräuterbuschns zu Mariä Himmelfahrt. Tabernaemontanus (1522–1590) vermutet: „Es wird die Stabwurtz von den alten Weibern auch zu den Würtzwischen gesamlet, damit sie dann mancherley aberglaubische Fantaseyen treiben, welches wir als ein unnütz Fabelwerck fahren lassen."

In Liebes- und Übergriffs-Zaubereien wurde die Stabwurz häufig verwendet: Wer seiner Angebeteten unbemerkt ein Eberrauten-Zweiglein zusteckt, dem könne sie nicht mehr widerstehen. Doch weil nur angezaubert, würde diese Liebe nicht lange halten.

Unter den Kräuterkundigen besteht ab dem 16. Jahrhundert Einigkeit darüber, dass die Eberraute aphrodisierende Wirkung habe. So heißt es beim oben zitierten Tabernaemontanus etwas weiter unten in seiner Eberrauten-Beschreibung: „Ein Büschlein Stabwurtz under das Hauptküssen geleget, sol den Menschen zu fleischlicher begierde der Unkeuschheit reitzen, unnd eine gewisse Hülffe seyn wider alle Gespenst unnd Zauberey, das solch Werck verhindern soll."

Solches Wissen hielt sich offenbar sehr lange in der Bevölkerung. So übermittelte mancherorts die Eberraute noch in den 50-er Jahren des letzten Jahrhunderts geheime Nachrichten unter Eheleuten: Wenn der Vater abends ganz unauffällig ein aufmunterndes Eberrautenzweiglein in Händen hielt, dann war der Mutter klar, dass später noch eheliche Werke auf sie warteten.

Getrocknete Eberrautenzweiglein finden sich aber auch in alten Gebetsbüchern zur Unterstützung gegen das Abschweifen der Gedanken und um einen wach zu halten.

Verwendung – gestern und heute

Eberrauten sind aus den mittelalterlichen Gärten nicht wegzudenken. So verwundert es nicht, dass die Eberraute auch im „Capitulare de villis vel curtis imperii" einen prominenten Platz einnimmt. Dieses Wirtschaftsmanual für Königshöfe wurde von Kaiser Karl dem Großen (747–814) um das Jahr 800 erlassen und schloss im 70. Kapitel mit einer Pflanzenliste von 73 Kräutern und Gemüsesorten die im pfalznahen Königsgarten anzubauen waren. Die Eberraute ist als „abrotanum" an der siebenten Stelle angeführt.

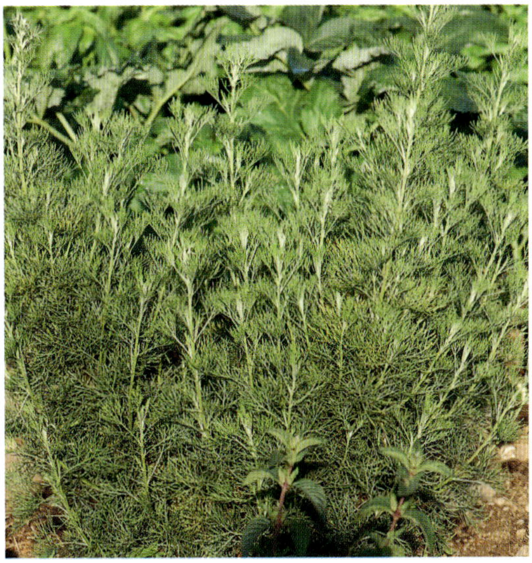

Wuchsform der Eberraute

In Walahfrid Strabos (808–849) Gartengedicht „Hortulus", einer lyrischen Beschreibung der wichtigsten Gewächse im Klostergarten auf der Insel Reichenau im Bodensee, findet sich die Eberraute nach Salbei und Weinraute an dritter Stelle. Ein deutlicher Hinweis auf die Wichtigkeit in jenen Zeiten. So endet seine Beschreibung mit den Worten: „Zudem besitzt die Eberraute ebenso viel Kräfte wie haarfeine Blätter."

Über die letzten 2300 Jahre, aus denen uns Beschreibungen der Eberraute vorliegen, gibt es wohl keinen Körperteil, den man nicht versucht hätte mit Eberrauten-Anwendungen zu behandeln: Hippokrates (460–370 v. Chr.) verwendete sie zur Geburtsbeschleunigung, Hildegard von Bingen (1098–1179) braute mit ihr einen Magenwein, Paracelsus (1493–1541) empfahl sie bei Asthma, Hüftweh und Nervenschmerzen und Nicholas Culpeper (1616–1654) beschrieb Anwendungen mit Eberrauten-Asche, um den Haar- und Bartwuchs anzuregen. Das getrocknete Kraut gilt als wirksames Mottenmittel und gehört heute mit seinem angenehmen Geruch in Schränke und Wäscheladen.

Eisenkraut

Lat. Name: *Verbena officinalis*
Pflanzenfamilie: Lippenblütler

Kein Duft, nur Gewicht – Das wohl wichtigste Zauberkraut der antiken Welt besticht durch seine saturnale Reduziertheit bei gleichzeitig unheimlichem Gewicht! Das Eisenkraut ist seit Jahrtausenden ein menschlicher Kulturbegleiter.

Durch seine Zurückhaltung beim Frühjahrsaustrieb kommt es auf meinem Acker schon vor, dass ich es übersehe, dass ich denke, es sei nicht über den Winter gekommen. Dabei hockt ein dicker Wurzelstock knapp unter der Oberfläche, der Kraft sammelt und sich bis zu einem halben Meter tief verankert hat. Anfänglich kam es vor, dass ich auf den scheinbar freien Platz direkt neben dem versteckten Wurzelstock andere Pflanzen setzte. Aber auch wenn es eng wird – das Eisenkraut gibt nicht auf und überragt mit seiner drahtigen Gestalt spätestens im Juli die übrigen Beetgenossen deutlich.

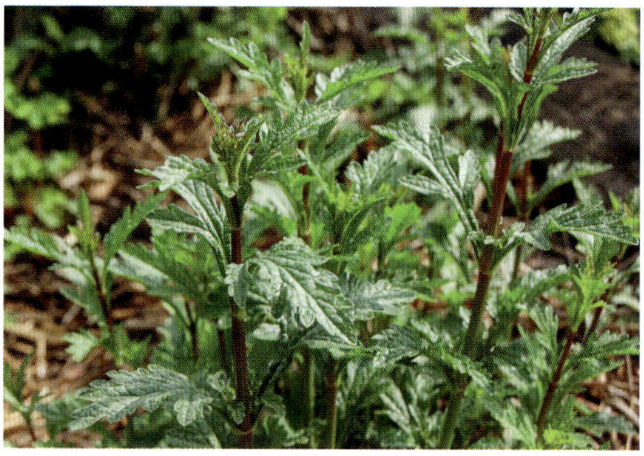
Blätter des Eisenkrauts

Rauch

Verwendete Pflanzenteile: Das ganze blühende Kraut.

Beste Sammel- und Erntezeit: Aufgrund der sehr langen Blühdauer des Eisenkrauts kann es den ganzen Sommer über geschnitten werden.

Wirkung, Wahrnehmung: Reinigend, stressreduzierend, allgemein belebend und aufbauend. Starkes Abwehrmittel gegen geistige Übergriffe und dunkle Mächte. Kopf- und Stresskraut: vertreibt negative Gedanken, hilft neuen Mut zu fassen und hebt das Selbstvertrauen in Zeiten großer Erschöpfung. Schutz gegen alles Negative; bei anspruchsvoller Kopfarbeit, fördert die Konzentration und Kreativität. Der Rauch vertreibt depressive Phasen und kann die dunkle Klammer der Migräne durchlichten.

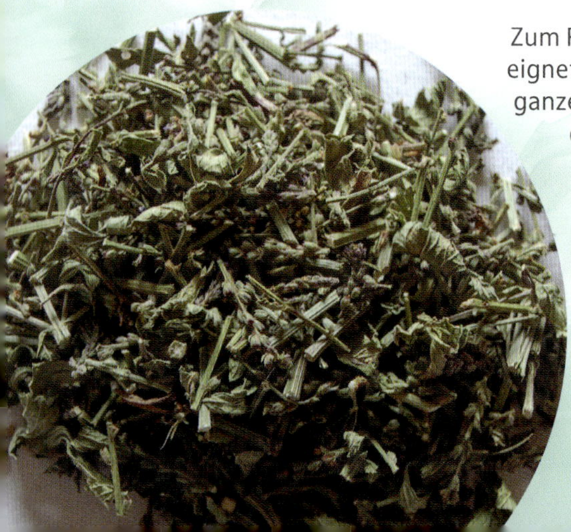
Zum Räuchern eignet sich das ganze blühende Kraut.

Magisches zum Rauch: Eisenkraut ist eines der zwölf magischen Kräuter der Rosenkreuzer, um Hellsichtigkeit und göttliche Inspiration zu erlangen. Der Rauch solle Menschen fröhlich und beliebt machen.

Schwerpunkt, Anwendungen, Rezepte: Für Abwehr- und Anrufungsräucherungen zusammen mit Engelwurz-Samen und Mistel (Harz kombinieren).

Mythologie und magische Praktiken

Unser Wissen über die Verwendung von Eisenkraut bei verschiedenen Ritualen und Zeremonien reicht bis ins alte Ägypten zurück. Die „Träne der Isis" war in allen großen Kulturen Europas stets mit religiösen Praktiken, ja mit dem Göttlichen verbunden und galt in der gesamten Antike als heilig!

Mit ihm wurden Kultstätten gereinigt, sein Rauch half, die Bitten angemessen der angerufenen Gottheit vortragen zu können. Ein Büschel lag stets auf dem Altar Jupiters, der höchsten römischen Gottheit. Kriegern verlieh es Unsterblichkeit, wenn derjenige noch kurz vor dem Ableben mit dem Kraut in Kontakt treten konnte. Man glaubte, es besäße die Kraft Eisen und Ketten zu sprengen, genauso wie auch Schwerter zu härten.

Die keltischen Druiden stellten aus ihrem heiligsten Kraut das Lustralwasser her. Dieses Wasser besaß nach ihrem Glauben eine große Zauberkraft und wurde für magische Rituale ebenso verwendet wie für Weissagungen. Insbesondere vertreibe es aber Dämonen, berichtet Plinius Secundus (23–79).

Eisenkraut wird auch als beliebte Amulettpflanze am Körper getragen: Es schütze vor allem Unheil und lasse den Träger nicht müde werden. Außerdem vertreibe es Albträume und sorge für einen entspannten Schlaf. Kindern hängte man ein Eisenkraut-Amulettsäckchen gegen schmerzhaftes Zahnen um, welches sie auch gegen jegliches Berufen schützen sollte.

Hieronymus Bock (1498–1554) vermerkt kurz und knapp: „Das Kraut Verbena würt noch heüttigs tags mehr zu der Zauberey dann zu der Arznei gesamlet und auffgehoben, mag aber in leib und ausserhalb genommen werden."

Eisenkraut-Pulver aufs Butterbrot gestreut mache Kindern und vielleicht auch Studenten Lust aufs Lernen!

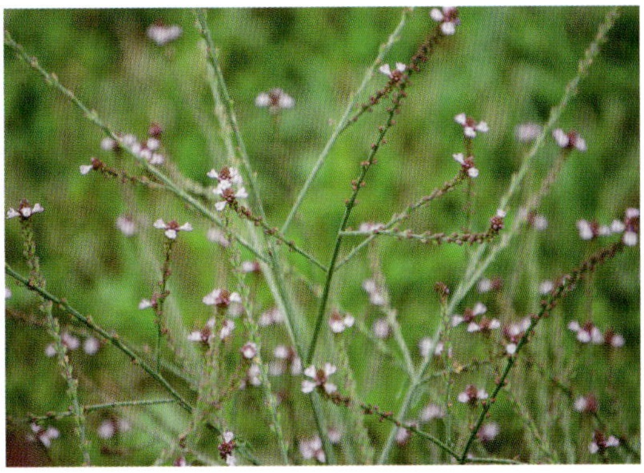

Blühendes Eisenkraut

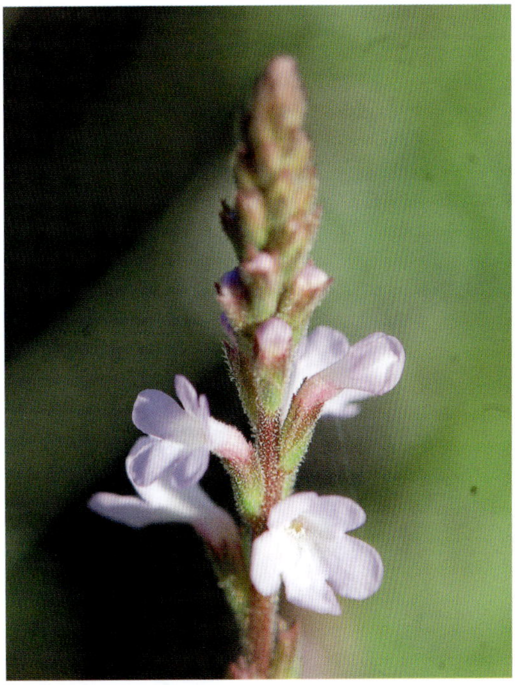

Blüte des Eisenkrauts

Verwendung – gestern und heute

Nach einem mittelalterlichen Rezept verhalf ein Trank aus der Eisenkraut-Wurzel dem „mann, der nit minnen mag" wieder zu gewohnter Stärke.

Bachblüte Nr. 31 „vervain" – Eisenkraut – hilft, damit man seine positive Energie zielgerichteter einzusetzen lernt; auch gegen Schlaflosigkeit, Spannungsgefühle im Zusammenhang mit Überanstrengung und Stress.

Als geburtsbeschleunigender Tee noch heute gebräuchlich, wobei in neueren Untersuchungen eine nervenberuhigende Wirkung belegt werden konnte.

Fenchel

Lat. Name: *Foeniculum vulgare var. dulce*
Botanischer Name: Gewürz-Fenchel
Pflanzenfamilie: Doldenblütler

Wenn ich meinen Gewürz-Fenchel mit seiner imposanten Höhe von über 1,80 m im Hochsommer im Garten bewundere, muss ich oft an seinen wackligen Start im Frühling denken: Direkt auf den getrockneten braunen kurzen Stängeln des Vorjahres wagt sich sein zartes Grün recht früh heraus. Doch fasst man es an, hat man den wurzellosen alten Stängel samt neuem Austrieb in der Hand. Also bloß nicht berühren und warten, bis sich der grüne Trieb aus eigener Kraft neu verankert. Der Gewürz-Fenchel sät sich sehr freizügig aus und so hat man immer ganz neue und ältere, mehrjährige Bestände im Garten.

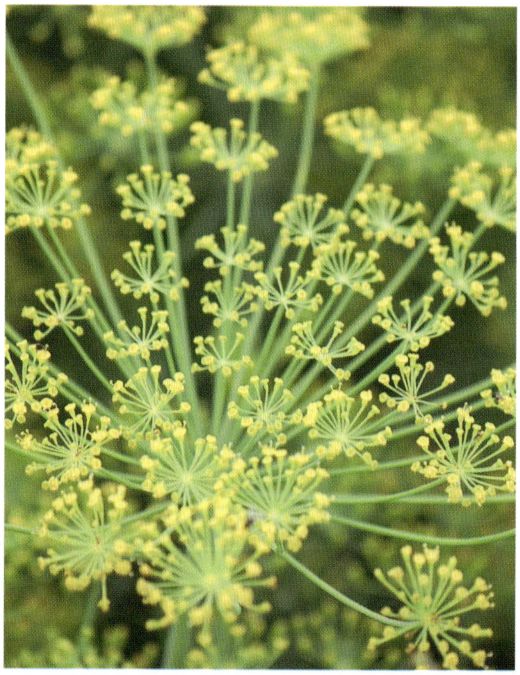

Blüten des Fenchels

Rauch

Verwendete Pflanzenteile: Das zarte Grün, die blühende Dolde und die Fenchel-Samen.

Beste Sammel- und Erntezeit: Das Grün ab Mai, die Blüten im Anschluss ab Ende Juni und die Samen von Anfang September, wenn sie noch grün sind, bis Ende November, nachdem sie auf der Pflanze getrocknet sind.

Wirkung, Wahrnehmung: Positiv polend! Generell desinfizierend, erfrischend, befreiend. Symbol für Glück und Erfolg; Freude und Hoffnung; leichtfüßiger Neuanfang wird möglich. Bedrückendes kann leichter losgelassen und überwunden werden. Nimmt eingebildete Lasten von den Schultern, vertreibt die lähmende Kraft der inneren Dunkelheit. Lässt wieder lebensbejahende Gedanken aufkommen.

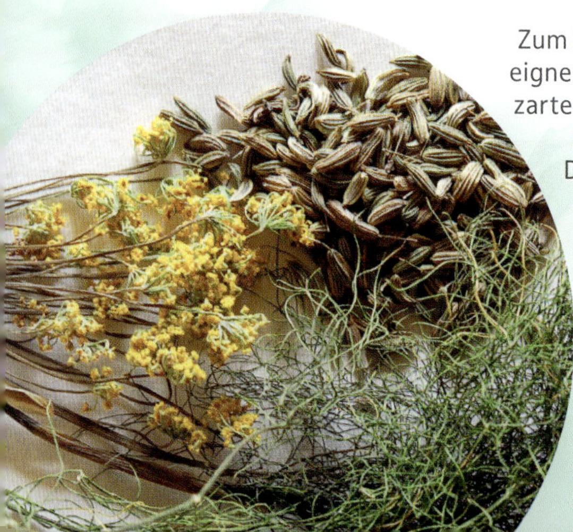

Zum Räuchern eignen sich das zarte Grün, die blühende Dolde und die Fenchel-Samen.

Schwerpunkt, Anwendungen, Rezepte: Räuchermischungen für einen guten Beginn, zur Befreiung von geistiger Unterdrückung, zum Heraustreten aus seelischem Schatten: zusammen mit Birkenblättern, Eberraute und Rosmarin. Neue Lebensabschnitte mit Rauch aus Fenchel, Rosenblüten und Eschenblättern bewusst feiern. Räuchermischungen mit Harz ergänzen.

Verwendung – gestern und heute

Seit es schriftliche Aufzeichnungen von Kräutern gibt, nimmt der Fenchel eine zentrale Stellung ein. Karl der Große (747–814) verordnet den verpflichtenden Anbau von Fenchel „fenicolum“ im „Capitulare des villis vel curtis“ um 800 n. Chr. auf seinen Königshöfen an 36. Stelle unter den insgesamt 73 Kräutern und Gemüsen. Für Hildegard von Bingen (1098–1179) ist der Fenchel wohl eine ihrer Lieblingspflanzen. Sein Genuss stärke allgemein die Gesundheit, mache eine gute Gesichtsfarbe und fördere eine optimistische Lebenseinstellung! Tabernaemontanus (1522–1590) überschlägt sich schier vor Bewunderung für die Fenchelkräfte und listet lange Seiten voller Rezepturen auf. Viele davon drehen sich um die Erhaltung der Sehkraft. Abschließend meint er, dass man den Fenchel nicht nur als Heilkraut verwenden solle, sondern auch als Gewürz in der Küche, um „die Speisen damit zu condiren und abzuwürzen, würde es nicht allein unseren Leibern zur Gesundheit und Wolfahrt gereichen, sondern es würde ein grosses Geld, daß man umb frembde und außländeische Specerey geben muß, erspahret werden." Noch heute hilft Fencheltee zuverlässig allen vom Baby bis ins hohe Alter.

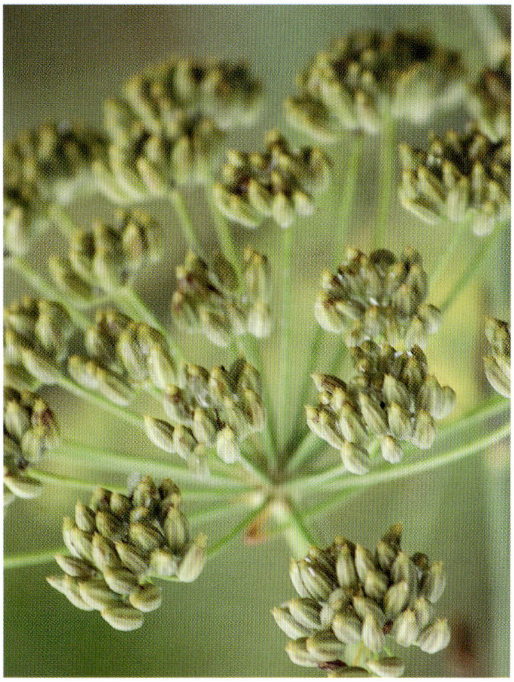

Samenstände des Gewürzfenchels

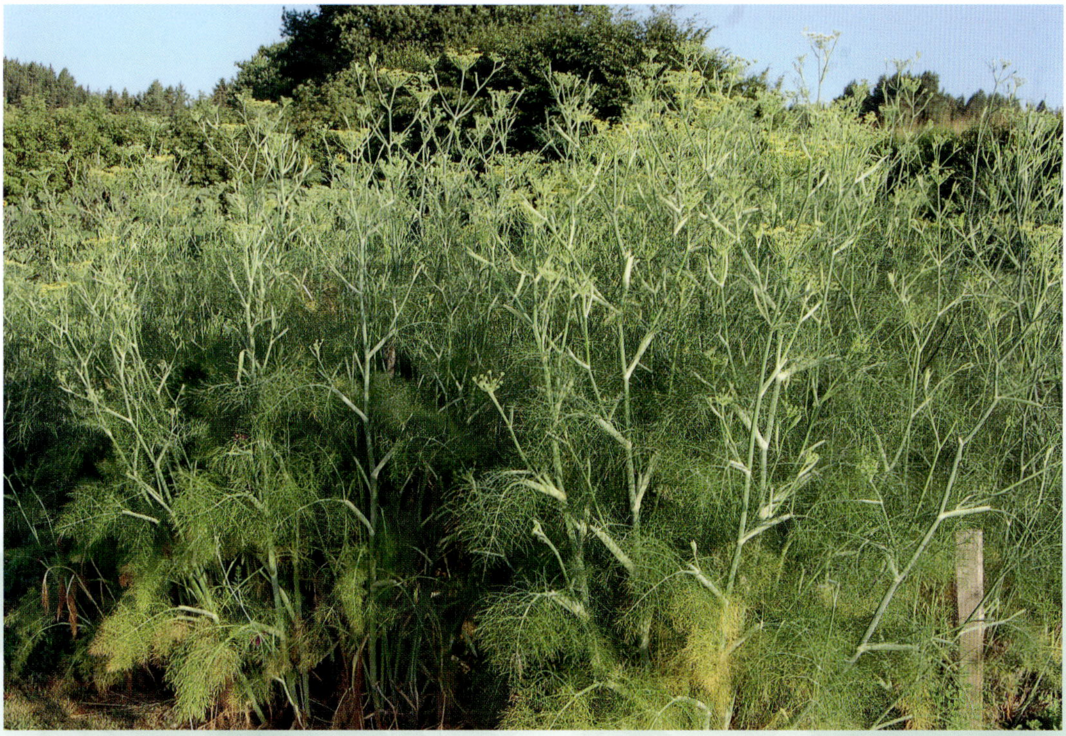

Blühender Fenchel

Goldrute

Lat. Name: *Solidago virgaurea*
Botanischer Name: Echte Goldrute
Pflanzenfamilie: Korbblütler

Die „goldene Jungfrau“ zeigt sich ab Sommermitte am Waldrand, auf Lichtungen und Wegrainen und blüht bis in den September/Oktober hinein. Sie ist von den antiken Kräuterkundigen des Mittelmeerraumes nicht beschrieben, da sie kühlere Gefilde bevorzugt.

Im Vergleich zur eingewanderten nordamerikanischen Verwandtschaft, der Kanadischen und der Riesen-Goldrute, ist die echte Goldrute ein zartes Geschöpf, das lieber vereinzelt vorkommt. Sie ist eine unwiderstehliche Köstlichkeit für Tiere des Waldes, denn der starke Mitteltrieb ist meist schon vor der Blüte verbissen.

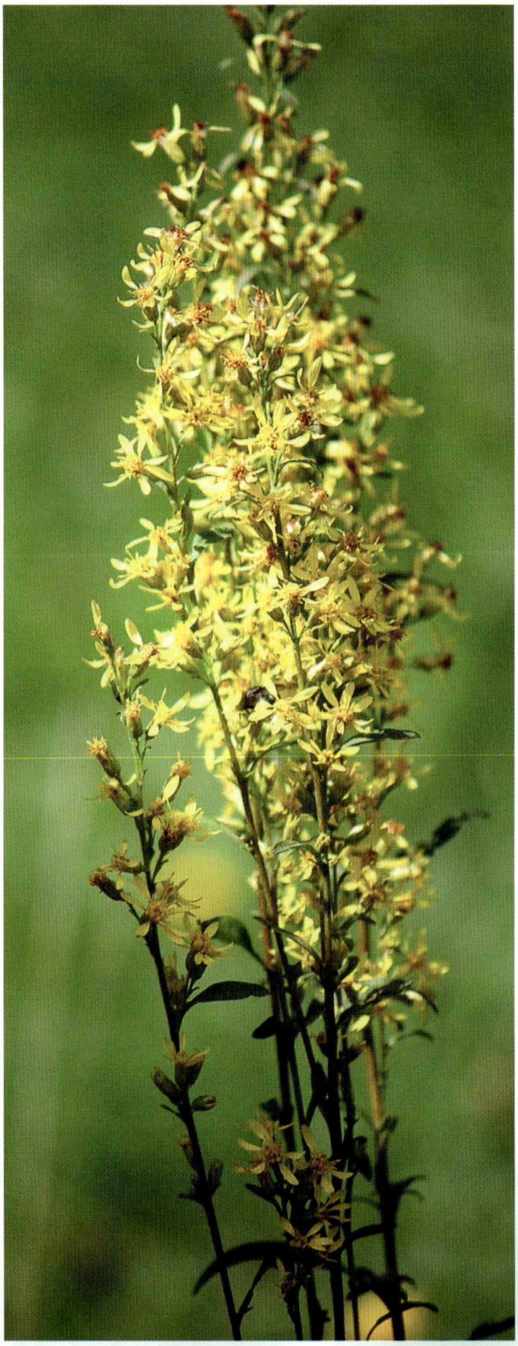

Blühende Goldrute

Rauch

Verwendete Pflanzenteile: Blätter, Stängel und noch geschlossene Blüten; die Blüten vervielfachen durch die Trocknung ihr Volumen und fliegen wie schwerelose Wattebällchen bei der geringsten Bewegung davon. Hier zeigt sich deutlich die scheue Jungfrau!

Beste Sammel- und Erntezeit: Ende Juni, Anfang Juli ist die Pflanze bereits erkennbar groß, hat die Blüten angesetzt, blüht aber noch nicht (Erntezustand). Wie am Foto erkennbar, sind die komplett geschlossenen Blüten in der Trocknung aufgeblüht. Sie haben sich jedoch noch nicht vom Stängel gelöst und können so gut verräuchert werden.

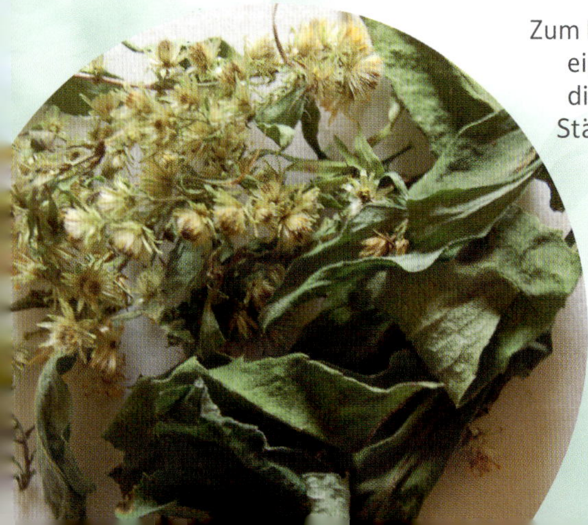

Zum Räuchern eignen sich die Blätter, Stängel und Blüten.

Wirkung, Wahrnehmung: Pflanze des geistigen Umschwungs. Positiv polend! Der wichtigste Impuls: ihr Rauch macht Schweres leicht. Segens- und Anrufungsräucherungen. Hat öffnende Wirkung auf der Gefühlsebene; unterstützt Umstimmungsprozesse und verhilft zu neuer Hoffnung. In belastenden, leidvollen und kränkenden Lebensphasen kann der Rauch der Goldrute wie ein wahrer Seelenbalsam wirken. Der Rauch holt uns aus der dunklen Ecke und spendet uns Wärme und Licht. Energetisch aufbauend bei Mangel an psychischer Energie und Antriebslosigkeit. Besonders stärkend für Menschen mit Bindungsängsten. Unterstützt die innere Harmonie. Der Rauch stärkt unsere Verbindung zu den schützenden Wesenheiten der uns umgebenden Natur.

Magisches zum Rauch: Mit der Kraft der goldenen Rute wird seit jeher Geld- und Liebesmagie in unterschiedlichen Ritualen betrieben.

Schwerpunkt, Anwendungen, Rezepte: Räucherungen zur Aufarbeitung alter Verstrickungen und Schuldmuster sowie von vergangenen stark belastenden Eintragungen in eine Raumenergie: zusammen mit Ysop, Rosenblüten und Heidekraut kombiniert mit Harz.

Mythologie und magische Praktiken

Im alpenländischen Brauchtum wird die Goldrute zur Wünschelrute, die ihren Besitzer zu Schätzen führen kann: Dazu braucht man ein reines Herz und die Hilfe von Zwergenwesen, die die Schätze der Erde hüten und sich der Kraft der „goldenen Jungfrau" nicht entziehen können.

Verwendung – gestern und heute

Eine Beschreibung der gewöhnlichen Goldrute als Heilkraut findet spät statt. Erst Matthiolus (1501–1578) erkennt ihre „gewaltig den Harn treibende und den Stein brechende" Kraft. Diese Eigenschaften der Pflanze werden noch heute in Apotheken-Präparaten genutzt.

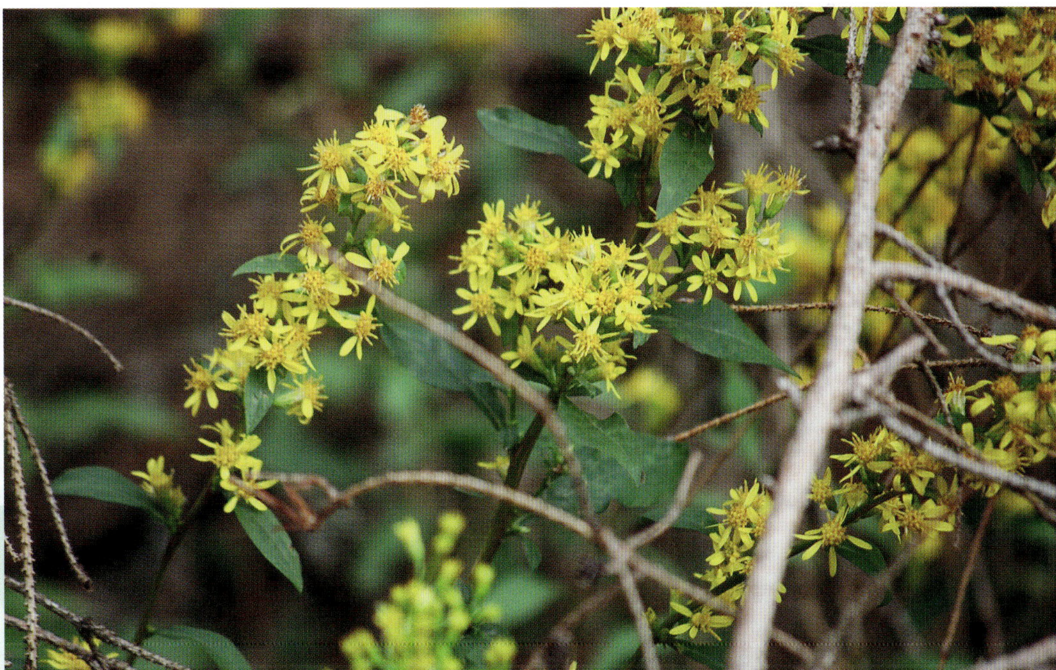

Blüten der Goldrute

Heilziest

Lat. Name: *Betonica officinalis*
Pflanzenfamilie: Lippenblütler

Jedes Jahr das gleiche Schauspiel: Irgendwann zwischen Anfang und Mitte Juli blüht im Garten der Heilziest auf. Mit dem Öffnen der ersten Blüte umschwirren ihn schlagartig zahllose Schmetterlinge, die man bis zu diesem Zeitpunkt im Garten kaum gesehen hat. Ich frage mich, wie diese sagenhafte Abstimmung zwischen Pflanze und Schmetterling funktioniert. So perfekt aufeinander abgestimmt sind diese beiden Lebensläufe, dass man nicht sagen könnte, wer wen mehr braucht. Rund um den Ziest blühen in diesen Tagen zahllose andere Kräuter in ebenfalls verführerischen Farben und Düften. Doch für die Schmetterlinge muss es der Heilziest sein, den sie bis zur letzten Blüte treu begleiten. Dann ist der Ziest verblüht und die Schmetterlinge sind verschwunden, so unbemerkt wie sie gekommen waren.

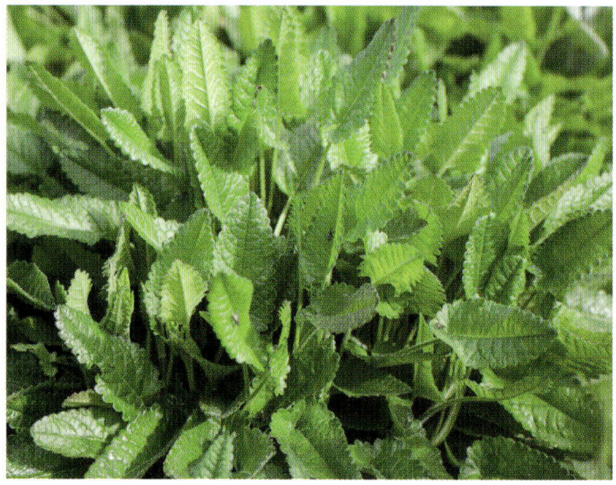

Blätter des Heilziest

Rauch

Verwendete Pflanzenteile: Das ganze blühende Kraut: Stängel, Blätter und Blüten. Die Blütenstängel können zur Gänze getrocknet werden, um dann als Trägerstab für selbst hergestellte Räucherstäbchen zu dienen.

Beste Sammel- und Erntezeit: Der Heilziest blüht meist ab Anfang Juli bis Ende August.

Wirkung, Wahrnehmung: Sehr angenehmer, balsamischer Duft, der gleich entspannend und entkrampfend wirkt. Der Rauch lindert Spannungskopfschmerzen, stressbedingte Unruhe sowie andere Spannungszustände in Körper, Geist und Seele. Großes Schutz- und Abwehrkraut: bewahrt vor negativem Zauber, Verwünschungen, Flüchen und dämonischen Überlagerungen. Stärkend und innerlich aufrichtend; hilft wieder zurück in einen heilsamen Rhythmus zu finden; sich selbst zu verzeihen, wenn es notwendig geworden ist. Segen und Schutzschild zugleich: verhilft bei tiefen seelischen Wunden langsam wieder seinen Seelenfrieden zu finden.

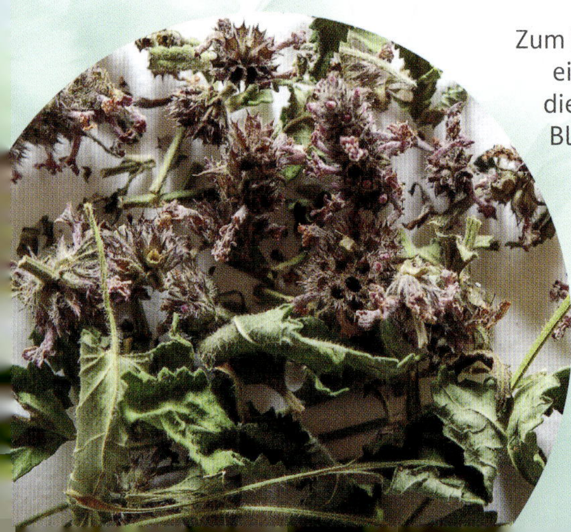

Zum Räuchern eignen sich die Stängel, Blätter und Blüten.

Magisches zum Rauch: Die große Kraft des Heilziestes verleitet auch dazu, ihn als Beschreikraut im negativen Sinne zu verwenden und mit dem Rauch der gebündelten Stängel schlechte Energien auf die Reise zu schicken. Zu bedenken wäre, dass solches Tun immer auch auf den Absender zurückfällt.

Schwerpunkt, Anwendungen, Rezepte: Zum Thema Mobbing-Abwehr hat sich eine einfache Räuchermischung mit Heilziest, Odermennig und Wermut in Kombination mit Harz bewährt.

Mythologie und magische Praktiken

Kinder, die als „verhext" galten, wurden in einem Absud der ganzen Pflanze gebadet, um den Fluch zu brechen. Hildegard von Bingen

(1098–1179) empfiehlt ein Betonica-Schlafkissen gegen „falsche Träume" und hat noch folgenden Rat für uns: „Wer dumm und einfältig ist", der solle Betonienkraut zu einem Pulver zerstoßen, einen Brei anrühren und diesen auf die Brust auftragen, mit einem Tuch festbinden; der Verstand würde dann nach und nach wieder zurückkommen!

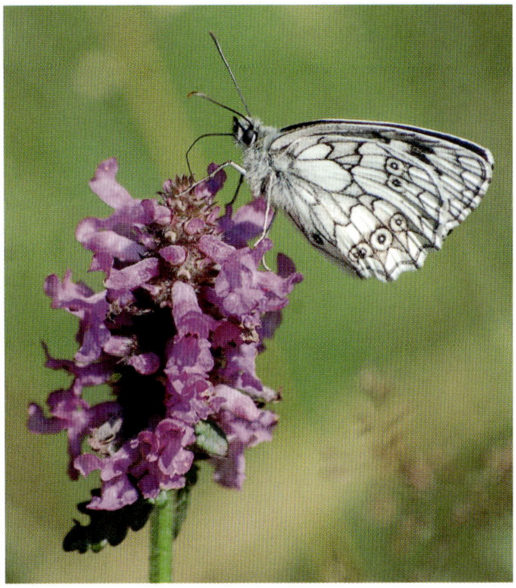
Blüte des Heilziestes

Verwendung – gestern und heute

Der Star früherer Zeiten: Seit der Antike wird der Heilziest als mächtiges Universalheilmittel eingesetzt, das sowohl innere als auch äußere Verletzungen heilen kann. Besonders der Arzt Dioskurid hob im 1. Jahrhundert n. Ch. die große Heilkraft der Betonica hervor! „Verkaufe deinen Mantel und kaufe Ziest dafür", lautete demnach eine Empfehlung.

Im 16. Jahrhundert schreibt Hieronymus Bock (1498–1554): „Bethonien Kreüter seind nützlich beinahe zu allen presten (Gebrechen), inwendig des leibs und auch ausserhalb zu geniessen."

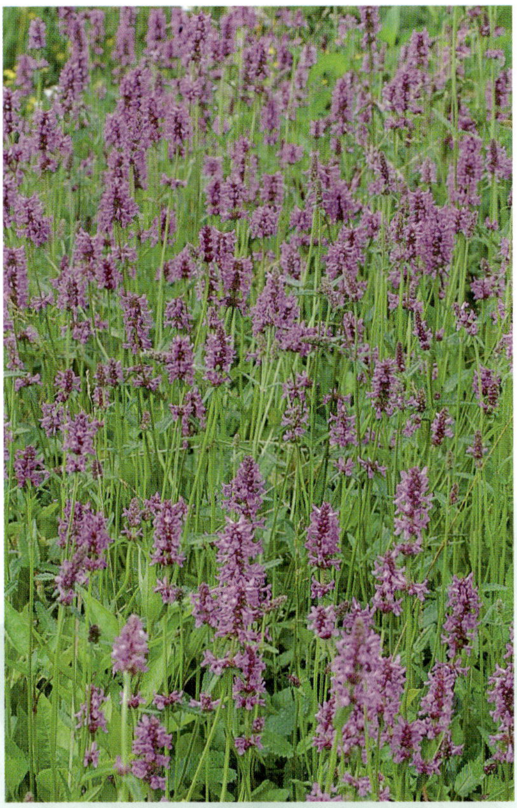
Blühender Heilziest

Im 17. Jahrhundert zitiert Nicholas Culpeper (1616–1654) in seinem Werk „Complete herbal" Antonius Musa, den Leibarzt von Kaiser Augustus (63 v. Ch. bis 14 n. Chr.), der geschrieben hatte: „Die Betonie schützt Leber und Leib vor Seuchen und schützt auch vor Zauberei." Und Culpeper fügt hinzu, um die Wirkung seines Zitates zu unterstreichen: „Es war nicht üblich, dass der Kaiser Narren in seinem Dienst hatte!" Dieser Antonius Musa (23 v. Chr. bis 1. Jhdt. n. Chr.) schrieb übrigens ein ganzes Buch über die ausserordentliche Heilkraft dieser Pflanze und gab unter anderem folgende Heilanzeigen: bei Dauerkopfschmerz, Epilepsie, Lähmungen, Sodbrennen, Krämpfen, Gicht, Leberleiden, Milzbeschwerden.

Der Heilziest zählt zu den ältesten bekannten Wundheilpflanzen: Die frischen Blätter werden als Art Pflaster auf kleinere Wunden aufgelegt. Für fiebernde Kinder werden die Essig-Patscherln in Heilziest-Essig getränkt.

Herzgespann

Lat. Name: *Leonorus cardiace*
Pflanzenfamilie: Lippenblütler

Das Herzgespann entfaltet seine ganze Pracht gerne ungehindert: Dafür verdrängt es schon einmal niedrigere Pflanzen, mäandert durch meinen Garten, wie es ihm gefällt und selbst am schotterigen Wegesrand findet es noch genug Halt, um bis zu 1,70 m hoch zu werden. Sein liebliches Rosa täuscht Friedfertigkeit vor – kaum greift man aber danach, spürt man auch schon die unbeugsamen, spitzen Kelch-Nadeln, die sich in die Finger bohren und die das blühende Kraut so geschickt unter dem in der Blütezeit leicht herabhängenden Blattwerk versteckt hält. Jede Blüte ist vielfach umstachelt, die rosa Verlockung löwenartig verteidigt. Es lässt sich Zeit mit dem Blühen, zelebriert über Wochen ein langsames Wachsen und Voranschieben des Blütenbereiches. Es ist, als hielte das Herzgespann den Sommer an, um nicht zu früh an die kommende Bitterkeit und das Vergehen denken zu müssen.

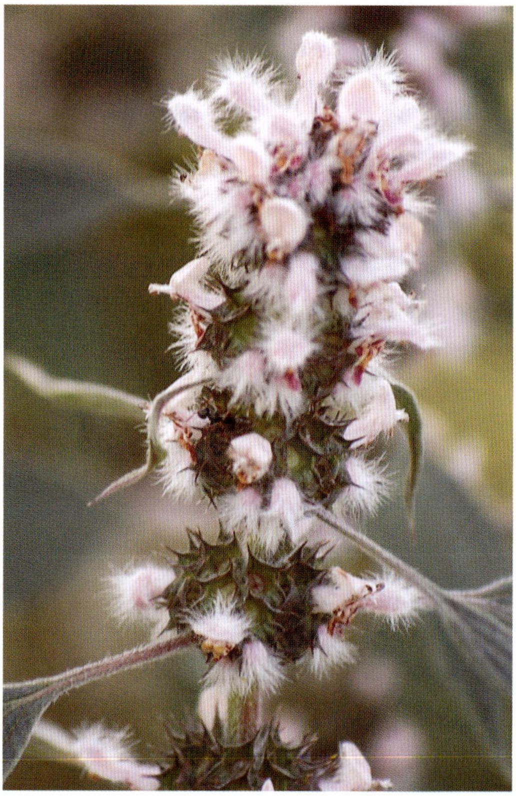

Blüte des Herzgespanns

Rauch

Verwendete Pflanzenteile: Das ganze blühende Kraut.

Beste Sammel- und Erntezeit: Ab Mitte Juni blüht die prächtige, im Blütenbereich stachelige Staude.

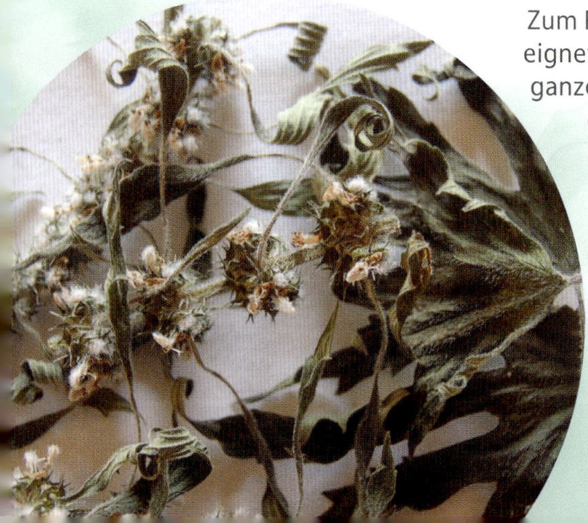

Zum Räuchern eignet sich das ganze blühende Kraut.

Wirkung, Wahrnehmung: Eine dumpfe Duftwolke scheint mit einem Atemzug alles Hochfliegende, alles Stressige, alle Unruhe auf den Boden zu zwingen. Man ist erstaunt ob der Mächtigkeit dieser klaren Information: Ruhe und Rhythmus. Man kann sich hinsetzen und will rasten, auch schlaffördernd. Wenn einem alles über den Kopf zu wachsen droht, setzt der Rauch des Herzgespannes einen Kontrapunkt. Innehalten wird möglich. Zurückfinden in den eigenen, heilsamen Rhythmus! Wie eine Notbremse, die einen nicht schont, aber zum Stehen bringt. Wenn man sich kräftemäßig verausgabt hat, aber dennoch nicht zur Ruhe kommen kann. Wenn sich alles nur mehr um das Wohl der anderen dreht und man das Gefühl hat, immer noch nicht genug zu leisten.

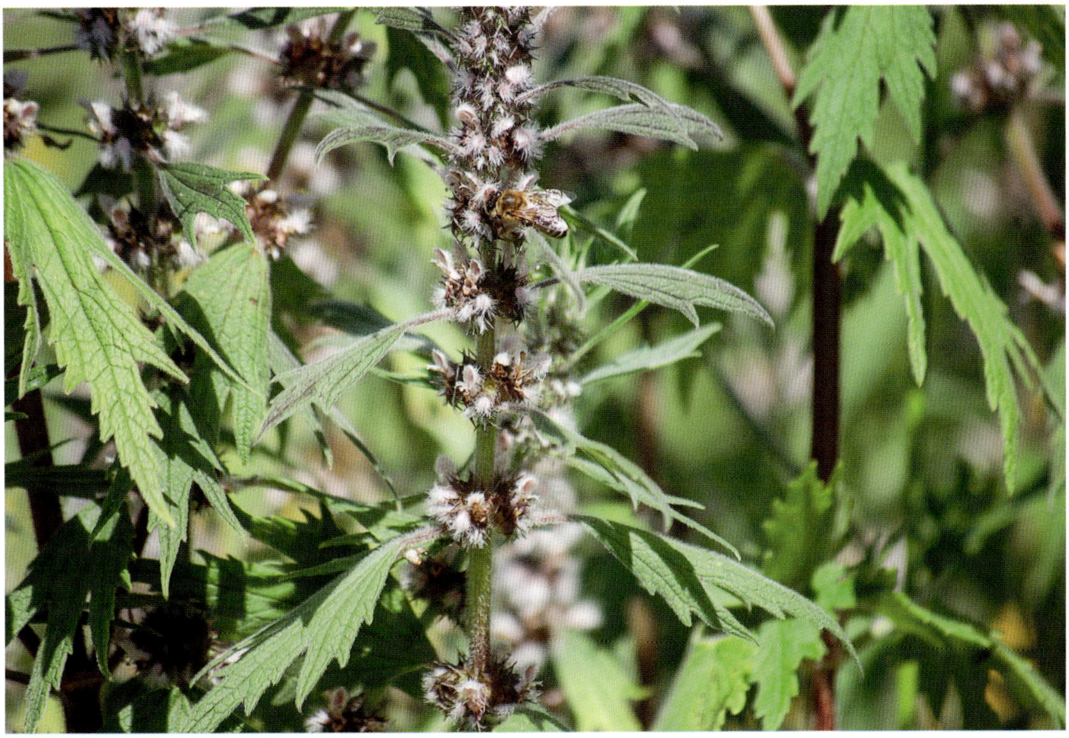

Blühendes Herzgespann

Schwerpunkt, Anwendungen, Rezepte: Um Botschaften ans Herz zu senden oder in Liebe die eigenen Ziele zu überprüfen, eignet sich folgende Räuchermischung: Herzgespann mit Johanniskraut und Diptam mit Harz kombiniert.

Verwendung – gestern und heute

Erst durch die Werke der Kräuterväter, Anfang bis Mitte des 16. Jahrhunderts, erfahren wir von heilsamen Anwendungen des Herzgespann-Krauts. So verweist Leonhart Fuchs (1501–1566) erstaunlich ungenau darauf, dass es überall dort einzusetzen wäre, wo mit bitteren Mitteln geheilt werden müsse: „Herzgespan ist fürtreffenlich gut zu dem klopffen des herzens. Item zu dem krampff und lemung der glider… und in summa vermag alles das, so den bittern dingen würt zugeeygnet."

Nicolas Culpeper (1616–1654) schreibt, dass es kein besseres Kraut gäbe, um die melancholischen Gedanken des Herzens zu zerstreuen und das Herz zu stärken. Heute ist eine Wirkung des Herzgespanns bei nervösen Herzbeschwerden bestätigt.

Johanniskraut

Lat. Name: *Hypericum perforatum*
Botanischer Name: Tüpfel-Johanniskraut
Pflanzenfamilie: Johanniskrautgewächse

Das Johanniskraut ist eine der großen Schutz- und Heilpflanzen und es ist mein mitteilsamer Lehrmeister im Reich der Kräuter!

Am Beginn meines Kräutergartens pflanzte ich die einzelnen Gewächse nach Beeten getrennt, schön eine Art neben der anderen. So auch in Beet Nr. 5 das Johanniskraut. Nach anfänglich gutem Gedeihen wurde es plötzlich rostig, verkrümmte sich und verschwand, noch ehe ich etwas ernten konnte. Klar, Wildkraut eben, dachte ich und machte keine neuen Anpflanzversuche. Es verschwand aber nicht ganz aus meinem Garten, sondern vagabundierte in den nächsten Jahren durch alle anderen Beete und zeigte mir so, wo es sich vielleicht wohlfühlen würde. Nur Beet Nr. 5 wurde geflissentlich gemieden! Zehn Jahre später staunte ich nicht schlecht, als ich in Beet Nr. 5 dicht gedrängt Johanniskraut aufgehen sah, das nicht rostig wurde und mir eine gute Ernte bescherte.

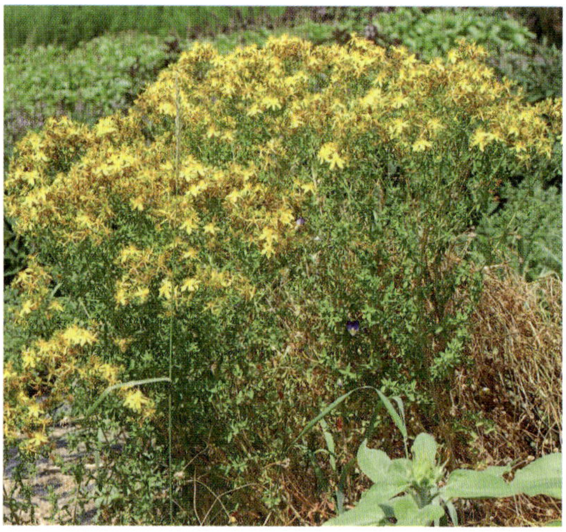

Blühendes Johanniskraut

Das Johanniskraut ist ein hoch emotionales heimisches Wildkraut, das zwar Sonnenkraft in sich trägt und diese auch über sein Blütengold nach außen zeigt, das aber einen noch viel stärkeren Bezug zum Wasserelement hat. Zwischen zwei Fingern zerrieben, färbt jede einzelne Blüte diese rot. Sein umfassendes lunares Wesen erkennt man erst im Trocknungsverhalten so richtig: Johanniskraut an Wassertagen geerntet, trocknet nicht zur Gänze! Es vervielfacht sogar seine Mondkräfte, lässt sich nicht geschlossen lagern und beginnt schließlich zu schimmeln. Sein Festhalten des Wassers ist ungleich größer als seine Hingabe an die Hitze der Sonne. Und es ist nicht bereit seinen Wesenskern der Sonnenglut zu opfern! So hilft es äußerlich gegen Verbrennungen und andere Wunden und innerlich gegen das Ausgebrannt-Sein.

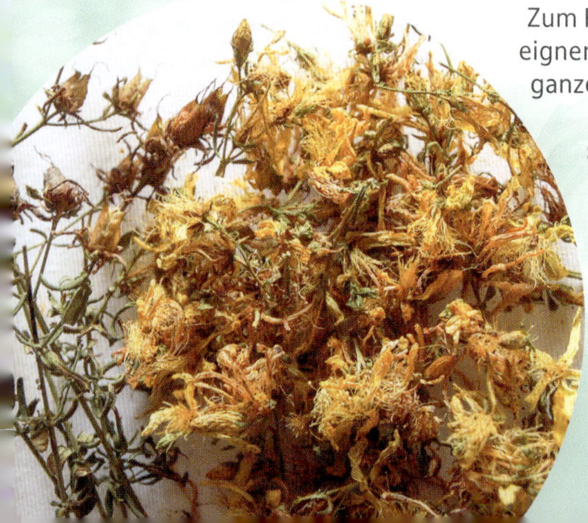

Zum Räuchern eignen sich das ganze blühende Kraut sowie die Samenstände.

Rauch

Verwendete Pflanzenteile: Das ganze blühende Kraut sowie die Samenstände.

Beste Sammel- und Erntezeit: Das Johanniskraut blüht ab dem 24. Juni, dem Johannistag und kann noch im August vereinzelt blühen, sodass es in die Kräuterbuschn am 15. August genommen werden kann; ab August/September werden die Samenstände dunkelrot und somit räucherisch sehr wertvoll.

Wirkung, Wahrnehmung: Besonderer Rauch der Sonnenwenden: zur Sommersonnenwende als spannungsabbauendes Wetterkraut; zur Wintersonnenwende als erster goldener Lichtbringer und Dämonenschreck. Heilsames Abwehr- und Segenskraut. Altes Wetterkraut; geist- und seelenschützender Burn-out-Rauch! Wenn Gewitter drohten streute man früher Johanniskrautblüten direkt auf die heiße Herdplatte, so dass viele kleine Rauchfahnen emporstiegen und sich, einen halben Meter oberhalb des Herdes, eine weißliche Rauchschicht in der Luft formierte.

Nach Streit und Ungemach, wenn in einem Raum, an einem Ort „dicke Luft" herrscht, überlagert der Johanniskraut-Rauch zuverlässig diese negativen Eintragungen. Dieser „fuga daemonum"-Rauch holt uns aus innerer Bedrängnis und Dunkelheit und kann mit seinem Sonne-Mond-Potenzial genau an unsere Ängste, Depressionen und innere Dämonen andocken, um diese mit Lebenskraft und Sonnenwärme auszugleichen und zu verfüllen. Der intensive Rauch der dunklen Samenstände macht eine sorgenbrechende Beruhigung möglich und lässt neue Hoffnung aufkeimen.

Hilfreich, um geistige Überanstrengung oder Erstarrung zu überwinden und negative Stressgefühle abzubauen. Bei ungenauen Ängsten vor Veränderungen, negativen Vorahnungen, Schlaflosigkeit, Gedankenkarussell, das einen nicht zur Ruhe kommen lässt. Wirkt stimmungsaufhellend und holt uns auf die lebensbejahende Seite zurück. Die Sonnenglut des Sommers, die in den goldgelben Blüten eingefangen ist, spendet uns wärmendes Licht im Winter. Überlagert und klärt zuverlässig jede aufgeladene Raumatmosphäre.

Magisches zum Rauch: In den Folterkammern der Inquisition wurde während der „peinlichen Befragungen" ständig Hartheu geräuchert – ob aus Angst der Folterer selbst vor dem Teufel, oder davor, dass dieser den Gemarterten zu Hilfe kommen könnte.

Zahllose wetterzauberische Sprüche und Räuchermischungen rund um das Johanniskraut, auch Hartheu oder Hartenau genannt, sind überliefert: „Hartenau und dill macht´s gewitter still", oder „Brennt eisenkraut und hartenau, dass sich das Gewitter stau."

Schwerpunkt, Anwendungen, Rezepte: Johanniskraut-Rauch erhellt die dunklen Tage und Umbrüche im persönlichen Lebenslauf wie auch die Sonnenwenden, die Übergänge im Jahreslauf. Zur Stärkung des seelischen Gleichgewichts kann folgende Räuchermischung beitragen: Johanniskraut, Kiefer (Harz), Salbei und Engelwurz.

Mythologie und magische Praktiken

Das Johanniskraut blüht zur Sommersonnenwende bzw. um den Johannistag, 24. Juni, und reicht so die höchste Kraft der Sonne an uns Erdlinge weiter. Eine Sage erzählt, dass der Teufel

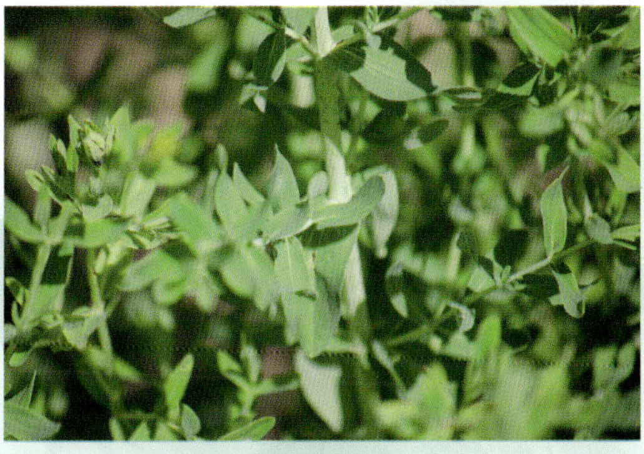

Blätter des Johanniskrauts

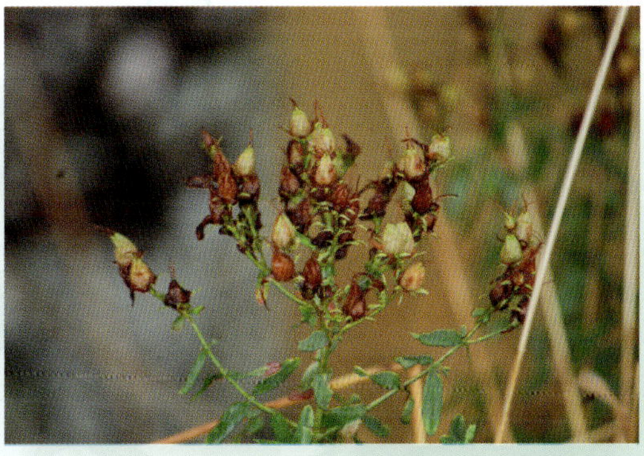

Samenstände des Johanniskrauts

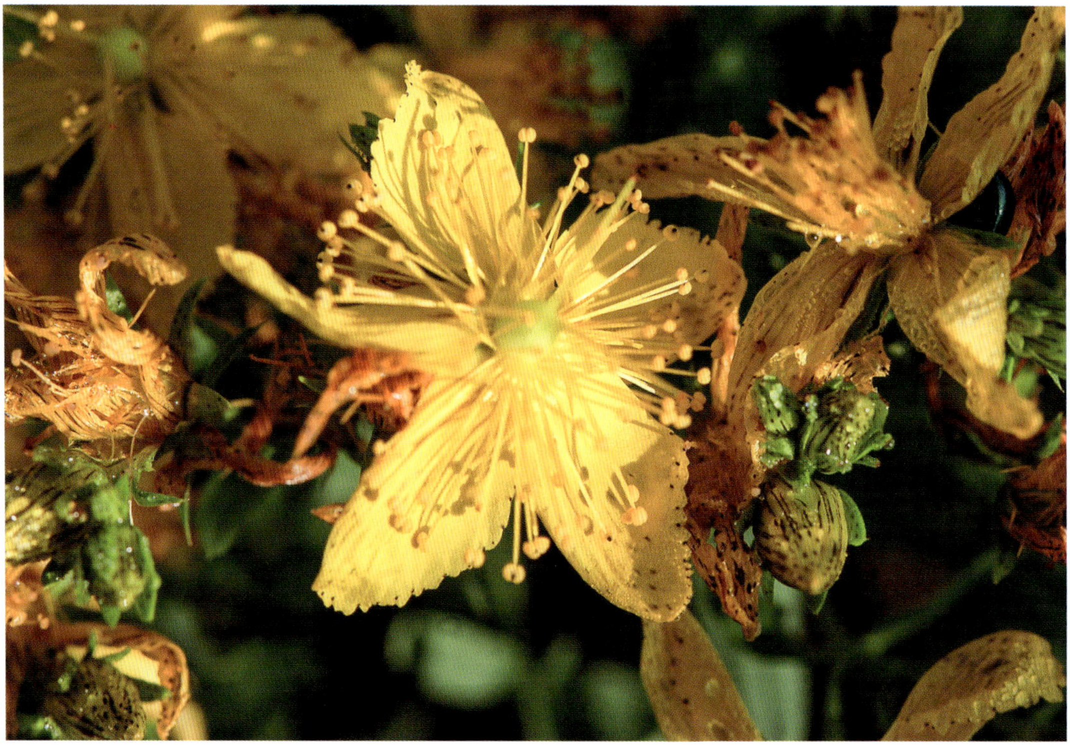

Blüte des Johanniskrauts

die grünen Blätter tausendfach durchstochen habe, weil er so erzürnt gewesen sei über die große Heilkraft dieser Pflanze.

Die fünfblättrige Blüte und die bei Zerreiben einer Blüte austretende rote Farbe signalisierten unseren Vorfahren die außergewöhnliche Abwehrkraft des Krauts: Der Fünfstern oder Drudenfuß ist die heidnische magische Abwehrzahl und muss in jedem Abwehrritual vorkommen.

Büschel und Kränze aus dem blühenden Johanniskraut wurden auf Dächern, Stalltüren, Getreidegarben oder auf dem eigenen Kopf festgemacht und sollten vor Blitz und Feuersbrunst schützen und teufels- und dämonenabwehrend wirken. Zum Auflösen von angezauberter Liebe wurde Johanniskraut in Wein gesotten und heiß getrunken: „So einer durch zauberische Liebe von Sinnen gekommen und unsinnig geworden ist."

Verwendung – gestern und heute

Paracelsus (1493–1541) schreibt in seinem „Buch von den natürlichen Dingen" von dem Sankt-Johannes-Kraut: „Die Adern auf den Blättern sind ein Zeichen, dass Perforata alle Phantasiegebilde (Phantasmata) im Menschen und auch außerhalb austreibt. Denn, die Phantasiegebilde rufen Erscheinungen hervor, so dass der Mensch Geister und Gespenster sieht und Phantasien hört…", und weiter: „Es ist eine Universalmedizin für den ganzen Menschen!"

Im 17. Jahrhundert verwendete man es äußerlich als Wundöl und innerlich „gegen Schwindel und gegen die fürchterlichen melancholischen Gedanken." Johanniskraut zählt zu den am besten erforschten Pflanzen. Seine Wirkung bei depressiven Verstimmungen ist in zahlreichen Studien nachgewiesen, das Johanniskraut-Öl ein Klassiker der Kräuterheilkunde.

Rosmarin

Lat. Name: *Salvia rosmarinus*
Pflanzenfamilie: Lippenblütler

Durch DNA-Sequenzierung wurde festgestellt, dass es kaum Unterschiede zwischen Rosmarin und Salbei-Arten gibt. Daraufhin wurde 2021 festgelegt, dass der Rosmarin keine eigene Gattung mehr darstelle, sondern zur Gattung der Salbei-Arten zähle. Diese Verwirrung zwischen Schein und Sein gefällt der Pflanze offensichtlich, fing sie doch bereits mit ihrer Namensgebung an: Die alten Griechen nannten den Rosmarin „Libanotis" was soviel heißt wie „vom Libanon stammend" und weihten sie der aus dem Meeresschaum geborenen Aphrodite, ihrer Göttin der Liebe und Schönheit. Die Römer hatten bei ihrer Namensgebung wohl die griechische Aphrodite vor Augen, wie sie den Wellen entsteigt, und nannten sie „ros marinus", „Tau des Meeres." Und das bei einer Pflanze, die trockene Standorte mit viel Hitze und Sonnenglut bevorzugt und himmelblaue Blüten hervorbringt. Aber blau ist ja bekanntlich auch das Meer an seinen schönsten Stränden. Rund ums Mittelmeer war der Rosmarin allen Völkern heilig und galt als Sinnbild für Liebe und Treue und deren Unvergänglichkeit. In diesen Gebieten kann der Rosmarin zu beeindruckender Größe heranwachsen.

Rauch

Verwendete Pflanzenteile: Das ganze Kraut. Die Stängel können zur Gänze getrocknet werden um dann als Trägerstab für selbst hergestellte Räucherstäbchen zu dienen.

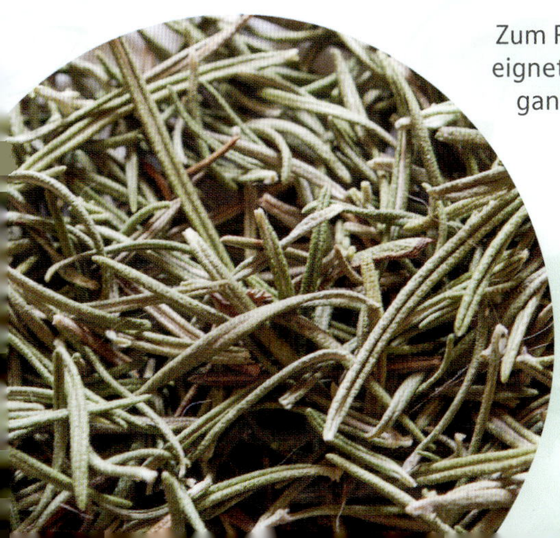

Zum Räuchern eignet sich das ganze Kraut.

Beste Sammel- und Erntezeit: Kann das ganze Jahr über geschnitten und getrocknet werden.

Wirkung, Wahrnehmung: Rosmarin, das auch „Weihrauchkraut" genannt wird, kann ohne Harz-Zugabe verräuchert werden und erzeugt einen warmen, entkrampfenden Duft. Reinigungsrauch mit desinfizierender Kraft; wurde während des Ersten Weltkrieges zur Desinfektion in den Lazaretten geräuchert; meist zusammen mit Wacholderbeeren. In Räumen, in denen sich erkaltete, negative Energien festgesetzt haben, sorgt er mit seinem „heiligen Feuer" für Bewegung und hilft dem Räuchernden selbst dabei, in Bewegung zu bleiben, um gelöste Energien schadlos abziehen zu lassen.

Gute Räucherung für Arbeitsräume, in denen hauptsächlich Kopfarbeit stattfindet. Hilfreich, wenn negative Energieeinträge produktive Gedanken blockieren. Als Pflanze des Feuers unterstützt ihr Rauch besonders die geistige Klarheit, ist förderlich zur Konzentration auf das Hier und Jetzt.

Nach belastenden Erfahrungen, negativen Erlebnissen in Beruf und Familie kann man sich mit Rosmarin, Salbei, Thymian wirkungsvoll frei räuchern. Der Rauch hilft, Veränderungen leichter anzunehmen und zu lernen, sie zu akzeptieren.

Magisches zum Rauch: Plinius (23–79) schreibt, dass der Rosmarin den römischen Hausgöttern geweiht war, weil die verräucherten Blätter wie Weihrauch duften und weil ihr Rauch böse Geister vertreibe. Leonhart Fuchs vermerkt 1543 in seinem „Neuen Kräuterbuch": „Das hauß zur zeit der Pestilentz mit Roßmarin gereücht / vertreibt darinn die bösen lüfft." Unzählige magische Räucherungen rund um Liebeszauber und Fruchtbarkeit sind belegt.

Schwerpunkt, Anwendungen, Rezepte: Räuchermischung bei schmerzenden Gelenken:

Wacholderbeeren, Rosmarin sowie Fichten- oder Tannennadeln mischen und das Räuchergefäß unter den Stuhl stellen, so dass der Rauch den ganzen sitzenden Menschen umfassen kann.

Um kalte Energien aus Räumen, von Gegenständen oder Orten zu lösen: Räuchermischung aus Rosmarin, Ysop und Holunderblüten.

Mythologie und magische Praktiken

Mit den Römern kam der Rosmarin recht früh in unseren Kulturraum und steht für den ewigen Zyklus des Lebens. Der Rosmarin begleitet den Menschen von der Geburt an, in allen Liebesangelegenheiten, bei der Hochzeit und selbst noch im Tode. Man glaubte, dass die bösen Geister, die uns umgeben, bei diesen markanten Ereignissen im Lebenslauf eines Menschen besonders gefährlich und übergriffig werden könnten. So entwickelten sich rund um diese Lebensphasen zahllose, je nach Region unterschiedliche Rosmarin-Zauber: Zur Taufe wurde Geld gesammelt, in ein Säcklein gegeben und oben drauf ein Rosmarinzweig gelegt. Um für den Täufling Glück und Reichtum herbei zu wünschen, wurde das Taufgeschenk mit folgenden Worten überreicht: „Hier bring ich vom Paten einen Strauß herein, der riecht nach lauter Rosmarein, die Wurzel wird wohl das Beste sein."
Der Rosmarin ist in Europa wohl das am meisten verwendete Kraut wenn es um Liebezauber, Liebesorakel, Treuezauber geht. Über Jahrhunderte war der Rosmarin das Pflichtkraut bei jeder Hochzeit. Der Bräutigam trug ein Zweigerl an der Brust, die Braut hatte den Rosmarin im Brautstrauß und ins Haar geflochten. Wenn eines davon herunterfiel, war es ein schlechtes Zeichen. Nach der Hochzeit steckte das neue Ehepaar die Zweiglein in die Erde, wo sie hoffentlich bewurzelten, was wiederum als gutes Zeichen für die junge Ehe galt.

Auch bei den Totenritualen war der Rosmarin omnipräsent. Er wurde im ägyptischen Totenkult verwendet und Ovid (43 v. Chr. bis 17 n. Chr.) berichtet, dass Tote stets mit Rosmarin- und Olivenzweigen eingeäschert wurden. Be-

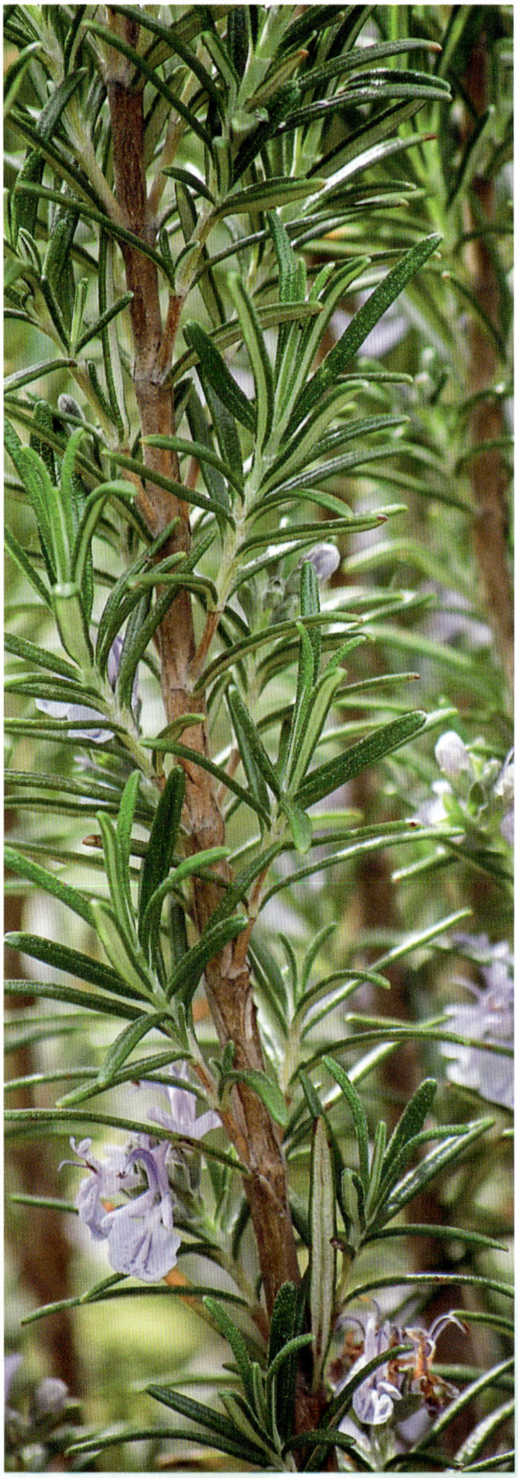

Blühender Rosmarin

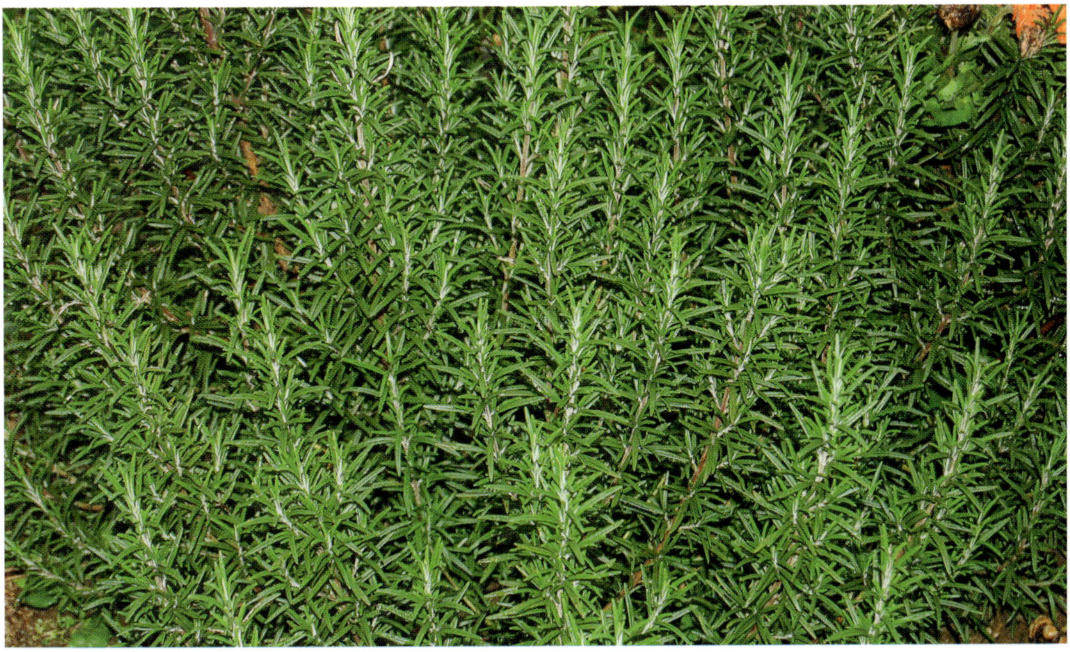

Rosmarinblätter

sonders im angelsächsischen Raum wurden die Toten mit Rosmarin bestreut, wurden Rosmarinzweige mit in den Sarg gegeben und ebenso an die Trauernden verteilt.

Der Rosmarin hat aber auch eine magische Verbindung zu Schülern und Studenten: In der Antike wurde er ihnen ins Haar geflochten, um das Lernen zu erleichtern und das Gedächtnis zu steigern.

Diese geistige Komponente, dass nämlich Rosmarin ein Kraut sei, das das Erinnerungsvermögen stärke, findet sich auch in Shakespeares (1564–1616) „Hamlet". Da zählt Ophelia (4. Akt, 5. Szene) in ihrem Wahn sieben Kräuter auf und beginnt dabei mit dem Rosmarin: „There´s rosemary, that´s for rememberance; pray, love, remember...."

Zu den „Engelländern" weiß Balthasar Ehrhart (1700–1756) in Verbindung mit dem Rosmarin zu berichten: „In catharrosen Kranckheiten hat das Rosmarin-Thee auch gehörigen Platz, als welches von denen Engelländern sehr geliebt wird."

Verwendung – gestern und heute

Kaiser Karl der Große (741–814) verfügt um das Jahr 800 in seinem „Capitulare de villis vel curtis imperii" an 13. Stelle von 73 Pflanzen, den Anbau von „rosmarinum" auf seinen Königshöfen. Hieronymus Bock (1498–1554) meint in seinem „New Kreütterbuch": „Roßmarein die wurtz, gehört in unserm land auch in die kuchen und keller, darumb das alle kost, speiß und tranck mit Roßmarein bereit, lieblich wol schmecken und beinahe zu allen presten gesundt seind." Er empfiehlt auch eine Art Rosen-Zucker mit den Blüten anzusetzen, da dieser als „krafft unnd sterckung der onmacht gebraucht" werde.

Rosmarin ist ein Muntermacher, aktiviert den Kreislauf und fördert die Durchblutung. Wertvoll auch als Tee, der besonders gut Fastentiefs ausgleichen kann.

Lavendel

Lat. Name: *Lavandula angustifolia*
Botanischer Name: Echter Lavendel
Pflanzenfamilie: Lippenblütler

Schon Perser, Griechen und Römer verbrannten Lavendel, um ihre Krankenzimmer zu reinigen. Er ist durch und durch eine Pflanze des Ausgleichs. Seine blaue Seelenfarbe und der unvergleichliche Duft haben den Lavendel zu einem der bewährtesten Volksheilmittel gemacht. In Töpfen und in Beeten spendet er über Wochen Freude fürs Auge, betörenden Duft für die Nase und Beruhigung für die Seele. Manchmal kommt es mir so vor, als gäbe es eine direkte Beziehung zwischen der Zunahme von Lavendel in Töpfen und Gärten und dem hektischen Lebensstil, der unsere Zeit prägt. Das ständige „mehr und schneller" braucht einen Ausgleich und der Lavendel scheint unsere Herzen mit der richtigen Botschaft zum kurzen Verweilen zu erreichen.

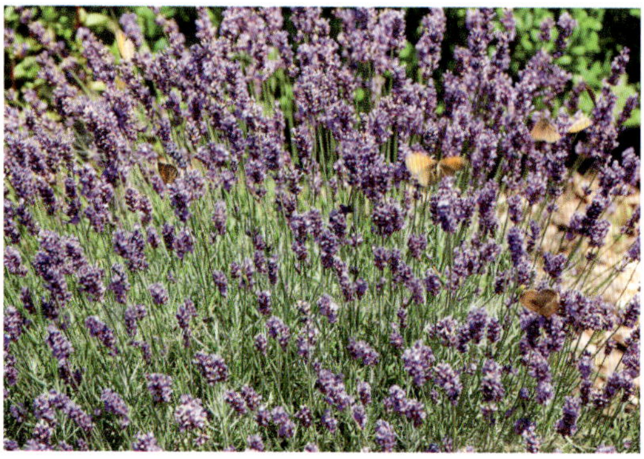

Blühender Lavendel

Rauch

Verwendete Pflanzenteile: Das ganze blühende Kraut: Blüten, Blätter, Stängel. Es können alle Lavendel-Sorten verräuchert werden. Die Blütenstängel können zur Gänze getrocknet werden, um dann als Trägerstab für selbst hergestellte Räucherstäbchen zu dienen.

Beste Sammel- und Erntezeit: Stängel und Blätter das ganze Jahr über, die Blüten ab Blühbeginn bis oft in den Oktober hinein.

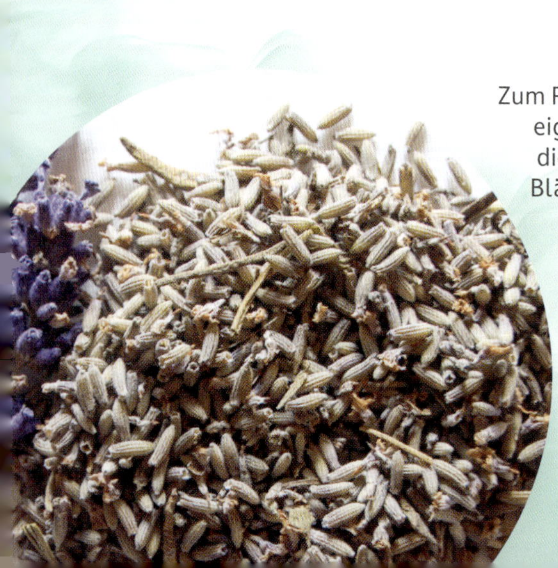

Zum Räuchern eignen sich die Blüten, Blätter und Stängel.

Wirkung, Wahrnehmung: Ganzheitlicher Reinigungsrauch mit starkem Bezug zu Geist und Seele. Große weißmagische Kraft, die Abwehr und Schutz vermittelt. Lavendel kann allein verräuchert werden. Die besondere Gnade des Lavendel-Rauches besteht aber darin, dass er viele Räuchermischungen unterstützt und abrundet, ohne dabei selbst dominant in den Vordergrund zu treten. Man spürt lediglich den sanften Flügelschlag einer unvergleichlichen und so auch schwer zu beschreibenden Wesenheit.

Vermittelt merkurielle Leichtigkeit: Lavendel-Rauch überlagert aktuelle, negative Raumeintragungen durch Streit, andere belastete Raumenergien und chaotische Rauminformationen, die durch mehrere Strahlungsquellen verursacht werden. Gibt in allen seelischen Notlagen Klarheit und ermöglicht so zu einer neuen Ordnung zu finden. Auf geistiger Ebene: verhindert Fixierungen; verhilft zu neuer Beweglichkeit im Denken und schärft die Kombinationsgabe im Lernen. Lässt einen wieder aufatmen und lächeln.

Magisches zum Rauch: Der Rauch des Lavendels, der am 24. Juni, dem Johannistag, geerntet wird, soll besondere Kräfte entfalten und vor bösen Zaubern, Flüchen und Verwünschungen schützen. Auch dunkle Gestalten und Angstschatten sollen durch diesen Rauch ferngehalten werden. Dem Lavendel wurden Zauberkräfte gegen das Verschreien, Verfluchen zugeschrieben.

Schwerpunkt, Anwendungen, Rezepte: Der Rauch fürs Kinderzimmer: glättet kindliche Unruhe, unbestimmte Ängste, vermindert das Nicht-einschlafen-Können; beseitigt Stolpersteine der pubertären Entwicklung. Der Rauch im Sterbezimmer, der den Zurückbleibenden einen liebevollen Abschied ermöglicht, aber vielmehr noch der scheidenden Seele den Übergang in ihre neue Welt erleichtert. Räuchermischung zum Stressabbau: Lavendel, Rosenblüten, Fichte (Harz), Weißdorn, Eberesche.

Mythologie und magische Praktiken

Die Abwehrkraft dieses Krauts soll so groß sein, dass es sogar Übeltäter und böse Geister schützt, wenn sie vom Teufel verfolgt werden: Durch bloßes Anfassen oder Draufsetzen auf einen Lavendelstrauch seien sie in Sicherheit.

Verwendung – gestern und heute

„lavare", das lateinische Wort für „waschen", bezeichnet die Hauptverwendung des Lavendels bei den Römern: Sie schätzten seinen Geruch und setzten Lavendel dem Badewasser zu – wie dies von Julius Cäsar (100–44 v. Chr.) bekannt ist.

Hildegard von Bingen (1098–1179) sieht im Lavendel eine „Mutter-Gottes-Pflanze", die unkeusche Gelüste vertreibe: „Lavendel wäscht Körper und Seele rein, vertreibt böse Geister und unreine Gedanken, stärkt das ICH und ist ein bitterer Trank gegen Leberleiden".

Aller Lavendel-Sackerln Anfang liegt vermutlich im 16. Jahrhundert, als eine Vielzahl von Empfehlungen verschriftlicht wurde, dass Lavendel gegen Motten, Schaben und anderes Ungeziefer im Haushalt wirksam sei. So schreibt beispielsweise Lonicerus (1528–1586) unter der Bezeichnung „Lavendel, Lavendula": „Lavendel in Wasser gesotten, in dem Wasser ein Hemd genetzt, von sich selbst getrucknet und angethan, fängt und behält keine Läuß, so lang es den Geruch von Lavendel hat."

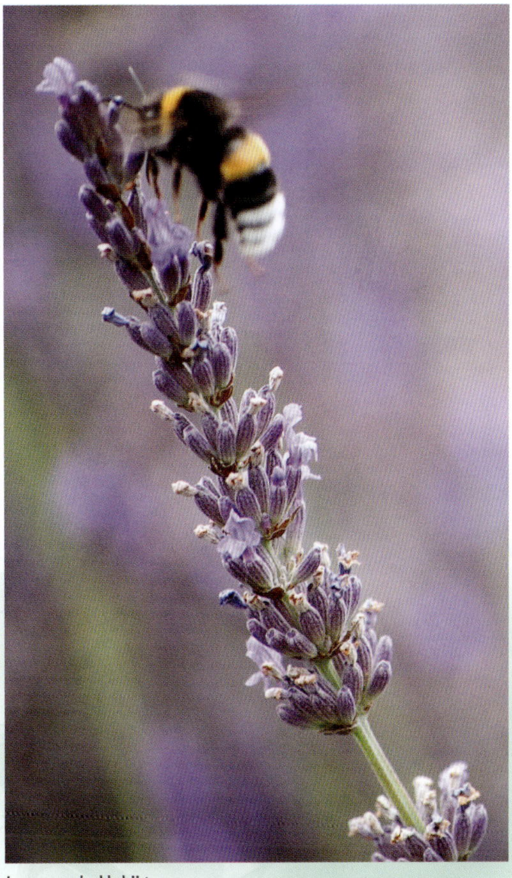

Lavendelblüte

Mädesüß

Lat. Name: *Filipendula ulmaria*
Pflanzenfamilie: Rosengewächse

Im Hochsommer finde ich das Mädesüß, die „Wiesenkönigin", stets schmal und hochaufragend am Sumpfrand oder entlang des Flusses Gurk oder an feuchten Stellen irgendwo entlang des Straßenrandes – bevorzugt absonnig, die Füße im kühlen Nass, umweht von unbändigem Wohlgeruch und in derart strahlendem Weiß, dass mir ganz warm ums Herz wird. Immer höher steigen die wattebauschähnlichen Blüten, wie transparente Etagen eines Wolkenkratzers und meine Augen fahren staunend auf und ab.

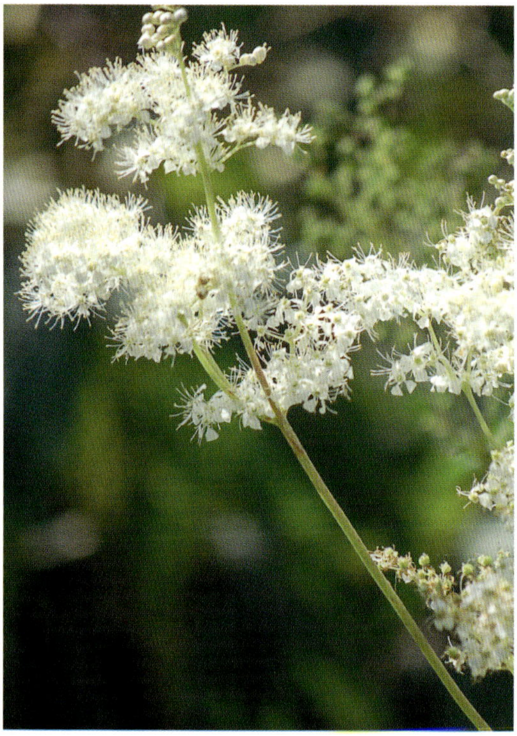
Blühendes Mädesüß

Rauch

Verwendete Pflanzenteile: Das ganze blühende Kraut: Blüten, Blätter, Stängel.

Beste Sammel- und Erntezeit: Ab Mitte Juni blüht das Mädesüß.

Wirkung, Wahrnehmung: Als Kraut der Sommersonnenwende und altes Wetterkraut trägt sein Rauch zur Entspannung und Entkrampfung von negativ überladenen Raumatmosphären und geistiger Überspanntheit bei. Zu den Sonnenwenden und anderen Übergängen soll dieser Rauch Dämonen und dunkle Wesenheiten abwehren und fernhalten.

Hilfreich bei allen Neuanfängen und Lebensübergängen: unterstützt und bekräftigt die schon vorhandenen positiven Erwartungen und soll Glück ins neue Haus, in die neue Beziehung, in den neuen Beruf ziehen. Es ist, als wandle sich das gleißende Weiß der Blüten im Rauch zu warmem Sonnenlicht, das einen einhüllt, aufbaut und träumen lässt.

Magisches zum Rauch: Mädesüß wurde für viele wetterwenderische Rituale eingesetzt: in Räuchermischungen mit Johanniskraut, Beifuß, Eisenkraut oder Rainfarn. In einigen Teilen Nordeuropas sollte der Mädesüß-Rauch den Dieb entlarven, wenn dieser auch nur in die Nähe des Rauches kam.

Schwerpunkt, Anwendungen, Rezepte: Mit Beifuß und Harz verräuchert, fördert der Rauch die Weitsicht und hilft, über den Dingen zu stehen.

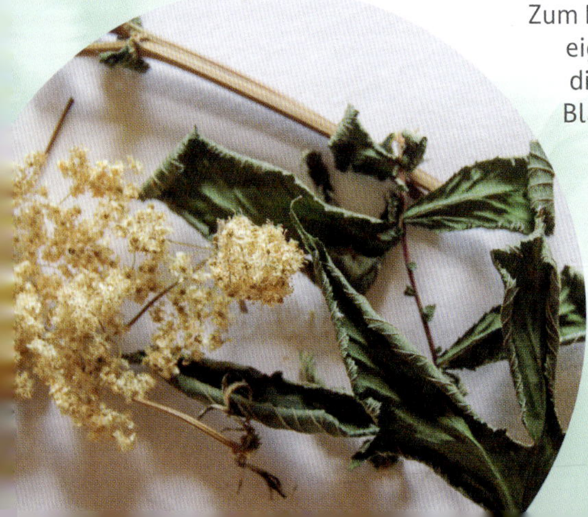
Zum Räuchern eignen sich die Blüten, Blätter und Stängel.

Mythologie und magische Praktiken

Mädesüß zählte zu den unheilabwehrenden Pflanzen, wurde um die Sommersonnenwende geerntet und gebüschelt auf Dachböden und in Ställen gegen Feuersbrunst, Unwetter und Krankheiten von Mensch und Vieh aufgehängt. Besonders beliebt waren Mädesüß-Kränze für Liebesmagie sowie Mädesüß-Blüten als Streukraut bei Hochzeiten, über welches das Brautpaar schreiten musste, um deren Wohlgeruch und die unheilabwehrende, schützende Kraft aufzunehmen.

Verwendung – gestern und heute

Neben Mistel, Eisenkraut und Brunnenkresse zählte das Mädesüß zu den vier heiligen Pflanzen der keltischen Druiden. Vor allem im englischen Bereich erkennt man eine durchgängige Verwendung der Pflanze ob als Streukraut am Hof von Königin Elisabeth I. (1533–1603) oder als fruchtig-süße Geschmacksverbesserung von Weinen.

Nicolas Culpeper (1616–1654) stellt die Wiesenkönigin, „queen of the meadows", unter die Herrschaft der reinen Venus. Er schreibt, dass sie verwendet werde, um alle Arten von Blutungen, Erbrechen und andere Bauchflüsse zu stillen. Sie mache „a merry heart", ein fröhliches Herz, wofür manche die Blüten und andere die Blätter verwendeten. Bereits 1839 isolierten zwei deutsche Chemiker, K. J. Löwig und S. Weidemann, Salicylsäure aus dem Mädesüß. Nach diesem Bauplan wurde die magenverträglichere Acetylsalicylsäure synthetisch hergestellt, heute besser bekannt als „Aspirin".

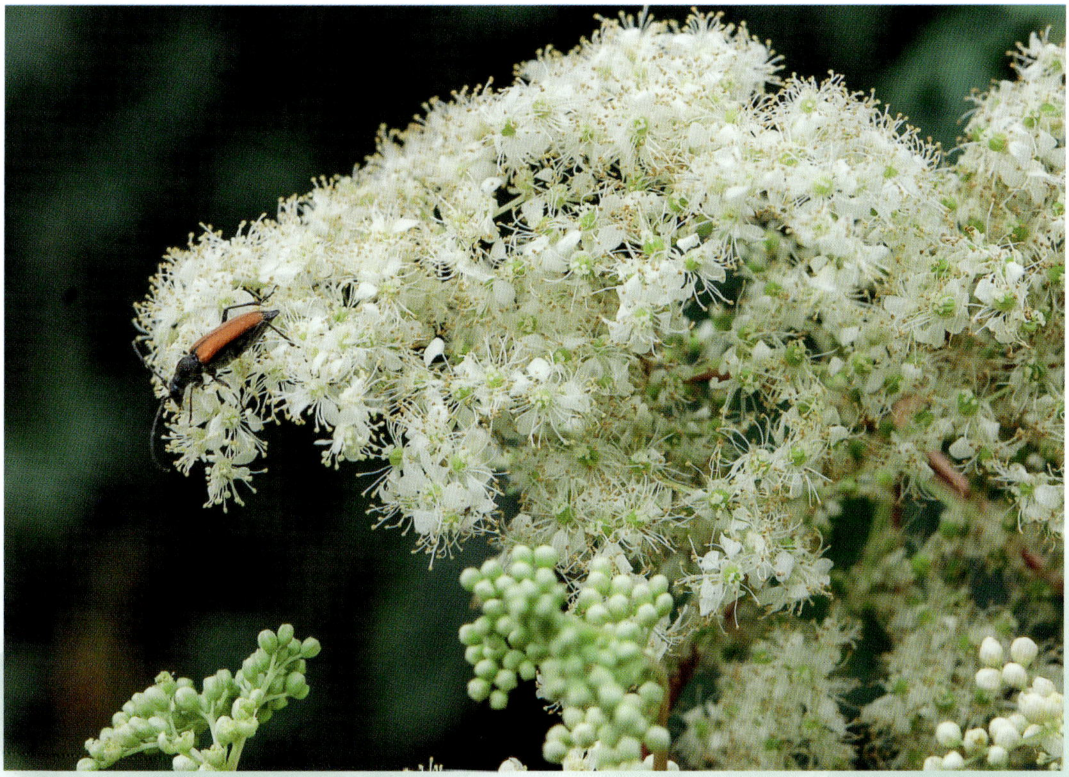

Blüte von Mädesüß

Rainfarn

Lat. Name: *Tanacetum vulgare*
Pflanzenfamilie: Korbblütler

Die Aufgabe von Rainfarn ist wohl die energetische Entflechtung seiner Umgebung. Er sucht geradezu Orte mit viel Unruhe, hält sich an den spannungsgeladensten Straßenrändern auf, nimmt diese verqueren Energieströme auf und wandelt sie in eine verträglichere Atmosphäre, leitet sie durch seine dunklen harten Stängel bis hinauf in die prallen gelben Knöpfe, die wie gespannte, feuerbereite Geschosse vor Dynamik zu bersten scheinen. Hier heroben ist das gelbe Ziel, die sonnenhafte Mächtigkeit tausendfach in kugelige Blütenköpfe verpackt. Nicht von ungefähr ist der Rainfarn auch eine taugliche Färbepflanze, die mit Alaun vorbehandelte Wolle intensiv dunkelgelb färbt.

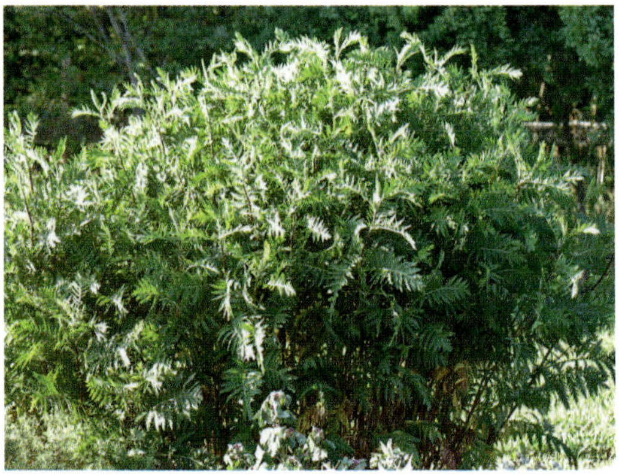

Blätter des Reinfarns

Rauch

Verwendete Pflanzenteile: Blätter, Blüten. Die Blütenstängel können zur Gänze getrocknet werden um dann als Trägerstab für selbst hergestellte Räucherstäbchen zu dienen.

Beste Sammel- und Erntezeit: Ab dem Blühbeginn, meist Ende Juli.

Wirkung, Wahrnehmung: Reinigungs- und Abwehrrauch; starkes Wetterkraut, das gegen Blitze und schlimme Gewitter geräuchert wurde. Man nennt den Rainfarn auch Donner- und Blitz-Kraut. Der Rainfarn-Rauch kann in Häusern und einzelnen Räumen hohe Spannungen abmildern und ausgleichen, genauso wie er auch belastenden Elektrosmog spielend überlagert.

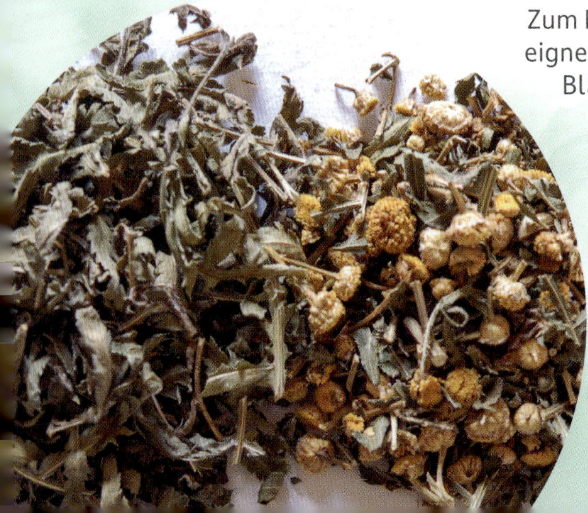

Zum Räuchern eignen sich die Blätter und Blüten.

Lässt Orte und Plätze in Häusern und in freier Natur ihren eigentlichen Genius spüren, legt diesen frei. Auf stark negativ belasteten Stellen reicht die Rainfarn-Energie meist nur für ein kurzes Aufblitzen; hier sollte mit einem stimmigen Ritual gearbeitet werden, um die Verstrickungen für länger, vielleicht sogar ganz, aufzulösen. Bei personenbezogenen Rainfarn-Räucherungen wird die emotionale und geistige Abwehrkraft gestärkt. Der Rauch wirkt gegen böse Geister, dunkle Dämonen und unbestimmte Ängste. Rainfarn kann bei allen Schwächezuständen verräuchert werden; macht Mut und hebt das Selbstwertgefühl und fokussiert ein positives Ich-Gefühl. Die kleinen Sonnenknöpfe springen wie Räuchertabletten in die Räucherschale und helfen gegen Verzagtheit, innere Unruhe, Unsicherheit und versuchte Übergriffe Dritter auf unsere Persönlichkeit.

Unterstützt eine klare Abgrenzung gegenüber anderen; befreit das Ego von fremden Lasten und hilft, auch wieder allein Fuß zu fassen; wirft einen Anker in die Seele, der das „bis hierher und nicht weiter“ in Erinnerung hält und immer besser umsetzen lässt.

Magisches zum Rauch: Am 28. März 1485 erscheint unter dem Titel „Gart der Gesundheit“ das erste gedruckte Kräuterbuch in deutscher Sprache, verfasst vom Arzt Johann Wonnecke von Kaub. Zum Rainfarn wird folgendes vermerkt: „Welche frawe yr kinder lyphafftig und frysch behalten wollen, di sollen die kinder über den rauch halten diß kruts: der benympt yn alle zufelligen sucht und alle böse gespenst des düfels und mat yn nit geschaden.“

Tabernaemontanus (1522–1590) notiert: „Der Rauch von Reynfahrn macht die jungen Kinder lustig unnd frölich, behütet sie vor Kranckheit unnd soll darneben alle Fantaseyen unnd Gespenst vertreiben, derowegen man die Kinder unnd Kindbetterinnen damit zu beräuchern pfleget.“

Schwerpunkt, Anwendungen, Rezepte: Zusammen mit Wermut, Dost und Johanniskraut ergibt der Rainfarn einen guten Abwehrrauch für die Raunächte und schützt uns so vor der Trud und anderen furchterregenden Wesen. Das Donner- und Blitz-Kraut soll starker Gewitterspannung entgegenwirken können: Dazu mischt man Rainfarn mit Königskerze und Beifuß oder Salbei. Harz kombinieren.

Mythologie und magische Praktiken

Den schwächlichen Kindern wurde ein Rainfarn-Säckchen unter das Kopfkissen gelegt, um sie zu kräftigen. Die offensichtliche große Kraft des Krauts verführte auch immer wieder zur Liebes-Zauberei, wobei es sich vor allem um Rituale zum Erzwingen von Liebe handelte.

Verwendung – gestern und heute

In der, um das Jahr 800 erlassenen Anbauverfügung Kaiser Karls des Großen (747–814), dem „Capitulare de villis vel curtis imperii“, werden 73 Kräuter und Gemüsesorten zum Anbau auf allen Königshöfen des Reiches vorgeschrieben. Der Rainfarn steht als „tanazitam“ an der 44. Stelle.

Hildegard von Bingen (1098–1174) beschreibt sehr ausführlich eine Anwendung für Frauen, die an „verstopftem Monatsfluss“ leiden. Weiters empfiehlt sie seinen Gebrauch gegen Husten, bei Magen-Schwere und -Drücken, sowie all jenen, „die den Harn nicht lassen“ können.

Tabernaemontanus (1522–1590) überliefert seitenweise Anwendungen des Rainfarns. Darunter auch ein äußerlich anzuwendendes Blüten-Öl: „Den Kindern, die Würm haben, soll man dieses Öl warm in Nabel reiben, das tödtet die Würm unnd treibet sie aus.“ Auch Balthasar Ehrhart (1700–1756), deutscher Mediziner, Apotheker und Botaniker vermerkt im Jahr 1737 in seinem Kommentar zum Kräuterbuch des Lonicerus (1528–1586) zum Rainfarn: „Zu Pag. 346, vom Rhainfarn. Dieses Kraut gehöret sonderlich unter diejenigen, welche wenig aestimiret werden und doch viel vermögen.“

Das alte Wurmkraut ist heute als **leicht giftig** einzustufen und nicht mehr für den innerlichen Gebrauch zu verwenden. Auszüge des Krauts helfen hingegen im Garten gegen Schadinsekten.

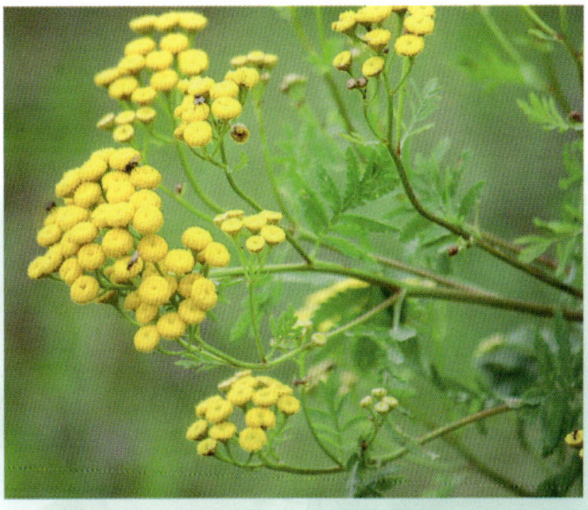

Blüte des Rainfarns

Salbei

Lat. Name: *Salvia officinalis*
Botanischer Name: Echter Salbei
Pflanzenfamilie: Lippenblütler

Der Name Salbei leitet sich vom lateinischen ab: „salvare" bedeutet retten, erlösen, „salvere" gesund sein, „salvus" wohlbehalten, heil und „Salvia" ist das Heilsame. Mit dem Gruß „Salve" wünscht man bei den Römern Gesundheit – und zwar „Sei gesund", auch „Sei willkommen!" Allein durch die Namensgebung zeigt sich die besondere Stellung des Salbeis unter den Heilkräutern: Er galt in den letzten zwei Jahrtausenden als Inbegriff heilsamer Kräuterkraft, weil er die menschliche Konstitution gegen den Verschleiß durch die Zeit zusammenhalten und das Wohlbefinden, vor allem im Alter, wirkungsvoll unterstützen kann. Der Lehrspruch lautete: „Contra vim mortis, crescit salvia in hortis!" Gegen die Kraft des Todes wächst Salbei im Garten; oder: „Wer auf Salbei baut, den Tod kaum schaut."

Im deutschen Sprachraum hieß es auch: „Treibt der Salbei üppig aus, herrscht nicht mehr der Mann im Haus!"

Rauch

Verwendete Pflanzenteile: Blätter, auch Blüten.

Beste Sammel- und Erntezeit: Den ganzen Sommer über bis spätestens Anfang September. Dann sollte der Salbei zurückgeschnitten sein und in Ruhe gelassen werden, damit er gut über den Winter kommt.

Getrocknete Salbeiblätter

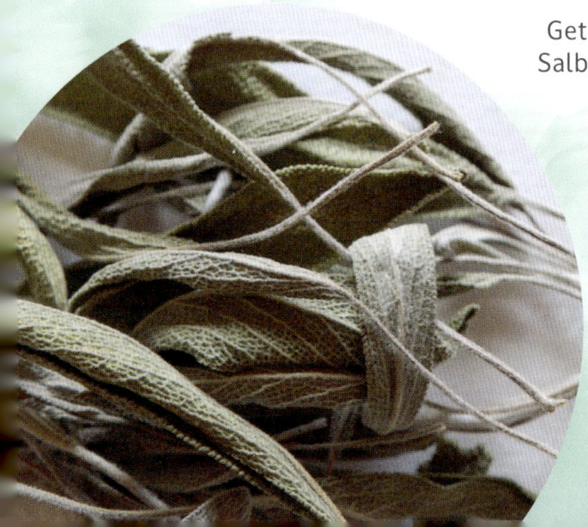

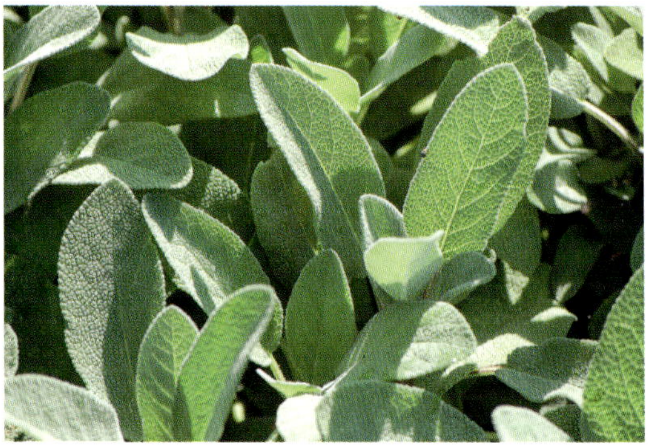

Salbeiblätter

Wirkung, Wahrnehmung: Die stark reinigende Kraft. In Räumen und an Orten löst und überlagert sein Rauch negative Eintragungen und als unangenehm empfundene, unbeweglich lauernde, kalte Energien. Der Salbei-Rauch kann stressbeladene Energie-Hinterlassenschaften wirkungsvoll verändern.

Unterstützt den Selbstschutz und die Abgrenzung gegenüber belastenden Energien, die von Orten, Gegenständen oder Menschen ausgehen; klärt und schützt die Aura. Abwehrrauch mit dämonenverscheuchender, geisterbannender Kraft, die stark lichtförderlich wirkt und uns im Innersten stabilisieren kann. Stimmungsausgleich; aufbauender, stark seelenschützender, klärender Rauch, der augenblicklich das Gefühl von Sicherheit und Geborgenheit auslösen kann.

Mutter-Schützerin-Pflanze, deren Rauch Übergänge erhellt, Veränderungen positiv begleitet und uns bei allen Arten von Unsicherheiten, erdet. Lebensübergänge und Phasen aufwühlender Lebensveränderungen können positiv gebildert und überdacht werden. In solchen Phasen hält der Salbei-Rauch Körper, Geist und Seele zusammen! Bringt verloren gegangene Energien zurück, hilft dabei, sich zu konzentrieren und sich unter veränderten Bedingungen neu auszurichten.

Magisches zum Rauch: Mit dem Kraut der Aphrodite wurden viele liebeszauberische Rituale durchgeführt: Um Liebe zu erwecken, um Liebe abzuwehren, um Liebe zwischen zwei Menschen auszulöschen. Stets wurde dazu Salbei verräuchert, um die Flüche und Bannungen auch in der geistigen Welt zu verankern. Indem man neun Salbeiblätter unter Rauch und Gebeten verzehrte, glaubte man vor jedem Fieber gefeit zu sein.

Schwerpunkt, Anwendungen, Rezepte: Die schnelle Reinigungsräucherung für zwischendurch: Ein getrocknetes Salbeiblatt anzünden, das Feuer ausblasen und am Stängel haltend mit dem feinen Duftfaden den gewünschten Bereich oder sich selbst abräuchern. Für gute Energie sowie zur Abgrenzung und Hebung des Selbstwertgefühles: Eine Räuchermischung aus Salbei, Weinraute, Rainfarn und Wermut kombiniert mit Harz herstellen.

Mythologie und magische Praktiken

Nach griechischer Mythologie habe ein Salbeistrauch der Göttin Aphrodite als Zuflucht und Versteck vor dem sie verfolgenden Zeus gedient. Als dieser davon erfuhr, wollte er die Pflanze vernichten und ließ die Sonne auf den Salbei herunterbrennen. Aphrodite jedoch schützte den Salbei, indem sie ihm samtig dicke Blätter verlieh und zudem noch große Heilkraft und betörenden Duft schenkte.

In der christlichen Version dieser Geschichte wird der Salbei zur Marienpflanze: Auf ihrer Flucht vor Herodes habe Maria alle Blumen um Schutz gebeten. Nur der Salbei habe sie hinter seinen schützenden Blättern versteckt. Als die Gefahr vorüber war, habe Maria gesagt: „Ich gebe dir die Kraft, die Menschen zu heilen von jeder Krankheit, errette sie vom Tode, wie du es auch mir getan hast."

Bei Ausgrabungen in Caesarea, im heutigen Israel, wurden 60 Fluchtäfelchen gefunden: Es handelte sich um Verwünschungen der gegnerischen Wagenlenker, damit diese im Wagenrennen scheiterten oder gar verunglückten. Diese Fluchtäfelchen waren gerollt, so groß wie ein Geldschein und enthielten drinnen ein Salbeiblatt!

Jahrhundertelang glaubten die Menschen, dass dem Salbei nicht nur große Heilkräfte, sondern auch große Zauberkräfte innenwohnten: Mit Salbeistängel und dem entsprechenden Ritual könnten Türen und Schlösser geöffnet und sogar Gewässer ausgetrocknet werden.

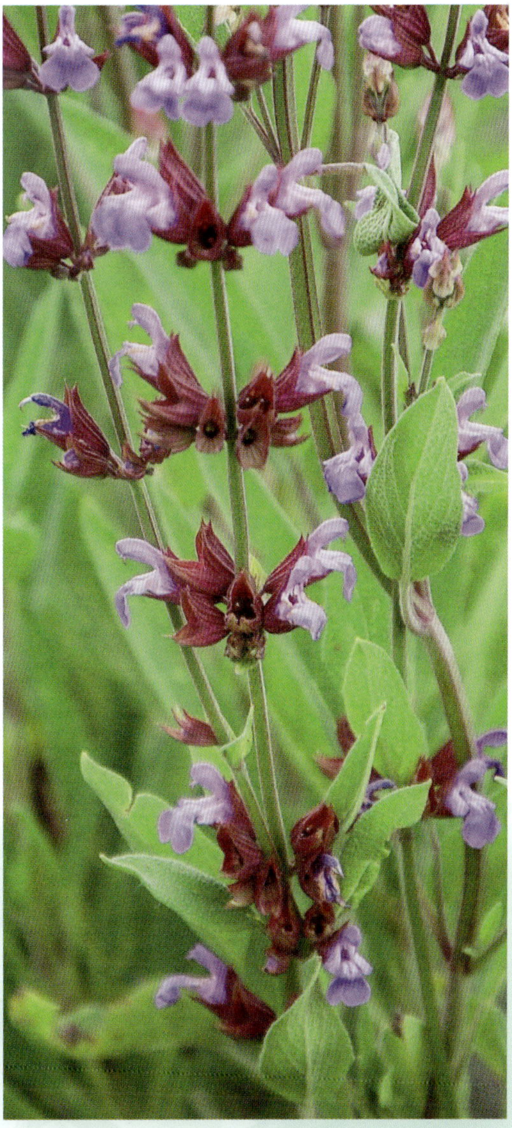

Salbeiblüten

Unter dem Salbeistrauch lauert die große Kröte, das Symbol für unheimliche, schwarzmagische Praktiken. Zwei Beispiele für diese weit verbreitete Salbei-Überhöhung: Nach einer Erzählung im „Decamerone" des Giovanni Boccaccio (1313–1375) hat Hans Sachs (1494–1576) ein Stück gereimt: „Historia, wie zwey liebhabende von einem salvenblatt sturben." Als die Gendarmen unter dem Salbeistock nachschauten, von dem die beiden Verliebten je ein Blatt als Zahnbürste verwendet hatten und daran gestorben waren, saß da eine dicke Kröte. Der Autor zieht am Ende seiner moralisierenden Geschichte den Schluss: „Auss dem ein Mensch sol lernen wol, das er sich fleißig hüten soll vor der lieb außerhalb der ee, die alzeit bringet ach und wee…".

Selbst ein aufgeklärter Geist wie Bartholomäus Ehrhart (1700–1756) ist sich hinsichtlich der dunklen Seite der Salbeikräfte nicht so ganz sicher: „Zu Pag. 280. Vom Salbey. Die uralte Erzehlung, dass die Blätter dieses Gewächs oft vergifft befunden worden, und zwar von denen Schlangen, verificiret sich heutiges Tages dahin, dass weilen die Blätter auf der untern Seiten sehr rauch, löcherig und ungleich seyn, so setzet sich sehr gern ein vergiffter Saamen von vielerley kleinem Geschmeiß, Raupen oder Spinnen hinein, daher gekommen, dass einem Chirurgo nur vom abschneiden eine vergiffte Geschwulst der Hand aufgefahren: und ein bleichsüchtiges Fräulein gar vom Salbey essen gestorben (wiewohl dieses auch andere Ursachen mit gehabt haben mag)."

Verwendung – gestern und heute

In Westeuropa wird der Salbei zur Nummer eins der mittelalterlichen Klostermedizin! Auch Kaiser Karl der Große (747–814) schreibt den Salbei zwingend zum Anbau auf seinen Königsgütern vor: „salviam" an fünfter Stelle von insgesamt 73 Pflanzen.

Um 840 stellt Walahfrid Strabo (808–849), Abt des Klosters Reichenau, den Salbei an die erste Stelle seines Gartengedichtes „Hortulus" und schreibt: : „Leuchtend blühet Salbei ganz vorn am Eingang des Gartens, süß von Geruch,

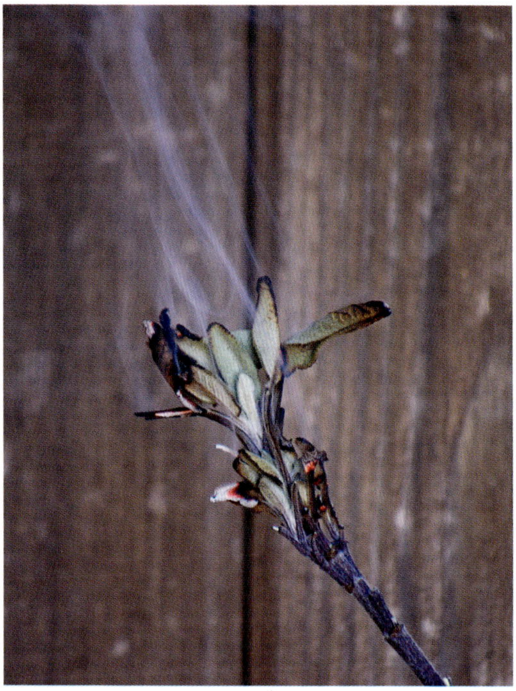

Salbei eignet sich für Reinigungsräucherungen.

voll wirkender Kräfte und heilsam zu trinken…" Hieronymus Bock (1498–1554) meint: „Under allen stauden ist kaum ein gewächs uber die Salbei, dann es dienet dem artzet, koch, keller, armen und reichen. Ist ein sonderlich wurz, denen so nit gen Franckfurt unnd Venedig haben zufaren, von denen es billich im garten als edelst Teütsch wurz gepflanzet solt werden." Einen besonderen Rat hat Leonhart Fuchs (1501–1566): „Die bletter und aest in wein gesotten unnd darmit gewaschen vertreiben das iucken an den gemechten."

Das alte Kräftigungs- und Stärkungsmittel wird auch heute wegen seiner zusammenziehenden, krampflösenden, schweißreduzierenden Wirkung geschätzt und als Gurgeltee bei Halsweh sowie in vielen Auszügen mit Alkohol oder Essig verwendet – allerdings nur in Maßen wegen seines Inhaltsstoffes Thujon.

Gelber Salbei

Lat. Name: *Salvia glutinosa*
Botanischer Name: Klebriger Salbei
Pflanzenfamilie: Lippenblütler

Auf feuchten, absonnigen Waldstellen an denen man sich nicht lange aufhalten möchte, auf alten Hohlwegen und anderen menschenfernen unruhigen Orten, trifft man unverhofft auf den klebrigen Salbei – eine verwunschene Pflanze mit einer besonderen Anziehungskraft. Die großen Blüten scheinen zangenartig nach einem zu greifen und es ist nicht klar, ob es sich um ein hilfreiches Entgegenstrecken, ein schützendes Angebot handelt oder doch um eine dunkel bedrohliche Verlockung aus einer anderen Welt. Doch dann kommt noch ein anderer Gedanke auf: Grimms „Goldene Gans“ oder Bechsteins „Schwan kleb an“ mag wohl auch so verführerisch gestrahlt haben.

Rauch

Verwendete Pflanzenteile: Das ganze blühende Kraut: Stängel, Blätter, Blüten.

Beste Sammel- und Erntezeit: Ab dem Hochsommer bis in den Herbst hinein.

Wirkung, Wahrnehmung: Heilige Pflanze der Kelten; das klebrige Verhalten der Pflanze bleibt auch nach der Trocknung erhalten. Die Pflanze setzt im Verglühen einen klärenden Rauch frei und fährt tief in die Seele ein. Notfall-Rauch: hilfreich bei gefühlter, ungewisser geistig-seelischer Bedrohung. Große Lösungsenergie bei negativen Andockungen. Gibt neue Zuversicht und kann Verwünschungen und deren Last, die auf die Brust drückt, abschwächen. Ich-stärkende Kraft, hilft zurück zu den eigenen Wurzeln, unterstützt die eigene Identität und Besonderheit.

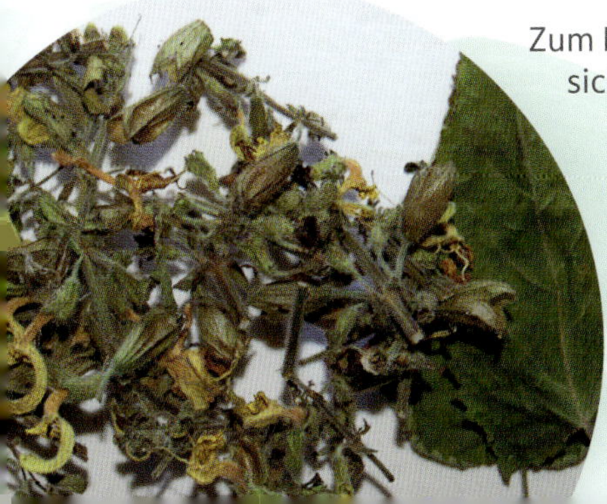

Zum Räuchern eignet sich das ganze blühende Kraut.

Magisches zum Rauch: Diesem Rauch werden große bipolare Kräfte zugeschrieben. Die Pflanze zählt zu den großen alten „Hexenpflanzen“ mit weiß-magischem, aber auch großem schwarz-magischen Potenzial (Verwendung für Bindezauber, Verwünschungen und Bannungen). Ihr Einsatz ist eine Gratwanderung und erfordert weiß-magisch ein reines Herz!

Schwerpunkt, Anwendungen, Rezepte: Für eine fluchbannende Räuchermischung wird Gelber Salbei, Farnkraut und Odermennigwurzel zusammen mit Harz vermörsert.

Mythologie und magische Praktiken

Der gelbe Salbei wird, wie auch der Wasserdost, mit dem Hirsch in Verbindung gebracht, weil diese Pflanzen dessen bevorzugtes Futter sind. Bei den Kelten gab es ein göttliches Wesen, das mit Hirschgeweih dargestellt wurde: Cernunnos, der Gehörnte, die Gottheit der Natur, des Waldes, der Tiere und der Fruchtbarkeit. Im Laufe der Christianisierung wurde er zum gehörnten Dämon und schließlich zum paganen Gegenspieler der christlichen Gottheit, zum Teufel.

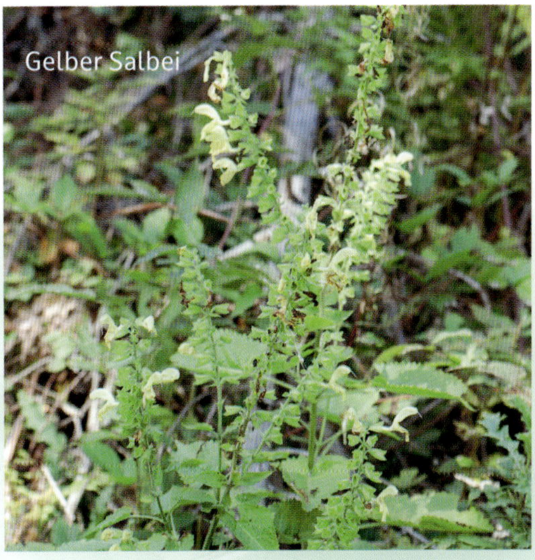

Gelber Salbei

Muskateller-salbei

Lat. Name: *Salvia sclarea*
Pflanzenfamilie: Lippenblütler

Von antiker Party-Droge über mittelalterliches Heilkraut bis in die gegenwärtige Bedeutungslosigkeit führt der Weg des Muskatellersalbeis. Selbst Walahfrid Strabo (808–849) konstatiert in seinem Gartengedicht „Hortulus" zur Pflanze: „Da sie nur selten zur Hilfe in Krankheit irgend verlangt wird, möchte man glauben, sie sei wohl den Händen der Ärzte entgangen."

Mit dem Muskatellersalbei sind in meinem Garten plötzlich Holzbienen aufgetaucht. Über die Jahre ist ihre Kolonie offensichtlich gewachsen und es gibt ein spannendes jährliches Wiedersehen, wenn der Muskatellersalbei zu blühen beginnt. Die zwei- bis mehrjährige Pflanze versät sich zuverlässig selbst im Garten und bildet richtige Horste, in die kein anderes Kraut einziehen möchte! Das Markanteste an ihm ist, neben den herrlich zart-lila Blüten, sein einzigartiger Geruch, der je nach Wetterlage und Tageszeit zwischen verführerisch duftend und abstoßend stinkend schwankt!

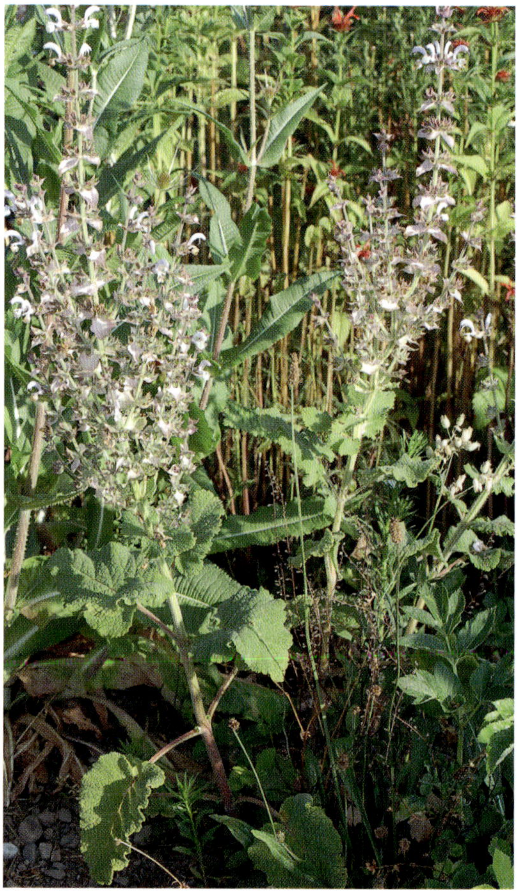

Blühender Muskatellersalbei

Rauch

Verwendete Pflanzenteile: Das ganze blühende Kraut: Stängel, Blätter, Blüten.

Beste Sammel- und Erntezeit: Da der Muskatellersalbei wochenlang blüht, ist den ganzen Sommer über Zeit ihn zu ernten.

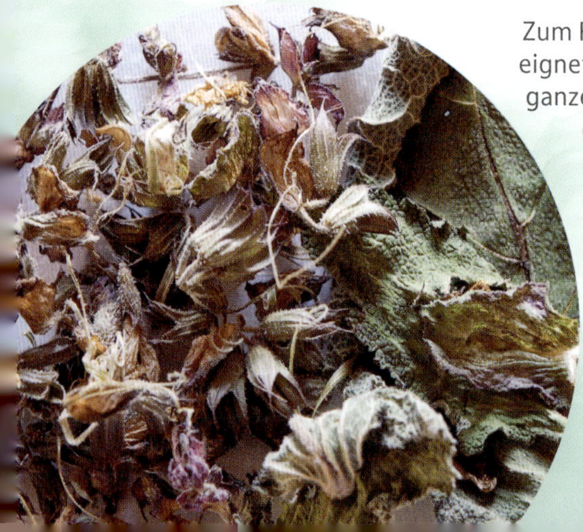

Zum Räuchern eignet sich das ganze blühende Kraut.

Wirkung, Wahrnehmung: Bereits nach den ersten Atemzügen merkt man, wie dieser Rauch einen aus dem tristen Alltag abholt, entspannt und für die schönen Dinge des Lebens öffnet. Der narkotisch krautige Duft wirkt aphrodisierend, euphorisierend und stimmungsaufhellend. Wenn man in einem stressigen Alltag gedanklich blockiert ist, dann setzt der Muskatellersalbeirauch den Funkenflug der Gedanken wieder in Gang. Mit seinem Rauch kann man negative Gedankenspiralen stoppen; er lässt uns lockerer werden und durchatmen. Sorgt für einen positiven Stimmungsausgleich; die aufbauende Wirkung kann besonders förderlich für kreative und schöpferische Arbeiten sein. Wirkt entspannend, baut körperliche und seelische Spannungen ab und sorgt für Lebensfreude; versetzt uns in eine sinnliche Stimmung. Passt auch zu Themen, wo es um Erdung, Schutz, Geborgenheit und neue Hoffnung geht.

Magisches zum Rauch: Muskatellersalbei wurde bei antiken Gastmahlen geräuchert, um die Anwesenden in eine lockere Stimmung zu versetzen. So waren sie wohl eher zu sinnlichen Ausschweifungen bereit. Auch in mittelalterlichen Badehäusern heizte man die Ungezwungenheit und die Freizügigkeit der Badenden mit Muskatellersalbeirauch noch weiter an.

Schwerpunkt, Anwendungen, Rezepte: Zum Überwinden von schöpferischen Blockaden wird eine Räuchermischung mit Muskatellersalbei, Beifuß und Rosenblüten mit Harz gemischt.

Verwendung – gestern und heute

Von Dioskurides (1. Jhdt.) wurde der Muskatellersalbei hochgelobt und bei Kopfschmerzen und als entspannendes Schlafmittel empfohlen. Im „Capitulare de villis vel curtis imperii“, der Anbauverordnung, die Kaiser Karl der Große (747–814) um das Jahr 800 erlassen hatte, findet sich an der 72. Stelle von insgesamt 73 aufgezählten Pflanzen, unter der Bezeichnung „sclareiam“, der Muskatellersalbei, der auf den karolingischen Königshöfen angebaut werden musste.

Hildegard von Bingen (1098–1179) nennt ihn „Scharleya“ und stellt fest: „Der Muskatellersalbei ist warm und er ist gut gegen Gift.“ Weiters meint sie: „Aber auch wer Kopfweh hat, der koche Muskatellersalbei in Wasser, und nach Auspressen des Wassers lege er es so warm um seinen Kopf und bedecke den Kopf mit einem Tuch und schlafe so, und es wird ihm besser gehen.“ Ein Sclarea-Trank wird noch heute in der Hildegard-Medizin zubereitet.

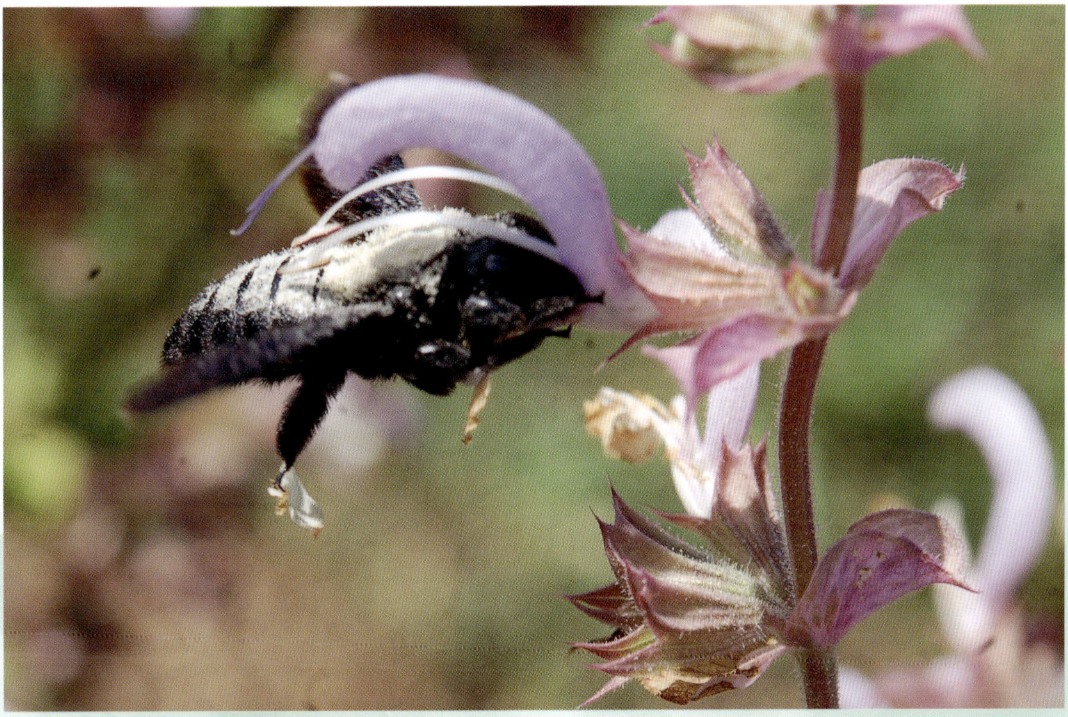

Muskatellersalbeiblüte

Thymian

Lat. Name: *Thymus vulgaris*
Botanischer Name: Echter Thymian
Pflanzenfamilie: Lippenblütler

Der wärmeliebende Halbstrauch braucht in unseren Breiten schon Unterstützung im Garten: einen voll sonnigen Platz, vielleicht einen großen Stein, der die Tageswärme speichert und in der Nacht an ihn weitergibt und – ganz wichtig – einen durchlässigen Boden, damit die Wurzeln nicht in Staunässe absterben. Das Kranzlkraut oder Herrgottskraut besticht durch seinen bescheidenen Habitus, dahinter pulsiert aber ein wirkmächtiger Kräutergeist!

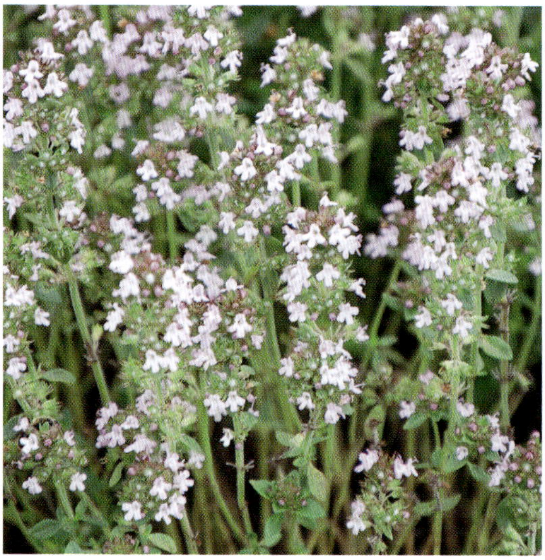
Thymianblüten

Rauch

Verwendete Pflanzenteile: Das ganze Kraut.

Beste Sammel- und Erntezeit: Im Sommer, wenn die Kraft des Thymians am größten ist.

Wirkung, Wahrnehmung: Einer der ganz frühen Räucherstoffe; hat eine kräftig reinigende Wirkung; in Häusern verräuchert, werden negative Raumeintragungen rasch überlagert und ausgeglichen. Wirkt aufbauend in Häusern, in denen Trauer herrscht und alles bedrückt ist, wo der Lebenswille nur schwach pulsiert oder wo lange Zeit Krankheiten und Siechtum den Alltag beherrschten.

Im Mittelalter häufig in der dunkeln Jahreszeit verräuchert, um den Lebenswillen und die Durchhaltekraft zu stärken. Bringt eine tiefe innere Beruhigung, entkrampft und stärkt das Gefühl gut aufgehoben zu sein. Aktivierender Rauch, anregend, aphrodisierend. Hilft Erschöpfungszustände zu überwinden, motivierend, steigert die Konzentrationsfähigkeit und die Lust, Dinge in Angriff zu nehmen. Glücksbringender Rauch, der freundliche Wesen anzieht.

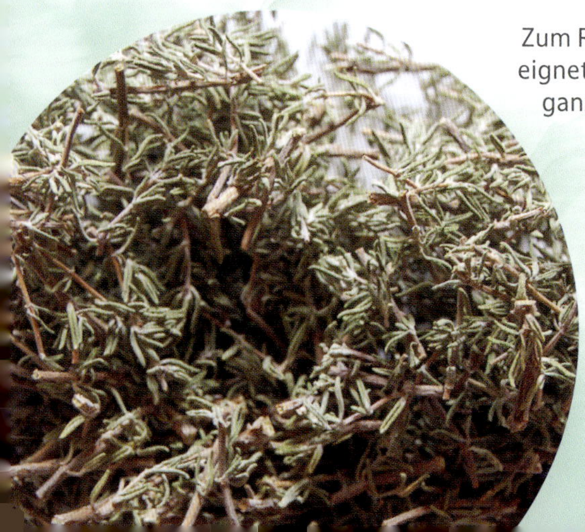
Zum Räuchern eignet sich das ganze Kraut.

Magisches zum Rauch: Die Römer glaubten, der Thymianrauch sei so heilig, dass durch ihn alle giftigen Kreaturen in die Flucht geschlagen werden können. Sie räucherten deshalb auch in Krankenzimmern. Nach den Römern wurde auch bei uns jahrhundertelang Thymian bei verschiedenen Krankheiten verräuchert, um lebenskraftsaugende Wesen zu verscheuchen. Thymian oder Quendel wurde als Kraut der Sommersonnenwende im Juni zusammen mit Beifuß verräuchert, um die Ernte-Dämonen zu vertreiben.

Schwerpunkt, Anwendungen, Rezepte: Für eine dämonenverscheuchende Räucherung mischt man Thymian mit Eberraute und Rainfarn (Harz kombinieren). Für einen Motivationsrauch Thymian, Tanne (Harz) und Rosmarin mischen. Zum Abräuchern von Kranken hilft eine Räuchermischung von Thymian, Rosmarin, Mistel und Wacholderbeeren.

Mythologie und magische Praktiken

Die Räucherspuren des Thymians reichen bis in die Antike zurück. Bei den Griechen bedeutete „thyein" zu räuchern und ein Opfer darzubringen. Mit dem Rauch von Thymianbündeln wurden Tempel und heilige Orte geweiht. Noch bei den Römern wurde mit dem griechischen Wort „thymiaterion" das Räuchergestell vor dem Hausaltar bezeichnet. In der christlichen Welt durfte in Notzeiten anstelle von Weihrauch Thymian in den Kirchen geräuchert werden.

Der Thymian war der griechischen Aphrodite geweiht, danach der römischen Venus, anschließend wird der Feldthymian oder Quendel der nordischen Freya, auch in der Gestalt der Frau Holle, zugeschrieben und schließlich wird er zum Marienkraut und gehört als solches in den Kräuterbuschn der zu Mariä Himmelfahrt am 15. August gebunden wird.

Nach einer griechischen Legende spross der Thymian zum ersten Mal aus der Erde, die von den Tränen der schönen Helena benetzt worden war. Bevor die Römer in den Krieg zogen, badeten sie in einem Thymian-Absud und tranken mit Thymian gewürzten Wein. Das sollte ihnen Mut und Tapferkeit verleihen. Um Mut und Tapferkeit ging es auch im Mittelalter, wenn edle Damen dem Ritter ihrer Gunst ein Tüchlein überreichten, auf welches sie zuvor einen Thymianzweig und eine Biene gestickt hatten. Machtbewusste Bräute steckten sich vor der Hochzeit einen Thymianzweig in den Schuh und murmelten dabei: „Ich tret, ich tret´ auf Thymian, schau mir keine andere an!"

In die Kränze, die in Bayern mit der Fronleichnamsprozession mitgetragen werden, wird Thymian eingeflochten, damit er später, wenn die Kränze in Stall und Haus verteilt werden, alle Dämonen, Teufel und böse Geister abwehren und in die Flucht schlagen könne. In England wurden Thymian-Kränze auch Schwerkranken auf den Kopf gesetzt, um den Tod abzuwehren!

Verwendung – gestern und heute

Hildegard von Bingen (1098–1179) widmet sich im 1. Buch der „Physica" intensiv dem Thymian und empfiehlt ihn in verschiedenen Rezepten gegen Lepra, als ausleitendes Sitzbad gegen schlechte Säfte, bei Gliederlähmung und zu einer Salbe verarbeitet, die Läuse am Menschen abtöten soll.

Der Thymian wird auch heute als wertvolles Mittel bei allen Atemwegserkrankungen genutzt. Darüber hinaus ist er ein besonderes Stärkungsmittel in der zweiten Lebenshälfte.

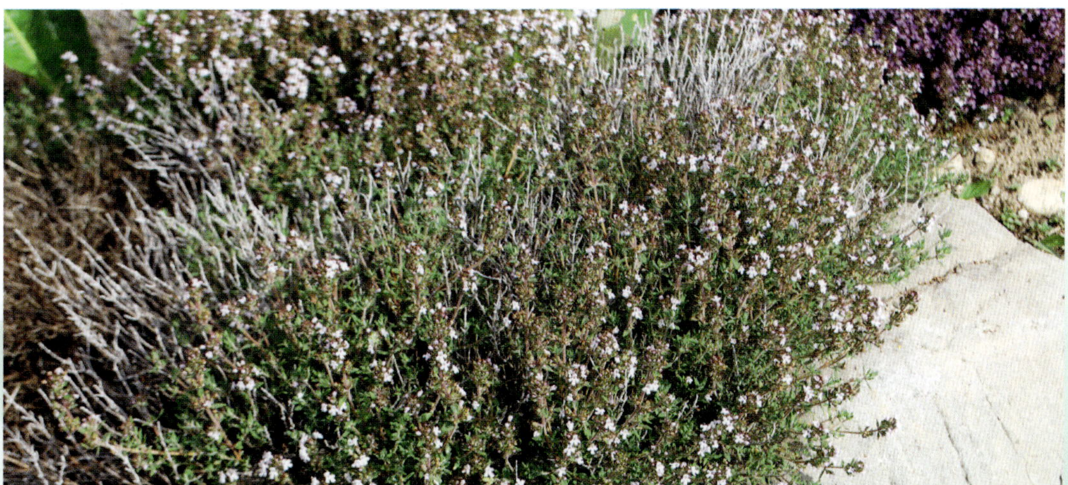

Blühender Thymian

Wald-Geißbart

Lat. Name: *Aruncus dioicus*
Pflanzenfamilie: Rosengewächse

Elfenhaft schwingen die langen Stängel am Waldrand. Tausendfache Leichtigkeit, ganz dem Wind hingegeben, in alle Richtungen strebend und strahlend wie eine neu geborene Galaxie. Apotropäisches Weiß, als machte er den Waldrand dicht, beschützte den Wald dahinter vor allem Ungemach. Jedes Jahr begeistert mich das Erscheinen des Wald-Geißbarts erneut. In seiner Erscheinung vereinigt sich erdenhafte Festigkeit mit überirdischer Eleganz.

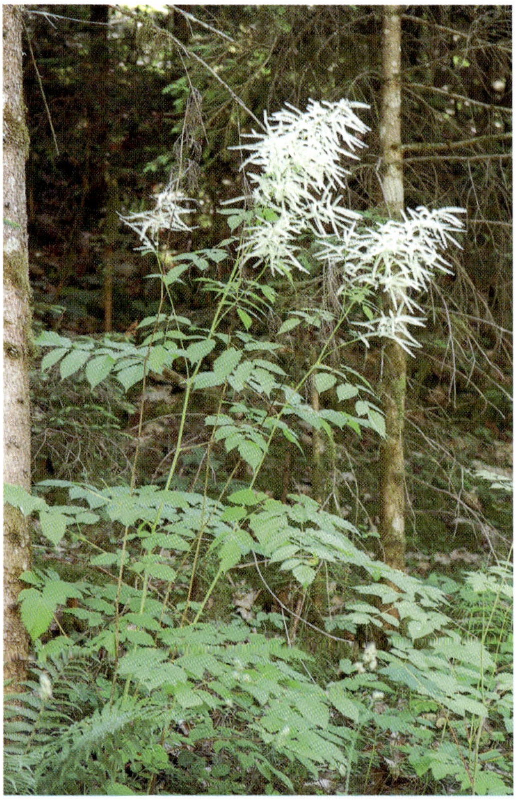
Blühender Wald-Geißbart

Rauch

Verwendete Pflanzenteile: Das ganze blühende Kraut.

Beste Sammel- und Erntezeit: Der Wald-Geißbart wächst gerne auf Feen-Plätzen, im schattigen Bäume-Überhang am Waldrand und blüht von Ende Mai bis Ende Juni.

Wirkung, Wahrnehmung: Ein mächtiges Schutzkraut, das als Räucherstoff kaum bekannt ist. Positiv stimmungsausgleichend; der Blütenrauch legt einen feinen Schutzmantel um gekränkte Seelen; man nimmt die durch den Rauch entstehende Atmosphäre als samtig weich wahr. Wirkt tröstend und leicht euphorisierend; man gleitet in ein leichtes Sein, kann die Schwere der Sorgen, des Alltags für kurze Zeit hinter sich lassen. Heilsam für sehr zurückgezogene Menschen, die anderen gegenüber eher misstrauisch begegnen. Im Schutzraum dieses Rauches können sie frei durchatmen. Wohltuender und aufbauender Rauch für Menschen, die viel alleine sind.

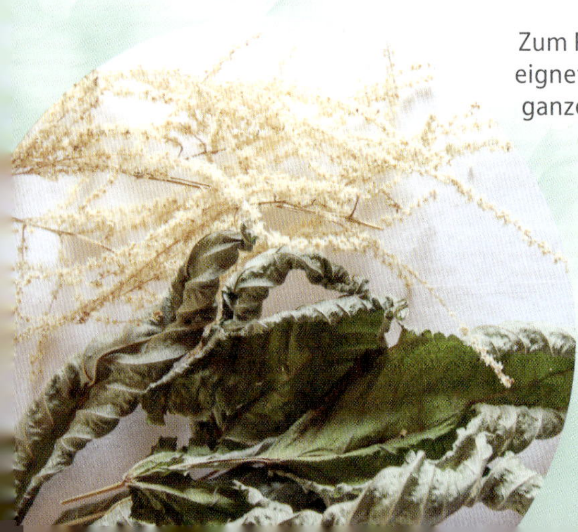
Zum Räuchern eignet sich das ganze blühende Kraut.

Magisches zum Rauch: In Vollmondnächten kann mit einer Räuchermischung aus Wald-Geißbart und Eberesche ein wertschätzender Kontakt zur Welt der Naturwesen gelingen.

Schwerpunkt, Anwendungen, Rezepte: Die Leichtigkeit des Lebens spüren: Räuchermischung aus Wald-Geißbart, Vogelkirsche und Apfelblüten sowie Harz.

Als Bestandteil von Räucherstäben, die man mit Farnkraut, Beifuß und Birkenzweigen bindet, um die Atmosphäre in frequentierten Räumen frei von belastenden Eintragungen zu halten. Auch zur wohltuenden Unterstützung und Erhellung in Burn-out-Phasen.

Mythologie und magische Praktiken

Die Beziehung des Wald-Geißbartes zum Brauchtum rund um die Sommersonnenwende zeigt sich in der landläufigen Bezeichnung „Johanniswedel". Er sollte mit seiner Feenkraft die Zeit bis zur Ernte unwetterfrei halten.

Verwendung – gestern und heute

In der europäischen Kräuterliteratur findet man nur vereinzelt knappe Besprechungen des Wald-Geißbartes. So beschreibt Hieronymus Bock (1498–1554): „Die blumen mit langen zaseln als ein schneeweisser bart. Auß disen blumen werden lange zapffen, wie an den haselhecken…". Hinsichtlich der Heilkraft meint er kurz: „… mögen in leib genommen und äusserlich auffgelegt werden."

Die jungen Triebe wurden früher als Waldspargel in der Küche gesammelt. Heute wird die Pflanze für homöopathische Mittel verwendet.

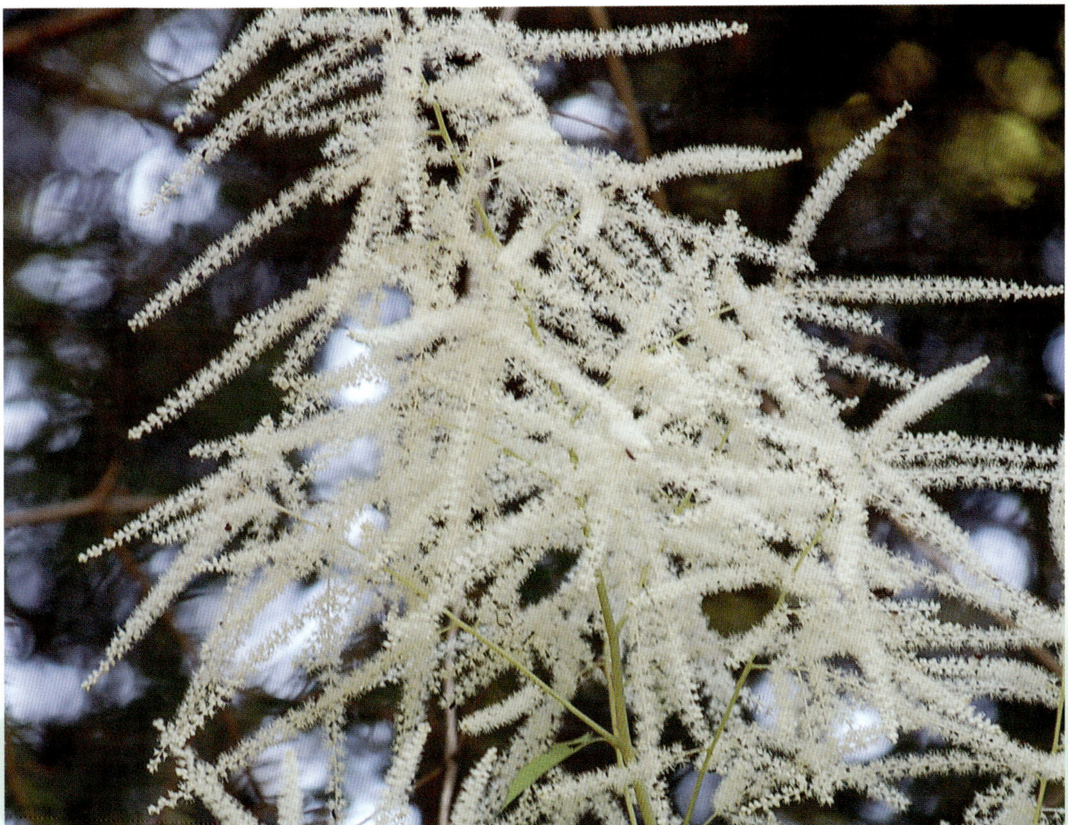

Blüte des Wald-Geißbarts

Wasserdost

Lat. Name: *Eupatorium cannabinum*
Botanischer Name: Gewöhnlicher Wasserdost
Pflanzenfamilie: Korbblütler

Die imposante Staude ist ein heiliges Wetterkraut alter Zeiten und als Räucherstoff in Vergessenheit geraten. Das Kunigundenkraut ist offenbar mit den Vögeln in meinen Garten gekommen. Es hat sich gleich in die vorderste Beetreihe gesetzt und ist mir über viele Jahre ein treuer Begleiter. Ich genieße und schätze seine große Schutzkraft und seine Mitteilsamkeit. Bemerkenswert finde ich, die Resonanzfähigkeit dieses Krauts: Wenn es wahrgenommen, angesprochen und gebraucht wird, kommt es auch mit ungünstigen Standortbedingungen zurecht, wiewohl es lieber seine Wurzeln im Feuchten hätte. Der Wasserdost wird auch Donnerkraut genannt, was auf seine ehemalige Zuschreibung zum germanischen Donnergott Thor bzw. Donar hinweist.

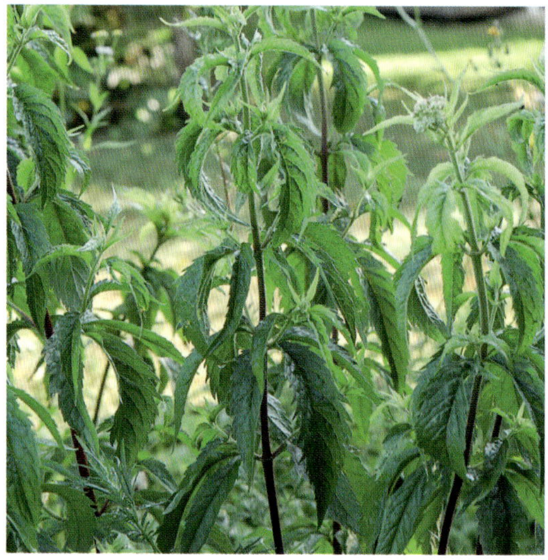

Blätter des Wasserdosts, der auch als Kunigundenkraut bezeichnet wird.

Rauch

Verwendete Pflanzenteile: Das ganze blühende Kraut.

Beste Sammel- und Erntezeit: Der Blühbeginn des Kunigundenkrauts ist meist Mitte/Ende Juli.

Wirkung, Wahrnehmung: Große weißmagische Kraftpflanze! Heilige Pflanze der Kelten; Abwehr- und Schutzkraut, Verschrei-Kraut gegen magische Übergriffe; Wetterkraut; intensiv klärende Wirkung. Abwehrrauch gegen negative Energien und hinterlistige Übertragungen durch Dämonen, dunkle Geister oder andere Menschen. Hilfreich, um sich vor schwarzer Magie, Verfluchungen, Bannungen, jeglichen Schadenszauber sowie die Auswirkungen von Neid und Missgunst zu schützen.

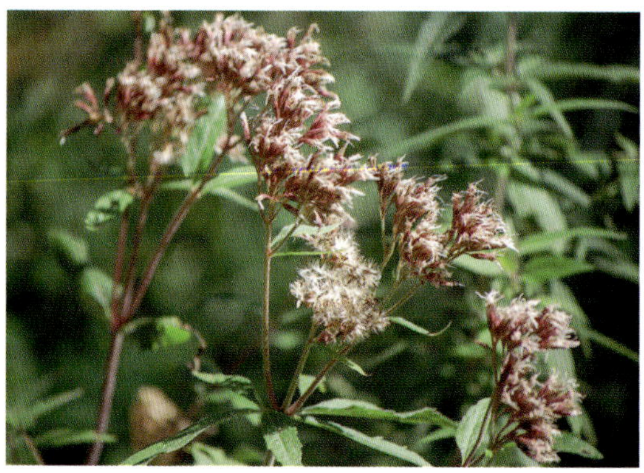

Blüten des Wasserdosts

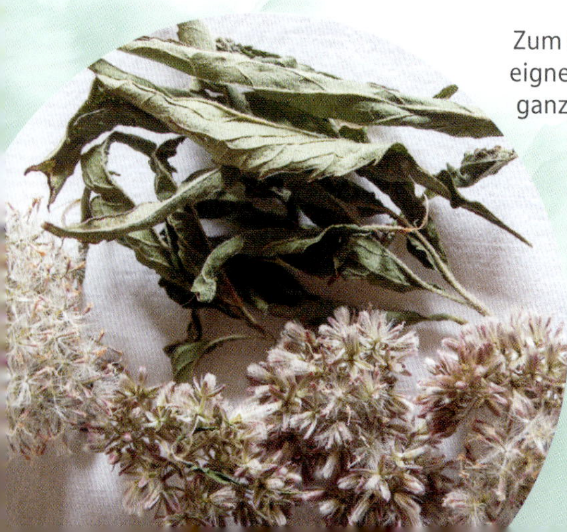

Zum Räuchern eignet sich das ganze blühende Kraut.

Der Rauch gehört in unsere Tage, um in der geistigen Welt gegen Mobbing, soziale Diskriminierung oder Unterdrückung einen Anker zu setzen.

Abwehrkraftsteigernder, teufelsscheuchender Kopf-hoch-Rauch! Klärender Rauch, der negative Gedanken verscheucht. Herzöffnend, fördert das Bewusstsein ein Teil der Natur zu sein.

Magisches zum Rauch: Wie Hieronymus Bock (1498–1554), meint auch Leonhart Fuchs (1501–1566) wortgleich: „Ein rauch von disem gedörrten kraut gemacht, vertreibt alle gifftigen gewürm."

Bock fügt jedoch hinzu: „Andere Stück, so ettlich mit disem kraut treiben, lassen wir anstehn." Was auf die häufige Verwendung von Wasserdostrauch zu verschiedenen magischen Zwecken im 16. Jahrhundert hindeutet. Als Wetterzauber wurde der Wasserdost zusammen mit anderen Wetterkräutern, wie Rainfarn oder Johanniskraut, zum Schutz von Haus und Hof vor Unwetter und Hagelschlag geräuchert. Dadurch versuchte man Donar, gerade zur Erntezeit, günstig zu stimmen. Wie beim Wald-Geißbart kann auch mit Wasserdostrauch den Naturwesen eine Freude gemacht werden.

Schwerpunkt, Anwendungen, Rezepte: Abwehrrauch bei Mobbing: Räuchermischung aus Wasserdost, Königskerze, Eisenkraut und kleinem Habichtskraut. Eine abwehrende Räuchermischung mit Wasserdost, Rainfarn und Wermut gegen Energieräuber und andere gefühlte seelisch-geistige Übergriffe (Harz nicht vergessen!).

Mythologie und magische Praktiken

Der Wasserdost wird, wie auch der gelbe Salbei, mit dem Hirsch in Verbindung gebracht, weil diese Pflanzen dessen bevorzugtes Futter sind. Die Hirsche galten ebenfalls als heilig, da sie für Boten der Anderswelt gehalten wurden. Bei den Kelten gab es ein göttliches Wesen, das mit Hirschgeweih dargestellt wurde: Cernunnos, der Gehörnte, die Gottheit der Natur, des Waldes, der Tiere und der Fruchtbarkeit. Eine alte Saga erzählt, dass kranke Hirsche Wasserdost zu sich nahmen, um auch den Menschen aufzuzeigen, welche Heilwirkung in dieser Pflanze zu finden sei.

Da die Bevölkerung unverrückbar am wetterzauberischen Tun mit dem Wasserdost festhielt, weihte man im 13. Jahrhundert diese Pflanze der Heiligen Kunigunde und gab ihr den Namen „Kunigundenkraut". Am Tag der Heiligen Kunigunde, am 13. Juli, durfte dann auch wieder Wetterzauber praktiziert werden, um die Ernte zu schützen. In vielen Gegenden wird der Wasserdost noch heute in die Kräuter-Buschn zu Mariä Himmelfahrt gebunden, um Haus und Hof vor Wetterschäden, Blitz- und Hagelschlag zu bewahren.

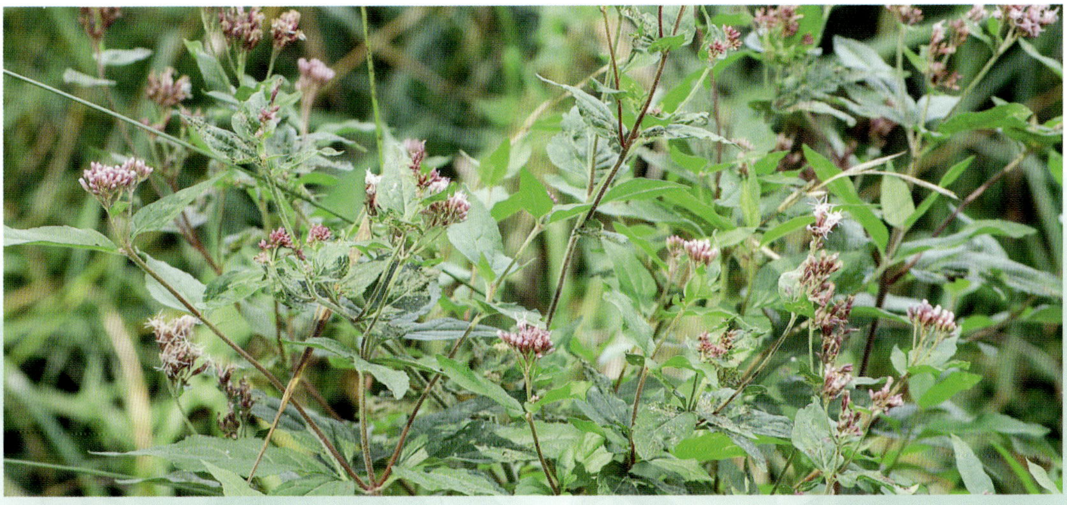

Blühender Wasserdost

Weinraute

Lat. Name: *Ruta graveolens*
Pflanzenfamilie: Rautengewächse

Die Weinrauten in meinem Garten erfreuen mich bis spät ins Jahr hinein, blühen immer wieder, tragen gleichzeitig die gekreuzten prallen Samenkapseln und leuchten aus den Beeten. Aber sie halten mich auf Abstand, wollen für sich sein. Sollte ich doch in einem unbedachten Moment an ihren Blättern ankommen, schießen an der Hautstelle nach zwei Tagen heftig schmerzende Brandblasen auf! Die Pflanze ist phototoxisch und manche Menschen reagieren heftig, andere gar nicht. Aber, das ist ja nichts Neues, wie uns bereits der Römer Columella in seinen Büchern „de re rustica", über die Landwirtschaft, wissen lässt: „... die Raute sät man im Herbst aus, verpflanzt sie im März auf sonniges Land, umhäufelt sie mit Asche, jätet das Unkraut, solange sie heranwächst, damit sie nicht von diesem erdrückt wird. Doch muss man beim Jäten die Hand schützen: Denn wenn man sie nicht bekleidet, entstehen verheerende Geschwüre. Hat man trotzdem aus Unkenntnis mit bloßer Hand gejätet und ist ein Ausschlag oder eine Schwellung entstanden, dann soll man sich sofort mit Öl einreiben..."

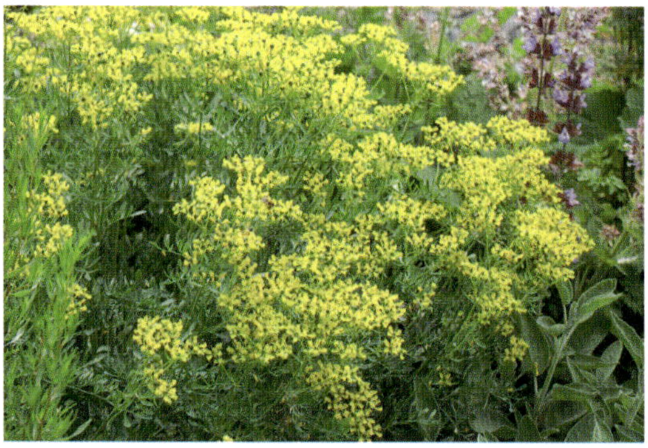

Blühende Weinraute

Rauch

Verwendete Pflanzenteile: Das ganze blühende Kraut: Blätter, Stängel, Blüten sowie die Samen.

Beste Sammel- und Erntezeit: In der Sommerzeit wird das blühende Kraut geerntet, die Samenkapseln können bis zum ersten Frost gesammelt werden.

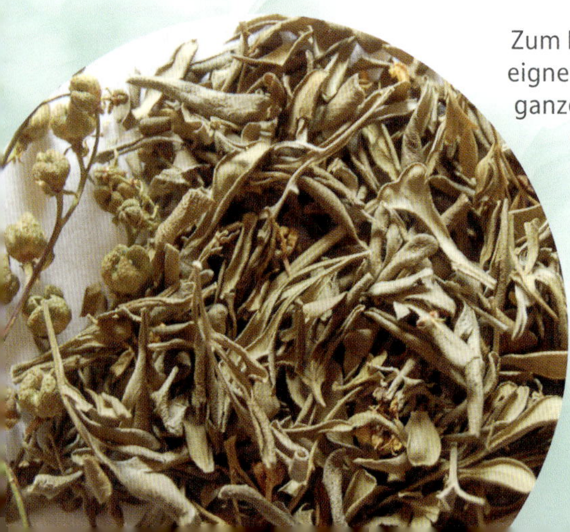

Zum Räuchern eignet sich das ganze blühende Kraut.

Wirkung, Wahrnehmung: Extremer Abwehr- und Schutzrauch. Der Rauch der Weinraute schützt Stall, Tiere, Haus und Menschen vor allen Verwünschungen anderer, die aus Neid und Zorn herausgeschleudert werden. Der Rauch überlagert das Gift der verfluchenden Worte und schützt vor dem bösen Blick der Nachbarn oder Kollegen. Stärkste Abwehrkraft gegen geistige Übergriffe dunkler Wesenheiten, die einem nichts Gutes wollen. Wenn man das Gefühl hat, da dockt etwas an. Der Rauch der Raute hat die Kraft Verwünschungen nicht nur abzuwehren, sondern sie auch aufzulösen, Mobbing abzumildern und alle, mit Nadeln durchgeführten Übergriffe, zu bannen.

Magisches zum Rauch: Paracelsus (1494–1541) schreibt über „Abwehrmittel für Haus und Hof", IV/320: „... was aber die Abwehrmittel betrifft, so wisset, dass es ihrer etliche gibt, deren ein jedes für sich selbst diese Kraft hat und stark genug ist. So erstens Beifuß, Johanniskraut, Raute, Abbiss und dergleichen Kräuter und Wurzeln mehr, insbesondere wenn sie auch in der rechten Influenz ausgegraben werden, wie in der Influenz des Jupiters und der Venus..."

Im persischen Kulturkreis werden Rautensamen als glücksbringendes Räucherwerk bei Festen und Feiern verräuchert. Der Rauch der Rautensamen wird in magischen Ritualen gegen den bösen Blick und zur Abwehr bzw. Auflösung von Verwünschungen und Flüchen verräuchert.

Schwerpunkt, Anwendungen, Rezepte: Schutzräucherung für die Aura: Man stellt sich in den Rauch der Mischung aus Weinraute, Wermut und Rainfarn kombiniert mit Harz und lässt den Rauch an sich hochsteigen, wobei die Hände geöffnet sein sollen, nicht geballt.

Der Apotheker und Botaniker und Rezeptesammler Tabernaemontanus (1522–1590) hält mehrere Räucherrezepturen mit Weinraute fest: „Weinrauthen aufgetrucknet, klein geschnitten, auff Kohlen geleget, und den jenigen so mit der grossen Kranckheit beladen, des Tages einmal oder drey damit geräuchert, und des Abends wann er zu Bette gehen will, das wird ihm fast dienlich und nutz sein."

Weiters: „Wann ein Kind das Fräsel oder Gegicht hat, so nimm ein Stück von einem Ziegelstein und mache das heiß, wirff darnach zerstossen oder zertriebene Rauten in Eßig darauf und lasse ihm den Rauch in die Nasen gehen. Dieses mag man auch den erwachsenen Menschen gebrauchen." Weiters: „Nimm Rauthenhaubtlein mit dem Saamen, wirff die auf glüende Kohlen, und lasse den rauch darvon dem Schlaffsüchtigen in die Nase gehen." Weiters: „Weinrauthen gedörret, auff glüent Kohlen geleget und damit geräuchert, vertreibt die Natteren, Viperschlangen und andere giftige Würm und Schlangen." Weiters: „Der Geruch der Weinrauthen vertreibet alle gifftige Thier, daß dieselben sich ihr nicht nahen: wann man sie aber vertreiben will von der Refier herum, so soll man nehmen Weinrauthen, gefeihlet Hirtzhorn, und des auffgetruckneten Galbensaffts, soll solche Stück wol vermischen, jedoch daß eines so viel sey als des andern, darvon mache einen Rauch in dein Hauß oder Garten, so fliehen alle gifftige Thier davon."

Mythologie und magische Praktiken

Im deutschen Sprachraum wurde die Weinraute fruchtbarkeitsmagisch rund um die Hochzeit und Ehe eingesetzt. Man dekorierte die Tische mit ihr, streute sie ins Ehebett oder an dessen vier Ecken. Hing das Eheglück einmal schief, dann sprengte man mit einem Rautenzweig Weihwasser aufs Ehebett, um die bösen Geister zu vertreiben, die die Beziehung vergiftet hatten.

Auch die Bezeichnung „Gnadenkraut" war geläufig, weil man bei Teufelsaustreibungen mit einem Rautenzweig das Weihwasser zum Ritual versprengte. Darüber hinaus legte man den Toten einen Rautenzweig auf die Brust oder legte ihnen einen Rautenkranz um den Hals, der sich nach der Auferstehung in pures Gold verwandeln sollte! In vielen Gegenden dienten frische Rautenzweige auch als abwehrendes Amulett, das gegen den bösen Blick schützen sollte.
Hieronymus Bock (1498–1554) hat einen anderen Rat: „In unsern landen setzt man Rauten und Salbey zusammen, ursach die Krotten haben ir wonung gern under den Salbeystöcken, vermeinen also ettliche mit der Rautten solch ungeziffer zu vertreiben."

In England lässt Shakespeare (1564–1616) in seinem Stück „Hamlet" Ophelia sagen: „There´s rue for you, and here´s some for me; we may call it herb of grace o´Sundays. O, you must wear your rue with a difference." (Da ist Raute für

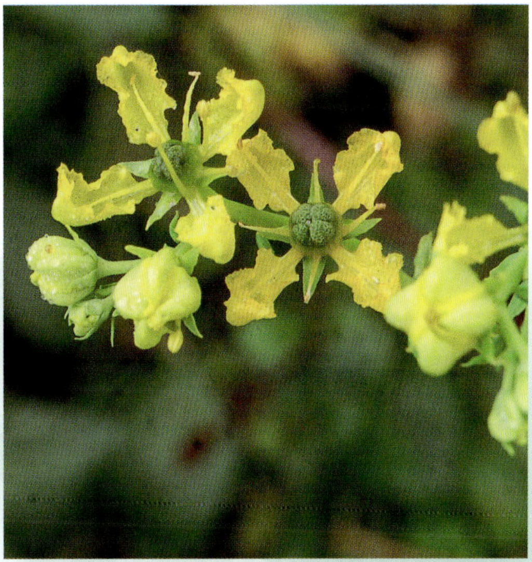

Blüte der Weinraute

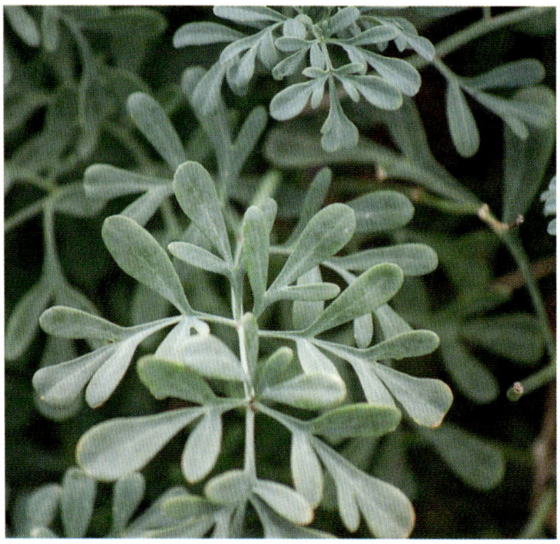

Blätter der Weinraute im Oktober

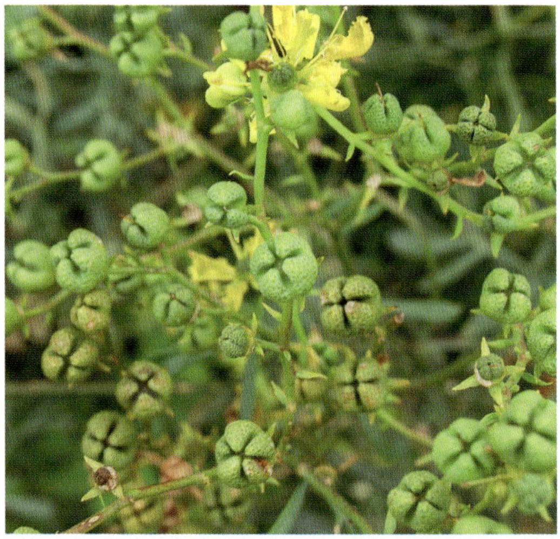

Samenkapseln der Weinraute

dich und eine für mich. An Sonntagen nennen wir sie Gnadenkraut. Oh, du musst deine Raute anders tragen.)

Überdies ist es noch nicht so lange her, dass man neben englischen Richtern Rautenbündel aufhängte, um sie vor dem sogenannten Knastfieber zu schützen!

Verwendung – gestern und heute

Die Weinraute war von der Antike bis in die Neuzeit eine hochgeschätzte Heilpflanze, die berühmt war für die Erhaltung der Sehkraft und im Ruf stand, ein wirksames Gegenmittel zu verschiedenen Giften zu sein: „Salvia cum ruta tibi faciunt pocula tuta!" – „Salbei und Raute vermengt mit Wein, lassen dir den Trunk nicht schädlich sein". Ein zuverlässiges giftwidriges Mittel parat zu haben, galt über Jahrhunderte als einzige Hoffnung, sollte man mit einem Giftanschlag zu Fall gebracht werden.

So verwundert es nicht, dass um das Jahr 800 die Weinraute auch im „Capitulare de villis vel curtis imperii", der Verordnung zur Bewirtschaftung von Königsgütern, ganz vorne auf der Pflanzenliste zu finden ist – gleich nach dem Salbei an 6. Stelle (siehe: salvia cum ruta). Diese Nähe von Salbei und Weinraute findet sich auch im Gartengedicht „Hortulus" von Walahfrid Strabo (808–849), dem Abt der Insel Reichenau im Bodensee. In der Abfolge der Pflanzen steht der Salbei an der ersten und die Weinraute an der zweiten Stelle: „Da die Raute vielfach wirkende Kraft im Innern trägt, sagt man, sie bekämpfe vor allem verborgene Gifte und vertreibe schädliche Stoffe aus befallenen Eingeweiden."

Alle großen Kräuterkundigen waren Rauten-Fans und haben uns seitenweise Lobgesänge und Rezepturen rund um das Allheil- und Pestmittel Weinraute hinterlassen. Schon Bartholomäus von Salerno (12. Jahrhundert) schrieb der Raute 34 Tugenden zu!

Hildegard von Bingen (1098–1179) rät zur Weinraute im Wechsel und bei Regulationsstörungen: „Die Weinraute ist gut gegen die trockenen Bitterkeiten, die in jenem Menschen wachsen, in dem die richtigen Säfte fehlen. Sie ist aber besser und nützlicher roh als pulverisiert zu essen." Das sieht auch Leonhart Fuchs (1501–1566) so, wenn er unter anderem schreibt: „Welcher rauten nüchter isset, der würdt denselbigen tag für allerley gifft sicher sein."

In Italien ist sie die Hauptzutat des Grappa. Frei nach dem italienischen Sprichwort: „Die Raute treibt das Übel rasch aus Haus und Leib!"

Wermut

Lat. Name: *Artemisia absinthium*
Pflanzenfamilie: Korbblütler

Der Wermut ist eine Pflanze der Extreme: Innerhalb kürzester Zeit wächst er zu einer gewaltigen Staude heran, er hält andere Pflanzen erfolgreich auf Abstand und präsentiert sich am liebsten alleinstehend. Er bildet eine einzigartige Bitterkeit mit einer alles durchdringenden Kraft aus, die noch dazu für Mensch und Tier heilsam sein kann.

In meinem Garten ist er ein Eroberer besonderer Art: Meist lässt er sich am Feldrand nieder oder er springt gleich unter einen Strauch oder Baum. Anfangs fand ich das noch recht nett, wie sich die graue Eminenz treffsicher vermehrte. Erst als mein geliebter Maulbeerbaum im zweiten Jahr seiner Wermutumfassung abzusterben begann, dämmerte es mir: Ich eleminierte den Wermut mit allem Wurzelwerk und kurze Zeit später hatte sich der Maulbeerbaum tatsächlich wieder erholt.

Rauch

Verwendete Pflanzenteile: Blätter, Blüten.

Beste Sammel- und Erntezeit: Die Blätter können ab April gezupft werden, die Blüten im Endstadium, wenn das erste Gelb bräunlich wird. Das ist meist Mitte bis Ende August der Fall.

Wirkung, Wahrnehmung: Reinigungsrauch, großer Abwehr- und Schutzrauch; Verschreikraut; Wetterkraut; Kraut der Sonnenwenden, das kraftvoll Übergänge und Umbrüche begleitet; neben dem Salbei ist der Wermut eines der beliebtesten Räucherkräuter. In Häusern, Räumen oder an Orten, an denen sich etwas Unheimliches manifestiert hat, hilft der Wermutrauch die kalte Energie zu durchdringen und zu überlagern. Klärender Reinigungsrauch für Räume, Gegenstände, Orte und emotional überlastete Menschen. Hilfreich, wenn am Arbeitsplatz nichts mehr geht, wenn die Gedanken kreisen, man den roten Faden verloren hat, wenn man bei geistigen Arbeiten keinen Anfang findet oder Themen nicht fassen kann. Insbesonders wirksam, wenn diese Blockaden einem von außen aufgebürdet wurden: durch Neid, den bösen Blick oder andere negative Übergriffe wie Mobbing.

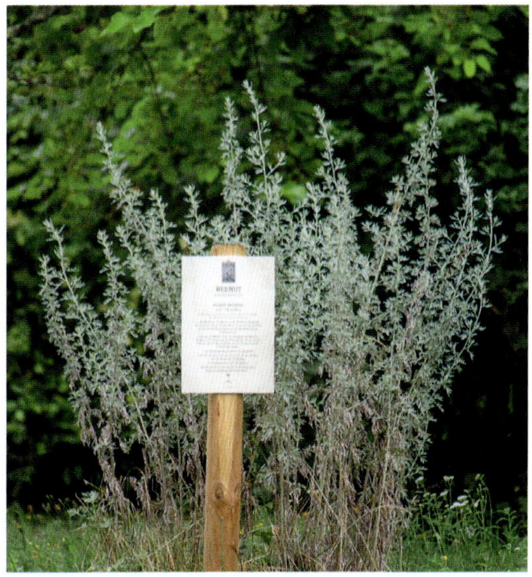
Wermut

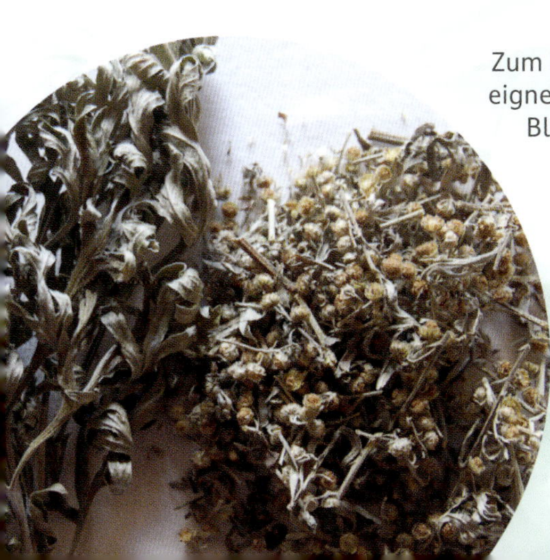
Zum Räuchern eignen sich die Blätter und Blüten.

Der Wermutrauch klärt die Atmosphäre und schützt so die Aura, das persönliche Kraftfeld. Die innere geistige Abwehrkraft wird gestärkt; man kann sich wieder motivieren, findet den Weg aus seinen düsteren Gedanken und Emotionen, entkommt den dunklen Dämonen und der

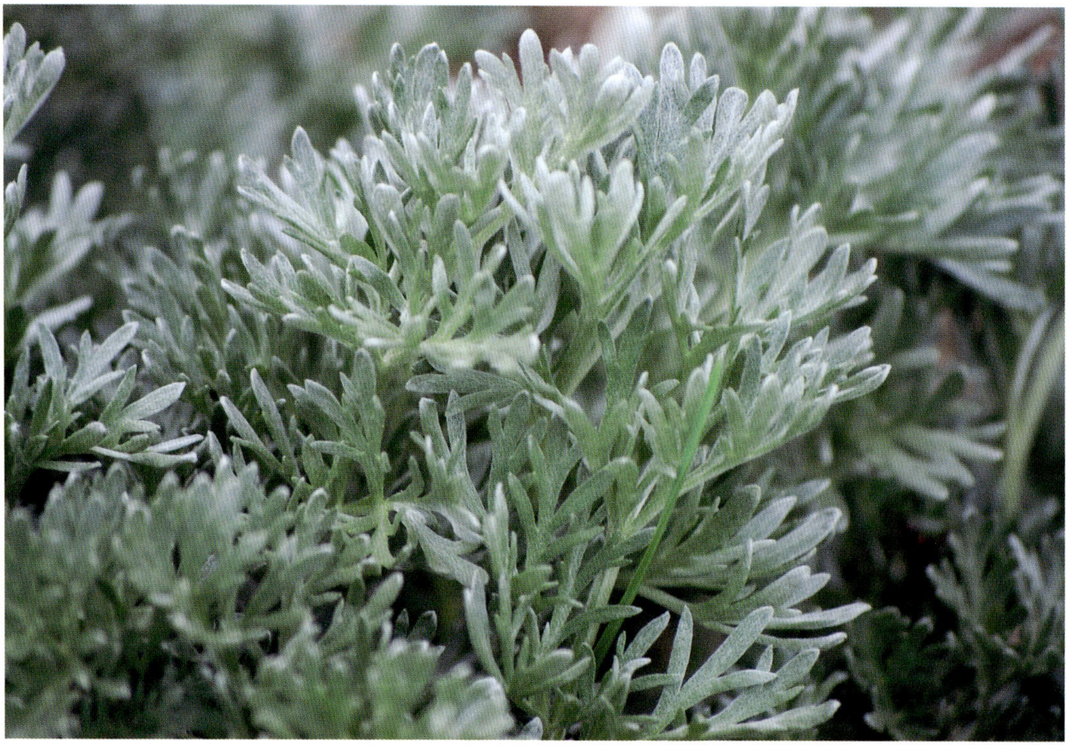

Wermutblätter

Bannkraft von negativen Geistern. So etwas wie Mut, Lebensmut wird möglich. Die Ich-Stärkung durch eine Wermut-Räucherung kann Phasen der Lebensveränderung erhellen und erleichtern. In jedem Fall leistet der Wermutrauch was sein Name verspricht: Er hilft einem sich zu „wehren“ und macht „Mut“.

Magisches zum Rauch: Martin Luther (1483–1546) wettert gegen den Brauch, das Bett von Mutter und Neugeborenem mit Wermut abzuräuchern, um beide gegen die Angriffe des Teufels zu schützen, der danach das Kind nicht mehr auswechseln könne! Tabernaemontanus (1522–1590) rät: „Wermuth auff glüende Kolen gelegt, und die Gemach darmit geraucht, verbessert den faulen, vergifftet, pestillenzischen Lufft. Derween die recht unnd wol thun, die das Rindviech und die Schaff, in den Viechsterben, morgens und abends in den Ställen, mit Wermuth beräuchen.“

In slawischen Ländern wurde Wermutkraut auf der Herdplatte verräuchert, um Unwetter und Hagelschauer abzuwenden, die von bösen Geistern oder Hexen verursacht schienen. Europaweit wird Wermut wider das Berufen geräuchert und um negative Geister abzuwehren. In solchen Phasen wurde oft als zusätzlicher Schutz ein kurzer Wermutstängel bei sich getragen.

Schwerpunkt, Anwendungen, Rezepte: Siehe Weinraute: Schutzräucherung für die Aura: Man stellt sich in den Rauch der Mischung aus Weinraute, Wermut und Rainfarn und lässt den Rauch an sich hochsteigen, wobei die Hände geöffnet sein sollen, nicht geballt. In römischen Haushalten wurde oft Wermutkraut anstelle von Weihrauch verbrannt.

Eine Räuchermischung aus Wermut, Lavendel, Eberraute und Harz klärt die geistigen Blockaden, öffnet die mentale Verstopfung durch zu viele Ideen und leitet das Chaos in überschaubare Bahnen zurück. Ein neuer Anfang kann gefunden werden.

Mythologie und magische Praktiken

Auf die große magische Dimension des Wermutkrauts geht Tabernaemontanus (1522–1590) gleich zu Beginn seiner 20-seitigen Abhandlung ein: Er hebt hervor, dass der Wermut bei den Alten in hohem Wert stand, bei ihren heidnischen Gottesdiensten Verwendung gefunden hätte und weiter: „Welcher Gebrauch vielleicht auch von ihnen, auff unsere Weiber geerbt und herkommen, die noch heutigs Tags dieses Kraut in ihre Würtzwüsche mit andern Kräutern samlen, und viel selzamer abgöttischer Phantaseyen und Narrenwercke darmit treiben."

Nancy Arrowsmith (geb. 1950) berichtet: „Im Jahr 1483 versuchten 2136 Jungfrauen aus Erfurt, Dürre und Armut von der Stadt abzuwenden, indem sie sich mit Wermut schmückten und durch die Straßen der Stadt zogen."

In den Kräuterbuschn, die zu Mariä Himmelfahrt kirchlich gesegnet werden, findet sich auch heute noch vielerorts der Wermut. Ob aus Vertrauen auf seine antidämonische Wirkkraft oder lediglich weil er Mitte August meist reichlich blüht, sei dahingestellt.

Verwendung – gestern und heute

Die große Heilkraft, die in dieser Pflanze steckt, wurde bereits im alten Ägypten erkannt, wo sie vor 3.000 Jahren als wurmwidriges Mittel verwendet wurde. Plinius Secundus (23–79) schreibt in seiner „Naturalis historiae", Liber XXVI über des Vorzüge des Wermuts: „Über den Gebrauch des Wermuts, dieser sehr leicht aufzufindenden und wie wenige, äußerst nützlichen Pflanze ist man sich einig; außerdem ist er bei den feierlichen Anlässen des römischen Volkes besonders berühmt geworden: Denn beim LATINERFEST fahren die Viergespanne am Kapitol um die Wette, und der Sieger erhält einen Wermuttrank, weil, nach meiner Meinung, unsere Vorfahren glaubten, es sei eine Ehrung, Gesundheit als Belohnung zu geben."

Für Hildegard von Bingen (1098–1179) zählte der Wermut zu den wichtigsten Heilkräutern. Sie empfiehlt eine Mai-Kur, die jeden dritten Tag von Mai bis Oktober getrunken werden und vorbeugend gegen viele Leiden sein soll. Und überhaupt: „Der Wermut ist sehr warm und sehr kräftig und ist der wichtigste Meister gegen alle Erschöpfung." Wegen ihres Absinthin- und Thujon-Gehaltes ist die Absinth-Pflanze innerlich nur mit großer Zurückhaltung zu verwenden. Die jüngere Forschung konnte nachweisen, dass ein Extrakt des Wermutkrauts bei nachlassendem Gedächtnis Rezeptoren im Gehirn aktiviert. Schon vor 2500 Jahren hatte Hippokrates (460–370 v.Chr.) Wermut bei nachlassendem Gedächtnis empfohlen.

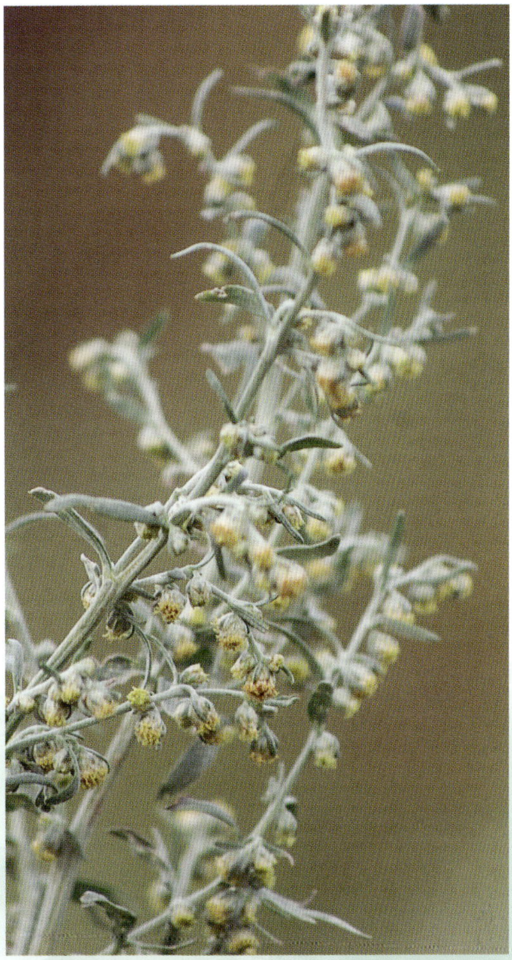

Wermutblüten

Wirbeldost

Lat. Name: *Clinopodium vulgare*
Botanischer Name: Gewöhnlicher Wirbeldost
Pflanzenfamilie: Lippenblütler

Als wäre ein Wirbelwind durch die Stängel gefahren, biegt sich der Wirbeldost in alle Richtungen. Bei seinem Anblick lächelt man automatisch, was für ein flauschiger, unaufgeregter kleiner Chaot. Beim Hingreifen weiß man gar nicht, wo man hinfassen soll – wo geht der Stängel weiter, ist alles nur eine polsterweiche rosarote Anhäufung von Blütenbällen. Hat man dann endlich ein paar Stängel in der Hand, sieht man, dass jeder unterschiedlich aufgeteilt ist, mal längere, mal wieder kurze Abstände zwischen den kugeligen Lampions hat. Man findet den Wirbeldost meist nahe am Waldrand, auf extensiv bewirtschafteten Rainen, aber auch auf Feuchtstellen in lichten Wäldern oder auf Waldwegen.

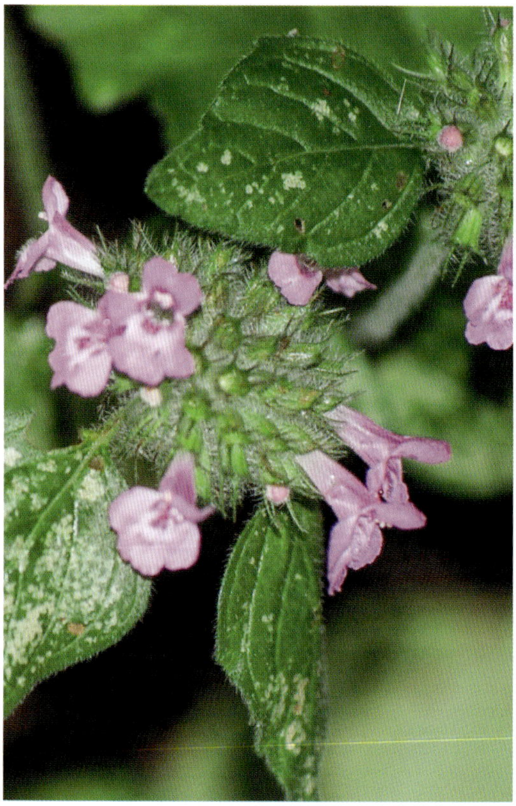

Blüten des Wirbeldosts

Rauch

Verwendete Pflanzenteile: Das ganz blühende Kraut: die Stängel, die Blätter und Blüten.

Beste Sammel- und Erntezeit: Im Spätsommer bis Frühherbst.

Wirkung, Wahrnehmung: Reinigungsrauch; vergessene weißmagische Räucherpflanze mit großer Schutzkraft. Klärt energetisch überladene Räume und bringt unruhige, chaotische Raumenergien wieder ins Lot. Überlagert negative Eintragungen, gleicht sie aus, so dass die Raumwahrnehmung deutlich angenehmer wird. Stark reinigende und lösende Kraft, wenn nichts mehr geht und alles zu kompliziert und undurchsichtige geworden ist. Durchtrennt den Gordischen Knoten mühelos, lässt die Gedanken wieder frei ziehen, löst Stockungen auf. Großes Schutzkraut gegen negative Beeinflussungen auf geistiger Ebene. Entgiftender Rauch, wenn man nur Negatives denkt und spricht! Stärkt das Vertrauen ins Leben; schenkt Herzenswärme und Einsicht in tiefere Zusammenhänge. Unterstützt den seelischen Ausgleich und lehrt uns, die Dinge so zu nehmen, wie sie sind.

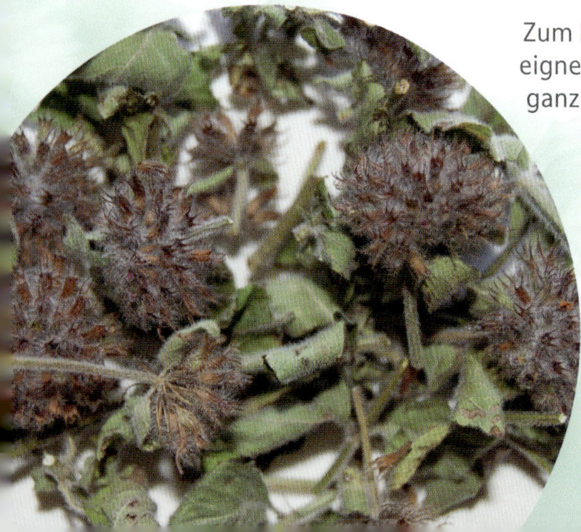

Zum Räuchern eignet sich das ganze blühende Kraut.

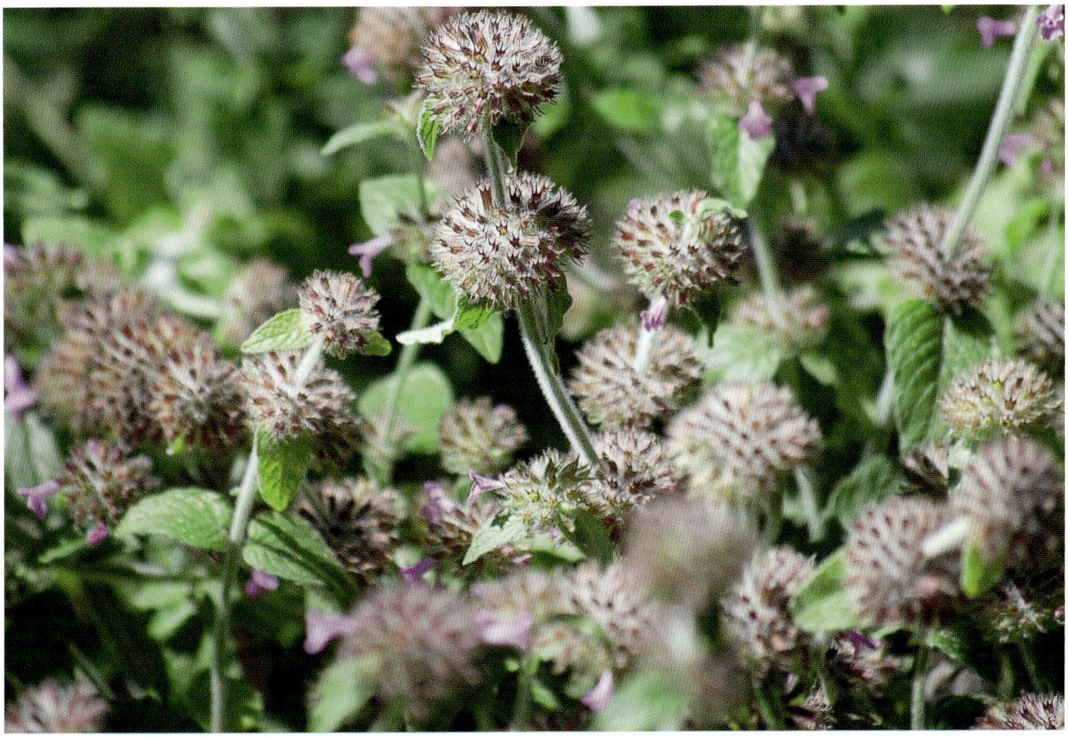

Wirbeldost zu Blühbeginn

Schwerpunkt, Anwendungen, Rezepte: Eine schützende Räucherung mit einer Mischung aus Wirbeldost, Wasserdost und Dost kombiniert mit Harz befördert positive Gedanken und Lösungen durch ihre dreifach weißmagische Kraft. Gehört in alle Räuchermischungen, mittels derer man den Wesenheiten der Natur näher kommen möchte.

Verwendung – gestern und heute

Dioskurides schreibt im 1. Jahrhundert, dass eine Abkochung von diesem Kraut gegen die Bisse giftiger Tiere, gegen Krämpfe, innere Brüche und Harnzwang genommen werde. Er verweist auch darauf, dass die Blüten Bettfüßen ähnelten.

Lonicerus (1528–1586) schreibt zum „Weberdost": „Es wächst dieses Kraut an steinichten Bergen, zwey Spannen hoch, die Blätter beynahe wie deß Quendels, die Blüth ist rings um den Stengel underschiedlich besetzt, wie am Andorn, wie ein Bethfuß formiert. Daher es bey den Griechischen den Nahmen „klinopodium" hat, welches so viel gesagt ist, als ein Bethfuß oder Bethstoll."

Findet in der Volksheilkunde kaum Verwendung, auch wenn wertvolle entzündungshemmende und antivirale Inhaltsstoffe belegt sind.

Ysop

Lat. Name: *Hyssopus officinalis*
Pflanzenfamilie: Lippenblütler

Der Ysop ist meine Pflanze der Unverdrossenheit: Egal wie herausfordernd der Jahreslauf auch sein mag, er verbreitet eine heitere laissez-faire-Stimmung. Er riecht gut, kommt jahrelang mit den kargsten Böden zurecht, leuchtet mir mit seinen blauen Blüten der Hoffnung freundlich entgegen und ist ein schier unerschöpfliches Labsal für viele liebgewonnene Insekten. Das wissen aber auch die Jäger und so ist mein Ysop-Beet ab Ende Juli nicht mehr zugänglich, weil da die Wespenspinnen neuerdings ihre versponnene Herrschaft übernehmen.

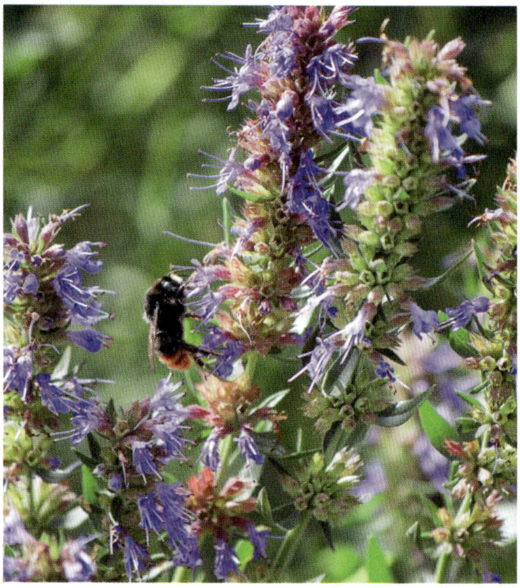
Blüten des Ysops

Rauch

Verwendete Pflanzenteile: Das ganze blühende Kraut: Stängel, Blätter, Blüten. Die stabilen Blütenstängel können zur Gänze getrocknet werden, um dann als Trägerstab für selbst hergestellte Räucherstäbchen zu dienen.

Beste Sammel- und Erntezeit: Der Ysop fängt im Juli zu blühen an. Die Blühdauer erstreckt sich bis Mitte, Ende August.

Wirkung, Wahrnehmung: Intensiver Reinigungsrauch; der Rauch des Ysops ist energetisch stark aufbauend und kann gut geistige Blockaden auflösen. Der Rauch räumt in Räumen und an Orten mit belastenden Hinterlassenschaften gründlich auf. Bei Reinigungsräucherungen in Häusern wird dieser Rauch oft wie ein energetischer Befreiungsschlag empfunden.

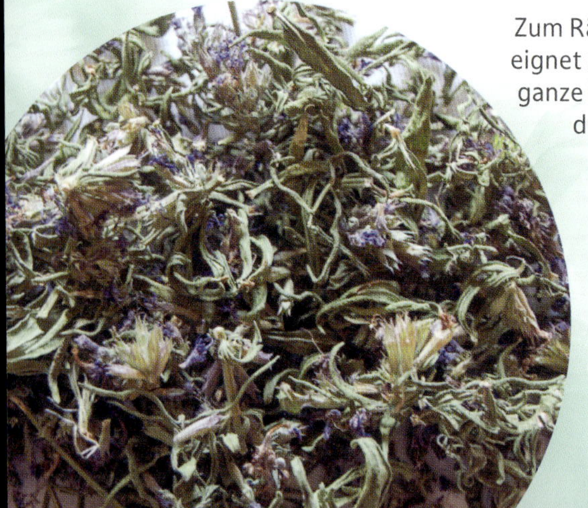
Zum Räuchern eignet sich das ganze blühende Kraut.

Reinigt und klärt die Atmosphäre in Krankenzimmern, in Räumen, in denen erkaltete Streitenergien zurückgeblieben sind. Nach Hausumbauten befinden sich belastete Stellen manchmal in Räumen mit neuer Verwendung, die jedoch durch die alte Eintragung nicht gut belebt werden können.

Ysop klärt die Eintrittspforten negativer Energien in Häusern, wie besonders zugige Ecken oder Fenster, die vielleicht von fremden, neidvollen Blicken belastet sind.

Der Rauch reinigt und klärt die eigenen Gefühle; wirkt anregend, macht den Kopf frei und fähig zur Konzentration, unterstützt das Durchhalten bei geistiger Arbeit. Hilft wilde und wirre Gedanken zu ordnen und sie mit mehr Gefühl zu betrachten; bricht das Eis, wenn die Seele vor inne-

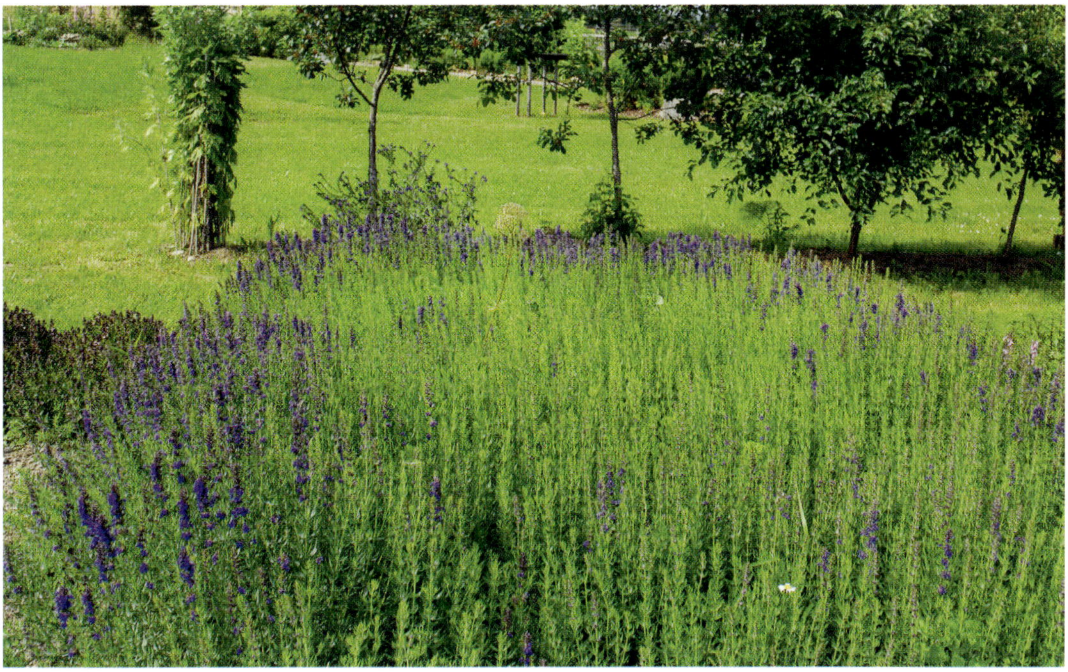

Blühender Ysop

rer oder äußerer Kälte erstarrt zu sein scheint. Der Rauch wärmt das kalte Herz; verhilft Menschen, die sich innerlich ganz zurückgezogen haben, zu mehr Offenheit und vielleicht auch neuer Hoffnung. Stärkt bei nervöser Erschöpfung; starker Impuls die Dinge zu überwinden, loszulassen und mit neuer Kraft weiterzugehen.

Schwerpunkt, Anwendungen, Rezepte: Räuchermischung für gute Energie in Räumen: Ysop, Rosmarin, Dost und Tanne (Harz). Für eine licht- und einsichtbringende Räucherung mischt man Ysop, Fenchel, Lavendel und Engelwurz-Samen mit Harz.

Verwendung – gestern und heute

Dioskurides hat im 1. Jahrhundert keine Rezepturen zum Ysop vermerkt, „da die Pflanze ja sowieso allseits bekannt sei". Hildegard von Bingen (1098–1179) zeigt ihre große Wertschätzung, indem sie schreibt: „Der Ysop ist von trockener Natur und gemäßigt warm, und er ist von so großer Kraft, dass sogar der Stein ihm nicht widerstehen kann, der dort wächst, wo der Ysop hingesät wird."

Lonicerus (1528–1586) schreibt über den „Isop oder Ispen": „Der Isop ist fast gleicher Tugend mit den Dosten... Welcher ein schön Angesicht haben will, der trincke von Isop, er sey grün oder dürr, der bekombt ein schön lauter Angesicht."

Ysop ist eine wunderbare Gewürz- und Kräutersalzpflanze. Die schleimlösende Kraft der Pflanze nutzt man am besten mit einem Ysop-Sirup, der mit Feigen und Honig gekocht wird.

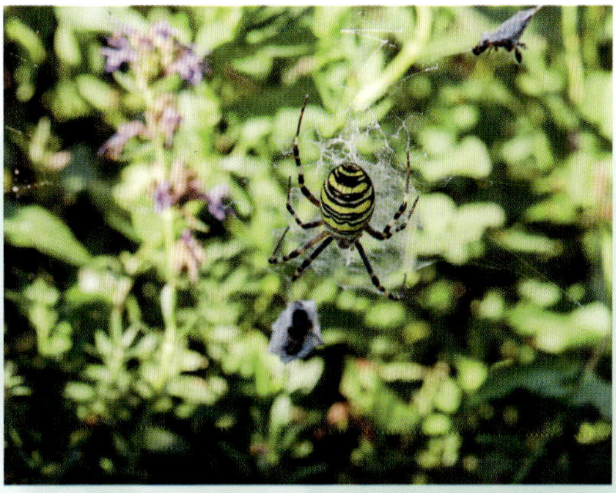

Wespenspinne auf Ysop

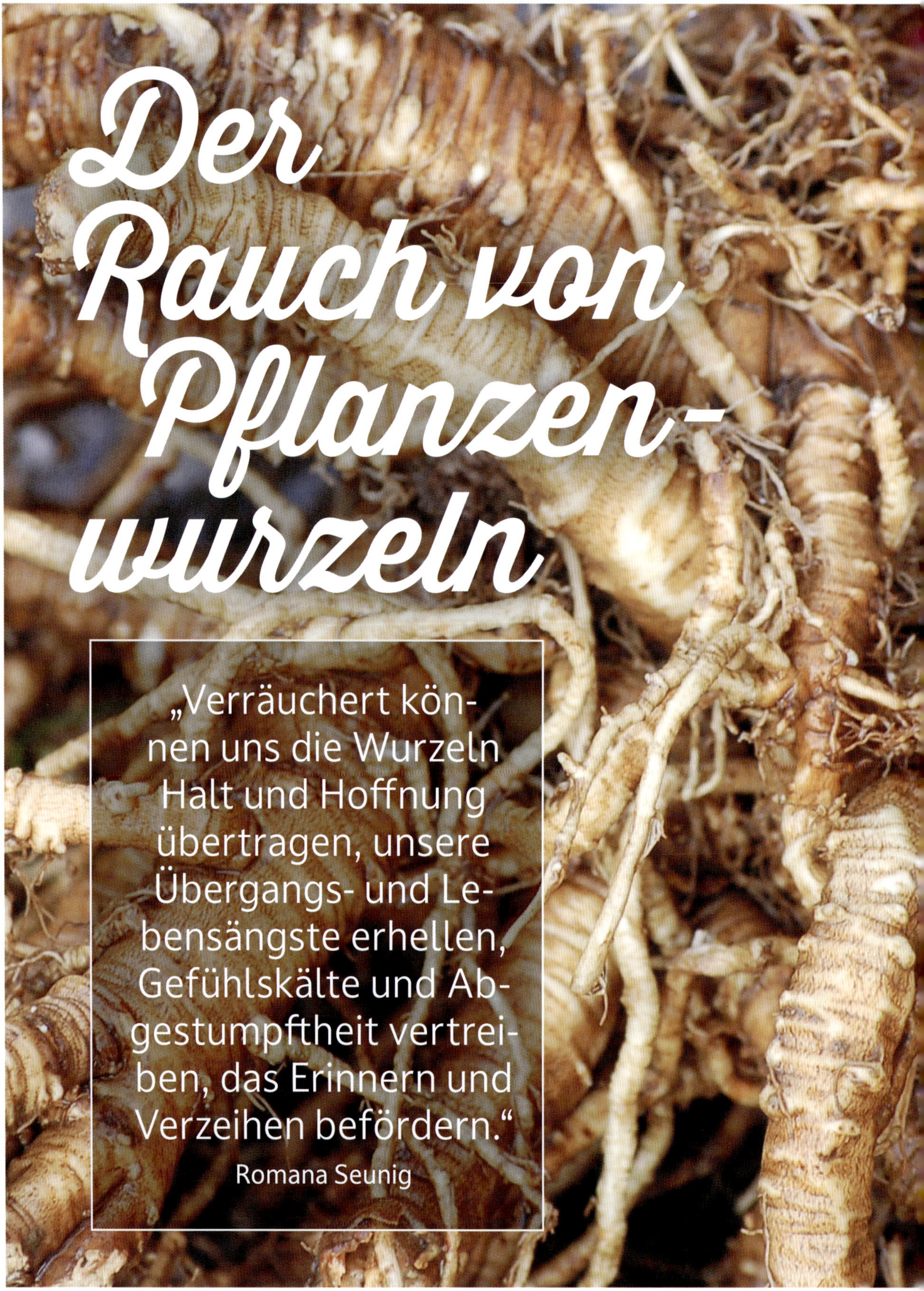

Der Rauch von Pflanzenwurzeln

„Verräuchert können uns die Wurzeln Halt und Hoffnung übertragen, unsere Übergangs- und Lebensängste erhellen, Gefühlskälte und Abgestumpftheit vertreiben, das Erinnern und Verzeihen befördern.“

Romana Seunig

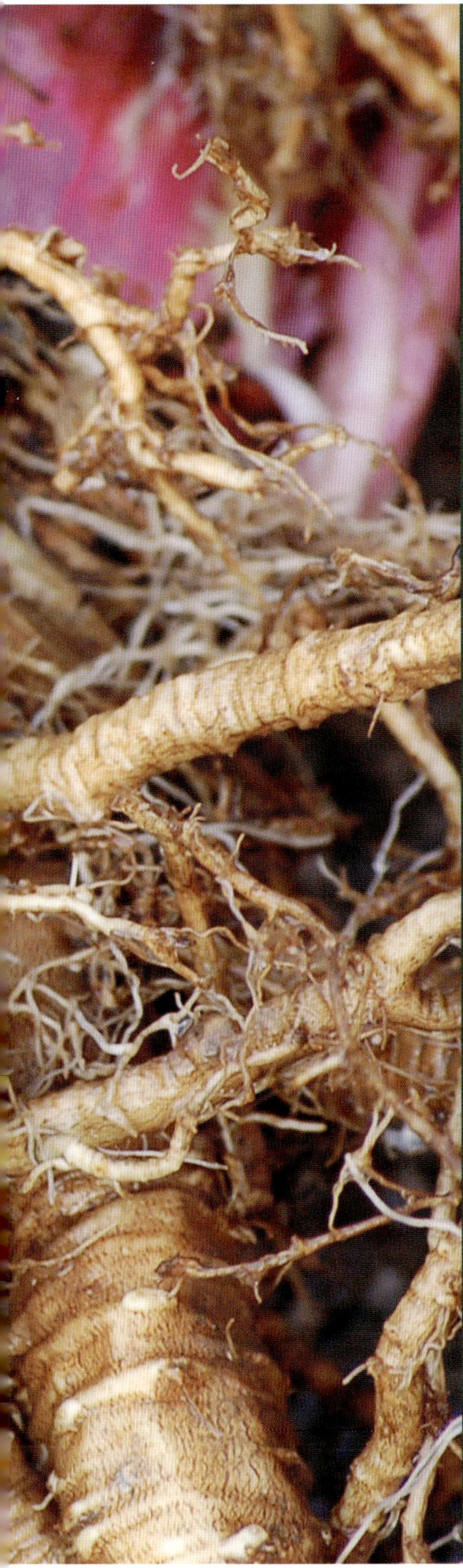

In den letzten Jahrzehnten habe ich zahllose Wurzeln von Pflanzen verräuchert und mich langsam ihrer Aussagekraft im Rauch angenähert. Dabei konnte ich feststellen, dass bei manchen Pflanzen die Wurzeln einen deutlich intensiveren Räucherstoff liefern als ihre oberirdischen Teile. Im Rauch sorgen sie für klare Impulse und umfassende starke geistige Eindrücke.

Ich möchte ein paar dieser ganzheitlichen Räucherpflanzen vorstellen, wobei die Wurzel immer das Haupträuchermittel ist. Aber mit den Wurzeln können und sollen natürlich auch andere Teile der jeweiligen Pflanze verräuchert werden.

Was sonst noch zum Wurzel-Rauch zu sagen wäre: Das Sichtbare entsteht im Nicht-Sichtbaren! Im Wurzelbereich schlägt das dunkle Herz der Pflanze. Hier fallen die Entscheidungen über eine gute Existenz oder frühes Vergehen! Es ist eine stille Welt, in der sich jede Veränderung doppelt auswirkt: in der Wurzel selbst, aber auch in der oberirdischen Gestalt der Pflanze.

Verräuchert können uns die Wurzeln Halt und Hoffnung übertragen, unsere Übergangs- und Lebensängste erhellen, Gefühlskälte und Abgestumpftheit vertreiben, das Erinnern und Verzeihen befördern. Ihr Rauch hilft uns beim Loslassen und erdet uns gleichzeitig auf unvergleichliche Weise. Manchmal scheint es als wäre ihr Rauch eine geistige Nahrung, der unser Denken öffnet und jeglichen geistigen Ansatz ins Positive lenkt.

Adlerfarn

Lat. Name: *Pteridium aquilinum*
Pflanzenfamilie: Adlerfarngewächse

Am Waldrand steht dicht an dicht das schützende Heer der Adlerfarne. Ihr geschickt verzweigtes Blätterdach lässt, von unten gesehen, für kleine Lebewesen schützende kathedralenartige Kuppelbögen entstehen, genug Raum, selbst für einen Fuchs, um aufrecht durchlaufen zu können. In manchen Wäldern findet sich an jeder lichten Stelle diese grüne Schutzdecke, die ein offenes Oben von einem geheimen Unten abdichtet. Es sind Palisadenfestungen mit unverzweigt dunkelglatten Wurzeln, auf Feen- und Nymphen-Plätzen in den Boden gerammt. Die Wurzelstämme unangreifbar mit Schwärze imprägniert. Doch innen strahlt ein wissendes Gesicht, erzählt von den Mühen, Schutz zu stellen für andere; erzählt von einer Welt, in der die Verbindung von schwarz und weiß ein unbezwingbares Grün ergibt.

Hieronymus Bock (1498–1554) sieht das anders: „Noch eins muß ich sagen, welchs mich an der farnwurzel ein sonderlich mirackel dunckt, nemlich sobald die wurzel durchschnitten, erscheint auff jeder seitten der zerschnittenen wurzel ein schwarzer auffgethoner vogel, anzusehen als ein Adler mit zweien köpffen in einem weissen feldt…"

Rauch

Verwendete Pflanzenteile: Wurzeln, Blätter.

Beste Sammel- und Erntezeit: Die Blätter bis zum Frühherbst. Die Pflanze wird behandschuht von Juni bis Oktober aus dem Boden gezogen.

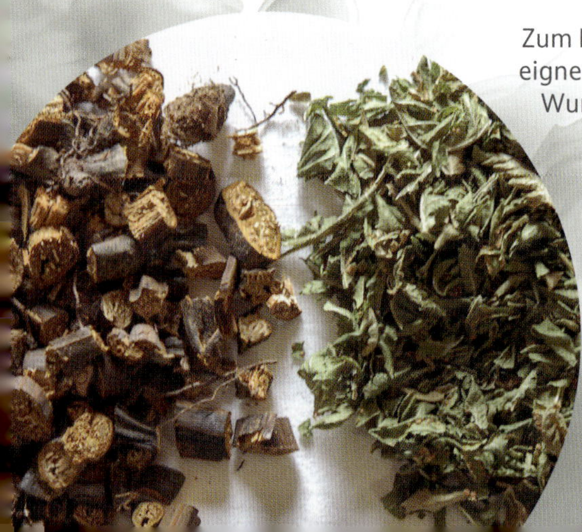

Zum Räuchern eignen sich die Wurzeln und Blätter.

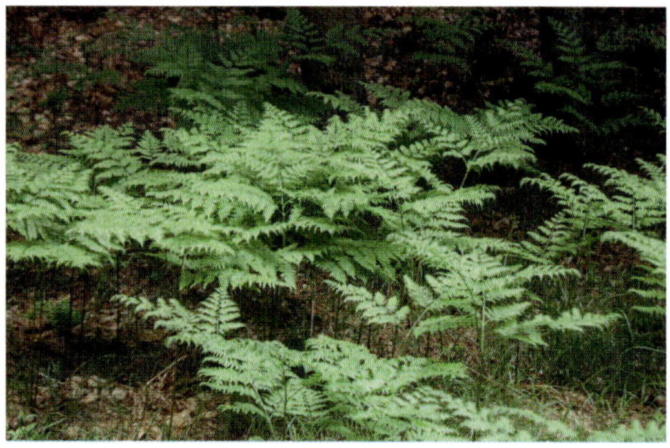

Adlerfarn

Die Wurzeln werden bis zu 5 cm in den hellen Bereich hinein abgeschnitten.

Wirkung, Wahrnehmung: Reinigungsrauch; Abwehrrauch – vor dem Rauch dieser Wurzel fliehen mißgünstige Wesenheiten und alles Negative. Reinigt und klärt belastete Orte; es kann sich wieder eine angenehme Atmosphäre durchsetzen. Auch in Vorbereitung auf wichtige Besprechungen oder andere Treffen, um die Räumlichkeiten sicher im positiven Energiebereich zu halten. Hilfreich bei der Auflösung von gefühlsmäßig wahrgenommenen Bedrohungen. Sollte stets mit anderen Wurzeln, Kräutern oder Blättern geräuchert werden.

Magisches zum Rauch: Für Abstand-Rituale zur inneren Abgrenzung und zum Schutz vor geistigen Übergriffen.

Schwerpunkt, Anwendungen, Rezepte: Räucherung, um das innere Gleichgewicht wieder zu finden: Adlerfarn, Mistel, Johanniskraut und Kiefer (Harz).

Mythologie und magische Praktiken

Am Johannistag, 24. Juni, wurden zahlreiche magische Werke vollbracht – so auch Farnkrautsamen gesammelt. Dies versuchte auch Hieronymus Bock (1498–1554), um damit gleichzeitig seine Lehrer zu widerlegen: „Alle Lehrer schreiben farnkraut trag weder blumen noch samen, jedoch so hab ich zum vierdten mal auff St. Johans nacht dem samen nach gangen unnd morgens frü ehe der tag anbrach, schwartzen kleinen samen auf düchern un breitten wulkraut blettern auffgehabet. Under einem stock mehr dann underm andern, es warn unter hunderten nit ein körnlin funden, dargegen hab ich unter einem stock mehr dann hundert körnlin funden... Wan ich den same hab wollen holen, bin ich nit allein gangen, es warn zwei zu mir genommen, und nachts in derselbe gegene (da nit vil überlauffens war) ein groß feur gemacht, und über nacht also lassen brennen. Wie nun solchs zugehe, oder was für ein geheimnuß die natur darmit gemein, ist mir verborgen. Das hab ich wollen anzeigen, seintemal alle lehrer den farn on samen beschreiben."

Verwendung – gestern und heute

Der oben zitierte Hieronymus Bock hat das Rezept für eine Brandsalbe überliefert, die helfen soll, wenn man sich mit Feuer, heißem Wasser, Öl oder dergleichen verletzt hat: „Nemet die wurzel von farnkraut, zerstossen, den safft heruß gedruckt, um das zu drucken, nemet darzu rosenwasser, kuhmistwasser oder Lyndenblüte oder ein gemein Brunnenwasser, darmit duchgestrichen, gibt ein zehen safft, der selbit ist nit zu bezalen für den brandt, dann wann nichts will helffen und leschen, ist gemelte arznei ein besonder erwölte arznei, des man sich billich muß verwundern."

Früher war der getrocknete Adlerfarn das Bettstroh der Holzknechte.

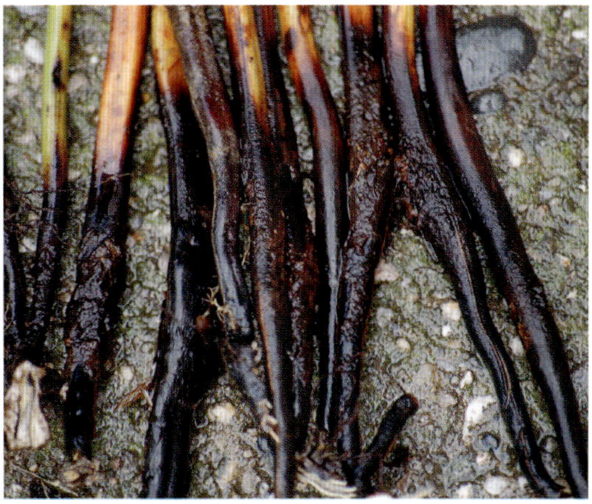

Adlerfarnwurzeln

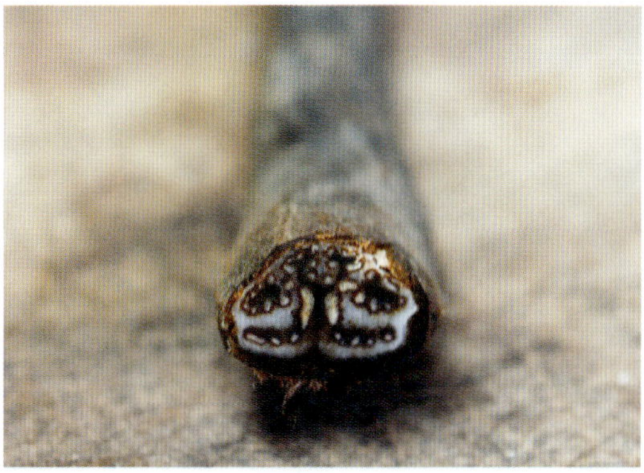

Aufgeschnittene Adlerfarnwurzel

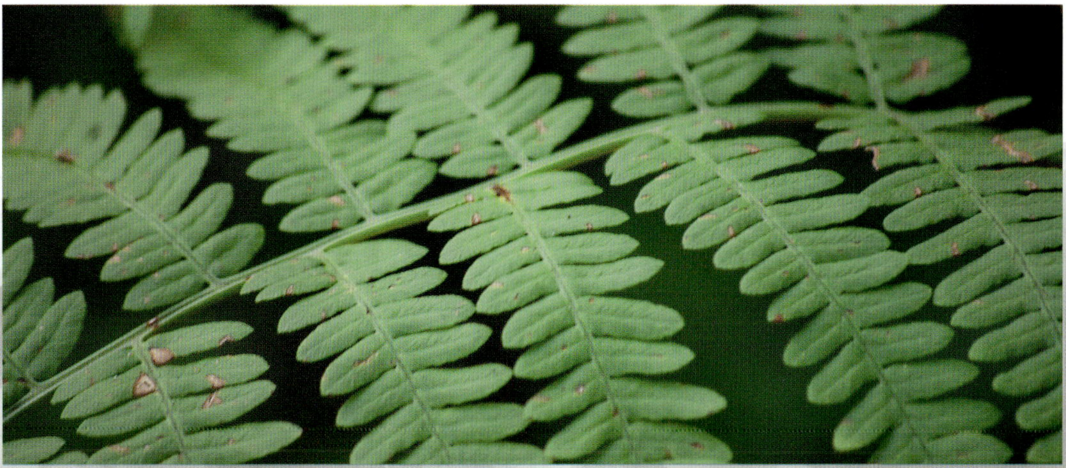

Gefiederte Blätter des Adlerfarns

Alant

Lat. Name: *Inula helenium*
Pflanzenfamilie: Korbblütler

Als die keltischen Söldner aus dem aufgelassenen Heer Alexanders des Großen (356–323 v. Chr.) um 323 v. Chr. wieder in ihre Heimat zogen – was aus dem vorderasiatischen Bereich bis zu drei Jahre gedauert haben dürfte – brachten sie von dort eine ganz besondere Wurzel mit, die ihnen Kraft und Ausdauer nicht nur im Kampf, sondern auch auf den langen Wegmärschen gegeben hatte. So oder so ähnlich dürfte es sich zugetragen haben, dass der Alant so früh nach Mitteleuropa gekommen ist und es vor allem so schnell zu höchstem Ansehen als Heilpflanze geschafft hat. Von diesem Bild sind dann die geheimen Zutaten des Zaubertrankes eines Asterix & Co. nur noch ein Gedankenwurf entfernt…

Tatsache ist, dass der griechische Arzt Theophrast (371–287 v. Chr.) den Alant als giftwidriges Mittel gepriesen, dass Plinius (23–79) den Alant hochgelobt hat und der gekochte Alant-Heilwein das gesamte Mittelalter über als Universalheilmittel unverzichtbar war.

Rauch

Verwendete Pflanzenteile: Wurzeln, Blüten, Blätter.

Beste Sammel- und Erntezeit: Die Wurzel wird im Herbst ausgegraben, zerteilt, gewaschen, gebürstet, sehr klein geschnitten und getrocknet. Wenn die Wurzelstücke sehr klein zusammengetrocknet sind, brauchen sie vor dem Räuchern nicht mehrt vermahlen zu werden. Die Blätter können das ganze Jahr über beerntet werden; die Zeit der Blüte reicht meist von Juli bis August.

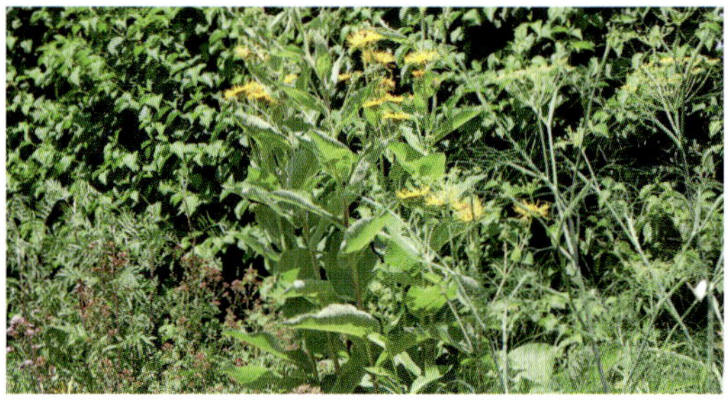

Wuchsform von Alant

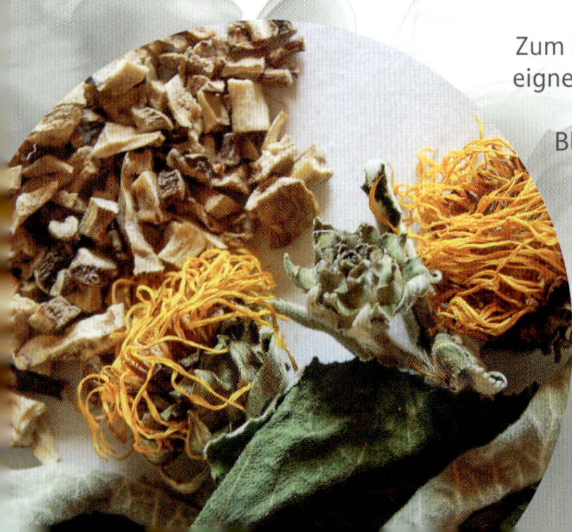

Zum Räuchern eignen sich die Wurzeln, Blüten und Blätter.

Wirkung, Wahrnehmung: Großer Abwehrrauch; Schutzrauch für Mensch und Tier; Reinigungsrauch. Abwehr von bösem Zauber und Dämonen der Dunkelheit; in angstvollen Stunden beruhigt der Alant-Rauch und wirkt aufbauend bei Niedergeschlagenheit, Depression und tiefsitzenden Zweifeln.

Die Kraft seiner kleinen Blütensonnen wird spürbar, was die Lebenskraft stärkt und neuen Mut in schweren Zeiten vermitteln kann. Rhythmusgebend in Veränderungsprozessen; hilft die Kraft der inneren Mitte wieder zu finden. Besonderes Räuchermittel bei emotionaler Erstarrung; balsamisch für „Kopfmenschen" und solche, die mehr in theoretischen Welten leben, um sich gut zu erden und um ihre körperliche Wahrnehmung zu unterstützen. Stress und Blockaden werden gelöst, geistige Klarheit und Ruhe können entstehen. Durchlichtet die Divergenz zwischen Sein und Schein. Weist den Weg zu geschärfter Aufnahme der persönlichen Umwelt und zum achtsamen Umgang mit anderen.

Magisches zum Rauch: Derwisch-Tänzer verräuchern Alant auf glühenden Kohlen, um sich noch schneller drehen zu können.

Schwerpunkt, Anwendungen, Rezepte: Aufbauende Räuchermischung für melancholische Gemüter: Zur Alantwurzel mischt man Ysop, große Klettenwurzel, Bibernellwurzel und Harz.

Mythologie und magische Praktiken

Mensch und Tier wurden seiner großen Schutzkraft unterstellt. So ist der Alant in vielen Gegenden unverzichtbarer Bestandteil des Kräuterbuschn zu Mariä Himmelfahrt am 15. August: Heinrich Marzell (1885–1970) schreibt, dass in Westfalen der Alant im Kräuterbuschn so viele Köpfe haben sollte, wie Pferde oder Kühe im Stall waren. In den Ställen wurden Alant-Büschel aufgehängt, um die Tiere vor magischen Schadensübergriffen zu schützen.

Zahlreiche magische Anwendungen reichen bis in die Gegenwart: So werden Alantwurzeln am Körper getragen, um Liebe anzuziehen oder um vor Verhexung zu schützen – was, wie man weiß, durchaus die zweite Seite derselben Medaille sein kann.

Verwendung – gestern und heute

Das hohe Ansehen des Alants reicht in der Antike weit zurück: So schreibt der Koch Apicius (25 v. Chr. bis 42 n. Chr.), dass „Alant als Gewürz in keinem römischen Haushalt fehlen dürfe."

Hildegard von Bingen (1098–1179) meint in ihrer „Physica": „Und das ganze Jahr über soll er sowohl dürr als auch grün in reinen Wein gelegt werden – und wer in der Lunge Schmerzen hat, der trinke ihn täglich mäßig vor dem Essen und nach dem Essen, und das Gift – das ist der Eiter – nimmt er aus seiner Lunge weg, und er unterdrückt die Migräne und reinigt die Augen... wenn du aber keinen Wein hast, um ihn einzulegen, dann mach mit Honig und Wasser eine reine Honigwürze und lege den Alant ein und trink wie oben gesagt wurde."

Ein Universalheilmittel des Mittelalters war die „Potio Paulina", das paulinische Getränk. Der ausgefallene Name bezieht sich auf eine Legende: Der Apostel Paulus hätte einst dem Timotheus gegen Magenschwäche und allerlei Krankheiten einen solchen Trunk empfohlen. Wohl ein kluger mittelalterlicher PR-Gag, denn mit einer Heiligenlegende im Gepäck verkaufte sich das Produkt gleich leichter. Der Alant-Heilwein wurde in Alant-Siedereien hergestellt (beispielsweise 1421 in Wörth an der Donau) und durch Händler über ganz Europa vertrieben.

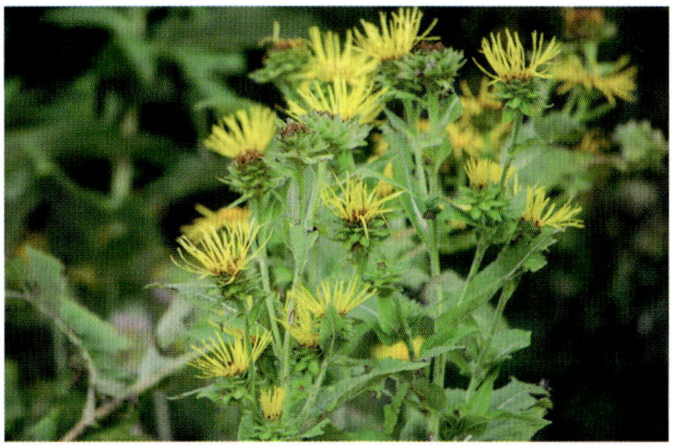

Blühender Alant

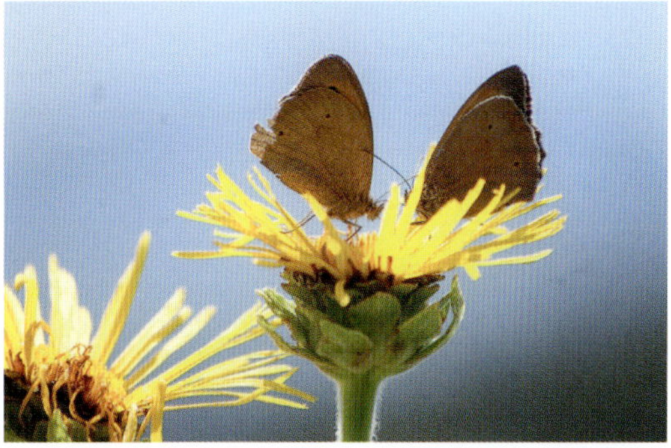

Alantblüte

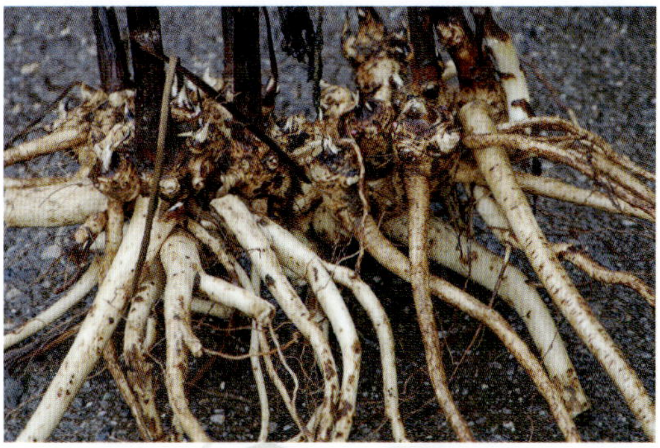

Alantwurzel

Hieronymus Bock (1498–1554) schreibt: „Alantwurzel ist ein köstlich arznei zu den Engbrüstigen und die ein kalten magen haben. Das pulver von der gedörte Alantwurz mit zucker od honig vermische zu einem latwerge. Ist ein gebenedeite arznei für das keichen und zehen husten."

Die Alant-Wurzel ist ein stoffwechsel- und rhythmusregulierendes Kräftigungsmittel, das als Einzeltee oder Heilwein gute Dienste leistet.

Ampfer

Lat. Name: *Rumex obtusifolius*
Botanischer Name: Stumpfblättriger Ampfer
Pflanzenfamilie: Knöterichgewächse

Ungeliebt, unverträglich, gefürchtet, bekämpft, verfolgt mit Gift und Spaten und doch obsiegender Platzräuber, eisenmächtiger Pfahlwurzler! Die beeindruckenden Überlebenskräfte des Ampfers offenbaren ein Pflanzenwesen, das von höchstem Wachstumsdruck sowohl in der Blatt- als auch in der Wurzelmasse beseelt ist. Einmal gekeimt, beschattet der Ampfer binnen kurzer Zeit seine Nachbarpflanzen und reißt wurzelseitig alles an Nährstoffen an sich. Dabei wehrt er etwaige Essensgelüste von Menschen und Tieren, ob seiner opulenten Erscheinung, sehr gezielt und nachhaltig ab: Er pumpt seine Blätter derart mit Oxalsäure voll, dass es bei Verzehr zu Unverträglichkeiten oder Mangel an Mineralstoffen kommen kann. Die Volksmedizin hatte sich aber nicht abhalten lassen und verwendete seit jeher die Wurzel bei Verdauungs- und diversen Hautproblemen.

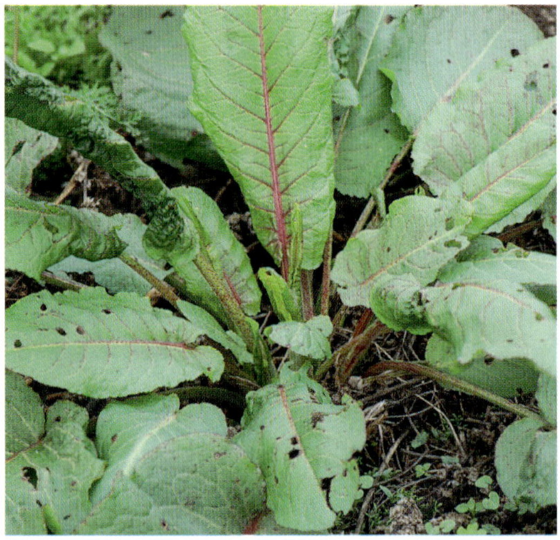
Blätter des stumpfblättrigen Ampfers

Rauch

Verwendete Pflanzenteile: Wurzel, Blätter.

Beste Sammel- und Erntezeit: Die Wurzeln werden in der zweiten Jahreshälfte gegraben, gewaschen und zerkleinert. Dabei Handschuhe tragen, da die Wurzeln sich stark gelb verfärben und gleichzeitig abfärben. Die getrockneten Wurzelstückchen werden vor dem Räuchern vermahlen. Die Blätter können das ganze Jahr über beerntet werden.

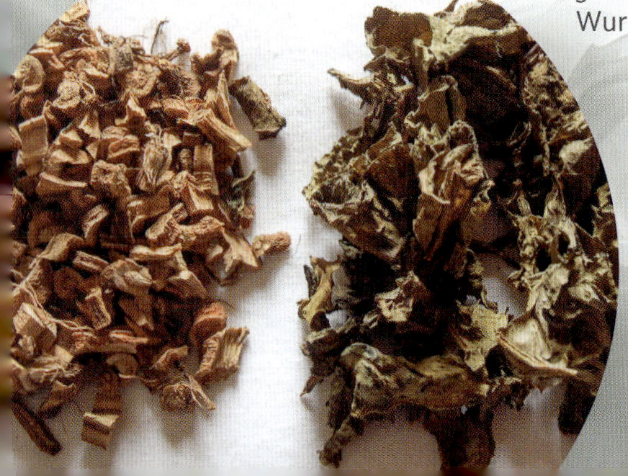
Zum Räuchern eignen sich die Wurzeln und Blätter.

Wirkung, Wahrnehmung: Die frische Wurzel verströmt einen extremen Duft, ähnlich wie die Wurzel der großen Klette. Abwehrrauch mit gleichzeitiger Kraft zum emotionalen Umschwung! Der Rauch stärkt die innere Kraft und den Widerstandswillen gegen äußere Anfeindungen – seien sie sozialer oder familiärer Natur. Vermittelt die Entschlossenheit durchzuhalten. Umschwungskraut mit Sonnen-, Jupiter- und Mars-Kräften die helfen, selbst in feindlicher Atmosphäre unversehrt und bei sich zu bleiben.

Das dreifache Feuer dieses Rauches verhilft zu neuem Lebensmut und klarer Abgrenzung gegenüber alten Lasten und Vereinnahmungen. Der Rauch klärt die Aura und ätzt Überflüssiges einfach weg. Die Wahrnehmung nach einer Ampfer-Räucherung ist eine sehr geradlinige und befreite. Das Gefühl, die Dinge selbst in der Hand zu haben, setzt sich durch. Die Dinge sind losgeeist und ins Fließen gebracht. Auch die Lebenslust steigt und unterstützt die bewusst gesetzten Aktionen: entweder um im Leben wieder Anker zu setzen, vom Blatt im Wind zum bestimmungsgemäß Sesshaften zu werden; oder um sich, endlich befreit, auf die große Suche zu machen.

Schwerpunkt, Anwendungen, Rezepte: Eine alte Räuchermischung sollte bei überbeanspruchten oder steifen Gelenken zu einer Schmerzlinderung führen, wenn die schmerzenden Stellen in den Rauch gehalten wurden: Ampferwurzel und -kraut mit Beifuß und Rosmarin vermischen und mit Harz fein mörsern. Räuchermischung zur inneren Umstimmung und um sich gegen depressive Phasen zu wappnen: Ampfer, Goldrute, Mistel und Salbei mit Harz kombinieren.

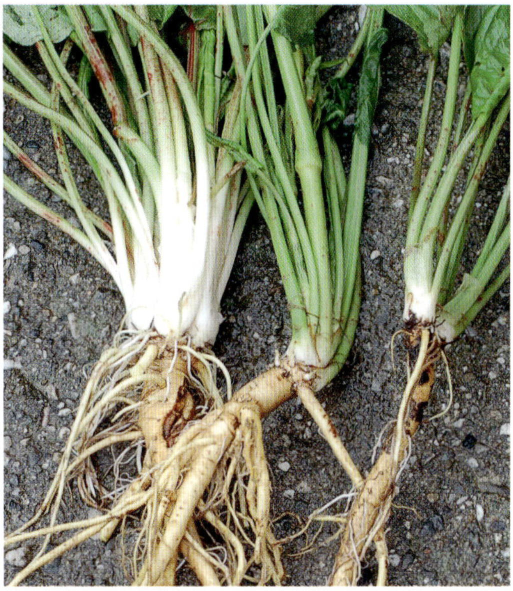
Ampferpflanze mit Wurzeln

Verwendung – gestern und heute

Hildegard von Bingen (1098–1179) stellt klar, dass der Ampfer zwar als Viehfutter nützlich sei, aber: „Der Ampfer ist weder warm noch kalt in richtigem Maße. Daher taugt der dem Menschen nicht zum Essen, da er gegen seine Natur erregt ist. Und wenn der Mensch ihn äße, würde er ihn traurig machen…"

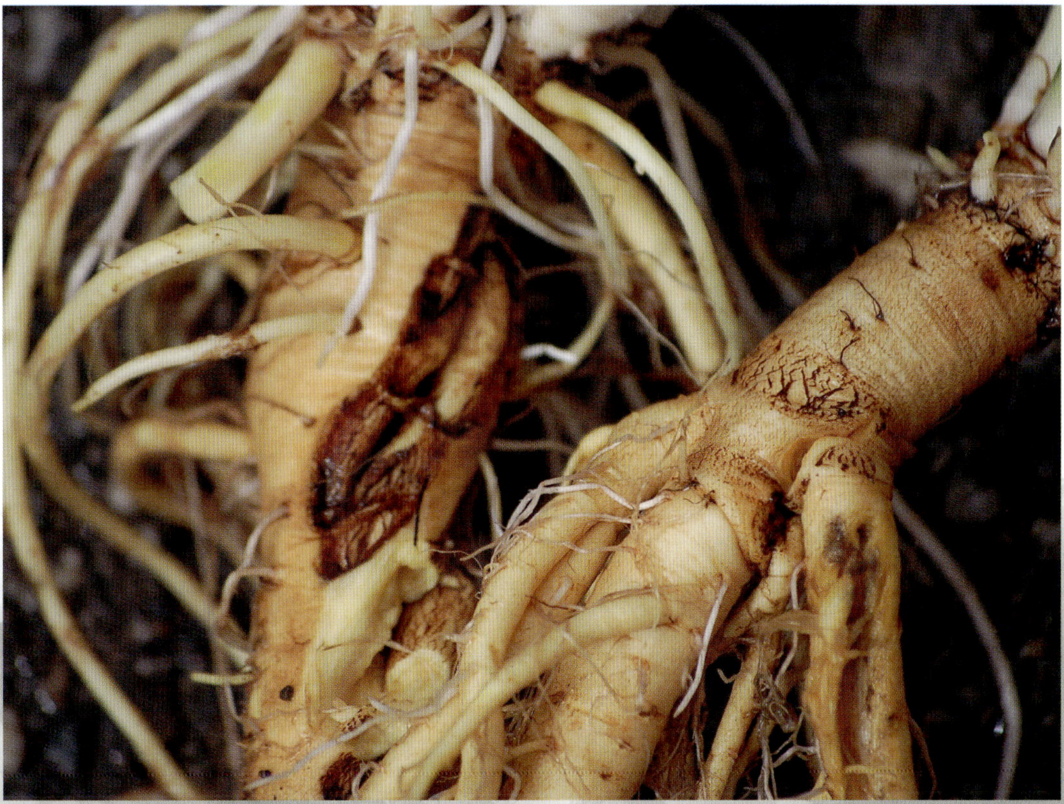
Speicherwurzel des Ampfers

Bärenschote

Lat. Name: *Astragalus glycyphyllos*
Pflanzenfamilie: Hülsenfrüchtler

Mit Bedacht und lange unbemerkt umrundet meine Bärenschote einen Haselnussstrauch, tanzt bodennah zum Wasserrhythmus der Haselnuss, indem sie viele kleine Wasserwirbel nachzuzeichnen scheint. Unterbrochen wird ihr Wasserballett immer wieder durch einige neugierige Gierschbegleiter, die in ihren Kreis drängen. Fröhlich locker die Blüte, extravagant, schwergewichtig und gleichzeitig federleicht wirkend, der frei nach oben stehende Samenstand. Die Süße der Blätter ist immer wieder überraschend. In der Traditionellen Chinesischen Medizin wird die Wurzel seit Jahrtausenden als Stärkungsmittel und Tonikum für Lebensenergie verwendet.

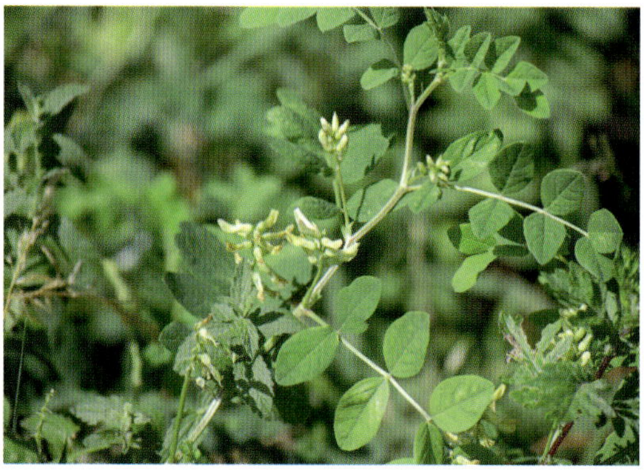

Blühende Bärenschote

Rauch

Verwendete Pflanzenteile: Wurzeln, Blätter, Samen.

Beste Sammel- und Erntezeit: Die Wurzeln werden in der zweiten Jahreshälfte, jedenfalls zur Zeit des Samenstandes, gegraben, gewaschen und fein aufgeschnitten. Nach der Trocknung dunkel verwahren und für die Räuchermischungen fein vermahlen. Die Blätter können das ganze Jahr über gesammelt werden. Die Samenstände sind ab Ende August verfügbar und werden zur Gänze getrocknet.

Wirkung, Wahrnehmung: Der frische Wurzelduft ist hell, grün, zitronig, erfrischend und entspannend zugleich. Schutzrauch; Kraut zur Begleitung der Sonnenwenden; die Wurzel eignet sich besonders für Abstreif-Räucherungen: Während langer Krankheiten und danach, in belastenden Lebensphasen, in und nach negativen Stresszeiten. Die Pflanze ist eine Botschafterin des Elementes Wasser und unterstützt verräuchert die Fähigkeit gelebtes Leben zu reflektieren, vielleicht sogar loszulassen. Der Rauch hilft einem dabei seine Rolle klar zu sehen, sie anzunehmen und – wenn notwendig – sich selbst zu vergeben.

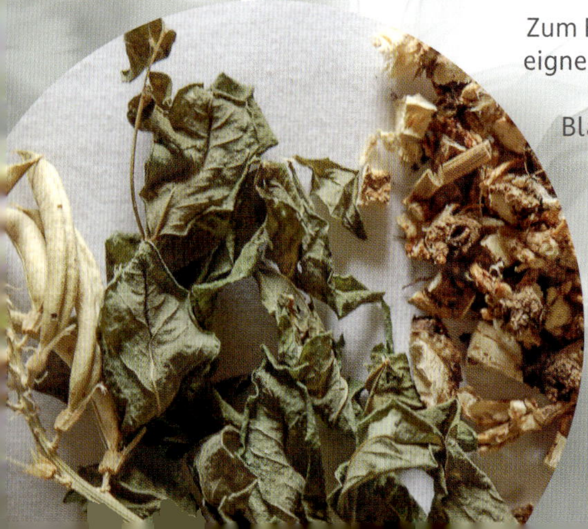

Zum Räuchern eignen sich die Wurzeln, Blätter und Samen.

Der Rauch führt zurück zur richtigen Ordnung, hilft beim Loslassen und Überwinden der eigenen Opferrolle. Unterstützt generell Veränderungsprozesse, hilft dabei solche anzunehmen und verhilft zur Erkenntnis, dass alles zu jeder Zeit in Bewegung und somit auch in Veränderung ist. Mit diesem räucherischen Potenzial passt die Bärenschote zu den Sonnenwenden im Jahr und hilft, sich neu auszurichten. Entspannungs-Räucherungen, die entkrampfend, beruhigend und erdend wirken und eine gewisse Zufriedenheit vermitteln können.

Schwerpunkt, Anwendungen, Rezepte: Ritual zum Abschließen negativer Phasen oder um den Übergang in eine heilsame Ordnung zu unterstützen, ist eine Räuchermischung aus Bärenschote, Beifuß, Engelwurz und Lavendel. Eine verzeihende Räuchermischung für sich selbst oder zur Bestärkung einer Versöhnung besteht aus Bärenschote, Ysop, Nelkenwurz und Kleinem Habichtskraut. Harz nicht vergessen!

Verwendung – gestern und heute

Lonicerus (1528–1586) erwähnt unter Astragalus eine „Christianwurtz" oder „Knollenkraut oder Erdmören" und schreibt bezüglich der Anwendung: „Christianwurtzel hat ein zusammenziehende stopffende Natur. Die Wurtzel mit Wein getruncken, stopffet den Bauchfluß, treibt den harn, und heilet die rothe Ruhr mit rothem Wein getruncken."

Die Bärenschote wird heute hinsichtlich ihres heilsamen Potenzials bei Heuschnupfen beforscht.

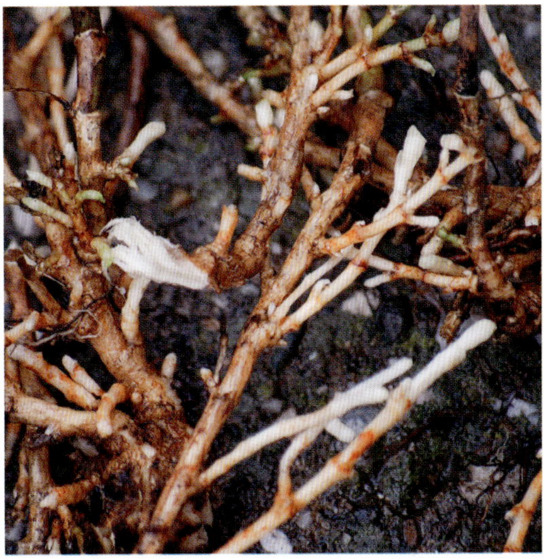

Wurzel der Bärenschote

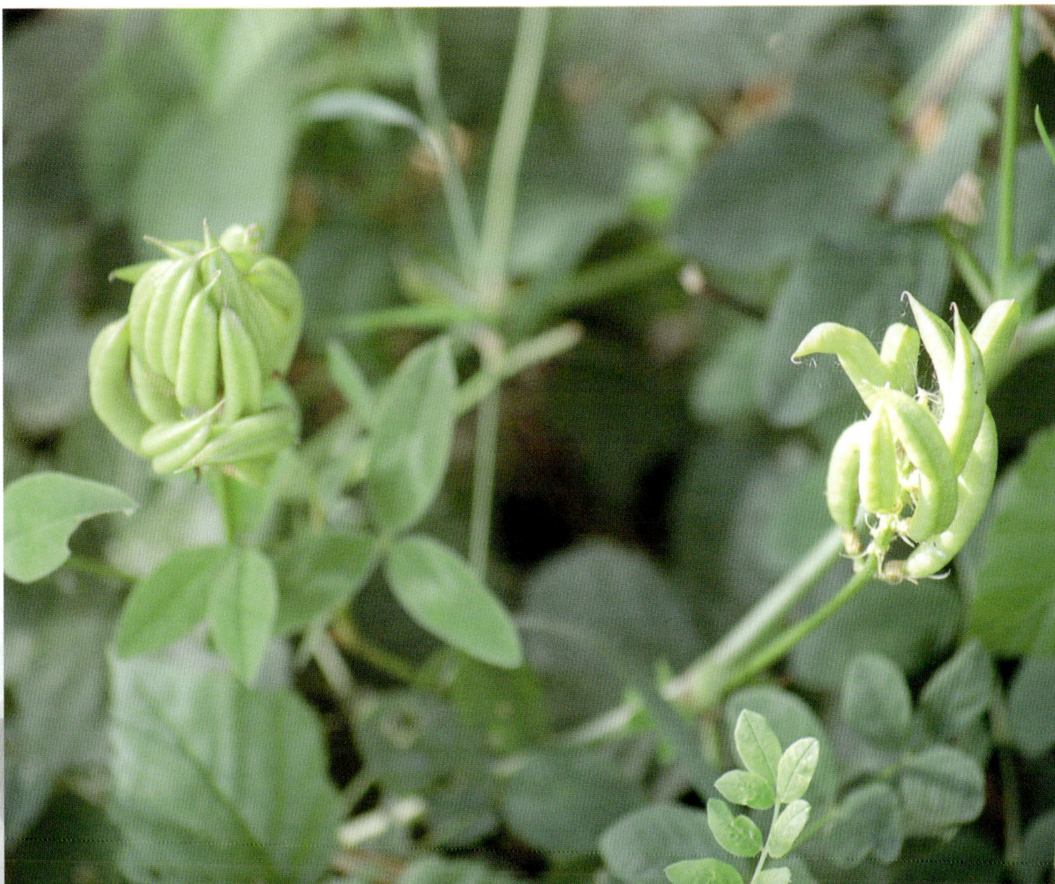

Samenstände der Bärenschote

Baldrian

Lat. Name: *Valeriana officinalis*
Botanischer Name: Arznei-Baldrian
Pflanzenfamilie: Baldriangewächse

Ausgestattet mit einem breiten Wirkspektrum zählte der Baldrian von Anfang der schriftlichen Aufzeichnungen an zur Kategorie der vielfältig einsetzbaren Heilpflanzen. Unzählige Reime rufen uns diese besonderen Kräfte ins Gedächtnis: „Trinkt Baldrian, sunst müsst ihr alle dran" oder „Esst Pimpinell und Baldrian, so gehet euch die Pest nit an", klang es in den Pestzeiten des Mittelalters. Das Kraut hat aber auch eine zarte Seite, die die eheliche Liebe beflügeln kann: „Macht holdselig eins und friedsam, wo zwei des wassers aus einem geschirr trinken", hieß es im 16. Jahrhundert.

In meinem Garten führt der Baldrian ein erstaunliches Eigenleben, wechselt von Beet zu Beet und entwickelt sich höchst unterschiedlich. Fast scheint es mir, als ließe er sich an dem einen Platz von seinen Nachbarpflanzen zu höchstem Wachstum, bis zu 1,90 m animieren und knapp daneben dümpelt er mühsam dahin und schleppt sich gerade einmal auf eine Höhe von 60 cm.

In manchen Jahren legen sich einige Baldriananstauden einen schwarzen Mantel aus Blattläusen um Stängel und Blüten, während andere wunderbar frei ihre rosa Blütenfarbe präsentieren. Und dann gibt es Jahre, in denen auf keiner einzigen Baldrianpflanze eine Blattlaus zu sehen ist. Es ist spannend zu sehen, wie der Baldrian in jedem Jahr seine ganz persönliche Wirklichkeit entwickelt, offensichtlich in stiller Interaktion mit den Elementen.

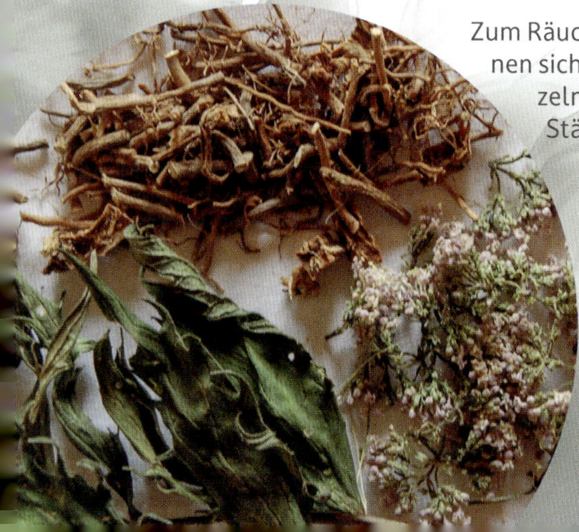

Zum Räuchern eignen sich die Wurzeln, Blätter, Stängel und Blüten.

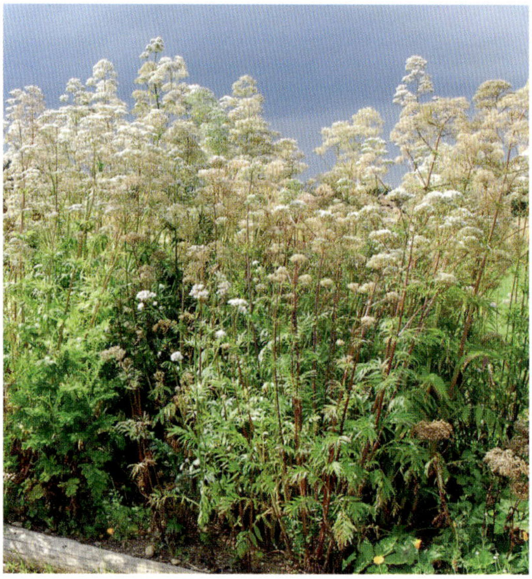

Blühender Baldrian

Rauch

Verwendete Pflanzenteile: Wurzeln, Stängel, Blätter, Blüten.

Beste Sammel- und Erntezeit: Die Wurzeln gräbt man am besten im Herbst, säubert und trocknet sie. Weil die Wurzeln so fein sind, kann man sie auch erst nach dem Trocknen mit der Hand zerkleinern. Die Blätter und Stängel erntet man zugleich mit der Wurzelernte, die Blüten im Frühsommer.

Wirkung, Wahrnehmung: Abwehrrauch; Verschreikraut gegen magische Übergriffe. Der Wurzelrauch unterstützt die Abwehrkraft gegen alle dunklen Mächte und Gefahren, gegen Dämonen, nächtliche Alpträume und ungenaue Bedrohungen.

Krankenzimmer wurden mit Baldrian ausgeräuchert, um den Kranken vor schwarzer Magie und lebenskraftsaugenden Wesenheiten zu schützen. Ebenso wurden kranke Kinder mit Baldrianwurzel abgeräuchert, um negative Anhaftungen zu lösen.

Unterstützt geistige Tätigkeiten, da er einem hilft, sich voll auf seine Aufgabe zu konzentrieren. Man kann die Außenwelt ausblenden und seine Geisteskraft fokussieren. Zum Freiräuchern von Verwünschungen, Bannungen und lähmenden Anhaftungen. Der Rauch erdet stark; hilft Hirngespinste zu erkennen und aufzulösen.

Vermittelt Selbstvertrauen bei innerer Unruhe und Angstzuständen. Der Rauch hat eine wohltuende Wirkung auf die Psyche, wird beruhigend und antidepressiv erlebt. Man kann endlich zur Ruhe kommen. Ängstliche Menschen können wieder durchatmen. Eine positive Gemütslage kann sich stabilisieren. Das Gefühl von Gelöstheit und Gelassenheit stellt sich manchmal jedoch erst Stunden später ein.

Magisches zum Rauch: Meditationsrauch, bei dem man sich leicht schwebend fühlt und die Gedanken ziehen lassen kann: Zur Vorbereitung trinkt man einen kalt angesetzten Wurzeltee und räuchert dann ganz wenig von der Wurzel pur, was zugegeben einen heftigen Geruch freisetzt, aber dafür wunderbar sinnlich entspannend wirkt. WICHTIG: Solange man in Räumen räuchert ganz wenig Wurzel nehmen! Zum abschließenden Abräuchern kann man im Freien vielleicht etwas mehr von der Wurzel nehmen.

Heinrich Marzell (1885–1970) verweist auf die besondere Stellung stark riechender Pflanzen im Volksglauben und setzt den heftigen Geruch in Beziehung zum Geisterglauben. Solche Räucherungen dienten stets „...zum Vertreiben der bösen Geister bei Natur- und Kulturvölkern..."

Wenn ein Pferd als verzaubert angesehen wurde, gab man ihm Freitag vor Sonnenaufgang Baldrian- und Beifußwurzeln. Dann hat man Koriander, Kampfer und Myrrhe vermischt und das Pferd durch den umgebundenen Maulsack hindurch beräuchert.

Schwerpunkt, Anwendungen, Rezepte: Bei Zorn und Uneinigkeit kann Baldrianrauch zu einem ausgleichenden Gemütszustand führen.

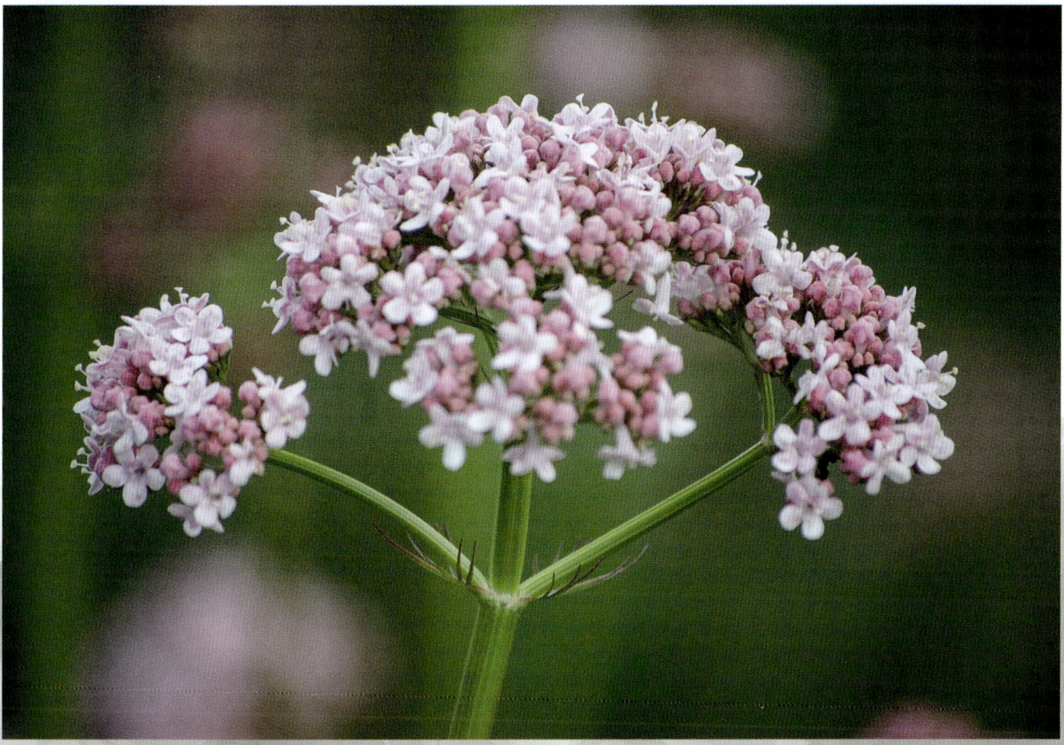

Baldrianblüte

Klärende Räuchermischung zur Abwehr und zum Lösen von angstvollen Blockaden: Baldrian, Wirbeldost, Wacholder und Weißdorn in Kombination mit Harz.

Mythologie und magische Praktiken

Sein intensiver, alles durchdringender Wurzelgeruch, der zudem für Katzen unwiderstehlich ist, brachte ihm seine Rolle als unverzichtbare hexen- und teufelsabwehrende Pflanze ein. Ob aufgehängt in Wohnräumen oder eingestreut in Ställen – überall sollte das Baldrianbüscherl vor Übergriffen dunkler Mächte schützen und die Seelen verängstigter Menschen trösten.

Verwendung – gestern und heute

Von der Antike weg galt er als Universalheilmittel bei Frauenleiden, vor allem als Bettstroh zur Geburt sowie im und nach dem Wechsel. Das gesamte Mittelalter diente er als Theriakkraut des kleinen Mannes, als Allheilmittel „gegen Pestilenz und allerhand Giffte“, das sich jeder leisten konnte, denn der Baldrian findet sich zuhauf in der freien Landschaft, begleitet Bäche und Rinnsale, schmiegt sich rund um Tümpel und Moore.

Hildegard von Bingen (1098–1179) empfiehlt „Kucheln“ oder Tabletten aus dem Baldrianpulver herzustellen: „Und wer an Brustfellentzündung oder an Gicht leidet, der pulverisiere Baldrian, füge pulverisierte Katzenminze hinzu, mache mit Mehl und Wasser Törtchen und Kucheln in einer Schüssel mit Fett und diese vorgenannten Pulver vermische er und so esse er es oft und die Brustfellentzündung und die Gicht werden in ihm weichen, sodass es ihm besser geht.“

Leonhart Fuchs (1501–1566) sagt zur Baldrianwurzel: „Sie würd under die arzneyen vermischt, so man für gifft braucht, darumb ist sie zu der zeit der Pestilentz seer gut, davon getruncken.“

Balthasar Ehrhart (1700–1756) ergänzt die Lonicerus-Empfehlung: „Der dritte und allerneueste Nutzen der Baldrian ist, daß mit dem continuirten Gebrauch des Pulvers derselben, fast durch den Winter durch, ein schon vieljährige und für incurable gehaltenen Ischiatique oder Hüfftweh, nach eines sehr vornebmen Leib.Medici experience, glücklich gehoben worden.“

Pfarrer Sebastian Kneipp (1821–1897) meint schließlich: „Alle Formen von nervösen Zuständen, ob im Krampf oder Schmerz, verlangen Baldrian.“ In der modernen Phytotherapie hat der Baldrian seinen fixen Platz als nervenberuhigendes und schlafförderndes Mittel. Die guten alten Baldriantropfen helfen rasch bei Unruhezuständen, Prüfungsängsten und geistiger Überanstrengung.

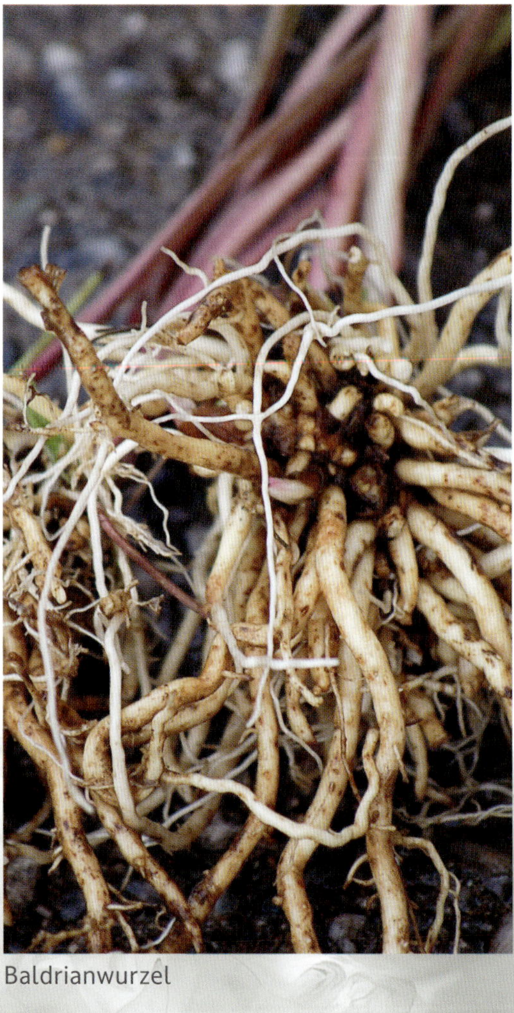

Baldrianwurzel

Beifuß

Lat. Name: *Artemisia vulgaris*
Botanischer Name: Gewöhnlicher Beifuß
Pflanzenfamilie: Korbblütler

Die „Mugwurz", die alte Machtwurz darf ungestört durch meinen Garten wandern. Sie wählt ihre Standorte mit Bedacht, bevorzugt exponierte Orte, wie zum Beispiel die Zeilenanfänge am Kräuteracker oder entlang des Hauptweges im Gemüsegarten. Der Beifuß schafft Ordnung – im Pflanzen- wie im Menschenreich!

Die „Mutter aller Kräuter" wie der Beifuß im *Macer floridus*, einem mittelalterlichen Heilpflanzen-Lehrgedicht aus dem 9./10. Jahrhundert genannt wird, ist ein herausragendes Kraut: Seine dreifache Macht liegt in der Wuchshöhe und äußeren Stärke, in der überragenden giftwidrigen Heilkraft, seiner Ausstrahlung und Präsenz und in der Kraft der Wurzel.

Rauch

Verwendete Pflanzenteile: Wurzeln, Blätter, Blüten.

Beste Sammel- und Erntezeit: Die Wurzel kann im Frühling oder im Herbst gegraben werden. Im Frühling werden die Blätter der ausgegrabenen Pflanze ebenfalls gesammelt und getrocknet. Anfang September, wenn die Beifußblüten eine rostbräunliche Färbung angenommen haben, wird die gesamte Pflanze ausgegraben und bis auf den Stängel, zerkleinert und getrocknet. Zusätzlich können die Blätter das ganze Jahr über gesammelt und getrocknet werden. Die Blüten können ab Blühbeginn im Sommer geerntet werden. Die stärkste räucherische Kraft haben die Blüten, wenn sie am Verblühen sind, also zu braunen beginnen.

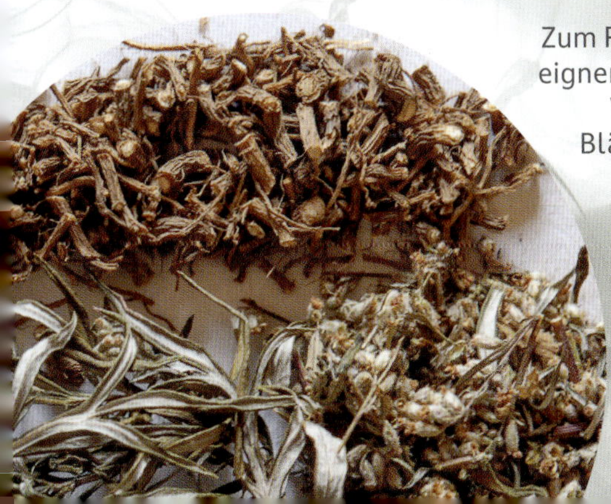

Zum Räuchern eignen sich die Wurzeln, Blätter und Blüten.

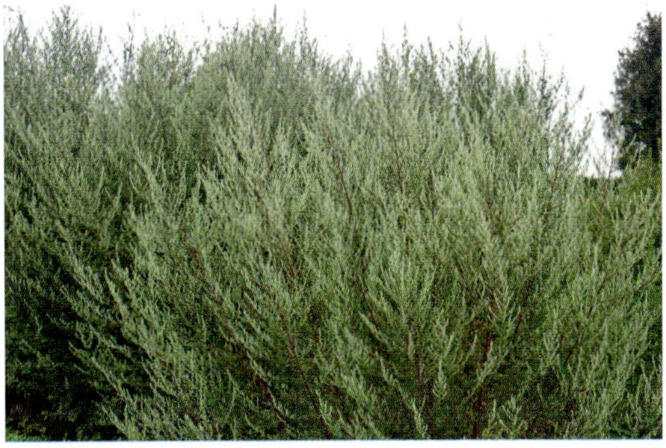

Gewöhnlicher Beifuß

Vor dem Räuchern die Wurzel vermahlen: Dabei wird das äußerliche Braun der Wurzelstückchen immer heller, bis es schließlich fast weiß anmutet. Die Blätter und Blüten sollten nur verrebelt werden, da sie sich beim Vermahlen gewölleähnlich verzahnen und nicht weiter mit anderen Räucherstoffen gemischt werden können. Die oberen Triebspitzen der Pflanze sind besonders geeignet zur Herstellung von Räucherstäben, die während des langsamen Trocknungsvorganges immer enger gebunden werden sollen.

Wirkung, Wahrnehmung: Die besondere Kraft dieser Universalentgiftungspflanze liegt darin, dass sie die Dinge des Lebens in Fluss halten kann, dass sie mit aller Macht körperlichen, geistigen, aber auch seelischen Verhärtungen, Blockaden oder Versteinerungen entgegenwirken kann.

Für eine derart mächtige Ordnungskraft gehören die Begleitung und der Schutz von Übergangsphasen im Leben zu den wichtigsten Aufgaben. Denn gerade in solchen Momenten, wo man Vertrautes verlässt, Neues aber noch nicht in Sicht ist, ist die Gefahr von negativen Einwirkungen am größten. Die einschneidenden Wendepunkte des Lebens begleitet der Beifuß mit seiner „Macht gegen das Übel, das über das Land hinfährt…"

Abwehrrauch für Menschen, Tiere, Haus und Hof; Schutzrauch und Geisterbanner; altes Wetterkraut. Wichtigstes Übergangskraut der beiden Sonnenwenden: Seine angstlösende Kraft verbindet die große sichtbare mit der übergroßen, unsichtbaren Welt und versinnbildlicht die kosmischen Wenden.

Reinigungsrauch zur Klärung der Raumatmosphäre. Stark lösende Kraft in Gebäuden, Räumen und an Orten, wo sich alte negative Eintragungen verfestigt haben und zu unbeweglichen, erkalteten Altlasten geworden sind. Teufelsscheuchende und stark positiv überlagernde Wirkung. Als Wetterkraut unterstützt sein Rauch den Abbau negativer Ladungen und Spannungen: in Räumen, wo Streit und Zwietracht herrscht, in elektrostatisch überladenen Arbeitsräumen oder allgemein in kabellos vernetzten Häusern.

Der Beifuß-Wurzelrauch überlagert sämtliche negative Raumenergien nachhaltig, seien sie schon alt und kalt oder jüngeren Datums, also noch „heiß". Verschreikraut zur Abwehr von Verwünschungen, negativen Bannungen und zur Neutralisierung von Flüchen. Geisterbannender Schutzrauch, der vor Behexungen und schlimmen Krankheitsgeistern schützt. Schützender Begleiter, wenn es über die Schwelle in die Dunkelheit geht. Rauch der Rauhnächte und in Phasen der inneren Dunkelheit und Veränderung.

Die oberirdische Mächtigkeit der Pflanze wächst aus einem sensiblen Wurzelwerk. Diese Wurzelform spiegelt die Vorsicht, die Behutsamkeit, aber auch die Zähigkeit und Klarheit im Moment des Übergangs. An kritischen Phasen und Wendezeiten im Leben Beifuß allein verräuchern, sich in den Rauch hineinsetzen und in den weichen Strudel hineinziehen lassen. Die Gedanken weiten sich und die schützende Kraft des Beifußes gibt neue Hoffnung, neuen Halt.

Magisches zum Rauch: Beifuß wurde und wird in allen Kulturen von Heilkundigen, Naturheilern, Schamanen geräuchert, wenn sie sich auf der Suche nach den Wurzeln von Krankheiten in Beifuß-Trance an die Schwelle zur Anderswelt begeben. Der Beifußrauch ist dabei der Schutzmantel für eine gute Rückkehr und eine heilsame Erkenntnis. Ist ihnen die passende Heilpflanze erschienen, können sie in dieser Welt mit der Heilung beginnen.

Schwerpunkt, Anwendungen, Rezepte: Abendräucherung bei Schlaflosigkeit und seelischer Erschöpfung: Räuchermischung aus Beifußwurzel, Eberesche, Rosenblüten und Harz.

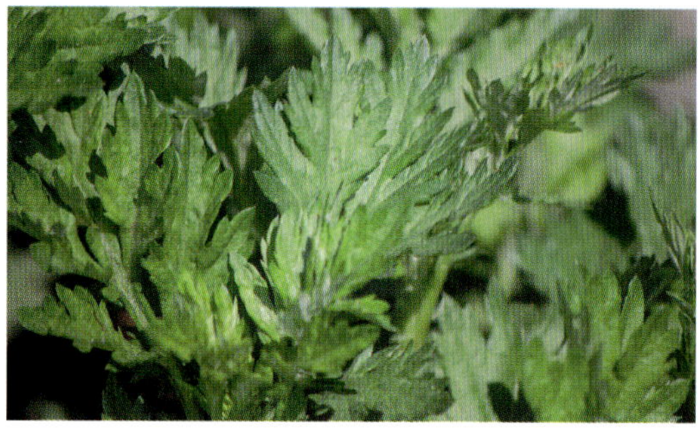
Beifußblätter

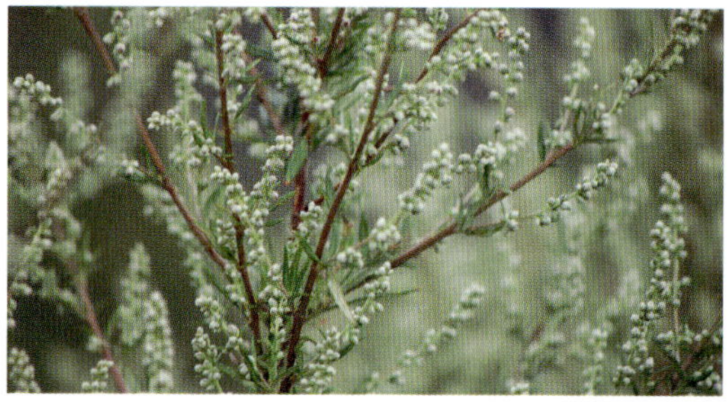
Beifußblüten

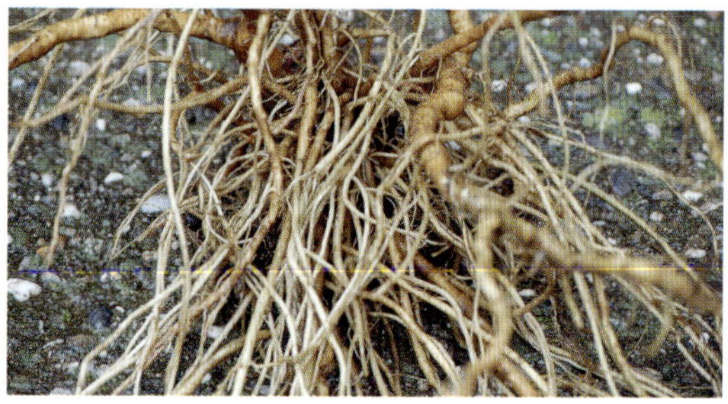
Beifußwurzeln

Mythologie und magische Praktiken

Seit Jahrtausenden steht der Beifuß in mannigfaltigem schutzmagischem Gebrauch, begleitet rituelle Handlungen in allen Kulturen, wird besungen, bedichtet und intensiv genutzt: Davon erzählen die geburtsbegleitenden Beifußbüschel, die die Keltenfrauen an die Innenseiten der Oberschenkel gepresst hielten, um ihrem Kind den Übergang in diese Welt zu erleichtern. Davon erzählen aber auch die Beifußsamen, die man an einer Begräbnisstätte der Neanderthaler gefunden hat, hingestreut, um den Toten den Übergang in die andere Welt zu ermöglichen.

In der Lacnunga, einem altenglischen heilkundlichen Manuskript aus dem 10./11. Jahrhundert, ist ein Neunkräutersegen überliefert. Hier steht der Beifuß an erster Stelle und wird gebührend verehrt: „Erinnere dich, Beifuß, was du verkündest hast, was du bekräftigt hast, bei der großen Verkündung. „Una" heißt du, ältestes Kraut. Du hast Macht für drei und gegen dreißig! Du hast Macht gegen Gift und gegen das fliegende Gift, du hast Macht gegen das Übel, das über das Land hinfährt!"

Im *Macer floridus* wird weiters empfohlen: „... die Wurzel (des Beifuß) um den Hals gehängt, soll Schlangen, die in Hecken leben und allen bösen Kröten widerstehen". Mit „bösen Kröten" sind die Schadens-Zauberinnen und negativen Dämonen gemeint, denen man überall begegnet. Wer also Beifußwurzel bei sich trägt, den kann kein böser Blick bannen, es kann ihn keine Hexe verrufen und er ist geschützt gegen Besessenheit.

Der Beifuß wird auch als Gürtlerkraut bezeichnet: Zur Sommersonnenwende wird aus den, im Juni schon hoch gewachsenen, aber noch biegsamen Beifußstängeln ein Gürtel um die Körpermitte gebunden. So gegürtet springt man über das Feuer, macht die Übergangskräfte des Krauts unmittelbar sichtbar und versichert sich seines Schutzes. Der aufgeklärte Arzt Tabernaemontanus (1522–1590) wettert: „Es treiben nicht allein die alten Weiber, sondern auch viel hoher Leute, die doch sich vor sehr weiss unnd verständig halten, viel Aberglauben mit dem Beyfuss, welches viel mehr einer Zauberey, dann Natürlichen Künsten zu vergleichen. Etliche graben dieses kraut auff gewisse Tage unnd stundt, suchen Narrenkohlen oder Thorellenstein darunder, das hencken sie an vor das Fieber unnd andere Kranckheiten. Andere machen Kräntz darauss, unnd gürten es umb den Leib, werffen es darnach mit ihren besondern Reymen und Sprüch in S. Johanns Fewer auff S. Johannsen dess heiligen Täuffers Tag, vermeinen darmit alles ihres Unglücks entledigt zu werden."

Auch Hieronymus Bock (1498–1554) verweist auf die magischen Bräuche rund um die Sommersonnenwende, um den Johannis-Tag und erzählt, dass die Wurzel zu einer bestimmten Stunde ausgegraben werde: „... andere hencken es umb sich, machen kreutz darauß, folgens werffen sie das kraut mit irem unfal in S. Johans Fewer, mit iren sprüchen und reimen. Diß affenspiel und ceremonen treiben nicht die geringsten zu Pareiß in Franckreich. Andere haben von Plinio gelernet, wa sie Beifuß mit Salbei anhencken, sollen sie auff der reiß nicht müd werden, und des dings ist kein ende!"

Verwendung – gestern und heute

Im Admonter Bartholomäus, einer Medizinhandschrift aus dem 15. Jahrhundert, wird gereimt: „Nu das weib enphinde, daß si well gen zu chinde, dy nem das selbig chrautt, und leg es auf den pauch!"

Der Arzt, Naturforscher und Botaniker Lonicerus (1528–1586) schreibt zum Beifuß als Frauenkraut: „Diß Kraut hat Artemisia deß Königs Mausoli Haußfrau sich selbsten zu geeignet, und nach ihrem Namen genennet, oder nach der Göttin Diana, welche Artemis heißt. Dann es ist diß Kraut den gebärenden Frauen, wie bey den Heyden Diana, sehr behülfflich." Weiter unten führt er aus: „Beyfuß mit Wein oder Bier gesotten, und das getruncken, thut den Weibern in Kindsnöhten nicht geringe Hülff. Treibt auch die todte Geburt. Oder man bind ihr das gesotten Kraut an ihr rechte Weych, sie genießt bald. Man soll auch, so bald das Kind gebohren wird, das Kraut wieder abnemmen, sonst bringt es grossen Schaden."

Heute gilt der Beifuß als allergieauslösendes Kraut. Der bittere Beifuß wird als Gewürz zur besseren Fettverdauung eingesetzt und soll in Kräuterkissen für einen ausgeglichenen Schlaf sorgen und gegen das Schlafwandeln wirken.

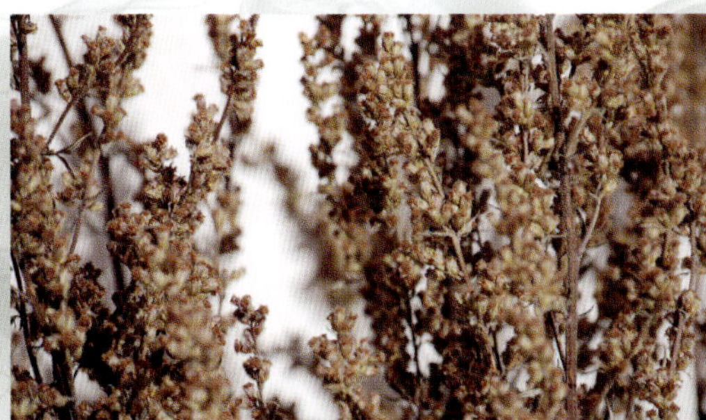

Beifußblüten getrocknet

Beinwell

Lat. Name: *Symphytum officinale*
Botanischer Name: Gewöhnlicher Beinwell
Pflanzenfamilie: Raublattgewächse

Eine Pflanze voller überbordender, unverwüstlicher Lebenskraft, die unsere Vorfahren zu allerlei magischen Handlungen anregt hat. So sollen junge Frauen ihre Jungfräulichkeit mit einem Bad im Wurzelabsud wiedererlangt haben. Seit der Antike wird die Wallwurz bei Knochenbrüchen und Wunden eingesetzt. Ihre Inhaltsstoffe verflüssigen die Wundsekrete, regen den Gewebsstoffwechsel an und fördern so die Heilung.

Die hilfsbereiten Talente des Beinwells äußern sich auch im Umgang mit anderen Pflanzen: Er folgt dem Ruf empfindsamerer Kräuter, um diese vor unangenehmen Gegebenheiten im Kräuterbeet zu schützen. Nachdem ich in meinem Kräutergarten die Blätter eines Gelben Enzians aus Versehen niedergemäht hatte, war dieser und nämlich nur dieser, im nächsten Jahr rundherum eingehüllt von kräftigen Beinwellpflanzen, deren plötzliche Herkunft nicht geklärt werden konnte.

Rauch

Verwendete Pflanzenteile: Wurzeln, Blätter, Blüten.

Beste Sammel- und Erntezeit: Die mindestens dreijährigen Wurzeln können im Frühjahr oder im Herbst gegraben werden. Sie werden gereinigt, klein geschnitten und getrocknet. Vor dem Verräuchern fein vermahlen. Die Blätter können

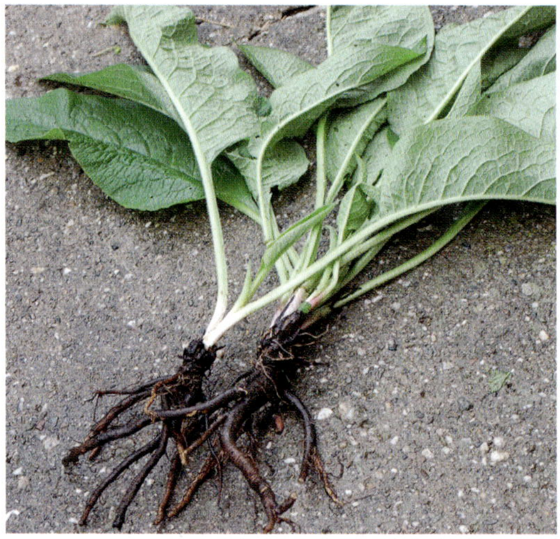

Beinwell mit Wurzel

das ganze Jahr über gesammelt und getrocknet werden. Die frühe Blütezeit des Beinwells beginnt oft schon im April.

Wirkung, Wahrnehmung: Reinigungsrauch, Schutzrauch. Der reine Wurzelrauch ist erdig und eher verhalten und erschließt sich erst zusammen mit anderen Räucherstoffen. Negativ überlastete Räume, Häuser und Orte erhalten einen Klärungsimpuls. Genauso werden Raumstrukturen, die durch zu viel komplizierende und widersprüchliche geistige Arbeit zugesponnen sind und keine Konzentration mehr zulassen, überlagert und langsam geöffnet.

Der Rauch vermittelt eine große Wandlungskraft, die in geistig-seelischen Belangen von Starre zu Bewegung führt: vom Verzetteln zum Zusammenschluss der Kräfte, von regloser Angst zu vertrauensvollem Tun. Geistige Teufelskreise werden durchbrochen; man ist wieder geerdet und kann den Blick auf Neues richten oder entspannen und sich einmal zurücklehnen.

Schwerpunkt, Anwendungen, Rezepte: Räuchermischung bei Kopfweh und geistiger Überlastung: Beinwell, Salbei und Heilziest kombiniert mit Harz.

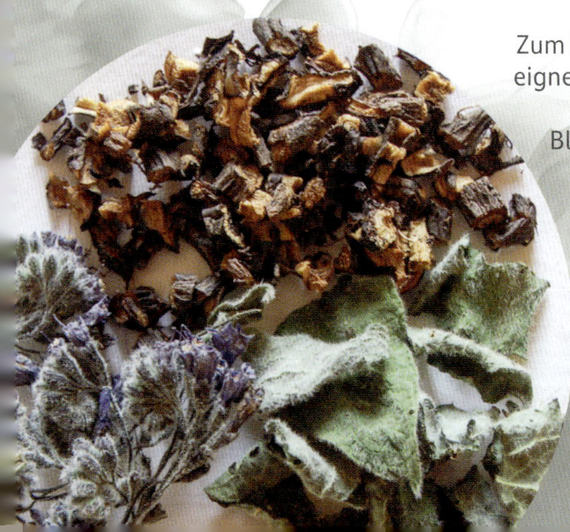

Zum Räuchern eignen sich die Wurzeln, Blätter und Blüten.

Verwendung – gestern und heute

Sämtliche Kräuterkundige loben die heilende Kraft der Wallwurz bei Knochenbrüchen. Lonicerus (1528–1586) weist noch auf eine andere Verwendung der Wallwurz hin: „Die Wurzel gekäuet, nimmt den Durst. Zehen Pfund Wallwurz in einem Eymer Wasser das halb Theil eingesotten, das Leder damit geschmiert, macht daß das Leder nit wieder hart wird. Dienet derowegen den Secklern wol."

Bei Gelenks-, Sehnen- und Knochenverletzungen hat sich die unterstützende Gabe homöopathischer Symphytum-Globuli bewährt.

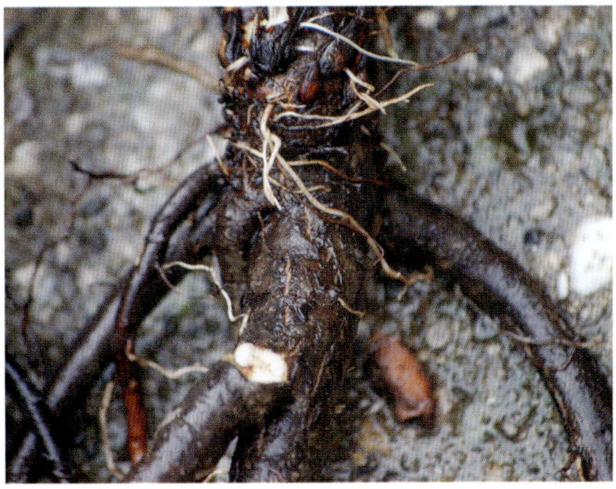

Beinwellwurzel

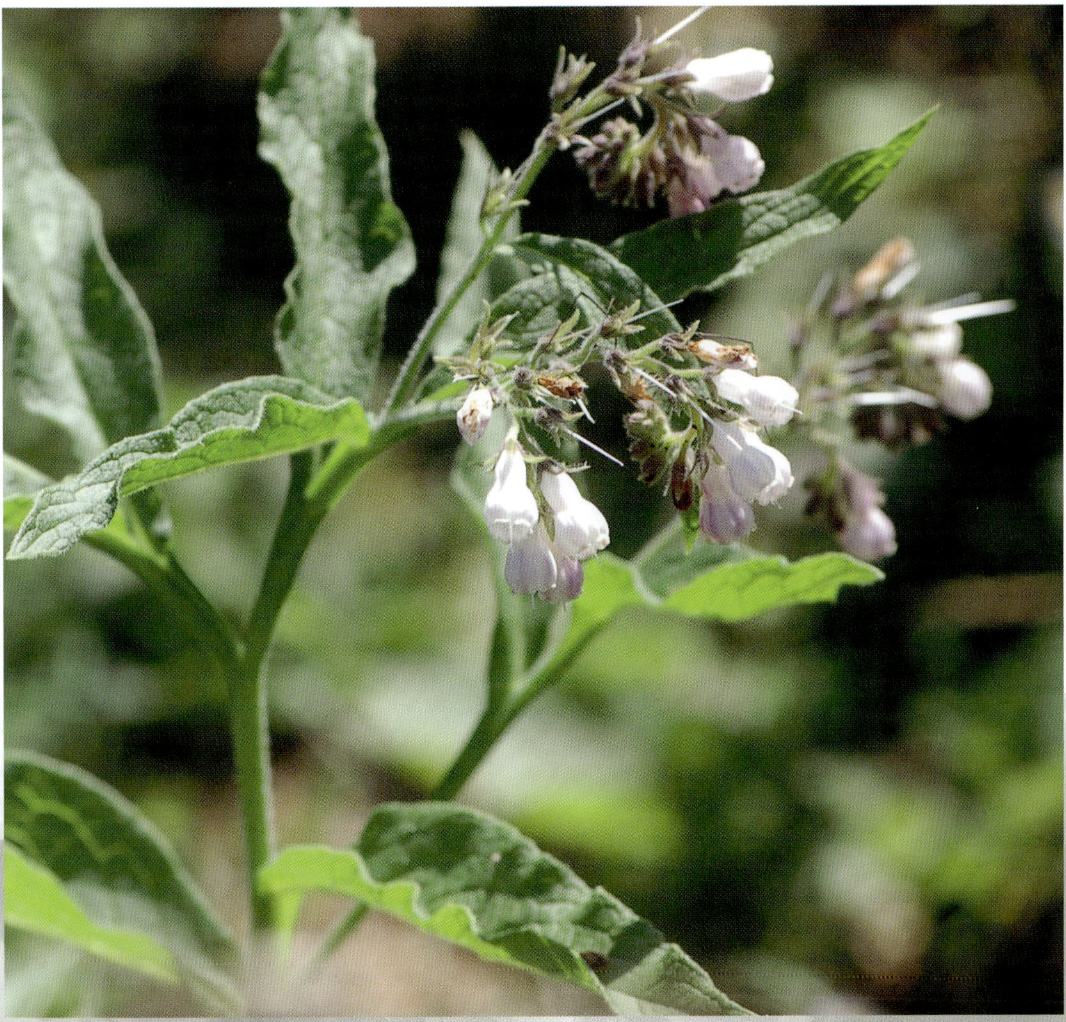

Blühender Beinwell

Bibernelle

Lat. Name: *Pimpinella* sp.
Botanischer Name: Kleine Bibernelle *(P. saxifraga)*, Große Bibernelle *(P. major)*
Pflanzenfamilie: Doldenblütler

In vielen Pestsagen wird die Bibernelle als geheimes Gegenmittel genannt, meistens zusammen mit Baldrian, um nicht so schnell dem schwarzen Tod zum Opfer zu fallen. Die mehrfach bekrönten weiß-roten Wurzelübergänge sind kräftige Vegetationsimpulse und lassen besondere Lebenskräfte erahnen, die die Bibernelle so wertvoll gemacht haben. Auch Bockwurz oder Pfefferwurz genannt, ist sie äußerst anspruchslos und verbreitet sich auf extensiv bewirtschafteten trockenen Flächen genauso gut wie in wasserreicherem Gelände. Heutzutage nimmt ihr jedoch das häufigere Mähen nach und nach den Lebensmut, sodass sie gebietsweise kaum noch zu finden ist. Im Garten kann man sie problemlos ansiedeln und aussamen lassen.

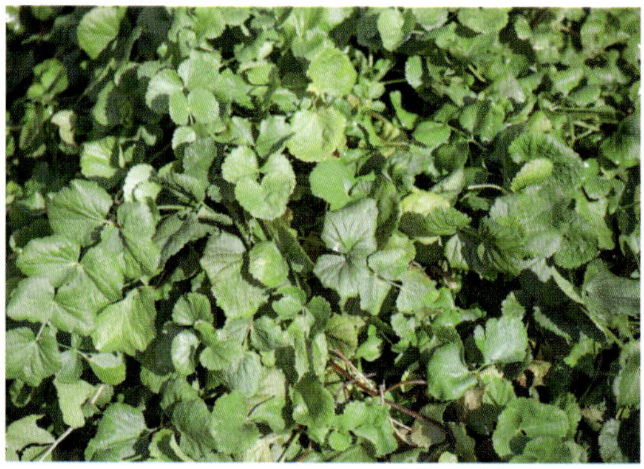

Kleine Bibernelle

Rauch

Verwendete Pflanzenteile: Wurzeln, Blätter.

Beste Sammel- und Erntezeit: Die Wurzeln werden im Frühling oder im Herbst gegraben, klein aufgeschnitten und getrocknet. Die Blätter können das ganze Jahr über geerntet werden.

Wirkung, Wahrnehmung: Schutz- und Segensrauch. Feenkraft für hoffnungsarme Lebensphasen. Engelflügel heben dich empor und richten dich innerlich wieder auf! Der Rauch hält einem im Positiven, gibt neue Kraft nach Durststrecken, in denen man zögerlich wird und depressiv zu werden droht.

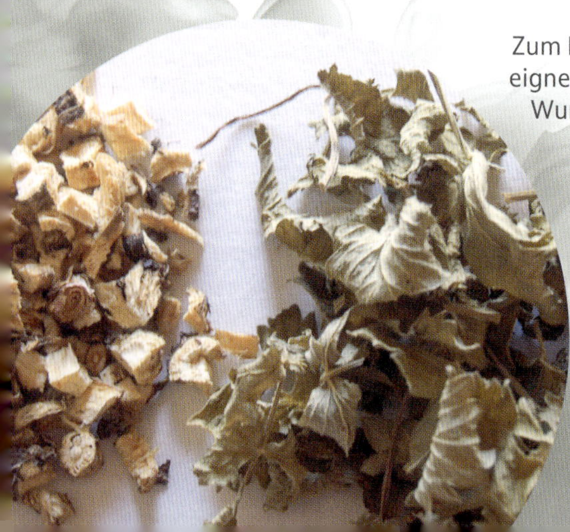

Zum Räuchern eignen sich die Wurzeln und Blätter.

Begleitet behutsam die Veränderungen und Umbrüche im Leben; hilft beim bildhaften Denken und Planen, lässt neues Licht am Ende des Tunnels erahnen. Stärkt die innere Gewissheit am richtigen Weg zu sein. Klärender Rauch, der die Ich-Findung unterstützt, strikt positiv polende Energie vermittelt und insgesamt aufbauend wirkt. Es entsteht eine warme, samtige, herzbesänftigende Atmosphäre, die das innere Auge öffnet. In Segensräucherungen wird die Verbindung zu Vegetationsgeistern mit der Bibernelle ermöglicht und für diejenigen, die reinen Herzens sind, auch gefestigt.

Schwerpunkt, Anwendungen, Rezepte: Zur Vorbereitung auf Meditationen oder Fragerituale werden anfänglich zwei bis drei kleine getrocknete Wurzelstückchen auf die Räucherkohle gegeben. Man lässt sich von diesem Wurzelrauch durchdringen, bis man sich gut konzentriert hat. Dann kann das Ritual mit einer entsprechenden Räuchermischung beginnen.

Mythologie und magische Praktiken

Hildegard von Bingen (1098–1179) stellt zwar fest, dass „der Bibernell" für den Menschen nicht viel tauge, hält es aber für wichtig, seine magische Kraft zu beschreiben: „Aber dennoch habe ihn stets an deinen Hals gehängt, und unterdessen wirst du nicht von Anrufungen der

Dämonen, von magischen Worten und nicht von Zauber, den du nicht gegessen und nicht getrunken hast, getäuscht werden können."

Verwendung – gestern und heute

Leonhart Fuchs (1501–1566), deutscher Arzt und Botaniker, meint in seinem „New Kreüterbuch" aus dem Jahr 1543: „Die wurtzel ist treffenlich gut zu der zeit der Pestilentz gebraucht, dann sie widerstrebt dem bösen lufft und bewart vor dieser grausamen plaag, auch so sie nur im mund gehalten würdt."

Lonicerus hält die kleine scharfe Wurzel für besonders giftwidrig. Im Übrigen schockiert er mit einem „Bibinell-Tier-Experiment", um zu zeigen, dass Bibernellsaft auch bei Menschen mit verletzter Hirnschale angewendet werden könne: „Zu einem Exempel: nimm einen Hanen, und stich ihm sein Hirnschal oben auf, doch nicht durch, nimm darnach daß Saffts von Bibinellenkraut, und tropffe es darein einmal oder zwey, so heilet sie wiederum zu."

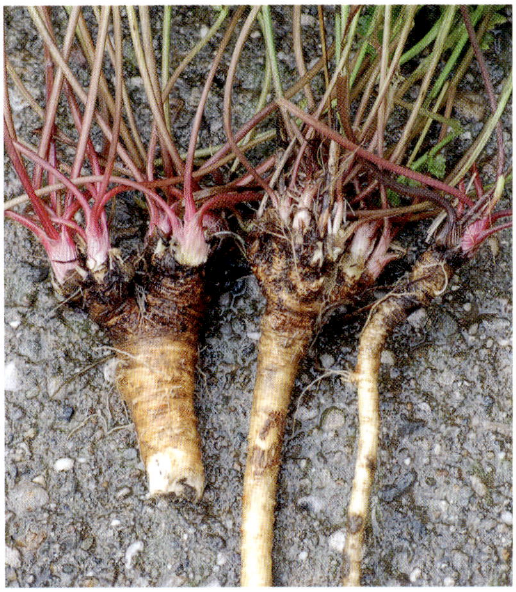
Wurzeln der Bibernelle

Volksheilkundlich wird ein Wurzeltee bei Müdigkeit und geschwächtem Allgemeinzustand empfohlen.

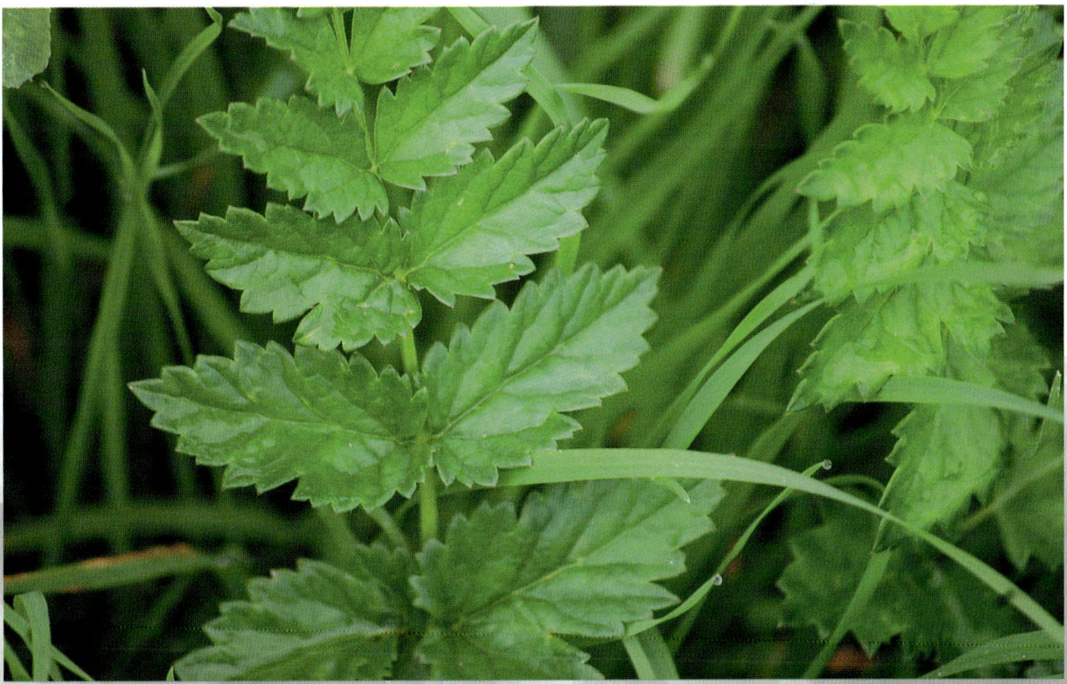
Große Bibernelle

Blutwurz

Lat. Name: *Potentilla erecta*
Pflanzenfamilie: Rosengewächse

Zartes Blattwerk und leuchtend gelbe Blüten, die die vier Himmelsrichtungen auszuleuchten scheinen, ziehen einen mit eigentümlicher Widersprüchlichkeit sofort in den Bann. Doch sie zu finden ist schwer, denn die machtvolle Pflanze liebt es, zurückgezogen zu leben. Ob mitten auf schattigen Waldwegen, entlang von Totholz in praller Sonne oder auf felsigem Untergrund immer gelingt es ihr, aus der spartanischen Kargheit ihres Lebensraumes ein Optimum an Wirkstoffen zusammenzutragen und in der Wurzel zu speichern. Bis diese allerdings blutrot leuchtet, braucht es etliche Jahre. Sie wächst ausschließlich auf äußerst mageren, nicht gedüngten Böden und breitet sich über Europa bis zum Altaigebirge im Osten aus.

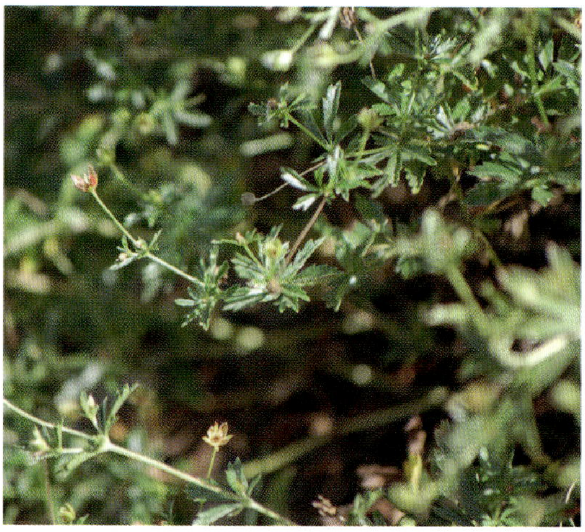

Blutwurzkraut

Rauch

Verwendete Pflanzenteile: Wurzeln.

Beste Sammel- und Erntezeit: Die Wurzel kann ganzjährig gegraben werden, die abgestorbenen Stellen alter Wurzelballen können im Räuchergut belassen werden und wirken im Rauch rhythmusgebend.

Wirkung, Wahrnehmung: Reinigungsrauch, Abwehr- und Schutzrauch, transformatorische Kraft. Der Rauch hat das Potenzial dichte und negativ empfundene Raumenergien zu überlagern und langsam aufzulösen. Der angenehme Rauch steigt sofort in den Kopf, man richtet sich unwillkürlich auf, horcht in sich hinein, wundert sich über die rinnende Nase. Aufbauender Rauch für eher dunkle Phasen, für Phasen des Selbstzweifels und der Unsicherheit. Stärkt die positive mentale Kraft und schützt vor Überforderung, wenn man sich zu viel vorgenommen hat und über längere Zeit dem eigenen Anspruch nicht genügen kann. Bringt einen in gemäßigte Bahnen zurück, stößt den richtigen Rhythmus wieder an und hilft dabei, Unwichtiges zu erkennen.

Große Abwehr- und Schutzkraft bei schwarzmagischen Übergriffen, Verwünschungen, hinterhältigen persönlichen Angriffen und Mobbing. Hilft dabei, sich abzugrenzen, auch einmal Nein zu sagen und hält vor allem das eigene Kraftfeld dicht. Der Rauch dieses roten Kraftbündels lehrt uns, den Blick aus einer gewissen Distanz prüfend auf uns selbst zu richten und vielleicht auch unser Verhalten zu reflektieren. Die Entschlusskraft wird gefördert und die Lust zu neuen Aktivitäten wird spürbar.

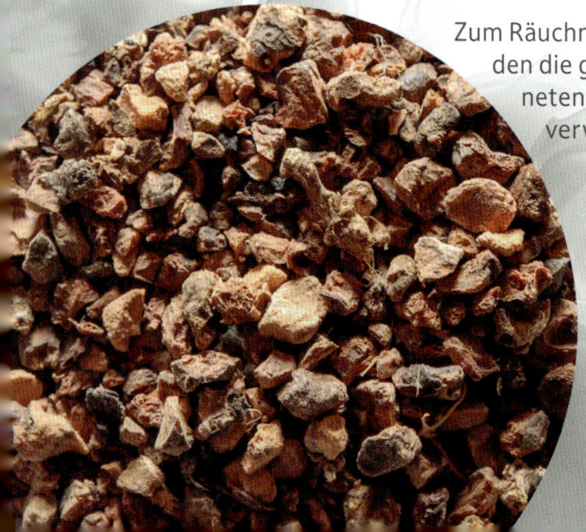

Zum Räuchnern werden die getrockneten Wurzeln verwendet.

Schwerpunkt, Anwendungen, Rezepte: Räuchermischung zur Hebung des Selbstbewusstseins, zur Erleichterung für Verzweifelte: Blutwurz, Eichenlaub, Hainbuche und Wermut in Kombination mit Harz.

Verwendung – gestern und heute

Tabernaemontanus (1522–1590), ein deutscher Arzt und Apotheker, rät: „Tormentillwurtzel gepülvert, unnd deß Morgens nüchtern eine Haselnuss groß eyngenommen mit einem Trüncklein Weins im Winter, im Sommer aber mit Essig oder Ampfferwasser, verhütet den Menschen denselben Tag, daß ihme kein Pestilentzische vergifftung schaden mag." Unter zahlreichen weiteren Empfehlungen findet sich auch diese: „Wann die Pferdt oder das Rindtviech sehr keichen unnd Lungensüchtig sind, soll man inen Tormentillkraut und Wurtzel in ihrem Futer unnd Trincken zu essen unnd zu trincken geben, unnd auch bißweilen das Pulver darvon mit warmem Wasser eynschütten."

Ihre breite volksmedizinische Nutzung sind den verträglichen Gerbstoffen der Wurzel zuzuschreiben, die nicht nur Durchfälle lindern helfen, sondern auch bei aufgesprungenen Mundwinkeln, rissigen Fingern und Händen die Abheilung beschleunigen können.

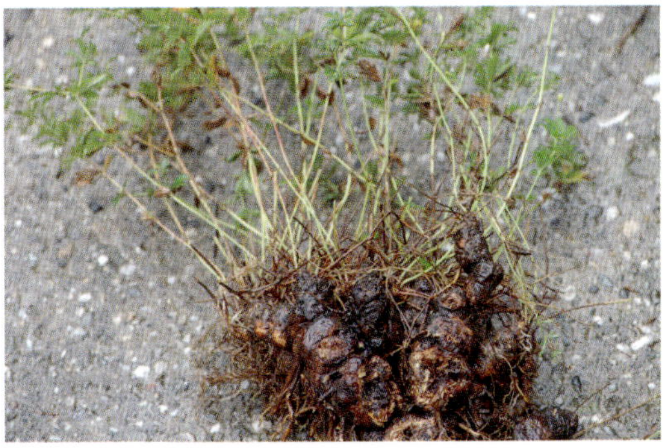

Ausgegrabene Blutwurz

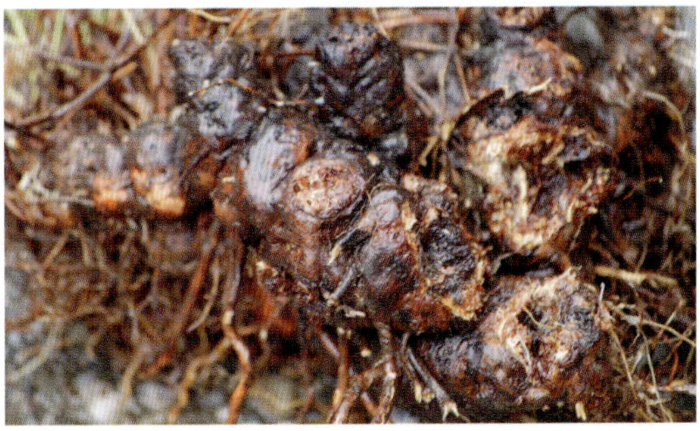

Wurzel der Blutwurz

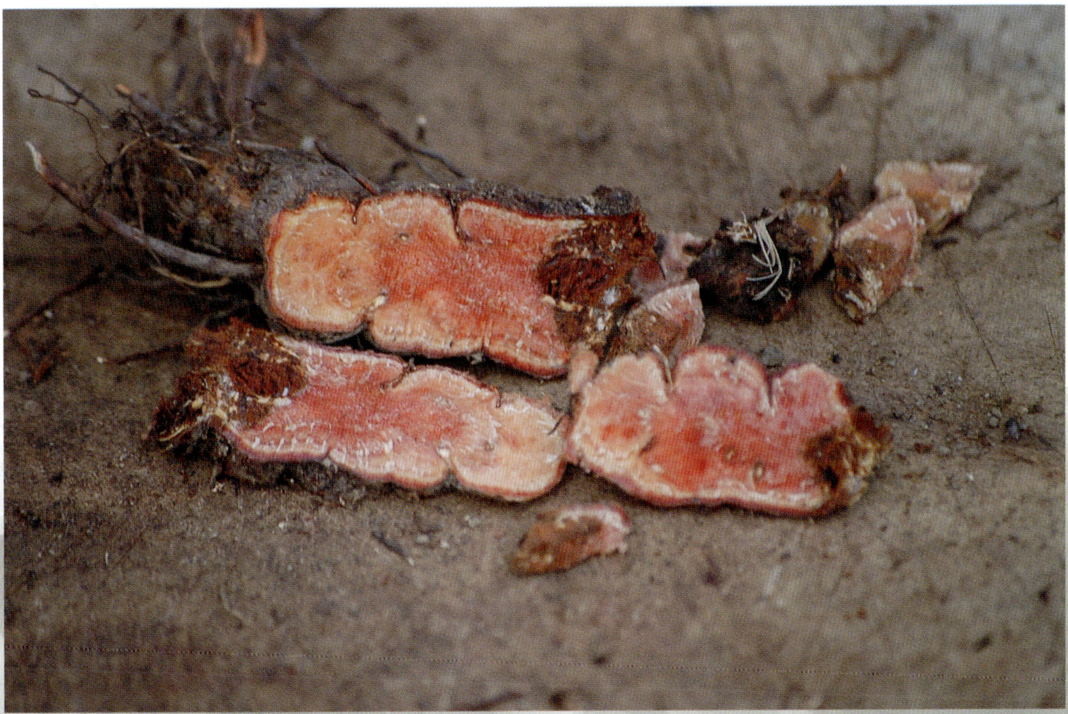

Aufgeschnittene Blutwurzwurzel

Braunwurz

Lat. Name: *Scrophularia* sp.
Botanischer Name: Knotige Braunwurz (*S. nodosa*), Hunds-Braunwurz *(S. canina)*
Pflanzenfamilie: Braunwurzgewächse

Die Braunwurz ist keine Pflanze, die einem sofort ins Auge sticht, im Gegenteil, sie ist von einer heilsamen Unaufdringlichkeit, meist am Waldrand oder auf Rainen zu finden, fast immer auf sich kreuzenden Wasseradern. Es ist meist schon August und sie trägt schon ihre tropfenähnlichen kleinen Samenkapseln, wenn sie mir auffällt und ich mich frage, warum ich sie nicht schon früher wahrgenommen habe.

Die Ruhe, die den oberirdischen Teil der Pflanze umgibt ist unendlich wohltuend. Man ist versucht, sich am Stängel festzuhalten, die Augen zu schließen und sich wegzuträumen. Gräbt man dann, unter vielen Entschuldigungen, doch tiefer, schwimmen plötzlich helle, fischartige Wurzelwesen seitwärts, die mit unzähligen größeren und kleineren Knoten übersät sind und an denen lange Tentakel hängen.

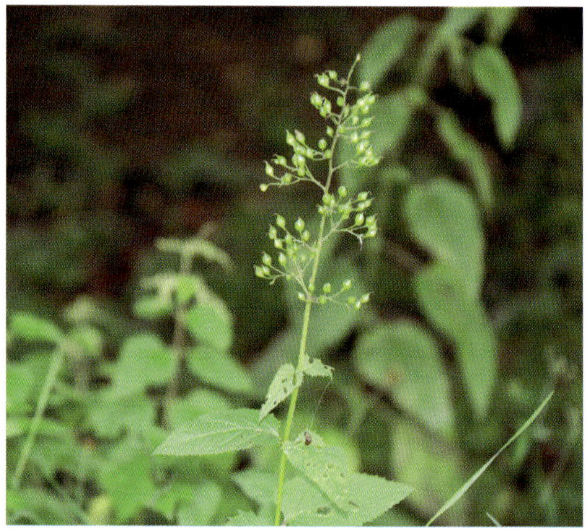

Braunwurz im Juli

Rauch

Verwendete Pflanzenteile: Wurzel, Blätter, Samenkapseln.

Beste Sammel- und Erntezeit: Die Wurzel wird im Frühherbst gegraben, wenn ein Teil der Blüten schon Samen trägt und ein Teil noch bräunlich blüht. Sämtliche Wurzeln, Knoten und Wurzelfäden klein schneiden und rasch trocknen lassen. Vor dem Räuchern vermahlen. Die Blätter können das Jahr über gesammelt werden. Die Samenkapseln anlässlich der Wurzelernte.

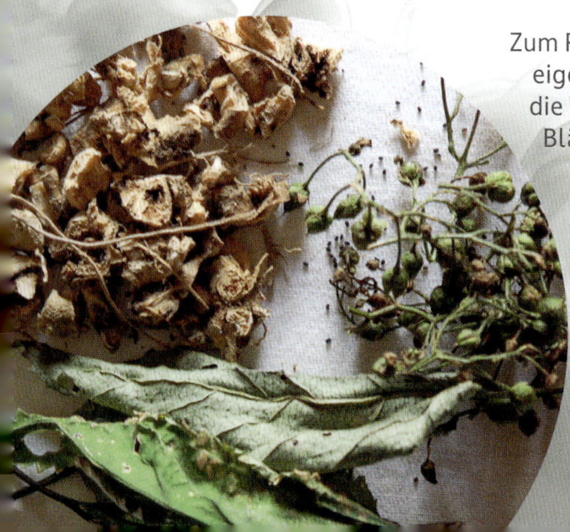

Zum Räuchern eigenen sich die Wurzeln, Blätter und Samen.

Wirkung, Wahrnehmung: Die frische Wurzel hat einen strengen Geruch, der beim Trocknen fast ganz verschwindet, sich im Rauch dann aber lieblich entwickelt. Abwehrrauch, Reinigungsrauch, Segensrauch. Geheimer alter Abwehrrauch gegen schwarzmagischen Krankheitszauber! Der Wurzelrauch reinigt die emotionale Ebene von Beziehungsgiften und anderen Anhaftungen. Der Rauch konfrontiert uns mit unserem blinden Fleck; stärkt die Bereitschaft auch schwierige Dinge, erstarrte Beziehungen, leidvolle Zurückweisungen im Leben aufzuarbeiten und emotional zu durchwärmen. Schafft Klarheit für Menschen, die zu viel denken, im Theoretischen verhaftet bleiben und dadurch nicht zu Lösungen kommen. Fördert die Hinwendung zum Tun, zum friedvollen Aufbruch. Schenkt uns manchmal die Erkenntnis, dass die ersten Schritte auf einem neuen Weg nicht unbedingt geradeaus gehen müssen, sondern dass der Beginn, der Keim des Neuen, oft schon weit zurück liegt, uns nur nicht bewusst gewesen war.

Schwerpunkt, Anwendungen, Rezepte: Durch ihre klärende Wirkung eignet sich die Braunwurz gut für abendliche Segensräucherungen: Braunwurz, Lavendel, Ysop und Harz.

Mythologie und magische Praktiken

Als alte Amulettpflanze soll die Wurzel am Hals getragen werden, um vor schädlichem Zauber zu schützen.

Hieronymus Bock (1498–1554) schreibt: „Die weiber binden die Braunwurtzel dem vihe an, vertreiben maden unnd würm darmit, treiben seltsame superstition mit gedachter Braunwurtz."

Verwendung – gestern und heute

1543 schreibt Leonhart Fuchs (1501–1566), deutscher Arzt und Botaniker, zur Gestalt der Braunwurz: „Die stengel tragen ihre kleine braune blümlin am gipffel, wie die hole scheckenheüßlin, oder helm, die werden zu runden gespitzten köpflin, voller samen. Die wurtzel ist weiß mit vilen knoden und zincken." Lonicerus (1528–1586) bevorzugt Braunwurzeln, die auf Kreuzungen von Wasseradern stehen für folgendes Rezept: „Der Saame der Braunwurtz, so auf den Wassergestaden ihre Wohnung hat, zerstossen, mit Honig gemischt, und Pflasterweiß über die Stirn gelegt, stillet das Trieffen der Augen."

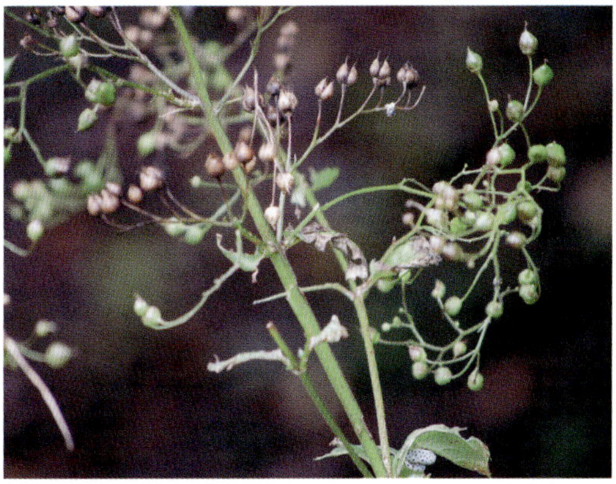
Samenstand der Braunwurz

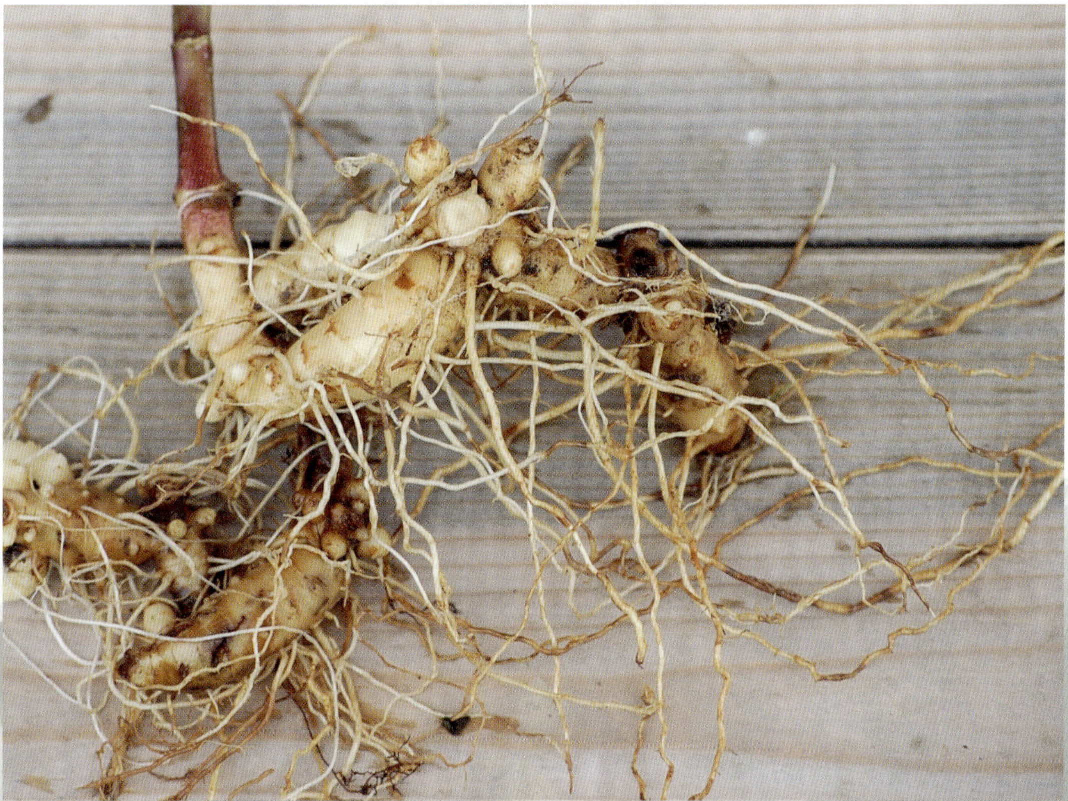
Braunwurzwurzeln

Brennnessel

Lat. Name: *Urtica dioica*
Botanischer Name: Große Brennnessel
Pflanzenfamilie: Nesselgewächse

Wehrhaft, wurzelsperrig, expansiv sind nur einige Eigenschaften, die die „Königin der Beikräuter“, die vielseitige Brennnessel an den Tag legt. Dementsprechend bunt und lang ist auch ihre Verwendungsliste: als Färbekraut für Gelbfärbungen nach Alaun-Vorbeize, als Faserkraut für Taue, Fischernetze, Decken und Rucksäcke, als Düngerveredler in Form der allgemein bekannten Brennnesseljauche, als Haarwuchs- und Schönheitsmittel, als Zauberkraut für allerlei magische Liebesrituale, als Futterpflanze für etliche Arten von Schmetterlingsraupen, als Gemüsepflanze für vitamin- und mineralstoffstrotzende Köstlichkeiten und letztendlich natürlich auch als wichtiges Heilkraut zur Blutreinigung und Entgiftung sowie zur Überwindung von Erschöpfungszuständen.

Mit ihrer Abwehrkraft hat wohl jeder schon einmal Bekanntschaft gemacht und dann noch stundenlang daran denken müssen. Man mag es sich gar nicht vorstellen: Die in Britannien stationierten Römer versuchten sich durch Urtifikation, das Abschlagen des ganzen Körpers mit einem frischen Brennnessel-Buschn, im feucht-kalten nordischen Klima vor rheumatischen Schmerzen und Gliedersteifigkeit zu schützen. Durch Urtifikation trieben die Bauern früher auch ältere Hengste und Stiere zur Paarung an.

Rauch

Verwendete Pflanzenteile: Wurzeln, Blätter, Stängel, Samen.

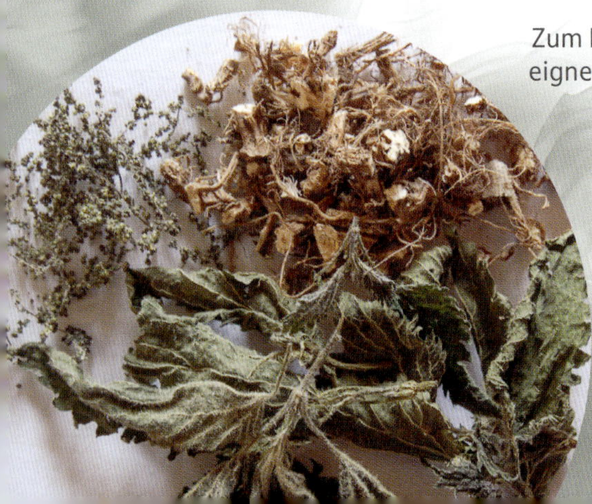

Zum Räuchern eignen sich die Wurzeln, Blätter, Stängel und Samen.

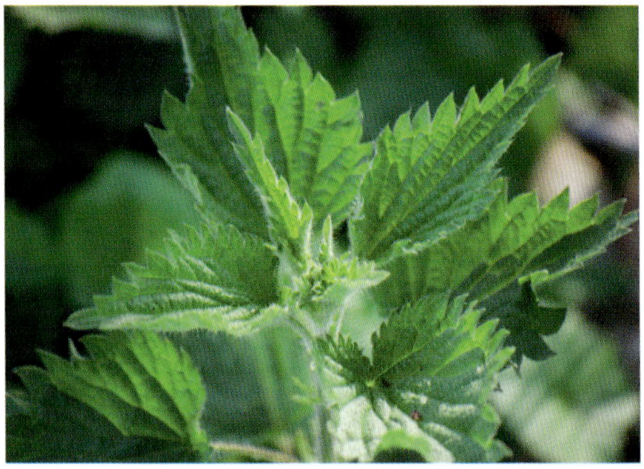

Blätter der Großen Brennnessel

Beste Sammel- und Erntezeit: Die Wurzeln können ganzjährig beerntet werden; werden die Brennnesseln regelmäßig geschnitten, dann kann man auch die Blätter und Stängel das ganze Jahr über ernten. Die Samen zeigen die weiblichen Brennnesseln meist erst im Sommer oder Frühherbst. Für Räucherungen im Freien einen Räucherstab aus Brennnesseln binden. Wenn dieser halbtrocken ist, fester zusammenbinden und durchtrocknen lassen.

Wirkung, Wahrnehmung: Die verräucherte Wurzel gibt die Brennnesselbotschaft am intensivsten wieder: Abwehrkraft und nachhaltige Klärung von verkopften Belastungen. Rauch der Sonnenwenden zur rituellen Abwehr von gefühlten Bedrohungen und negativen Wesenheiten. Der reine Wurzelrauch der Brennnessel hilft in kritischen Situationen, in denen man sich machtlos und ausgeliefert erlebt. Wenn man sich in diesen Rauch setzt, formieren sich die Seilschaften der geistigen Abwehrkräfte neu, die Angriffsflächen werden abgeschottet und die unklaren Ängste werden durchlichtet. Die Bereitschaft zur mentalen Überwindung von Krisen steigt.

Die Blätter, Samen und Wurzeln gemischt ergeben einen starken Abwehr- und Reinigungsrauch. Altes Wetterkraut. Liebesräucherungen. Der Rauch fährt gleich heftig in den Kopf und kann aggressive Gedanken auslösen. Wenn dieser Impuls nicht gleich wieder vorbei ist, sollte man gleich aufhören an diesem Tag Brennnessel zu räuchern! Der Rauch geht in Resonanz zu unserer Aura, wird durchgelassen oder komplett abgelehnt. Sollte gar keine Annahme der lösenden Kraft möglich sein, ist hier ebenfalls Schluss mit der Brennnessel-Räucherung.

Wird der Rauch als angenehm erlebt, können erstarrte seelische Altlasten abgeschwächt werden. Der Rauch klärt die Aura von jedweden Anhaftungen und erdet allzu vergeistigte Zeitgenossen. Der Rauch weckt das Bewusstsein für die eigene Einzigartigkeit und thematisiert zuweilen auch die persönliche Durchsetzungskraft; vermittelt das Gefühl, dass es in Ordnung sei, Abstand zu halten und auf die Einhaltung dieses Abstandes zu bestehen. Durch die stark klärende, reinigende Wirkung kann eine Brennnessel-Räucherung neue Energien übertragen und freisetzen. In einem Brennnesselrauch zu stehen, kann wie ein Jungbrunnen empfunden werden und einen nachhaltig mit neuer Kraft stärken. In jedem Fall verlangt eine Brennnessel-Räucherung emotionale Präsenz und Aufmerksamkeit, um eine Veränderung der Befindlichkeit zu erspüren und gegebenenfalls die Räucherung zu beenden.

Magisches zum Rauch: Am Gründonnerstag, in der Walpurgisnacht (30. April/1. Mai) und in der Sonnwendnacht wurden die Ställe mit Brennnesselkraut und -wurzeln ausgeräuchert, um das Vieh vor Hexen und Teufeln und deren schädlichen Milchzauber zu schützen.

Schwerpunkt, Anwendungen, Rezepte: Brennnessel-Buschn-Ritual im Freien: Zur Vertreibung von dunklen Geistern, nachbarlichen Ein- und Übergriffen und anderem Ungemach wird der getrocknete Brennnessel-Stab verräuchert. Herzurichten sind eine feuerfeste Schale sowie getrocknete Weißdorn- und Haselnussblätter und

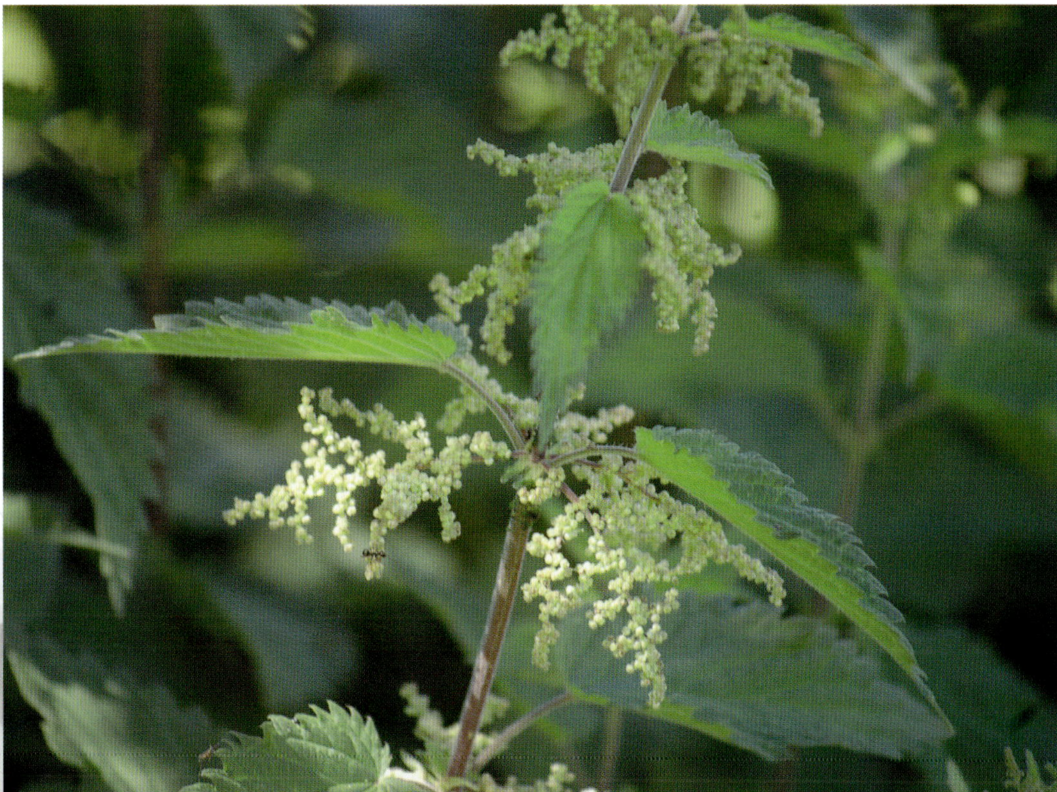

Blühende Brennnessel

etwas trockenes Erlengeäst. Man sollte sich dazu einen Ablauf überlegen, mit dem man seine innere Absicht, seinen Schutzbedarf, am besten zum Ausdruck bringt. Beispielsweise die Räucherungen nach den Himmelsrichtungen auszurichten oder nach den Lebensphasen zu personalisieren. Sobald der Buschn um die Hälfte abgebrannt und verräuchert ist, sollte er vorneüber auf die Erde gedrückt und so gelöscht werden. Dies an einem Ort, von dem aus man seine Räucherung begonnen hat. Als Abschluss sollte der restliche Brennnessel-Stab mit getrockneten Weißdorn- und Haselnussblättern sowie feinem Erlengeäst endgültig verbrannt – nicht geräuchert – werden.

Mythologie und magische Praktiken

In Frankreich glaubte man, wer Brennnessel und Schafgarbe in der Hand hielte, würde jede Angst überwinden. Brennnesselbüsche wurden im Stall und in den Häusern aufgehängt und sollten gegen fliegende Hexen helfen, die sich ja vor Eisen fürchteten, und gegen die Ausbreitung von Krankheiten und Seuchen in der Nachbarschaft.

Die Brennnessel wurde als Liebespflanze der besonderen Art angesehen: Man meinte, dass in den Brennnesselhorsten kleine hässliche Erdmännlein wohnten, die hübschen Mädchen nachstellen würden. Wurde die Liebe nicht gleich erwidert, zauberte man sie der/dem Angebeteten einfach an: Dazu musste man erst einmal an einem Freitag vor Sonnenaufgang, heimlich auf eine Brennnesselstaude urinieren, dabei den Namen der/des Begehrten aufsagen und danach die Pflanze mit Salz bestreuen. Nach Sonnenuntergang desselben Tages musste die Pflanze ausgegraben und in der Glut verbrannt werden, während man drei Dämonen beschwor: „Öl, Ammel und Ingrimm, so wie die Nessel brennt, so brenne auch ihr/sein Herz nach mir!" Der Erfolg blieb abzuwarten. Sollte jedoch die/der Angebetete Johanniskraut oder Wegerichwurzel bei sich getragen haben, konnte ihr/ihm der Zauber nichts anhaben!

Alltagstauglicher hingegen Ovids (43 v. Chr. bis 17 n. Chr.) Empfehlung, zur Steigerung der Liebeskraft den „Pfeffer wohl mit dem Samen der Nessel" zu mischen. Auch Otto Brunfels (1488–1534), Theologe, Botaniker und Arzt, wusste, wie man den ehelichen Pflichten nachkommen konnte. Er empfahl Nesselsamen, Zwiebel, Eigelb und Pfeffer, um den „menschlichen Körper zur Unzucht anzustacheln."

Verwendung – gestern und heute

Während Plinius (23–79) die Brennnessel als „die am meisten verhasste aller Pflanzen" titulierte, wurde sie von allen anderen Kräuterkundigen hoch geschätzt. Im *Macer floridus, einem mittelalterlichen Lehrgedicht aus dem 9./10. Jahrhundert, das die damals gebräuchlichsten Heilkräuter aufzählt, heißt es zur Brennnesselwurzel, diesem wahren Wundermittel an Heilkraft: „In Starkwein gestampft bezähmt die Wurzel jede Milzschwellung, lindert auch Fußgicht und hilft bei allen Leiden der Gelenke."*

Hieronymus Bock (1498–1554) stellt die Brennnessel an den Anfang seines großen Kräuterbuches und wundert sich: „Auß der kalten rauhen erden schlieffen vil hitziger gewechs, des man sich wol mag verwundern, als fürnehmlich die gemeine brennende Nessel". Balthasar Ehrhart (1700–1756) hielt die Fertigung von Nesselstoffen für erwähnenswert: „Einer Gattung feiner Leinwand oder das Nesseltuch daraus verfertigen, welches mir sehr glaublich, weilen auch der Hanff in Gestalt und Artzney-Krafft in nächster Gleichheit mit der Nessel ist. Dergleichen Nessel-Tuchfabriquen haben sie in Dreßden nachmachen wollen."

Zur Erinnerung: Eine handvoll Brennnesselblätter enthält mehr Eisen, Calcium, Eiweiß und Vitamin C als eine ganze Schüssel Kopfsalat!

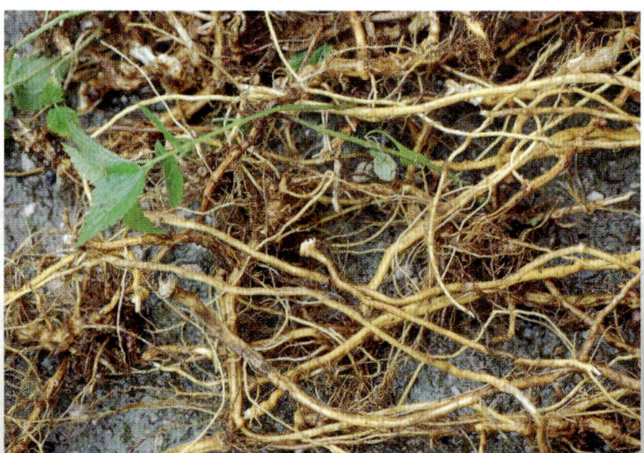

Brennnesselwurzeln

Diptam

Lat. Name: *Dictamnus albus*
Pflanzenfamilie: Rautengewächse

Weiße Fee und brennender Busch und Deiweilspflanze – das scheinen die harten Gegensätze zu sein, die in diesem Pflanzenwesen zutage treten. In seiner Jugend scheint der Diptam eher dahinzukümmern, lässt sich zwei, drei Jahre Zeit mit dem richtigen Fußfassen und auch mit dem Blühen. In dieser Zeit gibt er auch manchmal einfach auf, verschwindet aus dem Beet. Hat er jedoch diese Phase überwunden, entschädigt er uns mit betörend duftenden Blüten und faszinierenden Samensternen und wird von Jahr zu Jahr schöner.

Ist die Pflanze erst ausgewachsen, lässt sie sich nicht mehr versetzen. Sie kann mit noch so viel Umsicht ausgegraben werden, sie nimmt keinen neuen Standort mehr an. So eigensinnig der Diptam mit seiner Lebenskraft umgeht, so speziell sind auch seine Inhaltsstoffe, die von hautreizenden Furano-Cumarinen und vorsichtig zu beurteilenden Alkaloiden bis hin zu wertvollen Bitterstoffen, Anthocyanen und Flavon-Glykosiden reichen.

Rauch

Verwendete Pflanzenteile: Wurzel, Samensterne.

Beste Sammel- und Erntezeit: Die Wurzel wird an bedeckten Tagen bei abnehmendem Mond gegraben, ausreichend gewässert, gesäubert und dann klein geschnitten und im Schatten getrocknet. Die Samensterne werden Ende August gesammelt. Zusammen mit der Wurzel werden sie für die Räucherung fein vermahlen.

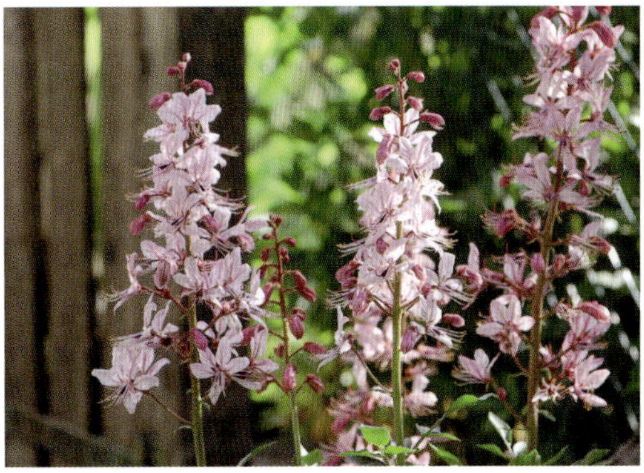

Blüten des Diptams

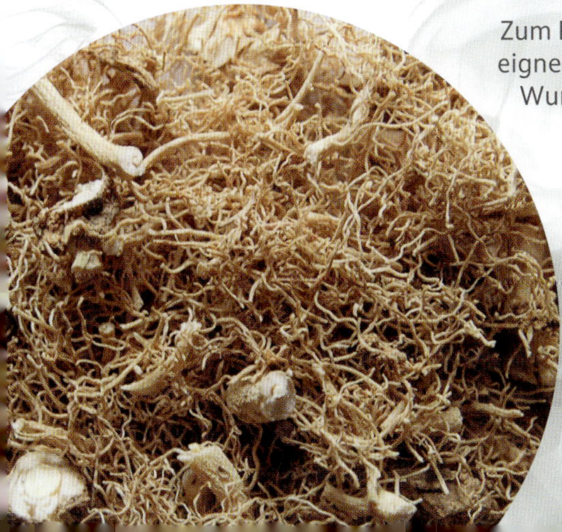

Zum Räuchern eignen sich die Wurzeln und Samensterne.

Wirkung, Wahrnehmung: Allein der Geruch der Wurzel und des Krauts sei so mächtig, dass alle „gifftige thier vom geruch müssen weichen unnd räumen", hält Hieronymus Bock (1498–1554) fest. Abwehrrauch. Reinigungsrauch. Verschreikraut und Kraut der Sonnenwenden. In der Antike verwendete man eine Diptam-Wurzelräucherung, um mit den Göttern in Verbindung zu treten und dabei gleichzeitig einen Blick in die Zukunft zu erhaschen. Der Wurzelrauch begleitet die Sonnenwenden mit seiner unheilabwehrenden, lichtmehrenden Kraft aus der weißen Wurzel. Auch innere „Sonnenwenden" werden hilfreich begleitet, wenn es darum geht, durch das zunehmende Licht einen Ausweg aus der Dunkelheit der Depression oder Verzweiflung zu finden. Oder wenn es darum geht, geschützt und heil eine Phase des abnehmenden Lichtes, der Trennungen, Lebenskrisen durchzustehen. Der Rauch des teufelsbannenden Drudensterns gemischt mit der apotropäisch wirkenden, weißen Feenwurzel macht die Aura und das weitere energetische Umfeld dicht. Das eigene Kraftfeld wird aufgepolstert.

Hat im Rauch die größte Kraft Verwünschungen, Flüche, Bannungen und andere Anhaftungen zu neutralisieren und nachhaltig zu überlagern. Der Diptamrauch ist auch ein Abwehrrauch für Partnerschaften, um das Miteinander frei zu halten von negativen Übertragungen anderer. Eine starke Abgrenzungswahrnehmung von innen und außen, von wichtig und unwichtig, drängt sich auf. Abwehr von Fremdbestimmung und manipulativen Übergriffen. Die Konzentration wird gestärkt, man kann sich ganz auf ein Thema fokussieren. Die Vorstellungskraft wird gestärkt; vielschichtige Gedankenreisen eröffnen neue Sichtweisen, bei denen ein Gedanke kettenartig zum nächsten führt.

Magisches zum Rauch: Unsere Vorfahren waren überzeugt, dass der Rauch von Diptam jeden Nestel- und Knotenzauber lösen könne. Begleitet wurden solche zauberischen Handlungen von geheimen Sprüchen und einem zentralen Wasser-Ritual mit Sprengung und Waschung. Hieronymus Bock hält überdies fest: „Dictamkraut treibt nit allein den weibischen fluß, sondern auch die ander geburt und die todten kinder. Ein rauch von Dictamkraut gemacht thut dergleichen."

Schwerpunkt, Anwendungen, Rezepte: Räuchermischung zur Stärkung der Durchsetzungskraft und vor Prüfungen: Diptam, Eisenkraut, Thymian, Baldrian. Räuchermischung zur persönlichen Abgrenzung und Abwehr von Fremdbestimmung: Diptam, Königskerze, Rainfarn und Weinraute. Jeweils mit Harz kombinieren.

Mythologie und magische Praktiken

Hieronymus Bock schreibt: „Ettlich melden der Dictam ziehe alle eingeschossene pfeil herauß nit allein dem menschen darauff gelegt, sonder aiuch wann das vihe von Dictam isset sollen die pfeil herauß fallen."

Verwendung – gestern und heute

Um das Jahr 800 erlässt Kaiser Karl der Große (747–814) mit der Verordnung „Capitulare de villis vel curtis imperii" eine Betriebsvorschrift für seine Königshöfe. Als Anhang ist eine Pflanzenliste erhalten, die 73 Kräuter und Gemüsesorten aufzählt, die in den hofnahen Gärten

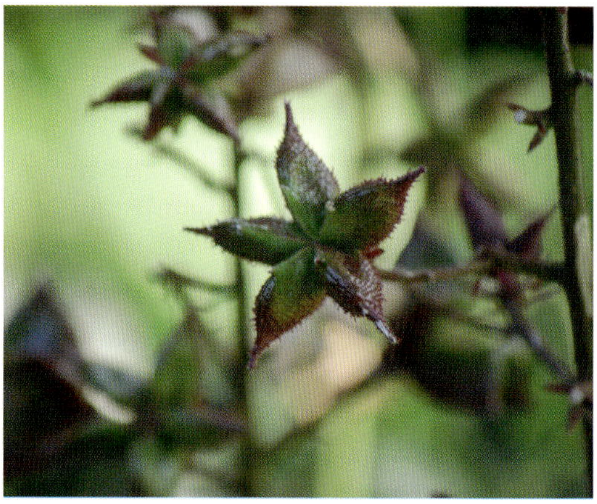

Fruchtstand des Diptams

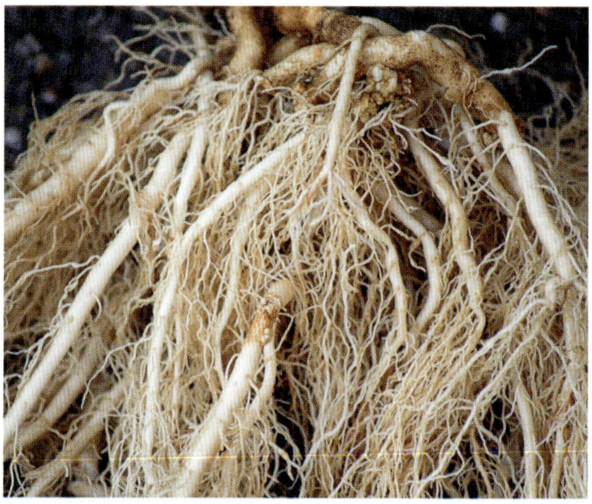

Diptamwurzeln

ausschließlich für den Herrscher anzubauen sind. An der 38. Stelle dieser Liste steht der Diptam als „diptamnum".

Lonicerus (1528–1586) stellt das Rezept für ein „Diptamwasser" zur Verfügung: „Das beste Theil weissen Diptam zu destillieren ist, die Wurtzel zwischen den zweyen unsern Frauen Tagen, gehackt und gebrannt. Dieses Wasser Abends und Morgens jedes mal auf drey Loth getrunken, ist gut für die Pestilenz. Auf sechs Loth getruncken, vertreibet alles Gifft."

In der Hildegard-Medizin (Hildegard von Bingen) wird heute noch ein Diptam-Pulver gegen Steinbildungen und Ablagerungen in den Gefäßen hergestellt.

Engelwurz

Lat. Name: *Angelica archangelica*
Botanischer Name: Echte Engelwurz
Pflanzenfamilie: Doldenblütler

Ursprünglich in Nordeuropa beheimatet gilt die Engelwurz als Universalheilmittel und von Engeln verkündete absolute Schutzpflanze für Körper, Geist und Seele, deren Hauptkraft auf die Wiederherstellung der Ordnung gerichtet ist. Um das Jahr 1000 wird sie bereits in nordischen Gärten angebaut. Im 12. Jahrhundert wird in Skandinavien verfügt, dass ein Pächter eines Gartens, bei Pachtauflösung die Angelika-Wurzeln in jedem Fall ausgraben und mitnehmen dürfe.

In meinem Garten darf die Engelwurz sich frei bewegen, darf sich in jedem Beet breitmachen, darf jede Zeile sprengen. Oft hocken die kleinen Engelwurzen mehrere Jahre am Acker, wachsen kaum, scheinen zu überlegen, wie es wohl weitergeht oder welche von ihnen einmal die höchste und schönste würde. Wenn sie sich entschließen, ihren zweijährigen Zyklus bis zur Aussamung zu starten, vervielfachen sie im ersten Jahr einmal das bodennahe Grün. Im darauffolgenden Jahr wird dann die ganze Kraft aus der Wurzel gezogen und für ein Wachstum in schwindelnde Höhen verwendet – 2,5 m und mehr können es da schon werden!

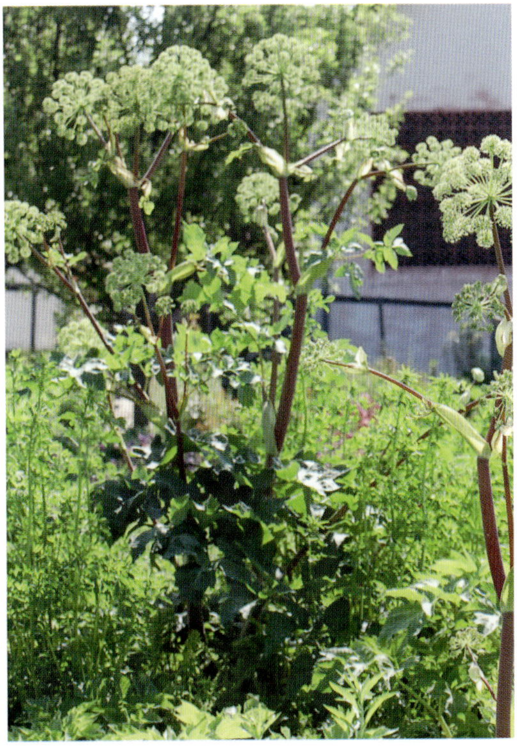
Blühende Engelwurz

Jede Blütendolde wird langsam zur hell leuchtenden Samendolde, perfekt rund geformt wie eine neue Sonne. Zu diesem Zeitpunkt im Jahr hat die Engelwurz bereits keinen Wurzelstock mehr und steht immer noch aufrecht, mit den beiden Seitendolden, die wie zwei nach oben gestreckte Arme die größere Mitteldolde überragen. Und wo immer dieses wunderbare Geschöpf in meinem Garten seine Samen ausstreut, dort darf sie wachsen und ihre Bestimmung finden.

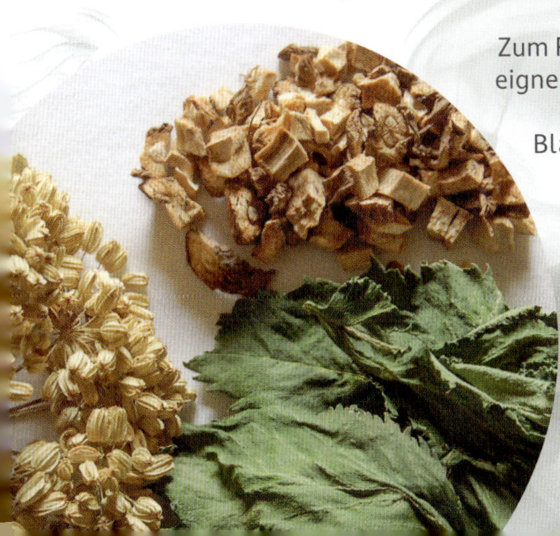
Zum Räuchern eignen sich die Wurzeln, Blätter und Samen.

Rauch

Verwendete Pflanzenteile: Wurzeln, Blätter, Samen.

Beste Sammel- und Erntezeit: Um von der Engelwurz Wurzeln zu ernten, müssen sie im Herbst jenes Jahres gegraben werden, in dem die Pflanze eine dichte Blattmasse entwickelt, aber noch keine Blütenstängel getrieben hat. Die Wurzel und auch das feine, bräunliche Wurzelhaar werden gewaschen, klein geschnitten und getrocknet. Die Blätter können das ganze Jahr über gesammelt werden; die Samen im Herbst des zweiten Jahres.

Wirkung, Wahrnehmung: Im Rauch werden die höchsten Kräfte aus der Wurzel sowie aus den getrockneten Samen freigesetzt: Die Samen stärken das „Bauchgefühl", heben den verlorenen sechsten Sinn, unterstützen auch den seelischen Schutzbedarf, vertreiben Angst und Unsicherheit. Die Wurzel ist kopfgerichtet, gibt Mut und Kraft, sorgt für festen Stand und klare Gedanken. Ihr Rauch überträgt aber auch stark erdende Impulse an Aura und Orte. Reinigungs- und Schutzrauch für Mensch, Haus und Hof; rein weißmagische Kraft, unter deren Schutz sich die Dinge gedeihlich entwickeln können. Die Kraft der Wandlung ins Sonnenlicht! Der Rauch ermöglicht Einsichten, Erkenntnisse und lässt alles Positive wachsen und größer werden. Die Mächte der Finsternis, wie Melancholie, Niedergeschlagenheit, depressive Zustände, werden wirkungsvoll gelindert.

Die Botin des Lichts bringt Sonne ins Herz und schenkt uns Vertrauen in den eigenen Lebensweg; sie baut uns innerlich auf, so dass wir Existenz- und Verlustängste sowie Mutlosigkeit hinter uns lassen können. Schock und Trauer können durchlichtet werden und so in Lösung gehen. Die starke Schutzwirkung ihres Rauches wirkt insgesamt kräftigend auf Immunsystem und Psyche. Der Rauch fördert die innere Ruhe und Klarheit der Gedanken ebenso wie die Entscheidungsfähigkeit und das Selbstvertrauen. In Räumen, Häusern und an Orten vermag der Wurzelrauch energetisch verdichtete Ecken und Stellen positiv zu überlagern und zu entflechten. Danach ist die entspannte Atmosphäre deutlich spürbar. Die Wandlungskraft des Wurzelrauches kann unrastende Verstorbene aus unserer materiellen Welt lösen helfen und sie mit wärmendem Licht in eine andere Welt begleiten. Der Rauch von Samen und Wurzel der Engelwurz verbindet uns ganz stark mit der Anderswelt und macht, hin und wieder in längeren Räuchersessions, diesen Existenzhintergrund wie ein beruhigendes Auffangnetz spürbar.

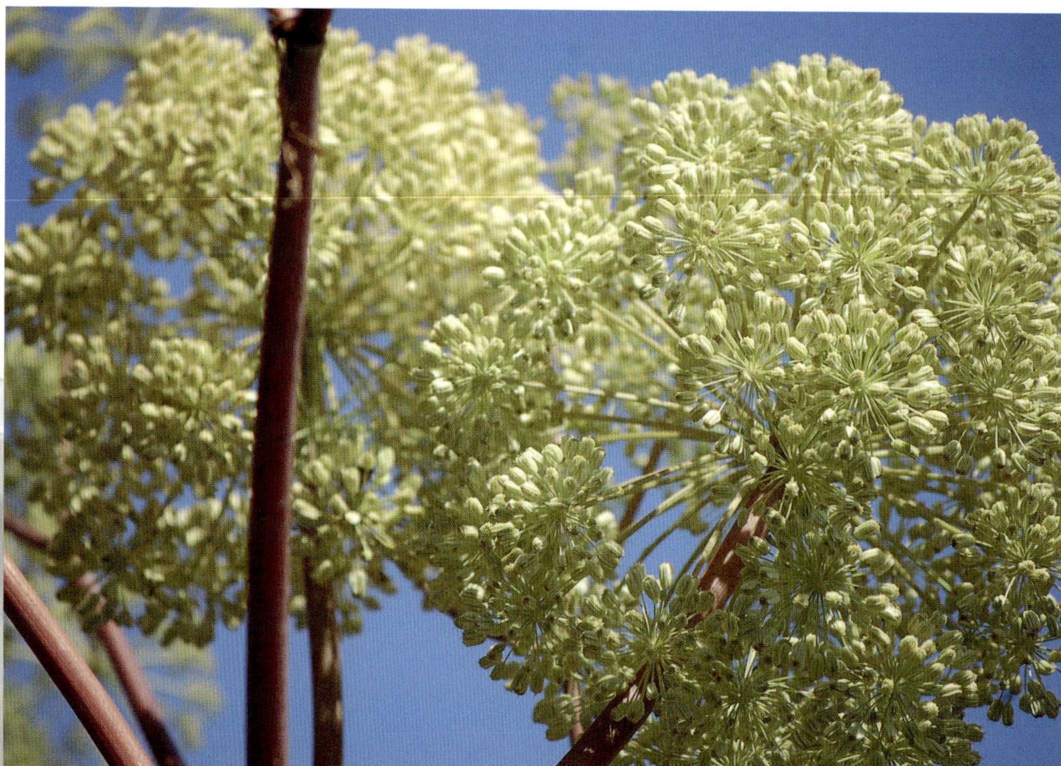

Blüte der Engelwurz

Magisches zum Rauch: Hausräucherung vor Umbautätigkeiten, nach dem Kauf bzw. Verkauf eines Hauses, oder wenn sich im Haus ein Todesfall ereignet hat: Hier sollen Alt- und Fremdenergien neutralisiert und abgeleitet werden. Zuerst wird eine Räuchermischung hergestellt: Man mischt Tannennadeln, Engelwurz, Heidekraut, Hollerblüten, Rosmarin und Ysop.

Der Ablauf beginnt und endet im energetisch ruhigsten Teil des Hauses und könnte so aussehen: Kerze und Räucherung entzünden, ein Wurzelstück der Engelwurz bei sich tragen, eines auf den Räucherrundgang durchs Haus mitnehmen und eines am Ausgangs- und Endpunkt dieses Räucherrituals neben die angezündete Kerze legen. Danach werden die zwei raumbezogenen Wurzelstücke in der Nacht, das heißt im Dunkeln unter einer Dachableitung vergraben, das persönliche Wurzelstück wird angezündet und im Freien abgebrannt bzw. verräuchert.

Schwerpunkt, Anwendungen, Rezepte: Räuchermischung zum Schutz vor Ansteckung und Übergriffen: Engelwurzsamen, Beifuß, Wacholderbeeren. Bei Stressbelastung mischt man einen Rauch aus Engelwurzwurzel und -samen, Königskerze, Eisenkraut und Ahornblättern. Für eine Räuchermischung, die überreizte Seelen beruhigt, tröstend und aufbauend erlebt wird, mischt man Engelwurzsamen, Mistel, Mädesüß, Lavendel und Rosenblüten. Dazu Harz kombinieren.

Mythologie und magische Praktiken

Als potente Amulett-Pflanze schützt sie einen überall vor körperlicher Ansteckung und geistiger Vereinnahmung. Tabernaemontanus (1522–1590) versucht den legendären Namen zu erklären: „Angelick, Heiligengeistwurz, Brustwurz und Engelwurz, und das umb seiner fürtrefflichen Krafft und tugend willen, als wann der H. Geist selber, oder die lieben Engel dem menschlichen Geschlecht dieses Gewächs und heylsame Wurzel geoffenbart hetten, derwegen es dann auch nicht unbillich von etlichen Panaces Angelicum (= Allheilkraut der Engel) genannt wird."

Verwendung – gestern und heute

Paracelsus (1493–1541) sieht in ihrem Saft die „höchste Arznei gegen innere Infektionen durch die Luft und ein Schutzmittel gegen die Pestilenz": Nach dem Erscheinungsbild der Pflanze wiesen deren dicken Blattumhüllungen auf ihre Heilkraft bei geschwollenen Lymphknoten und aufgetriebenen Pestbeulen hin. Auch Hieronymus Bock (1493–1554) und Leonhart Fuchs (1501–1566) sind sich über die Wirkkraft der Engelwurz einig und schreiben wortgleich: „So bewart und behüt sie den menschen vor der pestilentz."

Balthasar Ehrhart (1700–1756) meint in seinem Lonicerus-Kommentar: „Wir müssen von einem heilsamen erroris gedencken, da man einsten statt der Attich-Blätter, die grünen Blätter von einem wilden Angelica Geschlecht gefunden, und wider das Podagra (= Gicht) aufgelegt, ist solches heilsam gelindert und gestillet worden."

Maurice Messegué (1921–2017), berühmter französischer Kräuterkundler des 20. Jahrhunderts, meinte, dass die Engelwurz so wertvoll für den Menschen sei, dass sie mit Gold aufgewogen werden müsste. Über Jahrhunderte ist die Engelwurz Pflichtbestandteil in sämtlichen Theriak-Rezepturen bis herauf zum „Klosterfrau Melissengeist" und zum „Schwedenbitter". Auch heute gilt sie als Stärkungsmittel bei allen Schwächezuständen körperlicher oder seelischer Art.

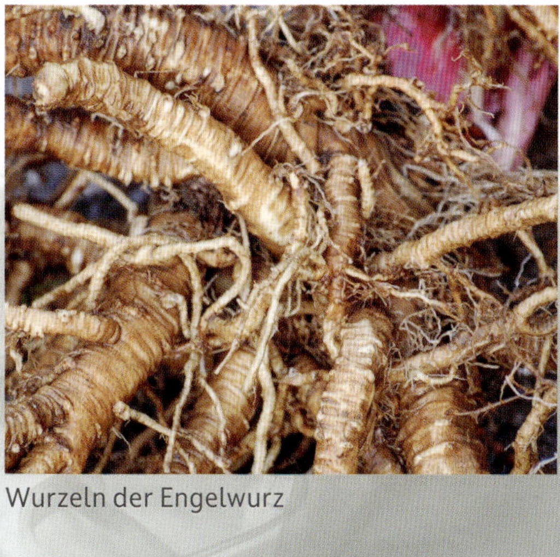

Wurzeln der Engelwurz

Eibisch

Lat. Name: *Althaea officinalis*
Pflanzenfamilie: Malvengewächse

Der Eibisch ist ein treuer Begleiter in jedem Garten, der scheinbar gegensätzliche Eigenschaften in sich vereint: höchste Empfindlichkeit bei gleichzeitiger extremer Zähigkeit. Zur Empfindlichkeit: Meine Eibischpflanzen haben mich in den letzten Jahrzehnten dazu erzogen, sie in den ersten Monaten ihres Jahreswachstums bis zur Blüte, wertschätzend und bewusst wahrzunehmen. Ich gehe also durch meinen Garten und spreche meine Eibische an, zolle ihnen meine Bewunderung, lobe ihre Schönheit, streife da und dort über die Blätter. Dann ist alles in Ordnung und die Luft ist erfüllt von einer erhebenden Resonanz aus dem Beet. Meine Eibische lächeln und es geht ihnen gut. Wenn ich dies jedoch unterlasse, stürzen sich einige von ihnen in Läuse, biegen sich nach unten, kräuseln ihre Blätter und stehen wie frierend mit hochgezogenen Schultern im Beet. Werden sie dann, unter tausend Entschuldigungen angesprochen, dauert es keine zwei Wochen und sie sind lausfrei und wieder wohlauf. Die Missachtung ist vergessen und vergeben. Zur Zähigkeit: Ein aufgelassener Bauerngarten findet sich heute mitten auf einer Pferdekoppel. Man wüsste es gar nicht mehr, wäre da nicht der Eibisch, der überlebt hat. Das ständige Getrampel der Pferdehufe versetzt Pflanzen in Dauerstress. Zwei Walnussbäume haben bereits resigniert und sind abgestorben. Aber jedes Jahr schießt der Eibisch, gut gedüngt, mitten auf der Pferdekoppel in die Höhe, dass es nur so eine Freude ist und widersetzt sich gelassen dem äußeren Stress.

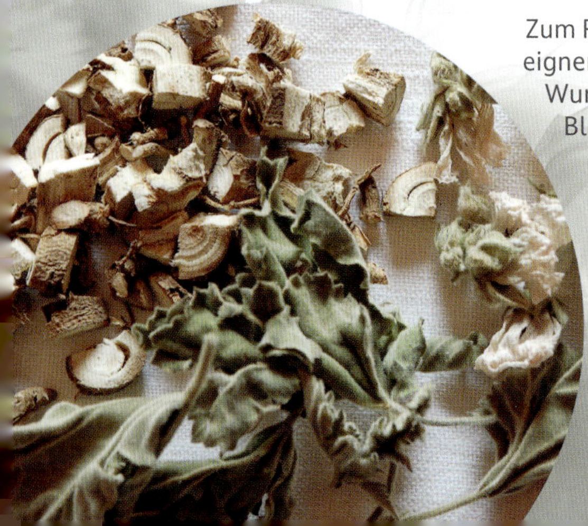

Zum Räuchern eignen sich die Wurzeln und Blätter, die Stängel und Blüten.

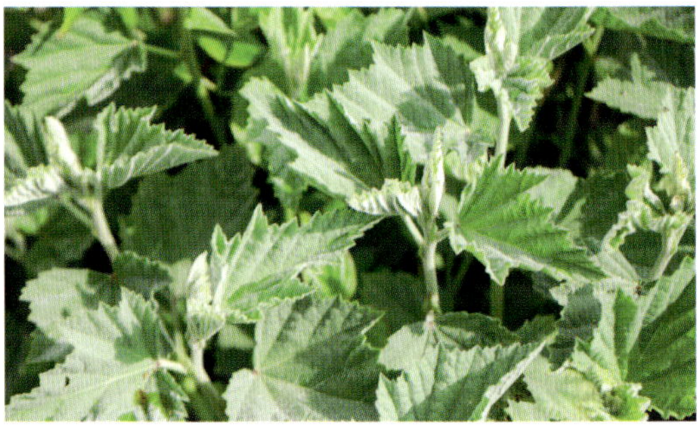

Eibischblätter

Rauch

Verwendete Pflanzenteile: Wurzel, Blätter, Stängel, Blüten.

Beste Sammel- und Erntezeit: Die Wurzel kann ganzjährig, am besten aber im Herbst, herausgestochen werden. Die gereinigte Wurzel besonders klein schneiden, da sie im getrockneten Zustand steinartig hart wird. Die Blätter werden ganzjährig beerntet, oder zur Blütezeit gemeinsam mit den Blüten.

Wirkung, Wahrnehmung: Schutzrauch für Haus und Hof. Mit dem Rauch der gesamten Pflanze tut sich sehr schnell eine schützende Höhle auf. Die Besinnung auf körperliche Nähe und Zusammenrücken wird gefördert. Rundum schützender Rauch, der förderlich für das Verständnis untereinander sein kann. Mit dem Wurzelrauch kommen wohlwollende Geister ins Haus; es bleibt eine geklärte Atmosphäre zurück, in der man zur Ruhe kommen und entspannt sein kann. Mit dem Rauch einfach die Seele baumeln lassen und sich wohlfühlen.

Magisches zum Rauch: In der Zeit der Hexenverfolgungen war dem Eibisch, wie anderen Kräutern auch, eine traurige Rolle zugedacht: Unter Folter gestanden die der Hexerei Angeklagten jene Kräuter, mit denen sie ihren angeblichen Schadenszauber betrieben hätten. Der Eibisch war dabei eines, von neun am häufigsten genannten Kräutern.

Hin und wieder denke ich mit folgender Räuchermischung an das unsagbare Leid, das unzähligen Menschen in der Inquisitionszeit zugefügt wurde. Inkriminierte Neun-Kräuter-Räuchermischung: Eibisch – Wermut – Vogelknöterich – Mutterkraut – Odermennig – guter Heinrich – Baldrian – Eberraute – Pestwurz.

Schwerpunkt, Anwendungen, Rezepte: Räuchermischung für Herzenswärme und ein gutes Miteinander: Eibisch, Wald-Geißbart, Mistel, Königskerze und Harz.

Verwendung – gestern und heute

In der Antike galt der Eibisch als Allheilmittel. Schon Hippokrates (460–370 v. Chr.), der berühmteste Arzt des Altertums, rühmt den Eibisch für seine wundheilende Kraft. Plinius (23–79) rät: „Wer täglich einen halben Kyathos (ein Schöpfbecher, ca. 45 ml) voll von dem Saft des Eibisches trinkt, wird gegen jede Krankheit immun sein". Darüberhinaus hält er fest: „Seine, vor Sonnenaufgang ausgegrabene Wurzel hüllt man in sogenannte naturfarbene Wolle, und zwar von einem Schaf, das ein weibliches Lamm geworfen hat, und legt sie auf Beulen oder Vereiterungen." Karl der Große (747–814) verfügt um das Jahr 800 den Eibisch verpflichtend zum Anbau auf all seinen Königsgütern: „altaea" an 50. Stelle der 73 Kräuter und Gemüsesorten umfassenden Liste.

Hildegard von Bingen (1098–1179) hebt die „Ybischa" als Allheilmittel hervor und hat ein besonderes Mittel bei Kopfweh anzubieten: „Wer Kopfweh hat, nehme Eibisch, füge etwas weniger Salbei bei und dies zerstoße er gleichzeitig und dem mische er etwas Baumöl (Olivenöl) hinzu und dann wärme er es nur neben dem Feuer in seiner Hand und so lege er es auf seine Stirn und binde ein Tuch darum und so schlafe er ein und es wird ihm besser gehen."

Über die Klöster kam der Eibisch in die Bauerngärten und war eine unverzichtbare Heilpflanze des Mittelalters und in der Volksheilkunde bis heute. In Notzeiten wurde die schleimstoffreiche Wurzel gedünstet und als Gemüse gegessen. Die Eibisch-Hustenzuckerl kennt man aus der Apotheke. Bei Erkältungen tut auch ein Kaltansatz der Eibischwurzel gut.

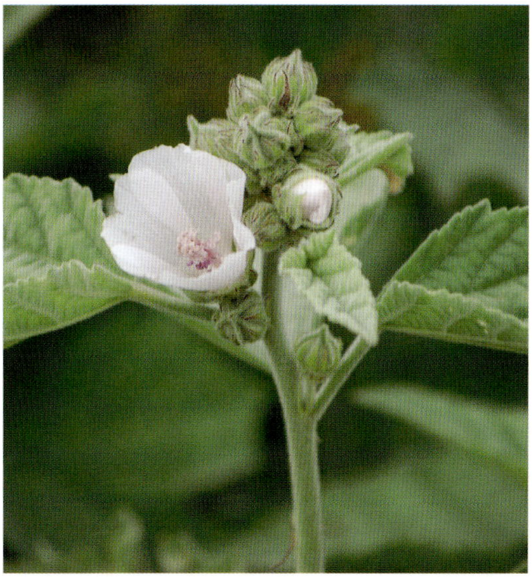

Eibischblüte

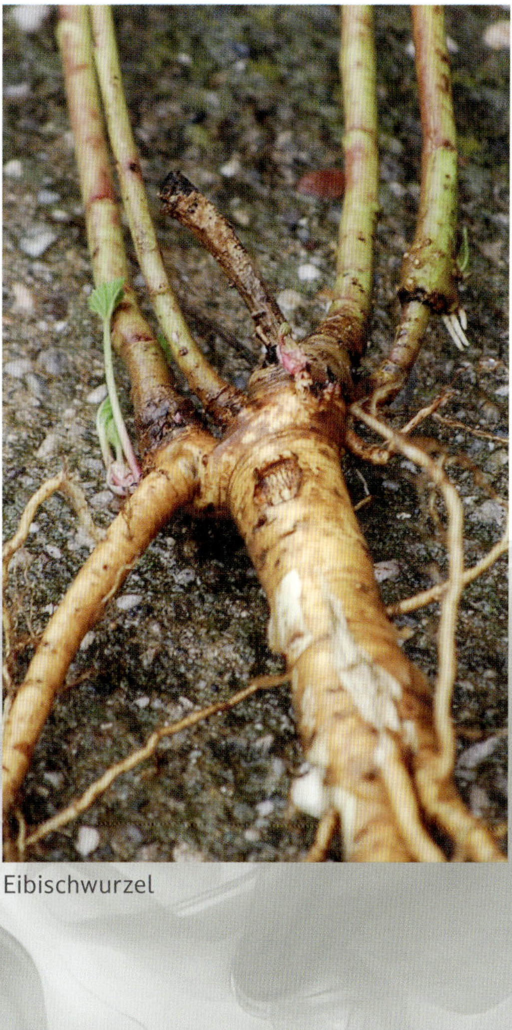

Eibischwurzel

Giersch

Lat. Name: *Aegopodium podagraria*
Pflanzenfamilie: Doldenblütler

„…es hat eine kleine weisse Wurtzel mit wenig Zaseln, die kreucht in dem Erdreich hin und her, unnd nimpt in kurtzer Zeit ein gantzen garten eyn, dann wo sie einmal eynwurtzelt, ist sie nicht leichtlich mehr auszurotten…“, klagt Tabernaemontanus (1522–1590) vor 500 Jahren und spricht damit Generationen von nachfolgenden Gartenbesitzern aus der Seele, die mit dem quicklebendigen und expansionsfreudigen Giersch dieselben Erfahrungen gemacht haben.

Bei all dem Ungemach, den er durch seine Aufdringlichkeit verursacht, übersieht man oft, dass der Giersch seit Jahrtausenden als wertvolles Heilkraut verwendet wurde und oft genug für einen vollen Teller und einen satten Magen sorgte. Pünktlich im Frühjahr liefert er reinstes Vitamin C, Provitamin A, Magnesium, Calcium, Mangan und Kupfer frei Haus, um nur einige seiner wertvollen Inhaltsstoffe zu nennen.

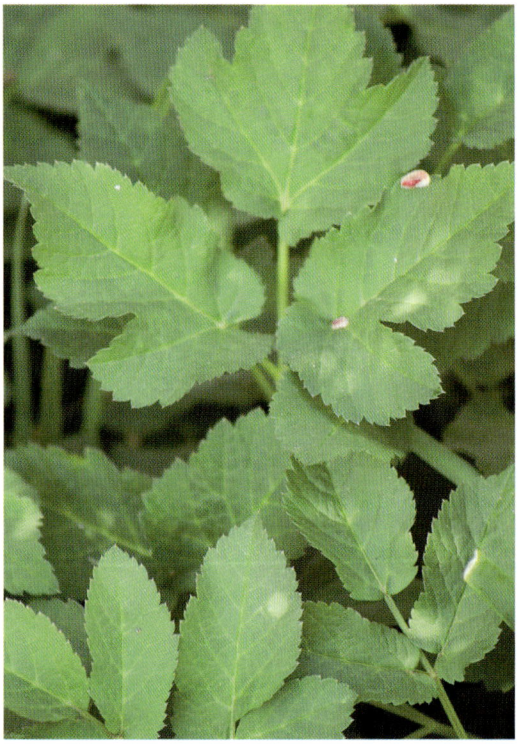

Gierschblätter

Rauch

Verwendete Pflanzenteile: Wurzeln sowie das ganze blühende Kraut.

Beste Sammel- und Erntezeit: Die Wurzeln können ganzjährig gesammelt werden. Man schneidet sie klein und trocknet sie. Auch die Blätter sind ganzjährig zu sammeln, die Blüten im Mai/Juni.

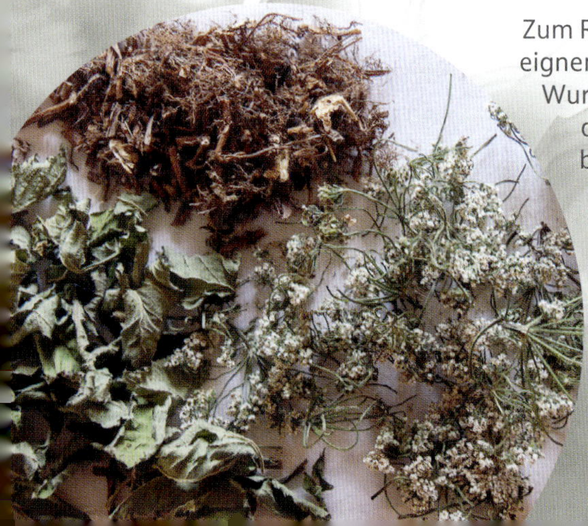

Zum Räuchern eignen sich die Wurzeln und die ganze blühende Pflanze.

Wirkung, Wahrnehmung: Reinigungsrauch. Stark positiv polende Kraft. Klärt die Raumatmosphäre für den Moment, wirkt jedoch nicht nachhaltig lösend. Verdichtete Raumstrukturen in Häusern, Räumen oder an Orten werden mit dem Rauch aus der weißen Wurzel zügig überlagert und in eine angenehmere Form gewandelt. Der Gierschrauch bewirkt einen geistigen und nachfolgend auch stimmungsmäßigen Umschwung von kraftlos zu neuer Energie, von überfordert zu aufnahmebereit und positiv ausgerichtet. Befreiung aus lähmendem Stillstand, aus beklemmender Enge, aus ungewollter Umklammerung. Fegt geistige Hemmschwellen hinweg, erleichtert den Weg von innen nach außen. Hilfreich für zurückhaltende Menschen. Stimuliert die Selbstheilungskräfte, hebt das Selbstbewusstsein und vermittelt neuen Mut.

Schwerpunkt, Anwendungen, Rezepte: Aufbauende Räuchermischung, die die Entschlusskraft stärkt: Giersch, Alant, Birke, Rosmarin, Mistel und Harz.

Verwendung – gestern und heute

Die mittelalterlichen Kräuterkundigen verwendeten den „Witscherlenwetsch" vor allem als Gicht- und Wundkraut. Wie wir jedoch heute von seinen sekundären Inhaltsstoffen her wissen, reichen seine Heilkräfte viel weiter: Er kann beispielsweise vor Allergien schützen und das Nerven- und Immunsystem nach der kalten Jahreszeit stärken.

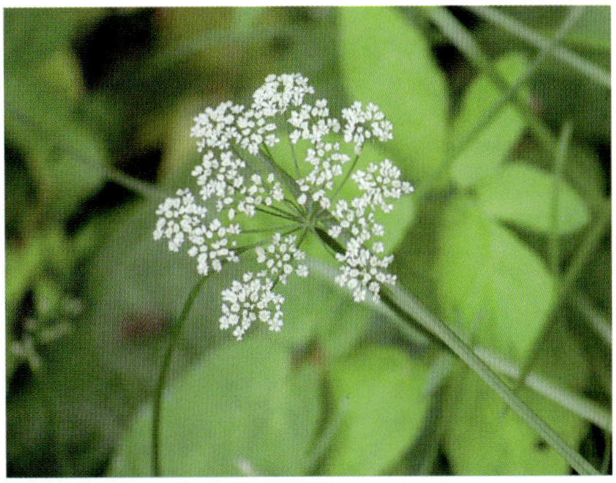

Blühender Giersch

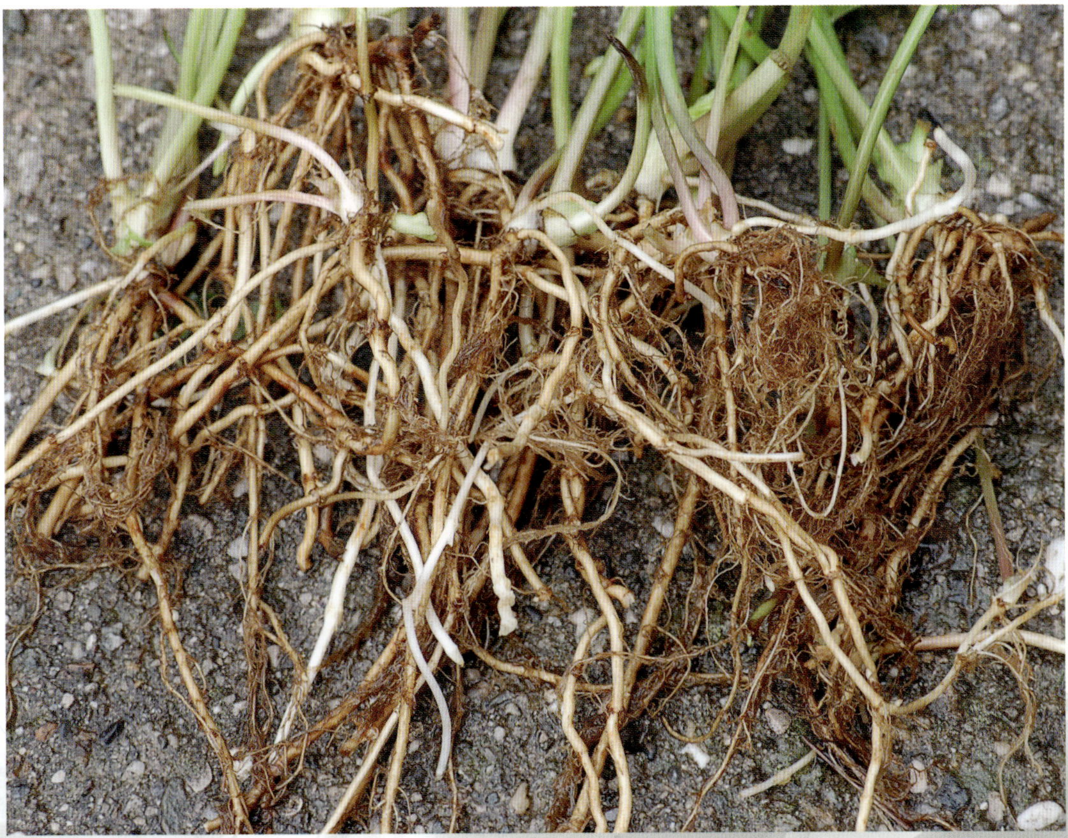

Gierschwurzeln

Große Klette

Lat. Name: *Arctium lappa*
Pflanzenfamilie: Korbblütler

Der kraftstrotzende Götterbär begleitete mit seiner imposanten Erscheinung sowohl die magische als auch die heilkundliche Vorstellungswelt unserer Vorfahren. Arctos, altgriechisch der Bär, wurde europaweit verehrt – als Krafttier und als besonderer Kenner von Kräutern und Wurzeln.

Alles an dieser Pflanze ist mächtig – die riesigen Blätter im ersten Jahr, die über zwei Meter emporragende Pflanzengestalt im zweiten Jahr, ihre über einen Meter lange und entsprechend dicke Pfahlwurzel, ihre große Heilkraft und ihre erstaunliche Entschlossenheit. Als ich vor vielen Jahren wie gewohnt zur Klettenwurzel-Ernte in unserer Pferdeweide anrückte, staunte ich nicht schlecht: Alles war niedergefressen, kein einziger Stängel mehr sichtbar. Das hatten die Pferde noch nie getan, aber offensichtlich hatten sie einen Bedarf und machten das mächtige Kraut nieder. Wie erstaunt war ich, als mir im darauffolgenden Jahr mitten auf meinem Kräuteracker eine kleine Klettenpflanze entgegenstrahlte. Da war sie, erstmals in meinem Garten und hat sich gleich zur „Leberklette", zum Odermennig gesetzt! Es schien mir, als wäre sie vor einer neuerlich zu befürchtenden Fressattacke der Pferde geflohen und hatte sich über hunderte Meter, bergauf und über zwei Zäune hinweg, in Sicherheit gebracht. Bis heute wachsen Klettenpflanzen auf meinem Acker. In der Pferdeweide ist keine einzige mehr nachgekommen!

Zum Räuchern eignen sich die Wurzeln und Blätter.

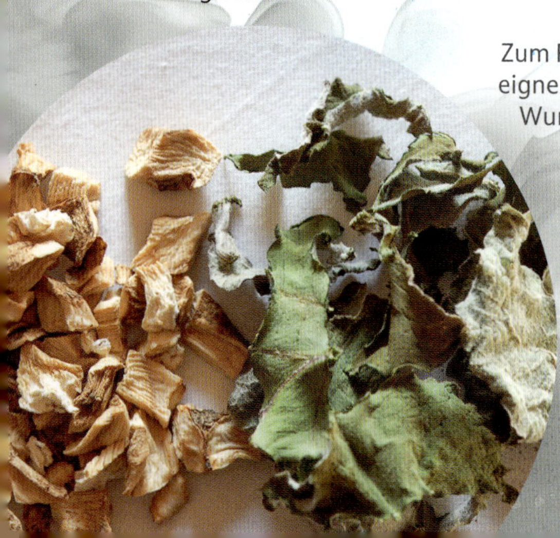

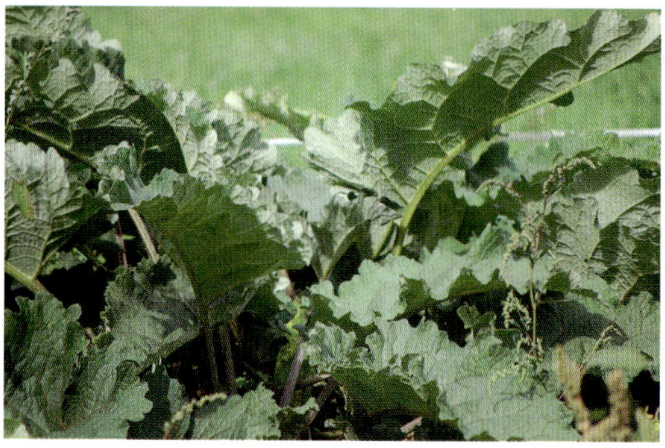

Blätter der Großen Klette

Rauch

Verwendete Pflanzenteile: Wurzel, Blätter.

Beste Sammel- und Erntezeit: Die Wurzeln werden im Herbst so tief wie möglich ausgegraben, gereinigt und klein geschnitten. Die Blätter können ebenfalls getrocknet und mit verräuchert werden. Die Klettenfrüchte sollten nicht verräuchert werden, sie sind wohl Türöffner für Anhaftungen!

Wirkung, Wahrnehmung: Abwehrrauch mit großer dämonenvertreibender Kraft; Reinigungsrauch; Kraut der Sonnenwenden. Reinigungsrauch in Räumen, um energetische Schieflagen auszugleichen; man räuchert unter Betten bei Schlafstörungen, unter und rund um Schreibtische bei Gedankenblockaden und geistiger Sprunghaftigkeit, die keine Arbeit konsequent zu Ende bringen lassen. Wehrt negative Energien, die von außen auf uns einwirken, zuverlässig ab. Ebenso werden magische Angriffe gestoppt, schlechte Vereinnahmungen enttarnt und die Kraft zum Gegensteuern mobilisiert. Wirkt auf Körper, Geist und Seele gleichermaßen befreiend, hilft Schwermütigkeit und Bedrücktheit zu überwinden, entmachtet die übergriffigen Einwirkungen durch andere, indem sie uns bewusst werden.

Magisches zum Rauch: Zur indirekten Räucherung wurde eine Klettenwurzelpflanze samt Wurzel als magischer Schlafbringer über dem

Herd aufgehängt. Wird zur Wintersonnenwende mit Beifußwurzel und Fichtennadeln verräuchert, um Bedrohungen, die aus der Dunkelheit kommen, Dämonen und mißgünstige Wesen zu bannen. Diese Räucherung sollte drei Mal erfolgen: am Tag der Sonnenwende, am Tag zuvor und am Tag danach.

Schwerpunkt, Anwendungen, Rezepte: Befreiende Räuchermischung nach Enttäuschungen: Klettenwurzel, Alantwurzel, Brennnesselwurzel, Engelwurzsamen. Wurzelräucherung zu den Sonnenwenden, um sich leichter neu auszurichten: Klettenwurzel, Meisterwurz, Bärenschotenwurzel, Bibernellwurzel. Jeweils mit Harz kombinieren.

Verwendung – gestern und heute

Die entzündungshemmende Wirkung der Großen Klette war bereits in der Antike bekannt. Auch noch im Mittelalter nahm sie in der volksheilkundlichen Praxis eine unverzichtbare Rolle ein. So veranlasste Kaiser Karl der Große (747–814) in seiner Anbauverfügung „Capitulare de villis vel curtis imperii" um das Jahr 800, den verpflichtenden Anbau der Großen Klette auf all seinen Königsgütern: „parduna" an 28. Stelle von 73 genannten Pflanzen.

Hieronymus Bock (1498–1554) beispielsweise schreibt: „Die gewächs so wir gemein und für unkreütter halten, seind in der artzenei vil

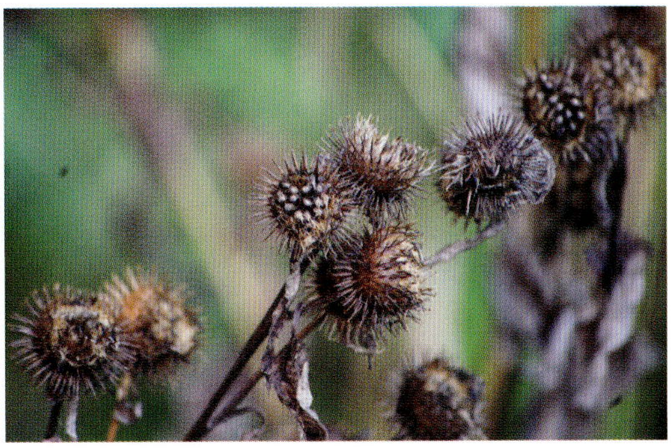

Samenstände der Großen Klette

mal die besten, das mag man an disem Kletten gewächs warnemen, dann sie seind nutz in leib und ausserhalb zu brauchen." Auch Sebastian Kneipp (1821–1897) stellte 300 Jahre später erneut klar: „Die Klette ist eine unter dem Unkraut hervorragende Pflanze. Sie steht häufig am Wege wie ein verkommener Handwerksbursche; mancher Wanderer hat eine Freude, wenn er mit seinem Stocke dieser Pflanze einen Hieb versetzen kann. Die muthwilligen Kinder treiben damit viel Unfug, indem sie die Fruchtkapseln der Klette einander in die Haare oder in ein wollenes Kleid bringen. So sehr aber diese Pflanze als Unkraut verachtet ist, ebenso sehr ist sie als Heilpflanze aller Achtung werth." Die moderne Wissenschaft forscht zu Arctigenin, einem Inhaltsstoff der Großen Klette, bei welchem antivirale und antitumorale Wirkungen beobachtet werden konnten.

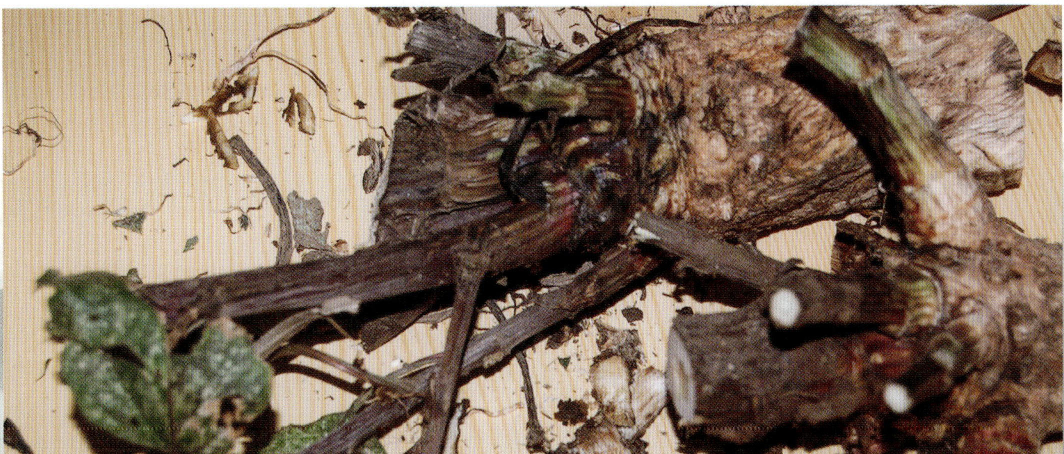

Wurzel der Großen Klette

Habichtskraut

Lat. Name: *Hieracium pilosella*
Botanischer Name: Kleines Habichtskraut
Pflanzenfamilie: Korbblütler

Hat das Habichtskraut erst einmal Fuß gefasst in einem Beet, kann man davon ausgehen, dass es sich fast unmerklich der ganzen Fläche bemächtigen wird. Dazu geht es stets in geschlossener Formation vor, ähnelt dabei einer antiken Schlachtaufstellung, wo die Schilde vorne dicht an dicht die Masse der Soldaten schützten. Mit atemberaubender Zähigkeit schiebt es sich über die Beete und weiter in die Wiese. Auch dort wächst es immer in Gruppen, besetzt einen Fleck, plättet ihn mit bodennahen Blättern und lässt dazwischen kein Gras hochkommen. Erst im Wurzelbereich erkennt man die ausgefeilte Eroberungstaktik dieser Pflanze: Tausendfach verweben sich weiße, ganz lange Wurzelfäden, die von dicken Wurzel-Pipelines wegführen, zu einem undurchdringlichen, ja unbeweglichen Fundamentteppich, was ein Ausjäten unmöglich macht. Nach dem Eisberg-Effekt steht auch hier das bescheidene oberirdische Erscheinungsbild in krassem Gegensatz zur unterirdischen Mächtigkeit.

Unnachgiebig sein, sich nicht unterkriegen lassen, stets nach vorwärts zu streben, Größe ist nicht so wichtig – mit all diesen Zuschreibungen kann das Kleine Habichtskraut bedacht werden. Und mit diesen Eigenschaften wurde es zu einem vielfältig verwendeten Heil- und Abwehrmittel der Volksheilkunde und vor allem als Stärkungsmittel für schwächliche Kinder und alte Menschen dringend gebraucht. Mit ca. 750 Arten ist es ja auch in ganz Europa verfügbar.

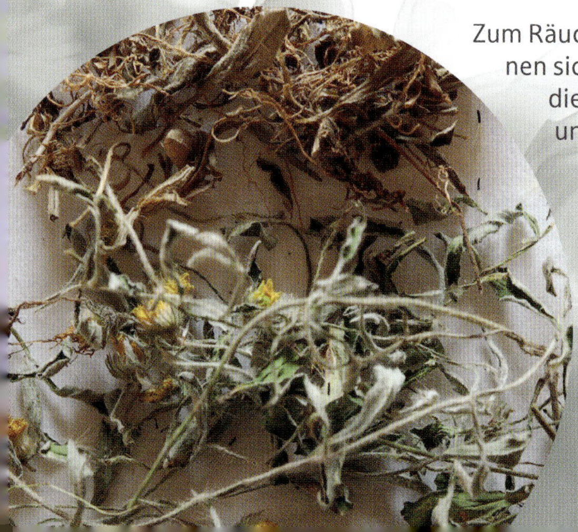

Zum Räuchern eignen sich sowohl die Wurzeln und Blätter als auch die Blüten und Stängel.

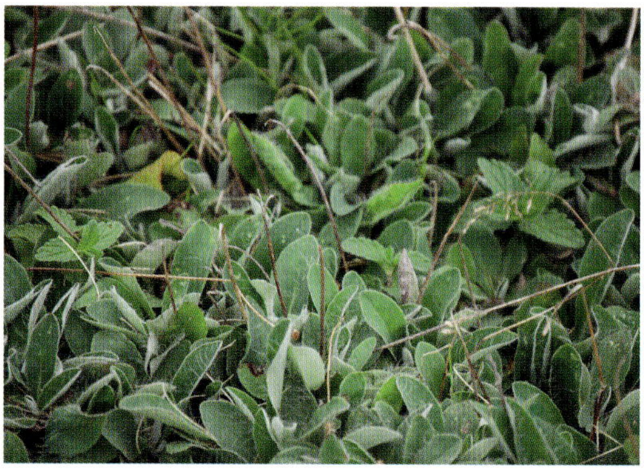

Blätter des Kleinen Habichtkrauts

Rauch

Verwendete Pflanzenteile: Die gesamte Pflanze: Wurzeln, Blätter, Stängel, Blüten.

Beste Sammel- und Erntezeit: Die Pflanze kann das ganze Jahr über gesammelt werden, die Wurzelteile werden gewaschen, gesäubert und dann die ganze Pflanze klein geschnitten und getrocknet.

Wirkung, Wahrnehmung: Abwehrkraut; Verschreikraut. Schutzkraut der Sommersonnenwende, das Überspannungen atmosphärischer Art und auch im persönlichen Umfeld abzuschwächen hilft; Reinigungsrauch der Aura. Abwehrrauch bei unerwarteten Angriffen, bei sozialen Hinterhalten und Mobbing. Der Rauch stärkt die Körper-Geist-Seele-Einheit, hilft bei derart negativen Erfahrungen, sich zu biegen, um nicht zu zerbrechen. Überlagert und neutralisiert der Aura anhaftende Verwünschungen, Verfluchungen, Bannungen. Schützt vor negativen magischen Praktiken und zerstörerischen Wesenheiten.

Durch die große Abwehrkraft wirkt der Rauch reinigend und klärend an persönlichen Sitzplätzen, gewohnten bzw. bevorzugten Aufenthaltsorten innerhalb der Wohnung bzw. des Hauses und befreit sie von negativen Eintragungen. Der klärende Rauch wirkt krampflösend und stimmungsaufhellend, sodass sich die Belastungen und Anforderungen des Alltags relativieren. Im Rauch stehend kann man gut neue Energie schöpfen, Selbstvertrauen zurückgewinnen. Hilft voran zu kommen. Belastende Gedanken verschwinden, man kann wieder zielgerichtet und konzentriert nach vorne blicken.

Man erdet sich gut in dem Habichtskraut-Rauch; besonders verkopfte Ängste lösen sich auf. Man wird insgesamt gelassener den Anforderungen des Alltags gegenüber. Wohlbefinden und tiefste Entspannung können erlebt werden; bis hin zu Traumbildern, die einen in Balance und Harmonie zurückführen. Man kann sich mit sich selbst versöhnen! Ausgeglichene Menschen versetzt der Rauch in eine euphorische Stimmung, man fühlt sich sehr wohl, irgendwie außerhalb von Raum und Zeit und kann, tief entspannt und beruhigt, Träumen und anderen Vorstellungen nachhängen.

Magisches zum Rauch: Mit dem Rauch können Amulette und andere persönliche Schutzgegenstände gestärkt und energetisch aufgeladen werden.

Schwerpunkt, Anwendungen, Rezepte: Um dem Alltag zu entfliehen und sich wegzuträumen, dient folgende Räuchermischung: Habichtskraut, Wermut, Traubenkirsche, Vogelkirsche. Stärkende Räuchermischung, wenn man sich ausgegrenzt fühlt und darunter leidet, Mobbing-Rauch: Habichtskraut, Löwenzahnwurzel, Wacholderbeeren, Wirbeldost. Jeweils mit Harz kombinieren.

Mythologie und magische Praktiken

Der deutsche Name „Habichts-Kraut" weist auf die ausgezeichnete Sehstärke dieses Tieres hin. Und so trug man vielerorts den dicken Teil der Habichtskrautwurzel um den Hals, um die Sehkraft zu erhalten oder wiederzubringen.

Verwendung – gestern und heute

Dioscurid (1. Jahrhundert) hielt es wegen seiner saturnalen Dominanz für kühlend, austrocknend und zusammenziehend und setzte es bei

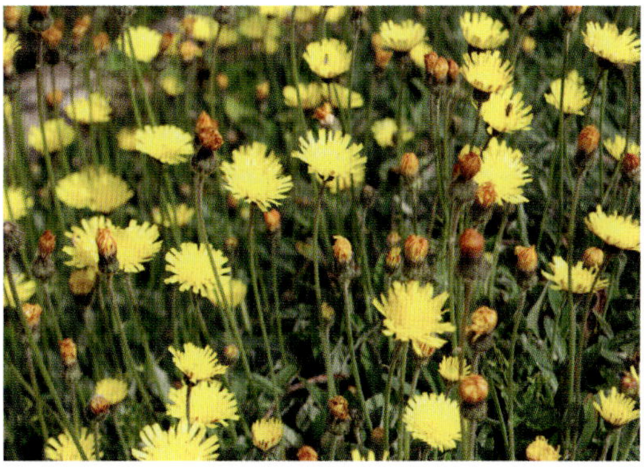

Blüten des Kleinen Habichtkrauts

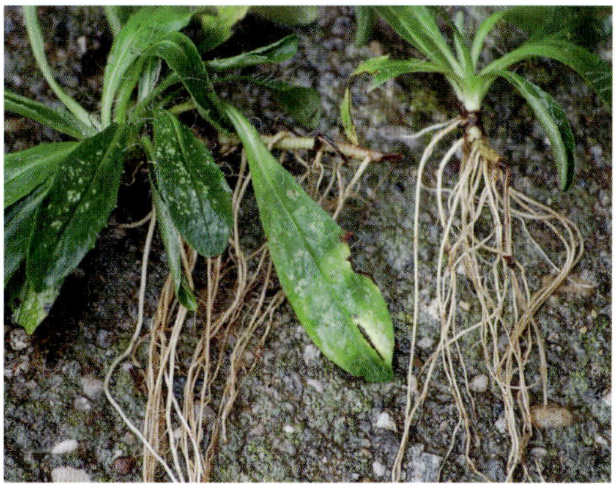

Wurzeln des Kleinen Habichtkrauts

Fieber, Magenproblemen und verschiedenen Entzündungen ein. Leonhart Fuchs (1501–1566) beschreibt die großen Stärken des Krauts so: „Es seind ettlich die so sagen, das diese Habichkreüter also krefftig zu den gebresten der augen seind, dass sie auch klarheyt derselbigen machen, so einer allein die wurtzel an hals gehenckt bey ihm trage".

Nicholas Culpeper (1616–1654), englischer Arzt und Astrologe, hebt eine Anwendung der frischen Blätter hervor: Die Blätter mit wenig Salz verrieben auf Brandwunden gelegt, noch ehe eine Blase aufgetreten ist, fördern die rasche Abheilung der Wunde. Als „legal high" wird das Kraut bezeichnet, wenn man es in Kräuterzigaretten raucht, denn so wirkt es psychoaktiv und führt zu tiefen Entspannungszuständen und Träumen.

Hauhechel

Lat. Name: *Ononis spinosa*
Botanischer Name: Dornige Hauhechel
Pflanzenfamilie: Schmetterlingsblütler

Mitten im Frauenmantelbeet zeigt sich eine schüchterne, rosarote Blüte. Wie schön, denke ich im ersten Jahr, im zweiten Jahr dann zeigt mir der „Weiberkrieg" was er kann: Im harten Erdreich ist seine Wurzel mittlerweile derart verholzt und verzweigt, dass sie sich mit der größten Anstrengung nicht mehr ganz entfernen lässt: Weil die „dicken groben holtzechtigen Wurtzeln unter der Erden durcheinander geflochten und weyt ausgebreytet seind", wusste schon Tabernaemontanus (1522–1590).

Ein derbe Wurzeleroberin also, die über Jahrhunderte in allen Ackerkulturen Europas gefürchtet war: Sie führte zu Ernteeinbußen, brachte die Pflüge zum Stehen, beschädigte die Sensen der Schnitter, „darumb die baurß-leüt disem kraut seer feind seindt", resümierte Leonhart Fuchs (1501–1566).

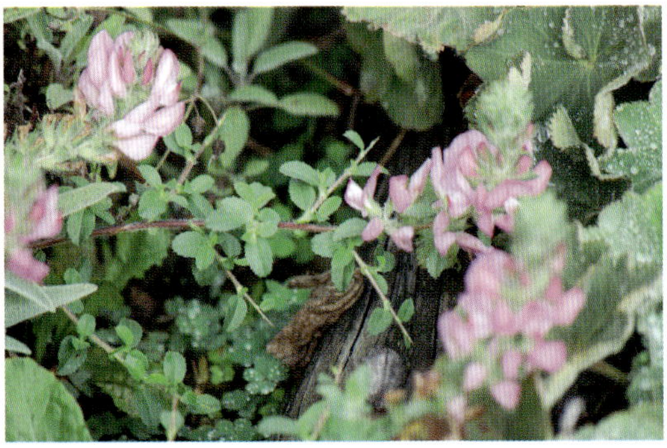

Blühende Hauhechel

Rauch

Verwendete Pflanzenteile: Die gesamte Pflanze: Wurzel, Blätter, Stängel, Blüten, Dornen.

Beste Sammel- und Erntezeit: Die Wurzel kann das ganze Jahr über gegraben werden. Meist wird man lediglich einen Teil der Wurzel herausbringen, die man anschließend wäscht und sofort klein aufschneidet, da sie ab dem Freilegen sofort auszuhärten beginnt! Sobald die Pflanze freigelegt ist, entwickelt sie einen äußert heftigen, bockartigen Geruch.

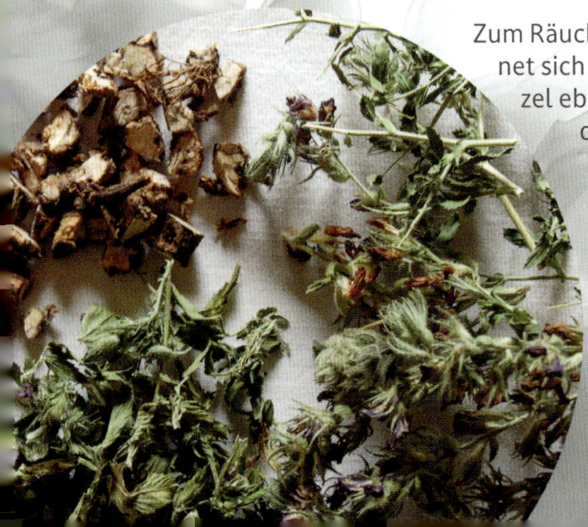

Zum Räuchern eignet sich die Wurzel ebenso wie die ganze oberirdische Pflanze.

Achtung: Bei der Bearbeitung kann die Wurzel plötzliche kurze Emotionsblitze übertragen: Aufregung, Aggression, Verachtung, Herzklopfen, Enge! Während man also die Wurzel wäscht, sollte man sie besprechen (= positiv auf sie einreden), um dadurch ihr sparriges Wesen etwas zu entspannen und zu beruhigen.

Wirkung, Wahrnehmung: Teufelsabwehr und stärkster Abwehrrauch! Wetterkraut. Abwehr- und Reinigungsrauch für Haus und Hof, mit dem negative Eintragungen und belastende kalte Energien mit schmerzhaften Hinterlassenschaften abgewehrt, überlagert und neutralisiert werden können. Als Wetterkraut kann die Hauhechel im Rauch gut Überspannungen in Räumen abbauen und auch in Krankenzimmern die sprichwörtlich „dicke Luft" und Krankheitsdämonen auflösen.

Starke geisterbannende Kraft, die in lange nicht genutzten Räumen oder Häusern oder an Orten, die aktuell bebaut worden sind, eine Klärung der energetischen Balance herbeiführt. Hier sollte nur geräuchert werden, wenn man diese Dissonanz oder Bedrückung auch tatsächlich wahrnimmt. Als Abwehrrauch auch in den Schlafräumen hilfreich: bei anhaltenden Schlafstörungen oder wiederholten Alpträumen.

Magisches zum Rauch: Die Kraft des Hauhechelrauchs vermag immer wiederkehrende Störungen in Räumlichkeiten nachhaltig aufzulösen. Dazu ist eine längere Räucher-Session mit vorher bedachtem Ablauf notwendig. Bei mir hat sich eine wiederholte Durchkreuzung des belasteten Raumes mit dem Rauch, das heißt x-förmiges Durchschreiten des Raumes bis zu den Raumecken, bewährt. Das klärt auch Räume, in denen lange Zeit Krankheit und Siechtum herrschten, die mit großen negativen Abladungen einhergegangen sind.

Schwerpunkt, Anwendungen, Rezepte: Die extremen Kräfte der Pflanze prädestinieren sie für alle Abwehrräucherungen, die man in der dunklen Jahreszeit und in den Raunächten vornimmt. In Stallungen säubert der Hauhechelrauch zusammen mit Wacholder die Luft und verhindert die Eintragung von Krankheiten.

Verwendung – gestern und heute

Leonhart Fuchs (1501–1566) erwähnt eine weitere Verwendung: „Es würt auch Stallkraut von den reüttern geheyssen, darumb das es die pferde stallen macht, so es gesotten würt, unnd den pferden ingegossen." Lonicerus (1528–1586) schreibt über das „Questenkraut": „Dieses Kraut ist der fürnemsten Steinkräuter eins, so den Stein und Harn im Menschen und im Viehe, außtreiben, daher es auch Steinwurtzl genennet wird. Die Alten haben dieses Kraut, in dem es noch jung war, eingebeizt, und zur Speiß über Jahr behalten, wird in der Artzney hoch gepriesen." Von der Hauhechel gibt es heute homöopathische Produkte.

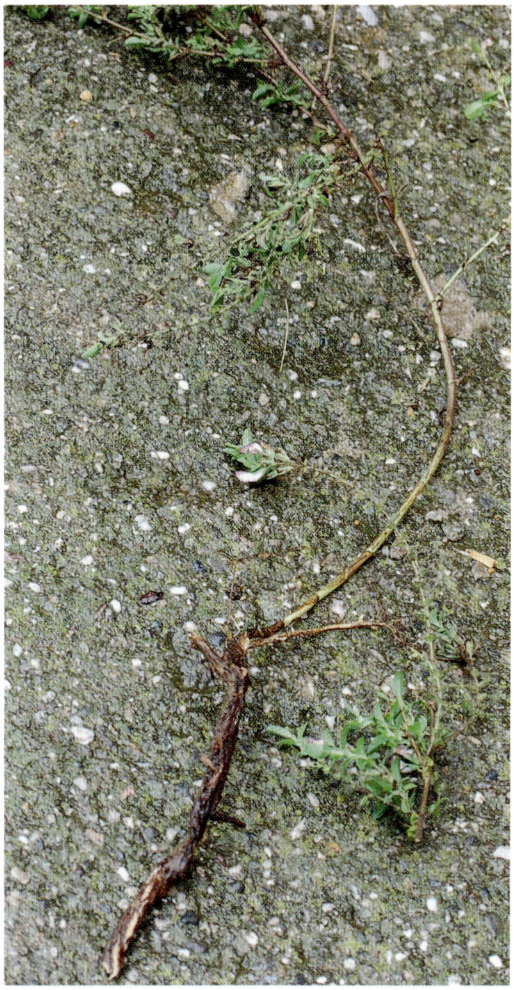

Hauhechel mit Wurzel

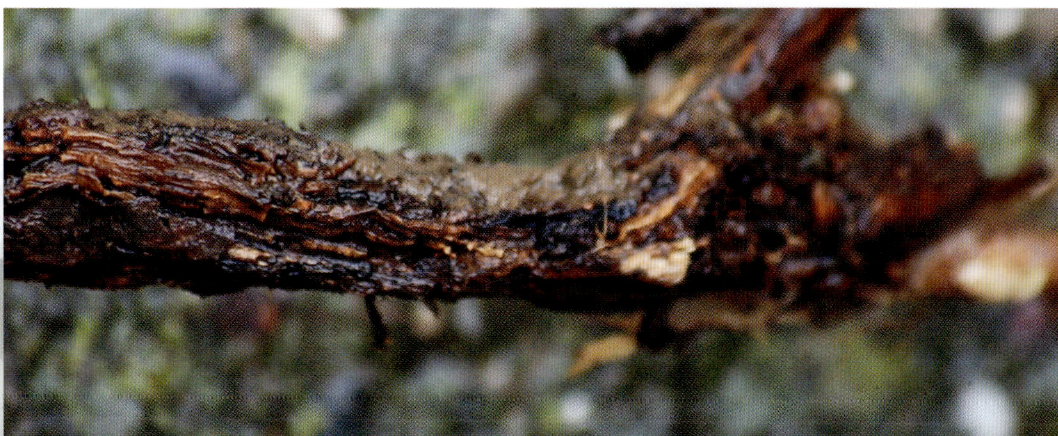

Hauhechelwurzel

Wilde Karde

Lat. Name: *Dipsacus fullonum*
Pflanzenfamilie:
Geißblattgewächse

Die mächtige Karde ist eine pflanzliche Grenzgängerin, ein Wesen, das sich nur unter tausendfacher Absicherung auf diese Welt wagt. Sie ist ein Lehrbeispiel von vorausschauenden Strategien zum Überleben unter erwarteten widrigen Bedingungen. Verdrängung ist ihr Lebensmotto, Abwehr auf allen Ebenen ihre Überlebensstrategie. Von unbändiger Lebenskraft getrieben fährt sie mit höchster Bewaffnung in die Beete: Sie lässt an der Blattunterseite Haken wachsen, die gegen eine wahrscheinliche Griffrichtung angeordnet sind und somit einen möglichen Angreifer in jedem Fall verletzen. An der Blattoberseite fährt sie spitzige Finger-Fänger auf. Sie bedornt jeden Dorn noch einmal weiter, wie in einem Spiegelkabinett, ist in Ewigkeit Abwehr. Sogar die stängelumfassenden Blattachseln sammeln tagelang Regenwasser und werden so zu Fallen für unvorsichtige Insekten. Die Wehrhaftigkeit der Wurzel zeigt sich in ihrer karussellartigen Ausbreitungstendenz –dabei scheint sie zu sagen: „Mich bekommt man nicht so leicht aus dem Boden und wenn, nehme ich alles rund um mich herum mit."

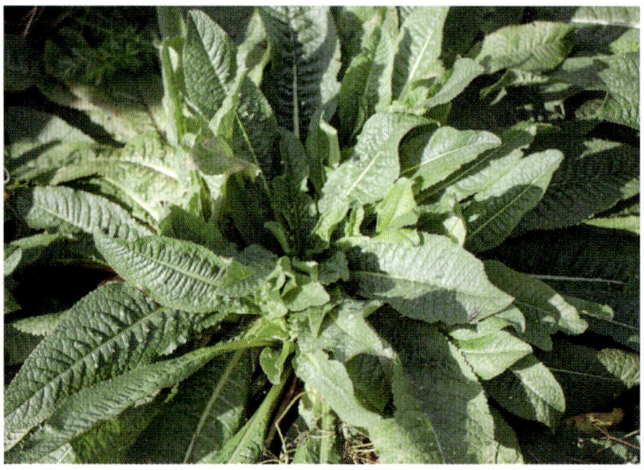

Blätter der Wilden Karde

Rauch

Verwendete Pflanzenteile: Wurzel, Blätter.

Beste Sammel- und Erntezeit: Die Wurzel wird im ersten Vegetationsjahr meist vom Frühjahr bis zum Herbst gegraben. Obwohl die Pflanze in diesem Stadium noch niedrig ist, sollte man sich vor den vielen Abwehrpfeilen gut schützen. Die Wurzel rasch zerkleinern und trocknen; ebenso die Blätter.

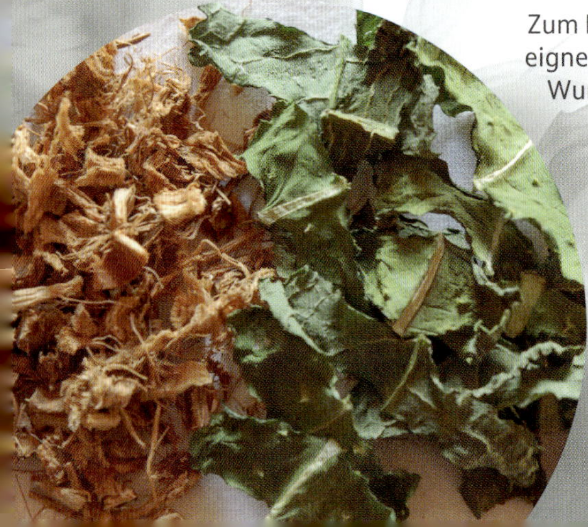

Zum Räuchern eignen sich die Wurzeln und Blätter.

Wirkung, Wahrnehmung: Abwehrrauch in seiner reinsten Form! Reinigungsrauch. Die überschießende Aggression der Pflanze macht sich im Verglühen in einem deutlichen Knistern bemerkbar, was sofort ein Befreiungsgefühl hervorruft. Es ist als hörte und spürte man, wie Ketten gesprengt werden, wie die Beengung kurz und klein geschlagen wird. Mit dem Rauch der Karde wird jeder geistige Übergriff, jede Manipulation bewusst gemacht und – in Resonanz zur eigenen Abwehrbereitschaft – radikal abgewehrt. Hilfreicher Wegbegleiter in geistigen Abnabelungsprozessen.

Die Kardenwurzel ist auch eine Angstwurzel, die mit ihrem Rauch die Angst, entwurzelt zu werden, heilen kann. Geistige und seelische Altlasten können überwunden werden! Reinigt Räume, in denen unangenehme Ereignisse stattgefunden haben und macht sie geistig wieder „begehbar".

Schwerpunkt, Anwendungen, Rezepte: Schmerzende Gelenke über einen Rauch aus Kardenwurzel, Löwenzahnwurzel und Rosmarin kombiniert mit Harz halten, solange es als angenehm empfunden wird.

Verwendung – gestern und heute

Plinius (23–79) überliefert ein ausführliches Rezept: „Schrunden am Gesäß, ebenso Fisteln und Warzen aller Art heilt sie, wenn man die Wurzel so lange in Wein kocht, bis sie die Dicke des Wachses erreicht hat, damit sie als Salbe in die Fisteln gebracht werden kann." Leonhart Fuchs (1501–1566) hat wohl bei Plinius nachgelesen und offensichtlich auch im Kräuterbuch des Hieronymus Bock (1498–1554), das 1539 erschienen war, vier Jahre vor seinem New Kräuterbuch (1543), denn er empfiehlt an erster Stelle: „Die wurtzel in wein gesotten, darnach gestossen biß sie ein pflaster gleich würdt, über die fistel und den zerschrundenen affter gelegt, heylet sie." Weiters schreibt er: „Das wasser so zwischen den blettern gefunden würdt, ist gut den trüben augen, darmit gewaschen." Als Kardentinktur bei bakteriellen Infektionen hat die Wilde Kardenwurzel heutzutage wieder von sich reden gemacht.

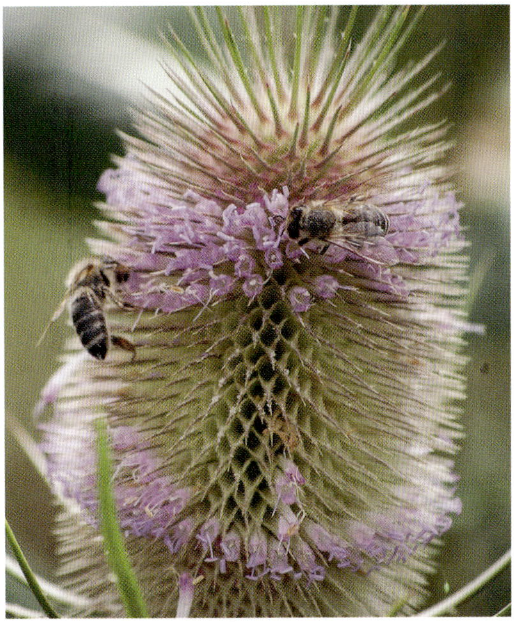

Blüte der Wilden Karde

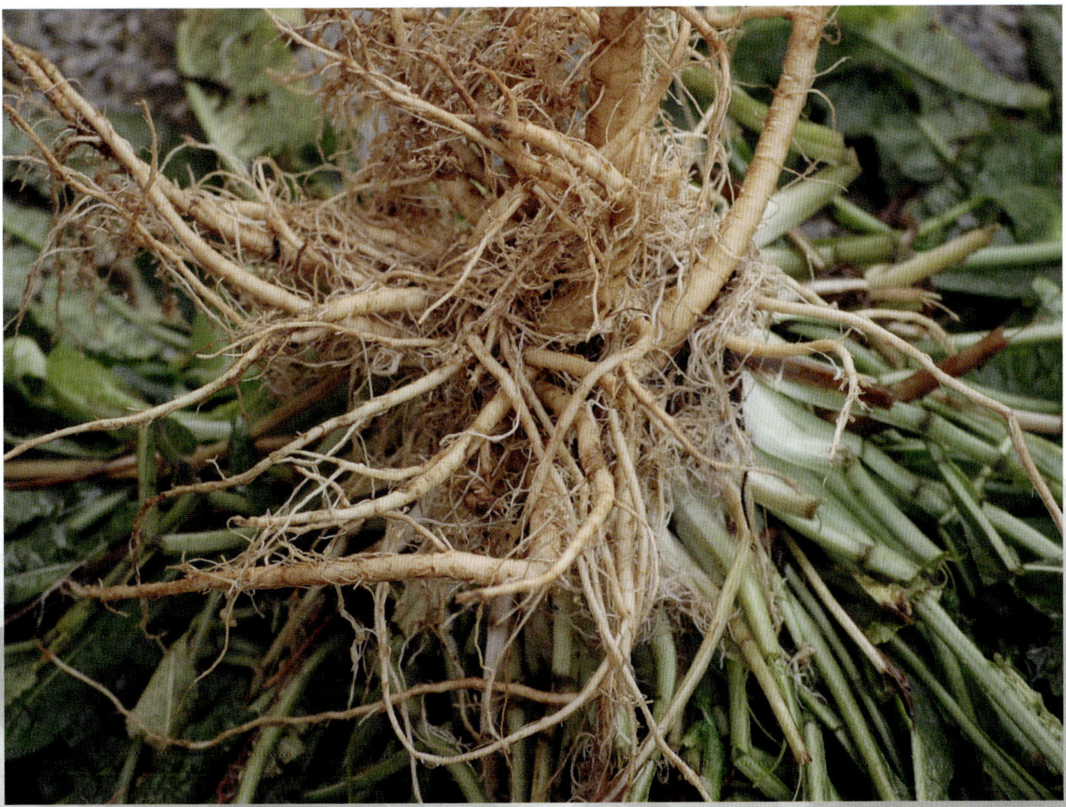

Kardenwurzel

Königskerze

Lat. Name: *Verbascum* sp.
Botanischer Name: Großblütige Königskerze (*V. densiflorum),* Gewöhnliche Königskerze *(V. phlomoides)*
Pflanzenfamilie: Braunwurzgewächse

Wenn im Hochsommer die Königskerzen meine Gartenbühne betreten, bin ich immer wieder fasziniert von ihrer Wuchskraft. Im tiefsten Vertrauen auf das Wohlwollen der Elemente schießen sie empor, werden die Stängel verstärkt, wird das Blattwerk optimiert, um gerade und für sich alleine stehen zu können. Dann aber nimmt sich der Himmelsbrand, wie man die Königskerze früher nannte, Zeit zum Blühen und öffnet eine Blütensonne nach der anderen. Über Wochen geht das so – bis sie ganz oben angekommen ist und in schwindelnder Höhe alle anderen Pflanzen überragt. Was diesem krönenden Abschluss vorangeht sind zwei bis drei Jahre Vorbereitungsarbeit, in denen die kleine Königskerzenpflanze ihren Standplatz austestet, sich nach und nach eine sichere Verankerung im Boden aufbaut und versucht, sich ein tragfähiges Fundament zu erschließen. „Wer hoch bauen will, muss tief graben" – das wussten schon die Dombaumeister des späten Mittelalters. Die Königskerze nimmt sich also genügend Zeit, um ihr Werk zu beginnen und es blühend zu vollenden.

Ob der Götterbote Hermes, unter anderem Schutzgott der Magie, tatsächlich dem Odysseus einen Königskerzenstängel zur Abwehr der Zaubermacht und der Zaubersprüche der Kirke gegeben hat, muss wohl offenbleiben. Es ist jedenfalls ein schönes Bild, das die ganze Hochachtung zeigt, die diesem imposanten Gewächs entgegengebracht wurde.

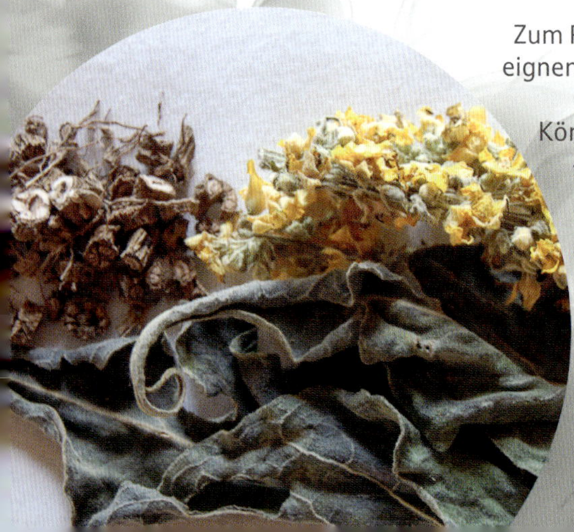

Zum Räuchern eignen sich alle Teile der Königskerze – von der Wurzel bis zur Blüte.

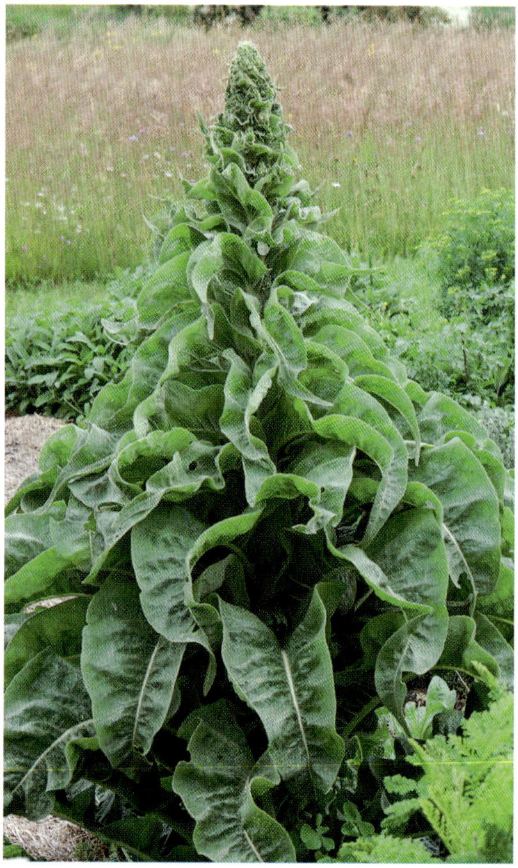

Blätter der Königskerze

Ein weiterer Hinweis auf die große abwehrzauberische Kraft der Königskerze findet sich auch im Pseudo Apuleius, einem frühen Kräuterbuch aus dem 4. Jahrhundert: Nichts erschrecke den Träger eines Königskerzenstängels, nichts Böses werde ihm begegnen.

In vielen Gegenden des Alpenraumes bildet ein Königskerzenstängel auch heute die Mitte der Kräuterbuschn, die zu Mariä Himmelfahrt in der Kirche gesegnet werden. Ihre wetterwenderische Kraft soll Haus und Hof vor Blitzschlag schützen – reißt man allerdings eine Königskerze grundlos ab und nimmt diese mit nach Hause, dann wird dort der Blitz einschlagen.

Rauch

Verwendete Pflanzenteile: Alle Teile der Königskerze können verräuchert werden: Wurzeln, Blätter, Blüten.

Beste Sammel- und Erntezeit: Die Blätter und die wohlriechende Wurzel sollte man von einer Pflanze ernten, die sich in ihrem ersten Vegetationsjahr befindet, das heißt, noch ehe die Pflanze zur Blüte nach oben schießt. Von einer weiteren Königskerze können dann die Blüten geerntet und rasch getrocknet werden, damit sie nicht verbraunen.

Wirkung, Wahrnehmung: Abwehr- und Schutzrauch. Wichtiges altes Wetterkraut. Zwei polare Kräfte – Sonne und Saturn – sind in der Königskerze miteinander verbunden. Und so symbolisiert der Wurzelrauch gleichzeitig den obersten goldenen Blütenkranz, der direkt in den Himmel zeigt.

Der Sonnenrauch vom saturnalen Zeitpfahl lehrt uns die komplexe gedankliche Gleichzeitigkeit von Vergangenheit, Gegenwart und Zukunft zu beachten und stärkt dadurch unsere Lebenskraft! Er wirkt innerlich aufrichtend und stärkt das Selbst und das Bewusste.

Der Abwehrrauch aus Wurzel und Blüten umhüllt einen mit einem spürbaren Schutzschild, das Bedrohungen von außen ausgleicht und Verwünschungen, Flüche, Nadelungen oder Bannsprüche überlagert und so neutralisiert. Negative Energien werden abgebaut und eigene dunkle Gedanken wieder heilsam durchlichtet. Der Wurzelrauch spiegelt das Ich! Saturn, der große Begrenzer der Zeit, lehrt uns Einfachheit, Geduld und Demut und führt uns zu innerer Ruhe. Vielleicht gelingt es mit diesem Rauch, Schuldmuster zu durchbrechen, sie aufzulösen und so zu innerem Frieden zu finden.

Als Wetterrauch hilft der Rauch der Königskerze Spannungen in der Raumatmosphäre abzubauen, Elektrosmog zu neutralisieren und so das Raumklima zu verbessern. Belastende atmosphärische Überbleibsel nach Streit und anderen Ärgernissen werden klärend überlagert.

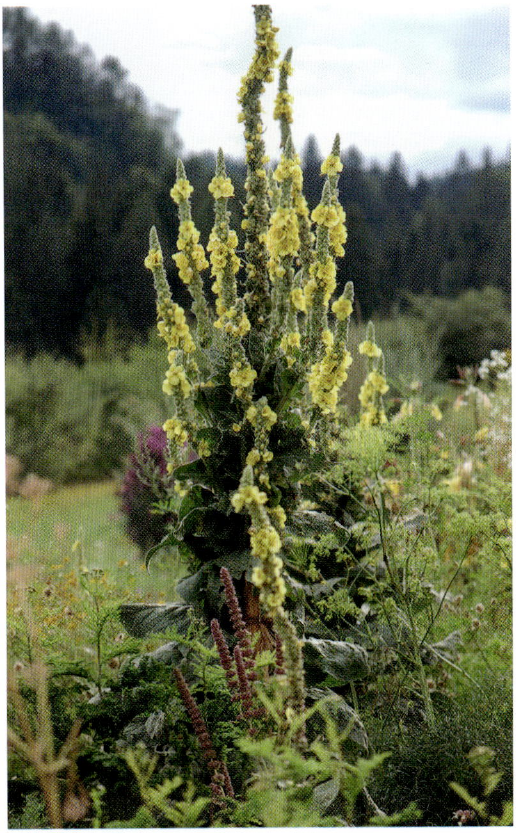

Blühende Königskerze

Der Sonnenrauch der Königskerze stärkt die lebensbejahende Seite in uns, lässt uns den Moment genießen und nicht an morgen denken. Schutz, Erdung, neue Hoffnung und geistige Fruchtbarkeit können sich durch den Rauch der Königskerze übertragen. Die große Sonnenkraft holt einen aus jeder depressiven Verstimmung, lässt Katastrophentage versöhnlich ausgehen.

Magisches zum Rauch: Abt Antonius II. (1718–1751) von Stift Admont hinterließ folgendes Räucherrezept gegen Zauberei, dessen Anfang hier wiedergegeben wird: „Rauch wider alle zaubery, Verschreyen von menschen und viech. Rauche Palm Käzl von feldern die an dem wasser wachsen, drei geweichte Kränzl von dem Hochw. guet in fronleichnams dägen (kleine Kränze, die am Fronleichnamstag mit dem Allerheiligsten mitgetragen werden), humel Kraut (Königskerze)…“

Schwerpunkt, Anwendungen, Rezepte: Königskerzen-Räucherungen stärken uns das Rückgrat, lassen uns wieder Haltung annehmen und die Dinge sonnendurchflutet und positiv sehen. Dazu setzt man sich entspannt auf einen Stuhl und stellt die Räucherschale hinter dem Stuhl auf den Boden, so dass der Rauch das Rückgrat entlang aufsteigen kann. Schon nach kurzer Zeit streckt man sich und räkelt sich angenehm hoch. Königskerze räuchert man bei Jugendlichen in schwierigen Entwicklungsphasen zusammen mit Beifuß und Lavendel. Zum Spannungsabbau bei Gewitter oder in der Familie oder einfach als entspannende Abendräucherung hilft eine Mischung aus Königskerze, Johanniskraut, Kunigundenkraut, Rainfarn. Jeweils mit Harz kombinieren.

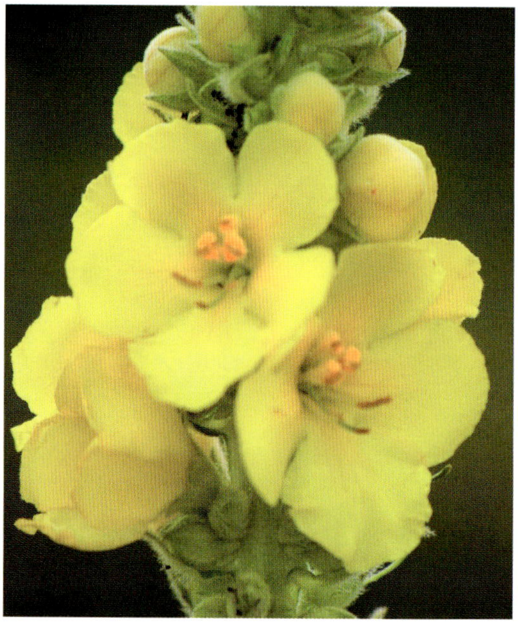

Blüte der Königskerze

Mythologie und magische Praktiken

Die Wurzel wird an besonderen Wendetagen im Jahr (Sommersonnenwende, Mariä Himmelfahrt, Allerheiligen) gegraben und soll als Amulett-Pflanze gegen Krankheiten schützen und vor Ansteckung bewahren.

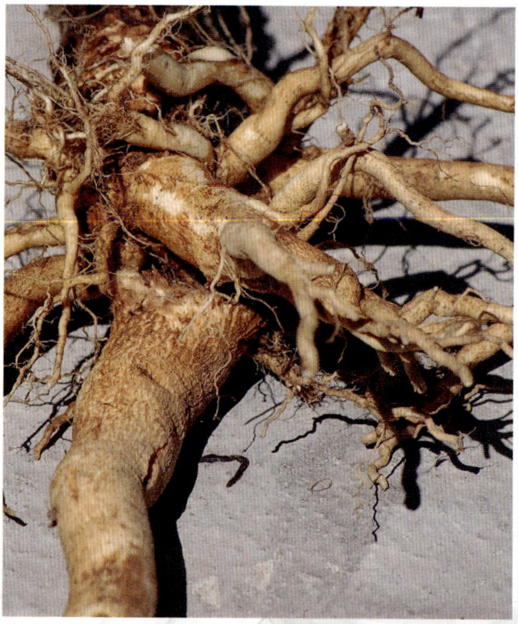

Wurzel der Königskerze

Verwendung – gestern und heute

Hildegard von Bingen (1098–1179) sieht die besondere geistig-seelische Heilkraft und empfiehlt die „Wullena“ auch solchen Menschen, die ein „schwaches und trauriges Herz“ haben. 400 Jahre später stellt Lonicerus (1528–1586) folgende Empfehlung an die erste Stelle seiner Abhandlung: „Das gemeine Wullkraut mit andern Kräutern bey Fleisch oder besonder in Gemüß gekocht, und gessen, benimbt alle Kranckheiten deß Herzens.“ Wiederum 300 Jahre später sieht Sebastian Kneipp (1821–1897) dies wohl ähnlich, wenn er Königskerze als herzstärkendes Mittel empfiehlt und dazu ihre Blätter in Fleischbrühe auskochen lässt. Hoch geschätzt ist weiterhin der schleimlösende und reizmildernde Königskerzen-Blütentee.

Meisterwurz

Lat. Name: *Peucedanum ostruthium*
Pflanzenfamilie: Doldenblütler

Heil aller Schäden, Kaiserwurz, Magisterwurz, Wurzel aller Wurzeln – so und ähnlich tönt es über Jahrhunderte aus allen Kräuterbüchern. Die Meisterwurz, ureuropäisch, alpenbezogen steht im Mittelpunkt der traditionellen europäischen Medizin: Sie wird im 11. Jahrhundert erstmals als Universalmittel gegen alle Leberschäden erwähnt und gilt bis Anfang des 20. Jahrhunderts als Allheilmittel gegen verschiedenste Giftwirkungen.

Die Meisterwurz wächst eher im Verborgenen, in geschützten, feuchten Bereichen, im schattigen Unterholz von Stauden. In Südtirol ist sie treue Begleiterin der Wale, jener Wasserrinnen, die das Wasser von den Bergen in die Anbauflächen leiten.

Die unbändige Lebenskraft dieser Wurzel lernte ich noch von einer ganz anderen Seite kennen: Im Herbst muss die Wurzelernte immer schnell gehen. Einmal vergaß ich so eine ausgegrabene Meisterwurz mit fein säuberlich frei geklopften Wurzeln neben dem Beet. Dann schneite es und die ganze Kraft des Winters fuhr über dieses ungeschützte heimatlose Wesen. Beim Frühjahrsputz wunderte ich mich über den unkenntlichen Erdhocker neben dem Beet. Erst als der Erdhocker genau von der Mitte aus zu treiben begann, erinnerte ich mich wieder an sie! Freundlicherweise hat sie meine tausendfachen Entschuldigungen angenommen, ließ sich wieder einsetzen und wohnt noch heute, absonnig unterm Dirndlstrauch.

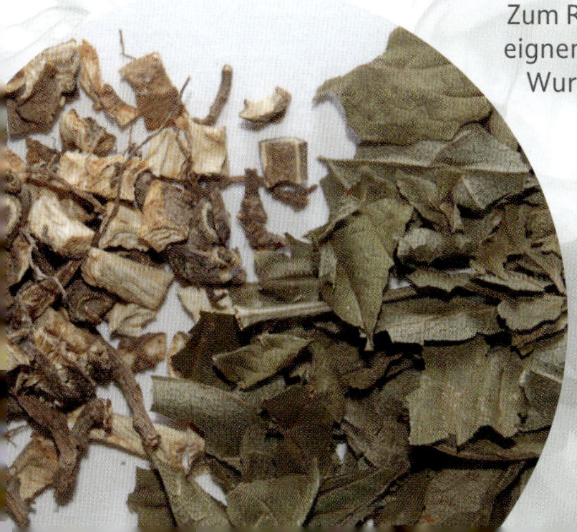

Zum Räuchern eignen sich die Wurzeln und Blätter.

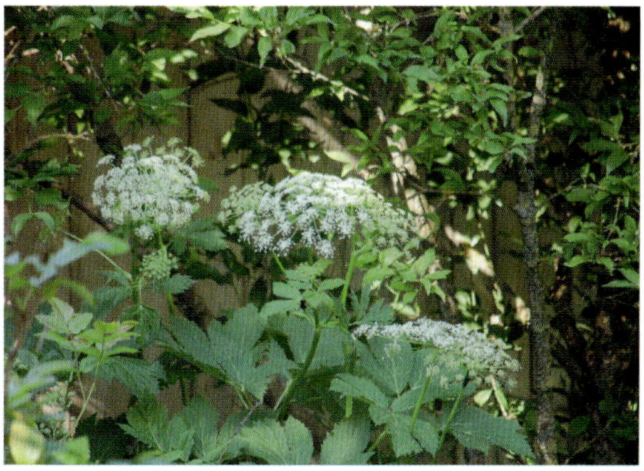

Blühende Meisterwurz

Rauch

Verwendete Pflanzenteile: Wurzeln und Blätter.

Beste Sammel- und Erntezeit: Die Wurzel wird im Herbst gegraben, gereinigt und fein geschnitten. Achtung: Da die Blätter Furanocumarine enthalten, die bei empfindlichen Menschen Verbrennungen auf der Haut auslösen können, sollte man sich beim Kontakt mit der Pflanze entsprechend schützen. Die Brandblasen treten, wie bei der Weinraute, erst einige Tage nach dem Kontakt auf und sind anfangs äußerst schmerzhaft. Meist weiß man gar nicht, woher die Verbrennungen stammen könnten.

Wirkung, Wahrnehmung: Abwehrkraut. Großer Schutzrauch! Sonnwendkraut und Lichtbringerin. Als Abwehrrauch wird die Wurzel in den Raunächten verwendet, wenn es darum geht befürchtete Bedrohungen aus dem Dunklen abzuwehren, dämonisches Treiben zu unterbinden und gleichzeitig Menschen, Tiere, Haus und Hof zu schützen. Abwehrrauch gegen geistiges Gift und dessen zwischenmenschliche Auswirkungen. Schutzrauch, der bei mangelnder innerer Sicherheit das Selbstbewusstsein steigert und die psychische Widerstandskraft stärkt. So können sich die belastenden Phasen der Übergänge im Leben verkürzen. Man wird schneller bereit, alten Ballast abzuwerfen und wieder nach vorne zu blicken.

Eine Meisterwurz-Räucherung erlebt man oft als befreiend, als würde man durch eine Tür ins Freie treten. Die Meisterwurz ist eine Beschützerin in dunklen Zeiten – ob innerlich oder im Jahreslauf. Mit ihrem wohltuenden Rauch hilft diese Lichtbringerin unsere dunklen Ängste zu besiegen, bringt Hoffnung und die rechte Energie in Stall und Haus.

Magisches zum Rauch: Meisterwurz war als „Hexenpulver" Bestandteil von Abwehrräucherungen, wenn schwarzmagische Übergriffe befürchtet wurden und in der Walpurgisnacht (30. April).

Schwerpunkt, Anwendungen, Rezepte: Für eine angstlösende und aufbauende Räuchermischung zu den Sonnenwenden mischt man zur Meisterwurz noch Klettenwurzel, Johanniskraut und Wacholderbeeren. Eine hilfreiche Räuchermischung, die Phasen tiefster Verzweiflung abmildern kann, wird aus Engelwurz, Meisterwurz und Birke kombiniert mit Harz gemischt. Hier verbinden sich große Lichtkräfte zu einem Appell an das Unterbewusste, das gegebene Leben dankbar anzunehmen und wertzuschätzen.

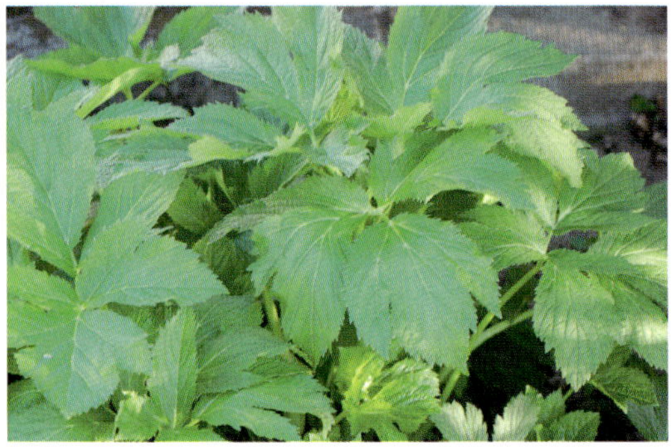
Blätter der Meisterwurz

Mythologie und magische Praktiken

Paracelsus (1493–1541) hält sie für ein großes Pestprophylaktikum und trug selbst stets eine Meisterwurz-Wurzel als Amulett gegen Schlaganfall und Pest um den Hals. Zahlreiche magische Handlungen wurden mit der Meisterwurz durchgeführt, vorwiegend zur Abwehr von bösen Geistern und ihren schädlichen Streichen und Verwünschungen. In einem Stallzauber wurde die Wurzel an bestimmten Tagen gegraben und an den Querbalken gehängt, um die Pferde ruhig zu halten, wenn sie mit ihren großen Augen einen Dämon sehen würden.

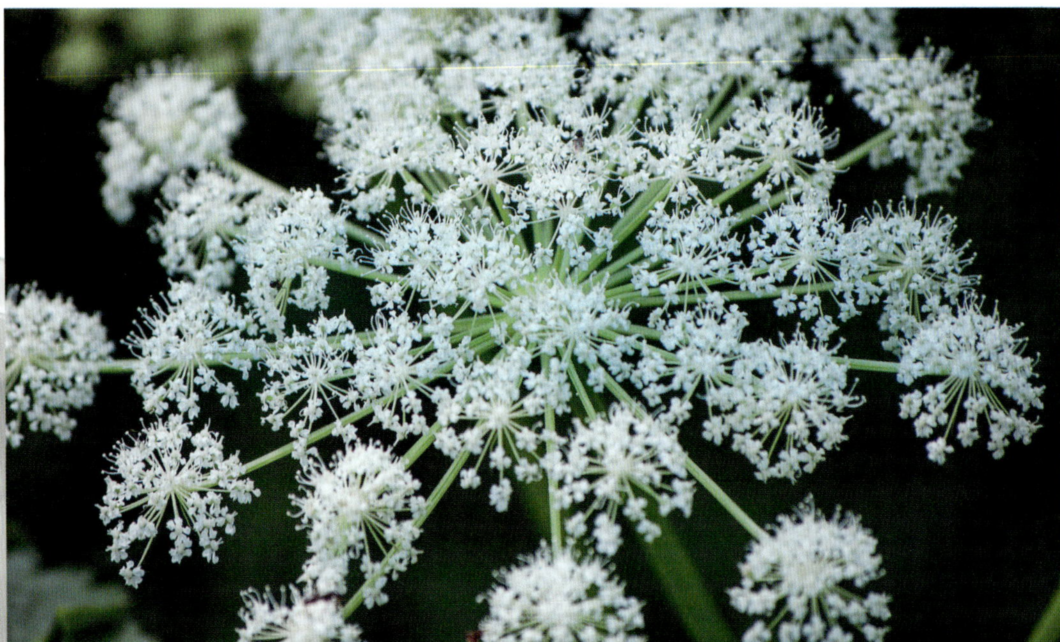
Blüte der Meisterwurz

Gegen langwieriges Husten wurde eine bei zunehmendem Mond gegrabene Meisterwurz auf den Rücken des Leidenden gebunden und bei Besserung in den Fluss geworfen.

Verwendung – gestern und heute

Paracelsus (1493–1541) weist auf die stark psychische Heilkraft der Meisterwurz hin: „Peucedanum ist die beste Arznei zur Erhaltung des Lebensgeistes im Kopfe, auch gegen Mania, Phrenesis, Melancholia, Phantasia, Ebrietas (Wahnsinn) und gegen die Krankheit des heiligen Veit." Leonhart Fuchs (1501–1566) meint: „Die wurtzel, der samen, kraut unnd safft der Meisterwurtz seind treffenlich nütz und gut wider allerley gifft. Sollen in sonderheyt zu der zeit der Pestilentz wider den vergifften bösen lufft gebraucht werden."

Über die potenzsteigernde Qualität der Meisterwurz berichten Matthiolus (1501–1578): „Hilfft dem unvermügigen kalten mann widerumb auff den gaul!", und etwas feiner auch Tabernaemontanus (1522–1590): „für ungeschickte Männer." Überrascht von ihrem Geschmack schreibt Hieronymus Bock (1498–1554): „Die Meisterwurtz hat mich schier verderbt, also übel brant mich der zähe gal safft auff der zungen. Der grün pfeffer ist nit so scharpff, als die grün Meisterwurtz." Und zur äußeren Wirkung schreibt er: „Meisterwurtz übertrifft Angelicam und Liebstöckel mit der hitz und außtreibenden krafft, seind sonst einander gleich, wunden und gifftige schäden zu heilen, eüßerlich auffgelegt, den safft in die wunden gelassen, oder mit dem gebranten wasser gereiniget."

Die weiße feingliedrige Wurzel trägt eine Schärfe in sich, die von einer einzigartigen Bitterstoff-Gerbstoff-Kombination herrührt und das Immunsystem anzuregen und gegen Infektionskrankheiten zu schützen vermag. Ob Tee oder Wurzel-Elixier – immer hilft die Imperatoria die Abwehrkraft zu stärken und Altersbeschwerden zu lindern.

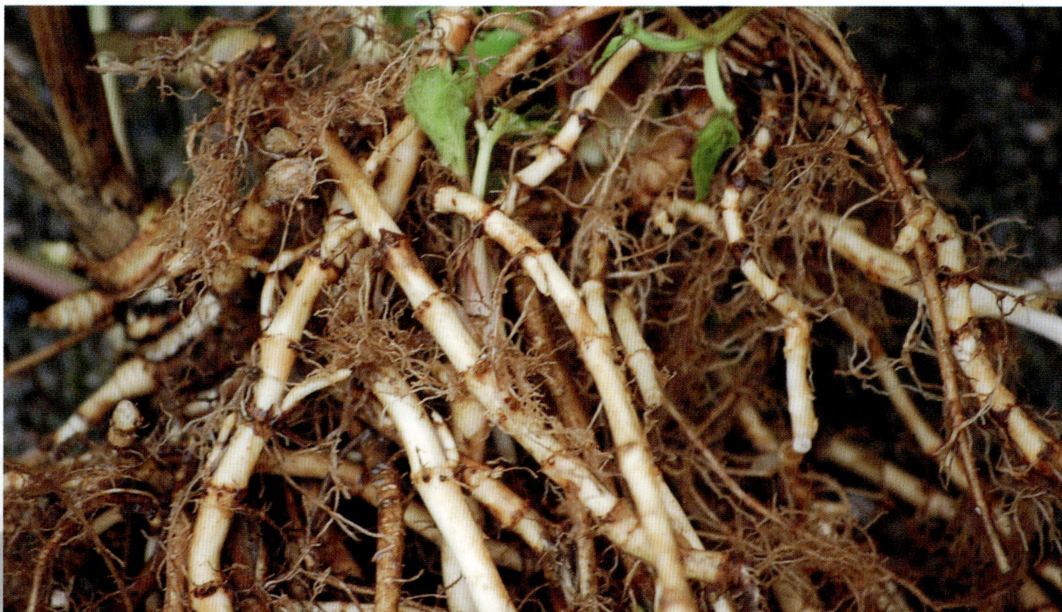

Wurzel der Meisterwurz

Liebstöckel

Lat. Name: *Levisticum officinale*
Botanischer Name: Garten-Liebstöckel
Pflanzenfamilie: Doldenblütler

Seit fast zwei Jahrzehnten steht mein Liebstöckel am Garteneingang gleich rechts und ist immer noch voller Triebkraft. Andere Pflanzen kamen und gingen, er freut sich des Lebens und begrüßt mich bei jedem Gartengang! Heilsam und nährend von der Wurzel über die hohlen Stängel bis zu den Blättern und den Samen – ein wahrer Menschenfreund und großer Pflanzenschutzgeist wohnt dem Liebstöckel inne.

Das in Wasser eingeweichte Liebstöckelkraut verleiht ihm magisch reinigende Kräfte, was dem Liebstöckel den Beinamen „Badkraut" einbrachte und dazu führte, dass in alten Zeiten Mütter ihren Töchtern von Jugend an Liebstöckel ins Badewasser gaben, damit diese später einmal die Gunst eines Mannes erlangen könnten. Soweit die aphrodisische Seite des Liebstöckels, auch Luststock genannt. Sogar Walahfrid Strabo (808–849) schwärmt im Jahr 827 in seinem Gartengedicht „Hortulus" von ihm: „Liebstöckel, kräftiges Kraut, dich zu nennen im duftenden Dickicht / heißt mich die Liebe, mit der ich im Gärtchen alles umfasse".

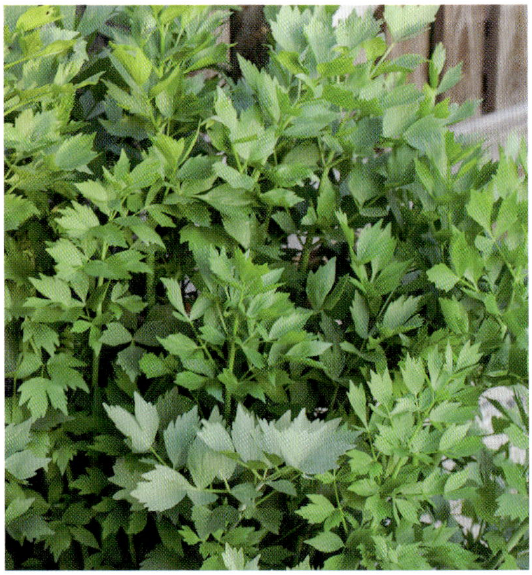

Liebstöckelblätter

Rauch

Verwendete Pflanzenteile: Wurzel, Blätter, Stängel, Blüten, Samen.

Beste Sammel- und Erntezeit: Die Wurzel wird im Herbst kurz vor Neumond besonders schonend gegraben, da die Pflanze sehr empfindlich auf jegliche Art von Wurzeleinwirkung reagiert. Soll die Pflanze im nächsten Jahre weiterwachsen, nur wenig Wurzel entnehmen und mit den Händen, nicht mit der Schaufel, die Wurzel wieder mit Erde bedecken. Blätter, Stängel, Blüten und Samen werden im Laufe des Jahres gepflückt, so wie sie erscheinen.

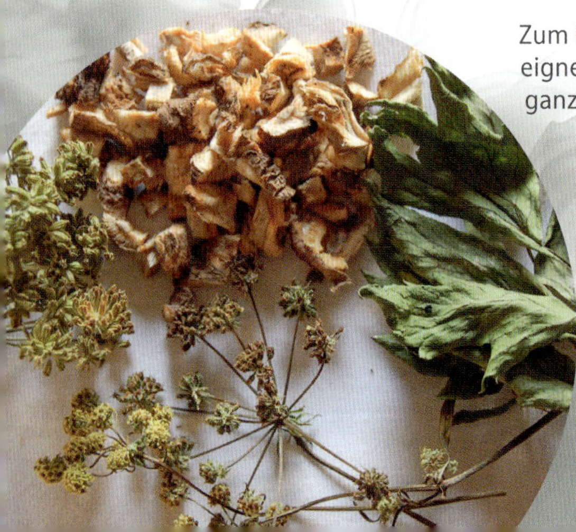

Zum Räuchern eignet sich die ganze Pflanze inklusive der Wurzel.

Wirkung, Wahrnehmung: Schutzrauch und Segensrauch. Große weißmagische Kraft. Pflanze des geistigen Umschwungs! Der Rauch legt sich schützend über die Raumluft und hinterlässt ein angenehmes Raumklima. Alle negativen Eintragungen werden überlagert, geklärt und aufgelöst.

Durch den Rauch einer stark weißmagischen Pflanze werden Nachsicht, Geduld und Segen vermittelt. Die Stimmung wird ausgeglichen und undurchdringlich für negative Botschaften. Niedergeschlagenheit und jede düstere Stimmung wird durchlichtet. Erdende, sinngebende und beruhigende Themen und Gedanken werden möglich – und Schweres wird leicht! Liebstöckel-Räucherungen eignen sich besonders für Balance-,

Ausgleichs-, Harmonie- und Friedens-Themen. Der Rauch der Wurzeln und der erblühten Dolde passt gut zu einem liebevollen Beginn von Meditationen, Gebetsstunden, für Anrufungen. Für Segensräucherungen und Meditationen, die dazu beitragen sollen, Verständnis und Nachsicht in uns und unserer Lebensumwelt wachsen zu lassen.

Magisches zum Rauch: Mit dem Liebstöckelrauch wurden teils bizarre Rituale für bindezauberischen Erfolg in der Liebe durchgeführt.

Schwerpunkt, Anwendungen, Rezepte: Räuchermischung zur besseren Einstimmung in Gruppen oder Familien: Liebstöckelwurzel, Eibischwurzel, Beinwellwurzel und Harz.

Mythologie und magische Praktiken

Am Johannistag, dem 24. Juni, wurde Liebstöckelkraut in jeden Trank gegeben, damit die dunklen Geister, Dämonen und neidvollen Wesenheiten Mensch und Tier in der Zeit der Sommersonnenwende sowie für den Rest des Jahres nichts anhaben konnten.

Verwendung – gestern und heute

Bereits für Plinius (23–79) ist der Liebstöckel ein alter Hut: „Einige nennen es auch Heilwurz, ist dem Magen von Nutzen, ebenso bei Krämpfen und Blähungen.“ Liebstöckel gehörte auch in jeden karolingischen Königsgarten: Um das Jahr 800 verordnete Kaiser Karl der Große (747–814) im „Capitulare de villis vel curtis imperii“ den Anbau von 73 Pflanzen, an 33. Stelle „levisticum“.

Hildegard von Bingen (1098–1179) empfiehlt gegen Halsschmerzen und geschwollene Mandeln heiße Milch durch hohle Liebstöckel-Stängel zu schlürfen, was vor allem bei Kindern rasch zu einer Besserung der Beschwerden führte. Die Kräuterväter des frühen 16. Jahrhunderts stellen die äußere Ähnlichkeit des Liebestöckels mit der Engelwurz fest und Hieronymus Bock (1498–1554) meint: „Lybstöckel die wurtzel gedörrt und gepulvert, ist ein edle wurtz zu der speiß, dient wol dem kalten magen, hilfft da-

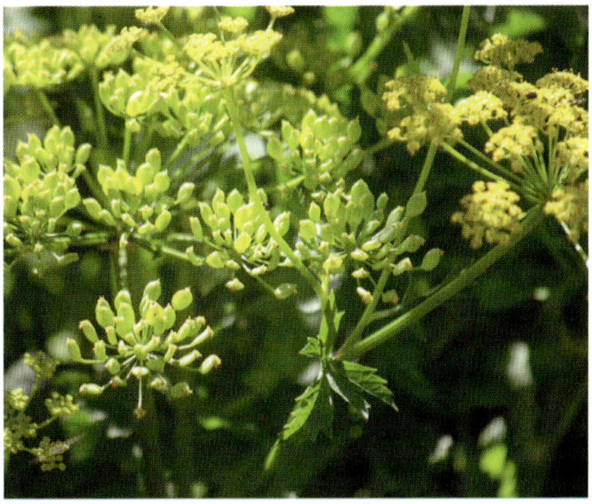

Blühender Liebstöckel

wen, und verzert alle uberflüßige feüchtigkeit, unnd dient zu allen presten, wie von Angelica beschriben ist.“ Auch Lonicerus (1528–1586) pflichtet bei: „.. .hat die Krafft wie Angelica.“ Er ergänzt: „Die Wurtzel samt dem Saamen in Wein gesotten, getruncken, treibt die Geelsucht und schwarze Melancholey auß dem Leib.“

Liebstöckel ist das klassische Gewürzkraut, das jeder Suppe ihren besonderen Geschmack verleiht. Früher hat man aus einem Wurzel-Öl-Auszug mit Bienenwachs eine Salbe gerührt und diese äußerlich bei Halsschmerzen aufgetragen.

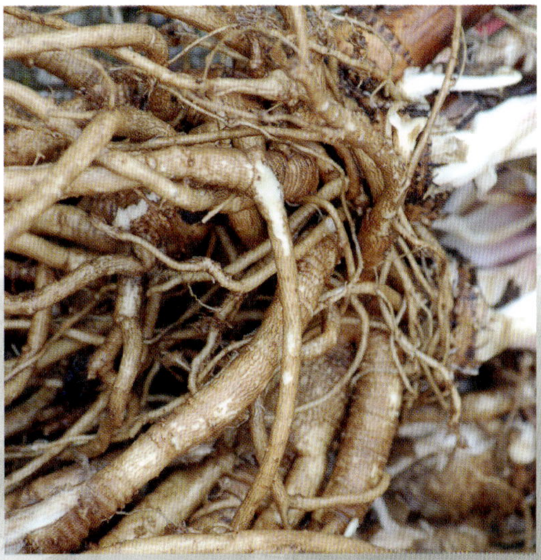

Liebstöckelwurzel

Löwenzahn

Lat. Name: *Taraxacum officinale*
Pflanzenfamilie: Korbblütler

Vom Frühjahr bis in den Spätherbst bietet sich der Löwenzahn als Gemüse und Heilpflanze an: Als Lichtgestalt des Frühlings leuchtet er kraftvoll aus allen Ecken, überflutet Wiesen und Felder mit seiner Lebenskraft und lädt uns zu häufiger Verwendung ein. Als frischer Salat, in vielen gekochten Speisen, in überraschenden Nachspeisen und natürlich in Gelees und Sirupen für den Winter.

Wenn es dann mehr als zwölf Stunden lang hell ist, hört er mit dem Blühen auf. Gegen Ende des Sommers, wenn man wieder etwas nachlässiger im Gemüsegarten werden kann, sollte man den Löwenzahn in die abgeernteten Beete einladen: Ende Oktober können so die schönsten Wurzeln geerntet werden. Diese haben zudem die höchste Konzentration an Inulin und Bitterstoffen. Sie können getrocknet und vermahlen den ganzen Winter über unser Wohlbefinden unterstützen.

Heinz Erhardt (1909–1979), der bekannte deutsche Schauspieler, Komponist und Kabarettist dichtete: „Löwenzahn ist schon seit jeher als höchst kriegerisch verschrien, denn er lässt bei gutem Winde Fallschirmtruppen feindwärts ziehen – und ich sitz auf der Veranda und verzehre meine Suppe und entdecke in derselben zwei Versprengte dieser Truppe“.

Rauch

Verwendete Pflanzenteile: Wurzeln, Blüten oder nur die abgeblühten Blütenböden.

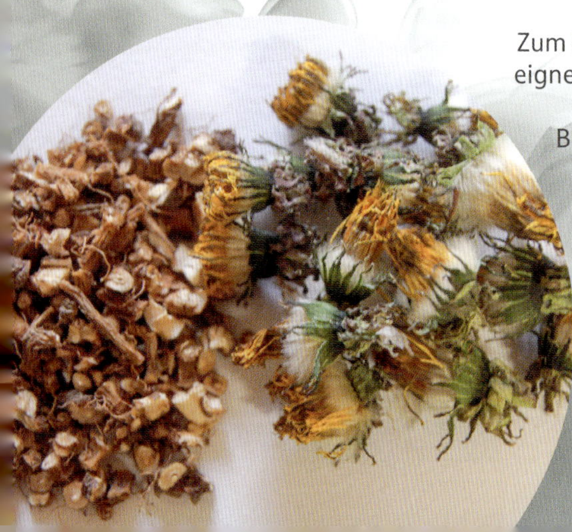

Zum Räuchern eignen sich die Wurzeln, Blüten und Blütenböden.

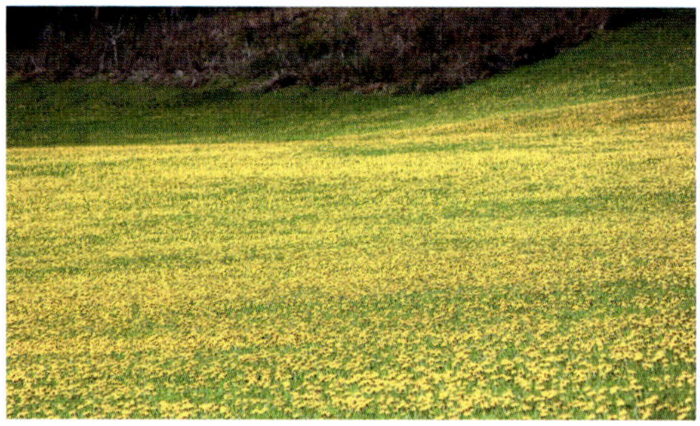

Löwenzahnwiese

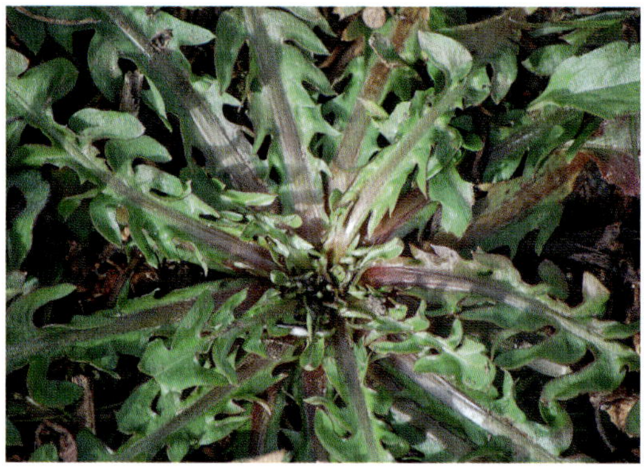

Löwenzahnblätter

Beste Sammel- und Erntezeit: Die Blüten im April bis Mai, die Wurzeln können ganzjährig, am ergiebigsten jedoch im Herbst geerntet werden. Da sie abfärben sollte mit Handschuhen gearbeitet werden. Die Wurzeln waschen, klein schneiden und trocknen.

Wirkung, Wahrnehmung: Reinigungsrauch. Abwehrkraft. Glücksrauch! Pflanze des geistigen Umschwungs, mit der Kraft der Sonne wird Erstarrtes und Aufgestautes durchbrochen. Kraut der Sonnenwenden. Stark positiv polend. Der Wurzelrauch ist ein mächtiger Reinigungsrauch, der Eintragungen und erkaltete Hinterlassenschaften in der Raumenergie wie ein starker Besen in Bewegung bringen, überlagern und schließlich lösen kann. Klärender Rauch für das Krankenzimmer, für das Schlafzimmer bei Schlafstörungen und Alpträumen, auch fürs Büro, wenn Überlastung droht oder bereits eingetreten ist. Die unbezwingbare Lebenskraft aus der Wurzel vermittelt besonders im Rauch positive Impulse in unsere Umgebung, so dass dunkle Schatten, Blockaden und andere übelwollende Dämonen überwunden werden können. Wohltat für eine verletzte oder geschwächte Seele. Belastende Anhaftungen werden beseitigt und lösen sich aus dem persönlichen Kraftfeld, das dadurch wieder dicht und widerstandsfähig wird.

Hilfreich für Menschen, die sich täglich überfordert fühlen oder im Burn out sind oder davor stehen. Auch für Menschen, die aggressive Phasen durchleben oder bereits in der Verbitterung gelandet sind. Bringt Klarheit ins Gefühlsleben und hat eine stark aufbauende, positive Einwirkung auf die geistige Ebene. Im Rauch wird Schweres leicht, neuer Schwung zieht ein, die Motivation steigt und Sorgen können abdanken. Unterstützt Übergangsphasen: Das Zutrauen in das Gelingen wird gefestigt. Wandlungs- und Entwicklungsprozesse werden einem bewusst und erscheinen bewältigbar. Man steht im Licht, es kann wieder aufwärts gehen!

Magisches zum Rauch: Zur Erfüllung von Wünschen wurde ein magischer Rauch aus Löwenzahn, Goldrute und Thymian/Quendel bereitet und die Räucherung mit verschiedenen Zaubersprüchen begleitet.

Schwerpunkt, Anwendungen, Rezepte: Räuchermischung für einen intensiven Motivationsrauch, der auch hilft, ungeliebte Aufgaben lustvoll in Angriff zu nehmen: Löwenzahnwurzel, Brennnessel, Weißdorn und Beifuß. Bei Gelenksschmerzen kann eine Räuchermischung aus Löwenzahn, Ampferwurzel und Rosmarin Hilfe bringen. Man hält die schmerzende Stelle über den Rauch oder setzt sich auf einen Sessel und gibt die Räucherschale darunter. Jeweils mit Harz kombinieren.

Verwendung – gestern und heute

Hieronymus Bock (1498–1554), deutscher Arzt und Botaniker, erzählt von einer besonderen Anwendung des „Wassers“, das aus den Blättern und der Wurzeln des Löwenzahnes gebrannt wird: „Die weiber pflegen sich auch under augen mit disem wasser zu weschen, verhoffen dadurch ein lautter angesicht zu erlangen und die rote purpur oder bläterlein damit zu vertreiben“.

In der Frühlingsküche wird wohl kein anderes Wildkraut so intensiv und vielseitig genutzt. Die Bitterstoffe in den Blättern fördern die Sekretion der Verdauungsdrüsen und bringen uns nach dem Winter wieder in Schwung.

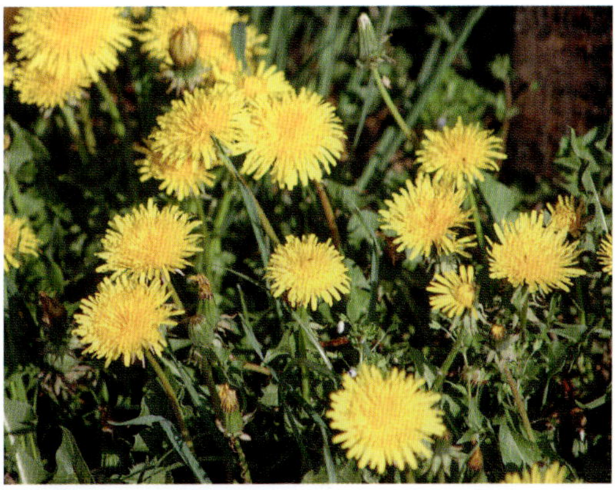

Blühender Löwenzahn

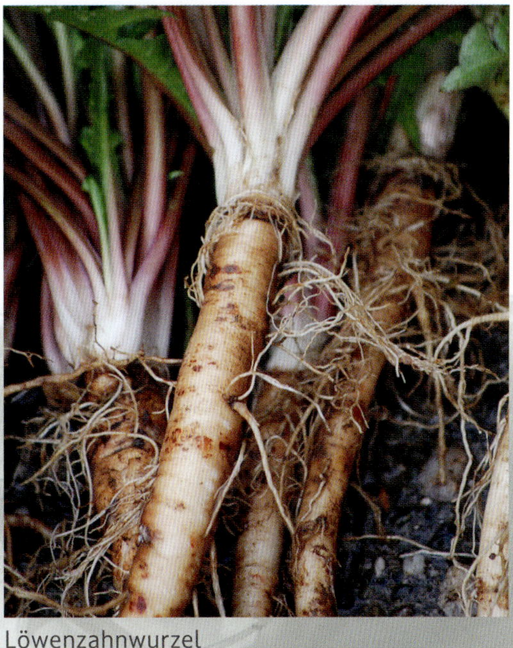

Löwenzahnwurzel

Nelkenwurz

Lat. Name: *Geum urbanum*
Botanischer Name: Echte Nelkenwurz
Pflanzenfamilie: Rosengewächse

Die Nelkenwurz ist ein Phänomen von Pflanzenintuition. Sie kommt gern als Besucherin wie eine gute Fee in den Garten, siedelt entlang der Gartenwege und scheint jeden noch so leisen Gedanken zu hören und zu spiegeln: Es hat den Anschein als führten negative Gedanken zur Verdichtung ihrer vegetativ-einfühlsamen Kraft, als mobilisierten sie die Abwehrkraft der Pflanze, was sich im darauffolgenden Jahr in einem vervielfachten Bestand zeigt, obwohl sie normalerweise keine großen expansiven Neigungen zeigt.

Sie eilt zu Hilfe, ist zu gemeinsamer Abwehr bereit, mit ihren dunklen Frühlingsblättern, mit ihren stacheligen Samenkugeln, die, Wurfgeschossen gleich, sich von langen Speerstangen in die Welt hinauskatapultieren, mit ihrem stark riechenden, feurigen Wurzelstock.

Die Bezeichnungen „herba benedicta" oder „Heil aller Welt" weisen aber auch auf das große heilsame Potenzial hin, das Kräuterkundige über die Jahrhunderte hinweg dieser Pflanze zugeschrieben haben. Überwiegend wurde sie als universelles giftwidriges Mittel bei Verdauungsproblemen und als Lebermittel eingesetzt.

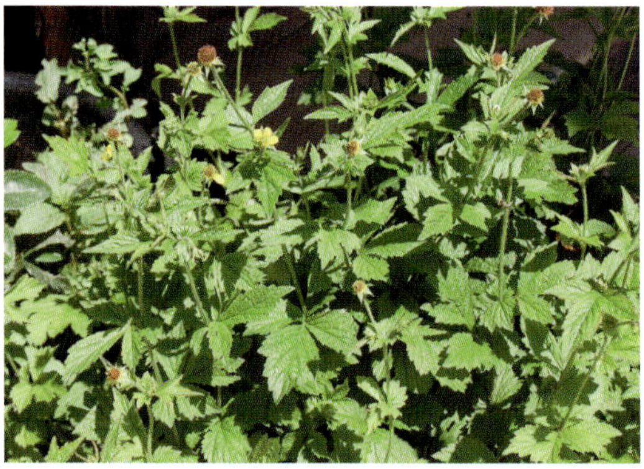

Blühende Nelkenwurz

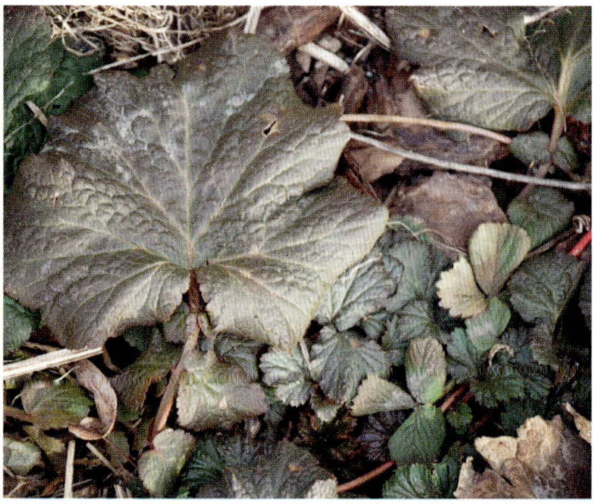

Nelkenwurzblätter

Rauch

Verwendete Pflanzenteile: Wurzeln, sowie die Blüten, Blätter und Fruchtstände.

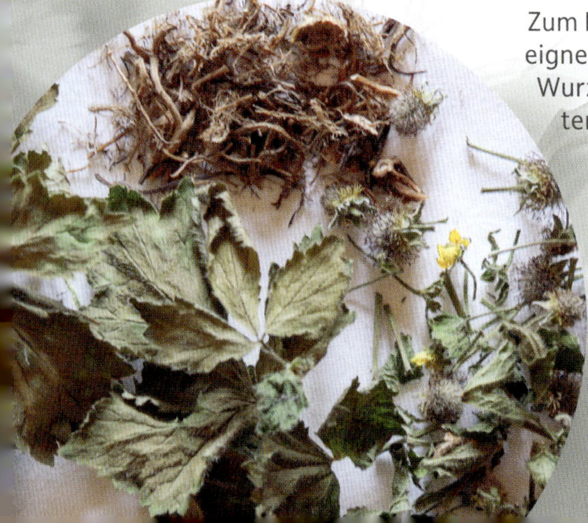

Zum Räuchern eignen sich die Wurzeln, Blüten, Blätter und Fruchtstände.

Beste Sammel- und Erntezeit: Die Wurzeln eher im Herbst sammeln; Blüten und Fruchtstände sind im Mai/Juni eine Zeit lang gemeinsam auf der Pflanze. Die Blätter können ganzjährig geerntet werden. Die Wurzel ist jedoch die bestimmende Kraft im Rauch.

Wirkung, Wahrnehmung: Abwehrrauch. Schutzkraut! Anrufungs- und Segensräucherungen. Große weißmagische Kraft! Schützt vor Angriffen im geistig-seelischen Bereich und wirkt dabei stark antidämonisch. Hilfreich in Mobbing-Phasen, weil der Rauch auch einhüllend und schutzgebend wirkt. Der Rauch der Nelkenwurz schwächt schwarzmagische Übergriffe und Nadelungen ab;

wirkt gegen neidvolle und missgünstige Wesen in der Menschen-, wie auch in der Geisterwelt. Schenkt einem einen distanzierten Blick auf Zerwürfnisse und emotionale Belastungen, hilft Abstand zu nehmen und auch zu halten. Sorgt für ein Gefühl von Sicherheit, Geborgenheit. Der Wurzelrauch breitet sich schützend über jene, die sich zu viel zugemutet haben und jetzt damit nicht fertig werden. Die Einsicht, dass auch Umwege zum Ziel führen können, nimmt den Druck weg und bezähmt den eigenen Ehrgeiz. Unbelastete genießen einen beruhigenden Rauch, bei dem man sich ganz entspannen, die Augen schließen und genießen kann.

Magisches zum Rauch: Mit Malefizräucherungen versuchte man dunkle Mächte abzuwehren. Dazu wurde eine Räuchermischung hergestellt aus Nelkenwurzwurzel, Johanniskraut, Beifußwurzel, Wacholderbeeren und Weinraute. Der „Neidstock", wie die Nelkenwurz vielerorts bezeichnet wird, hilft mit seinem Rauch mißgünstige Verwünschungen und jeglichen Schadenszauber abzuwehren.

Schwerpunkt, Anwendungen, Rezepte: Eine segnende Räuchermischung soll das reine Herz stärken: Nelkenwurz, Bibernell, Goldrute und Berg-Bohnenkraut kombiniert mit Harz.

Mythologie und magische Praktiken

Man vertraute seit jeher auf ihre antidämonische Kraft und nutzte sie zu vielen magischen Handlungen. In der Zeit der Hexenverfolgung (ca. 1450–1750) wurde die pulverisierte Nelkenwurz-Wurzel zum Hauptbestandteil des Malefizpulvers, mit dem man sich vor Hexen und Dämonen zu schützen versuchte. Es finden sich Empfehlungen zu zahllosen körperlichen Leiden, bei denen auf die rein äußerliche Übertragung ihrer Kräfte vertraut wird. So soll beispielsweise die Nelkenwurz-Wurzel als „Augenbündel" um den Hals gehängt und bei Heilung des Augenleidens in den fließenden Bach geworfen werden. Als „Mannskraftwurzel" wird ebenfalls die Nelkenwurz-Wurzel um den Hals gehängt, um andere Schwächen auszugleichen.

Verwendung – gestern und heute

Hildegard von Bingen (1098–1179) hat ganz klare Vorstellungen von diesem Kraut: „Das Benediktenkraut ist warm und wenn jemand es im Trank einnimmt, entbrennt er in begehrlicher Liebe. Aber wenn es einem Menschen am ganzen Körper an seinen Körperkräften gebricht, dann koche er Benediktenkraut in Wasser, und dieses Wasser trinke er oft so warm, und er wird die Körperkräfte wieder erlangen, und nachdem es mit dem Körper besser geworden ist, meide er es."

Leonhart Fuchs (1501–1566) schreibt: „Die Benedicten wurtzel haben vilerley gebrauch. Ettlich seubern diese wurtzel, dörrens, und besprengens mit essig, legens also in die kisten und truhen zu den kleydern das sie wol davon schmecke." Überdies meint er: „Diese wurtzel gedörrt und zu pulver gestossen, darnach in wein ingenommen, ist gut wider allerley gifft." Die frische Wurzel enthält das ätherische Öl Eugenol, das entzündungshemmend wirkt und früher bei Zahnfleischproblemen gekaut wurde.

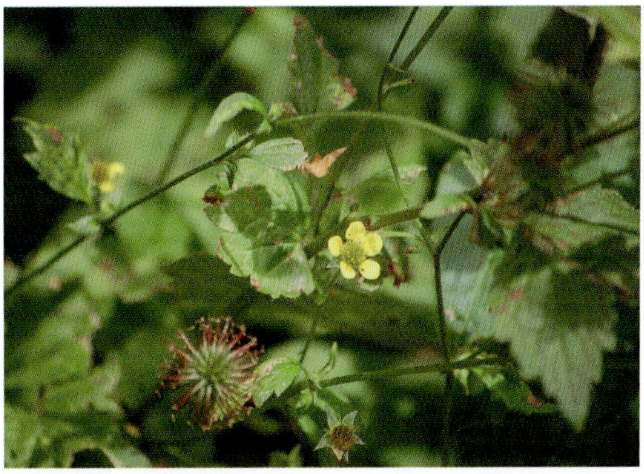

Blüte der Nelkenwurz

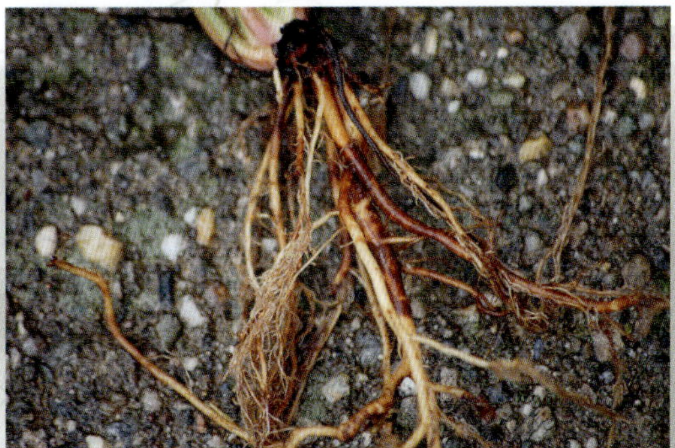

Nelkenwurzwurzel

Odermennig

Lat. Name: *Agrimonia eupatoria*
Pflanzenfamilie: Rosengewächse

Ein Kraut höchster Heilkraft für Körper, Geist und Seele ist der gern bescheiden und zurückgezogen auf hartgefahrenen Wegen am Waldrand lebende Odermennig. Der „König aller Heilkräuter" wird bereits im Papyrus Ebers, ca. 1600 v. Chr., erwähnt und als Augenheilmittel gepriesen. Bei den Römern wurde er Minerva, der Göttin des Verstandes zugeordnet und seine zerquetschten Wurzeln sollten jene heilen, die unter Gedächtnisschwund litten.

Auffällig sind die zahlreichen Superlativ-Bezeichnungen, mit denen man versuchte, das Kraut adäquat darzustellen und gleichzeitig dem Pflanzengeist näherzukommen, ihn gewogen zu machen: Heil aller Schäden, Heil aller Welt oder Heilandskraut – abgesehen von den komplizierten sprachlichen Her- und Ableitungen, um von „arge mone", Plage des Auges, auf Odermennig zu kommen. In der Gegend um Grafenstein in Kärnten hat sich im bäuerlichen Umfeld ein weiterer Name erhalten: „s`Besserle" – das sagt schon alles.

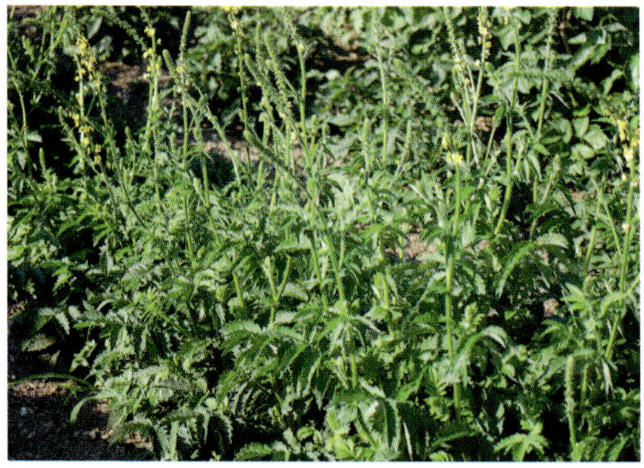

Odermennig im Garten

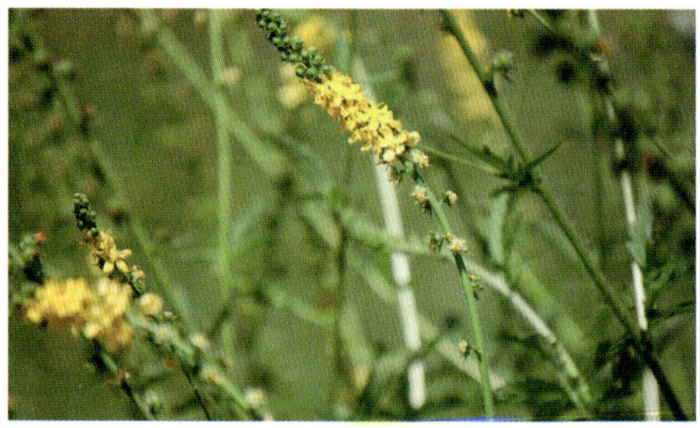

Blühender Odermennig

Rauch

Verwendete Pflanzenteile: Das ganze blühende Kraut, speziell die Wurzel.

Beste Sammel- und Erntezeit: Die Wurzel kann mit dem blühenden Kraut im August gegraben werden. Sie wird gesäubert, klein aufgeschnitten und getrocknet.

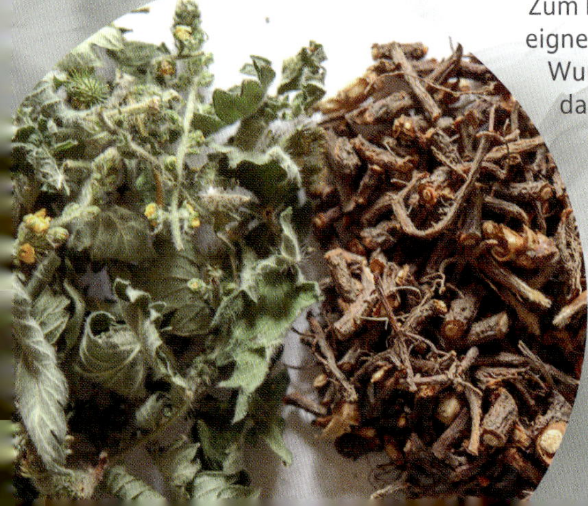

Zum Räuchern eignen sich die Wurzeln und das blühende Kraut.

Wirkung, Wahrnehmung: Abwehrrauch. Großes Schutzkraut! Reinigungsrauch. Verschreikraut! Reinigende und klärende Kraft des Rauchs für jede belastete Raumatmosphäre. Große auflösendes Potenzial bei Schadenszauber und kopfbezogenen Bannungen. Negative Anhaftungen durch Flüche, Verwünschungen, schwarzmagische Handlungen und Nadelungen werden überlagert, somit entkräftet und schließlich vom Rauch davongetragen.

Die große Schutzkraft des Odermennigrauches beruhigt Kinder, die Angst haben im Dunkeln einzuschlafen. Der reinigende Rauch stärkt bei Mobbing und hilft zu sich zu stehen. Die ausgleichende Wirkung dieses Rauches verhilft zu mehr Offenheit und Mut, sich einzubringen und durchzusetzen. Die Angst vor seelischen Verletzungen kann kleiner werden.

Der Wurzelrauch des Odermennigs besänftigt sämtliche angstbesetzten Bereiche, unterlegt sie mit seiner Schutzkraft und durchlichtet sie, so dass die Ängste langsam schwinden. Der Rauch ermutigt dazu, seine Handlungen in kritischen Situationen zu reflektieren, nachsichtig mit sich selbst umzugehen und sich, gegebenenfalls, das eigene Versagen zu verzeihen.

Magisches zum Rauch: Beim rituellen Heilen durch Abbeten wird eine Mischung aus Odermennig, Beifuß und Thymian geräuchert.

Schwerpunkt, Anwendungen, Rezepte: Räuchermischung für eine angenehme Abendräucherung und zur Beruhigung nach aufregenden Ereignissen: Odermennig, Eibischwurzel und Lavendel. Hilfe bei der seelischen Verarbeitung von belastenden Ereignissen: Odermennig, Kleines Habichtskraut, Bärenschote und Ysop. Jeweils mit Harz kombinieren.

Verwendung – gestern und heute

Walahfrid Strabo (808–849), Abt des Klosters Reichenau am Bodensee, nennt ihn in seinem Gartengedicht „sarcocolam": sarx, Fleisch und cola, Leim. Diese Bezeichnung geht wohl zurück auf den Pseudo-Apuleius, ein illustriertes Kräuterbuch, dessen Urtext vermutlich aus dem 4. Jahrhundert stammt. Sie veranschaulicht die Kraft des Odermennigs, innere und äußere Wunden zu heilen. Hieronymus Bock (1498–1554) führt an: „Odermeng ist ein recht glider gewächs, zu den verruckten spannadern und nerven, die bringt es wider zurecht, soll in leib und eüsserlich genützet werden." Auch Leonhart Fuchs (1501–1566) meint: „Die bletter der Odermenig mit alltem schweinemschmalz oder schmär warm auffgelegt, heylet die wunden so sich nit leicht zu heylung schicken wollen." Matthiolus (1501–1577), italienischer Arzt und Botaniker, Leibarzt Kaiser Maximilians II., fasst zusammen: Es handle sich um das „fürnembst kraut der alten zu allem verstopfften lebern".

Bachblüte Nr. 1 „agrimony" – Odermenning – ist die Ehrlichkeitsblüte, für sehr höfliche Menschen, die Scheinharmonie einer Konfrontation vorziehen.

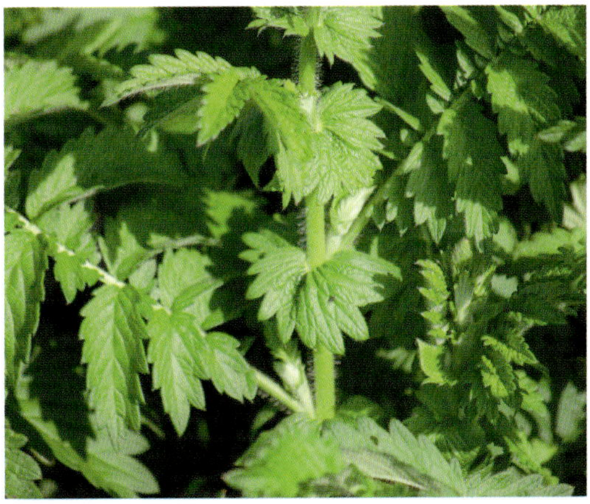

Odermennigblätter

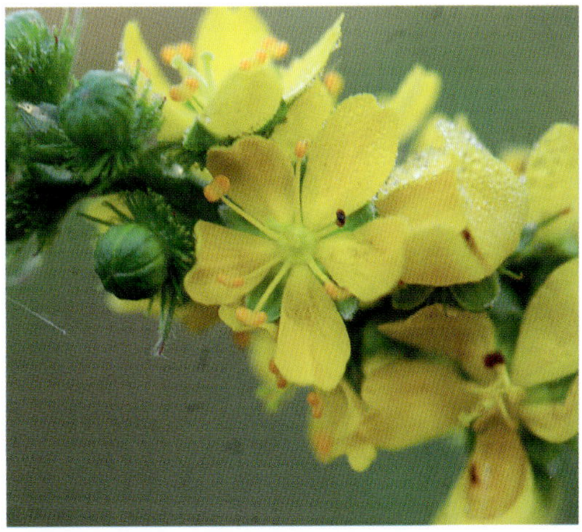

Blüte des Odermennigs

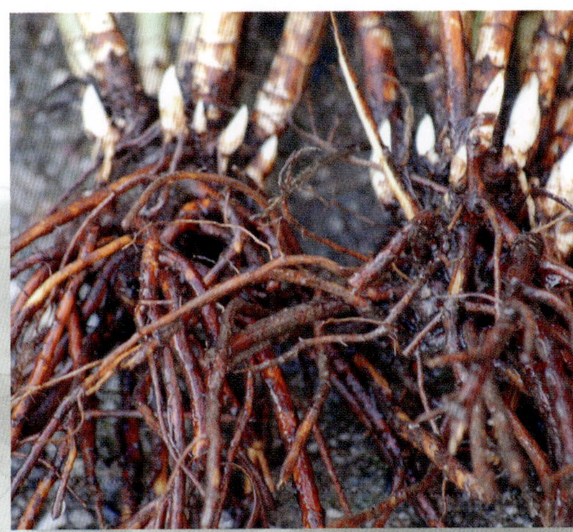

Odermennigwurzel

Quecke

Lat. Name: *Elymus repens*
Botanischer Name: Gewöhnliche Quecke
Pflanzenfamilie: Süßgräser

Auf lockeren Ackerböden hat sich die Quecke mit ihren rasch wachsenden Wurzelausläufern nicht gerade beliebt gemacht. Ihre Wurzeln scheiden überdies eine Substanz aus, die andere Pflanzen in ihrem Wachstum bremst. Zudem ist sie Wirtspflanze für Viren und jenen Pilz, der das giftige Mutterkorn im Getreide bildet. Nährstoffreiches Tierfutter könnte sie sein, aber mit diesem Steckbrief – wer will sich da schon mit ihr einlassen? Lediglich in den Staaten der ehemaligen Sowjetunion wird die Quecke mancherorts als Nahrungsmittel angebaut, die getrockneten Wurzeln zum Strecken von Mehl oder geröstet als Kaffeeersatz verwendet.

Sie will erobern, will Pionierin sein und gleichzeitig Herrscherin nach außen. Geschwindigkeit und Oberflächlichkeit sind ihre Attribute. Dazu errichtet sie ein horizontales Baugerüst, dessen Bauplan dezentral in den Knoten entschieden werden muss, weil die zentrale Wurzel so schwach ist, dass sie die Pflanze gerade einmal in der Erde festzuhalten vermag. Wer so rasch wächst, muss Kompetenz abgeben, muss sich auf sein verbindendes Netz und die Verknüpfungen verlassen können. Jeder Knoten setzt sofort Bodenanker als Sicherungsmaßnahme des Gebietsgewinnes. Hier pulsieren Mut und Rücksichtslosigkeit.

Rauch

Verwendete Pflanzenteile: Die gesamte Pflanze: Wurzeln, Halme.

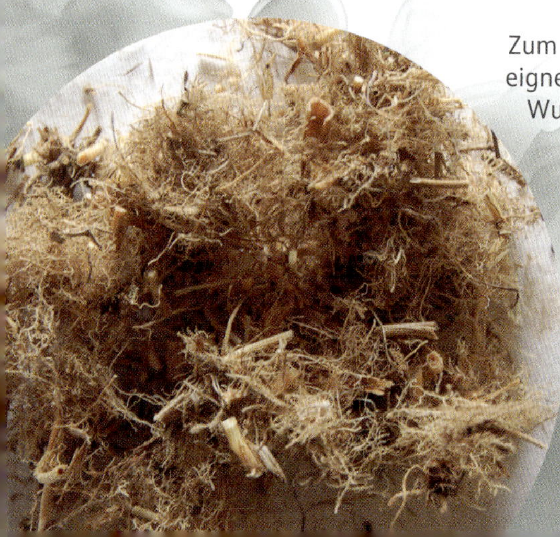

Zum Räuchern eignen sich die Wurzeln und Halme.

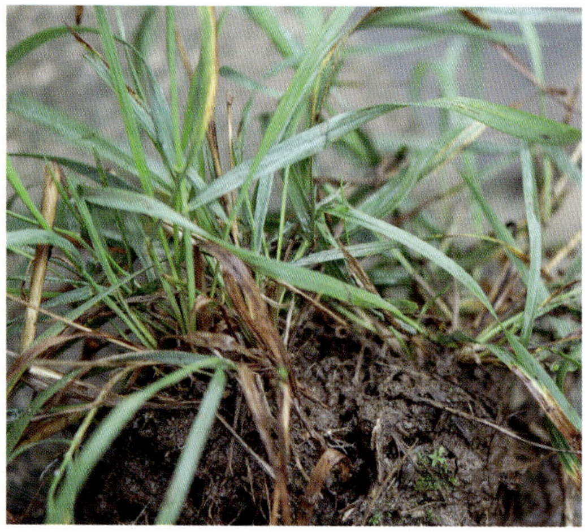

Die Quecke ist eine Pionierpflanze.

Beste Sammel- und Erntezeit: Das ganze Jahr über kann die Wurzel mit ihren weißen Wurzelausläufern und den oberirdischen Grasschäften gestochen, entflochten, gereinigt und getrocknet werden.

Wirkung, Wahrnehmung: Reinigungsrauch. Pflanze des geistigen Umschwungs! Klärender Reinigungsrauch, der einen aus tunnelartigen Gedankenverengungen befreit. Kraftvolle Auflösung von zu einfach Gedachtem! Der Queckenrauch macht geistig lebendig, setzt die Gestaltungskraft der Natur gegen eindimensionale Menschenlogik. Geistiger Umschwung im Sinne von erweitertem Denken wird möglich. Hilfreich für ausschließlich geistig arbeitende Menschen: Mit dem Rauch heben sich die Nebel der Ungenauigkeit der geistigen Arbeit, man kann die wichtigen letzten Meilensteine seiner Arbeit wie neu durchdenken.

Schutz für jede geistige Arbeit! Lässt uns erkennen, dass wir uns wesentliche Erkenntnisse nur etappenweise erarbeiten können. Nimmt gleichzeitig die Ungeduld aus oberflächlichen Denkprozessen, die zu keinem Ergebnis führen können. Nach einer Quecken-Räucherung ist man zufriedener mit sich selbst.

Schwerpunkt, Anwendungen, Rezepte: Eine Wurzel-Räuchermischung für „Workaholics“, um geistig bei Kräften zu bleiben: Quecke, Giersch, Diptam und Bärenschote in Kombination mit Harz.

Verwendung – gestern und heute

Gelenksheilsame Rezepturen von Süßgräsern sind bis ins 4. vorchristliche Jahrhundert vorhanden. Eine konkrete Zuordnung zur Quecke lässt sich aber erst mit den Aufzeichnungen der Kräuterväter des frühen 16. Jahrhunderts nachvollziehen. Bei Tabernaemontanus (1522–1590) findet man die Quecke, wenn er „von den graskreutern“ spricht. Die Quecke, so meint er unter anderem in seitenlangen Anwendungsvorschlägen, „eröffnet die verstopffung der leber, ist erfahren wider alle gebrechen der nieren unnd blasen, wider das grieß, den stein, schwerlich und tröpfflingen harnen…“ An anderer Stelle rät er, die Wurzel bei abnehmendem Mond nur drei Knoten weit abzureißen und um den Hals zu hängen, was die Hitze der Augen stillen möge.

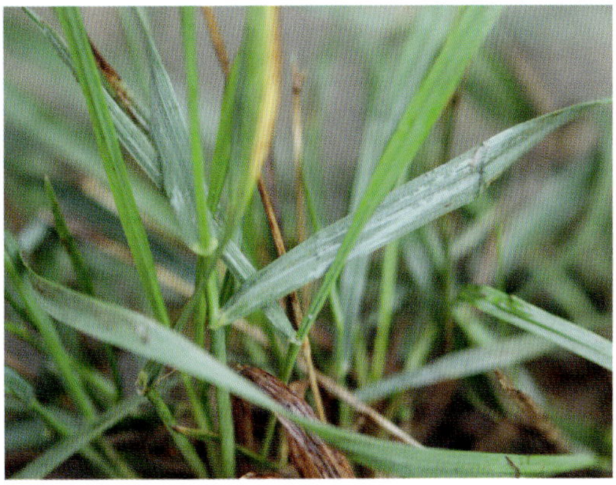

Queckenblätter

Hieronymus Bock (1498–1554) schreibt, nach langer Herleitung aus verschiedenen Gräsern, die dem Vieh als Futter dienen, zur Quecke: „Die weisse lange wurtzel von den Quecken mögen inn leib genützt werden, ein hand vol dieser wurtzeln in einer maß weissen weins gesotten und gedruncken etliche tag, treiben on zweiffel die würm auß dem leib und ist ein recht bewert kinder artznei!“

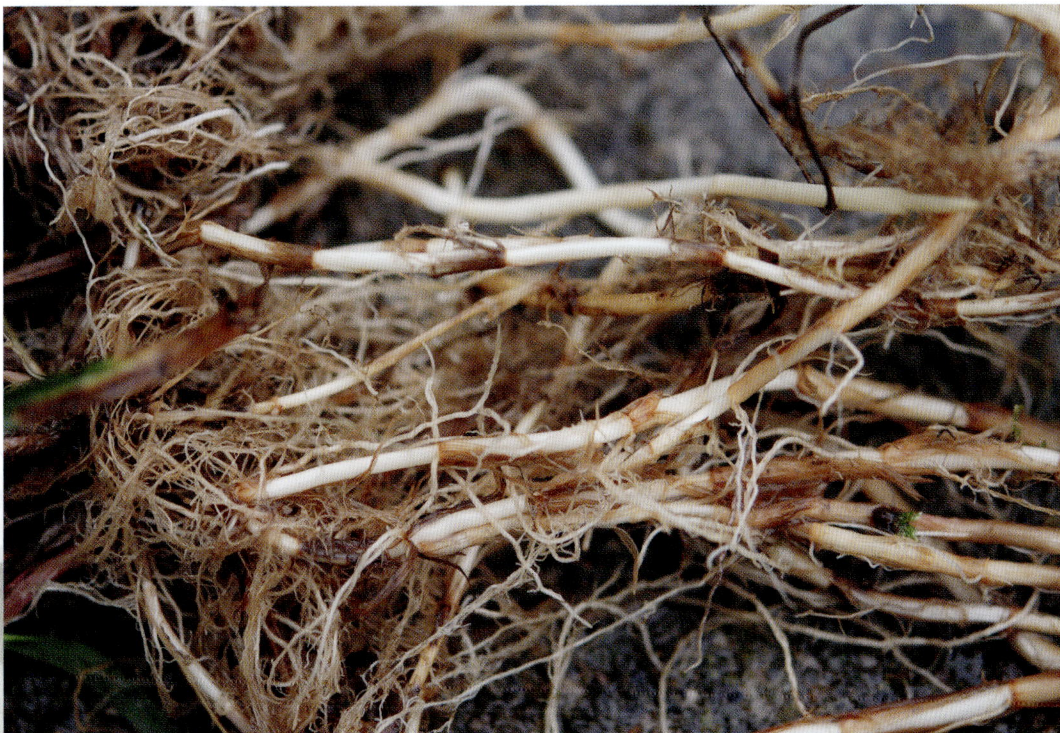

Queckenwurzel

Seifenkraut

Lat. Name: *Saponaria officinalis*
Botanischer Name:
Gewöhnliches Seifenkraut
Pflanzenfamilie: Nelkengewächse

Über Jahrtausende diente die Wurzel des Seifenkrauts zur Reinigung von Wäsche und Gerätschaften. Leonhart Fuchs (1501–1566) bezeichnete sie beispielsweise als altes Kraut der Walker, das die Kleider reinigt. Im Garten wuchert das anspruchslose Seifenkraut gern, füllt ganze Beete aus und verdrängt respektlos andere Pflanzen. Es fängt ganz harmlos mit zarten rosafarbenen Blüten an, die wie Windräder ihre Flügel in alle Himmelsrichtungen spreizen. Aus den dicken örtlichen Wurzeln der Stammpflanzen schlagen dann rötlich glänzende Eroberungswurzeln peitschenartig kreuz und quer durchs Beet, gehen einmal tiefer, dann wieder nahe an der Oberfläche, als wollten sie anderen Pflanzen den Lebensraum vermiesen.

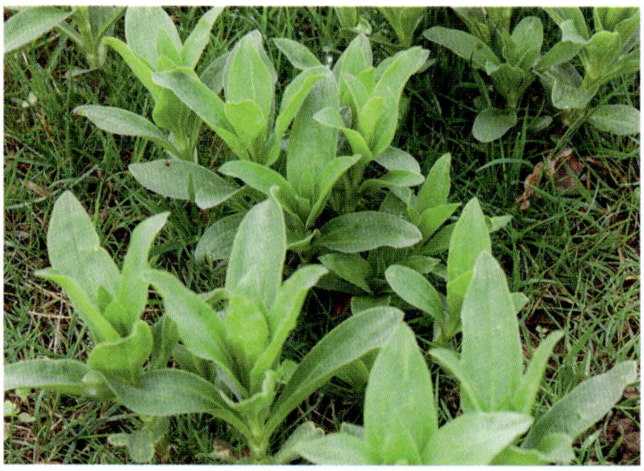

Blätter des Seifenkrauts

Rauch

Verwendete Pflanzenteile: Das ganze blühende Kraut: Wurzel, Blätter, Stängel, Blüten.

Beste Sammel- und Erntezeit: Die Wurzeln können das ganze Jahr über gegraben werden. Sie werden gewaschen, kleingeschnitten und getrocknet. Die Blätter, Stängel und Blüten werden zur Blütezeit gesammelt.

Wirkung, Wahrnehmung: Klärender Rauch; Familienrauch. Seelenrauch! Die Wurzel entwickelt im Rauch einen eigentümlichen Geruch, der nicht unangenehm, aber etwas fremdartig wahrgenommen wird. Die Räucherung bringt die Dinge ins Fließen, entstaut geistige und seelische Blockaden. Wird dadurch entlastend und aufbauend erlebt. Die Kraft der Wurzel zielt stets in die engsten Lebenskreise, in die Familie; fördert das Zusammengehörigkeitsgefühl und die eigene innere Öffnung hin zur Gemeinschaft. Unausgesprochene Probleme und nicht ausgetragenen Konflikte können im beruhigenden Rauch überdacht werden. Die Liebesbereitschaft innerhalb der Gruppe und die Verbundenheit mit der Familie werden gestärkt.

Der Rauch kann in Situationen hilfreich sein, in denen man starke Zweifel an der eigenen Kraft hat, in denen man befürchten muss, von Ereignissen überrollt zu werden, mit Vorkommnissen nicht fertig zu werden: Beruhigung, Nervenentlastung, Rückzug auf das Wesentliche können erfühlt werden.

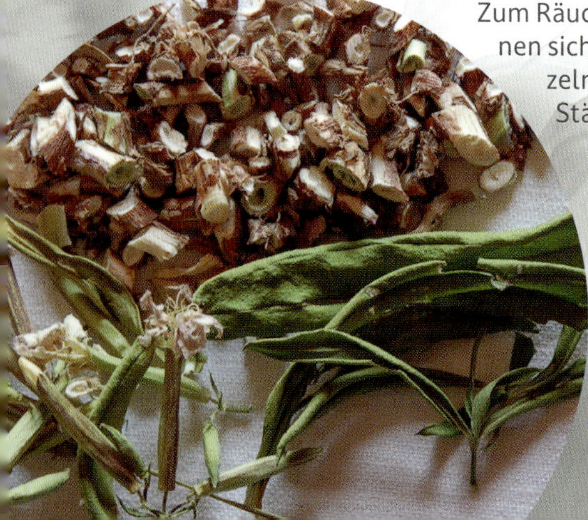

Zum Räuchern eignen sich die Wurzeln, Blätter, Stängel und Blüten.

Schwerpunkt, Anwendungen, Rezepte: Ausgleichender Familienrauch für Groß und Klein ist eine Räuchermischung mit Seifenkraut, Braunwurz, Lavendel und Hagebutten oder Rosenblüten und Harz.

Verwendung – gestern und heute

Hieronymus Bock (1498–1554) schreibt über den Namen der „Speichelwurtz oder Seiffenkraut“: „Zu Teütsch Weschkraut, Seiffenkraut, darumb das etlich Klosterleüt ire kappen und gerete mit disem gewächs seübern und weschen, sparen hiermit Seiffen unnd Alaun, haben des gelts nicht Seiffen zu kauffen oder wescherin zu dingen, wie sich dann die arme brüder sanct Francisci höchlich beklagen." Zu den innerlichen Wirkungen führt er auswurffördernde und leberreinigende Qualitäten an und meint abschließend: „Sol auch den schwachen kalten mennern wider auff helfen!"

Die heilsamen, schleimlösenden Qualitäten dieses Krauts waren wohl früh bekannt und wurden bei Hautproblemen genauso eingesetzt wie bei zähem Hustenschleim. Wichtigster Inhaltsstoff des Seifenkrauts ist das Saponin, das im menschlichen Körper vor allem die Entgiftung von Schleimen und Schlacken vorantreiben und Cholesterin binden kann.

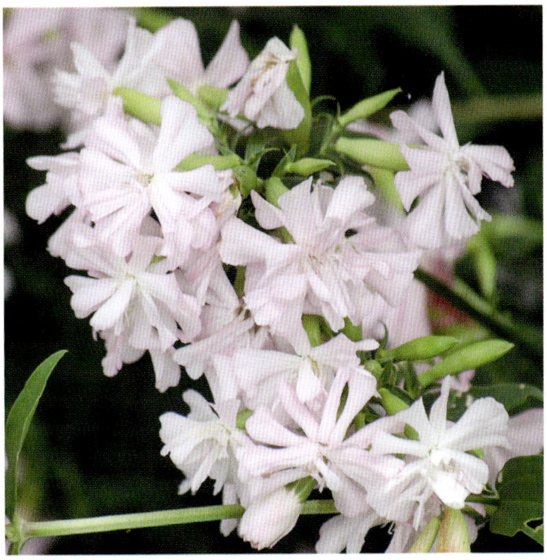

Blüte des Seifenkrauts

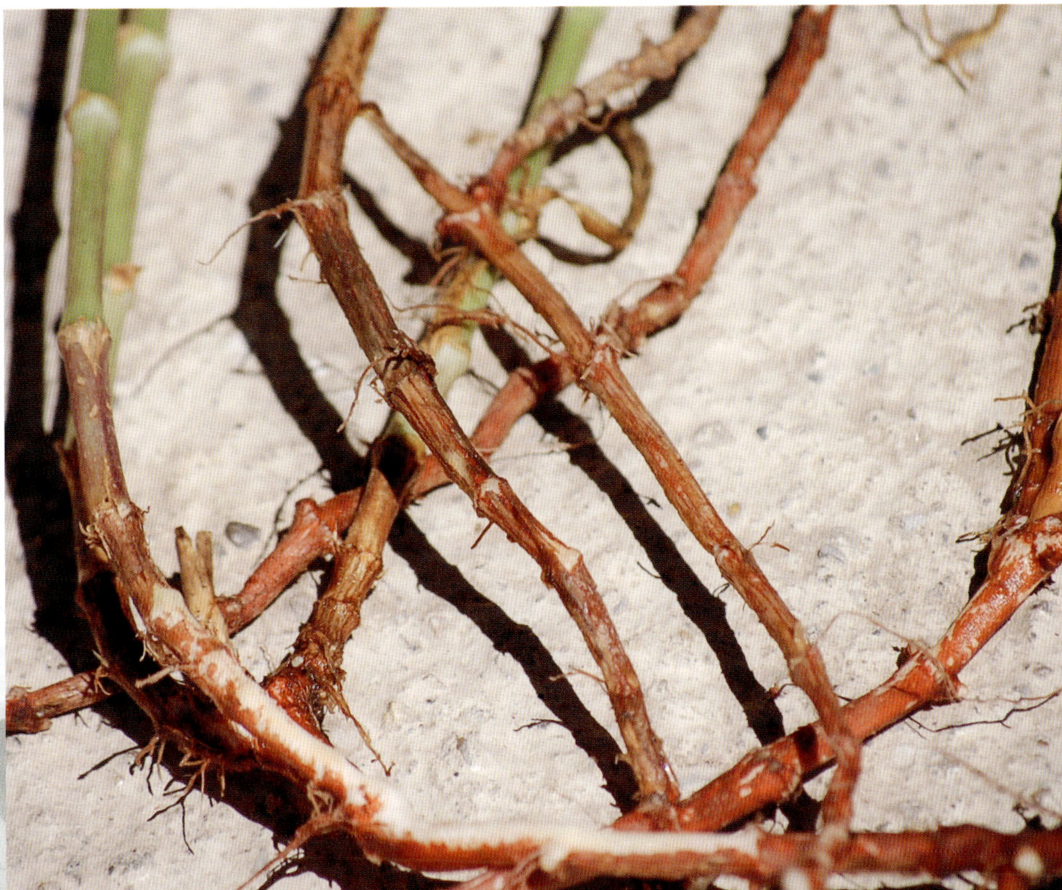

Seifenkrautwurzel

Wegwarte

Lat. Name: *Cichorium intybus*
Pflanzenfamilie: Korbblütler

Seit sechs Jahrtausenden im Einsatz für Liebe und Treue! Unerreicht scheinen die magischen Kräfte der Wegwarte – auch als Zichorie bekannt – zu sein, wenn man sich die zahllosen seherischen Zuschreibungen und zauberischen Rituale ganzer Völkerschaften vor Augen hält. Dann komme ich und frage mich Jahr für Jahr: Kommt sie oder kommt sie nicht? Innerlich bin ich überzeugt, dass sie es bald schaffen wird! Sie hört mich ja rufen! Vor zehn Jahren waren die wenigen Wegwartenpflanzen in meiner Umgebung noch bergab und gemessene zwei Kilometer von meinem Garten entfernt. Letztes Jahr dann hat sich ein schüchternes Wegwartengeschöpf tatsächlich in die Nachbarwiese neben der Straße gesetzt. Entlang des Straßenverlaufes ist sie deutlich vorangekommen. Ob sie heuer wohl kommt? Vielleicht ist sie schon da, unterm Schnee!

Die Zähigkeit sämtlicher Pflanzenteile und die Kompromisslosigkeit mit der sie straßennahe schwierige Standorte auswählt, lassen eine unbeugsame Pflanzenpersönlichkeit erkennen. Sie ist die große Einzelgängerin, die auch unter ihresgleichen lieber einen räumlichen Abstand einhält. Simon & Garfunkels Lied „I am a rock, I am an island…" scheint wie für sie geschrieben. In meinem Garten wäre jedenfalls genug Platz für die schöne Eigenbrötlerin und auch harte Wegflächen hätte ich anzubieten.

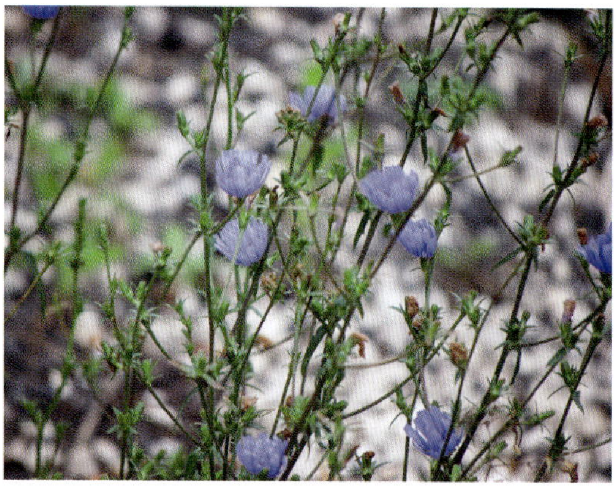

Blühende Wegwarte

Rauch

Verwendete Pflanzenteile: Die ganze blühende Pflanze: Wurzel, Blätter, Blüten.

Beste Sammel- und Erntezeit: Wenn die Pflanze blüht, kann sie zur Gänze ausgegraben werden. Die Wurzel sollte sofort gereinigt und klein aufgeschnitten werden, da sie, wie die Hauhechelwurzel, von Haus aus besonders zäh ist und sofort beginnt sich auszuhärten! Die sparrigen Stängel ergeben im Rauch sehr verwirrende Botschaften, so dass ich sie nicht zur Trocknung für Räucherungen empfehle. Man könnte sie jedoch gut zu einem Wetterbuschn binden, den man bei Gewitter im Ofen oder im Freien verbrennt, nicht verräuchert.

Wirkung, Wahrnehmung: Schutzrauch. Seelenrauch. Die blaue Kraft des Verstandes! Wetterkraut. Die große räucherische Vereinfacherin! Die Räucherung führt Herz und Verstand zusammen, sorgt für einen klaren Verstand und unterstützt einen, um sich von Altem besser und im Guten lösen zu können. Allerdings werden überdrehte Gedanken mit erdhaftem Ernst zur sicheren Landung gebracht und übersteigerte Erwartungen auf den Boden der Realität zurückgeholt. Der Rauch ist für schnelllebige und gestresste Menschen eine Herausforderung, weil er sie unerwartet abbremst.

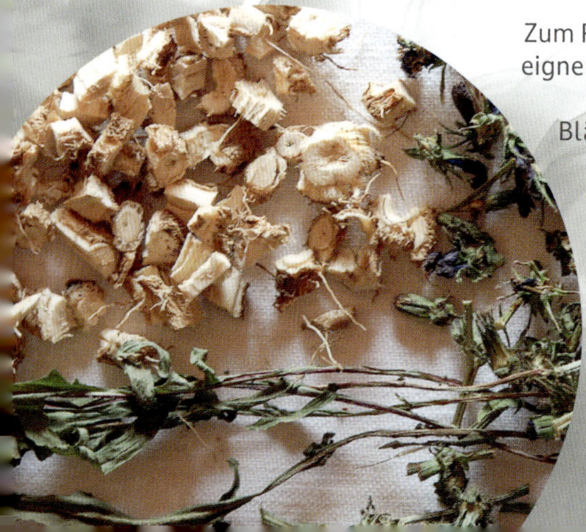

Zum Räuchern eignen sich die Wurzeln, Blätter und Blüten.

Die reinigende Kraft der Wurzel schärft den Blick fürs Wesentliche und hält negative Kräfte fern. Sie hilft, das Leben leichter zu nehmen und auch Hindernisse zu überwinden. Die Pflanzen mit blauen Blüten helfen verräuchert gegen Schwermut und Melancholie. Der blaue Himmel, der sich in ihnen widerspiegelte, überträgt im aufsteigenden Rauch einen Impuls der Liebe und Freude. So kann die Schwere überwunden werden. Stabilisiert Menschen, die sich zu sehr für andere aufgeopfert haben und sich jetzt leer und überflüssig fühlen. Seelenrauch – zeigt den Weg zum Herzen, tröstet die verletzte Seele und hilft den richtigen Abstand zu anderen zu finden. Als Wetterkraut ist der Rauch der Wegwarte in der Lage, Spannungen auszugleichen – mögen sie in Räumen herrschen oder Menschen um sich herum aufgebaut haben.

Magisches zum Rauch: Die meisten der unten angeführten magischen Praktiken wurden, wo immer es ging, auch von Räucherungen mit der Wegwarte und anderen zauberischen Gewächsen, begleitet. Um sich von angezauberter Liebe zu befreien, wurde unablässig Wegwarten-Wurzel geräuchert.

Schwerpunkt, Anwendungen, Rezepte: Für eine spannungsabbauende Räucherung werden gemischt: Wegwarte, Königskerze, Brennnesselwurzel und Harz.

Mythologie und magische Praktiken

Die erste Beschreibung der Wegwarte als Zauberpflanze findet sich auf einem ägyptischen Papyrustext aus dem 4. Jahrtausend vor Christus. Bereits in der Antike erfüllte die Wegwarte die Hoffnung eifersüchtiger Ehefrauen, die ihren Ehemännern, wenn diese verreisen mussten, die gepulverte Wurzel verabreichten oder Wurzelstücke in ihre Kleidung einnähten, um sie so von ehelichen Verfehlungen abzuhalten. Komplizierter waren da schon die Handlungsanweisungen, um die Wurzel zu zwingen, den Namen oder das Gesicht des zukünftigen Ehemannes preiszuge-

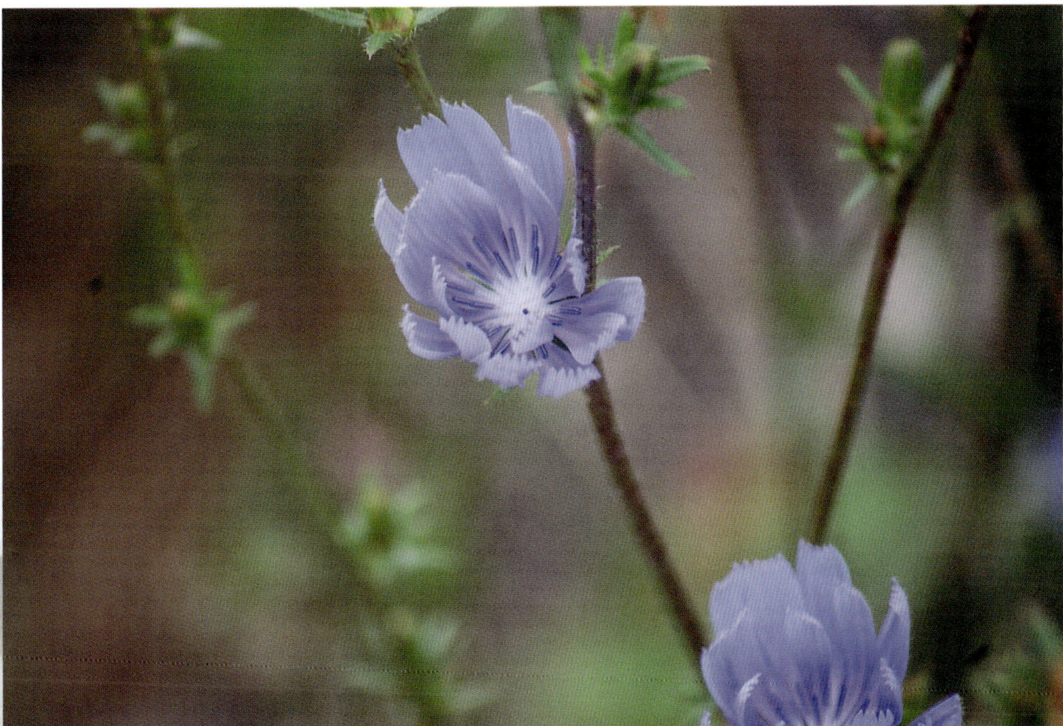

Blüte der Wegwarte

ben. Um einen Dieb zu entlarven, wurde die Wurzel unter den Schlafpolster gegeben und zwingend erschien einem der Dieb im Traum.

Männern half die Wurzel am Jakobitag (25. Juli) „hieb- und stichfest" zu werden, so sie mit goldenem Werkzeug mit dem Gesicht nach Osten in der Frühe ausgegraben wurde. Die Saligen Frauen aus dem Wald brachten den Gebärenden das Kräutlein „Nimmerweh", wenn diese zu verbluten drohten. Es gibt unzählige lokale Liebeszauber, die heiratswillige Frauen früher ausprobierten und ebenfalls unzählige Treuezauber der verheirateten Frauen, die an gewisse Tage im Jahr oder an gewisse nächtliche Uhrzeiten gebunden waren und bestimmter Utensilien wie Silbermünzen, Hundszähne oder Hirschgeweihe bedurften.

Hildegard von Bingen (1098–1179) beginnt ihre „Sunnewirbel"-Betrachtung ebenfalls magisch: „Die Wegwarte neigt in ihrer Natur zum Anstand, und sie ist erdentsprossen. Wer sie jedoch bei sich trägt, wie jener der über andere zu herrschen trachtet, wird von anderen Menschen gehasst." Paracelsus (1493–1541) behauptete, dass sich die Wegwarten-Wurzel alle sieben Jahre in einen Vogel verwandle! Selbst in die Weltliteratur hat sie es geschafft – als blaue Blume der Romantik taucht sie erstmals auf in „Heinrich von Ofterdingen", einem Romanfragment von Novalis (1772–1801). Darin wartet eine Prinzessin Jahr für Jahr allein am Wegesrand und blickt nach Osten, in die Richtung, in welche ihr Geliebter einst davongeritten war, in der Hoffnung, dass er von dort auch wiederkommen werde…

Verwendung – gestern und heute

Im „Capitulare de villis vel curtis imperii" Karls des Großen (747–814), erlassen um das Jahr 800, werden 73 Pflanzen zum Anbau auf den karolingischen Königsgütern vorgeschrieben: an 37. Stelle von insgesamt 73 Pflanzen findet sich unter „intubas", die Wegwarte. Sebastian Kneipp (1821–1897) führte die Wegwarten-Euphorie auf den heilenden Aspekt zurück und meinte, die Wegwarte warte wirklich an jedem Weg auf dich, um dich gesund zu machen.

Bachblüte Nr. 8 „cichory" – Wegwarte – gilt als Blüte der Mütterlichkeit, die helfen soll sich zurückzunehmen, wenn man andere überbemuttert.

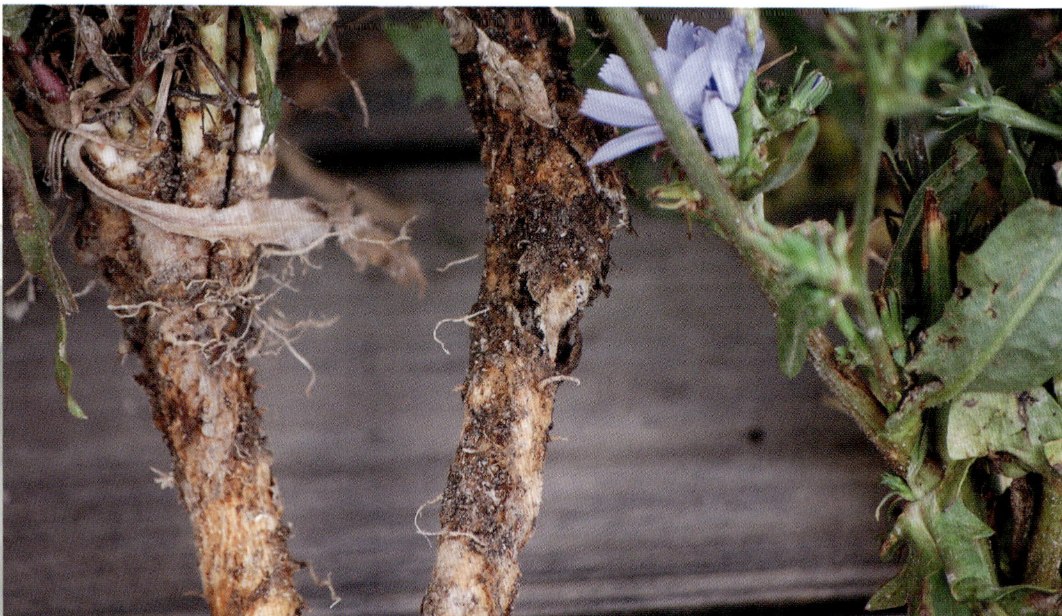

Wegwartenwurzel

Anhang

Weiterführende Literatur

Arrowsmith, N., Herbarium Magicum, Allegria by Ullstein Buchverlage GmbH, Berlin, 2004

Aschner, B. Dr., Paracelsus – sämtliche Werke, Band I bis IV; Anger Verlag Eick, 1993

Bach, E. Dr., Gesammelte Werke – von der Homöopathie zur Bach-Blüten-Therapie; Aquamarin Verlag, Grafing, 2003

Beiser, R., Geheimnisse der Hecken; Ulmer Verlag, 2019

Bingen, H. v., Heilkraft der Natur – Physica; Verlag Herder, Freiburg im Breisgau, 1991

Bock, H., Kreuter Buch darinn underscheidt Namen unnd Wurckung der Kreutter, Stauden; Josias Rihel, Book Renaissance

C. Plinius Secundus d. Ä., Naturkunde, Buch XX; Roderich König und Gerhard Winkler Herausgeber; Heimeran Verlag, München, 1979

Columella, L.I.M., Zwölf Bücher über Landwirtschaft; Will Richter Herausgeber; Artemis Verlag, 1981

Culpeper, N., Culpeper`s Complete Herbal; Arcturus Publishing Limited, London, 2009

Cunningham, S., Enzyklopädie der magischen Kräuter; Schirner Verlag, Darmstadt, 2006

Fischer-Rizzi, S., Medizin der Erde; AT Verlag, Baden, Schweiz, 2005

Fuchs, L., Le nouvel herbier de 1543, New Kreüterbuch; Taschen GmbH, Köln, 2001

Haag, St., Liebeskraut und Zauberpflanzen; Kosmos Verlag, Stuttgart, 2010

Hasitschka, J., Admonter Herbarium; Schnell und Steiner GmbH, Regensburg, 2001

Hertzka, G. Dr. und Strehlow, W. Dr., Große Hildegard-Apotheke; Christiana Verlag, Stein am Rhein, 2005

Kalbermatten, R., Wesen und Signatur der Heilpflanzen; AT Verlag, Aarau und München, 2002

Kalbermatten, R. und Kalbermatten H., Psyche des Menschen und Signatur der Heilpflanzen, AT Verlag, Aarau und München, 2020

Klikovits, P. M. Mag., Was wir vom Gänseblümchen lernen können; Neusiedl am See, 2008

Künzle, J., Das grosse Kräuter-Heilbuch; Unveränderter Nachdruck der Erstausgabe von 1945, Verlag Otto Walter AG Olten, 1995

Laudert, D., Magie der Bäume; BLV Buchverlag, München, 2017

Lonicerus, A., Kreuterbuch; Reprint des Kräuterbuches 1679 von Adamo Lonicero by Verlag Konrad Kölbl, Grünwald bei München, 1962

Madaus, G., Lehrbuch der biologischen Heilmittel, Band I bis III; Georg Olms Verlag, Hildesheim, 2016

Marzell, H. Prof. Dr., Geschichte und Volkskunde der deutschen Heilpflanzen; Nachdruck der Ausgabe 1938, Reichl Verlag, St. Goar, 2002

Perger, Anton Ritter von; Der deutsche Mythos und unsere Pflanzen; Vortrag gehalten am 07.02.1872; Ver. zur Verbr. naturwiss. Kenntnisse; Download unter www.biologiezentrum.at

Rippe, O. und Madejsky M., Die Kräuterkunde des Paracelsus; AT Verlag, Baden und München, 2006

Schmeil-Fitschen, Die Flora Deutschlands und angrenzender Länder; Gerald Parolly und Jens G. Rohwer; 97. Auflage, Quelle & Meyer Verlag GmbH & Co, Wiebelsheim, 2019

Van Wyck, Wink, Wink, Handbuch der Arzneipflanzen; Wissenschaftliche Verlagsgesellschaft mbH, Stuttgart, 2004

Von Nettesheim, A., Die magischen Werke; herausgegeben von Marco Frenschkowski; Marix Verlag, Wiesbaden, 2008

Wood, M., Die Weisheit der Pflanzen; AT Verlag, Aarau und München, 2012